Yearbook of Intensive Care and Emergency Medicine 2005

Edited by J.-L. Vincent

With 168 Figures and 71 Tables

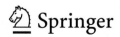 Springer

Prof. Jean-Louis Vincent
Head, Department of Intensive Care
Erasme Hospital, Free University of Brussels
Route de Lennik 808, B-1070 Brussels, Belgium

ISBN 3-540-23476-4 Springer-Verlag Berlin Heidelberg New York

ISSN 0942-5381

Springer is a part of Springer Science+Business Media
springeronline.com

Typesetting: K + V Fotosatz, Beerfelden
Printing: Strauss Offsetdruck, Mörlenbach
Bookbinding: J. Schäffer, Grünstadt

SPIN 11371182   21/3130-5 4 3 2 1 0 – Printed on acid-free paper

Table of Contents

Cardiac Crises

Circulatory Shock

Sepsis and MOF: Basic Mechanisms

Sepsis: Clinical Aspects

Blood Transfusions

Metabolic Alterations

Sedation

Quality Issues

List of Contributors

Appendini L
Salvatore Maugeri Foundation
IRCCS
Scientific Institute of Veruno
Division of Pneumology
Via Revislate 13
28010 Veruno
Italy

Arnold JH
Department of Anesthesia
Division of Critical Care Medicine
Children's Hospital
300 Longwood Ave
Boston, MA 02115
USA

Azoulay E
Department of Intensive Care
Medicine
Hôpital Saint-Louis
10, avenue Claude Vellefaux
75010 Paris
France

Baer A
Department of Internal Medicine
University of Virginia School of
Medicine
Charlottesville, VA
USA

Bickenbach J
Department of Anesthesiology
Universitätsklinikum Aachen
Pauwelsstraße 30
52074 Aachen
Germany

Bjertnaes LJ
Department of Anesthesiology
and Intensive Care Medicine
University Hospital
9038 Tromso
Norway

Bogers AJJC
Department
of Cardiothoracic Surgery
Erasmus MC
PO Box 1738
3000 DR Rotterdam
The Netherlands

Boldt J
Department of Anesthesiology
and Intensive Care Medicine
Klinikum der Stadt Ludwigshafen
Bremserstraße 79
67063 Ludwigshafen
Germany

Bollaert PE
Department
of Intensive Care Medicine
Hôpital Central
29 bld Maréchal de Lattre
de Tassigny
54035 Nancy
France

Böttiger BW
Department of Anesthesiology
University of Heidelberg
Im Neuenheimer Feld 110
69120 Heidelberg
Germany

Brady WJ
Department of Internal Medicine
University of Virginia School of
Medicine
Charlottesville, VA
USA

Brendolan A
Department of Nephrology
San Bortolo Hospital
Viala Rodolfi 37
3610 Vicenza
Italy

Buyse S
Department
of Intensive Care Medicine
Hôpital Saint-Louis
10, avenue Claude Vellefaux
75010 Paris
France

Byhahn C
Department of Anesthesiology
and Intensive Care Medicine
J.-W.-Goethe-University Hospital
Center
Theodor-Stern-Kai 7
D-60590 Frankfurt
Germany

Carney D
Department of Surgery
Upstate Medical University
750 E Adams St
Syracuse, NY 13210
USA

Choi G
Department
of Intensive Care Medicine
Academic Medical Center, University
of Amsterdam
Meibergdreef 9
1105 AZ Amsterdam
The Netherlands

Christ-Crain M
Department of Internal Medicine
University Hospital
Petersgraben 4
4031 Basel
Switzerland

Colpaert K
Department
of Intensive Care Medicine
Ghent University Hospital
185 De Pintelaan
9000 Ghent
Belgium

Combes A
Department
of Intensive Care Medicine
Institute of Cardiology
Groupe Hospitalier Pitié-Salpêtrière
47, boulevard de l'Hôpital
75651 Paris cédex 13
France

Curtis JR
Division of Pulmonary
and Critical Care Medicine
Harborview Medical Center,
Box 359762
325 Ninth Avenue
Seattle, WA 98104-2499
USA

Deeren D
Department of Internal Medicine
University Hospital Gasthuisberg
Herestraat 49
3000 Leuven
Belgium

Decruyenaere J
Department
of Intensive Care Medicine
Ghent University Hospital
185 De Pintelaan
9000 Ghent
Belgium

Dembinski R
Anesthesiology Clinic
Universitätsklinikum Aachen
Pauwelsstraße 30
52074 Aachen
Germany

De Potter TJR
Department of Cardiology
Cardiovascular Center
OLV Hospital
Moorselbaan 164
9300 Aalst
Belgium

Determann RM
Department
of Intensive Care Medicine
G3-228
Academic Medical Center
Meibergdreef 9
1105 AZ Amsterdam
The Netherlands

DiRocco J
Department of Surgery
Upstate Medical University
750 E Adams St
Syracuse, NY 13210
USA

Doddoli C
Department of Thoracic Surgery
Hôpital Ste Marguerite
13009 Marseille
France

Donati SY
Department
of Intensive Care Medicine
Hôpital Ste Marguerite
13009 Marseille
France

Donner CF
Salvatore Maugeri Foundation
IRCCS
Scientific Institute of Veruno
Division of Pneumology
Via Revislate 13
28010 Veruno
Italy

Drabek T
Department
of Critical Care Medicine
Safar Center for Resuscitation
Research
University of Pittsburgh School
of Medicine
3434 Fifth Avenue
Pittsburgh, PA 15260
USA

Enkhbaatar P
Department of Anesthesiology
University of Texas Medical Branch
610 Texas Avenue
Galveston, TX 77555-0833
USA

Ely EW
Division of Allergy, Pulmonary,
Critical Care Medicine
Center for Health Sciences Research
6th Floor Medical Center East #6109
Vanderbilt University Medical Center
Nashville, TN 37232-8300
USA

Esmat E
The Liver Unit
3rd Floor Nuffield House
Queen Elizabeth Hospital
Birmingham B15 23TH
United Kingdom

Ferreyra G
Department of Anesthesiology
Ospedale S. Giovanni Battista
Corso Dogliotti 14
10126 Torino
Italy

Ferrer LE
Regions Hospital
640 Jackson Street
St. Paul, MN 55101
USA

Fertmann JM
Department of Surgery
Ludwig-Maximilians-University
of Munich-Großhadern
Marchioninistraße 15
81377 München
Germany

Gattinoni L
Institute of Anesthesiology
and Intensive Care Medicine
IRCCS
Ospedale Maggiore di Milano
Via F. Sforza 35
20122 Milan
Italy

Georgopoulos D
Department
of Intensive Care Medicine
University Hospital
Heraklion
Greece

Ghaemmaghami CA
Department of Internal Medicine
University of Virginia School of
Medicine
Charlottesville, VA
USA

Gibot S
Department
of Intensive Care Medicine
Hôpital Central
29 bld Maréchal de Lattre
de Tassigny
54035 Nancy
France

Giebelen IAJ
Laboratory of Experimental
Internal Medicine
Academic Medical Center
University of Amsterdam
Meibergdreef 9, C2-321
1105 AZ Amsterdam
The Netherlands

Ginsberg F
Robert Wood Johnson Medical
School at Camden
University of Medicine
and Dentistry of New Jersey
One Robert Wood Johnson Place
New Brunswick, NJ 08901-1977
USA

Girard TD
Division of Allergy, Pulmonary,
Critical Care Medicine
Center for Health Sciences Research
6th Floor Medical Center East #6109
Vanderbilt University Medical Center
Nashville, TN 37232-8300
USA

Gottschalk A
Department of Anesthesia
and Intensive Care Medicine
Academic Hospital of the University
of Cologne
Goten Straße 1
42653 Solingen
Germany

Groeneveld ABJ
Department
of Intensive Care Medicine
Vrije Universiteit Medical Centre
De Boelelaan 1117
1081 HV Amsterdam
The Netherlands

Handy JM
The Magill Department
of Anesthesia and Intensive
Care Medicine
Chelsea and Westminster Hospital
369 Fulham Road
London
United Kingdom

Hansen M
Department of Anesthesiology
Robert-Bosch-Krankenhaus
Auerbachstraße 110
70376 Stuttgart
Germany

Hart MHL
Sanquin Research
Central Laboratory for Blood
Transfusion Services
Plesmanlaan 125
1066 CX Amsterdam
The Netherlands

Hoffmann JN
Department of Surgery
Ludwig-Maximilians-University
of Munich-Großhadern
Marchioninistraße 15
81377 Munich
Germany

Huang SJ
Department
of Intensive Care Medicine
University of Sidney
Nepean Campus
PO Box 63
Penrith NSW 2751
Australia

Ince C
Department of Physiology
Academic Medical Center
Meibergdreef
1105 AZ Amsterdam
The Netherlands

Ishizaka A
Division of Pulmonary Medicine
Department of Medicine
Keio University School of Medicine
35 Shinanomachi, Shinjuku-ku
Tokyo 160-8582
Japan

Jardin F
Department
of Intensive Care Medicine
Hôpital Ambroise Paré
9 avenue Charles-de-Gaulle
92104 Boulogne cédex
France

Jonas M
Department
of Intensive Care Medicine
Southampton Hospitals University
Trust
Tremona Road
Southampton SO16 7BQ
United Kingdom

Kellum JA
Department
of Critical Care Medicine
University of Pittsburgh Medical
Center
3550 Terrace Street
Pittsburgh, PA 15216
USA

Kirov MY
Department of Anesthesiology
and Intensive Care Medicine
Northern State Medical University
Troitsky Avenue 51
163000 Arkhangelsk
Russian Federation

Kochanek PM
Department
of Critical Care Medicine
Safar Center for Resuscitation
Research
University of Pittsburgh School
of Medicine
3434 Fifth Avenue
Pittsburgh, PA 15260
USA

Kostner K
Department of Medicine
University of Queensland
Princess Alexandra
& Wesley Hospitals
Brisbane, Queensland 4102
Australia

Krueger WA
Department of Anesthesiology
University Hospital
Hoppe-Seyler-Str. 3
72076 Tübingen
Germany

Kruger P
Department of Intensive Care
University of Queensland
Princess Alexandra
& Wesley Hospitals
Brisbane, Queensland, 4102
Australia

Kuhlen R
Department of Anesthesiology
Universitätsklinikum Aachen
Pauwelsstraße 30
52074 Aachen
Germany

Kuzkov VV
Department of Anesthesiology
and Intensive Care Medicine
Northern State Medical University
Troitsky Avenue 51
163000 Arkhangelsk
Russian Federation

Labaien F
Department
of Intensive Care Medicine
Santiago Apostol University Hospital
Olaguibel 29
01004 Vitoria
Spain

Lachmann B
Department of Anesthesiology
Erasmus MC
PO Box 1738
3000 DR Rotterdam
The Netherlands

Lamia B
Medical Intensive Care Unit
CHU de Bicêtre
78, Av du général Leclerc
94275 Le Kremlin Bicêtre Cedex
France

Lebuffe G
Department
of Intensive Care Medicine
Hôpital Claude Huriez
Centre Hospitalier Universitaire
Rue Michel Polonowski
59037 Lille Cedex
France

Lehmann A
Department of Anesthesiology
and Intensive Care Medicine
Klinikum der Stadt Ludwigshafen
Bremserstr. 79
67063 Ludwigshafen
Germany

Levi M
Department of Internal Medicine
Academic Medical Center
University of Amsterdam
Meibergdreef 9
1105 AZ Amsterdam
The Netherlands

Levy B
Department
of Intensive Care Medicine
Hôpital Central
29 bld Maréchal de Lattre
de Tassigny
54035 Nancy
France

Lindeboom JAH
Department of Oral
and Maxillofacial Surgery
Academic Medical Center
Meibergdreef
1105 AZ Amsterdam
The Netherlands

Lombardo A
Department
of Intensive Care Medicine
Ospedale di Circolo
e Fondazione Macchi
Viale Borri 57
21100 Varese
Italy

Luyt CE
Department
of Intensive Care Medicine
Institute of Cardiology
Groupe Hospitalier Pitié-Salpêtrière
47, boulevard de l'Hôpital
75651 Paris Cedex 13
France

Madjdpour C
Department of Anesthesiology
University Hospital
1011 Lausanne
Switzerland

Malbrain MLNG
Department
of Intensive Care Medicine
ZiekenhuisNetwerk
Campus Stuivenberg
Lange Beeldekensstraat 267
2606 Antwerpen 6
Belgium

Marcucci C
Department of Anesthesiology
University Hospital
1011 Lausanne
Switzerland

Marik P
Department of Medicine
Thomas Jefferson University
Philadelphia, PA
USA

Marini JJ
Department of Pulmonary Medicine
and Critical Care
Regions Hospital
640 Jackson Street
St. Paul, MN 55101
USA

Mathura KR
Department of Physiology
Academic Medical Center
Meibergdreef
1105 AZ Amsterdam
The Netherlands

Mayer SA
Division of Stroke and Critical Care
Neurological Institute
710 West 168th Street
New York, NY 10032
USA

Maynar J
Department
of Intensive Care Medicine
Santiago Apostol University Hospital
Olaguibel 29
01004 Vitoria
Spain

McLean AS
Department
of Intensive Care Medicine
University of Sidney
Nepean Campus
PO Box 63
Penrith NSW 2751
Australia

Mebazaa A
Department of Anesthesiology,
Critical Care and SMUR
Lariboisière University Hospital
University Paris VII
2 rue Ambroise Paré
75475 Paris Cédex
France

Mehta NM
Department
of Intensive Care Medicine
Children's Hospital
30 Longwood Avenue
Boston, MA 02115
USA

Mehta S
Division of Critical Care Medicine
and Respirology
Department of Medicine
Mount Sinai Hospital
600 University Avenue, Suite 1825A
Toronto, Ontario M5G 1X5
Canada

Menger MD
Institute for Clinical
and Experimental Surgery
University of Saarland
66421 Homburg
Germany

Michard F
Surgical Intensive Care Unit
Marie Lannelongue Hospital
University Paris XI
133 avenue de la Résistance
92350 le Plessis Robinson
France

Mirza DF
Liver Unit
3rd Floor Nuffield House
Queen Elizabeth Hospital
Birmingham B15 23TH
United Kingdom

Monaco F
Medical Intensive Care Unit
Department of Surgical
and Anesthesiological Sciences
Federico Secondo of Naples
Via Pansini 5
80100 Naples
Italy

Monnet X
Medical Intensive Care Unit
CHU de Bicêtre
78, Av du général Leclerc
94275 Le Kremlin Bicêtre Cedex
France

Müller B
Department of Internal Medicine
University Hospitals
Petersgraben 4
4031 Basel
Switzerland

Nieman G
Department of Surgery
Upstate Medical University
750 E Adams St
Syracuse, NY 13210
USA

Opal SM
Infectious Disease Division
Brown University School
of Medicine
Providence, RI
USA

Papazian L
Department
of Intensive Care Medicine
Hôpital Sainte-Marguerite
13009 Marseille
France

Parkinson J
Department of Immunology
Berlex Biosciences
Richmond, CA
USA

Parrillo JE
Cardiovascular
and Critical Care Services
Cooper University Hospital
One Cooper Plaza
Camden, NJ 08103
USA

Patessio A
Salvatore Maugeri Foundation
IRCCS
Scientific Institute of Veruno
Division of Pneumology
Via Revislate 13
28010 Veruno
Italy

Pearse RM
Department
of Intensive Care Medicine
1st Floor St James' wing
St. George's Hospital
Blackshaw Road
London SW17 0QT
United Kingdom

Pelosi P
Department
of Intensive Care Medicine
Ospedale di Circolo
e Fondazione Macchi
Viale Borri 57
21100 Varese
Italy

Pepe PE
Department of Emergency Medicine
University of Texas Southwestern
Medical Center
5323 Harry Hines Boulevard
Mail Code 8579
Dallas, TX 75390-8579
USA

Pinsky MR
Department
of Critical Care Medicine
University of Pittsburgh School
of Medicine
606 Scaife Hall
3550 Terrace Street
Pittsburgh, PA 15213
USA

Pirracchio R
Department of Anesthesiology,
Critical Care and SMUR
Lariboisière University Hospital
University Paris VII
2 rue Ambroise Paré
75475 Paris Cédex
France

Polderman KH
Department
of Intensive Care Medicine
VU University Medical Center
PO Box 7057
1007 MB Amsterdam
The Netherlands

Potolidis E
Department
of Intensive Care Medicine
University Hospital
Heraklion
Greece

Ranieri VM
Department of Anesthesiology
Ospedale S. Giovanni Battista
Corso Dogliotti 14
10126 Torino
Italy

Ratanarat R
Department of Nephrology
San Bortolo Hospital
Viala Rodolfi 37
3610 Vicenza
Italy

Rhodes A
Department
of Intensive Care Medicine
1st Floor St James' wing
St. George's Hospital
Blackshaw Road
London SW17 0QT
United Kingdom

Ronco C
Department of Nephrology
St. Bortolo Hospital
Viale Rodolfi
36100 Vicenza
Italy

Roppolo LP
Department of Surgery
University of Texas Southwestern
Medical Center
5323 Harry Hines Boulevard
Mail Code 8579
Dallas, TX 75390-8579
USA

Samy Modeliar S
Department of Intensive Care
Nephrology
CHU Sud
80054 Amiens Cedex 1
France

Schlemmer B
Department
of Intensive Care Medicine
Hôpital Saint-Louis
10, avenue Claude Vellefaux
75010 Paris
France

Schroeder TH
Department of Anesthesiology
University Hospital
Hoppe-Seyler-Str. 3
72076 Tübingen
Germany

Schultz MJ
Department of Intensive Care
and Laboratory of Experimental
Medicine
Academic Medical Center, University
of Amsterdam
Meibergdreef 9
1105 AZ Amsterdam
The Netherlands

Severgnini P
Department
of Intensive Care Medicine
Ospedale di Circolo
e Fondazione Macchi
Viale Borri 57
21100 Varese
Italy

Sevestre-Pietri MA
Department of Intensive Care
Nephrology
CHU Sud
80054 Amiens Cedex 1
France

Silva MA
Liver Unit
3rd Floor Nuffield House
Queen Elizabeth Hospital
Birmingham B15 23TH
United Kingdom

Slama M
Department of Intensive Care
Nephrology
CHU Sud
80054 Amiens Cedex 1
France

Spahn DR
Department of Anesthesiology
University Hospital
1011 Lausanne
Switzerland

Spöhr F
Department of Anesthesiology
University of Heidelberg
Im Neuenheimer Feld 110
69120 Heidelberg
Germany

Squadrone V
Department of Anesthesiology
Ospedale S. Giovanni Battista
Corso Dogliotti 14
10126 Torino
Italy

Standl T
Department of Anesthesia
and Intensive Care Medicine
Academic Hospital
of the University of Cologne
Goten Straße 1
42653 Solingen
Germany

Sun S
Institute of Critical Care
1695 North Sunrise Way, Bldg. #3
Palm Springs, CA 92262
USA

Tacx AN
Department
of Intensive Care Medicine
VU Medical Centre
De Boelelaan 1117
1081 HV Amsterdam
The Netherlands

Tang W
Institute of Critical Care
1695 North Sunrise Way, Bldg. #3
Palm Springs, CA 92262
USA

Tasaka S
Division of Pulmonary Medicine
Department of Medicine
Keio University School of Medicine
35 Shinanomachi, Shinjuku-ku
Tokyo 160-8582
Japan

Teboul JL
Medical Intensive Care Unit
CHU de Bicêtre
78, Av du général Leclerc
94275 Le Kremlin Bicêtre Cedex
France

Traber DL
Department of Anesthesiology
University of Texas Medical Branch
610 Texas Avenue
Galveston, TX 77555-0833
USA

Trouillet JL
Department
of Intensive Care Medicine
Institute of Cardiology
Groupe Hospitalier Pitié-Salpêtrière
47, boulevard de l'Hôpital
75651 Paris cédex 13
France

Vakouti E
Department
of Intensive Care Medicine
University Hospital
Heraklion
Greece

Valenza F
Institute of Anesthesiology
and Intensive Care Medicine
Ospedale Maggiore di Milano
IRCCS
Via F. Sforza 35
20122 Milan
Italy

Vallet B
Clinic of Anesthesiology
and Intensive Care Medicine
Hôpital Claude Huriez
Centre Hospitalier Universitaire
Rue Michel Polonowski
59037 Lille cédex
France

van der Kaaij NP
Department
of Cardio-Thoracic Surgery
Erasmus MC
PO Box 1738
3000 DR Rotterdam
The Netherlands

van der Poll T
Department of Infectious Diseases,
Tropical Medicine & AIDS
Academic Medical Center
University of Amsterdam
Meibergdreef 9, C2-321
1105 AZ Amsterdam
The Netherlands

van der Voort PHJ
Department
of Intensive Care Medicine
Leeuwarden Medical Center
P.O. Box 888
8901 BR Leeuwarden
The Netherlands

van Westerloo DJ
Laboratory of Experimental
Internal Medicine
Academic Medical Center
University of Amsterdam
Meibergdreef 9, C2-321
1105 AZ Amsterdam
The Netherlands

van Zanten ARH
Department
of Intensive Care Medicine
Gelderse Vallei Hospital
Willy Brandtlaan 10
6710 HN Ede
The Netherlands

Varon J
The University of Texas Health
Science Center
St. Luke's Episcopal Hospital
2219 Dorington
Houston, TX 77030
USA

Venkatesh B
Department
of Intensive Care Medicine
University of Queensland
Princess Alexandra
& Wesley Hospitals
Brisbane, Queensland, 4102
Australia

Vieillard-Baron A
Department
of Intensive Care Medicine
Hôpital Ambroise Paré
9 avenue Charles-de-Gaulle
92104 Boulogne cédex
France

Vroom MB
Department
of Intensive Care Medicine
G3-228
Academic Medical Center
Meibergdreef 9
1105 AZ Amsterdam
The Netherlands

Walsh TS
Department of Anesthetics,
Critical Care, and Pain Medicine
Edinburgh Royal Infirmary
Little France Crescent
Edinburgh EH16 2SA
Scotland

Wartenberg KE
Division of Stroke and Critical Care
Neurological Institute
710 West 168th Street
New York, NY 10032
USA

Weil MH
Institute of Critical Care
1695 North Sunrise Way, Bldg. #3
Palm Springs, CA 92262
USA

Westphal K
Department of Anesthesiology
J.-W.-Goethe-University
Hospital Center
Theodor-Stern-Kai 7
D-60590 Frankfurt
Germany

Wiel E
Clinic of Anesthesiology
and Intensive Care Medicine
Hôpital Claude Huriez
Centre Hospitalier Universitaire
Rue Michel Polonowski
59037 Lille Cedex
France

Wigginton JG
Department of Surgery
University of Texas Southwestern
Medical Center
5323 Harry Hines Boulevard,
Mail Code 8579
Dallas, TX 75390-8579
USA

Wolf GK
Department of Anesthesia
Division of Critical Care Medicine
Children's Hospital
300 Longwood Ave
Boston, MA 02115
USA

Wu X
Department
of Intensive Care Medicine
Safar Center for Resuscitation
Research
University of Pittsburgh School
of Medicine
3434 Fifth Avenue
Pittsburgh, PA 15260
USA

Zwissler B
Department of Anesthesiology
and Intensive Care Medicine
J.-W.-Goethe-University Hospital
Center
Theodor-Stern-Kai 7
60590 Frankfurt
Germany

Common Abbreviations

ALI	Acute lung injury
AMI	Acute myocardial infarction
APC	Activated protein C
ARDS	Acute respiratory distress syndrome
ATP	Adenosine triphosphate
BAL	Bronchoalveolar lavage
CHF	Congestive heart failure
CNS	Central nervous system
COPD	Chronic obstructive pulmonary disease
CPB	Cardiopulmonary bypass
CPR	Cardiopulmonary resuscitation
CRP	C-reactive protein
CT	Computed tomography
CVP	Central venous pressure
DIC	Disseminated intravascular coagulation
DNA	Deoxyribonucleic acid
DO_2	Oxygen delivery
EDV	End-diastolic volume
EKG	Electrocardiogram
EVLW	Extravascular lung water
FiO_2	Inspired oxygen fraction
HFOV	High frequency oscillatory ventilation
HIV	Human immunodeficiency virus
IAP	Intraabdominal pressure
ICU	Intensive care unit
IFN	Interferon
IL	Interleukin
LPS	Lipopolysaccharide
MAP	Mean arterial pressure
MOF	Multiple organ failure
MRI	Magnetic resonance imaging
NAD	Nicotinamide adenine dinucleotide

NF-κB	Nuclear factor kappa-B
NIV	Non-invasive ventilation
NO	Nitric oxide
NOS	Nitric oxide synthase
PAC	Pulmonary artery catheter
PaO$_2$	Partial pressure of oxygen
PAOP	Pulmonary artery occlusion pressure
PEEP	Positive end-expiratory pressure
pHi	Gastric intramucosal pH
RBC	Red blood cell
RNA	Ribonucleic acid
ROS	Reactive oxygen species
SaO$_2$	Arterial oxygen saturation
ScvO$_2$	Central venous oxygen saturation
SvO$_2$	Mixed venous oxygen saturation
SVR	Systemic vascular resistance
TBI	Traumatic brain injury
TEE	Transesophageal echocardiography
TGR	Transforming growth factor
TLR	Toll-like receptor
TNF	Tumor necrosis factor
VAP	Ventilator-associated pneumonia
VILI	Ventilator-induced lung injury
VO$_2$	Oxygen uptake
WBC	White blood cell

Respiratory Failure

Exacerbations of COPD:
The Role of Invasive Mechanical Ventilation

L. Appendini, A. Patessio, and C. F. Donner

▍ Introduction

The severity of exacerbations of chronic obstructive pulmonary disease (COPD) ranges from a mild increase in usual symptoms to overt acute respiratory failure [1] represented by an increase in $PaCO_2$ above 45 mmHg or above previous stable hypercapnia, if present, and by the consequent respiratory acidosis (pH <7.36) [2, 3]. In patients with ventilatory failure, optimal medical therapy and adequate oxygenation may be insufficient, and mechanical ventilation may be required in the presence of unbearable breathlessness at rest, signs of respiratory distress (tachypnea with a respiratory rate >30 breaths/min, evident use of accessory respiratory muscles, paradoxical breathing), and laboratory findings of worsening of hypercapnia and acidosis.

The aims of mechanical ventilation, whatever the modes and settings selected, are:
- ▍ to support the overloaded ventilatory pump,
- ▍ to improve arterial blood gases and pH,
- ▍ to relieve dyspnea and unload the respiratory muscles, and
- ▍ to 'buy time' for the patient, by allowing adequate minute ventilation notwithstanding a failing ventilatory pump, until the causes of the exacerbation are resolved by medical therapy.

Mechanical ventilation can be administered in different modes:
- ▍ invasively through an endotracheal tube bypassing the upper airways through nasal-orotracheal tubes, tracheostomy, or laryngeal cannulae, and
- ▍ non-invasively through interfaces applied externally on the body surface (NIV). NIV can be delivered in the form of positive pressure ventilation (NPPV) through nasal/face masks and helmets, or in the form of negative pressure ventilation (NPV), placing the patient inside an iron lung or applying ponchos or cuirasses.

The indications for initiating some form of ventilatory assistance and the choice between conventional mechanical ventilation and NIV, as well as the mode and settings of mechanical ventilation, depend not only on the severity of the exacerbations and respiratory acidosis, but also on many other factors such as the timing of the intervention, patient characteristics, the skill of the team, available monitoring facilities, etc. [4–6]. Notwithstanding the complexity of this clinical problem, there is now little doubt that NIV represents an effective treatment for ventilatory failure resulting from acute exacerbations of COPD, with a number of randomized controlled trials and at least four meta-analyses more than strongly attesting its effectiveness [7–10]. In fact, NIV has been shown to reduce the need for endotracheal intubation and mechanical ventilation, with a concomitant improved survival, and reduced complication rates and length of both intensive care unit (ICU) and hospital stay [8–10] compared to standard medical therapy. In particular, the higher rate of infectious complications observed during mechanical ventilation with respect to NIV seems a key factor in the worse survival and ICU length of stay reported in reference to mechanical ventilation [11–14].

On the basis of the published evidence, it has been suggested that NIV be considered as the gold standard mode of ventilatory support for exacerbations of COPD, and endotracheal intubation and mechanical ventilation as second-line therapy [15]. The present chapter, however, will focus on the indications for invasive mechanical ventilation on the premise that NIV and mechanical ventilation should not be considered as competing alternatives, but rather as complementary tools in the comprehensive treatment of ventilatory failure due to acute exacerbations of COPD.

▌ Mechanical Ventilation as a First-line Intervention

For many years mechanical ventilation was the only mode of ventilatory assistance for treating ventilatory failure, i.e., there was no choice; hence all patients were exposed to the discomfort and the well-known and potentially harmful side effects of endotracheal intubation [16]. Nowadays, mechanical ventilation and NIV are both available to treat COPD patients who develop ventilatory failure after failure of medical treatment. A randomized prospective study by Conti et al. compared mechanical ventilation vs NIV in this clinical condition [17]. This study showed that COPD patients treated with either mechanical ventilation or NIV had similar length of ICU stay, number of days on mechanical ventilation, overall complications, ICU mortality, and hospital mortality. Moreover, the subgroup of patients treated with NIV who avoided endotracheal intubation (48% of the total) had a better survival rate, shorter duration of ICU stay, and a lower hospital readmission rate (65 vs 100%) in the year following their discharge to home. On one hand, the favorable results obtained by Conti et al. in the subgroup of patients who received NIV and avoided endotracheal intubation [17] strengthen the current recommendation to attempt a trial of NIV in the vast majority of patients who are acidotic as the result of an acute exacerbation of COPD [7–11, 15]. On the other hand, these results suggest that mechanical ventilation can be used without increasing the overall risk and with the same probability of success as NIV if the former is applied in the general population of COPD patients with acute respiratory failure. This supports the use of endotracheal intubation and mechanical ventilation whenever an elective indication to tracheal intubation co-exists with the need to deliver ventilatory assistance because of exacerbation of COPD, such as in the presence of:

▌ respiratory arrest;
▌ factors that prevent the proper positioning of the patient-ventilator interface (recent facial surgery, fixed nasopharyngeal abnormality);
▌ extreme obesity;
▌ primary indication to protect airways from aspiration (coma, coexistent neurological illness impairing swallowing, recent gastro-esophageal surgery, risk of vomiting, etc.);

▌ need for airway aspiration because of copious and tenacious secretions associated with inefficient cough.

A present or impending clinical indication for endotracheal intubation and mechanical ventilation does not imply that these latter should always be adopted. The patient's resulting quality of life and prognosis, the prospects of short- and long-term benefits, the possibility of becoming ventilator-dependent (and, hence, undergoing tracheostomy), the patient's and/or family's views and expectations regarding treatment, may discourage use of mechanical ventilation. Precise guidelines on these issues are lacking. Pending such directives, advice from senior team members may be useful.

A recent prospective survey performed over a period of 3 weeks among 42 ICUs in French-speaking countries [11] provides valuable data on the current use of NIV and mechanical ventilation. In the 42 ICUs, mechanical ventilation was always used for patients in coma, and was the first attempted ventilatory technique in 50% of patients with hypercapnic acute respiratory failure, despite the favorable results reported in the literature for this group of patients without recourse to mechanical ventilation (see above). The authors' feeling was that the present incidence of mechanical ventilation in hypercapnic respiratory failure is unduly high. The high intubation rate in Emergency Departments and outside the hospital was reported as a cause of this abnormally high number of COPD patients undergoing mechanical ventilation [11]. However, two studies in which NIV was started in the Emergency Department failed to show any advantage of NIV over conventional therapy [18, 19], and no data are available on the use of NIV and mechanical ventilation outside the hospital. In conclusion, the optimal number of patients who really can benefit from endotracheal intubation and mechanical ventilation as a first choice intervention (i.e., that minimizes NIV failure and institution of mechanical ventilation) is largely unknown, and further research is required.

▌ Mechanical Ventilation as 'Rescue' Intervention

Studies on NIV, used for the treatment of acute respiratory failure due to exacerbations of COPD, have reported variable percentages of failure ranging from 5 to 40% [11, 19–25]. Mechanical ventilation is always considered the rescue treatment for NIV failure, insofar as endotracheal intubation and institution of mechanical ventilation are included in the definition of all types of failure (early and late) if death during NIV is excluded [25]. In fact, early failure is defined as the need for intubation due to lack of improvement in arterial blood gas tensions and clinical parameters after a few hours of ventilation (usually 1–3 hours), and late failure as clinical deterioration and subsequent intubation during hospital stay [25]. Data on the efficacy of mechanical ventilation as a rescue treatment after late failure of NIV are provided in a recent paper by Moretti et al. [25]. They show that more than 20% of COPD patients mechanically ventilated with NIV because of acute exacerbations experience a new episode of acute respiratory failure. Among these patients, a higher mortality rate (91.6%) was found in patients continuing with NIV compared to those who were switched to endotracheal intubation and mechanical ventilation (52.6%). The authors concluded that the in-hospital prognosis of such patients is very poor, especially if NIV is continued and endotracheal intubation avoided.

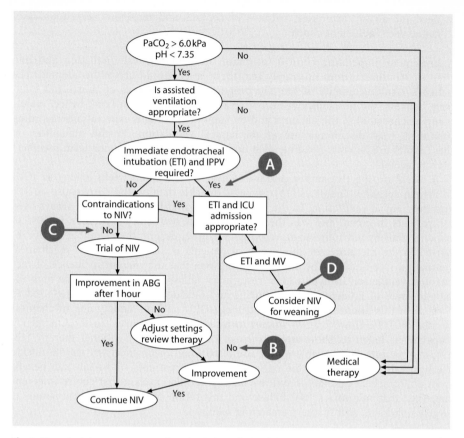

Fig. 1. Flow chart for management of mechanical ventilation (MV) in acute exacerbation of COPD. Legend: A→ = invasive mechanical ventilation considered as first choice intervention; B→ = invasive mechanical ventilation considered as rescue intervention; C→ = non-invasive mechanical ventilation (NIV) main pathway; D→ = NIV used to speed liberation from mechanical ventilation. IPPV: intermittent positive pressure ventilation; ETI: endotracheal intubation; ABG: arterial blood gases. Redrawn from [31] with permission

Data on the efficacy of mechanical ventilation started after early NIV failure are indirect. In a study by Nava et al., in which NIV was tested during weaning of patients with acute respiratory failure due to COPD, 44% of patients (n = 22) underwent invasive mechanical ventilation for 24–48 hours because of early failure of NIV [26]. Most of those who were extubated after this period and treated again with NIV were eventually weaned from ventilatory assistance. This suggests that mechanical ventilation allowed the patients to improve sufficiently to take advantage of a treatment (NIV) previously ineffective [26]. Unfortunately, this evidence is based on a very small number of patients, and further research is needed, but the study is innovative in suggesting a true integration between mechanical ventilation and NIV.

The paper of Nava et al. addresses a further major issue of mechanical ventilation in COPD: What is the optimal duration [26]? It is well known that prolonged mechanical ventilation has associated risks [16, 27] and a high mortality rate [28–

30]. In particular, the presence of COPD and duration of mechanical ventilation longer than 3 days has been demonstrated to be associated with an increased risk of nosocomial pneumonia [28]. Nava et al. provided evidence that a reduction in mechanical ventilation duration below this time limit (by using NIV) can result in shorter durations of mechanical ventilation, and of ICU stay, a reduced rate of nosocomial pneumonia and better 60-day survival rates [26].

▌ Conclusion

In conclusion, both mechanical ventilation and NIV seem to mutually reinforce each other, if considered as part of an integrated approach to acute respiratory failure due to acute exacerbations of COPD. Figure 1 reproduces a flow chart for mechanical ventilation management in this clinical situation [31]. The evidence outlined above indicates that mechanical ventilation still has a number of indications for which it should be considered as a first choice intervention (condition A in Fig. 1) even if it seems overused at the present [11]. Moreover, mechanical ventilation is the sole rescue intervention effective and available when NIV fails (condition B in Fig. 1). On the other hand, NIV plays a key role in the management of acute respiratory failure due to acute exacerbations of COPD. Given its potential advantages [8–15], it should be attempted whenever possible (conditions C and D in Fig. 1), keeping mechanical ventilation facilities readily available as a precaution (condition B in Fig. 1). In spite of its advantages, NIV seems widely underused in most settings, especially when it should be employed as a first line intervention [11, 15].

In light of the above considerations, effort and research is warranted to define the most effective indications and boundaries of use for mechanical ventilation and NIV in order to obtain the best results in terms of patient survival and quality of life. Competition between mechanical ventilation and NIV will result only in a waste of energy.

Acknowledgements. We thank Rosemary Allpress for her help in the preparation of the manuscript.

References

1. Stoller GK (2002) Acute exacerbations of COPD. N Engl J Med 346:988–994
2. Barbera JA, Roca J, Ferrer A, Felez MA, Diaz O, Roger N (1997) Mechanisms of worsening gas exchange during acute exacerbations of chronic obstructive pulmonary disease. Eur Respir J 10:1285–1291
3. Schmidt GA, Hall JB (1989) Acute on chronic respiratory failure. Assessment and management of patients with COPD in the emergency setting. JAMA 261:3444–3453
4. BTS Guideline (2002) Non invasive ventilation in acute respiratory failure. British Thoracic Society Standards of Care Committee. Thorax 57:192–211
5. Evans TV, Albert RK, Angus DC, et al (2001) International Consensus Conference in intensive care medicine: non-invasive positive pressure ventilation in acute respiratory failure. Am J Respir Crit Care Med 163:283–291
6. Pauwels RA, Buist AS, Calverley PMA, Jenkins CR, Hurd SS (2001) Global strategy for the diagnosis, management, and prevention of chronic obstructive pulmonary disease. NHLBI/WHO global initiative for chronic obstructive lung disease (GOLD). Workshop summary. Am J Respir Crit Care Med 163:1256–1276

7. Keenan SP, Kernerman PD, Cook DJ, Martin CM, McCormack D, Sibbald WJ (1997) Effect of non-invasive positive pressure ventilation on mortality in patients admitted with acute respiratory failure: a meta-analysis. Crit Care Med 25:1685–1692

8. Peter JV, Moran JL, Phillips-Hughes J, Warn D (2002) Noninvasive ventilation in acute respiratory failure – A meta-analysis update. Crit Care Med 30:555–562

9. Keenan SP, Sinuff T, Cook DJ, Hill NS (2003) Which patients with acute exacerbation of chronic obstructive pulmonary disease benefit from non-invasive positive-pressure ventilation? A systematic review of the literature. Ann Intern Med 138:861–870

10. Lightowler JV, Wedzicha JA, Elliott MW, et al (2003) Non invasive positive pressure ventilation to treat respiratory failure resulting from exacerbations of chronic obstructive pulmonary disease: chocrane systematic review and meta-analysis. BMJ 326:185–189

11. Carlucci A, Richard JC, Wysocki M, et al (2001) Noninvasive versus conventional mechanical ventilation: an epidemiologic survey. Am J Respir Crit Care Med 163:874–880

12. Girou E, Schortgen F, Delclaux C, et al (2000) Association of non-invasive ventilation with nosocomial infections and survival in critically ill patients. JAMA 284:2361–2367

13. Guerin C, Girard R, Chemorin C, De Varax R, Fournier G (1997) Facial Mask non-invasive mechanical ventilation reduces the incidence of nosocomial pneumonia. A prospective epidemiological survey from a single ICU. Intensive Care Med 23:1024–1032

14. Nourdine K, Combes P, Carton MJ, Beuret P, Cannamela A, Ducreux JC (1999) Does non-invasive ventilation reduce the ICU nosocomial infection risk? A prospective clinical survey. Intensive Care Med 25:567–573

15. Elliott MW (2002) Non-invasive ventilation in acute exacerbations of chronic obstructive pulmonary disease: a new gold standard? Intensive Care Med 28:1691–1694

16. Stauffer JL (1994) Complications of translaryngeal intubation. In: Tobin MJ (ed) Principles and Practice of Mechanical Ventilation. McGraw-Hill Inc, New York, pp 711–747

17. Conti G, Antonelli M, Navalesi P, et al (2002) Noninvasive vs conventional mechanical ventilation in patients with chronic obstructive pulmonary disease after failure of medical treatment in the ward: a randomised trial. Intensive Care Med 28:1701–1707

18. Barbe F, Togores B, Rubi M, Pons S, Maimo A, Agusti AGN (1996) Noninvasive ventilatory support does not facilitate recovery from acute respiratory failure in chronic obstructive pulmonary disease. Eur Respir J 9:1240–1245

19. Wood KA, Lewis L, Von Harz B, Kollef MH (1998) The use of non-invasive positive pressure ventilation in the Emergency Department. Chest 113:1339–1346

20. Brochard L, Mancebo J, Wysochi M, et al (1995) Noninvasive ventilation for acute exacerbations of chronic obstructive pulmonary disease. N Engl J Med 333:817–822

21. Bott J, Carroll TH (1993) Randomized controlled trial of nasal ventilation in acute ventilatory failure due to chronic obstructive airways disease. Lancet 341:1555–1557

22. Kramer N, Meyer TJ, Meharg J, et al (1995) Randomized, prospective trial of noninvasive positive pressure ventilation in acute respiratory failure. Am J Respir Crit Care Med 151:1799–1806

23. Celikel T, Sungur M, Ceyhan B, et al (1998) Comparison of non-invasive positive ventilation with standard medical therapy in hypercapnic acute respiratory failure. Chest 114:1636–1642

24. Meduri GU, Abou-Shala N, Fox RC, et al (1991) Non-invasive face mask ventilation in patients with acute hypercapnic respiratory failure. Chest 100:445–454

25. Moretti M, Cilione C, Tampieri A, Fracchia C, Marchioni A, Nava S (2000) Incidence and causes of non-invasive mechanical ventilation failure after initial success. Thorax 55:819–825

26. Nava S, Ambrosino N, Clini E, et al (1998) Noninvasive mechanical ventilation in the weaning of patients with respiratory failure due to chronic obstructive pulmonary disease: a randomised, controlled trial. Ann Intern Med 128:721–728

27. Stauffer JL, Olson DE, Petty TL (1981) Complications and consequences of endotracheal intubation and tracheotomy. A prospective study of 150 critically ill adult patients. Am J Med 70:65–76

28. Torres A, Aznar R, Gatell JM, et al (1990) Incidence, risk, and prognosis factors of nosocomial pneumonia in mechanically ventilated patients. Am Rev Respir Dis 142:523–528

29. Craven DE, Kunches LM, Kilinsky V, Lichtenberg DA, Make BJ, McCrabe WR (1986) Risk factors for pneumonia and fatality in patients receiving continuous mechanical ventilation. Am Rev Respir Dis 133:792–796
30. Fagon JY, Chastre J, Hance AJ, Montravers P, Novara A, Gilbert C (1993) Nosocomial pneumonia in ventilated patients: a cohort study evaluating attributable mortality and hospital stay. Am J Med 94:281–288
31. Simonds AK (2001) Starting NIPPV: practical aspects. In: Simonds AK (ed) Non-invasive Respiratory Support, 2nd edn. Arnold, London, pp 58–75

Acute Respiratory Failure after Abdominal Surgery

G. Ferreyra, V. Squadrone, and V. M. Ranieri

▌ Introduction

Each year, millions of patients undergo abdominal surgery. Despite advances in anesthesia and surgical care, postoperative pulmonary complications are still a major problem in modern practice. Over the last three decades, extensive research has been focused on their prevention; however, they continue to produce increase in length of hospital stay, overall increased health care costs, and it is estimated that they account for 24% of all deaths occurring within 6 days of surgery [1]. The incidence rate of postoperative pulmonary complications in abdominal patients depends on the surgical site, presence of predictive risk factors, and the criteria used to define them. Unfortunately, there is no homogeneity to determine the frequency and variety of events due to a lack of uniform definition of postoperative pulmonary complications among different studies. Postoperative pulmonary complications are usually defined as events occurring in the postoperative period producing clinical disease or dysfunctions that adversely affect the clinical course (Table 1). The literature reports postoperative pulmonary complication rates of 6 to 80% [1–9].

The most severe form of postoperative pulmonary complication is acute respiratory failure, a condition in which the respiratory system fails in one or both of its gas exchange functions: oxygenation and/or elimination of carbon dioxide. Acute respiratory failure due to postoperative pulmonary complications involves 10 to

Table 1. Some postoperative pulmonary complications

▌ Hypoxemia
▌ Hypoventilation (analgesic and/or residual neuromuscular blockade)
▌ Bronchospasm
▌ Atelectasis
▌ Pleural effusion
▌ Chemical pneumonitis (aspiration of gastric contents)
▌ Nosocomial pneumonia
▌ Pulmonary edema
▌ Exacerbation of underlying pulmonary conditions (COPD)
▌ Embolic phenomena (thrombus, fat, air)
▌ ARDS
▌ Tracheal laceration or rupture

25% of postoperative abdominal patients and is associated with a 40 to 65% mortality rate [7–9]. Acute respiratory failure has been mostly defined as need for mechanical ventilation. The data regarding the time at which mechanical ventilation is instituted vary broadly from a few hours after surgery to 5 days postoperatively [3, 4]. Patients who develop acute respiratory failure and require endotracheal intubation and prolonged mechanical have an increased morbidity and mortality [6].

Hypoxemia is the most common phenomenon responsible for acute respiratory failure and mechanical ventilation in postoperative abdominal patients. Most studies have documented severe episodes of arterial oxygen desaturation in the early postoperative period that may persist for several days [10]. There are many definitions used depending on its severity. The incidence ranges from 41 to 68% [11]. The criteria for starting mechanical ventilation vary from a PaO_2 lower than 60 mmHg [5] to a PaO_2/FiO_2 lower than 200 mmHg. Atelectasis and pneumonia are the most common underlying mechanisms responsible for postoperative hypoxemia. Atelectasis is defined as closure or collapse of alveoli and is often described in relation to radiologic findings and clinical symptoms. Pneumonia is usually addressed with atelectasis together because many of the pathological changes with atelectasis may predispose a patient to pneumonia [12]. The incidence of pneumonia, considered as presence of clinical features consistent with collapse or consolidation plus an otherwise unexplained temperature above 38 °C and either a positive chest radiograph or evidence of infection from sputum microbiology, ranges between 2 and 19% [5, 13, 14].

Development of atelectasis within the perioperative period ranges between 80–85%; in the postoperative period 20–70% of the episodes of severe hypoxemia are due to atelectasis [9, 13]. Development of postoperative atelectasis and pneumonia are associated with a 30 to 50% increased risk of developing acute respiratory failure requiring mechanical ventilation [9, 15]. Atelectasis is considered one of the important mechanisms responsible for the development of acute lung injury (ALI) by reducing local alveolar lung tissue oxygen tension and increasing lung permeability. Recent data indicating that alveolar hypoxia may result in pulmonary vascular leak and increased lung inflammation through macrophage recruitment support

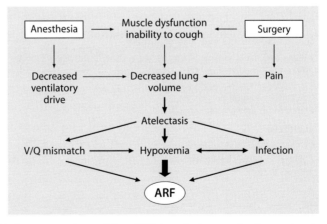

Fig. 1. Mechanisms responsible for acute respiratory failure (ARF) in patients recovering from major abdominal surgery

this contention [16]. Moreover, atelectasis formation promotes both bacterial growth in the lung and translocation from the lung into the blood stream [12] (Fig. 1).

Etiology of Postoperative Acute Respiratory Failure

The outcome of the surgical procedure depends on the correct management of the pre-, intra- and postoperative periods.

Preoperative Factors

Risk factors in the preoperative period that may predispose to acute respiratory failure are listed in Table 2. In a case-control study in patients undergoing abdominal surgery, a multivariate analysis found, in order of importance, abnormal chest examination, abnormal chest radiograph, high cardiac-risk index, and presence of relevant co-morbidities were independently associated with an increased risk of acute respiratory failure [17].

Table 2. Preoperative risk factors for postoperative acute respiratory failure

General health and nutritional status:
- age: (the risk increases over 70 years old)
- ASA class
- co-morbidity
- obesity
- low albumin
- loss of body weight

Respiratory status:
- COPD, asthma
- smoke
- sputum production
- sleep disorders
- presence of naso-gastric tube

Surgical incision site and type of surgery:
- Upper abdominal surgery: when the site is close to the diaphragm the risk is 10 to 40% more than in other sites
- abdominal aortic aneurysm repair
- emergency surgical procedures
- open versus laparoscopic surgical approach

Anesthesia:
- longer than 2 hours
- general vs peripheral anesthesia

Perioperative Factors

Anesthesia. Around 90% of all patients who are anesthetized develop atelectasis. Moreover, these lesions occupy 15–20% of the lung before any surgery is performed [18]. Atelectasis produced by anesthesia is predominantly due to three factors:

- loss of diaphragm muscle tone which no longer acts as a rigid wall between abdomen and thoracic cavity; the abdominal pressure is hence transmitted to the thorax compressing the lung and causing compression atelectasis
- breathing with high inspiratory fraction of oxygen (FiO_2) may promote atelectasis formation because of gas re-absorption
- surfactant seems to be impeded during anesthesia reducing alveolar stability [3, 19, 20].

Surgery. Surgical manipulations cause structural abnormalities with increased permeability and bowel wall edema, and motility disorders with accumulation of secretions and gas, both resulting in abdominal distension and increase in abdominal pressure [21].

Postoperative Factors

Pulmonary complications in the first hours after abdominal surgery are predominantly due to atelectasis in the dependent regions of the lung, which are produced due to several factors during surgery. One of the basic mechanisms of development of atelectasis is the reduction in lung inflation, which is invariably affected after abdominal surgery. Despite that, there is no change in the percentage of forced expired volume in the first second (FEV1) thus indicating the presence of a restrictive process [22]. There is an important reduction in inspiratory and expiratory reserve volume during the first days [23, 24] with a 30 to 40% reduction in functional residual (FRC) [24, 25] and total lung (TLC) [26] capacities. All these factors are emphasized by a prolonged recumbent position and residual pain producing impaired mucociliary clearance that combined with a weak cough effectiveness increases the risk of atelectasis and infections [27].

It has been suggested that chest wall and diaphragmatic dysfunction may be important in the genesis of postoperative pulmonary complications. They contribute to the altered lung function due to a restriction in diaphragm movement. Ford et al. and others noted a decrease in trans-diaphragmatic pressure and diaphragm contribution to tidal volume after surgery, which did not reach the normal value even with active maximal inspirations and incentive spirometry done by the patient [23, 28]. Furthermore, the marked diaphragmatic dysfunction concomitant with a paradoxical movement of the diaphragm may persist for up to one week after upper abdominal surgery [23, 29]. In a recent study conducted in patients with supra-umbilical laparotomy, modifications in the diaphragm in the three days consecutive to surgery were found. These were compatible with an altered diaphragmatic excitability and or reduced central drive [30]. To date it is not clear if optimum control of postoperative pain by regional anesthesia may result in greater respiratory excursion or improvement in lung function [31]. This suggests that respiratory muscle dysfunction and respiratory failure may be produced by an alteration in central drive, even in the presence of enhanced pain control. It has been demonstrated that when animals breathe against severe inspiratory resistive loads, no changes are observed in diaphragm force output, despite development of progressive hypercapnia and respiratory acidosis [32].

Pain is one of the factors responsible for decreased lung volumes provoking diminished respiratory performance. Optimum pain control using postoperative epidural analgesia may result in several benefits through a reduction in the incidence of pulmonary complications [33].

Hypoventilation, the result of a reduction in carbon dioxide elimination and eventually oxygenation is the consequence of a depression in respiratory drive caused by any anesthetic agent, an increase in abdominal pressure due to surgery, reduction of FRC and vital capacity, reduced respiratory muscle function, pain provoked from an abdominal incision, and an analgesic regime involving opioids [34, 35]. Although there has been a significant decrease in the incidence of respiratory depression and hypoventilation over the course of the last two decades, a recent report found that the incidence of respiratory depression and consequent hypoventilation continue to be the same using patient controlled anesthesia vs epidural analgesia [36].

▌ Treatment

Preoperative

Considerable time and effort are devoted to prevention and treatment of acute respiratory failure. There is no absolute consensus as to the most appropriate and effective therapy, and considerable controversy exists. The goal is to identify patients with preexisting pathologies or predisposing factors that may affect the postoperative course. Smokers have a high risk of postoperative pulmonary complications even when they are not affected by chronic obstructive pulmonary disease (COPD). It has been shown that 8 weeks smoking abstinence is beneficial [37]. The treatment for COPD patients before surgery should include a combination of bronchodilators, physical therapy, and corticosteroids. The use of preoperative antibiotics does not prevent the risk of postoperative pulmonary complications unless there is a current respiratory infection. Asthma patients should be free of wheezing, and if necessary the patient should receive corticosteroids [38]. A strict follow up should be done in patients with a diagnosis or suspicion of obstructive sleep apnea.

Preoperative physiotherapy has been demonstrated to have beneficial effects on postoperative pulmonary complications [8]. In a recent randomized control trial, Fagevik Olsen and colleges studied the effect of preoperative chest physiotherapy vs no respiratory therapy in patients with and without high risk factors. The treatment, including breathing exercises with pursed lips, huffing, coughing and resistive training during inspiration and expiration, was associated with a reduction in postoperative pulmonary complications and improvement in oxygen saturation after abdominal surgery [7].

Intraoperative

A recent study showed that reduction in oxygen concentration from 100 to 60% decreased atelectasis [39]. Also, the application of positive end-expiratory pressure (PEEP) in the intraoperative period may play an important role in reopening the collapsed lung [40]. However, there is no evidence that it improves arterial oxygenation or lung function postoperatively [41].

Postoperative

Early treatment. In the postoperative period, there is evidence in favor of chest physiotherapy [42]. However, in many studies there is no definition of the specific chest physiotherapy intervention, which makes the evaluation of outcome difficult. Lung expansion maneuvers are the mainstay to reduce postoperative pulmonary complications. The techniques of percussion and postural drainage have shown no value as routine interventions; they may be of benefit in patients with established atelectasis or diseases causing secretion management problems [43]. Data regarding deep breathing and incentive spirometry are conflicting. Incentive spirometry is the technique to sustain maximal inspirations through a device. It is a widely used technique for prophylaxis and treatment of postoperative pulmonary complications [44], although there is not enough evidence to support its use. Most of the randomized trials [45–47] have shown no effectiveness or at least no superiority of deep breathing, chest physiotherapy, or continuous positive airway pressure (CPAP).

Oxygen therapy is usually successful in preventing both continuous and episodic hypoxemia and can reduce tachycardia, particularly in the most hypoxemic patients [48]. However, oxygen therapy is rarely continued after the second postoperative night and the apparent incidence of hypoxemia may be greater in subsequent nights. A recent meta-analysis showed that although postoperative hypoxemia is more closely controlled with better oxygenation, there are no benefits regarding morbidity and mortality nor evidence of reduction in the incidence of acute respiratory failure [49].

Although the use of CPAP in post-abdominal surgery is rational, its effects on the treatment of atelectasis and on clinical outcomes are still not clear. From the 330 articles related to CPAP, only six randomized trials fit into the category of postoperative abdominal patients and most of them studied a small population. There is evidence that the application of CPAP in comparison with conservative physiotherapy and other techniques and when used for consecutive days after surgery, improves residual lung capacity and lung volumes in general more rapidly [24, 47, 48]. Furthermore, it may also diminish the development of atelectasis [43, 45, 46]. Stock et al. in a randomized study confirmed that after 72 hours of treatment only 22% of the CPAP group had atelectasis compared to 41% with physiotherapy and 42% with incentive spirometry [45]. In two subsequent randomized trials, the authors were not able to confirm a better outcome in physiologic effect or a reduction in clinically relevant variables like pneumonia or a reduction in length of ICU stay in patients treated with CPAP [50, 51]. All these trials were characterized by the fact that treatment was applied only for a few hours and by the small number of patients included. Bohner et al. in a more recent study with a larger number of patients undergoing vascular abdominal surgery also found no correlation between CPAP and improvement in postoperative pulmonary complications [52]. However, there was a trend to a lower intubation rate in the group treated with CPAP. The limited scope of the foregoing randomized trials leaves unanswered questions about the utility of CPAP as a preventive treatment in acute respiratory failure. Delclaux and coworkers conducted a multicenter, randomized controlled trial comparing

CPAP with standard medical treatment. Although the authors reported better gas exchange in the CPAP group in the first hours, no other benefit in reduction of endotracheal intubation rate and length of ICU and hospital stay was demonstrated thereafter. It may be that as these patients already had ALI they were more likely to require prolonged ventilator support and develop pulmonary complications [53]. Data addressing the use of non-invasive ventilation (NIV) in patients developing postoperative acute respiratory failure are sparse [53–58].

Conclusion

Postoperative pulmonary complications remain a significant problem after abdominal surgery. Efforts should be focused on optimizing patient condition before and immediately after surgery when signs of acute respiratory failure are still not evident. Physiotherapy, CPAP, and NIV seem to have a strong physiological rationale for reducing the development of atelectasis and increasing lung volumes to prevent acute respiratory failure when they are instituted early. Carefully conducted controlled clinical trials are necessary to draw valid conclusions relative to the clinical efficacy of these interventions in preventing and treating postoperative pulmonary complications in patients recovering from abdominal surgery.

References

1. Arozullah AM, Conde MV, Lawrence VA (2003) Preoperative evaluation for postoperative pulmonary complications. Med Clin North Am 87:153–173
2. Doyle RL (1999) Assessing and modifying the risk of postoperative pulmonary complications. Chest 115(Suppl 5):77S–81S
3. Thompson JS, Baxter BT, Allison JG, Johnson FE, Lee KK, Park WY (2003) Temporal patterns of postoperative complications. Arch Surg 138:596–602
4. Arozullah AM, Daley J, Henderson WG, Khuri SF (2000) Multifactorial risk index for predicting postoperative respiratory failure in men after major noncardiac surgery. The National Veterans Administration Surgical Quality Improvement Program. Ann Surg 232:242–253
5. Hall JC, Tarala RA, Hall JL (1996) Respiratory insufficiency after abdominal surgery. Respirology 1:133–138
6. Epstein SK, Ciubotaru RL, Wong JB (1997) Effect of failed extubation on the outcome of mechanical ventilation. Chest 112:186–192
7. Fagevik Olsen M, Hahn I, Nordgren S, Lonroth H, Lundholm K (1997) Randomized controlled trial of prophylactic chest physiotherapy in major abdominal surgery. Br J Surg 84:1535–1538
8. Celli B (1984) A control trail of intermittent positive pressure breathing, incentive spirometry and deep breathing exercises in preventing pulmonary complications after abdominal surgery. Am Rev Respir Dis 130:12–15
9. Brooks- Brunn JA (1995) Postoperative atelectasis and pneumonia. Heart Lung 24:94–115
10. Reeder MK, Goldman MD, Loh L, et al (1992) Postoperative hypoxaemia after mayor abdominal vascular surgery. Br J Anaesth 68:23–26
11. Moller JT, Wittrup M, Johansen SH (1990) Hypoxemia in the postanesthesia care unit: an observer study. Anesthesiology 73:890–895
12. van Kaam AH, Lachmann RA, Herting E, et al (2004) Reducing atelectasis attenuates bacterial growth and translocation in experimental pneumonia. Am J Respir Crit Care Med 169:1046–1053
13. Golfieri R, Giampalma E, Morselli Labate AM, et al (2000) Pulmonary complications of liver transplantation: radiological appearance and statistical evaluation of risk factors in 300 cases. Eur Radiol 10:1169–1183

14. Blankensteijn JD, Lindenburg FP, Van der Graaf Y, Eikelboom BC (1998) Influence of study design on reported mortality and morbidity rates after abdominal aortic aneurysm repair. Br J Surg 85:1624–1630
15. Mermel LA, Maki DG (1990) Bacterial pneumonia in solid organ transplantation. Semin Respir Infect 5:10–29
16. Duggan M, McCaul CL, McNamara PJ, Engelberts D, Ackerley C, Kavanagh BP (2003) Atelectasis causes vascular leak and lethal right ventricular failure in uninjured rat lungs. Am J Respir Crit Care Med 167:1633–1640
17. Lawrence VA, Dhanda R, Hilsenbeck SG, Page CP (1996) Risk of pulmonary complications after elective abdominal surgery. Chest 110:744–750
18. Gunnarsson L, Tokics L, Gustavsson H, Hedenstierna G (1991) Influence of age on atelectasis formation and gas exchange impairment during general anaesthesia. Br J Anaesth 66:423–432
19. Hedenstierna G (2003) Alveolar collapse and closure or airways: regular effects of anaesthesia. Clin Physiol Funct Imaging 23:123–129
20. Otis DR Jr, Johnson M, Pedley TJ, Kamm RD (1993) Role of pulmonary surfactant in airway closure: a computational study. J Appl Physiol 75:1323–1333
21. Mirza K, Baig MD, Steven D, Wexner MD (2004) Postoperative ileus: a review. Dis Colon Rectum 47:516–526
22. Meyers JR, Lembeck L, O'Kane H, Baue AE (1975) Changes in functional residual capacity of the lung after operation. Arch Surg 110:576–583
23. Ford GT, Whitelaw WA, Rosental TW, Cruse PJ, Guenter CA (1983) Diaphragm function after upper abdominal surgery in humans. Am Rev Respir Dis 127:431–436
24. Lidner KH, Lotz P, Ahnefeld F (1987) Continuous positive airway pressure effect on functional residual capacity, vital capacity and its subdivisions. Chest 92:66–70
25. Fagevik Olsen M, Wennberg E, Johnsson E, Josefson K, Lonroth H, Lundell L (2002) Randomized clinical study of the prevention of pulmonary complications after thoracoabdominal resection by two different breathing techniques. Br J Surg 89:1228–1234
26. Zikria BA, Sencer JL, Kinney JM, Broell JR (1974) Alterations in ventilatory function and breathing patterns following surgical trauma. Ann Surg 179:1–7
27. Bartlett RH, Gazzaniga AB, Geraghty T (1973) Respiratory maneuvers to prevent postoperative pulmonary complications: a critical review. JAMA 224:1017–1021
28. Chuter TA, Weissman C, Mathews DM, Starker PM (1990) Diaphragmatic breathing maneuvers and movement of the diaphragm after cholecystectomy. Chest 97:1110–1114
29. Simonneau G, Vivien A, Sartene R, et al (1983) Diaphragm dysfunction induced by upper abdominal surgery. Role of postoperative pain. Am Rev Respir Dis 128:899–903
30. Berdah SV, Picaud R, Jammes Y (2002) Surface diaphragmatic electromyogram changes after laparotomy. Clin Physiol Funct Imaging 22:157–160
31. Rodgers A, Walker N, Schug S, et al (2000) Reduction of postoperative mortality and morbidity with epidural or spinal anaesthesia: results from overview of randomised trials. BMJ 321:1493
32. Radell PJ, Eleff SM, Traystman RJ, Nichols DG (1997) In vivo diaphragm metabolism comparison: comparison of pace and inspiratory resistive loaded breathing in piglets. Crit Care Med 25:339–345
33. Block BM, Liu SS, Rowlingson AJ, Cowan AR, Cowan JA Jr, Wu CL (2003) Efficacy of postoperative epidural analgesia: a meta-analysis. JAMA 290:2455–2463
34. Catley DM, Thornton C, Jordan B, Lehane JR, Royston D, Jones JG (1985) Pronounced episodic oxygen desaturation in the postoperative period: its association with ventilatory pattern and analgesic regimen. Anesthesiology 63:20–28
35. Motamed C, Spencer A, Farhat F, Bourgan L, Lasser P, Jayr C (1998) Postoperative hypoxemia: continuous extradural infusion of bupivacaine and morphine vs patient-control analgesia with intravenous morphine. Br J Anaesth 80:742–747
36. Cashman JN, Dolin SJ (2004) Respiratory and haemodynamic effects of acute postoperative pain management: evidence from published data. Br J Anaesth 93:212–223
37. Moller AM, Villebro N, Pedersen P (2002) Effect of preoperative smoking intervention on postoperative complications: a randomized clinical trial. Lancet 359:114–117

38. Warner DO, Warner MA, Barnes RD (1996) Perioperative respiratory complications in patients with asthma. Anesthesiology 85:460–467
39. Edmark L, Kostova-Aherdan K, Enlund M, Hedenstierna G (2003) Optimal oxygen concentration during induction of general anesthesia. Anesthesiology 98:28–33
40. Brismar B, Hedenstierna G, Lundquist H, Strandberg A, Svensson L, Tokics L (1985) Pulmonary densities during anesthesia with muscular relaxation – a proposal of atelectasis. Anesthesiology 62:422–428
41. Lotz P, Heise U, Schaffer J, Wollinsky KH (1984) The effects of intraoperative PEEP ventilation and postoperative CPAP breathing on postoperative lung function following upper abdominal surgery. Anaesthesist 33:177–188
42. Thoren L (1954) Postoperative pulmonary complications. Observation on their prevention by means of physiotherapy. Acta Chir Scand 107:194–205
43. Stein M, Cassava EL (1970) preoperative pulmonary evaluation and therapy for surgery patients. JAMA 211:787–790
44. O'Donohue WJ Jr (1985) National survey of the usage of lung expansion modalities for the prevention and treatment of postoperative atelectasis following abdominal and thoracic surgery. Chest 87:76–80
45. Stock MC, Downs JB, Gauer PK, Alster JM, Imrey PB (1985) Prevention of postoperative pulmonary complications with CPAP, incentive spirometry and conservative therapy. Chest 87:151–157
46. Ricksten SE, Bengtsson A, Soderberg C, Thorden M, Kvist H (1986) Effects of periodic Positive airway pressure by mask on postoperative pulmonary function. Chest 89:6:774–781
47. Overend TJ, Anderson CM, Lucy SD, Bhatia C, Jonsson BI, Timmermans C (2001) The effect of incentive spirometry on postoperative pulmonary complications: a systematic review. Chest 120:971–978
48. Rosemberg-Adamsen S, Lie C, Bernhard A, Kehlet H, Rosemberg J (1999) Effect of oxygen treatment on heart rate after abdominal surgery. Anesthesiology 90:380–384
49. Pedersen T, Dyrlund Pedersen B, Moller AM (2003) Pulse oximetry for perioperative monitoring. Cochrane Database Syst Rev CD002013
50. Denehy L, Carroll S, Ntoumenopoulos G, Jenkins S (2001) A randomized control trial comparing periodic mask CPAP with physiotherapy after abdominal surgery. Physiother Res Int 6:236–250
51. Carlsson C, Sonden B, Thylen U (1981) Can postoperative continuous positive airway pressure (CPAP) prevent pulmonary complications after abdominal surgery? Intensive Care Med 7:225–229
52. Bohner H, Kindgen-Milles D, Grust A (2002) Prophylactic nasal continuous positive airway pressure after mayor vascular surgery: results of a prospective randomized trial. Arch Surg 387:21–26
53. Delclaux C, L'Her E, Alberti C (2000) Treatment of acute hypoxemic non hypercapnic respiratory insufficiency with continuous positive airway pressure delivered by face mask: a randomized controlled trial. JAMA 284:2352–2360
54. Antonelli M, Conti G, Bufi M, et al (2000) Noninvasive ventilation for treatment of acute respiratory failure in patients undergoing solid organ transplantation. A randomized trial JAMA 283:235–241
55. Kilger E, Briegel J, Haller M, et al (1999) Effects of noninvasive pressure ventilatory support in non-COPD patiens with acute respiratory insufficiency after early extubation. Intensive Care Med 25:1374–1380
56. Antonelli M, Conti G, Rocco M, et al (1998) A comparison of Noninvasive positive pressure ventilation and conventional mechanical ventilation in patients with acute respiratory failure. N Engl J Med 339:429–435
57. Keenan SP, Powers C, McCormack DG, Block G (2002) Noninvasive positive pressure ventilation for postextubation respiratory distress. A randomized control trial. JAMA 287:3238–3244
58. Esteban A, Frutos-Vivar F, Ferguson ND, et al (2004) Noninvasive positive pressure ventilation for respiratory failure after extubation. N Engl J Med 350:2452–2460

Tracheostomy in Critically Ill Patients:
The Right Technique in the Right Patient

P. Pelosi, A. Lombardo, and P. Severgnini

Introduction

Tracheostomy is one of the most frequent procedures carried out in critically ill patients [1, 2]. Translaryngeal endotracheal intubation, oral or nasal, can cause lesions to the vocal cords if prolonged, difficulties in oral nursing, tube obstruction with an increase in airway resistance, and increased patient intolerance [3]. Orotracheal translaryngeal intubation can also be associated with kinking of the tube, while nasotracheal translaryngeal intubation can be associated with anatomical fractures of nasal bones and sinusitis. Tracheostomy can provide several theoretical advantages compared to translaryngeal endotracheal intubation such as reduced laryngeal anatomical alterations, better patient tolerance, reduced inspiratory load, and easier nursing. Thus, tracheostomy is indicated for prolonged ventilatory support and long-term airway maintenance, making patient care and the process of weaning from mechanical ventilation easier. Furthermore, recently percutaneous tracheostomy has gained increasing popularity as an alternative to conventional surgical tracheostomy [4–6]. Moreover, percutaneous tracheostomy can be safely performed at the bedside after previous tracheostomy [7]. Different percutaneous techniques have been developed, but data are lacking about the specific indication and clinical management of each of them. Finally, a multidisciplinary approach has been suggested to improve care of patients with tracheostomy. These dedicated teams, comprised of doctors, nurses, speech therapists, physiotherapists and dietetic staff, have to work closely and in a co-ordinated collaborative manner to assure that all the needs of these patients are met and outcomes are optimized [8]. In this chapter, we will discuss:
- percutaneous and open surgical tracheostomy;
- different percutaneous techniques;
- tracheostomy timing and patient selection;
- complications of percutaneous techniques.

Percutaneous Versus Surgical Tracheostomy

Comparing percutaneous tracheostomy with historical data of complications for surgical tracheostomy is erroneous and may give a biased picture. Furthermore, due to different definitions of complications used by authors, these figures should be interpreted cautiously. Percutaneous tracheostomy can be performed immediately once the decision is made and few personnel are needed. In contrast, surgical tracheostomy requires more organization and if it is to be done in the operating

Table 1. Comparison between surgical (ST) and percutaneous (PDT) tracheostomy techniques: Randomized trials

	Type	pts (n)	Type of pts.	Length of intub/ tracheo (days)	Bleeding (pts. n)	Infections (pts. n)	Intraop. compl.* (pts. n)	Postop. compl.** (pts. n)
Holdgaard [11]	ST/PDT	60	medical/ trauma	6.7/9.9	36/9	19/3	26/19	30/7
Heikkinen [12]	ST/PDT	56	medical/ trauma	NA	1/5	0/0	0/1	NA
Freeman [13]	ST/PDT	80	medical/ surgical	14.1/NA	2/0	NA	NA	1/0
Friedman [14]	ST/PDT	53	medical	19.2/21.5	7/5	4/0	11/9	12/3
Crofts [15]	ST/PDT	53	medical/ trauma	11.5/NA	3/3	1/0	NA	10/6
Hazard [16]	ST/PDT	46	medical/ trauma	8.4/19.4	4/1	8/1	NA	11/3
Porter [17]	ST/PDT	53	medical/ trauma	11.1/NA	0/0	0/0	1/5	0/0
Gysin [18]	ST/PDT	70	N/A	6.6/NA	4/4	3/4	4/14	1/6
Massick [19]	ST/PDT	100	miscel- laneous	9.7/NA	0/2	0/1	1/4	1/9

* Intraoperative complications: Hypotension; hypoxia; subcutaneous emphysema; cuff puncture; difficulties in tube placement
** Postoperative complications: Accidental decannulation; cannula obstruction; tracheitis; tracheal stenosis; pneumothorax
NA: not available; Length of intubation and tracheo mean the average period of time of intubation before tracheostomy and the period of time with tracheostomy, respectively

room, time scheduling. The time required for percutaneous tracheostomy is generally shorter than that for the surgical route, which implies less stress to the patient and better use of resources. Although cost analysis between percutaneous and surgical tracheostomies is not easy because of varying reimbursment systems and hospital structures, available studies show that percutaneous tracheostomy is considerably cheaper than the surgical route. It is common sense that if fewer personnel and no operating room time are required and the patient need not be moved, then the overall cost of percutaneous tracheostomy has to be lower than that of surgical tracheostomy [9, 10]. In Table 1, we show the prospective randomized trials comparing percutaneous and surgical tracheostomies. The majority of the prospective randomized trials show that the potential advantages of percutaneous technique relative to surgical tracheostomy include ease of performance, and lower incidence of peristomal bleeding and postoperative infection associated with lower costs [11–16]. Some prospective randomized trials have confirmed that percutaneous tracheostomy is a simpler and quicker procedure compared to surgical tracheostomy, with lower early postoperative complications. Nevertheless late tracheal complications were more frequent in the percutaneous group [17, 18]. Other prospective randomized trials reported that the percutaneous technique was associated with an increased postoperative complication incidence and costs, suggesting that surgical procedures should represent the standard of care in bedside tracheostomy placement providing a more secure airway at a markedly reduced patient charge [19, 20]. Finally, four recent meta-analyses have reported conflicting results when percutaneous and surgical tracheostomies were compared: two were in favor of percutaneous techniques [21, 22], one against [23], and one reported similar complications and costs between both techniques [24]. However, the real clinical impact of the results of these meta-analyses is limited by the heterogeneity of the patients and the percutaneous techniques included in the studies cited.

▌ Percutaneous Techniques

A percutaneous dilatational technique was proposed by Ciaglia et al. in 1985 [25] using progressive dilatation with blunt tipped dilators. Since then several other methods have been proposed to perform percutaneous tracheostomy at the bedside [26–29]. The major problem related to the use of progressive dilatation with blunt tipped dilators is the time factor, potentially increasing the risk of traumatic and infective complications. Thus, newer techniques have been developed, some of them characterized by the insertion of the tracheostomy cannula from outside the trachea:

▌ modified original Ciaglia technique ("single step" Blue-Rhino) [26];
▌ guide wire dilator forceps technique proposed by Griggs [27];
▌ the Percu-twist as proposed by Frova and Quintel [28];

while another is characterized by the fact that the tracheostomy cannula is inserted from inside the trachea, the translaryngeal technique proposed by Fantoni [29].

The Blue-Rhino is characterized by a modification of the original Ciaglia technique simplified with only one single dilator. The preferred site of entry is now between the first and the second or the second and the third tracheal rings. Initial skin incision and blunt preparation of the pretracheal tissue may be helpful to identify the tracheal rings, thus avoiding either too high or too low tracheal puncture. After dilatation with the maximal available dilator, a tracheal cannula (inner diameter up to 9 mm) can be inserted whilst mounted on a corresponding dilator. The average time required to perform the dilational tracheostomy is 10–15 min. Although Ciaglia's technique has been carried out successfully on children [30], there are still reservations on its use in this age group due to marked elasticity of the tracheal tissue. The main problems related to this technique are: a) difficult ventilation; b) bleeding; c) rupture or dislocation of tracheal rings.

Grigg's technique is characterized by the use of forceps for blunt dilatation of the pretracheal and intercartilagineous tissue after insertion of the guide wire into the trachea and skin incision. The average time required for a tracheostomy is about 5 min. Applying this method on patients with a short and/or thick neck may be difficult, if not dangerous, particularly while attempting to perform intercartilaginous dilatation. Although not widely investigated, this method could possibly be applied in emergency situations [31] and in hematologic patients at risk of bleeding [32], following proper patient selection. The main problems of this technique are:

▌ the dilation with forceps is not easily calibrated with cannula diameter;
▌ rupture or dislocation of tracheal rings;
▌ difficult ventilation.

The Percu-twist technique is characterized by a controlled rotating dilation performed by an external spiral, which should reduce the tracheal wall collapse during the maneuver. The problem with this technique is rupture or dislocation of tracheal rings. All these percutaneous techniques are characterized by the dilation of the tissues and applied of forces from outside to inside the tracheal wall.

The translaryngeal technique [29] is different from the others because the cannula is stripped from inside to outside. In contrast to the other techniques, the initial puncture of the trachea is carried out with the needle directed cranially and the tracheal cannula inserted with a pull through technique along the orotracheal route. This modification in the direction of the forces should favor:

- much less injury to the tissues and tracheal wall itself, both in the anterior and posterior wall;
- reduced bleeding;
- possibility to ventilate during the maneuver;
- the possible application of this technique in pediatric patients in which all other techniques are often contraindicated.

The major problems related to the technique are:
- the difficulty to intubate the patients with a rigid fiberscope;
- need of several intubations and extubations (thus this technique is contraindicated in patients with difficult intubation and in those in whom neck extension has to be avoided);
- difficulties in ventilation during the maneuver;
- not indicated for emergency procedures.

While performing percutaneous tracheostomy, independent of the technique, several tools have been suggested to improve the safety of the maneuver:
- the use of bronchoscopy with simple endoscopy or videoassisted endoscopy to facilitate and reduce possible complications [33–36];
- previous evaluation by chest radiography, magnetic resonance imaging (MRI) and ultrasound assessment prior to percutaneous dilatational tracheostomy in patients with altered neck and tracheal anatomy [37];
- chest radiograph following dilatational percutaneous tracheostomy after procedures noted to be difficult by the physician [38].

In particular clinical situations, ultrasound-guided control and the use of laryngeal mask have also been reported to be useful [39, 40]. However, we discourage the routine use of laryngeal mask due to the unnecessary increased risks related to the lack of optimal airway control.

Finally, the standardization of a correct ventilatory procedure in pressure control, oxygen fraction 1.0, and positive end expiratory pressure (PEEP) of 0 cmH$_2$O, associated with capnography has been suggested to make the procedure safer [41]. Other studies have demonstrated the safety of the procedure even with the use of high PEEP in patients with severe respiratory failure [42].

A few studies in small groups of patients have been performed to evaluate possible differences between each technique. In Table 2, the prospective randomized trials comparing different percutaneous techniques are reported. The major limitations of these studies are the heterogeneity of the patients included and the different learning curves of the operators. With all the limitations of these studies it is possible to summarize:

Table 2. Comparison between different percutaneous tracheostomy techniques: Randomized trials

	Type	pts (n)	Type of pts.	Intub/ tacheo length (days)	Bleeding (pts. n)	Infections (pts. n)	Intraop. compl.* (pts. n)	Postop. compl.** (pts. n)
Johnson [43]	Ciaglia/ CBR	50	miscel- laneous	NA	3/4	0/0	11/8	0/0
Byhahn [26]	Ciaglia/ CBR	50	miscel- laneous	7.3/17.2	1/7	0/1	6/11	1/6
Nates [44]	CBR/ Griggs	100	miscel- laneous	6.2/NA	1/7	0/1	0/5	1/6
Anón [45]	CBR/ Griggs	53	miscel- laneous	18.8/NA	2/1	0/1	0/5	1/6
Heurn [46]	CBR/ Griggs	127	miscel- laneous	14/14.5	4/7	0/0	3/13	0/0
Ambesh [47]	CBR/ Griggs	50	miscel- laneous	8.5/11.5	1/5	0/0	14/19	5/3
Cantais [48]	Griggs/ Fantoni	100	miscel- laneous	18.5/NA	12/2	NA	1/20	NA
Byhahn [49]	Griggs/ Fantoni	100	medical	NA	9/0	0/0	1/2	NA
Westphal [50]	CBR/ Fantoni	80	medical/ surgical	11/NA	3/0	0/0	2/0	2/0
Byhahn [51]	CBR/ PercuTw	70	medical/ surgical	9.5/NA	3/2	4/9	0/1	1/6

* Intraoperative complications: Hypotension; hypoxia; subcutaneous emphysema; cuff puncture; difficulties in tube placement
** Postoperative complications: Accidental decannulation; cannula obstruction; tracheitis; tracheal stenosis; pneumothorax
CBR: Ciaglia Blue-Rhino percutaneous technique; PercuTw: Percutwist percutaneous; Fantoni: Translayngeal percutaneous technique; Griggs: forceps percutanepus technique; Length of intubation and tracheo mean the average period of time of intubation before tracheostomy and the period of time with tracheostomy, respectively

▌ the 'single step' Blue-Rhino technique presents advantages compared to the conventional Ciaglia technique in terms of time consumed and complications [26, 43]
▌ there is no clear difference between Blue-Rhino and Griggs' technique. One study [44] reported a lower complication rate, less operative and postoperative bleeding and less overall technical difficulties with Blue-Rhino compared to Griggs. Two other studies [45, 46] reported no substantial differences between these two techniques. Finally a third study [47] reported equal efficiency of both techniques, but Blue-Rhino was associated with rupture of tracheal rings in one-third of patients, whereas the Griggs' technique was associated with under- or over-formation of the tracheal opening, each in one third of patients
▌ no clear advantages of the translaryngeal technique compared to the Blue-Rhino or Griggs' techniques. One study found that Griggs' technique was superior to translaryngeal in terms of shorter time spent for the procedure, fewer technical

difficulties, and fewer complications [48], while another study reported no significant differences [49]. No differences were reported between Blue-Rhino and Fantoni [50]

▌ the Percutwist appears to be comparable to the Blue Rhino and Griggs, although more severe complications were observed with the former technique [51].

Thus it does not appear that any one percutaneous technique is much better than another, but that the right choice of patient and the personal experience of the operators is crucial.

Some complications have been reported for all percutaneous techniques. Among them the most frequent are: the intermittent obstruction of the cannula caused by swelling and irritation of the posterior tracheal wall, emphysema pneumothorax due to posterior tracheal wall laceration, tracheal ring fracture, tracheo-esophageal fistula, tracheal stenosis and obliteration above the tracheostoma, and acute fatal hemorrhage [52]. Sometimes, a partial occlusion of the tracheostomic cannula is possible, due to the protrusion of the tip of the cannula in the posterior membranous part of the trachea. In this case a modification of the shape of the tip of the cannula (from flat to angled) can help to reduce the incidence of partial airways obstruction [53].

▌ Timing and Patient Selection

The majority of pathologies can be managed both by conventional endotracheal intubation or tracheostomy, thus the timing of tracheostomy is still controversial. There is general agreement that translaryngeal endotracheal intubation should be the first approach and only subsequently is evaluation for possible tracheostomy necessary. In particular, translaryngeal intubation has been recommended for an anticipated need of up to 10 days and a tracheostomy if an artificial airway is anticipated to be needed for more than 21 days [54]. Recently, the use of early tracheostomy has been recommended by several authors in different categories of patients. We believe that early tracheostomy is mandatory in severe maxillofacial or neck trauma, burns to the head, neck and airways, and presence of altered swallowing. However, no beneficial effects of early tracheostomy on outcome in burn patients or in earlier extubation has been reported, except for better patient comfort and security [55]. In a recent prospective randomized trial performed in medical patients the effects on outcome of early (within 48 hours) and delayed (at 14–16 days) percutaneous tracheostomy was assessed [56] showing a significant reduction in mortality, incidence of ventilator-associated pneumonia (VAP), days spent on ventilatory support, and days sedated in the early tracheostomized group. The authors hypothesized that the benefits of early tracheostomy are the direct result of the reduction in VAP which in turn resulted from early cessation of sedation, a reduction in time spent on ventilatory support, and the ability to change the tracheostomy inner cannula on a daily basis thus preventing the accumulation of infected secretions in the tube. This study would provide compelling evidence to consider early tracheostomy in those patients who seem likely to require prolonged ventilatory support. In other studies performed in surgical patients resolving from acute respiratory failure and in trauma patients, early tracheostomy has been found to be effective at reducing intensive care stay and resource utilization, but not hospital length of stay or mortality [57, 58]. From these studies, enthusiasm is growing for early tracheostomy in critically ill patients [59], but further studies in selected categories of patients are needed.

Unfortunately, tracheostomy per se does not reduce the incidence of VAP. In fact the presence of tracheostomy has been associated with a six fold increased risk for developing VAP [60]. Moreover, several studies found that the presence of tracheostomy was not associated with a decreased ICU and hospital length of stay and lower mortality [61, 62]. We believe that the decision on the timing of a tracheostomy should be made on an individual basis and should depend on prognostic evaluation. In fact, there are some general contraindications such as presence of large masses in the neck, usually due to the thyroid alterations, or the presence of infections in the tracheostomy area, which can preclude tracheostomy.

It is important to emphasize that the introduction of different percutaneous techniques has reduced the contraindications to tracheostomy in selected patients. Patients with neurologic or maxillofacial trauma are at particular risk of infection and difficult airway management; thus tracheostomy may be favored compared to other categories of patients. After the acute phase and once satisfactory weaning parameters have been achieved, the patient's impaired level of consciousness and inability to protect their airway represent strong reasons to delay extubation. However, appropriate timing in these patients must be considered in view of the risk of intracranial hypertension. In other words, even if early tracheostomy would appear reasonable, delaying tracheostomy until brain physiology is stabilized may be preferred [63]. Recently it has been reported that, in head trauma patients with reduced risk of intracranial hypertension, surgical, percutaneous dilatational, and translaryngeal tracheostomy were tolerated equally [64, 65]. Moreover, the percutaneous dilatational technique has been shown to be quicker and to be associated with fewer late infections of the stoma compared to surgical tracheostomy in patients with anterior cervical spine fixation [66]. In spine injured patients, we believe that Blue-Rhino, Griggs, and Percutwist techniques should be preferred due to the lesser need to move the neck in the optimization of the maneuver.

In cardiothoracic patients, with mediastinal wounds, percutaneous techniques should be considered as first choice due to the marked reduction in tracheostomy-associated risk of mediastinitis. Tracheostomy in these patients has been reported to be correlated with a reduction in the duration of mechanical ventilation and faster weaning [67]. Furthermore the routine use of percutaneous tracheostomy has been associated with a reduction in the risk of mediastinitis after thoracic and cardiovascular surgery [68]. Of the percutaneous techniques, we believe that the translaryngeal technique should be preferred in patients with coagulation problems due to hematologic disorders or iatrogenic causes, although it is always wise to temporarily interrupt any heparin infusion before the procedure. Finally, percutaneous techniques can be safely used in patients with severe respiratory failure who need high levels of PEEP [42]. It is also important to emphasize that after the operation careful clinical monitoring of patients is mandatory, as well as a bronchoscopy to clean airway secretions and blood. Thus, we believe that tracheostomy should be individualized both in terms of timing and of technique, depending on the clinical characteristics of each patient and not on global rules [69].

▮ Conclusion

In conclusion, tracheostomy can offer several advantages in the management of critically ill patients who need control of airways and/or long-term mechanical ventilation. The right timing of tracheostomy remains controversial, however it appears that early tracheostomy in selected patients, such as severe trauma and neurological patients, could be effective to reduce intensive care stay and costs. Further studies are warranted to better define the role of early tracheostomy in different categories of patients. Percutaneous tracheostomy techniques are becoming the procedure of choice in the majority of cases. This is due to the fact that percutaneous techniques are safe, easy and quick, and complications are minor, compared with surgical tracheostomies. In particular, percutaneous techniques are generally characterized by a reduction in stomal infections, and cheaper costs. However, percutaneous tracheostomies should always be performed by experienced physicians to avoid unnecessary additional complications. Surgical techniques should be considered when contraindications for percutaneous techniques are present, such as anatomical difficulties or in the presence of a previous failed percutaneous technique. The superiority of one percutaneous technique compared to another is unclear, but the experience of the operator and individual clinical, anatomical, and pathophysiological characteristics of the patient should always be considered.

References

1. Zetouni A, Kost K (1994) Tracheostomy: a retrospective review of 281 cases. J Otolaryngol 23:61–66
2. Fischler L, Erhart S, Kleger GR, Frutiger A (2000) Prevalence of tracheostomy in ICU patients. A Nation-wide survey in Switzerland. Intensive Care Med 26:1428–1433
3. Alberti PW (1984) Tracheostomy versus intubation: a 19th century controversy. Ann Otol Rhinol Laryngol 93:333–337
4. Petros S (1999) Percutaneous tracheostomy. Crit Care 3:R5–R10
5. Moe KS, Stoeckli SJ, Schmidt S, Weymulller EA Jr (1999) Percutaneous tracheostomy: a comprehensive evaluation. Ann Otol Rhinol Laryngol 108:384–391
6. DeBoisblanc BP (2003) Percutaneous dilational tracheostomy techniques. Clin Chest Med 24:399–407
7. Meyer M, Critchlow J, Mansharamani N, Angel LF, Garland R, Ernst A (2002) Repeat bedside percutaneous dilational tracheostomy is a safe procedure. Crit Care Med 30:986–988
8. Russell C, Matta B (ed) (2004) Tracheostomy-A multiprofessional handbook. Greenwich Medical Media Limited, San Francisco, CA
9. Kaylie DM, Andersen PE, Wax MK (2003) An analysis of time and staff utilization for open versus percutaneous tracheostomies. Otolaryngol Head Neck Surg 128: 109–114
10. Grover A, Robbins J, Bendick P, Gibson M, Villalba M (2001) Open versus percutaneous dilatational tracheostomy: efficacy and cost analysis. Am Surg 67:297–301
11. Holdgaard HO, Pedersen J, Jensen RH, et al (1998) Percutaneous dilatational tracheostomy versus conventional surgical tracheostomy: a clinical randomized trial. Acta Anesthesiol Scand 42:545–550
12. Heikkinen M, Aarnio P, Hannukainen J (2000) Percutaneous dilatational tracheostomy or conventional surgical tracheostomy? Crit Care Med 28:1399–1402
13. Freeman BD, Isabella K, Cobb JP, et al (2001) A prospective, randomized study comparing percutaneous with surgical tracheostomy in critically ill patients. Crit Care Med 29:926–930
14. Friedman Y, Fildes J, Mizock B, et al (1996) Comparison of percutaneous and surgical tracheostomies. Chest 110:480–485
15. Crofts SL, Alzeer A, Mc Guire M, et al (1999) A comparison of percutaneous and operative tracheostomies in intensive care patients. Can J Anaesth 42:775–779

16. Hazard P, Jones C, Benitone J (1991) Comparative clinical trial of standard operative tracheostomy. Crit Care Med 19:1018–1024
17. Melloni G, Mattini S, Gallioli C, et al (2003) Surgical tracheostomy versus percutaneous dilatational tracheostomy. A prospective randomized study with long term follow-up. J Cardiovasc Surg 43:113–121
18. Gysin C, Dulguerov P, Guyot JP, Perneger TV, Abajo B, Chevrolet JC (1990) Percutaneous versus surgical tracheostomy: a double blind randomized trial. Ann Surg 230:708–714
19. Massick DD, Yao S, Powell DM, et al (2001) Bedside tracheostomy in the intensive care unit: a prospective randomized trial comparing open surgical tracheostomy with endoscopically guided percutaneous dilatational tracheotomy. Laryngoscope 111:494–500
20. Porter JM, Ivatury RR (1999) Preferred route of tracheostomy-percutaneous versus open at the bedside: a randomized, prospective study in the surgical intensive care unit. Am Surg 65:142–146
21. Freeman BD, Isabella K, Lin N, Buchnan TG (2000) A meta-analysis of prospective trials comparing percutaneous and surgical tracheostomy in critically ill patients. Chest 118:1412–1418
22. Cheng E, Fee WE Jr (2000) Dilatational versus standard tracheostomy: a meta-analysis. Ann Otol Rhinol Latyngol 109:803–807
23. Dulgerov P, Gysin C, Perneger TV, Chevrolet JC (1999) Percutaneous or surgical tracheostomy: a meta-analysis. Crit Care Med 27:1617–1625
24. Lams E, Ravalia A (2003) Percutaneous and surgical tracheostomy. Hosp Med 64:36–39
25. Ciaglia P, Firshing R, Syniec C (1985) Elective percutaneous dilatational tracheostomy: a new simple bedside procedure: preliminary report. Chest 87:715–719
26. Byhahn C, Wilke HJ, Halbig S, Lische V, Westphal K (2000) Percutaneous tracheostomy: Ciaglia Blue Rhino versus the basic Ciaglia technique of percutaneous dilatational tracheostomy. Anesth Analg 91:882–886
27. Griggs WM, Worthley LIG, Gilligan JE, Thomas PD, Mayburg JA (1990) A simple percutaneous tracheostomy technique. Surg Gynec Obstet 170:543–545
28. Frova G, Quintel M (2002) A new simple method for percutaneous tracheostomy: controlled rotating dilating. A preliminary report. Intensive Care Med 28:299–303
29. Fantoni A, Ripamonti D (1997) A non derivative, non-surgical tracheostomy: the translaryngeal method. Intensive Care Med 23:386–392
30. Toursarkissian B, Fowler CL, Zweng TN, Kearney PA (1994) Percutaneous dilational tracheostomy in children and teenagers. J Pediatr Surg 29:1421–1424
31. Ben-Nun A, Altman E, Best LA (2004) Emergency percutaneous tracheostomy in trauma patients: an early experience. Ann Thorac Surg 77:1045–1047
32. Kluge S, Meyer A, Kuhnelt P, Baumann HJ, Kreymann G (2004) Percutaneous tracheostomy is safe in patients with severe thrombocytopenia. Chest 126:547–551
33. Oberwalser M, Weis H, Nehoda H, et al (2004) Videobronchoscopic guidance makes percutaneous dilational tracheostomy safer. Surg Endosc 18:839–842
34. Ciaglia P (1999) Video-assisted endoscopy, not just endoscopy, for percutaneous dilatational tracheostomy. Chest 115:915–916
35. Hinerman R, Alvarez F, Keller CA (2000) Outcome of bedside percutaneous tracheostomy with bronchoscopic guidance. Intensive Care Med 26:1850–1856
36. Jefferson P, Ball DR (2002) Endoscopy is useful during percutaneous tracheostomy. BMJ 324:977–978
37. Muhammad JK, Major E, Patton DW (2000) Evaluating the neck for percutaneous dilatational tracheostomy. J Craniomaxillofac Surg 28:336–342
38. Datta D, Onyirimba F, McNamee MJ (2003) The utility of chest radiographs following percutaneous dilatational tracheostomy. Chest 123:1603–1606
39. Rustic A, Zupan Z, Antoncic I (2004) Ultrasound-guided percutaneous dilatational tracheostomy with laryngeal mask airway control in a morbidly obese patients. J Clin Anesth 16:121–123
40. Dosemeci L, Yilmaz M, Gurpinar F, Ramazanoglu A (2002) The use of the laryngeal mask airway as an alternative to the endotracheal tube during percutaneous dilatational tracheostomy. Intensive Care Med 28:63–67

41. Mallick A, Venkatanath D, Elliot SC, Hollins T, Nanda Kumar CG (2003) A prospective randomized controlled trial of capnography vs bronchoscopy for Blue Rhino percutaneous tracheostomy. Anesthesia 58:864–868
42. Beiderlinden M, Groeben H, Peters J (2003) Safety of percutaneous dilatational tracheostomy in patients ventilated with high positive end expiratory pressure (PEEP). Intensive Care Med 29:944–948
43. Johnson JL, Cheatham ML, Sagraves SG, Block EF, Nelson LD (2001) Percutaneous dilational tracheostomy: a comparison of single-versus multiple-dilator techniques. Crit Care Med 29:1251–1254
44. Nates NL, Cooper DJ, Myles PS, Scheinkestel CD, Tuxen DV (2000) Percutaneous tracheostomy in critically ill patients: a prospective, randomized comparison of two techniques. Crit Care Med 28:3734–3739
45. Anon JM, Escuela MP, Gomez V, et al (2004) Percutaneous tracheostomy: Ciaglia Blue-Rhino versus Grigg's guide wire dilating forceps. A prospective randomized trial. Acta Anesthesiol Scand 48:451–456
46. Van Heurn LW, Mastboom WB, Scheeren CI, Brink PR, Ramsay G (2001) Comparative clinical trial of progressive dilatational and forceps dilatational tracheostomy. Intensive Care Med 27:292–295
47. Ambesh SP, Pandey CK, Srivastava S, Agarwal A, Singh DK (2002) Percutaneous tracheostomy with single dilatation technique: a prospective, randomized comparison of Ciaglia Blue Rhino versus Grigg's guide wire dilation forceps. Anesth Analg 95:1739–1745
48. Cantais E, Kaiser E, Le Goff Y, Palmier B (2002) Percutaneous tracheostomy: prospective comparison of the translaryngeal technique versus the forceps-dilational technique in 100 critically ill adults. Crit Care Med 30:815–819
49. Byhahn C, Wilke HJ, Lische V, Rinne T, Westphal K (2001) Bedside percutaneous tracheostomy: clinical comparison of Griggs and Fantoni techniques. World J Surg 25:296–301
50. Westphal K, Byhahn C, Rinne T, Wilke HJ, Wimmer-Greinecker G, Lische V (1999) Tracheostomy in cardiosurgical patients: surgical tracheostomy versus Ciaglia and Fantoni methods. Ann Thorac Surg 68:486–492
51. Byhahn C, Westphal K, Meininger D, Gurke B, Kessler P, Lische V (2002) Single-dilator percutaneous tracheostomy: a comparison of Percutwist and Ciaglia Blue Rhino techniques. Intensive Care Med 28:1262–1266
52. Briche T, Le Manach Y, Pats B (2001) Complications of percutaneous tracheostomy. Chest 119:1282–1283
53. Trottier SJ, Ritter S, Lakhsmanan R, Sabaku SA, Troop BR (2002) Obstruction of the tracheostomy tube during percutaneous tracheostomy. Chest 4:27–31
54. Plummer AL, Gracey DR (1989) Consensus conference on artificial airways in patients receiving mechanical ventilation. Chest 96:178–180
55. Saffle JR, Morris SE, Edelman L (2002) Early tracheostomy does not improve outcome in burn patients. J Burn Care Rehabil 23:431–438
56. Rumbak MJ, Newton M, Truncale T, Schwartz SW, Adams JW, Hazard PB (2004) A prospective randomized study comparing early percutaneous dilational tracheotomy to prolonged translaryngeal intubation (delayed tracheotomy) in critically ill medical patients. Crit Care Med 32:1689–1694
57. Boynton JH, Hawkins K, Eastridge BJ, O'Keefe GE (2004) Tracheostomy timing and the duration of weaning in patients with respiratory failure. Crit Care 8:R261–R267
58. Arabi Y, Haddad S, Shirawi N, Al Shimemeri A (2004) Early tracheostomy in intensive care trauma patients improves resources utilization: a cohort study and literature review. Crit Care Med 8:R347–R352
59. Croshaw R, McIntire B, Fann S, Nottingham J, Bynoe R (2004) Tracheostomy: timing revisited. Curr Surg 61:42–48
60. Ibrahim EH, Tracy L, Hill G, Fraser VJ, Kollef MH (2001) The occurrence of ventilator associated pneumonia in a community hospital: risk factors and clinical outcome. Chest 120:555–561
61. Livingston DH (2000) Prevention of ventilator associated pneumonia. Am J Surg 179:12–17
62. Esteban A, Frutos F, Anzueto A, et al (2001) Impact of tracheostomy on outcome of mechanical ventilation. Am J Respir Crit Care Med 163(Suppl):A129 (abst)

63. Mascia L, Corno E, Terragni PP, Stather D, Ferguson N (2004) Pro/con clinical debate: Tracheostomy is ideal for withdrawal of mechanical ventilation in severe neurological impairment. Crit Care 8:327–330
64. Stocchetti N, Parma A, Lamperti M, Songa V, Tognini L (2000) Neurophysiological consequences of three tracheostomy techniques: a randomized study in neurosurgical patients. J Neurosurg Anesthesiol 12:307–313
65. Stocchetti N, Parma A, Lamperti M, Songa V, Tognini L (2000) Early translaryngeal tracheostomy in patients with severe brain injury. Intensive Care Med 26:1101–1107
66. Sustic A, Krstulovic B, Eskinja N, Zelic M, Ledic D, Turina D (2002) Surgical tracheostomy versus percutaneous dilational tracheostomy in patients with anterior cervical spine fixation; preliminary report. Spine 27:1942–1945
67. Gatti C, Cardu C, Bentini C, Pacilli P, Pugliese P (2004) Weaning from ventilator after cardiac operation using the Ciaglia percutaneous tracheostomy. Eur J Cardiothorac Surg 25:541–547
68. Patel NC, Deane J, Scawn N (2002) Reduction in tracheostomy-associated risk of mediastinitis by routine use of percutaneous tracheostomy. Am Thorac Surg 73:2033
69. Pelosi P, Severgnini P (2004) Tracheostomy must be individualized! Crit Care 8:322–324

Percutaneous Tracheostomy: Past, Present, and Future Perspectives

C. Byhahn, K. Westphal, and B. Zwissler

▌ Introduction

"Tracheostomy: A useful, but dangerous intervention" – was the title of a lecture given by the German anesthesiologist Erich Rügheimer in 1963. At that time, percutaneous techniques for tracheostomy were not available, and conventional tracheostomy, according to Jackson [1], was frequently associated with serious, even fatal complications [2, 3]. Intensivists avoided tracheostomy, and patients remained intubated for weeks and even months to forgo the potential risks of conventional tracheostomy. However, in 1985, Bishop and colleagues published a well-designed experimental study on the consequences of long-term intubation [4], and Pasquale Ciaglia, a 73-year-old surgeon from Syracuse, NY, had a paper published in *Chest* entitled "Elective percutaneous dilatational tracheostomy. A new simple bedside procedure; preliminary report" [5]. Independent of each other, these articles launched a new era of long-term airway management in the intensive care unit (ICU).

It is now proven that percutaneous tracheostomy provides many advantages over long-term intubation *and* conventional tracheostomy, and a recent meta-analysis of five prospective, randomized trials comparing percutaneous with surgical tracheostomy in ICU patients found that postoperative complications, perioperative bleeding, and stoma infection were far less likely with percutaneous techniques [6].

Recent postal surveys in the United Kingdom [7], Germany [8], Switzerland [9], the Netherlands [10], and Spain [11] revealed a prevalence of percutaneous techniques in the ICU of 52–82%. If the ICU is run by anesthesiologists, minimally invasive tracheostomy represents the technique of choice [9]. Percutaneous tracheostomy has undoubtedly gained widespread acceptance and represents the artificial airway of choice in ICU patients on long-term ventilation.

▌ The Era of Seldinger

The foundation for modern percutaneous tracheostomy was laid in 1953, when the Swedish radiologist Sven Ivar Seldinger reported a new technique of vessel catheterization, in which a guidewire was introduced through the puncture needle into the vessel, the needle withdrawn, and a catheter inserted via the guidewire [12]. Salesman Bill Cook from Indiana, USA, and his cousin Van Fucilla, a radiologist, were the first to manufacture and distribute sets for vascular catheterization. Since its first use at the Illinois Masonic Hospital, Chicago, IL, USA, in autumn 1963, Seldinger's technique has become part of medicinal history [13].

Table 1. Currently available techniques of percutaneous tracheostomy

Technique	Characteristics	Manufacturer
▌PDT (Percutaneous dilational tracheostomy)	Antegrade, multi-step dilation with up to 7 dilators	Cook Critical Care, Bloomington, IN, USA
▌GWDF (Guidewire dilating forceps)	Antegrade, two-step dilation with modified Howard-Kelly forceps	SIMS Portex Ltd., Hythe, Kent, United Kingdom
▌TLT (Translaryngeal tracheostomy)	Retrograde, single-step dilation with the cannula itself	Tyco Healthcare, Athlone, Ireland
▌CBR (Ciaglia Blue Rhino)	Antegrade, single-step dilation with a conically shaped, hydrophilically coated dilator	Cook Critical Care, Bloomington, IN, USA

All techniques for percutaneous tracheostomy currently available – five in total – are based on Seldinger's technique. The trachea is punctured either blind or under bronchoscopic visualization, and a guidewire is introduced into the tracheal lumen. Afterwards, the trachea is dilated in one or multiple steps in either antegrade or retrograde direction, and a cannula is finally inserted. The methods of dilation and cannula insertion is mainly what distinguishes the different techniques. Table 1 gives an overview of the principal technical properties of the different systems currently in use. A detailed description of the respective technique is beyond the scope of this chapter and can be found in the literature [5, 14–17].

▌ Tracheostomy Timing

A number of clinically important advantages of tracheostomy over prolonged endotracheal intubation are summarized in Table 2, of which two aspects are of utmost importance when tracheostomy timing is discussed. The shape of the endotracheal tube is contrary to the natural shape of the human airway, resulting in enormous pressure of up to 100 mmHg exerted on the vulnerable laryngotracheal structures when the tube is bent to fit into the patient's airway. Inflammation is induced within the first seven days of endotracheal intubation already, and may result in permanent airway injury [4, 18].

To facilitate weaning, airway resistance in the intubated patient should be reduced to the physiologic level. The endotracheal tube's internal diameter must be between 8.5 and 9.4 mm, depending on its length, to allow spontaneous ventilation without increasing the work of breathing. Large-bore short tracheal cannulas contribute significantly to weaning the patient off the ventilator by reducing airway resistance and work of breathing.

Regardless of the huge number of reports investigating almost all facets of percutaneous tracheostomy, evidence-based recommendations for the optimal timing of tracheostomy still do not exist. Two reports published independently in 2004 sought to investigate whether early tracheostomy could be beneficial in terms of earlier weaning, ICU length of stay, and ventilator-associated pneumonia (VAP) [19, 20]. Arabi and colleagues found in a retrospective study in trauma patients who either underwent early tracheostomy around day 6 of ventilation or late tracheos-

Table 2. Evidence-based advantages of percutaneous over conventional tracheostomy

General
▌ Reduced airway resistance and work of breathing
▌ Improved oral hygiene and airway toilet
▌ Oral feeding
▌ Verbal communication
▌ Less sedative and analgesic requirements

In case of early tracheostomy
▌ Reduced incidence and severity of laryngotracheal injury
▌ Less nosocomial sinusitis
▌ Improved and faster weaning
▌ Shortened ICU length of stay

tomy at about day 13 of intubation, that the time from tracheostomy to definitive weaning was identical in both groups. This implies that early tracheostomy was crucial to shorten ventilator dependency and ICU length of stay [19]. Rumbak et al. prospectively randomized 120 medical ICU patients projected to need ventilation longer than 14 days to either early (within 48 hrs) or late tracheostomy at days 14–16. The early tracheostomy group showed significantly less mortality, pneumonia, and spent significantly less time in the ICU and on mechanical ventilation [20]. In an editorial accompanying Rumbak's study the authors state that "the current standard of day 10–14 for tracheostomies has little to support its practice. A real concern in terms of the current standard of delayed tracheostomy may be the committing of the classic type I error – accepting a practice that is incorrect" [21]. Even if more studies are required to confirm these obvious results, the time has arrived to entirely revise the current practice of tracheostomy timing.

▌ Contraindications

Only a few, but important contraindications exist and should be strictly observed. Digital identification of cricoid cartilage and trachea is essential, because accidental injury to the cricoid cartilage may result in circumferential shrinking of the cricoid and thus in subglottic stenosis that is difficult to repair. Other contraindications include emergency airway access and patient's age < 16–18 years.

In the eventual case of intraoperative airway loss, as well as in the case of accidental decannulation during the first 7 to 10 days after any percutaneous tracheostomy, immediate oral reintubation is mandatory to secure the airway. Therefore, it is essential not to perform percutaneous tracheostomy – regardless of the particular technique – in patients with known or expected difficult airway, because severe morbidity and even fatalities have been reported as a result of airway loss and subsequent difficult reintubation [22, 23].

Relative contraindications are summarized in Table 3. Personal skills in tracheostomy and airway management should be taken into consideration, and a thorough risk-benefit analysis should be made if percutaneous tracheostomy is planned in these patients.

Table 3. Absolute and relative contraindications of percutaneous tracheostomy

Absolute
▌Emergency airway access
▌Known or anticipated difficult endotracheal intubation
▌Age < 16–18 years
▌Cricoid cartilage not identified

Relative
▌Severe coagulopathy
▌Severe respiratory insufficiency
▌Difficult cervical anatomy (short neck, unstable cervical spine, large goiter, etc.)
▌Morbid obesity

▌ Is there a 'Best Technique'?

Answering the question, which percutaneous tracheostomy technique should be the one of choice, requires focusing on a number of variables, of which the perioperative complication rate is the most important. In contrast to other topics in medicine, guidelines for Good Clinical Research Practice do not yet exist for percutaneous tracheostomy. Dulguerov and co-workers were the first to subdivide complications during tracheostomy systematically into three groups: serious, intermediate, and minor [24]. 'Serious' complications were defined as potentially life-threatening, requiring immediate surgical intervention, while 'intermediate' complications should not result in significant morbidity, when recognized and treated appropriately. Finally, complications were considered 'minor' when no specific treatment was required, and the respective problem was without clinical relevance (Table 4) [24].

Clinical studies comparing two or more percutaneous techniques are rare. Table 5 gives an overview of comparative clinical trials and the respective complication rates of the techniques used, while Table 6 summarizes all data.

An incidence of less than 5% of clinically important complications makes the percutaneous route a reliable alternative to surgical tracheostomy. Regarding complication rates, percutaneous dilational tracheostomy (PDT), translaryngeal tra-

Table 4. Definition of perioperative complications according to Dulguerov et al. [24]

Serious	Minor
▌Death	▌Hemorrhage
▌Cardiac arrest	▌Difficult cannula placement
▌Pneumothorax	▌Subcutaneous emphysema
▌Pneumomediastinum	
Intermediate	
▌Oxygen desaturation	
▌Arterial hypotension	
▌Posterior tracheal wall injury	
▌Cannula false placement	
▌Unplanned conversion to surgical tracheostomy	
▌Aspiration	

Table 5. Overview of clinical trials comparing two or more percutaneous techniques (for abbreviations see Table 1)

Author and year	Technique	Patients (n)	Complications		
			Serious	Intermediate	Minor
van Heerden et al. [25]	PDT	29	–	1 (3.5%)	5 (17.2%)
1996	GWDF	25	–	–	5 (20.0%)
Ambesh and Kaushik [26]	PDT	40	–	–	9 (22.5%)
1998	GWDF	40	–	–	12 (30.0%)
Walz and Peitgen [27]	PDT	25	–	–	–
1998	TLT	25	–	1 (4.0%)	–
Westphal et al. [28]	PDT	45	–	1 (2.2%)	4 (8.9%)
1999	TLT	45	–	–	–
Nates et al. [29]	PDT	50		1 (2.0%)	4 (8.0%)
2000	GWDF	50		7 (14.0%)	15 (30.0%)
MacCallum et al. [30]	PDT	13	–	–	1 (7.7%)
2000	TLT	37	–	1 (2.7%)	–
Byhahn et al. [16]	PDT	25	1 (4.0%)	3 (12.0%)	–
2000	CBR	25	–	2 (8.0%)	–
Johnson et al. [31]	PDT	25	–	4 (16.0%)	8 (32.0%)
2001	CBR	25	–	5 (20.0%)	6 (24.0%)
Byhahn et al. [32]	GWDF	50	1 (2.0%)	1 (2.0%)	9 (18.0%)
2001	TLT	50		2 (4.0%)	–
Cantais et al. [22]	GWDF	50	–	1 (2.0%)	2 (4.0%)
2002	TLT	50	–	9 (18.0%)	12 (24.0%)
Ambesh et al. [33]	GWDF	30	–	–	17 (56.7%)
2002	CBR	30	1 (3.3%)	2 (6.7%)	3 (10.0%)
Goepfert et al. [34]	PDT	35	–	–	2 (5.7%)
2002	GWDF	35	–	–	2 (5.7%)
	TLT	35	–	–	1 (2.9%)
	CBR	35	–	–	–
Byhahn et al. [35]	CBR	35	–	–	6 (17.1%)
2002	PercuTwist	35	2 (5.7%)	1 (2.9%)	8 (22.9%)
Anon et al. [36]	CBR	27	–	–	2 (7.4%)
2004	GWDF	26	–	5 (19.3%)	1 (3.8%)

cheostomy (TLT), and Ciaglia Blue Rhino (CBR) did not differ substantially. However, many minor complications occurred during guidewire dilating forceps (GWDF), most of which consisted of a higher bleeding rate. Because data regarding PercuTwist are still limited, no final statement can be made regarding its perioperative safety.

In summary, there is no 'best technique'. Because the rate of clinically important complications was low with any technique, the choice of procedure should be based upon the specific features of both the particular technique and the particular patient.

Table 6. Incidence of perioperative complications reported in the clinical trials shown in Table 5. Complications are classified according to Dulguerov et al. [24]. For abbreviations see Table 1

Technique	Patients (n)	Complications			
		Overall	Serious	Intermediate	Minor
PDT	287	43 (15.0%)	1 (0.3%)	9 (3.1%)	33 (11.5%)
GWDF	306	78 (25.5%)	1 (0.3%)	14 (4.6%)	63 (20.6%)
TLT	242	28 (11.6%)	–	15 (6.2%)	13 (5.4%)
CBR	177	27 (15.2%)	1 (0.6%)	9 (5.1%)	17 (9.6%)
PercuTwist	35	11 (31.4%)	2 (5.7%)	1 (2.9%)	8 (22.9%)
Total	1047	187 (17.9%)	5 (0.5%)	48 (4.4%)	134 (12.3%)

▌ Infectious Complications and Late Outcome

The risk of stomal infection after percutaneous tracheostomy is far less than 1% [6, 24]. Because the stoma is only dilated, tissue tension against the cannula seems to seal the lower airway from the skin. In contrast to conventional tracheostomy, there is no communication between body surface and lower airway, making cross-contamination of the stoma with bacteria from the airway unlikely. On the other hand, bacteria are unlikely to migrate from the body's surface alongside the cannula into the trachea. This fact might explain the low incidence of pneumonia after percutaneous tracheostomy to some extent. As a matter of fact, percutaneous tracheostomy can be safely applied in patients with fresh surgical wounds (e.g., median sternotomy, anterior cervical spine surgery, etc.), as well as in immunodeficient patients (e.g., organ transplant recipients) without running an increased risk for infectious complications [37–39].

The reduction in the incidence and severity of subglottic laryngeal injury and tracheal stenosis is a major advantage of percutaneous tracheostomy over prolonged endotracheal intubation. However, the number of patients who underwent late outcome examinations is still low, and no late outcome studies are available for the Ciaglia Blue Rhino and PercuTwist techniques. Only eight studies have so far been performed to investigate the outcome at least 6 months after either PDT (n=213) [40–44], GWDF (n=35) [45, 46], or TLT (n=13) [47] (Table 7). Only Norwood et al. [40] and Walz et al. [42] showed tracheal narrowing of more than 50% in five patients after PDT. The degree of stenosis described in the remaining studies was less than 50% at all times, and in most cases less than 30%. Because clinical symptoms – shortness of breath at rest or exercise, cough and stridor are unlikely to occur unless the degree of stenosis exceeds 75%, most of these findings were of minor clinical importance. Finally, the question whether post-tracheostomy tracheal stenosis was primarily caused by the tracheostomy itself, previous endotracheal intubation, the tube or cannula cuff, or a combination of these factors, remains unanswered.

Table 7. Late outcome after percutaneous tracheostomy

Author	Technique	n	Method	Degree of stenosis
Fischler et al. [40]	PDT	10	LTC	No tracheal stenosis
Law et al. [41]	PDT	40	LTC	10–30% (n = 3) 40% (n = 1)
Norwood et al. [42]	PDT	48	CT+LTC	11–25% (n = 10) 26–50% (n = 4) >50% (n = 1)
Rosenbower et al. [43]	PDT	9	LTC	No tracheal stenosis
Walz et al. [44]	PDT	106	X-ray	<10% (n = 60) 11–25% (n = 19) 26–50% (n = 23) >50% (n = 4)
Leonard et al. [45]	GWDF	10	LTC	No tracheal stenosis
Steele et al. [46]	GWDF	25	CT	No tracheal stenosis Moderate tracheal dilation (n = 8)
Hommerich et al. [47]	TLT	13	LTC	<30% (n = 13)

CT: computed tomography; LTC: laryngotracheoscopy

▌ Conclusion

Percutaneous tracheostomy has become an integral part of airway management in the critical care setting. Four different techniques have been extensively studied and do not differ significantly in terms of overall complications. The fifth technique, PercuTwist, introduced in 2002, requires further research before a final statement can be made. Based on the data in the literature, no technique has significant advantages or disadvantages, not even in high-risk patients. Nevertheless, the tracheostomy team should include an experienced physician capable of handling eventual complications and being an expert in airway management, to further reduce both the incidence and adverse sequelae of perioperative complications.

▌ References

1. Jackson C (1909) Tracheotomy. Laryngoscope 18:285–290
2. Brown AH, Braimbridge MV, Panagopoulos P, Sabar EF (1969) The complications of median sternotomy. J Thorac Cardiovasc Surg 58:189–197
3. Stauffer JL, Olson DE, Petty TL (1981) Complications and consequences of endotracheal intubation and tracheotomy. Am J Med 70:65–76
4. Bishop MJ, Hibbard AJ, Fink BR, Vogel AM, Weymuller EA (1985) Laryngeal injury in a dog model of prolonged endotracheal intubation. Anesthesiology 62:770–773
5. Ciaglia P, Firsching R, Syniec C (1985) Elective percutaneous dilatational tracheostomy. A new simple bedside procedure; preliminary report. Chest 87:715–719
6. Freeman BD, Isabella K, Lin N, Buchman TG (2000) A meta-analysis of prospective trials comparing percutaneous and surgical tracheostomy in critically ill patients. Chest 118:1412–1418
7. Cooper RM (1998) Use and safety of percutaneous tracheostomy in intensive care. Report of a postal survey of ICU practice. Anaesthesia 53:1209–1212

8. Westphal K, Byhahn C (2001) Update 2000. Percutaneous tracheostomy in German intensive care units: a postal survey. Anaesth Intensivmed 42:70–74

9. Fischler L, Erhart S, Kleger GR, Frutiger A (2000) Prevalence of tracheostomy in ICU patients. A nation-wide survey in Switzerland. Intensive Care Med 26:1428–1433

10. Fikkers BG, Fransen GA, van der Hoeven JG, Briede IS, van den Hoogen FJ (2003) Tracheostomy for long-term ventilated patients: a postal survey of ICU practice in The Netherlands. Intensive Care Med 29:1390–1393

11. Anon JM, Escuela MP, Gomez V, Garcia de Lorenzo A, Montejo JC, Lopez J (2004) Use of percutaneous tracheostomy in intensive care units in Spain. Results of a national survey. Intensive Care Med 30:1212–1215

12. Seldinger SI (1953) Catheter replacement of the needle in percutaneous arteriography. Acta Radiol 39:368–376

13. McCullough P (2003) 40 years. The history of Cook®. Cook Inc., Bloomington, IN, USA

14. Griggs WM, Worthley LIG, Gilligan JE, Thomas PD, Myburgh JA (1990) A simple percutaneous tracheostomy technique. Surg Gynecol Obstet 170:543–545

15. Fantoni A, Ripamonti D (1997) A non-derivative, non-surgical tracheostomy: the translaryngeal method. Intensive Care Med 23:386–392

16. Byhahn C, Wilke HJ, Halbig S, Lischke V, Westphal K (2000) Percutaneous tracheostomy: Ciaglia Blue Rhino versus the basic Ciaglia technique of percutaneous dilational tracheostomy. Anesth Analg 91:882–886

17. Frova G, Quintel M (2002) A new simple method for percutaneous tracheostomy: controlled rotating dilation. Intensive Care Med 28:299–303

18. Weymuller EA, Bishop MJ, Fink BR, Hibbard AW, Spelman FA (1983) Quantification of intralaryngeal pressure exerted by endotracheal tubes. Ann Otol Rhinol Laryngol 92:444–447

19. Arabi Y, Haddad S, Shirawi N, Shimemeri A (2004) Early tracheostomy in intensive care trauma patients improves resource utilization: a cohort study and literature review. Crit Care 8:R347–R352

20. Rumbak MJ, Newton M, Truncale T, Schwartz SW, Adams JW, Hazard PB (2004) A prospective, randomized study comparing early percutaneous dilational tracheotomy to prolonged translaryngeal intubation (delayed tracheotomy) in critically ill medical patients. Crit Care Med 32:1689–1694

21. Ahrens T, Kollef MH (2004) Early tracheostomy – has its time arrived? Crit Care Med 32:1796–1797

22. Cantais E, Kaiser E, Le-Goff Y, Palmier B (2002) Percutaneous tracheostomy: Prospective comparison of the translaryngeal technique versus the forceps-dilational technique in 100 critically ill adults. Crit Care Med 30:815–819

23. Wang MB, Berke GS, Ward PH, Calcaterra TC, Watts D (1992) Early experience with percutaneous tracheotomy. Laryngoscope 102:157–162

24. Dulguerov P, Gysin C, Perneger TV, Chevrolet JC (1999) Percutaneous or surgical tracheostomy. A meta-analysis. Crit Care Med 27:1617–1625

25. Van Heerden PV, Webb SAR, Power BM, Thompson WR (1996) Percutaneous dilational tracheostomy – A clinical study evaluating two systems. Anaesth Intensive Care 24:56–59

26. Ambesh SP, Kaushik S (1998) Percutaneous dilational tracheostomy: The Ciaglia method versus the Rapitrach method. Anesth Analg 87:556–561

27. Walz MK, Peitgen K (1998) Puncture tracheostomy versus translaryngeal tracheostomy. Chirurg 69:418–422

28. Westphal K, Byhahn C, Wilke HJ, Lischke V (1999) Percutaneous tracheostomy: A clinical comparison of dilatational (Ciaglia) and translaryngeal (Fantoni) techniques. Anesth Analg 89:938–943

29. Nates JL, Cooper DJ, Myles PS, Scheinkestel CD, Tuxen DV (2000) Percutaneous tracheostomy in critically ill patients: A prospective, randomized comparison of two techniques. Crit Care Med 28:3734–3739

30. MacCallum PL, Parnes LS, Sharpe MD, Harris C (2000) Comparison of open, percutaneous, and translaryngeal tracheostomies. Otolaryngol Head Neck Surg 122:686–690

31. Johnson JL, Cheatham ML, Sagraves SG, Block EFJ, Nelson LD (2001) Percutaneous dilational tracheostomy: A comparison of single- versus multiple-dilator techniques. Crit Care Med 29:1251–1254

32. Byhahn C, Wilke HJ, Lischke V, Rinne T, Westphal K (2001) Bedside percutaneous tracheostomy: Clinical comparison of Griggs and Fantoni techniques. World J Surg 25:295–301
33. Ambesh SP, Pandey CK, Srivastava S, Agarwal A, Singh DK (2002) Percutaneous tracheostomy with single dilation technique: A prospective, randomized comparison of Ciaglia Blue Rhino versus Griggs' Guidewire Dilating Forceps. Anesth Analg 95:1739–1745
34. Goepfert A, Witter B, Gottstein P, Ennker IC, Ennker J (2002) Comparison of minimally invasive percutaneous techniques of tracheostomy. Intensivmed 39:595–603
35. Byhahn C, Westphal K, Meininger D, Gürke B, Kessler P, Lischke V (2002) Single-dilator percutaneous tracheostomy: a comparison of PercuTwist and Ciaglia Blue Rhino techniques. Intensive Care Med 28:1262–1266
36. Anon JM, Escuela MP, Gomez V, et al (2004) Percutaneous tracheostomy: Ciaglia Blue Rhino versus Griggs' Guide Wire Dilating Forceps. A prospective, randomized trial. Acta Anaesthesiol Scand 48:451–456
37. Sustic A, Krstulovic B, Eskinja N, Zelic M, Ledic D, Turina D (2002) Surgical tracheostomy versus percutaneous dilational tracheostomy in patients with anterior cervical spine fixation: preliminary report. Spine 27:1942–1945
38. Byhahn C, Rinne T, Halbig S, et al (2000) Early percutaneous tracheostomy after median sternotomy. J Thorac Cardiovasc Surg 120:329–334
39. Pirat A, Zeyneloglu P, Candan S, Akkuzu B, Arslan G (2004) Percutaneous dilational tracheotomy in solid-organ transplant recipients. Transplant Proc 36:221–223
40. Fischler L, Kuhn M, Cantieni R, Frutiger A (1995) Late outcome of percutaneous dilatational tracheostomy in intensive care patients. Intensive Care Med 21:475–481
41. Law RC, Carney AS, Manara AR (1997) Long-term outcome after percutaneous dilational tracheostomy. Endoscopic and spirometry findings. Anaesthesia 52:51–56
42. Norwood S, Vallina VL, Short K, Saigusa M, Fernandez LG, McLarty JW (2000) Incidence of tracheal stenosis and other late complications after percutaneous tracheostomy. Ann Surg 232:233–241
43. Rosenbower TJ, Morris JA Jr., Eddy VA, Ries WR (1998) The long-term complications of percutaneous dilational tracheostomy. Am Surg 64:82–87
44. Walz MK, Peitgen K, Thürauf N, et al (1998) Percutaneous dilatational tracheostomy – Early results and long-term outcome of 326 critically ill patients. Intensive Care Med 24:685–690
45. Leonard RC, Lewis RH, Singh B, van Heerden PV (1999) Late outcome from percutaneous tracheostomy using the Portex kit. Chest 115:1070–1075
46. Steele APH, Evans HW, Afaq MA, et al (2000) Long-term follow-up of Griggs percutaneous tracheostomy with spiral CT and questionnaire. Chest 117:1430–1433
47. Hommerich CP, Rödel R, Frank L, Zimmermann A, Braun U (2002) Long-term results after surgical tracheotomy and percutaneous dilatation tracheostomy. A comparative retrospective analysis. Anaesthesist 51:23–27

Acute Lung Injury

Role of iNOS-derived Excessive Nitric Oxide in the Pathogenesis of Acute Lung Injury

P. Enkhbaatar, J. Parkinson, and D. L. Traber

▌ Introduction

More than 1 million burn injuries occur every year in the United States, resulting in millions of dollars spent to treat patients and fund clinical and basic science research projects seeking to reduce mortality and morbidity associated with thermal injury. Over the past two decades, clinicians have greatly advanced the treatment of burn patients, developing effective surgical management strategies involving the excision the damaged soft tissues followed by immediate closure of wounds with autologous, allogenic, or artificial skin. This approach, combined with adequate fluid resuscitation therapy, has favorably reduced the mortality and morbidity associated with burn injury. Yet despite these major advances, patients with thermal injury are still subject to serious life-threatening complications such as multiple organ failure (MOF) including an acute lung injury (ALI) or acute respiratory distress syndrome (ARDS). Patients with extensive cutaneous burns in which the burned area exceeds 30% of the total body surface area, exhibit microvascular pressure and hyperpermeability increases not only at the injured site but also in regions distant from the injury, leading eventually to burn shock [1, 2]. This pulmonary vascular hyperpermeability leads to a large amount of fluid flux from the circulating plasma to the interstitial spaces, resulting in lung edema formation [3, 4].

All burn related pathologies appear to be more severe if the thermal damage sustained is combined with inhalation injury [5, 6]. Hot air flow, toxic components of smoke, or combination of both can cause damage to the airway columnar epithelium, increasing susceptibility to the secondary infection. It has been reported that approximately 35% of thermally injured patients have sustained an inhalation injury and that 38% of these patients develop subsequent pneumonia [7]. Smoke inhalation increases mortality in patients with thermal injury by 20%, and pneumonia increases mortality 40% [7]. Thus, understanding the pathophysiology of ALI and providing subsequent adequate therapy are crucial for managing patients with combined burn and smoke inhalation injury.

▌ Acute Lung Injury in Burn and Smoke Inhalation

To most closely mimic the clinical manifestation of ALI in humans, we previously developed, a sheep model of combined burn and smoke inhalation injury [8]. The injury model is advantageous to researchers in that it allows for continuous monitoring of cardiopulmonary variables and frequent, intermittent blood sampling.

The size of the animals insures that there is adequate blood volume for frequent sampling to insure adequate resuscitation. In addition, the lungs of sheep are similar to those of humans. More importantly, sheep accept positive-pressure ventilation without sedation. Finally, this model of injury allows for access to pulmonary lymphatic data, which is crucial for studying pulmonary microvascular fluid flux.

As mentioned earlier, thermal injury is often complicated by development of MOF including ARDS. Pulmonary dysfunction is more severe if the thermal injury is associated with smoke inhalation. Pulmonary gas exchange begins to decline 3 h after combined burn and smoke inhalation injury, progressively worsening up-to 48 h after injury, when the PaO_2/FiO_2 ratio falls below 200, a characteristic of ARDS [8, 9]. Sheep subjected to combined burn and smoke inhalation injury display a marked increase in pulmonary vascular permeability with formation of lung tissue edema [8, 9]. Pulmonary transvascular fluid flux, evaluated by measuring lung lymph flow, increases ~10 fold [8, 9]. Consequently, lung water content, evaluated by measuring lung wet-to-dry weight ratio, significantly increases 48 h after the insult [8, 9]. Pulmonary lung edema formation is confirmed by histological examination, which reveals a severe edema and congestion. Airway (trachea) blood flow, measured by microsphere injection technique, also increases (~ 20 fold) in sheep subjected to combined burn and smoke inhalation injury [9]. This increase in airway blood flow is associated with airway edema and airway obstruction caused by cast material, with subsequent increase in ventilatory pressures. All of these pathologies lead to poor pulmonary gas exchange, resulting in hypoxia of the multiple organs. Although the precise mechanism(s) of the ALI in burn and smoke inhalation injury is not completely known, a few pathogenic factors have been described. One of the critical factors involved in the pathological process is excessive nitric oxide (NO). In previous studies, we have reported that NO plays an important role in the pathogenesis of ALI in sheep subjected to combined burn and smoke inhalation injury [9, 10]. We obtained this evidence by inhibiting NO initially with L-NG-nitroarginine methyl ester, a non-selective NO synthase (NOS) inhibitor and later with mercapto-ethylguanidine (MEG, a partially selective inducible NOS [iNOS] inhibitor) [10]. We subsequently tested the effect of the potent and selective iNOS dimerization inhibitor, BBS-2, on the same model of ALI and reported the beneficial effects of selective inhibition of iNOS-derived excessive NO [9].

▌ Role of Excessive NO in Acute Lung Injury

NO is an important biological messenger involved in a variety of physiological processes [11]. It was first described in 1980 by Furchgott and Zavadzki as an endothelial-derived relaxing factor (EDRF) [12]. In 1987, Ignarro et al. reported that EDRF from artery and vein was either NO or a chemically related radical species [13]. In 1988, Moncada et al. reported that, among the endothelial factors, which include both vasodilators and vasoconstrictors, there was a free radical gas, i.e., NO (nitrogen monoxide), which fulfilled the properties of EDRF [14].

Biosynthesis of NO by NOS starts with the amino acid L-arginine [15]. There are three types of NOS, named neuronal NOS (nNOS), endothelial NOS (eNOS), and inducible NOS (iNOS) [16, 17]. eNOS and nNOS are forms of constitutive NOS (cNOS) and produce a basic amount of NO under normal conditions. It is believed that constitutively expressed NO has a good effect such as regulation of vascular tone and anti-inflammatory properties [18]. The third isoform, iNOS is induced by pro-inflammatory cytokines and bacterial substances and has been shown to play an important role in the pathogenesis of conditions such as sepsis and multiple trauma that are frequently complicated by ARDS. These cytokines and bacteria are present in combined burn and smoke inhalation injury. In this condition, cytokines such as interleukin-1 (IL-1) are upregulated in lung tissue [19]. In addition, translocation of endotoxin and bacteria from the intestine into the systemic circulation has been reported to occur after burn and smoke inhalation injuries [20, 21]. Both IL-1 and endotoxin activate nuclear factor kappa B (NF-κB), which induces synthesis of iNOS. iNOS catalyzes production of large amounts of NO and, under conditions of substrate or cofactor limitation, may also synthesize superoxide (O_2^-) [22]. We have previously reported an upregulation of NO in burn and smoke inhalation injury [8, 9] and noted that plasma nitrite and nitrate (NOx), a stable metabolite of NO, was increased $\sim$ 2–2.5 fold. We also have reported an upregulation of iNOS mRNA in lung tissues 48 h after burn and smoke inhalation injury in sheep [10]. The immunohistochemical intensity of iNOS started to increase 4 h after the burn and smoke inhalation injury and was gradually increased up to 24 h after insult [23]. These results strongly suggest that elevated levels of plasma NOx are mainly due to iNOS. In support of this hypothesis, we noted that plasma NOx was almost completely inhibited by the potent and truly selective iNOS dimerization inhibitor, BBS-2 [9], suggesting that iNOS is the dominant isoform producing an excessive amount of NO in our model of ALI. The selectivity of BBS-2 for iNOS is 1500 and 620 times greater than for eNOS and nNOS, respectively [24]. Thus, we believe that BBS-2 inhibited only iNOS-derived NO without acute effects on nNOS or eNOS activity.

The formation of NO in the lung results in the loss of hypoxic pulmonary vasoconstriction (HPV), the physiological process that diverts blood flow from alveoli that are not being ventilated and perfuses the alveoli that are being ventilated [25, 26]. When loss of HPV is present, vasodilation occurs in the low or non-ventilated areas of the lung, leading to ventilation/perfusion (V/Q) mismatching, which in turn results in poor oxygenation [27]. Hyperpermeability in dilated vessels leads to plasma leak into the interstitial spaces. We have previously shown an increase in pulmonary microvascular permeability to both fluid and protein in sheep with burn/smoke inhalation [8]. At high concentrations, NO becomes a potential pro-inflammatory and cytotoxic factor by reacting with superoxide to form the toxic product, peroxynitrite [28], which can oxidize/nitrate other molecules or decay and produce even more damaging species such as the hydroxyl radical. Peroxynitrite may damage the alveolar capillary membrane [29], resulting in additional pulmonary edema. We have previously reported the presence of peroxynitrite in the airway and parenchyma of the lungs of sheep subjected to burn and smoke inhalation injury [10] by measuring its stable product, 3-nitrotyrosine. We have also reported that the plasma concentration of L-arginine is markedly depleted after burn and smoke inhalation injury [30]. In conditions where arginine is depleted, NOS produces superoxide, which also can cause tissue injury. Monocytes, one of the major sources of iNOS, produce superoxide radicals. Previously, we have shown an accumulation of neutrophils in lung tissue from sheep subjected to combined burn and smoke inhalation injury by measuring lung tissue myeloperoxidase activity [31]. Activated neutrophils produce large amounts of superoxide. Post-treatment with potent iNOS dimerization inhibitor markedly improved the pulmonary gas exchange and significantly reduced the pulmonary transvascular fluid flux [9]. Lung water content was also reduced by the inhibitor. Taken together, the above-mentioned results strongly suggest a key role of iNOS-derived NO in the pathogenesis of ALI.

Of particular interest, peroxynitrite has been shown to induce DNA single-strand damage, which in turn, causes an activation of poly(ADP-ribose) polymerase (PARP), a nuclear DNA binding enzyme [32]. PARP is a constitutively expressed enzyme that plays a role in DNA repair [33]. However, over-activation of this enzyme results in reduced cellular content in NAD^+, slowing the rate of glycolysis, mitochondrial respiration, and high-energy phosphate generation and, ultimately leading to cell death. Shimoda et al. reported a marked increase of PARP immunoreactivity in sheep subjected to combined burn and smoke inhalation injury [31]. Interestingly, treatment with PARP inhibitor significantly inhibited plasma NOx in those animals, suggesting that PARP may upregulate iNOS, possibly through NF-κB. As mentioned previously, NO and reactive oxygen species (ROS) form peroxynitrite, which can damage DNA, thereby upregulating PARP, and initiating a positive feed back loop.

As mentioned previously, airway (trachea) blood flow increases ~ 20 fold in sheep subjected to combined burn and smoke inhalation injury [9]. Abdi et al. reported that bronchial blood flow was increased ~ 8 fold after smoke inhalation injury in sheep [34]. Bronchial blood flow enters into the pulmonary vasculature through the various bronchiopulmonary anastomoses. This evidence was obtained by noting that bronchial artery occlusion, either by ligation or ethanol injection after smoke inhalation injury, markedly improved pulmonary function. Reduced bronchial blood flow reversed the fall in pulmonary gas exchange, and most importantly, increased lung lymph flow and lung water content seen in sheep with smoke inhalation injury [35], suggesting that increased airway blood flow possibly contributes, at least in part, to pulmonary edema formation. Soejima et al. reported that iNOS inhibition significantly reduces smoke inhalation-induced increases in tracheal blood flow [36]. In support of these results, we have shown in recent studies that potent and selective iNOS dimerization inhibitor significantly reduced airway blood flow [9], suggesting that increased airway circulation might be mediated by NO derived from iNOS.

We have previously reported a possible role of airway obstruction in the pathogenesis of ALI. Cox et al. have shown obstruction with a mean reduction in cross-sectional area of about 29% in bronchi, 11% in bronchioles, and 1.2% in respiratory bronchioles in sheep 48 h after combined burn and smoke inhalation injury [37]. They also demonstrated in their study a correlation between the airway obstruction score and pulmonary gas exchange (PaO_2/FiO_2 ratio). The bronchial obstruction score was predictive of the PaO_2/FiO_2 (correlation coefficient of 0.76) [37]. We have also shown that aerosolized tissue plasminogen activator markedly reduced a degree of ALI in sheep with burn and smoke inhalation injury [38]. Thus, the role of airway obstruction is significant in the deterioration of pulmonary gas exchange. Near total obstruction of a few bronchi would prevent ventilation of individual lung segments [39], whereas partial obstruction would be expected to reduce ventilatory flow, thus producing hypoxia. The formation of NO in the lung results in the loss of HPV leading to V/Q mismatching. V/Q mismatching in occluded areas can result in pulmonary shunt formation leading to poor gas exchange. Since the columnar epithelium is lost shortly after the smoke and burn injury, increased airway blood flow could contribute to increased airway exudation containing various procoagulants, thereby resulting, in part, in increased airway

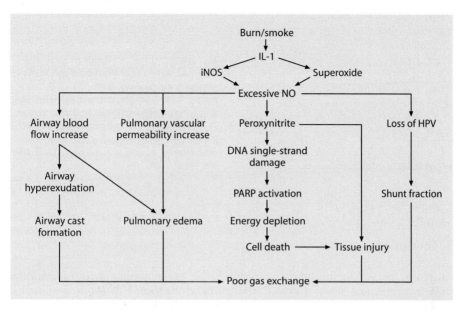

Fig. 1. Role of inducible nitric oxide (NO) synthase (iNOS)-derived NO in pathogenesis of acute lung injury induced by burn and smoke inhalation. IL-1: interleukin-1; PARP: poly(ADP-ribose) polymerase; HPV: hypoxic pulmonary vasoconstriction

obstruction. As reported previously, we have shown that post-treatment of sheep subjected to combined burn and smoke inhalation injury using a selective iNOS inhibitor reduced the increase in both airway blood flow and airway obstruction score. Thus, excessive NO may play a role in airway obstruction, possibly through increasing microvascular permeability in the airways.

Taking all of these findings into account, the role of iNOS-derived NO in the pathogenesis of ALI induced by burn and smoke inhalation is significant. In this chapter, we have described that iNOS-derived excessive NO may contribute to deterioration of the pulmonary gas exchange through:

▌ increase in pulmonary microvascular permeability,
▌ airway circulation changes,
▌ loss of HPV, and
▌ induction of PARP (Fig. 1).

This profound role of iNOS-derived NO in the pathogenesis of ALI is supported by findings that the potent and selective iNOS dimerization inhibitor, BBS-2 ameliorated ALI in our burn and smoke inhalation injury model. More importantly, we noted that treatment with BBS-2 markedly improved the survival rate of the animals in this model (Fig. 2).

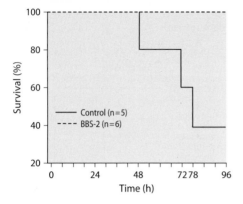

Fig. 2. Effect of iNOS inhibition on survival of sheep subjected to combined burn and smoke inhalation injury. Sheep given 40% total body surface flame burn and cotton smoke inhalation injury under deep anesthesia were post treated (1 h after injury) with potent and selective iNOS dimerization inhibitor BBS-2 (continuous, intravenous infusion) or vehicle and 5-day survival rate was monitored

▌ Conclusion

Currently, there is significant debate over whether the inhibition of NO is beneficial or detrimental, and whether excessive amounts of NO should be suppressed, and if excessive NO should be suppressed, what isoform should be targeted. Recently, it was reported that the non-selective NOS inhibitor 546C88 increased mortality in patients with septic shock. Non-specific NOS inhibitors inhibit all three isoforms of NOS, including eNOS, which adversely affects cardiovascular function. We have hypothesized that certain NOS isoforms could express at certain time points depending on the type of injury. More targeted and selective inhibition of NOS isoforms at their maximum activity level could be beneficial in managing MOF in this model. Our recent studies suggest that iNOS may dominate the pathophysiology of ALI in a combined burn and smoke inhalation model.

References

1. Bowen BD, Bert JL, Gu X, Lund T, Reed RK (1989) Microvascular exchange during burn injury: III. Implications of the model. Circ Shock 28:221–233
2. Lund T, Bert JL, Onarheim H, Bowen BD, Reed RK (1989) Microvascular exchange during burn injury. I: A review. Circ Shock 28:179–197
3. Isago T, Fujioka K, Traber LD, Herndon DN, Traber DL (1991) Derived pulmonary capillary pressure changes after smoke inhalation in sheep. Crit Care Med 19:1407–1413
4. Isago T, Noshima S, Traber LD, Herndon DN, Traber DL (1991) Analysis of pulmonary microvascular permeability after smoke inhalation. J Appl Physiol 71:1403–1408
5. Demling R, LaLonde C, Youn YK, Picard L (1995) Effect of graded increases in smoke inhalation injury on the early systemic response to a body burn. Crit Care Med 23:171–178
6. Navar PD, Saffle JR, Warden GD (1985) Effect of inhalation injury on fluid resuscitation requirements after thermal injury. Am J Surg 150:716–720
7. Shirani KZ, Jr Pruitt BA, Jr Mason AD (1987) The influence of inhalation injury and pneumonia on burn mortality. Ann Surg 205:82–87
8. Soejima K, Schmalstieg FC, Sakurai H, Traber LD, Traber DL (2001) Pathophysiological analysis of combined burn and smoke inhalation injuries in sheep. Am J Physiol Lung Cell Mol Physiol 280:L1233–L141
9. Enkhbaatar P, Murakami K, Shimoda K, et al (2003) The inducible nitric oxide synthase inhibitor BBS-2 prevents acute lung injury in sheep after burn and smoke inhalation injury. Am J Respir Crit Care Med 167:1021–1026

10. Soejima K, Traber LD, Schmalstieg FC, et al (2001) Role of nitric oxide in vascular permeability after combined burns and smoke inhalation injury. Am J Respir Crit Care Med 163:745–752
11. Kerwin, JF Jr, Lancaster JR, Feldman PL (1995) Nitric oxide: a new paradigm for second messengers. J Med Chem 38:4342–4362
12. Furchgott RF, Zavadzki JV (1980) The obligatory role of endothelial cells in the relaxation of arterial smooth muscle by acetylcholine. Nature 288:373–376
13. Ignarro LJ, Byrns RE, Buga GM, Wood KS (1987) Endothelium-derived relaxing factor from pulmonary artery and vein possesses pharmacologic and chemical properties identical to those of nitric oxide radical. Circ Res 61:866–879
14. Moncada S, Radamski MW, Palmer RM (1988) Endothelial-derived relaxing factor. Identification as nitric oxide and role in the control of vascular tone and platelet function. Biochem Pharmacol 37:2495–2501
15. Schmidt HH, Hofmann H, Schindler U, Shutenko ZS, Cunningham DD, Feelisch M (1996) No NO from NO synthase. Proc Natl Acad Sci USA 93:14492–14497
16. Jaffrey SR, Snyder SH (1995) Nitric oxide: a neural messenger. Annu Rev Cell Dev Biol 11:417–440
17. Alderton WK, Cooper CE, Knowles RG (2001) Nitric oxide synthases: structure, function and inhibition. Biochem J 357:593–615
18. Nathan C (1992) Nitric oxide as a secretory product of mammalian cells. FASEB J 6:3051–3064
19. Traber DL, Traber LD, Sakurai H (2000) Pulmonary microvascular changes seen with acute lung injury role of the bronchial circulation. JPN J Burn Inj 24:233–246
20. Tokyay R, Zeigler ST, Traber DL, et al (1993) Postburn gastrointestinal vasoconstriction increases bacterial and endotoxin translocation. J Appl Physiol 74:1521–1527
21. Baron P, Traber LD, Traber DL, et al (1994) Gut failure and translocation following burn and sepsis. J Surg Res 57:197–204
22. Xia Y, Dawson VL, Dawson TM, Snyder, SH, Zweier JL (1996) Nitric oxide synthase generates superoxide and nitric oxide in arginine-depleted cells leading to peroxynitrite-mediated cellular injury. Proc Natl Acad Sci USA 93:6770–6774
23. Burke AS, Oliveras G, Hunter GC (2004) Bronchial gland expression of pro-inflammatory mediators in an ovine model of smoke inhalation and burn injury. J Histochem Cytochem 52(Suppl 1):40 (abst)
24. Blasko E, Glaser CB, Devlin JJ, et al (2002) Mechanistic studies with potent and selective inducible nitric-oxide synthase dimerization inhibitors. J Biol Chem 277:295–302
25. Marshall BE, Hanson CW, Frasch F, Marshall C (1994) Role of hypoxic pulmonary vasoconstriction in pulmonary gas exchange and blood flow distribution. 2. Pathophysiology. Intensive Care Med 20:379–389
26. Sweeney M, Yuan JX (2000) Hypoxic pulmonary vasoconstriction: role of voltage-gated potassium channels. Respir Res 1:40–48
27. Hopkins SR, Johnson EC, Richardson RS, Wagner H, De Rosa M, Wagner PD (1997) Effects of inhaled nitric oxide on gas exchange in lungs with shunt or poorly ventilated area. Am J Respir Crit Care Med 156:484–491
28. Hughes MN (1999) Relationships between nitric oxide, nitroxyl ion, nitrosonium cation and peroxynitrite. Biochim Biophys Acta 1411:263–272
29. Miranda K, Espey MG, Jourd'heuil D, et al (2000) The chemical biology of nitric oxide. In: Ignarro LJ (ed) Nitric Oxide: Biology and Pathophysiology. Academic Press, San Diego, pp 41–45
30. Murakami K, Enkhbaatar P, Hecox S, et al (2003) L-arginine attenuates ovine model of acute lung injury following smoke inhalation and burn. Circulation 108:IV1041–IV1042 (abst)
31. Shimoda K, Murakami K, Enkhbaatar P, et al (2003) Effect of poly(ADP ribose) synthetase inhibition on burn and smoke inhalation injury in sheep. Am J Physiol Lung Cell Mol Physiol 285:L240–L249
32. Zhang J, Dawson VL, Dawson TM, Snyder SH (1994) Nitric oxide activation of poly(ADP-ribose) synthetase in neurotoxicity. Science 263:687–689
33. Ikai K, Ueda K (1983) Immunohistochemical demonstration of poly (adenosine diphosphate-ribose) synthetase in bovine tissue. J Histochem Cytochem 31:1262–1264

34. Abdi S, Herndon DM, Traber LD, et al (1991) Lung edema formation following inhalation injury: role of the bronchial blood flow. J Appl Physiol 71:727–743
35. Sakurai H, Traber LD, Traber DL (1998) Altered systemic organ blood flow after combined injury with burn and smoke inhalation. Shock 9:369–374
36. Soejima K, McGuire R, Snyder N, et al (2000) The effect of inducible nitric oxide synthase (iNOS) inhibition on smoke inhalation injury in sheep. Shock 13:261–266
37. Cox RA, Burke AS, Soejima K, et al (2003) Airway obstruction in sheep with burn and smoke inhalation injuries. Am J Respir Cell Mol Biol 29:295–302
38. Enkhbaatar P, Murakami K, Cox R, et al (2004) Aerosolized tissue plasminogen activator improves pulmonary function in sheep with burn and smoke inhalation injury. Shock 22:70–75
39. Thomas HM III, Garrett RC (1982) Strength of hypoxic vasoconstriction determines shunt fraction in dogs with atelectasis. J Appl Physiol 53:44–51

Ischemia-reperfusion Injury of the Lung: Role of Surfactant

N. P. Van der Kaaij, A. J. J. C. Bogers, and B. Lachmann

∎ Introduction: Lung Transplantation and Lung Ischemia-reperfusion Injury

Lung transplantation is an accepted treatment for patients with end-stage pulmonary disease. Despite refinement in lung preservation and improvement in surgical techniques and peri-operative care, lung ischemia-reperfusion injury remains a significant cause of early morbidity and mortality after lung transplantation [1]. Clinical symptoms will usually occur within the first 72 hours after lung transplantation and consist of non-cardiogenic lung edema, increased pulmonary artery pressure and resistance, decreased lung compliance and hypoxemia [2–7]. Microscopy shows diffuse alveolar damage with micro-atelectases. Although approximately 97% of the recipients show some degree of reperfusion edema on chest X-ray, severe lung ischemia-reperfusion injury occurs in 15–30% of lung transplant recipients [8]. The most severe form of lung ischemia-reperfusion injury is primary acute graft failure which clinically resembles the acute respiratory distress syndrome (ARDS); both conditions lead to increased utilization of intensive care resources, extended hospital stay and mortality [9–11].

The acute phase of ARDS can either resolve quickly or result in death. Already 4–7 days after onset of the clinical symptoms, the acute phase can develop into a 'chronic' fibroproliferative state, which is characterized by hyperplasia of alveolar type II (AT II) cells, infiltration of activated fibroblasts, collagen deposition, and re-modeling of lung architecture [12]. However, this fibroproliferative state was thus far not described after lung ischemia-reperfusion injury. We now confirm in an animal model that also after severe lung ischemia-reperfusion injury, impaired oxygenation capacity of the lung, decreased lung compliance, and a fibroproliferative pre-stage are observed months after reperfusion (van der Kaaij, et al., unpublished data).

Lung ischemia-reperfusion injury is the main cause for early morbidity and mortality after lung transplantation. Nevertheless, one-year survival after lung transplantation is about 75%. The long-term prognosis also remains limited, with a 5-year survival of less than 50% [1]. The major obstacle to long-term survival is the development of post lung transplant bronchiolitis obliterans syndrome, which is associated with chronic transplant dysfunction. This affects about 50% of patients who survive beyond 3 months after transplantation [13]. The exact etiology of the bronchiolitis obliterans syndrome is not fully understood but its pathogenesis appears to involve a 'response to injury' type of pattern, where multiple periods of injury may result in this syndrome (Fig. 1). Both donor characteristics (age,

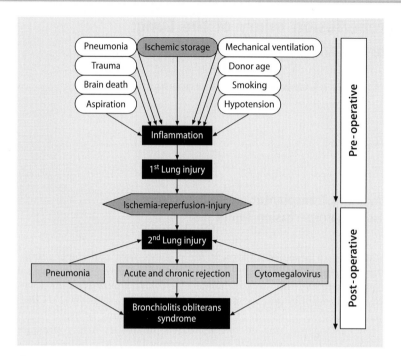

Fig. 1. Lung transplantation: A multiple hit theory for the development of bronchiolitis obliterans syndrome, which is associated with chronic transplant dysfunction of the lung

smoking years, cause of death) and complications during the donor procedure (ischemic time, hypotension, mechanical ventilation, aspiration) may result in early lung injury. Lung ischemia-reperfusion injury can aggravate this early lung injury, whereafter rejection and alloantigen independent factors (pneumonia, cytomegalovirus infection) can act as subsequent 'injuries' and increase the risk of bronchiolitis obliterans syndrome [10, 14, 15]. Because lung ischemia-reperfusion injury is an early contributor to lung injury, intervention at this stage may prove to decrease early morbidity and mortality after lung ischemia-reperfusion injury, but may also prevent or delay the onset of the bronchiolitis obliterans syndrome, thereby also influencing late morbidity and mortality after lung transplantation.

Several studies have highlighted the possibility that alterations in pulmonary surfactant (*surface active agent*) are present shortly after lung ischemia-reperfusion injury, contributing to early morbidity and mortality [2–4, 16–19]. Furthermore, in bronchoalveolar lavage (BAL) fluid from human lung transplant recipients, surfactant dysfunction was still visible up to seven years after transplantation [20]. The changes in pulmonary surfactant after lung transplantation resemble the changes seen in ARDS and contribute to a great extent to lung dysfunction [11]. Clinical trials studying the effect of exogenous surfactant on ARDS appear promising, providing a rationale to study the possibilities of surfactant treatment for lung ischemia-reperfusion injury.

∎ Surfactant

To facilitate normal breathing with minimal effort, pulmonary surfactant lowers the surface tension at the alveolo-capillary membrane. In addition, lowering of the surface tension is important for the fluid homeostasis across the alveolo-capillary membrane. Furthermore, surfactant serves as a functional barrier in the alveolus, so that the transfer of molecules across the alveolo-capillary membrane is limited. Finally, surfactant protects the lung against microorganisms [10, 21, 22].

Surfactant is composed of lipids (90%), of which dipalmitoyl-phosphatidylcholine (DPPC) is the most surface tension lowering lipid, and surfactant associated proteins (SP) (10%). The proteins of pulmonary surfactant can be divided into two groups: the hydrophilic proteins SP-A and SP-D, and the hydrophobic proteins SP-B and SP-C. SP-B, as well as SP-C, have been demonstrated to enhance lipid insertion into the monolayer at the air/liquid interface. In this way they maintain a low surface tension, thereby protecting the surface film from being contaminated by non-surfactant proteins, which can result in inactivation or degradation of the surfactant film. SP-A and SP-D are believed to be molecules of the innate immune system through their ability to recognize a broad spectrum of pathogens. Several studies have shown that SP-A and SP-D interact with a number of viruses, bacteria and fungi, and with inhaled glycoconjugate allergens, such as pollen grains and mite allergens [10]. Furthermore, SP-A has been suggested to play an important role in phospholipid secretion and recycling, formation of tubular myelin and blocking surfactant inhibition by serum proteins [21, 22].

Surfactant can be divided by ultra centrifugation into two subfractions, which differ in morphological appearance and density. The heavy subtype or large aggregate subform of surfactant is highly surface active, contains a high amount of SP and is made up of tubular myelin, lamellar bodies and large vesicles. The light subtype or small aggregate subform has a poor surface lowering capacity and consists of small vesicles [22].

Production and secretion of surfactant is done by the AT II cells. Both AT II cells and alveolar macrophages are important for recycling of surfactant lipids, which is essential for maintaining homeostasis of the endogenous surfactant pool [22, 23].

∎ Fluid Homeostasis in the Lung

As discussed previously, surfactant is essential for maintaining normal fluid homeostasis in the lung and preventing pulmonary edema. Fig. 2 presents a diagram of fluid balance across the lung. The normal plasma oncotic pressure of 37 cmH$_2$O is opposed by the capillary hydrostatic pressure of 15 cmH$_2$O, the oncotic pressure of interstitial fluid proteins of 18 cmH$_2$O and by the surface tension conditioned suction pressure of 4 cmH$_2$O. In general, alveolar flooding will not occur when the surfactant system is properly functioning. However, when the surface tension rises above a critical level, alveolar flooding will occur, leading to influx of proteins into the alveolar space which results in further inactivation of surfactant [10, 24].

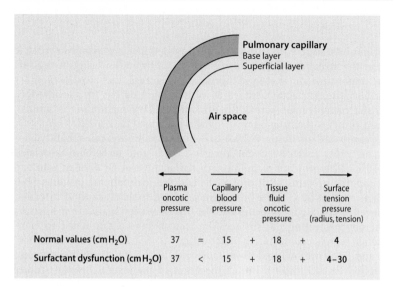

Fig. 2. Simplified diagram showing the factors influencing fluid balance in the lung (from [11] with permission)

▌ Lung Ischemia-reperfusion Injury: Pathophysiology

Lung ischemia-reperfusion injury, which occurs to a certain extent during lung transplantation, can damage the surfactant system. After the lung has been removed from the donor, the organ is hypothermically stored to reduce the rate of biochemical reactions, which results in a decreased degradation of important cellular components. Nevertheless, adenosine triphosphate (ATP) is depleted during ischemia, which ultimately causes inactivation of ATP-dependent membrane pumps, an increase in intracellular calcium, inflammation, the formation of reactive oxygen species (ROS), and cell death [10, 25] (Fig. 3).

Lung Ischemia-reperfusion Injury: Inactive ATP-dependent Membrane Pumps and Intracellular Calcium Accumulation

Under normal conditions, the action of the Na^+/K^+-ATPase pump sets up a gradient of high extracellular Na^+ relative to intracellular levels, which in turn drives the Na^+/Ca^{2+}-exchanger, so that Ca^{2+} is pumped out of the cell. During ATP depletion, the Na^+/K^+-ATPase pump becomes inactivated, leading to an increase in intracellular Na^+. As a result, the Na^+/Ca^{2+} pump will not function, causing Ca^{2+} to accumulate inside the cell. When ischemia is prolonged, the ionic balance may be so upset that the Na^+/Ca^{2+}-pump activity is reversed, resulting in import of Ca^{2+} in exchange for Na^+, thereby exacerbating calcium overload. Other mechanisms contributing to high intracellular Ca^{2+} levels are an inactive plasmalemmal ATP-dependent Ca^{2+}-pump, important to move Ca^{2+} out of the cell, liberation of stored cytoplasmic calcium due to the acidosis, and a decreased uptake by the sarcoplasmic/endoplasmic reticulum [10, 25].

Cytosol elevated Ca^{2+} activates phospholipase A_2, which results in the induction of arachidonic acid. Arachidonic acid is normally incorporated in the cell mem-

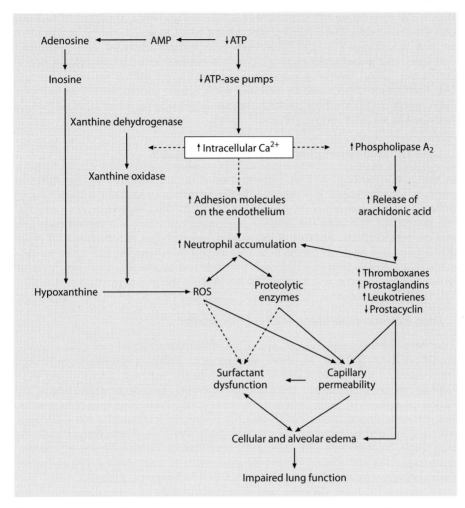

Fig. 3. Pathophysiology of lung ischemia reperfusion injury. See text for explanation. ATP: adenosine triphosphate; AMP: adenosine monophosphate; ROS: reactive oxygen species

brane and functions as a precursor for the production of eicosanoids, consisting of thromboxanes, leukotrienes, prostacyclin and prostaglandins. The effects of the eicosanoids due to tissue injury are various [10, 25].

While thromboxanes are predominantly produced by platelets, leukotrienes are formed by leukocytes (mostly neutrophils), prostacyclin by endothelial cells and prostaglandins by smooth muscle cells. Thromboxane A_2 has a potent vasoconstriction action, induces leukotriene production by neutrophils, and activates neutrophil adhesion receptors to facilitate interaction with the endothelium, which also expresses adhesion molecules due to the elevated Ca^{2+}. Leukotrienes too cause vasoconstriction, but may as well increase vascular permeability, and enhance neutrophil accumulation, adhesion and extravasation through the endothelium. Prostacyclin plays an important role in vascular function because it inhibits platelet adhesion to the vascular endothelium and is a strong vasodilator. Damaged endothelial cells do not produce PGI_2, thereby making the vessel more susceptible to thrombosis and vasospasm. Prostaglandins have both a vasoconstrictor and vasodilator function. Next to leukotrienes, prostaglandins can also make the vascular endothelium more 'leaky' thereby promoting edema formation during inflammation [10, 25]. Furthermore, increased intracellular Ca^{2+} causes transformation of xanthine dehydrogenase into xanthine oxidase, thereby facilitating the production of ROS, as described in the next section [10, 25].

Lung Ischemia-reperfusion Injury: Production of ROS

In the aerobic setting, ATP is converted to urea and xanthine by the effect of xanthine dehydrogenase. However, due to the formation of xanthine oxidase in lung ischemia-reperfusion injury, hypoxanthine is broken down into ROS. A second system to generate ROS is by the NADPH oxidase system, which is predominantly present on the membrane surfaces of monocytes, macrophages, neutrophils, and endothelial cells, and catalyzes the reduction of oxygen to superoxide and hydrogen peroxide. The superoxide anion, hydrogen peroxide and hydroxyl radical, which are all ROS, are very unstable and damage cell membranes by lipid peroxidation [10, 25].

Lung Ischemia-reperfusion Injury: Inflammation

After lung ischemia-reperfusion injury, pro-inflammatory cytokines (like interleukin [IL]-8, IL-10, IL-12, IL-18, tumor necrosis factor [TNF]-α, and interferon [IFN]γ) are released by macrophages due to activation during ischemia. Consequently, neutrophils and lymphocytes are recruited into the lung. Because of expression of adhesion molecules to both endothelium (E-selectin, P-selectin, intercellular-adhesion-molecule-1) and leukocytes (L-selectin, β-integrins), leukocytes roll (selectins), adhere (β-integrins, intercellular-adhesion-molecule-1), and extravasate into the lung tissue. Macrophages and neutrophils contribute to cellular damage by the production of ROS and several other mediators, such as proteolytic enzymes (gelatinases, collagenases and elastases), lysozyme, and lactoferrin [10, 25].

To summarize these different pathways: the increase in intracellular Ca^{2+} and Na^+ and the formation of ROS, eicosanoids, proteolytic enzymes and (phospho)lipases damage the lipid membrane of the cell, causing increased cellular permeability, the formation of cellular edema and eventually cell death. Finally all these pathways lead to a disturbed surfactant system [10, 25].

▌ Experimental Models of Lung Ischemia-reperfusion Injury

To study the complex pathophysiology of lung ischemia-reperfusion injury and to investigate surfactant treatment possibilities, an animal model is often used. Three major types of animal models have been reported: an isolated *ex vivo*, perfused lung system, a whole lung transplantation model, and an *in situ* warm ischemia model of the lung.

The isolated, perfused lung system is a model whereby the organ is taken out of the animal, hypothermically stored for a certain period of ischemia and subsequently reperfused by the use of a Langendorff system. Although this model has advantages (e.g., the use of lungs of knock-out mice), the most important disadvantage clearly is the *ex vivo* situation, disturbing normal physiological interactions. Furthermore, only short follow-up periods after reperfusion (hours) can be established [26].

Animal whole lung transplantation has the advantage that it best reflects human transplantation and allows the investigation of the effect of cold ischemic storage, the use of storage solutions, and the study of allo-antigen settings. However, disadvantages are that, especially in small animals, it is a time-consuming and technically difficult procedure with often high mortality rates, limiting the study of longer follow-up periods after transplantation [3, 4, 18, 19, 27]. Also, larger animals, like pigs and dogs have been used to avert the possible high mortality and the technical difficulties [6, 28–30]. Nevertheless, the limitations of this model are the difficulties in activating and blocking specific pathways (due to costs and receptor specificity) and the unavailability of genetically modified animals.

To overcome some of the disadvantages in transplantation models, an *in situ* warm ischemia model of the lung in small rodents has been developed, in which the ischemia is induced by clamping the pulmonary artery, veins and bronchus of (usually) the left lung. Clamping time generally ranges from 60 to 120 minutes (van der Kaaij, et al., unpublished data) [31, 32]. After declamping, reperfusion occurs. Although this *in vivo* model is technically much easier than the aforementioned transplantation models, there are some disadvantages. Firstly, warm ischemia is used, accompanied by a high metabolic rate. However, the use of short periods of warm ischemia is accepted as an accelerated model of ischemia-reperfusion injury of the lung [33]. Additionally, because of often long warm ischemic periods, severe ischemia-reperfusion injury is induced resulting in still high mortality. As a result, most studies still investigate short time periods (max. 6 hours) after the start of reperfusion. Only a few studies report long reperfusion times of about 1 week [27, 32]; however, in these studies mortality was still very high after extubation of the animals. We have recently developed a model of lung ischemia-reperfusion injury in which (by adjusting the anesthetic protocol and ventilator strategy) we are able to study intervals up to months after reperfusion, with acceptable mortality (van der Kaaij, et al., unpublished data).

▌ Surfactant Dysfunction and Lung Ischemia-reperfusion Injury

Using these experimental models, several research groups have gained valuable information on how specific parts of the surfactant system are affected by lung ischemia-reperfusion injury [2, 3, 16, 17, 34] (Fig. 4).

Surfactant Dysfunction: Alveolar Proteins

The presence of alveolar proteins after lung ischemia-reperfusion injury has been described in many studies [2–5, 16, 19, 28, 29, 35–40]. Both different warm (1–2 h [3, 36], van der Kaaij, et al., unpublished data) and cold (2–20 h [2, 4, 5, 19, 35]) ischemic intervals have resulted in increased levels of alveolar protein between 1 and 24 hours after reperfusion. Due to ROS, proteolytic enzymes and phospholipases, endogenous surfactant and the endothelial and epithelial membrane are damaged. This results in leakage of proteins into the alveolus and surfactant com-

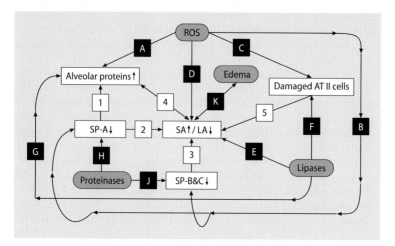

Fig. 4. *Reactive oxygen species* (ROS) directly damage **[A]** the alveolo-capillary membrane, thereby facilitating the influx of serum proteins into the alveolus, **[B]** the surfactant-associated proteins (SP), **[C]** the alveolar type II (AT II) cells, and **[D]** the large aggregate (LA) surfactant subform. *Phospholipases* cause degradation of **[E]** the surfactant phospholipids inside the alveolus, **[F]** the membranes of ATII cells and **[G]** capillary endothelium, resulting in the influx of serum proteins. *Proteinases* break down **[H]** SP-A and **[J]** SP-B and -C **[K]**. *Edema* results in dilution of the surfactant phospholipids inside the alveolus, which results in further formation of edema. A decrease in SP-A leads to **[1]** less inhibition of serum proteins, and **[2]** decreased phospholipid secretion, recycling, and formation of tubular myelin. **[3]** SP-B&C degradation causes less phospholipids to be inserted into the phospholipid monolayer lining the alveolar epithelium. **[4]** Once serum proteins have infiltrated the alveolus, they compete for a place at the air-liquid interface, thereby dose-dependently inhibiting surfactant function. Furthermore, once the phospholipid monolayer is damaged, the molecule transfer limiting function of surfactant is also impaired, resulting in further influx of serum proteins, so that a vicious circle has developed. **[5]** Finally AT II cells, important in the production, recycling and secretion of surfactant phospholipids are damaged, so that less LA is secreted and a smaller amount of SA is being recycled. Due to these factors, a decrease in LA and an increase in SA has been noticed after lung ischemia-reperfusion injury

ponents into the bloodstream. Since surfactant is rate limiting for the transfer of proteins across the alveolo-capillary membrane and is either inactivated or lost due to the increased endothelial permeability after lung ischemia-reperfusion injury, a further influx of proteins is facilitated. Because proteins, once accumulated in the alveolus, then dose-dependently inhibit surfactant, this results in a self-triggering mechanism of surfactant inactivation [24]. Under normal conditions, SP-A is able to counteract the inactivating effects of serum proteins on surfactant [41]. However, after lung ischemia-reperfusion injury, a decrease in SP-A was found in human lung transplant recipients and animal models of lung ischemia-reperfusion injury [19, 42].

Surfactant Dysfunction: Inactivation of Surfactant Associated Proteins

A decrease in SP-A was already visible after prolonged ischemic storage without reperfusion and decreased further after the start of reperfusion [2, 4, 19]. Moreover, in lung transplant recipients, the level of SP-A is still low more than one year after transplantation [42]. SP-A can be degraded by ROS and proteolytic enzymes. It was also shown that the levels of SP-A decreased with ascending severity of lung isch-emia-reperfusion injury, suggesting that preservation or amelioration of SP-A is es-sential for improvement after lung ischemia-reperfusion injury [19]. Besides the protein inhibiting function of SP-A, SP-A also plays a central role in phospholipid secretion and recycling, contributing to a decrease in surface activity of surfactant.

SP-B and SP-C have also been found to be decreased after lung ischemia-reperfu-sion injury [28]. Decreased levels or inactivation of SP-B and SP-C can result in a diminished quantity of phospholipids, but also in a changed composition of the surfactant on the surface of the alveolar epithelium, thereby impairing the surfac-tant lowering properties [28].

Studies have reported surfactant dysfunction without a change in the overall amount of phospholipids [2, 3]. Both a decrease in DPPC and phosphatidyl-glycerol and an increase in sphingomyelin have been described [2, 3, 17, 28]. DPPC, the sat-urated form of phosphatidylcholine, is the most important phospholipid known to reduce the minimum surface tension. Although Klepetko et al. demonstrated a cor-relation between an impaired oxygenation capacity of the lung and a decrease in DPPC (signifying the possible importance of this phospholipid in normal lung function), Veldhuizen et al. found no relationship between the changes in surfactant composition and surface lowering properties of surfactant, illustrating the complex pathophysiology of surfactant dysfunction [2, 17].

▍ Experimental Results of Surfactant Treatment in Lung Ischemia-reperfusion Injury

Several authors have examined the effect of the lung preservation protocol and sur-factant replacement therapy on surfactant function in experimental models of cold and warm lung ischemia-reperfusion injury [4–6, 16, 19, 27–29, 35–40, 43, 44]. By changing the lung preservation solution from Euro-Collins to low potassium dex-tran solution, and by flushing the graft retrograde instead of antegrade, the damag-ing effects of lung ischemia-reperfusion injury on pulmonary surfactant could be ameliorated [29, 37–40, 44]. Furthermore, it was demonstrated that when, in the case of replacement therapy, surfactant was administered just before, at or after re-perfusion, it improved lung compliance and PaO_2 and prevented an increase in the small aggregate/light aggregate ratio directly after lung ischemia-reperfusion injury [4, 35]. However, other studies have shown that treatment with exogenous surfac-tant before the onset of ischemia is more beneficial when compared to treatment at reperfusion [30, 35, 45, 46]. This can be explained by less complement activation, diminished membrane damage, and an enlarged surfactant phospholipid pool after donor treatment, thereby preventing deterioration of the entire endogenous surfac-tant pool [6, 46]. Also, surfactant given to the donor may result in a more homoge-neous distribution in the lung as compared to treatment after reperfusion, when al-veolar damage has already occurred [6].

Most studies investigating the effect of surfactant replacement therapy have only addressed the first hours (2–6) after reperfusion. Studies on the longer term effects of lung ischemia-reperfusion injury and surfactant treatment are scarce. In this re-gard, Erasmus and colleagues demonstrated that surfactant treatment just before reperfusion enhanced recovery from lung ischemia-reperfusion injury at one week postoperatively [27]. We confirm that lung ischemia-reperfusion injury resulted in the conversion of surfactant into less active surfactant, and impaired PaO_2 and lung compliance throughout the first week after reperfusion. However, even months after reperfusion, diffuse alveolar damage and decreased lung compliance were visible. Surfactant treatment before the induction of warm ischemia completely normalized these parameters from 3 to 90 days after reperfusion (van der Kaaij et al., unpublished data).

The rationale behind surfactant replacement therapy is to ameliorate the damage caused by ROS, to decrease the inhibitory effects of serum proteins, and to preserve the levels of surfactant protein and DPPC.

Surfactant Therapy: Decreasing the Inhibitory Effects of Serum Proteins

When the quantity of surfactant is low or its composition is changed, serum proteins (like albumin, fibrin, fibrinogen, C-reactive protein [CRP], and hemoglobin) leak into the alveolus [47]. This protein leakage can be ameliorated by surfactant therapy [4, 24, 26, 48] (van der Kaaij et al., unpublished data). However, some studies failed to show a decrease in leakage of serum proteins into the alveolus, which can probably be explained by the different treatment strategies [6, 35, 48]. We hypothesize that surfactant administration to the donor may be more beneficial in inhibiting serum protein leakage than treatment at the time of reperfusion. However, once alveolar proteins accumulate in the alveolus, the lung can resist against surfactant inactivation by the interference of SP-A. Cockshutt et al. showed *in vitro* a reversed inhibition of serum proteins on the surface lowering function of surfactant when SP-A was administered [41].

Surfactant Therapy: Preservation of Surfactant Composition

With surfactant treatment the surface tension in the lung remains low, thereby maintaining the ventilation and perfusion of the lung, resulting in optimal oxygenation [6]. As mentioned earlier, an increase in the small/large aggregate ratio occurs due to lung ischemia-reperfusion injury. Since most of the exogenous surfactant administered to lung is in the large aggregate subform, a larger pool of surface-active phospholipids (DPPC) is created, so that the rise in small/large aggregate ratio is prevented [6, 28]. Thus, the instilled exogenous surfactant protects the endogenous surfactant pool against damage. This is illustrated by the fact that the normal endogenous surfactant pool is about 10–15 mg lipid per kilogram, and that the amount of surfactant used for treatment is in the range of 50–400 mg lipid per kilogram [6].

Furthermore the preservation of SP-A, SP-B, and SP-C can result in normal phospholipid recycling and secretion [28]. As already mentioned, exogenous surfactant treatment preserves the endogenous surfactant, resulting in normal endogenous SP-A, SP-B, and SP-C. Moreover, it was shown that SP-A enriched surfactant was able to improve lung function after prolonged ischemia, whereas this was not possible to the same extent with SP-A deficient surfactant within one hour after reperfusion [19]. Also, a decrease of the large aggregate subform was found indicating an increased recycling capacity of the SP-A enriched surfactant compared with SP-A deficient surfactant [19].

Surfactant Therapy: Anti-inflammatory and Antioxidant Function

Surfactant has also been shown to inhibit cytokine release from activated mono-cytes and macrophages [49, 50]; the modulation of lymphocytes has also been sug-gested. Furthermore, surfactant is known to have antioxidant capacities, resulting in reduced ROS damage at the level of the alveolus [51]. Surfactant treatment can thus ameliorate the accumulation and adherence of inflammatory cells, so that en-dothelial and AT II injury is prevented, normalizing cell permeability and surfac-tant recycling. Semik and colleagues showed that the decreased function of AT II cells after lung ischemia-reperfusion injury is prevented by surfactant treatment [42].

∎ Clinical Studies of Surfactant Treatment after Lung Transplantation

Some investigators have used surfactant to treat lung transplant recipients who de-veloped severe lung ischemia-reperfusion injury after transplantation [52–54]. In a case report by Strüber and colleagues in 1995, a 26-year old woman who under-went right lung transplantation and developed severe reperfusion injury 5 hours after transplantation, was treated with intrapulmonary nebulized synthetic surfac-tant [53]. Shortly after surfactant therapy, lung compliance, PaO_2, and tidal volume increased. Moreover, 24 hours after therapy, the edematous infiltrate of the trans-planted lung on chest X-ray film was resolved. Another study in six lung transplant patients also suggested improvement in lung ischemia-reperfusion injury due to surfactant replacement. However, in 1 of the 6 recipients, surfactant therapy failed to improve dynamic lung compliance, which could be attributed to the application approach or the type of surfactant used (synthetic versus natural surfactant) [52].

Although the use of surfactant in human lung transplantation seems promising, no prospective randomized clinical trial has so far been set up to treat severe lung ischemia-reperfusion injury. Also, a clinical trial should investigate possible addi-tional effects of donor pretreatment as compared to treatment after reperfusion.

∎ Conclusion

In this chapter we have discussed the effects of lung ischemia-reperfusion injury on the surfactant system. Lung ischemia-reperfusion injury damages the endoge-nous surfactant system by the production of ROS, proteolytic enzymes, and (phos-pho)lipases. Surfactant is composed of phospholipids and associated proteins and its main function is to reduce the surface tension inside the alveolus, allowing nor-mal breathing. Impairment of the surfactant system will increase surface tension (leading to instability and collapse of alveoli), atelectasis formation, influx of serum proteins into the alveolus, pulmonary edema, decreased lung compliance, and im-paired gas exchange.

The use of surfactant replacement therapy (either before or after lung ischemia-reperfusion injury) ameliorates lung ischemia-reperfusion injury. Surfactant therapy restores the activity of the endogenous surfactant pool and reduces the inhibitory effect of serum proteins; possible other effects are that it serves as an anti-oxidant and an anti-inflammatory agent. Although human data on the use of surfactant in lung transplant patients are scarce, the positive results in experimental models and a few patient reports suggest that (pre)treatment with surfactant in lung transplantation patients could improve outcome. Future studies should further investigate the effect of surfactant on lung ischemia-reperfusion injury markers on both short and long term.

Acknowledgments. The authors thank Laraine Visser-Isles (Department of Anesthesiology) for English-language editing.

References

1. Hosenpud JD, Bennett LE, Keck BM, Boucek MM, Novick RJ (2000) The registry of the international society for heart and lung transplantation: Seventeenth official report-2000. J Heart Lung Transplant 19:909–931
2. Veldhuizen RA, Lee J, Sandler D, et al (1993) Alterations in pulmonary surfactant composition and activity after experimental lung transplantation. Am Rev Respir Dis 148:208–215
3. Erasmus ME, Petersen AH, Oetomo SB, Prop J (1994) The function of surfactant is impaired during the reimplantation response in rat lung transplants. J Heart Lung Transplant 13:791–802
4. Erasmus ME, Petersen AH, Hofstede G, Haagsman HP, Bambang Oetomo S, Prop J (1996) Surfactant treatment before reperfusion improves the immediate function of lung transplants in rats. Am J Respir Crit Care Med 153:665–670
5. Novick RJ, Gilpin AA, Gehman KE, et al (1997) Mitigation of injury in canine lung grafts by exogenous surfactant therapy. J Thorac Cardiovasc Surg 113:342–353
6. Novick RJ, Veldhuizen RA, Possmayer F, Lee J, Sandler D, Lewis JF (1994) Exogenous surfactant therapy in thirty-eight hour lung graft preservation for transplantation. J Thorac Cardiovasc Surg 108:259–268
7. Khan SU, Salloum J, O'Donovan PB, et al (1999) Acute pulmonary edema after lung transplantation: The pulmonary reimplantation response. Chest 116:187–194
8. King RC, Binns OA, Rodriguez F, et al (2000) Reperfusion injury significantly impacts clinical outcome after pulmonary transplantation. Ann Thorac Surg 69:1681–1685
9. Lee KH, Martich GD, Boujoukos AJ, Keenan RJ, Griffith BP (1996) Predicting icu length of stay following single lung transplantation. Chest 110:1014–1017
10. de Perrot M, Liu M, Waddell TK, Keshavjee S (2003) Ischemia-reperfusion-induced lung injury. Am J Respir Crit Care Med 167:490–511
11. Lachmann B (1987) The role of pulmonary surfactant in the pathogenesis and therapy of ARDS. In: Vincent JL (ed) Update in Intensive Care and Emergency Medicine. Springer, Heidelberg, pp 123–124
12. Ingbar DH (2000) Mechanisms of repair and remodeling following acute lung injury. Clin Chest Med 21:589–616
13. Boehler A, Kesten S, Weder W, Speich R (1998) Bronchiolitis obliterans after lung transplantation: A review. Chest 114:1411–1426
14. Fiser SM, Tribble CG, Long SM, et al (2002) Ischemia-reperfusion injury after lung transplantation increases risk of late bronchiolitis obliterans syndrome. Ann Thorac Surg 73:1041–1047
15. Tullius SG, Tilney NL (1995) Both alloantigen-dependent and -independent factors influence chronic allograft rejection. Transplantation 59:313–318
16. Andrade RS, Solien EE, Wangensteen OD, Tsai MY, Kshettry VR, Bolman RM, 3rd (1995) Surfactant dysfunction in lung preservation. Transplantation 60:536–541
17. Klepetko W, Lohninger A, Wisser W, et al (1990) Pulmonary surfactant in bronchoalveolar lavage after canine lung transplantation: Effect of l-carnitine application. J Thorac Cardiovasc Surg 99:1048–1058
18. Erasmus ME, Veldhuizen RA, Novick RJ, Lewis JF, Prop J (1996) The effect of lung preservation on alveolar surfactant. Transplantation 62:143–144
19. Erasmus ME, Hofstede GJ, Petersen AH, et al (2002) Sp-a-enriched surfactant for treatment of rat lung transplants with sp-a deficiency after storage and reperfusion. Transplantation 73:348–352

20. Hohlfeld JM, Tiryaki E, Hamm H, et al (1998) Pulmonary surfactant activity is impaired in lung transplant recipients. Am J Respir Crit Care Med 158:706–712
21. Haitsma JJ, Papadakos PJ, Lachmann B (2004) Surfactant therapy for acute lung injury/ acute respiratory distress syndrome. Curr Opin Crit Care 10:18–22
22. Griese M (1999) Pulmonary surfactant in health and human lung diseases: State of the art. Eur Respir J 13:1455–1476
23. Haitsma JJ, Lachmann RA, Lachmann B (2003) Lung protective ventilation in ards: Role of mediators, peep and surfactant. Monaldi Arch Chest Dis 59:108–118
24. Lachmann B, Eijking EP, So KL, Gommers D (1994) In vivo evaluation of the inhibitory capacity of human plasma on exogenous surfactant function. Intensive Care Med 20:6–11
25. Grace PA, Mathie RT (1999) Ischaemia-reperfusion Injury. Blackwell Science Ltd, London
26. Buchanan SA, Mauney MC, Parekh VI, et al (1996) Intratracheal surfactant administration preserves airway compliance during lung reperfusion. Ann Thorac Surg 62:1617–1621
27. Erasmus ME, Hofstede GJ, Petersen AH, Haagsman HP, Oetomo SB, Prop J (1997) Effects of early surfactant treatment persisting for one week after lung transplantation in rats. Am J Respir Crit Care Med 156:567–572
28. Gunther A, Balser M, Schmidt R, et al (2004) Surfactant abnormalities after single lung transplantation in dogs: Impact of bronchoscopic surfactant administration. J Thorac Cardiovasc Surg 127:344–354
29. Struber M, Hohlfeld JM, Kofidis T, et al (2002) Surfactant function in lung transplantation after 24 hours of ischemia: Advantage of retrograde flush perfusion for preservation. J Thorac Cardiovasc Surg 123:98–103
30. Koletsis E, Chatzimichalis A, Fotopoulos V, et al (2003) Donor lung pretreatment with surfactant in experimental transplantation preserves graft hemodynamics and alveolar morphology. Exp Biol Med (Maywood) 228:540–545
31. Krishnadasan B, Naidu B, Rosengart M, et al (2002) Decreased lung ischemia-reperfusion injury in rats after preoperative administration of cyclosporine and tacrolimus. J Thorac Cardiovasc Surg 123:756–767
32. Takeyoshi I, Otani Y, Koibuchi Y, et al (1999) Effects of fr167653 on pulmonary ischemia-reperfusion injury: Administration timing. Transplant Proc 31:1935–1936
33. Warnecke G, Sommer SP, Gohrbandt B, et al (2004) Warm or cold ischemia in animal models of lung ischemia-reperfusion injury: Is there a difference? Thorac Cardiovasc Surg 52:174–179
34. Oosting RS, van Greevenbroek MM, Verhoef J, van Golde LM, Haagsman HP (1991) Structural and functional changes of surfactant protein a induced by ozone. Am J Physiol 261:L77–83
35. Friedrich I, Borgermann J, Splittgerber FH, et al (2004) Bronchoscopic surfactant administration preserves gas exchange and pulmonary compliance after single lung transplantation in dogs. J Thorac Cardiovasc Surg 127:335–343
36. Warnecke G, Struber M, Fraud S, Hohlfeld JM, Haverich A (2001) Combined exogenous surfactant and inhaled nitric oxide therapy for lung ischemia-reperfusion injury in minipigs. Transplantation 71:1238–1244
37. Andrade RS, Wangensteen OD, Jo JK, Tsai MY, Bolman RM 3rd (2000) Effect of hypothermic pulmonary artery flushing on capillary filtration coefficient. Transplantation 70:267–271
38. Struber M, McGregor CG, Locke TJ, Miller VM (1990) Effect of flush-perfusion with euro-collins solution on pulmonary arterial function. Transplant Proc 22:2206–2211
39. Struber M, Ehlers KA, Nilsson FN, Miller VM, McGregor CG, Haverich A (1997) Effects of lung preservation with euro-collins and university of wisconsin solutions on endothelium-dependent relaxations. Ann Thorac Surg 63:1428–1435
40. Struber M, Hohlfeld JM, Fraund S, Kim P, Warnecke G, Haverich A (2000) Low-potassium dextran solution ameliorates reperfusion injury of the lung and protects surfactant function. J Thorac Cardiovasc Surg 120:566–572
41. Cockshutt AM, Weitz J, Possmayer F (1990) Pulmonary surfactant-associated protein a enhances the surface activity of lipid extract surfactant and reverses inhibition by blood proteins in vitro. Biochemistry 29:8424–8429

42. Semik M, Schnabel R, Bruske T, et al (1994) Ultrastructural studies of acute rejection following single lung transplantation in the rat–histological and immunohistological findings. Thorac Cardiovasc Surg 42:290–297

43. Hohlfeld JM, Struber M, Ahlf K, et al (1999) Exogenous surfactant improves survival and surfactant function in ischaemia-reperfusion injury in minipigs. Eur Respir J 13:1037–1043

44. Struber M, Wilhelmi M, Harringer W, et al (2001) Flush perfusion with low potassium dextran solution improves early graft function in clinical lung transplantation. Eur J Cardiothorac Surg 19:190–194

45. Novick RJ, MacDonald J, Veldhuizen RA, et al (1996) Evaluation of surfactant treatment strategies after prolonged graft storage in lung transplantation. Am J Respir Crit Care Med 154:98–104

46. Hausen B, Rohde R, Hewitt CW, et al (1997) Exogenous surfactant treatment before and after sixteen hours of ischemia in experimental lung transplantation. J Thorac Cardiovasc Surg 113:1050–1058

47. Casals C, Varela A, Ruano ML, et al (1998) Increase of c-reactive protein and decrease of surfactant protein a in surfactant after lung transplantation. Am J Respir Crit Care Med 157:43–49

48. Novick RJ, Gehman KE, Ali IS, Lee J (1996) Lung preservation: The importance of endothelial and alveolar type ii cell integrity. Ann Thorac Surg 62:302–314

49. Thomassen MJ, Meeker DP, Antal JM, Connors MJ, Wiedemann HP (1992) Synthetic surfactant (exosurf) inhibits endotoxin-stimulated cytokine secretion by human alveolar macrophages. Am J Respir Cell Mol Biol 7:257–260

50. Speer CP, Gotze B, Curstedt T, Robertson B (1991) Phagocytic functions and tumor necrosis factor secretion of human monocytes exposed to natural porcine surfactant (curosurf). Pediatr Res 30:69–74

51. Matalon S, Holm BA, Baker RR, Whitfield MK, Freeman BA (1990) Characterization of antioxidant activities of pulmonary surfactant mixtures. Biochim Biophys Acta 1035:121–127

52. Struber M, Hirt SW, Cremer J, Harringer W, Haverich A (1999) Surfactant replacement in reperfusion injury after clinical lung transplantation. Intensive Care Med 25:862–864

53. Struber M, Cremer J, Harringer W, Hirt SW, Costard-Jackle A, Haverich A (1995) Nebulized synthetic surfactant in reperfusion injury after single lung transplantation. J Thorac Cardiovasc Surg 110:563–564

54. Della Rocca G, Pierconti F, Costa MG, et al (2002) Severe reperfusion lung injury after double lung transplantation. Crit Care 6:240–244

Biomarkers for Pulmonary Injury in Critically Ill Patients

R. M. Determann, M. B. Vroom, and M. J. Schultz

▮ Introduction

The lungs of critically ill patients are at a constant threat of diverse inflammatory reactions. First, critically ill patients may develop acute lung injury (ALI) or the acute respiratory distress syndrome (ARDS), which can be the result of either a pulmonary insult (e.g., pneumonia) or an indirect insult (e.g., sepsis). Although frequently mandatory and life-saving, mechanical ventilation puts patients at additional risks for secondary inflammatory processes. Indeed, mechanically ventilated patients are prone to pneumonia (so-called ventilator-associated pneumonia, VAP), causing substantial additional morbidity and mortality [1]. Furthermore, mechanical ventilation may aggravate pulmonary inflammation (also known as ventilator-induced lung injury, VILI), which leads to a decreased chance of survival [2]. A recent report even suggests that mechanical ventilation by itself may initiate lung injury [3], i.e., VILI may develop without pre-existing lung disease. Early and adequate recognition of ARDS, VAP and VILI is required for intensive care physicians to take adequate actions at the right time (e.g., the use of so-called lung-protective mechanical ventilation or the initiation of antimicrobial therapy).

The problem is, however, that these entities are hard to differentiate in clinical practice. Clinical manifestations of ARDS include critical hypoxemia and new onset bilateral chest radiographic consolidations consistent with edema [4]. Unfortunately, these clinical criteria are either hard to recognize or subject to inter-observer variability. Indeed, the chest radiographic appearance does not differentiate well between edema, atelectasis and pleural fluid, thereby limiting inter-observer agreement [5]. In addition, radiographic abnormalities and hypoxemia are dependent on the level of positive end-expiratory pressure (PEEP) [6]. Comparable diagnostic problems apply for the diagnosis of VAP [1]. A presumptive clinical diagnosis of VAP is often made on the basis of presence of new radiographic infiltrates on the chest radiograph, fever, leukocytosis, hypoxemia and purulent tracheal secretions. Such a clinical approach, however, inevitably leads to overestimation of the incidence of VAP and subsequent unwanted extensive antibiotic (mis)use [7]. While results from the ARDS Network trial have underscored the potential importance of VILI in the management of ARDS [8] and it is now advised to use lower tidal volumes in patients with ARDS [9], it might be that lung-protective mechanical ventilation settings may differ from one patient to another. A non-injurious mechanical ventilation setting in one patient may be highly injurious in another patient. Unfortunately, neither chest radiograph findings, nor clinical parameters can be used to gauge the effects of the individual mechanical ventilation settings.

While clinical parameters are not sufficient to diagnose ARDS, VAP, or VILI, biomarkers might help intensive care physicians in making differential diagnoses when confronted with a clinical diagnostic problem. Biomarkers might also be valuable if they could predict development of ALI in separate patients who are at risk. In addition, biomarkers might help to determine which mechanical ventilation setting is least injurious in an individual patient. Recent research suggests a potential role for several biomarkers of pulmonary injury in critically ill patients in the near future. These include the triggering receptor expressed on myeloid cells (TREM)-1, the human alveolar type I cell-specific apical membrane protein HTI56, and surfactant proteins. In this chapter we will discuss the value of these potential biomarkers in critically ill patients with diverse pulmonary inflammatory processes.

▌ Triggering Receptor expressed on Myeloid Cells

Background

TREM-1, a 30 kDa glycoprotein, is a member of the immunoglobulin superfamily, and only weakly expressed on cells in tissues from patients with non-infectious inflammatory disorders [10]. Upon invasion of bacteria or fungi, tissues are infiltrated with neutrophils and monocytes that strongly express TREM-1 [11]. TREM-1 triggers the release of pro-inflammatory cytokines and chemokines, and increases surface expression of cell adhesion molecules [11]. TREM-1 is also shed by the membrane of activated neutrophils and monocytes and can be measured in this soluble form (sTREM-1) in different body fluids. Levels of sTREM-1 in bronchoalveolar fluid might thus serve as a biomarker for pulmonary infection.

sTREM-1 as a Biomarker for Pneumonia

TREM-1 is probably selectively expressed by neutrophils and alveolar macrophages in the lungs of patients with pneumonia caused by extra-cellular bacteria [12]. Indeed, TREM-1 expression by inflammatory cells was significantly higher in the lungs of patients with community-acquired pneumonia (CAP), as compared to cells in bronchoalveolar-lavage (BAL) fluid from patients with tuberculosis and patients with interstitial lung disease. In contrast, TREM-1 expression on peripheral blood neutrophils was not different among the three groups.

In a prospective study on mechanically ventilated patients, Gibot et al. determined the diagnostic value of measuring pulmonary levels of sTREM-1 [13]. For this, they determined sTREM-1 in pulmonary fluid (obtained by mini-lavage) by means of a rapid immunoblot technique. A final diagnosis of CAP was made in 38 patients and VAP in 46 patients. No pneumonia was diagnosed in 64 patients; in this group, either an alternative diagnosis was made or patients recovered without antibiotic treatment. Pulmonary lavage levels of sTREM-1 were significantly higher in both pneumonia groups, as compared to lavage levels in patients without pulmonary infection (Fig. 1). At a level of ≥ 5 pg/ml, sTREM-1 was detected in BAL fluid from 36/38 patients with CAP (sensitivity of 95%), 46/46 patients with VAP (sensitivity of 100%), and 6/64 patients without pneumonia. In the same samples tumor necrosis factor (TNF)-α and interleukin (IL)-1β were measured: levels of these pro-inflammatory cytokines showed the same trend but with a large overlap of values. The presence of sTREM-1 by itself was more accurate than any clinical finding or

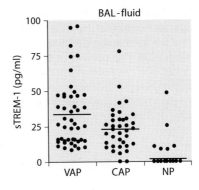

Fig. 1. Levels of soluble triggering receptor expressed on myeloid cells (sTREM-1) in bronchoalveolar lavage fluid from patients with ventilator-associated pneumonia (VAP), patients with community-acquired pneumonia (CAP), and patients without pneumonia (NP). The individual data are plotted, the horizontal line represents the mean sTREM-1 level. Differences are statistically significant for the comparison between the group of patients without pneumonia, and each group of patients with pneumonia. Modified from [13] with permission

laboratory value in identifying the presence of bacterial or fungal pneumonia. In a multiple logistic-regression analysis, the presence of sTREM-1 was the strongest independent predictor of pneumonia. It must be emphasized, however, that a significant number of patients in this study were considered not to have pneumonia even though they met the usual criteria for pulmonary infection; it can be questioned whether all patients with negative lavage cultures did indeed not have pneumonia.

sTREM-1 as a Biomarker for ARDS or VILI

At the present time, to our knowledge, there are no studies that have studied local levels of sTREM-1 in ARDS or VILI (see also "advantages and potential drawbacks").

Advantages and Potential Drawbacks

Determination of pulmonary levels of sTREM-1 in mini-lavages has some important advantages: mini-lavages are easily performed; the immunoblot technique is rapid, accurate, and inexpensive and can be used for small batches of specimens or even individual samples. Importantly, however, test materials are not yet commercially available, for research or for clinical use.

Some potential drawbacks exist, however. One problem is that it was not mentioned at which time point relative to the development of pneumonia mini-lavages were performed in the above-cited study by Gibot et al. [13]. It is thus unknown whether levels of sTREM-1 rise already before (all) signs and symptoms of pulmonary infection are present, and new studies are needed to reveal the exact relation in time between pulmonary levels of sTREM-1 and clinical signs of pneumonia, such as radiographic infiltrates and purulent secretions. Additional studies may also reveal whether sTREM-1 can be used to monitor efficacy of antimicrobial treatment, i.e., whether (and how fast) pulmonary levels of sTREM-1 decline after start of an (effective) antimicrobial therapy.

Furthermore, it is presently unknown whether pulmonary levels of sTREM-1 will adequately differentiate between pneumonia and other states of pulmonary inflammation, such as ARDS and VILI. ARDS is frequently present in patients with sepsis, in which both elevated concentrations of blood myeloid cells expressing TREM-1 and high systemic levels of sTREM-1 are found [14]. In addition, ARDS is characterized by massive pulmonary infiltration of neutrophils, and with many pulmonary disorders including ARDS or VILI, alveolar-capillary disruption is present. It can thus be speculated that neutrophils expressing TREM-1 may infiltrate pulmonary tissues during development of ARDS or VILI, after which TREM-1 is shed from these cells; otherwise, sTREM-1 present in the systemic compartment during sepsis might diffuse directly into the pulmonary compartment through the disrupted alveolar-capillary barrier. It is clear that additional studies are needed to learn more about the relation between systemic and pulmonary levels of sTREM-1 during different forms of pulmonary inflammation.

▌ Human Alveolar Type I Cell-specific Apical Membrane Protein

Background

The alveolar epithelium is composed of two morphologically distinct types of cells, alveolar type I and alveolar type II cells. The thin cytoplasmic extensions of alveolar type I cells cover more than 95% of the internal surface area of the lungs. HTI56 is a 56 kDa integral membrane protein of the apical membrane of human alveolar type I cells [15]. In the normal situation, small amounts of HTI56 are detectable in blood [16]. However, upon lung injury, concentrations of HTI56 rise both in blood and bronchoalveolar fluids. HTI56-levels in bronchoalveolar fluid or blood might thus serve as a biomarker for lung injury.

HTI56 as a Biomarker for Pneumonia

The hypothesis that the integral membrane protein of the apical membrane of alveolar type I cells would be effective as a marker of pneumonia has been tested in animals. Rat alveolar type I (RTI) cell-specific apical membrane protein 40, a 40–42 kDa integral membrane protein of rat alveolar type I cells has been used successfully as a marker of alveolar epithelial injury in a rat pneumonia model [17]. Indeed, instillation of *Pseudomonas aeruginosa* into the lungs of anesthetized, ventilated rats resulted in an 80-fold increase of pulmonary levels of RTI40 in comparison to control rats. This increase correlated with both morphological evidence of injury to alveolar epithelial type I cells and increased permeability of the alveolar epithelium to protein tracers. These findings indicate that the alveolar fluid content of a type I cell-specific protein can be used as a sensitive and specific biochemical marker of type I cell injury caused by pulmonary infection. At the present time however, to our knowledge, there are no human studies establishing the efficacy of HTI56 as a biomarker for pneumonia.

HTI56 as a Biomarker for ARDS or VILI

Newman et al. performed a prospective study in intensive care patients and healthy volunteers [16]. Of the intensive care patients, one group had a clinical diagnosis of ALI and one group suffered from hydrostatic pulmonary edema. Diagnosis of ALI was based on clinical criteria and an edema fluid protein/plasma protein ratio >0.75. Diagnosis of hydrostatic pulmonary edema was based on clinical criteria and an edema fluid protein/plasma protein ratio <0.65. Patients with a protein/plasma protein ratio between 0.65 and 0.75 were excluded. HTI56 was measured

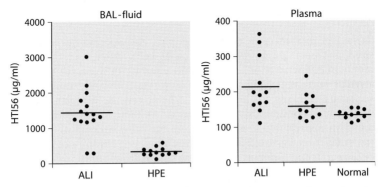

Fig. 2. Left graph: HTI56 content of undiluted pulmonary edema fluid from patients with acute lung injury (ALI) or hydrostatic pulmonary edema (HPE). Individual data are plotted, the horizontal line represents the mean HTI56 level. The average quantity of HTI56 was 4.3-fold higher in the ALI-group than in the HPE-group ($p < 0.0001$). Right graph: HTI56 content of plasma. Average quantity of HTI56 was 1.4-fold higher in the ALI group than in the HPE group ($p < 0.05$). Modified from [16] with permission

using a specific ELISA for HTI56. HTI56 was detectable in pulmonary edema fluid from both patient groups and in plasma from all patients and healthy volunteers. However, pulmonary levels of HTI56 from patients with ALI were significantly higher as compared with patients with hydrostatic pulmonary edema (Fig. 2). Of special interest was the fact that the systemic levels of HTI56 from ALI patients were also significantly higher compared with patients with hydrostatic pulmonary edema.

Advantages and Potential Drawbacks

Determination of systemic and/or pulmonary levels of HTI56 has some important advantages: the ELISA-technique is rapid, accurate, and inexpensive and can be used for small batches of specimens. In addition, HTI56 is specific for injury of lung tissue, and thus seems the ideal marker of lung injury. Furthermore, the fact that systemic levels of HTI56 are also elevated with pulmonary injury means that ALI possibly can be determined by means of a simple blood test (i.e., there is no need to obtain pulmonary samples). Very similar to the test materials for determination of sTREM-1, however, test materials for HTI56-ELISA are not yet commercially available, for research or for clinical use.

Similar to sTREM-1 determination, some potential drawbacks exist. First, it is presently unknown how local and systemic levels change in time, i.e., how quickly levels of this lung specific marker will rise when pneumonia or ARDS/VILI develops, and in the same way, how quickly levels will decline upon healing of lung tissue. What we also do not know is whether levels of HTI56 will adequately differentiate between pneumonia and other states of pulmonary inflammation, such as ARDS and VILI. Obviously, additional studies are needed to establish whether HTI56 is truly a useful biomarker of lung injury.

Surfactant Proteins

Surfactant is a mixture of phospholipids and specific surfactant proteins, synthesized and secreted by alveolar type II cells. After secretion, surfactant forms a monomolecular layer at the gas/liquid interface of the alveolus, where it reduces the alveolar surface tension. This monolayer is constantly being inactivated; inactive surfactant is taken up by alveolar type II cells or alveolar macrophages and new surfactant is continuously being released. Although surfactant proteins are normally found in appreciable amounts only in the lung, leakage of surfactant proteins into the circulation has been reported in a number of respiratory disorders [18–20]. Indeed, surfactant proteins can diffuse in small amounts into the circulation, a process which is dependent on a concentration gradient as well as the permeability of the alveolar-capillary barrier [20]. In addition, leakage is dependent on the size and molecular weight of the different surfactant proteins. Surfactant protein-A (SP-A) predominantly forms high-molecular-weight oligomers ($\sim$650 kDa). SP-B is a dimer normally intimately associated with complexes of surfactant phospholipids, possibly too large to readily breach the alveolar-capillary barrier. Some of the protein is secreted as a hydrophilic monomeric proprotein ($\sim$42 kDa) and processing intermediate ($\sim$26 kDa). These are the major immunoreactive forms found in plasma [20]. The surfactant protein-D is a dodecamer formed of hydrophilic 43-kDa glycoproteins. Since SP-B is considerably smaller than SP-A and SP-D, it possibly breaches the alveolar-capillary barrier more readily. Following diffusion into the circulation surfactant proteins are rapidly cleared from this compartment [21]. Higher concentrations of surfactant proteins are found in the blood after disruption of the alveolar-capillary barrier, and thus might serve as a marker of lung injury. However, surfactant synthesis, secretion, reuptake and catabolism might also be disrupted with pulmonary inflammation, leading to lower local concentrations. In this way, local levels of surfactant proteins might also serve as a biomarker of pulmonary inflammation.

Surfactant Proteins as Biomarkers for Pneumonia

Several studies on changes in local or systemic levels of surfactant proteins in patients with pulmonary infection have been performed in the last decade. Günther et al. demonstrated that SP-A concentrations, but not SP-B concentrations, in BAL-fluid were reduced in patients with pneumonia as compared with healthy controls [22]. Similar results were obtained by Baughman et al., who compared levels of SP-A in patients with bacterial pneumonia, patients with idiopathic pulmonary fibrosis and healthy controls [23]. While the amount of SP-A in BAL fluid was similar for the controls and patients with idiopathic pulmonary fibrosis, patients with pneumonia had significantly lower SP-A concentrations in their BAL fluid. Interestingly, there was significantly less SP-A in BAL fluid from patients with pneumonia caused by a Gram-positive pathogen, compared with patients with a Gram-negative pneumonia. Leth-Larsen et al. recently measured SP-D concentrations in blood samples from consecutive patients hospitalized for CAP of suspected bacterial origin [24]. In this study, at the day of admission to the hospital serum SP-D concentrations were significantly lower than in healthy subjects. At day 5, the SP-D concentration had increased on average three times the concentration on admission and then slowly returned toward normal levels.

Surfactant Proteins as Biomarkers for ARDS or VILI

Numerous studies have focused on alterations in alveolar surfactant protein concentrations in patients with ARDS [22, 25–29]. They all show more or less the same, i.e., local levels of surfactant proteins in patients with ARDS are lower as compared to levels in patients without ALI and/or healthy volunteers. For instance, Greene et al. determined serial changes in surfactant protein levels in BAL fluid in a prospective study in intensive care patients and healthy volunteers [28]. They found that the concentrations of SP-A and SP-B were low in the BAL fluid of patients at risk for ARDS. In patients with established ARDS, alveolar SP-A and SP-B concentrations were low during the entire observation period.

While local concentrations of surfactant proteins decline, plasma concentrations of surfactant proteins rise with pulmonary injury [19–21, 27, 28, 30]. Doyle et al. compared plasma concentrations of SP-A and SP-B in patients with ARDS, patients with acute cardiogenic pulmonary edema, mechanically ventilated patients with no cardiorespiratory disease, and normal subjects [19, 20]. They found that plasma SP-A and SP-B levels were significantly higher in ARDS-patients and patients with acute cardiogenic pulmonary edema, as compared with the other subjects. On average, plasma SP-levels were higher in ARDS-patients than in the patients with acute cardiogenic pulmonary edema. In addition, plasma SP-A and SP-B levels were inversely related to blood oxygenation and static respiratory system compliance. These data were in line with data from other studies by the same group, in which they showed that levels of SP-A and SP-B were related to the lung injury score [21], and that SP-A and SP-B plasma levels were elevated in cardiac patients [27]. In the above-cited study by Greene et al., in which alveolar concentrations of SP-A and SP-B were low in patients at risk for ARDS before the onset of clinically defined lung injury, as well as in patients with established ARDS, SP-A and SP-D were not increased in the serum of patients at risk for ARDS. However, plasma levels of both surfactant proteins increased after the onset of ARDS to a maximum on day 3 and remained elevated for as long as 2 weeks (Fig. 3) [28]. Unfortunately, these data are not completely confirmed in other studies: In a study by Cheng et al. it was found that plasma SP-A levels, but not SP-D levels, were higher in ARDS-patients with more severe lung injury [29]. Even more confusing, Bersten et al. showed that plasma levels of SP-A were not different between patients who developed ARDS and those who did not, and remained unchanged over the study period. In this study, however, at study entry plasma SP-B levels were higher in patients with a direct lung insult who developed ARDS than in those who did not. In patients with an indirect lung insult who developed ARDS, plasma SP-B was no different at study entry, but gradually increased, and was similar to plasma SP-B in patients with a direct lung insult by day 3 [30].

In a recent study, Eisner et al. [31] determined plasma levels of SP-A and SP-D in plasma samples from participants in the ARDSNet randomized trial [8]. Plasma levels of SP-A and SP-D were measured at baseline and on day 3 after the start of the mechanical ventilation-protocol. Baseline plasma SP-A levels were not related to any clinical outcome. In contrast, higher baseline plasma SP-D levels were associated with a greater risk of death, fewer ventilator-free days, and fewer organ failure-free days. While the lower tidal volume strategy had no effect on the rise in plasma SP-A levels, it attenuated the rise in plasma SP-D levels. These observations not only indicate that plasma SP-D may be a valuable biomarker in ALI/ARDS, but also that levels of systemic SPs may be useful in gauging the effects of treatment.

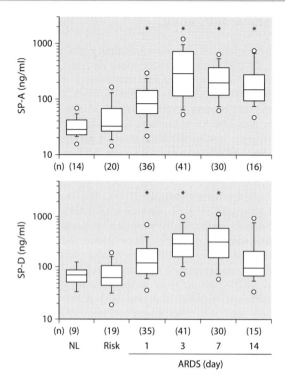

Fig. 3. Box plots of levels of surfactant protein-A and -D in plasma of normal volunteers (NL), patients at risk for ARDS, and patients with established ARDS at sequential days. The box encompasses 75% of the data; the central line indicates the median, and the error bars represent 90% confidence intervals. NL, normal lungs; Risk, patient at risk for ARDS; (n), number of patients; *, $p \leq 0.005$ versus normal subjects. Modified from [28] with permission

Advantages and Potential Drawbacks

While local and systemic levels of surfactant proteins were determined by means of ELISA in all cited studies, unfortunately, the described ELISAs for SP-A and SP-B are not yet commercially available, for research or for clinical use. ELISAs for SP-D have become available for research purposes recently.

An important drawback is that elevation of systemic levels of surfactant proteins can be seen with other pulmonary conditions. Indeed, several studies demonstrate that systemic concentrations of SP-A and SP-B are elevated in patients with congestive heart failure [19, 20]. A recent study even suggests the use of SP-B as a marker of chronic heart failure [32]. Although, on average, plasma surfactant protein levels were higher in ARDS patients than in patients with acute cardiogenic pulmonary edema in the above-cited studies by Doyle et al. [19, 20], it must be concluded that plasma levels of surfactant proteins rise with any form of pulmonary injury.

▌ Conclusion

Recent research shows that sTREM-1 (as measured in BAL fluid) can be used as a biomarker for pulmonary infection. Of course, these results need to be confirmed in other studies. At present, it is uncertain whether pulmonary levels of sTREM-1 can really discriminate VAP from other pulmonary conditions in critically ill patients. In addition, it is of importance to see how quick local concentrations of sTREM-1 rise in response to development of pulmonary infection as well as resolution of pneumonia in future research.

HTI56 (both measured in plasma and BAL-fluid) probably is another potentially valuable biomarker for determining the presence of ALI, whether infectious of origin or not. Unfortunately, similar to sTREM-1, additional studies are needed to determine the true value of this biomarker in critically ill patients.

Finally, numerous studies have shown the usefulness of plasma levels of surfactant proteins in determining (the extent of) pulmonary injury. These studies, however, show that plasma levels rise with any form of pulmonary injury. Thus, similar to the other biomarkers discussed in this manuscript, additional studies are needed to determine the true clinical value of these biomarkers. Interestingly, a recent study now suggests that plasma surfactant protein levels may be useful in gauging the effects of mechanical ventilation in individual patients.

References

1. Chastre J, Fagon JY (2002) Ventilator-associated pneumonia. Am J Respir Crit Care Med 165:867–903
2. Dos Santos CC, Slutsky AS (2004) Protective ventilation of patients with acute respiratory distress syndrome. Crit Care 8:145–147
3. Gajic O, Dara SI, Mendez JL, et al (2004) Ventilator-associated lung injury in patients without acute lung injury at the onset of mechanical ventilation. Crit Care Med 32:1817–1824
4. Bernard GR, Artigas A, Brigham KL, et al (1994) The American-European Consensus Conference on ARDS. Definitions, mechanisms, relevant outcomes, and clinical trial coordination. Am J Respir Crit Care Med 149:818–824
5. Meade MO, Cook RJ, Guyatt GH, et al (2000) Interobserver variation in interpreting chest radiographs for the diagnosis of acute respiratory distress syndrome. Am J Respir Crit Care Med 161:85–90
6. Estenssoro E, Dubin A, Laffaire E, et al (2003) Impact of positive end-expiratory pressure on the definition of acute respiratory distress syndrome. Intensive Care Med 29:1936–1942
7. Fagon JY, Chastre J, Hance AJ, Domart Y, Trouillet JL, Gibert C (1993) Evaluation of clinical judgment in the identification and treatment of nosocomial pneumonia in ventilated patients. Chest 103:547–553
8. The Acute Respiratory Distress Syndrome Network (2000) Ventilation with lower tidal volumes as compared with traditional tidal volumes for acute lung injury and the acute respiratory distress syndrome. N Engl J Med 342:1301–1308
9. Dellinger RP, Carlet JM, Masur H, et al (2004) Surviving Sepsis Campaign guidelines for management of severe sepsis and septic shock. Crit Care Med 32:858–873
10. Bouchon A, Facchetti F, Weigand MA, Colonna M (2001) TREM-1 amplifies inflammation and is a crucial mediator of septic shock. Nature 410:1103–1107
11. Bouchon A, Dietrich J, Colonna M (2000) Cutting edge: inflammatory responses can be triggered by TREM-1, a novel receptor expressed on neutrophils and monocytes. J Immunol 164:4991–4995
12. Richeldi L, Mariani M, Losi M, et al (2004) Triggering receptor expressed on myeloid cells: role in the diagnosis of lung infections. Eur Respir J 24:247–250
13. Gibot S, Cravoisy A, Levy B, Bene MC, Faure G, Bollaert PE (2004) Soluble triggering receptor expressed on myeloid cells and the diagnosis of pneumonia. N Engl J Med 350:451–458
14. Gibot S, Kolopp-Sarda MN, Bene MC, et al (2004) Plasma level of a triggering receptor expressed on myeloid cells-1: its diagnostic accuracy in patients with suspected sepsis. Ann Intern Med 141:9–15
15. Dobbs LG, Gonzalez RF, Allen L, Froh DK (1999) HTI56, an integral membrane protein specific to human alveolar type I cells. J Histochem Cytochem 47:129–137
16. Newman V, Gonzalez RF, Matthay MA, Dobbs LG (2000) A novel alveolar type I cell-specific biochemical marker of human acute lung injury. Am J Respir Crit Care Med 161:990–995

17. McElroy MC, Pittet JF, Hashimoto S, Allen L, Wiener-Kronish JP, Dobbs LG (1995) A type I cell-specific protein is a biochemical marker of epithelial injury in a rat model of pneumonia. Am J Physiol 268:L181–L186
18. Honda Y, Kuroki Y, Matsuura E, et al (1995) Pulmonary surfactant protein D in sera and bronchoalveolar lavage fluids. Am J Respir Crit Care Med 152:1860–1866
19. Doyle IR, Nicholas TE, Bersten AD (1995) Serum surfactant protein-A levels in patients with acute cardiogenic pulmonary edema and adult respiratory distress syndrome. Am J Respir Crit Care Med 152:307–317
20. Doyle IR, Bersten AD, Nicholas TE (1997) Surfactant proteins-A and -B are elevated in plasma of patients with acute respiratory failure. Am J Respir Crit Care Med 156:1217–1229
21. Doyle IR, Hermans C, Bernard A, Nicholas TE, Bersten AD (1998) Clearance of Clara cell secretory protein 16 (CC16) and surfactant proteins A and B from blood in acute respiratory failure. Am J Respir Crit Care Med 158:1528–1535
22. Gunther A, Siebert C, Schmidt R, et al (1996) Surfactant alterations in severe pneumonia, acute respiratory distress syndrome, and cardiogenic lung edema. Am J Respir Crit Care Med 153:176–184
23. Baughman RP, Sternberg RI, Hull W, Buchsbaum JA, Whitsett J (1993) Decreased surfactant protein A in patients with bacterial pneumonia. Am Rev Respir Dis 147:653–657
24. Leth-Larsen R, Nordenbaek C, Tornoe I, et al (2003) Surfactant protein D (SP-D) serum levels in patients with community-acquired pneumonia small star, filled. Clin Immunol 108:29–37
25. Gregory TJ, Longmore WJ, Moxley MA, et al (1991) Surfactant chemical composition and biophysical activity in acute respiratory distress syndrome. J Clin Invest 88:1976–1981
26. Pison U, Obertacke U, Seeger W, Hawgood S (1992) Surfactant protein A (SP-A) is decreased in acute parenchymal lung injury associated with polytrauma. Eur J Clin Invest 22:712–718
27. Bersten AD, Doyle IR, Davidson KG, Barr HA, Nicholas TE, Kermeen F (1998) Surfactant composition reflects lung overinflation and arterial oxygenation in patients with acute lung injury. Eur Respir J 12:301–308
28. Greene KE, Wright JR, Steinberg KP, et al (1999) Serial changes in surfactant-associated proteins in lung and serum before and after onset of ARDS. Am J Respir Crit Care Med 160:1843–1850
29. Cheng IW, Ware LB, Greene KE, Nuckton TJ, Eisner MD, Matthay MA (2003) Prognostic value of surfactant proteins A and D in patients with acute lung injury. Crit Care Med 31:20–27
30. Bersten AD, Hunt T, Nicholas TE, Doyle IR (2001) Elevated plasma surfactant protein-B predicts development of acute respiratory distress syndrome in patients with acute respiratory failure. Am J Respir Crit Care Med 164:648–652
31. Eisner MD, Parsons P, Matthay MA, Ware L, Greene K (2003) Plasma surfactant protein levels and clinical outcomes in patients with acute lung injury. Thorax 58:983–988
32. De Pasquale CG, Arnolda LF, Doyle IR, Aylward PE, Chew DP, Bersten AD (2004) Plasma surfactant protein-B. A novel biomarker in chronic heart failure. Circulation 110:1091–1096

Pharmacology of Acute Lung Injury

S. Tasaka and A. Ishizaka

▌ Introduction

The acute respiratory distress syndrome (ARDS) is a process of acute inflammatory lung injury resulting from a variety of predisposing conditions including severe pneumonia, sepsis, massive transfusion and trauma [1]. Recent reports showed substantial improvement in the prognosis of acute lung injury (ALI)/ARDS over the last 2 decades [2]. In the 1980s, mortality rates in excess of 50% were commonly reported, whereas the current mortality of ARDS seems to be in the 30 to 40% range. This improvement in clinical outcomes of ARDS is likely to be due to the advances in supportive therapy and ventilatory management, because it has occurred in the absence of specific new pharmacological intervention for this disease. Although a number of clinical trials have been performed, it is a frequent and unfortunate finding in this area that encouraging results from early studies are not replicated in larger, phase III studies [3]. This chapter, an update of the authors' 2002

Table 1. Possible pharmacological interventions for ARDS

Therapeutic agents for physiological abnormality in ARDS
▌ Alveolar surfactant
▌ β_2-agonists
▌ Diuretics and atrial natriuretic peptide
▌ Prostaglandins and other vasodilators
Therapeutic agents for acute inflammatory responses in ARDS
▌ Ketoconazole
▌ Neutrophil elastase inhibitor
▌ Monoclonal antibodies (endotoxin, cytokines, adhesion molecules, etc)
▌ TNF-α receptor fusion protein
▌ IL-1 receptor antagonist
▌ Pentoxifylline/Lisofylline
▌ Prostaglandin E_1
Therapeutic agents for abnormalities in coagulation system in ARDS
▌ Activated protein C
▌ Antithrombin
▌ Tissue factor pathway inhibitor
Therapeutic agents for fibroproliferative stage of ARDS
▌ Glucocorticoids

review [4], reviews the current status of pharmacological approaches to the treatment of ALI/ARDS (Table 1).

Anticytokine Therapy

Since ALI/ARDS is often associated with systemic inflammation such as sepsis, it is reasonable to assume that therapy directed against the putative mediators might reduce the incidence of the syndrome. Because tumor necrosis factor (TNF)-α is thought to play a central role in the pathogenesis of sepsis, various TNF-α neutralizing compounds (monoclonal antibodies against human TNF-α and soluble TNF-α receptors) have been produced. Recent clinical trials using anti-TNF antibody fragment (afelimomab) for septic patients seem favorable [5, 6]. A dose-ranging study using afelimomab failed to show any beneficial effect on 28-day survival, but a post hoc analysis of this trial suggested that patients with baseline increased serum interleukin (IL)-6 concentrations (> 1000 pg/ml) appeared to benefit from afelimomab [5]. In the patients with increased IL-6, a significant improvement in survival was observed in the afelimomab group after adjusting for the sepsis severity score [6].

Type I (55 kDa) and type II (75 kDa) TNF-α receptors (TNFR) have been identified and used to bind TNF-α in patients with sepsis. Pittet and colleagues assessed the impact of therapy with TNFR fusion protein (p55-IgG) on the incidence of end-organ failures in patients with severe sepsis. Patients treated with p55-IgG had more organ failure-free days and shorter ICU stay than those who received placebo [7].

IL-1 is another important mediator in the pathogenesis of sepsis syndrome. IL-1 receptor antagonist (IL-1ra) is a naturally occurring human protein produced by macrophages and other cells and prevents cellular responses mediated by IL-1. Although IL-1ra decreased mortality in experimental endotoxemia, randomized, double-blind trials failed to demonstrate a clinical benefit of IL-1ra in patients with sepsis syndrome [8, 9].

▌ Anti-adhesion Molecule Therapy

One of the initial steps in ALI/ARDS is an interaction between neutrophils and pulmonary endothelial cells, which is mediated by various adhesion molecules. A small clinical study showed that administration of monoclonal antibody against CD18, an adhesion molecule on neutrophils, to trauma patients with hemorrhagic shock less than 6 hours after onset may be beneficial [10]. Because the onset of trauma is more definite compared with other events such as onset of sepsis, this measure provides a potent new approach to prevent the development of ALI/ARDS in at-risk groups.

▌ Alveolar Surfactant

Surfactant dysfunction or deficiency is thought to be important in the development of ALI/ARDS. Surfactant can be delivered either by an in-line nebulizer or by direct intrabronchial instillation by means of bronchoscopy. Because, in the alveolar spaces of established ARDS, the leakage of circulatory proteins and the inflammatory exudates may adversely affect the administered surfactant, the lavage method of administering surfactant appears to offer advantages not experienced with the bolus method of administration.

Two phase II trials of animal-based surfactant products containing apoprotein demonstrated survival advantages in ARDS patients, but the quantity of exogenous surfactant necessary to treat ARDS patients may preclude the use of natural surfactant because of cost and resource requirement [11, 12]. Since the protein component appears to enhance surfactant activity, KL4-surfactant, an artificial preparation containing a synthetic 21-amino-acid peptide (KL4-peptide) with properties similar to those of surfactant protein B, was developed. Wiswell and colleagues reported that sequential bronchopulmonary segmental lavage with KL4-surfactant (Surfaxin®) improved oxygenation and outcome without any adverse effect in patients with ARDS [13].

Spragg and colleagues recently published the results of two phase III trials of a recombinant surfactant protein C-based surfactant (Venticute®) as treatment for ARDS [14]. Patients were prospectively randomized to receive either standard therapy or standard therapy plus up to four intratracheal doses of Venticute® given within a period of 24 hours. Although the exogenous surfactant did not improve survival of ARDS patients, those who received surfactant had a greater improvement in gas exchange during the treatment period [14].

▌ Albuterol

Pulmonary edema is a common cause for severe hypoxemia in ARDS patients, and β_2-agonists have been shown to accelerate edema clearance by regulating epithelial Na^+ channels (ENaC) and other key proteins of alveolar epithelial active Na^+ transport [15]. The ARDS Network plans to conduct the Albuterol versus Placebo in Acute Lung Injury (ALTA) study to test the safety and efficacy of aerosolized β_2-agonist (albuterol sulfate) for reducing mortality in patients with ALI.

▌ Pentoxifylline/Lisofylline

Pentoxifylline is a phosphodiesterase inhibitor that enhances intracellular levels of cyclic AMP. A derivative of pentoxifylline, lisofylline, is effective at down-regulating the inflammatory response in ALI [16]. In an NIH-sponsored ARDS Network study, 235 patients with ALI/ARDS were randomly assigned to receive either intravenous lisofylline (3 mg/kg every 6 hours) or placebo [17]. After the interim analysis, the trial was stopped, because the reported 28-day mortality for the lisofylline group was 31.9%, versus 24.7% in the placebo group. The trial also found no significant difference between lisofylline and placebo in ventilator-free days, resolution of organ failure, or infection-related mortality.

▌ Ketoconazole

Ketoconazole is an antifungal agent and is also a potent inhibitor of thromboxane A2, which has been implicated as an important mediator in septic shock and the development of ARDS. A multicenter trial, under the auspices of the ARDS Network, was undertaken using ketoconazole as therapy for ALI/ARDS, and no difference in survival or ventilator-free days was noted in this trial [18].

▌ Atrial Natriuretic Polypeptide

Atrial natriuretic polypeptide (ANP) is a polypeptide hormone that is primarily synthesized in the right atrium in response to atrial stretch. Besides producing natriuresis, ANP regulates vascular tone and may decrease vascular permeability in the lung. A prospective, randomized, study revealed that, in ALI patients, the measures of oxygenation and thoracic compliance were significantly improved at 24 h after initiating the ANP infusion, associated with decreases in lung injury score and shunt [19]. However, Bindels and co-workers compared ANP infusion and inhaled nitric oxide (NO) in ARDS and reported that, whereas inhaled NO reduced the mean pulmonary artery pressure and improved alveolar gas exchange, ANP infusion had no significant effects on these parameters [20].

▌ Prostaglandin E_1

Prostaglandin E_1 (PGE_1) is an arachidonic acid derivative which blocks platelet aggregation, causes vasodilation, and modulates inflammatory response. In a randomized, double-blinded trial of liposomal encapsulated PGE_1, it was noted that liposomal PGE_1 was associated with a significantly shorter time to reach a PaO_2/FIO_2 ratio of >300 mmHg and to off mechanical ventilation, although the 28-day mortality did not differ [21].

▌ Glucocorticoids

The disappointing results of a series of clinical trials using a short course of glucocorticoids in the 1980s have prevented the use of steroids especially in the acute phase of ALI/ARDS. More recently, Meduri and colleagues described a small randomized trial of glucocorticoid as treatment for the later or fibroproliferative stage of ALI/ARDS [22]. Among 24 patients randomized, 16 were treated with a glucocorticoid at 2 mg/kg per day, started 7 days after the diagnosis of ARDS and continued for 32 days, resulting in a significant reduction in lung injury and organ failure scores and improvement in oxygenation. Glucocorticoid treatment also decreased hospital-associated mortality from 62% in the placebo group to 12% in the treated group [22]. In 1997, the ARDS Network began the Late Steroid Rescue Study (LaSRS), a larger randomized, placebo-controlled, multicenter trial to compare the effect of corticosteroids with placebo in the management of late-phase ARDS. In the trial, ARDS patients between 7 and 28 days of onset and under continuous mechanical ventilation were enrolled. Patients in the treatment group received bolus injection of 2 mg/kg of methylprednisolone sodium succinate (mPSL), followed by 0.5 mg/kg every 6 hours for 14 days. LaSRS was designed to include 180 patients, and its primary endpoint is in-hospital mortality at 60 days. Secondary endpoints include ventilator free days and organ failure free days. In the 2004 international conference of the American Thoracic Society, the investigators presented an interim report of the LaSRS. Although there was no difference in 60-day in-hospital mortality between the mPSL and the placebo groups, the ventilator free days and ICU free days to day 28 were significantly longer in the mPSL group. There were no differences in ICU free days or hospital free days in the placebo versus the mPSL groups. Further analyses are in process to evaluate mortality and morbidity endpoints at 180 days.

▌ Coagulation System

Inflammatory cytokines, including TNF-α, IL-1β, and IL-6, are capable of activating coagulation and inhibiting fibrinolysis, whereas the procoagulant thrombin is capable of stimulating multiple inflammatory pathways [23]. Tissue factor is highly thrombogenic and occupies a central position in the extrinsic coagulation pathway. A recent phase II human study suggested that administration of tissue factor pathway inhibitor (TFPI), which regulates extrinsic pathway activity by suppressing tissue factor and factors VIIa and Xa, could reduce mortality associated with sepsis [24].

Antithrombin inhibits activated proteases, including factors IXa, Xa, and thrombin. Randomized, double-blind trials of antithrombin or antithrombin concentrates to septic patients revealed improvement in survival and sepsis-induced disseminated intravascular coagulation (DIC) [25, 26]. A large clinical trial with nearly 2500 patients enrolled is presently investigating this hypothesis.

Protein C is a vitamin K-dependent protein, which is activated by the thrombin-thrombomodulin complex on endothelial cells. Activated protein C (APC), with the cofactor protein S, cleaves and inactivates the procoagulant activity of activated factors V and VIII. Recently, the effect of recombinant human APC (drotrecogin alfa [activated]) was studied in a randomized, placebo-controlled trial of 1690 patients who had systemic inflammatory response syndrome (SIRS) and organ failure caused by suspected infection [27]. The two most common sites of infection reported were the lungs (53%) and abdomen (20%). Treatment with APC was associated with a significant reduction in the mortality at 28 days of approximately 6%. The relative risk of death was reduced by almost 20%. As the most important adverse effect reported was serious bleeding, the risks and benefits of APC therapy remain to be studied in patients at a higher risk of bleeding. The cost-effectiveness of the APC treatment has recently been evaluated, and it was noted that APC is relatively cost-effective when targeted specifically to patients who have severe sepsis, an APACHE II score higher than 25, and a long life expectancy if they survive the episode of sepsis [28].

▌ Neutrophil Elastase Inhibitor

Neutrophil elastase is a potent proteolytic enzyme, which decomposes various proteins including the extracellular matrix components, elastin, fibrinogen, proteoglycan and collagen. A randomized, double-blind trial with 230 SIRS patients in Japan revealed that high-dose sivelestat, a small molecular weight inhibitor of neutrophil elastase, significantly shortened ICU stay, although overall survival rate was not changed [29]. Since the methodological quality assessment score of the study is higher than the average, the sivelestat study in Japan is not considered methodologically inferior [30]. Recently, Zeiher and colleagues reported results of the STRIVE study, in which 492 mechanically ventilated patients with ALI were enrolled [31]. They found no effect of sivelestat on the primary end points of ventilator-free days or 28-day all-cause mortality. The STRIVE study group, however, concluded that their findings do not preclude benefit of sivelestat in ALI patients, because the patients in their study had more non-pulmonary organ failures and worse baseline measures of lung function [31].

▮ Future Direction

In the past few decades, there has been substantial progress in the understanding of ALI/ARDS. Although the progress in specific treatment has lagged behind basic research to date, a number of ongoing clinical trials of new ventilatory and pharmacological strategies should further reduce mortality from this common clinical syndrome.

References

1. Ware LB, Matthay MA (2002) The acute respiratory distress syndrome. N Engl J Med 342:1334–1349
2. Hudson LD, Steinberg KP (1999) Epidemiology of acute lung injury and ARDS. Chest 116:74S–82S
3. McIntyre RC Jr, Pulido EJ, Bensard DD, Shames BD, Abraham E (2000) Thirty years of clinical trials in acute respiratory distress syndrome. Crit Care Med 28:3314–3331
4. Tasaka S, Hasegawa N, Ishizaka A (2002) Pharmacology of acute lung injury. Pulm Pharmacol Ther 15:83–95
5. Reinhart K, Menges T, Gardlund B, et al (2001) Randomized, placebo-controlled trial of the anti-tumor necrosis factor antibody fragment afelimomab in hyperinflammatory response during severe sepsis: The RAMSES Study. Crit Care Med 29:765–769
6. Panacek E, Marshall J, Fischkoff S, Barchuk W, Teoh L, MONARCS Study Group (2000) Neutralization of TNF by a monoclonal antibody improves survival and reduces organ dysfunction in human sepsis: Results of the MONARCS trial. Chest 118:88S (abst)
7. Pittet D, Harbarth S, Suter PM, et al (1999) Impact of immunomodulating therapy on morbidity in patients with severe sepsis. Am J Respir Crit Care Med 160:852–857
8. Opal SM, Fisher CJ Jr, Dhainaut JF, et al (1997) Confirmatory interleukin-1 receptor antagonist trial in severe sepsis: a phase III, randomized, double-blind, placebo-controlled, multicenter trial. Crit Care Med 25:1115–1124
9. Fisher CJ Jr, Dhainaut JF, Opal SM, et al (1994) Recombinant human interleukin 1 receptor antagonist in the treatment of patients with sepsis syndrome. Results from a randomized, double-blind, placebo-controlled trial. Phase III rhIL-1ra Sepsis Syndrome Study Group. JAMA 271:1836–1843
10. Vedder N, Harlan J, Winn R (1997) Pilot phase 2 clinical trial of a humanized CD11/CD18 monoclonal antibody in hemorrhagic shock. In: Faist E (ed) 4th International Congress on the Immune Consequences of Trauma, Shock and Sepsis: Mechanisms and Therapeutic Approaches. Mondezzi editore, Bologna, pp 941
11. Gregory TJ, Steinberg KP, Spragg R, et al (1997) Bovine surfactant therapy for patients with acute respiratory distress syndrome. Am J Respir Crit Care Med 155:1309–1315
12. Kesecioglu JM, Schultz MJ, Lundberg D, Lauven PM, Lachmann B (2001) Treatment of acute lung injury (ALI/ARDS) with surfactant. Am J Respir Crit Care Med 163:A813 (abst)
13. Wiswell TE, Smith RM, Katz LB, et al (1999) Bronchopulmonary segmental lavage with Surfaxin (KL4-surfactant) for acute respiratory distress syndrome. Am J Respir Crit Care Med 160:1188–1195

14. Spragg RG, Lewis JF, Walmrath HD, et al (2004) Effect of recombinant surfactant protein C-based surfactant on the acute respiratory distress syndrome. N Engl J Med 351:884–892
15. Mutlu GM, Sznajder JI (2004) β_2-agonists for treatment of pulmonary edema: Ready for clinical studies? Crit Care Med 32:1607–1608
16. Hasegawa N, Oka Y, Nakayama M, et al (1997) The effects of post-treatment with lisofylline, a phosphatidic acid generation inhibitor, on sepsis-induced acute lung injury in pigs. Am J Respir Crit Care Med 155:928–936
17. The ARDS Clinical Trial Network (2002) Randomized, placebo-controlled trial of lisofylline for early treatment of acute lung injury and acute respiratory distress syndrome. Crit Care Med 30:1–6
18. The ARDS network (2000) Ketoconazole for early treatment of acute lung injury and acute respiratory distress syndrome. JAMA 283:1995–2002
19. Mitaka C, Hirata Y, Nagura T, Tsunoda Y, Amaha K (1998) Beneficial effect of atrial natriuretic peptide on pulmonary gas exchange in patients with acute lung injury. Chest 114:223–228
20. Bindels AJ, van der Hoeven JG, Groeneveld PH, Frolich M, Meinders AE (2001) Atrial natriuretic peptide infusion and nitric oxide inhalation in patients with acute respiratory distress syndrome. Crit Care 5:151–157
21. Abraham E, Baughman R, Fletcher E, et al (1999) Liposomal prostaglandin E1 (TLC C-53) in acute respiratory distress syndrome: a controlled, randomized, double-blind, multicenter clinical trial. Crit Care Med 27:1478–1485
22. Meduri GU, Headley AS, Golden E, et al (1998) Effects of prolonged methylprednisolone therapy in unresolving acute respiratory distress syndrome: a randomized controlled trial. JAMA 280:159–165
23. Hasegawa N, Husari AW, Hart WT, Kandra TG, Raffin TA (1994) Role of the coagulation system in ARDS. Chest 105:268–277
24. Laterre PF, Wittebole X, Dhainaut JF (2003) Anticoagulant therapy in acute lung injury. Crit Care Med 31:S329–S336
25. Balk R, Emerson T, Fourrier F, et al (1998) Therapeutic use of antithrombin concentrate in sepsis. Semin Thromb Hemost 24:183–194
26. Eisele B, Lamy M, Thijs LG, et al (1998) Antithrombin III in patients with severe sepsis. A randomized, placebo-controlled, double-blind multicenter trial plus a meta-analysis on all randomized, placebo-controlled, double-blind trials with antithrombin III in severe sepsis. Intensive Care Med 24:663–672
27. Bernard GR, Vincent JL, Laterre PF, et al (2001) Efficacy and safety of recombinant human activated protein C for severe sepsis. N Engl J Med 344:699–709
28. Angus DC, Linde-Zwirble WT, Clermont G, et al (2003) Cost-effectiveness of drotrecogin alfa (activated) in the treatment of severe sepsis. Crit Care Med 31:1–11
29. Tamakuma S, Shiba T, Hirasawa H, Ogawa M, Nakajima M (1998) A phase III clinical study of a neutrophil elastase inhibitor; ONO-5046·Na in SIRS patients. J Clin Ther Med (Japan) 14:289–318
30. Bellomo R, Uchino S, Naka T, Wan L (2004) Hidden evidence to the West: multicentre, randomised, controlled trials in sepsis and systemic inflammatory response syndrome in Japanese journals. Intensive Care Med 30:911–917
31. Zeiher BG, Artigas A, Vincent JL, et al. (2004) Neutrophil elastase inhibition in acute lung injury: results of the STRIVE study. Crit Care Med 32:1695–1702

The Mechanism of Ventilator-induced Lung Injury: Role of Dynamic Alveolar Mechanics

J. DiRocco, D. Carney, and G. Nieman

▌ Introduction

Supportive therapy with mechanical ventilation is critical for survival of all patients with the acute respiratory distress syndrome (ARDS) [1]. We now recognize ventilator-induced lung injury (VILI) as a potential complication of this therapy. VILI occurs when improper methods of mechanical ventilation exacerbate the primary lung injury in ARDS [2]. Indeed, VILI significantly increases mortality from ARDS, yet the mechanism of VILI remains ill-defined [2–4]. No proven remedy for the inflammatory response associated with ARDS has yet been developed. An improved understanding of VILI will limit mortality from ARDS. Known bedside measures to guide the clinician when adjusting mechanical ventilation to minimize VILI are crude and limited [5–8]. In order to investigate the mechanism of VILI, first the *dynamic* behavior of alveolar inflation and deflation (i.e., alveolar mechanics) during tidal ventilation in the normal and injured lung must be understood.

Currently, there are believed to be three mechanisms of VILI:
1) Atelectrauma is an alveolar shear stress-induced injury caused by alveolar recruitment-derecruitment
2) Volutrauma is an alveolar overexpansion injury caused by high lung pressures and volumes, and
3) Biotrauma is an alveolar, inflammatory injury caused by cytokine release from the pulmonary parenchyma secondary to mechanical injury induced by atelectrauma or volutrauma [9].

Since VILI-induced injury occurs mainly at the level of the alveolus or alveolar duct, understanding dynamic alveolar mechanics is critical to clarify the mechanism of VILI. Despite extensive research, the mechanics of alveolar inflation are poorly understood [10–39].

In this chapter, we will move from a review of the *dynamic* changes in alveoli during ventilation to postulates regarding changes in alveolar mechanics in the acutely injured lung. Finally we will discuss how improper ventilation with preservation of abnormal alveolar mechanics may cause VILI. We will not discuss the role of pulmonary surfactant, the elastin/collagen support tissue, or the three dimensional architecture of the alveolus, all of which may play an important role in normal and abnormal alveolar mechanics as discussed elsewhere [40].

Currently, there is no technique available to measure the three-dimensional changes in the alveolus and alveolar duct during tidal ventilation. However, it is possible to study two-dimensional dynamic alveolar mechanics in subpleural alveoli. Our laboratory utilizes *in vivo* microscopy to study the two-dimensional changes in subpleural alveoli in real-time with lung inflation and deflation. In order to assess dynamic mechanics in both the normal and acutely injured lung, we will integrate data from our *in vivo* microscopic assessment of alveolar mechanics with those generated from static models (histologic assessment at varying lung volumes) or surrogate measurements (quasi-static pressure/volume [P/V] curve, computed tomography [CT] scan, impedance tomography).

▌ Dynamic Alveolar Ventilation

Alveoli are not physically independent structures but rather are interconnected with shared walls containing elastin and collagen fibers [41]. This is disparate to common descriptions in current medical textbooks that depict alveoli as individual balloon-like structures bunched together as a cluster of grapes [42]. Histological studies have contributed substantially to our understanding of alveolar ducts and alveoli, but these studies have focused on two-dimensional static structures with little extrapolation to three-dimensional, dynamically moving structures. This is a critical oversight, for understanding dynamic change is essential to define normal alveolar mechanics and to interpret how alterations in alveolar mechanics in the acutely injured lung may lead to a VILI.

Numerous experimental techniques have been used to study dynamic alveolar mechanics. In the normal lung, four models of dynamic alveolar size change have been proposed (Table 1):

▌ isotropic balloon-like expansion and contraction of alveoli;
▌ expansion and contraction of the alveolar ducts with little change in alveolar volume;
▌ successive alveolar recruitment and derecruitment; and
▌ alveolar crumpling and un-crumpling along septa similar to a paper bag [18, 19].

There is no consensus as to which of the above mechanisms predominates [10–25].

Isotropic Balloon-like Alveolar Mechanics

Early depictions of alveoli as grape clusters led to a belief that each alveolus was a functionally independent unit. Therefore, it was thought that morphometric measurement of the change in alveolar surface area could be used to determine the mechanism by which alveoli change size during lung expansion [10, 12, 14, 16, 17, 21]. In addition, this thought would allow for mathematical verification since if alveoli truly expand isotropically (i.e., balloon-like stretching), the surface area of the lung should change predictably with change in lung volume. Indeed, early reports indicated that uniform, isotropic alveolar expansion and contraction were responsible for the majority of changes in lung volume [10, 12, 16]. Studies on fresh lung tissue frozen at various levels of inflation and deflation [10, 11, 14–17] indicate that alveolar shape remains relatively unchanged with changes in lung volume, supporting conventional morphometric data that alveoli change by means of isotropic expansion and contraction. Further mathematical interpretation came from Dunnill's comparison of the regression line of alveolar surface area/alveolar volume to the re-

Table 1. Measurement of dynamic alveolar ventilation

Species	Protocol	Methods	Conclusions	Reference
▌Rabbit	*In vivo* & Freezing	Point count & Lm	Isotropic alveolar expansion, Interior alveoli also isotropic	10
▌Rat	*In vivo* & Freezing	Dynamic 2 point count	Geometric hysteresis Subpleural alveoli same size *in vivo* and in frozen tissue	11
▌Dog	Formalin vapor	Lm	Isotropic alveolar expansion	12
▌Dog	Excised lungs	Alveolar septae and area with map reader	New method for calculating surface tension *in situ*	13
▌Guinea pig	Rapidly Frozen	Point count & Lm	Alveolar volume ↑ linear Duct volume ↑ at 40% V_L No alveolar folding Thickness of A-B barrier ↓ 33%	14
▌Cats	Freeze + Freeze dry	D/MD ratio	No Δ in alveolar shape FRC → TLC Alveoli collapse like a accordion	15
▌Cats	Freeze + Freeze dry	Alveolar microholes	Isotropic alveolar expansion Alveoli & duct Δ proportionally	16
▌Cats	Freeze + Freeze dry	Morphometry	Alveoli & duct Δ proportionally	17
▌Rat	Vascular perfusion	Morphometry Stereology	No Δ in alveolar diameter and alveolar walls pleat. R/D is a major mechanism of $V_L\Delta$ The entire alveolus does not collapse	18
▌Rabbit	Vascular perfusion	Morphometry	Multiple possible mechanisms of alveolar volume change: 1) Sequential alveolar derecruitment 2) Balloon-like reduction in size 3) Change in size and shape 4) Crumpling of alveolar surface	19, 20
▌Rat	Airway instillation	Morphometry	Anisotropic alveolar expansion	21
▌Dog	In vivo	Morphometry	Little change in alveolar volume Lung volume change by R/D	22
▌Dog	In vivo	Monodispersed Aerosol	Little change in alveolar volume Lung volume change by R/D	23
▌Gerbil	Freeze + Freeze dry	Lm	Little change in alveolar volume Lung volume change by R/D	24
▌Rat	Vascular perfusion	3D reconstruction	Alveolar shape Δs with deflation Little Δ in alveolar diameter until very low lung volume	25
▌Human	Excised lung	P/V curve Mathematical model	Alveolar collapse without Pflex Lung volume change by R/D	26
▌Rat	*In vivo* microscopy	Morphometry	11% Δ in alveolar diameter during tidal ventilation	27
▌Rabbits	Excised lung	P/V curve	Alveolar diameter ↓ with ↑ in lung volume, R/D important	28

Table 1 (continued)

Species	Protocol	Methods	Conclusions	Refer-ence
Rats	Excised lung	Microfocal X-ray tomography	Small airway ($<$ 300 μm) Δ length & diameter with lung volume Δ	29
Mice	Freeze substitution *In situ*	Lm P/V curve	Alveoli ↑ in size with lung volume Δ No maximum lung volume	30
Mice	Airway fixation	Lm	No Δ in alveolar size with Δ in lung volume	31
Rats	Airway fixation	Morphometry	Lung volume Δ due to ↑↓ in alveolar number not size	32
Human	Frozen section	Morphometry	Alveolar wall stretched and thus carry force. Alveolar ducts and alveolar walls in mechanical equailibrium	33
Rat	Glutaraldehyde	Morphometry Light & EM	At low lung volume alveoli expand either by unfolding or expansion of alveolar ducts. At high lung volumes the basement membrane and attached cells deform	34
N/A	Math model	Math P/V curve	Alveoli recruit throughout lung inflation not only at lower Pflex. The P/V curve did not predict optimal ventilator setting	35
N/A	Math model	Math P/V curve	Best compliance during decremental, but not incremental, PEEP is related to open-lung PEEP	36
Dog	Oleic acid lung injury	CT scan	Recruitment throughout lung inflation not just at Pflex. More alveoli open on expiration than inspiration at the same airway pressure	37
Human	ALI/ARDS	CT scan	Recruitment throughout lung inflation not just at Pflex. Derecruitment did not parallel deflation	38
Dog Rabbit Rat	Normal Excised Lungs	Morphometry	Lung folding appeared in all species with some protocols but absent in others. Folding depends on lung volume history	39

Lm: mean linear intercept; A-B: air-blood barrier; R/D: alveolar recruitment/derecruitment; P/V: lung pressure/volume curve; Pflex: inflection point on the P/V curve; N/A: not applicable; VL: Lung volume; FRC: Functional residual capacity; TLC: Total lung capacity; Δ: Change

gression line of alveolar surface area/lung volume [12]. His mathematical comparison supported uniform, isotropic alveolar expansion, however repeat calculations of his data could not distinguish either recruitment/derecruitment or isotropic alveolar volume change as the most important mechanism of lung inflation. Subtle modifications to the postulate of isotropic change followed including ideas that alveoli increase in volume in linear fashion with lung volume [14], alveoli undergo anisotropic expansion (i.e., unequal or asymmetrical alveolar expansion) [21], or a combination of isotropic expansion of the alveolus and alveolar duct [16]. None of these early postulates are easily defended.

Alveolar Folding

Rather than balloon-like elastic expansion and contraction, the alveolus could change size by folding and unfolding of the alveolar walls similar to an accordion. An early study by Forest suggested that alveoli did not fold [14]. This work was followed by several studies that disagreed and concluded that alveoli do indeed change volume by complex folding [15, 18–20, 34, 39]. In a theoretical model of complex alveolar folding, alveolar surface area would not significantly change with lung inflation and thus alveolar volume and alveolar surface area would not necessarily be related. If the alveolar surface area increased with lung expansion alveoli would change either be stretching or recruiting.

The first demonstration of septal folding in the rabbit was by Gil and Weibel who found "crumpling" of the alveolar surface and showed that the epithelium folds back onto adjacent epithelium [18]. Gil et al. demonstrated the presence of septal folding in fixed tissue [19]. Their photomicrographs showed heavy thickened septa with capillaries piled upon each other. This demonstrated the potential anatomic mechanism for alveolar septal folding. Klingele and Staub [15] demonstrated that there is no change in alveolar shape from functional residual capacity (FRC) to total lung capacity (TLC) but at low lung volumes alveoli collapse from side to side similar to folding of an accordion.

Oldmixon and Hoppin demonstrated that alveolar folding was seen in rat but not dog and rabbit lungs fixed over a range of inflation pressures and inflation histories [39]. They noted that the presence of septal folding was more related to lung volume history that lung pressure at fixation and that there was temporal component to the unfolding process. A transient inflation pressure of 22 cmH$_2$O did not resolve septal folding, but holding the pressure at 22 cmH$_2$O (or cycling the pressure at 30 cmH$_2$O) did eliminate folding. The possibility of septal folding is anatomically feasible since the curvature of the air-liquid interface in the corners of the alveolar space would allow enough "slackness" in the alveolus to allow septal folding [16].

Septal folding may be the prime mechanism causing distinctive inflection points (Pflex) on the quasi-static P/V curve that are the hallmarks of lung reopening. Tschumperlin and Margulies [34] found that at low volumes lung inflation is by either septal unfolding or expansion of the alveolar ducts without a change in alveolar volume. At high lung volume, their data suggests that the basement membrane and attached cells deform as the lung nears physiological limits. An electron microscope (EM) photomicrograph clearly demonstrates an alveolar fold at low lung volume (Fig. 1). This biphasic change in alveolar size by one mechanism at low lung volume (septal folding) and a different mechanism at high lung volume (alveolar stretching) was support by the data obtained by Klingele and Staub [15].

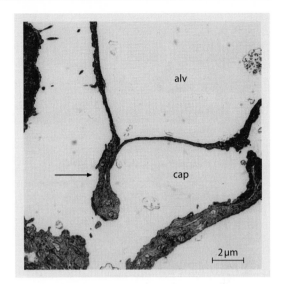

Fig. 1. Electron micrograph demonstrating septal folding (*arrow*) between an alveolus (alv) and capillary (cap) at low lung volume. Septal folding would allow alveoli to change volume greatly without a change in basement membrane surface area. An alternate interpretation is volume change exclusively in the alveolar duct without a change in alveolar volume or surface area. From [34] with permission

Alveolar Recruitment/Derecruitment

Another possibility is that the lung changes volume by recruitment and derecruitment of large populations of alveoli. Alveoli are either open or collapsed and do not change size with ventilation, other than by rapid opening or total collapse. To prove the above, it would have to be shown that open alveoli do not change size with ventilation and that there are more alveoli open at inspiration than at expiration. A number of studies have concluded that the lung changes volume primarily by alveolar recruitment/derecruitment [22–24, 26, 28, 32].

Smaldone and coworkers [23] developed a unique technique in which they filled excised lungs with a mono-dispersed aerosol and measured its deposition in alveoli at zero airflow. By evaluating the relationship of particle deposition and morphometric assessment of alveolar size, they concluded that the lung inflates by a progressive recruitment of alveoli and deflates by alveolar derecruitment. In addition they noted that at low lung volume alveoli were large and actually got smaller during inflation concomitant with an increase in alveolar number. Data from Lum and coworkers suggested that the predominant mechanism of lung volume change is alveolar recruitment. They also observed a temporal recruitment of alveoli with application of 30 cmH$_2$O airway pressure [24]. Specifically, alveoli recruit over time as long as elevated airway pressure was maintained. Although not directly observed with EM in this studies, the authors postulate that the anatomical mechanism of alveolar recruitment is septal pleating akin to previously described studies [18, 19]. Using data from postmortem, excised human lungs, Salmon et al. [26] created a mathematical model of a P/V curve and concluded that reopening of collapsed alveoli during lung inflation is responsible for the majority of hysteresis in the P/V curve. Boyle et al. [28] showed that the mean air space diameter declined with increased volume in rabbit lungs. This suggests that a significant amount of alveolar recruitment had occurred. Direct visualization of subpleural alveoli during large changes in lung volume in the living animal also suggests that the lung changes volume by alveolar recruitment/derecruitment [22]. *In vivo* photomicrographs

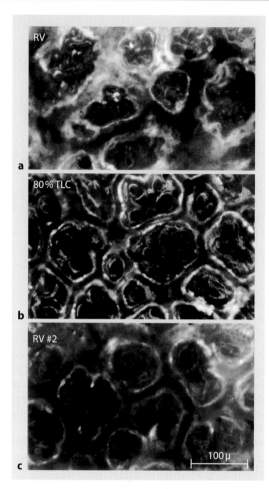

Fig. 2. *In vivo* photomicrographs of normal subpleural alveoli at residual volume (RV), inflation to 80% of total lung capacity (TLC) and deflation to a second RV (RV #2). The number of alveoli changed greatly with lung volume change whereas alveolar size changed very little. This suggests that the normal lung changes volume by alveolar recruitment/derecruitment rather than balloon-like expansion and contraction. From [22] with permission

showed that the size of alveoli at residual volume, as compared to 80% TLC, was not significantly different suggesting that lung volume change is due to either recruitment/derecruitment or changes in the alveolar duct (Fig. 2).

In a recent morphometric study, it was determined that changes in lung volume are due to changes in the number of alveoli (recruitment/derecruitment) without a change in alveolar size [32]. They further postulated that the mechanism of the hysteresis between the inflation and deflation limb of the P/V is due to a difference in the number of open alveoli.

Another method to determine if alveolar recruitment/derecruitment occurs is to measure the change in alveolar size with lung inflation. If alveoli do not change size then it can be inferred that recruitment/derecruitment may be taking place. Several studies looked at alveolar size change with lung inflation with variable results. Mercer et al. did a three-dimensional reconstruction of alveoli and found that there was little change in alveolar volume except at low lung volume [25]. In two recent studies by Soutiere et al., [30, 31] it was found that the observation of alveolar size change during lung inflation was dependent on whether fixation was by freezing (change) [30] or airway fixation (no change) [31]. Thus, these experiments yield variable results in support of the lung changing volume by alveolar recruitment.

Summary of Normal Alveolar Mechanics

Although there are excellent studies suggesting that alveoli change volume in a balloon-like fashion [10–12, 14–17], we believe the best available data support the theory that the lung changes volume by either alveolar folding [15, 18–20, 34, 39] or alveolar recruitment/derecruitment [22–24, 26, 28, 32]. Alveolar folding and recruitment/derecruitment need not be mutually exclusive. The studies investigating alveolar recruitment/derecruitment did not considered the mechanism by which the alveolus recruits and derecruits. It is very conceivable that lung volume change is by recruitment/derecruitment and the mechanism of alveolar collapse and opening is through septal folding. Hopefully, new techniques such as CT will yield dynamic three-dimensional images of alveoli and alveolar ducts to resolve this long standing controversy [29].

▌ Abnormal Alveolar Mechanics

Although we are still unsure of how the normal lung changes volume, most of the literature favors relatively stable alveoli and that other mechanisms (e.g., duct volume change, normal recruitment/derecruitment, crumpling and pleating) account for normal lung volume change. Thus, unstable alveoli that collapse and expand with each breath will be considered abnormal.

Early studies by both Gil et al. [19] and Bachofen et al. [20] demonstrated that derecruitment was the dominant mechanism of lung deflation in a surfactant deactivation model of ARDS. These data are supported by a mathematical model of the P/V curve that suggested that in ARDS the lung changes volume primarily by recruitment/derecruitment [35, 36]. Two studies measuring alveolar recruitment via a CT scan, one in a dog model of ARDS [37], the other in humans with ARDS [38], both support the above hypothesis that in the acutely injured lung volume change is predominately by alveolar recruitment/derecruitment.

More recently, alveolar recruitment/derecruitment has been shown to be the predominant mechanism of lung volume change in the acutely injured lung inflated to near TLC [18–22] as well as during tidal ventilation [43, 44]. Indirect techniques have been used to study dynamic alveolar stability during tidal ventilation [43, 44]. Dynamic alveolar collapse and recruitment following lung injury by oleic acid, saline lavage, and endotoxin was assessed utilizing CT [43]. In all three injuries, alveoli collapse and reopen rapidly (as fast as 0.6 seconds following a breath hold) (Fig. 3).

Grasso et al. utilized P/V curves during tidal ventilation and hypothesized that increase in slope indicated tidal alveolar recruitment, decrease in slope indicated tidal alveolar over-inflation and a linear curve indicates normal aerated alveoli [44]. These data support those of Neumann [43] and suggest that dynamic alveolar inflation is altered in acute lung injury (ALI) during tidal ventilation.

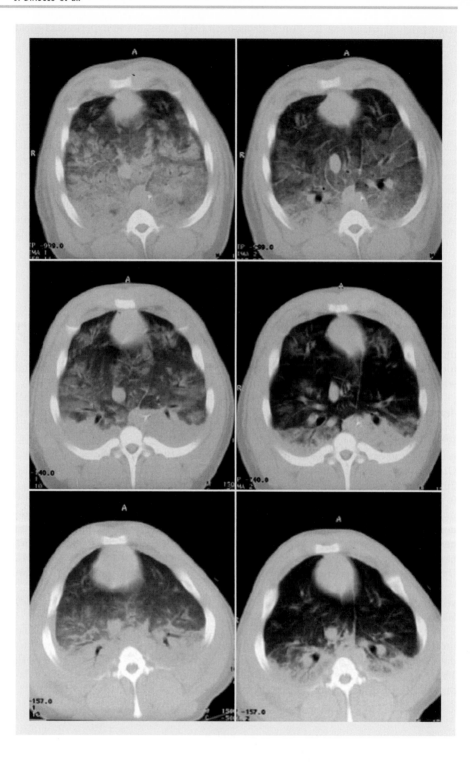

Ventilator Injury and Dynamic Alveolar Mechanics

Regardless of how normal alveoli change volume with tidal ventilation, in ALI dynamic alveolar mechanics are dramatically altered [43–46]. Atelectrauma is caused when unstable alveoli result in a shear stress induced lung injury [41]. Ventilator settings that presumably cause alveolar recruitment/derecruitment are known to cause VILI (i.e., high peak inspiratory pressure and low positive end-expiratory pressure [PEEP]) [47]. Reducing tidal volume, which presumably reduces alveolar recruitment/derecruitment has been shown to reduce mortality in patients with ARDS [1, 5]. Our lab directly measured dynamic alveolar mechanics utilizing *in vivo* microscopy and demonstrated that inappropriate ventilation of unstable alveoli results in VILI (Fig. 4) [46].

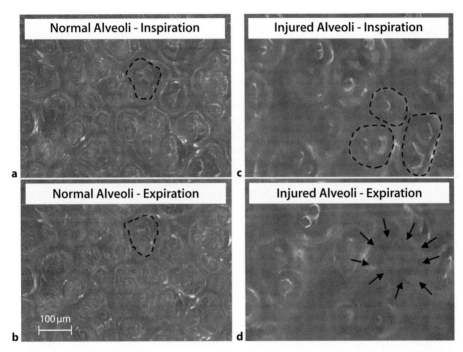

Fig. 4. *In vivo* photomicrographs of the same normal alveoli at peak inspiration (**a**) and end expiration (**b**). Normal alveoli are very stable with little change in size during tidal ventilation (dots). Injurious mechanical ventilation (High peak inspiratory pressure, low PEEP) causes a ventilator induced lung injury resulting in alveolar instability. Abnormal alveoli in an injured lung at peak inspiration (**c**) and end expiration (**d**) demonstrating severe instability with alveoli open on inspiration (*dots*) and collapsed on expiration (*arrows*)

Fig. 3. Computed tomography (CT) scans of lungs injured by 3 different mechanisms (Oleic acid, *top*; Saline Lavage, *middle*; Endotoxin, *bottom*). CT scans were obtained after 4 seconds of inspiratory hold (*right*) and 4 seconds of expiratory hold (*left*). Note that there was more collapse during both the expiratory and inspiratory hold in the oleic acid injured lungs (*top*). This suggests that the etiology of injury has an impact on alveolar instability. From [43] with permission

Altered dynamic alveolar mechanics may cause VILI by two mechanisms: 1) large gross tears could be ripped in the alveolar wall, or 2) the cell membrane maybe injured without gross tears [48–50]. In a patient subjected to very high-pressure mechanical ventilation during support for ARDS, Hotchkiss et al. found multiple large tears in the alveolar wall [48]. Gajic et al. demonstrated that injurious mechanical ventilation damaged pulmonary cell membranes and that the injury was reversible if injurious ventilation was discontinued [49]. Injury to the cell membrane was confirmed utilizing electron microscopy that revealed ultra-structural disruption to both pulmonary epithelium and endothelium [50]. VILI caused destruction of epithelial cells and denudation of the basement membrane. These studies suggest that altered alveolar mechanics are a primary mechanism of VILI and that alveolar injury ranges from gross tearing to ultrastructural damage.

▌ Conclusion

The exact mechanism of dynamic lung volume change at the alveolar level is unknown. Postulated mechanisms of alveolar mechanics include 'normal' alveolar recruitment/derecruitment, change in the size of the alveolar duct with little change in alveolar size, and crumpling/uncrumpling of the alveolus similar to a paper bag and balloon-like alveolar size change. It appears that normal alveoli are stable and that with ALI alveoli become unstable and will often collapse and re-open with every breath. This recruitment/derecruitment causes a shear stress injury that damages lung tissue leading to VILI.

More knowledge of normal and abnormal alveolar mechanics is necessary to better understand the mechanism of VILI. This knowledge will ultimately improve ventilator strategies leading to reduced morbidity and mortality associated with VILI.

References

1. Acute Respiratory Distress Syndrome Network (2000) Ventilation with lower tidal volumes as compared with traditional tidal volumes for acute lung injury and the acute respiratory distress syndrome. N Engl J Med 342:1301–1308
2. Rubenfeld GD (2003) Epidemiology of acute lung injury. Crit Care Med 31:S276–S284
3. Pinhu L, Whitehead T, Evans T, Griffths M (2003) Ventilator-associated lung injury. Lancet. 361:332–340
4. Dreyfuss D, Saumon G (1998) Ventilator-induced lung injury. Lessons from experimental studies. Am J Respir Crit Care Med. 157:294–323
5. Amato MBP, Barbas CSV, Medeiros DM, et al (1998) Effect of a protective-ventilation strategy on mortality in the acute respiratory distress syndrome. N Engl J Med 338:347–354
6. Putensen C, Baum M, Hormann C (1993) Selecting ventilator settings according to variables derived from the quasi-static pressure/volume relationship in patients with acute lung injury. Anesth Analg 77:436–447
7. Harris RS, Hess DR, Venegas JG (2000) An objective analysis of the pressure-volume curve in the acute respiratory distress syndrome. Am J Respir Crit Care Med 161:432–439
8. Victorino JA, Borges JB, Okamato, et al (2004) Imbalances in regional lung ventilation. A validation study on electrical impedance tomography. Am J Respir Crit Care Med 169:791–800
9. Slutsky AS (1999) Lung injury caused by mechanical ventilation. Chest 116 (Suppl): 9S–15S
10. Tangelo E (1972) Local alveolar size and Tran pulmonary pressure in situ and in isolated lungs. Respir Physiology 14:251–266

11. Daly BDT, Parks GE, Edmonds CH, Hibbs CW, Norman JC (1975) Dynamic alveolar mechanics as studied by videomicroscopy. Respir Physiol 24:217–232
12. Dunnill MS (1967) Effect of lung inflation on alveolar surface area in the dog. Nature 214:1013–1014
13. Flicker E, Lee JS (1974) Equilibrium of force of subpleural alveoli: implications to lung mechanics. J Appl Physiol 36:366–374
14. Forrest JB (1970) The effect of changes in lung volume on the size and shape of alveoli. J Physiol 210:533–547
15. Klingele TG, Staub NC (1970) Alveolar shape changes with volume in isolated, air-filled lobes of cat lung. J Appl Physiol 28:411–414
16. Kuno K, Staub NC (1968) Acute mechanical effects of lung volume changes on artificial microholes in alveolar walls. J Appl Physiol 24:83–92
17. Storey WF, Staub NC (1962) Ventilation of terminal air units. J Appl Physiol 17:391–397
18. Gil J, Weibel ER (1972) Morphological study of pressure-volume hysteresis in rat lungs fixed by vascular perfusion. Respir Physiol 15:190–213
19. Gil J, Bachofen H, Gehr P, Weibel ER (1979) Alveolar volume–surface area relation in air and saline-filled lungs fixed by vascular perfusion. J Appl Physiol Respir Environ Exercise Physiol 47:990–1001
20. Bachofen H, Gehr P, Weibel ER (1979) Alterations of mechanical properties and morphology in excised rabbit lung rinsed with detergent. J Appl Physiol Respir Environ Exercise Physiol 47:1002–1010
21. Forest JB (1976) Lung tissue plasticity: Morphometric analysis of anisotropic strain in liquid filled lungs. Respir Physiol 27:223–239
22. Carney DE, Bredenberg CE, Schiller HJ, et al (1999) The mechanism of lung volume change during mechanical ventilation. Am J Respir Crit Care Med 160:1697–1702
23. Smaldone GC, Mitzner W, Itoh H (1983) Role of alveolar recruitment in lung inflation: influence on pressure-volume hysteresis. J Appl Physiol Respir Environ Exercise Physiol 55:1321–1332
24. Lum H, Huang I, Mitzner W (1990) Morphological evidence for alveolar recruitment during inflation at high transpulmonary pressure. J Appl Physiol 68:2280–2286
25. Mercer RR, Laco JM, Crapo JD (1987) Three-dimensional reconstruction of alveoli in the rat lung for pressure-volume relationships. J Appl Physiol 62:1480–1487
26. Salmon RB, Primiano FP, Saidel GM, Niewoehner DE (1981) Human lung pressure-volume relationships: alveolar collapse and airway closures. J Appl Physiol Respir Environ Exercise Physiol 51:353–362
27. Moreci AP, Norman JC (1973) Measurements of alveolar sac diameters by incident-light photomicrography. Ann Thorac Surg 15:179–185
28. Boyle J, Englestein ES, Sinoway LI (1977) Mean air space diameter, lung surface area and alveolar surface tension. Respiration 34:241–249
29. Sera T, Fujioka H, Yokota H, et al (2004) Localized compliance of small airways in excised rat lungs using microfocal X-ray tomography. J Appl Physiol 96:1665–1673
30. Soutiere SE, Mitzner W (2004) On defining total lung capacity in the mouse. J Appl Physiol 96:1658–1664
31. Soutiere SE, Tankersley CG, Mitzner W (2004) Differences in alveolar size inbred mouse strains. Respir Physiol Neurobiol 140:283–291
32. Escolar JD, Escolar MA, Guzman J, Roques M (2002) Pressure volume curve and alveolar recruitment/derecruitment. A morphometric model of the respiratory cycle. Histol Histopathol 17:383–392
33. Yager D, Feldman H, Fung YC (1992) Microscopic vs macroscopic deformation of pulmonary alveolar duct. J Appl Physiol 72:1348–1354
34. Tschumperlin DJ, Margulies SS (1999) Alveolar epithelial surface area-volume relationship in isolated rat lungs. J Appl Physiol 86:2026–2033
35. Hickling KG (1998) The pressure-volume curve is greatly modified by recruitment. A mathematical model of ARDS lungs. Am J Respir Crit Care Med 158:194–202
36. Hickling KG (2001) Best compliance during a detrimental, but not incremental, positive end-expiratory pressure trial is related to open-lung positive end-expiratory pressure. A

mathematical model of acute respiratory distress syndrome lungs. Am J Respir Crit Care Med 163:69–78

37. Pelosi P, Goldner M, McKibben A, et al (2001) Recruitment and derecruitment during acute respiratory failure. An experimental study. Am J Respir Crit Care Med 164:122–130

38. Crotti S, Mascheroni D, Caironi P, et al (2001) Recruitment and derecruitment during acute respiratory failure. A clinical study. Am J Respir Crit Care Med 164:131–140

39. Oldmixon EH, Hoppin FG (1991) Alveolar septal folding and lung inflation history. J Appl Physiol 71:2369–2379

40. Gatto LA, Fluck RR, Nieman GF (2004) Alveolar mechanics in the acutely injured lung: Role of alveolar instability in the pathogenesis of ventilator-induced lung injury. Respir Care 49:1045–1055

41. Mead J, Takishima T, Leith D (1970) Stress distribution in lungs: a model of pulmonary elasticity. J Appl Physiol 28:596–608

42. West JB (2000) Respiratory Physiology – The Essentials, 6th ed Lippincott Williams & Wilkins, Philadelphia, p 83

43. Neumann P, Berglund JE, Mondejar EF, Magnusson A, Hedenstierna G (1998) Dynamics of lung collapse and recruitment during prolonged breathing in porcine lung injury. J Appl Physiol 85:1522–1543

44. Grasso S, Terragni P, Mascia L, et al (2004) Airway pressure-time curve profile (stress index) detects tidal recruitment/hyperinflation in experimental acute lung injury. Crit Care Med 32:1018–1027

45. Halter JM, Steinberg JM, Schiller HJ, et al (2003) Positive end-expiratory pressure (PEEP) after a recruitment maneuver prevents both alveolar collapse and recruitment/derecruitment. Am J Respir Crit Care Med 167:1620–1626

46. Steinberg J, Schiller HJ, Halter JM, et al (2004) Alveolar instability causes early ventilator-induced lung injury independent of neutrophils. Am J Respir Crit Care Med 169:57–63

47. Tremblay L, Valenza F, Riberio SP, Li J, Slutsky AS (1997) Injurious ventilatory strategies increase cytokines and c-fos m-RNA expression in an isolated rat lung model. J Clin Invest 99:944–952

48. Hotchkiss JR, Simonson DA, Marek DJ, Marini JJ, Dries DJ (2002) Pulmonary microvascular fracture in a patient with acute respiratory distress syndrome. Crit Care Med 30:2368–2370

49. Gajic O, Lee J, Doerr CH, Berrios JC, Myers JL, Hubmayr RD (2003) Ventilator-induced cell wounding and repair in the intact lung. Am J Respir Crit Care Med 167:1057–1063

50. Dreyfuss DP, Soler P, Basset G, Saumon G (1988) High inflation pressure pulmonary edema: respective effects of high airway pressure, high tidal volume an positive end-expiratory pressure. Am Rev Respir Dis 137:1159–1164

Ventilation-perfusion Distribution Analysis to Assess Ventilatory Modes

J. Bickenbach, R. Dembinski, and R. Kuhlen

▌ Introduction

Despite a better understanding of pathophysiological processes as well as implementation of new treatment options, the acute respiratory distress syndrome (ARDS) is still a life threatening disease with a high mortality [1]. ARDS is characterized by severe hypoxemia requiring mechanical ventilation [2]. The main reason for the impairment of gas exchange is a mismatching of ventilation and perfusion [3–5]. Large fractions of pulmonary blood flow are directed towards non-ventilated, atelectatic shunt regions or areas with low ventilation-perfusion (V/Q) ratios. In addition, increased dead space ventilation (Q_D/Q_T) may further worsen gas exchange. Therefore, in ARDS, hypoxemia occurs despite high inspiratory oxygen fractions. Consequently, the paramount target in ARDS is to recruit atelectatic lung regions in order to redirect pulmonary blood flow towards normally ventilated regions.

To determine the corresponding V/Q mismatch in ARDS, a large amount of information can be generated by the use of the multiple inert gas elimination technique (MIGET) [6, 7]. This technique allows exact analysis of V/Q distributions in ARDS and changes in the V/Q distribution in the different ventilation modalities can be assessed.

In this chapter, we will describe the approach to investigate gas exchange in experimentally induced lung injury and the assessment of different ventilatory modes.

▌ History and Background

Acute Respiratory Distress Syndrome

Since the first description by Ashbaugh et al. in 1967, ARDS has been a main focus in intensive care research [8]. After many years of uncertainty, the American-European Consensus Conference established specific criteria in 1994 (Table 1) which are still used to define ARDS [2].

ARDS can be caused by direct (e.g., pneumonia) or indirect (e.g., sepsis, shock) pulmonary injury [9]. The clinical syndrome is characterized by a distinctive dysfunction of pulmonary gas exchange as well as pulmonary edema visible on chest x-rays as diffuse infiltrations. A further main characteristic is the profound arterial hypoxemia due to V/Q mismatch, which is often resistant to increases in inspired oxygen tension. With growing knowledge about pathophysiological interactions and

Table 1. ARDS criteria after American-European consensus conference [2]

ARDS-Criteria

▌Timing

▌Oxygenation: $PaO_2/FiO_2 \leq 200$ mmHg

▌Chest radiograph: Bilateral infiltrates seen on frontal chest radiograph

▌$Paw \leq 18$ mmHg when measured or no clinical evidence of left atrial hypertension

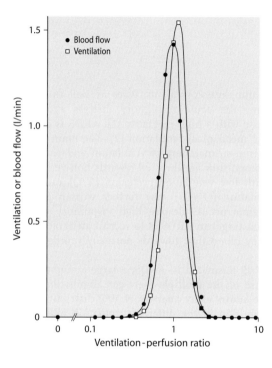

Fig. 1. Ventilation-perfusion distributions. Ventilation and perfusion are plotted against ventilation-perfusion (V/Q) ratio on a logarithmic scale in a resting young healthy subject breathing room air

with the possibility of describing them, e.g., using computed tomography (CT) or MIGET, the main therapeutic target today is to recruit atelectatic lung regions and therefore to improve pulmonary gas exchange by redirecting pulmonary blood flow towards normal V/Q regions without inducing further damage to the lung by the application of mechanical ventilation itself.

Multiple Inert Gas Elimination Technique

MIGET was a development carried out by Farhi [10] and further examined by the research group of Wagner et al. [6, 7] and others with the goal of analyzing the distribution of V/Q of the whole lung. MIGET describes the relations between gas exchange of inert gases in the lungs, the V/Q distribution, and the solubilities of the gases used. A simultaneous venous infusion of six inert gases (sulphur hexafluoride, ethane, cyclopropane, enflurane, ether and acetone) covering a broad spectrum of partition coefficients from 0.005 (sulphur hexafluoride) to 300 (acetone) characterize the distribution of the V/Q ratios within the whole lung.

According to the mass balance of gases, retention (the ratio of the gas concentration in arterial to that in mixed venous blood) and excretion (the ratio of the gas concentration in expired gas to that in mixed venous blood) depends on the solubility of the gas and the V/Q ratio of the lung unit. The retention of the six inert gases allows the determination of pulmonary blood flow distribution against V/Q ratios on a logarithmic scale (Fig. 1). Similarly, the excretion of the six inert gases facilitates an estimation of the alveolar ventilation against V/Q ratios.

To describe the method briefly, 45 min before the first blood sampling for V/Q calculation, an isotonic saline solution equilibrated with the six inert gases has to be infused into a peripheral vein at a constant rate of 2–4 ml/min. With samples of arterial and mixed venous blood and mixed expired gas, retention and excretion can be calculated for each inert gas, and V/Q distributions can be estimated by using the individual blood gas coefficients.

The key result of MIGET is a quantitative picture and a differentiation of functional lung units of particular V/Q ratio. Shunt (Q_S/Q_T) is defined as the fraction of pulmonary blood flow perfusing lung areas with a V/Q less than 0.005. 'Low' V/Q regions are defined as those with V/Q ratios betweeen 0.005 and 0.1 and 'normal' V/Q regions as those with V_A/Q ratios between 0.1 and 10. 'High' V/Q regions illustrate V/Q ratios between 10 and 100, whereas dead space ventilation (Q_D/Q_T) is defined as the fraction of gas entering unperfused lung units (V/Q > 100).

Assessment of Ventilatory Modes in Experimental Lung Injury Using MIGET

The primary goal of mechanical ventilation in ARDS is to restore gas exchange by recruiting atelectatic areas and thereby reducing intrapulmonary shunting without inducing further damage to the lung.

Although there are different approaches, the avoidance of ventilator-induced lung injury (VILI) has generally become a major goal when setting any mode of ventilator support. Two major factors contributing to the progress of lung injury have been clearly identified: overdistension of the lungs using tidal volumes which are too big for the diseased and therefore 'small' lung [11], and recurrent expiratory lung collapse leading to relevant sheer stress when these collapsed areas are reopened during the next inspiration [12, 13]. According to these pathophysiological findings it has been clearly demonstrated that the reduction of tidal volumes to 6 ml/kg body weight results in an improved outcome in acute lung injury (ALI) patients [14]. Smaller clinical studies suggest that the use of an adjusted positive end-expiratory pressure (PEEP) level, avoiding expiratory collapse might result in better clinical outcomes as well [15, 16].

By assessing ventilatory modes with MIGET, some more detailed insights into gas exchange can be observed when assessing lung protective ventilation. Some of the essential ventilatory modes used clinically and experimentally will be reviewed here.

Controlled Mechanical Ventilation

There are many clinical trials that have described changes in conventional gas exchange in ARDS after pressure-controlled or volume-controlled ventilation [17, 18]. Only a few of them determined changes in V/Q distribution. As a major finding,

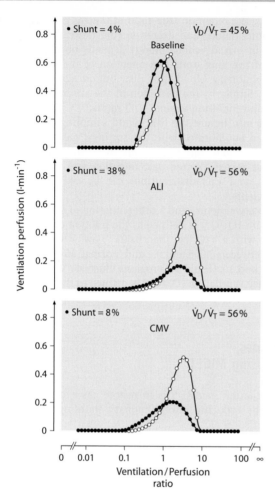

Fig. 2. Ventilation-perfusion /V/Q) distribution during controlled mechanical ventilation (CMV) in one animal. V/Q distributions were calculated by using the multiple inert gas elimination technique on one animal after 12 h with CMV exemplary for 4 animals in the CMV group with a decrease in shunt and an increase in blood flow to areas with low and normal V/Q ratios

V/Q distribution during controlled mechanical ventilation with a PEEP level of 10 cmH₂O showed a decrease in intrapulmonary shunt (Q_S/Q_T) in favor of an increase in Q_{normal} in a study with experimentally induced lung injury caused by surfactant washout. Thus, MIGET revealed an improvement in the distribution of pulmonary perfusion due to controlled mechanical ventilation [19, 29]. The changes of blood flow are attributable to recruitment of atelectatic lung areas (Fig. 2).

Regarding the effects of different flow patterns on pulmonary gas exchange, pressure-controlled mechanical ventilation (PCV) with decelerating inspiratory flow (V_{dec}) has been suggested to improve oxygenation when compared with volume-controlled mechanical ventilation with constant flow (V_{con}) [20]. In this study, however, changes in V/Q distribution were not taken into account. The prolonged effect of different flow patterns in controlled mechanical ventilation was examined by Dembinski et al. [21]. It was hypothesized that V_{dec} provides a more favorable V/Q distribution when compared with V_{con} due to an increase in Pmean at lower Ppeak levels, thereby increasing alveolar recruitment. In this study, the tidal volume as well as the PEEP level was kept constant for the different flow patterns. As a result Pmean increased with V_{dec} when compared with V_{con}. However, regarding MIGET, improved V/Q distribution due to increased perfusion to normal V/Q areas was observed with V_{con} only. The increase in Pmean was not associated with an increase in V_D/V_T and a decrease in Q_{high}, due to compression of alveolar vessels, as previously expected. These findings cannot be fully explained yet. These data demonstrate that gas exchange in ALI depends not only on the level of Pmean but also on the concomitant inspiratory flow pattern. Whereas V_{peak} is higher during ventilation with V_{dec}, end-inspiratory flow is higher during V_{con} than during V_{dec}. Thus, it can be speculated that after a phase of recruitment of atelectatic lung regions during inspiration a certain amount of end-inspiratory flow as with V_{con} is necessary to provide adequate ventilation to theses areas.

Concerning lung protective ventilation with low tidal volumes, it has been shown that high levels of Pmean might be associated with an increasing mortality rate [22]. In terms of clinical outcomes, V_{con} might be beneficial due to improved gas exchange when reducing Pmean compared to V_{dec}. This hypothesis should be investigated clinically.

High Frequency Oscillatory Ventilation (HFOV)

In HFOV, small tidal volumes of approximately 2 ml/kg body weight with a respiratory rate of 4.5 Hz are used. Gas exchange can be explained primarily by alveolar ventilation. In addition, clinical studies suggested that mechanisms of convection play a central role in HFOV as well [23].

Concerning V/Q distribution during HFOV, an improvement in pulmonary perfusion after oleic acid-induced lung injury has been found. Thus, shunt decreased and blood flow to normal V/Q areas increased, which was similar to the findings in a control group with controlled mechanical ventilation. Obviously, pulmonary recruitment is the main mechanism of improved gas exchange during HFOV. However, it is worth noting that equal improvements required a twofold higher mean airway pressure with HFOV when compared to controlled mechanical ventilation [24]. Moreover, the assessment of ventilation distribution by inert gas elimination has certain limitations: gas transport is different during HFOV, depending on the solubility of each gas. Consequently, higher excretion values result in the calculation of large amounts of dead space and high V/Q regions [25]. Therefore, the validity of excretion values and the analysis of the corresponding ventilation distribution may be reduced. In ARDS, V/Q mismatching is mainly characterized by intrapulmonary shunt and perfusion of low V/Q regions, though. Changes of perfusion distribution during HFOV can be precisely demonstrated by MIGET (Fig. 3).

Nevertheless, further investigations are needed to validate HFOV as an alternative, clinically useful ventilatory mode.

Biphasic Positive Airway Pressure (BiPAP)

Mechanical ventilation without spontaneous breathing efforts compromises venous return and cardiac output which in consequence leads to a decrease in organ perfusion. Steinhoff and Falke demonstrated that in intermittent mandatory ventilation (IMV) with some degree of spontaneous breathing activity, the renal water and sodium excretion was improved compared to controlled mechanical ventilation [26]. Obviously, even a small superimposed spontaneous breathing activity resulted in

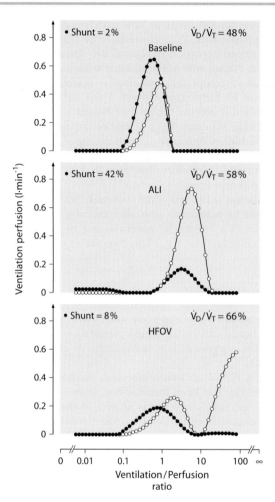

Fig. 3. Ventilation-perfusion (V/Q) distribution during high-frequency oscillatory ventilation (HFOV). V/Q distributions were calculated by the multiple inert gas elimination technique at baseline, oleic-acid induced lung injury (ALI) and HFOV

such a decrease in thoracic pressure that the renal perfusion as well as the excretion function was better preserved than during controlled mechanical ventilation [27]. Thus, the increasing use of partial support modalities is not only due to technological improvements but also to data showing that avoiding controlled mechanical ventilation by preserving some spontaneous breathing activity of the diaphragm might be beneficial for gas exchange, hemodynamics, and the clinical course of ALI.

BiPAP might be regarded as the cyclic change from a lower to a higher continuous positive airway pressure (CPAP) level with spontaneous breathing being possible on both levels using an active flow regulation. The machine part of ventilation is due to the cyclic shift from the lower level to the higher level and back whereas the patient might breathe spontaneously throughout the whole respiratory cycle. It has to be stressed that the setting of the two pressure levels during BiPAP follows the principal rules of a protective ventilation strategy: the lower pressure level should be set to keep a minimal lung volume in order to avoid repetitive lung collapse and reopening. The upper level should be set to avoid lung overdistension. Since a limited tidal volume of 6 ml/kg body weight has been found to result in a better clinical outcome than 12 ml/kg, the resulting tidal volume during BIPAP should also be around 6 ml/kg body weight. Hence, the pressure amplitude between lower and higher CPAP levels has to be adjusted properly.

It has been shown that BiPAP results in an improved gas exchange compared to controlled mechanical ventilation [28, 29]. Putensen and colleagues showed a clear redistribution of areas with low V/Q towards normal V/Q regions using superimposed spontaneous breathing in ARDS patients [28].

In an experimental study by our group, the effects of BiPAP with spontaneous breathing on V/Q distribution were investigated in experimentally induced lung injury [30]. We hypothesized that improvement in V/Q distribution in BiPAP was attributed to an increased transpulmonary pressure (Ptp) which can also be achieved by increasing airway pressure (Paw) during pressure-controlled ventilation to achieve the same Ptp as with BiPAP. As a major finding resulting from MIGET analysis, shunt decreased during BiPAP, and perfusion of normal V/Q regions increased. Improvements in oxygenation are explainable by effectively increased transpulmonary pressure in the dependent lung, since we could demonstrate equal effects on gas exchange if inspiratory pressures were increased to create the same transpulmonary pressure during controlled ventilation without spontaneous breathing. However, this resulted in increased airway pressures and tidal volumes, which are meant to worsen clinical outcome in ARDS patients [14]. Furthermore, the increase in Ptp with controlled mechanical ventilation was clearly associated with pronounced hemodynamic suppression.

The previously described effect of preserved diaphragm activity on the recruitment of atelectasis formation and a more homogeneous distribution of blood flow [31, 32] could not be demonstrated so clearly in this study. Although BiPAP could be useful in improving pulmonary gas exchange, further studies need to analyze the particular effect of spontaneous breathing activity on VILI in ARDS patients.

Further clinical studies need to clarify the role of different ventilatory modes allowing spontaneous breathing in the clinical setting.

Pressure Support Ventilation (PSV)

Pressure support was designed to support each inspiratory effort with flow to reach a preset pressure level. Originally, it was implemented in mechanical ventilators to compensate for a certain pressure drop during demand flow regulation due to non-ideal ventilator properties. It was further applied as an actual mode of ventilation that augmented each inspiratory effort of the patient. As a function of the applied level of pressure support, it is thereby possible to progressively unload a patient from an increased breathing workload. In a classic paper PSV was found to prevent the development of diaphragmatic fatigue [33] and, therefore, it is frequently applied as a weaning mode when the patient is recovering from respiratory failure. Depending on the level with which it is applied it might facilitate a fast, safe, and gradual weaning [34]. Being a widely accepted weaning tool, which has been extensively investigated, it has been recently shown that PSV might be successfully used as a primary support mode applied early in the course of acute respiratory failure in clinical practice as well [35].

Concerning V/Q distribution, Putensen et al. demonstrated that in patients with ARDS partial ventilatory support for 1h may result in an improvement in pulmonary gas exchange because of a redistribution of V/Q when spontaneous breathing is possible throughout the whole respiratory cycle in BiPAP [28]. Comparing PSV with BIPAP and controlled mechanical ventilation respectively, PSV did not improve V/Q distribution. Apparently, mechanical assistance of each inspiration during PSV was not sufficient to counterbalance the ARDS-induced V/Q-mismatch in this short-term-evaluation. It should be noted however, that tidal volumes with PSV were lower than with the other modes in this investigation.

Prolonged effects of PSV on V/Q distribution have been demonstrated in a study by Dembinski et al. [36]. V/Q distribution analysis with MIGET revealed a decrease in blood flow to normal V/Q areas and a decrease in shunt. It seems likely that the improvement in gas exchange was mainly caused by alveolar recruitment, which was attributed to the use of a PEEP level of 10 cmH$_2$O. However, compared with controlled mechanical ventilation, spontaneous breathing activity in PSV did not lead to additional improvement in gas exchange. One possible explanation might be the respirator setting: the tidal volume of approximately 4 ml/kg body weight during PSV compared to 10 ml/kg in controlled mechanical ventilation may have resulted in decreased gas exchange because of reduced alveolar ventilation and tidal recruitment as well as an increased Q$_D$/Q$_T$.

It was concluded that PSV does not provide beneficial prolonged effects on gas exchange in this experimental model. However, the hypothesis that long-term use of PSV in acute respiratory failure might prevent diaphragmatic fatigue at a level of gas exchange comparable to controlled mechanical ventilation has not yet been investigated.

▌ Conclusion

Severe impairment of oxygenation in ALI and ARDS is caused by a mismatch of ventilation-perfusion distribution with an increased fraction of shunt. One of the major therapeutic targets is to recruit atelectatic alveoli in order to improve V/Q distribution and to reduce shunt fraction. However, it has been shown several times, that mechanical ventilation itself might contribute to a further progress of lung injury. The avoidance of VILI and the implementation of lung protective ventilation modes play a key role when setting any ventilatory support modality.

With MIGET, the impaired pulmonary gas exchange in ARDS can be investigated very precisely. It allows an assessment of the V/Q distribution mismatch associated with ARDS as well as its improvement during mechanical ventilation with different settings. It can be clarified whether the improved gas exchange is caused by modulation of pulmonary blood flow or by increase in transpulmonal pressure. Thus, MIGET can be seen as an excellent diagnostic tool helping us to understand the complex pathophysiology in acute respiratory failure. Nevertheless, MIGET does not give information about clinical benefit of a given modality. Moreover, it has to be taken into account that mechanical ventilation can dramatically worsen the clinical course of ARDS. The avoidance of VILI has therefore become a major goal of any therapeutic concept. MIGET can help, as a basic science tool, to assess the specific effects of different ventilatory modes used in the treatment of ARDS on V/Q distribution.

References

1. Kraft P, Friedrich P, Pernerstorfer T, et al (1996) The acute respiratory distress syndrome: Definitions, severity, and clinical outcome: an analysis of 101 clinical investigations. Intensive Care Med 22:519–552
2. Bernard GR, Artigas A, Brigham KL, et al (1994) The American-European Consensus Conference on ARDS. Definitions, mechanisms, relevant outcomes and clinical trial coordination. Am J Respir Crit Care 149:818–824
3. Dantzker DR, Brook CJ, Dehart P, et al (1979) Ventilation-perfusion distribution in the adult respiratory distress syndrome. Am Rev Respir Dis 120:1039–1052
4. Gattinoni L, Bombino M, Pelosi P, et al (1994) Lung structure and function in different stages of severe adult respiratory distress syndrome. JAMA 271:1772–1779
5. Pelosi P, D'Andrea L, Vitale G, et al (1994) Vertical gradient of regional lung inflation in adult respiratory distress syndrome. Am J Respir Crit Care Med 149:8–13
6. Wagner PD, Saltzmann HA, West JB (1974) Measurement of continuos distributions of ventilation-perfusion ratios: theory. J Appl Physiol 36:588–599
7. Wagner PD, Naumann PF, Laravuso R (1974) Simultaneous measurement of eight foreign gases in blood by gas chromatography. J Appl Physiol 36:600–605
8. Ashbaugh DG, Bigelow DB, Petty TL, Levine BE (1967) Acute respiratory distress in adults. Lancet 2:319–323
9. Lewandowski K, Pappert D, Kuhlen R, Rossaint R, Gerlach H, Falke KJ (1996) Klinische Aspekte des akuten Lungenversagens des Erwachsenen (ARDS). Anästhesist 45:2–18
10. Farhi LE (1967) Elimination of inert gas by the lung. Respir Physiol 3:1–11
11. Dreyfuss D, Saumon G (1998) Ventilator-induced lung injury: lessons from experimental studies. Am J Respir Crit Care Med 157:294–323
12. Chiumello D, Pristine G, Slutsky AS (1999) Mechanical ventilation affects local and systemic cytokines in an animal model of acute respiratory distress syndrome. Am J Respir Crit Care Med 160:109–116
13. Muscedere JG, Mullen JB, Gan K, Slutsky AS (1994) Tidal ventilation at low airway pressures can augment lung injury. Am J Respir Crit Care Med 149:1327–1334
14. The Acute Respiratory Distress Syndrome Network (2000) Ventilation with lower tidal volumes as compared with traditional tidal volumes for acute lung injury and the acute respiratory distress syndrome. N Engl J Med 342:1301–1308
15. Amato MB, Barbas CS, Medeiros DM, et al (1998) Effect of a protective-ventilation strategy on mortality in the acute respiratory distress syndrome. N Engl J Med 338:347–354
16. Ranieri VM, Suter PM, Tortorella C, et al (1999) Effect of mechanical ventilation on inflammatory mediators in patients with acute respiratory distress syndrome: a randomized controlled trial. JAMA 282:54–61
17. Esteban A, Alia I, Gordo F, et al (2000) Prospective randomized trial comparing pressure-controlled ventilation and volume-controlled ventilation in ARDS. Chest 117:1690–1696
18. Lessard MR, Guerot E, Lorino H, et al (1994) Effects of pressure-controlled with different I:E ratios versus volume-controlled ventilation on respiratory mechanics, gas exchange, and hemodynamics in patients with adult respiratory distress syndrome. Anesthesiology 80:983–991
19. Dembinski R, Kuhlen R, Lopez F, et al (2000) Ventilation-perfusion distribution during controlled mechanical ventilation (CMV) and pressure support (PS). Intensive Care Med 26 (Suppl 3):S284 (abst)
20. Abraham E, Yoshihara G (1990) Cardiorespiratory effects of pressure-controlled ventilation in severe respiratory failure. Chest 98:1445–1449
21. Dembinski R, Henzler D, Bensberg R, Prusse B, Rossaint R, Kuhlen R (2004) Ventilation-perfusion distribution related to different inspiratory flow patterns in experimental lung injury. Anesth Analg 98:211–219
22. Eichacker PQ, Gerstenberger EP, Banks SM, et al (2002) Meta-analysis of acute lung injury and acute respiratory distress syndrome trials testing low tidal volumes. Am J Respir Crit Care Med 166:1510–1514
23. Smith BE (1990) High frequency ventilation: past, present and future? Br J Anaesth 65:130–138

24. Dembinski R, Max M, Bensberg R, Bickenbach J, Kuhlen R, Rossaint R (2002) High-frequency oscillatory ventilation in experimental lung injury: effects on gas exchange. Intensive Care Med 28:768–774
25. McEvoy RD, Davies NJ, Mannino FL, et al (1982) Pulmonary gas exchange during high-frquency ventilation. J Appl Physiol 52:1278–1287
26. Steinhoff H, Falke K, Schwarzhoff W (1982) Enhanced renal function associated with intermittend mandatory ventilation in acute respiratory failure. Intensive Care Med 8:69–74
27. Steinhoff H, Kohlhoff R, Falke K (1984) Facilitation of renal function by intermittend mandatory ventilation. Intensive Care Med 10:59–65
28. Putensen C, Mutz NJ, Putensen-Himmer G, Zinserling J (1999) Spontaneous breathing during ventilatory support improves ventilation-perfusion distributions in patients with acute respiratory distress syndrome. Am J Respir Crit Care Med 159:1241–1248
29. Putensen C, Zech S, Wrigge H, et al (2001) Long-term effects of spontaneous breathing during ventilatory support in patients with acute lung injury. Am J Respir Crit Care Med 164:43–49
30. Henzler D, Dembinski R, Bensberg R, Hochhausen N, Rossaint R, Kuhlen R (2004). Ventilation with biphasic positive airway pressure in experimental lung injury. Intensive Care Med 30:935–943
31. Putensen C, Rasanen J, Lopez FA (1994) Ventilation-perfusion distributions during mechanical ventilation with superimposed spontaneous breathing in canine lung injury. Am J Respir Crit Care Med 150:101–108
32. Sydow M, Buchardi H, Ephraim E, Zielmann S, Crozier TA (1994) Long-term effects of two different ventilatory modes on oxygenation in acute lung injury. Comparison of airway pressure release ventilation and volume controlled inverse ration ventilation. Am J Respir Crit Care Med 149:1550–1556
33. Brochard L, Harf A, Lorino H, Lemaire F (1989) Inspiratory pressure support prevents diaphragmatic fatigue during weaning from mechanical ventilation. Am Rev Respir Dis 139:513–521
34. Brochard L, Rauss A, Benito S, et al (1994) Comparison of three methods of gradual withdrawal from ventilatory support during weaning from mechanical ventilation. Am J Respir Crit Care Med 150:896–903
35. Cereda M, Foti G, Marcora B, et al (2000) Pressure support ventilation in patients with acute lung injury. Crit Care Med 28:1269–1275
36. Dembinski R, Max M, Bensberg R, Rossaint R, Kuhlen R (2002) Pressure support compared with controlled mechanical ventilation in experimental lung injury. Anesth Analg 94:1570–1576
37. The ARDS Clinical Trials Network (2004) Higher versus lower positive end-expiratory pressures in patients with the acute respiratory distress syndrome. N Engl J Med 351:327–336

Modulators of Ventilator-induced Lung Injury

L. E. Ferrer and J. J. Marini

▌ Introduction

Numerous experimental studies demonstrate the potential for adverse patterns of mechanical ventilation to initiate acute lung injury (ALI) that is characterized by proteinaceous edema, inflammation, and hemorrhage. The great majority of these investigations into ventilator-induced lung injury (VILI) have focused on the characteristics of the individual tidal cycle-tidal volume, inspiratory flow rate, and end-expiratory airway pressure. Although these features are of unquestioned importance, other characteristics of the clinical environment have been shown to modify the intensity and/or nature of the resulting damage.

In the largest and perhaps the most widely cited clinical trial of ventilator strategy in ALI yet undertaken, smaller tidal volumes were associated with reduced mortality [1]. This result was attributed to the generally lower peak alveolar pressures and reduced mechanical stresses associated with smaller tidal volumes. Analysis of the data pooled from both trial groups not only demonstrated a positive correlation between plateau pressure and mortality rate, but also revealed its monotonic, linear nature, without an obvious break point down to pressures that are considerably lower than those that are feasible to use in the management of acute respiratory distress syndrome (ARDS) [2] (Fig. 1). Although such an association does not confirm plateau pressure as the sole causative variable, it implies that

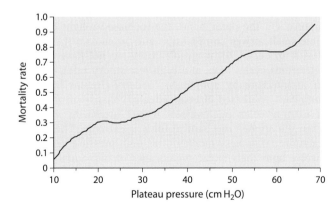

Fig. 1. Relationship of mortality to inspiratory plateau pressure on the first day after randomization in a clinical trial of tidal volume reduction in ALI. From [2] with permission

there may be no 'safe' plateau pressure below which mortality cannot be influenced by further pressure reduction. This observation underscores the need to identify any cofactors that influence VILI expression.

To this time, almost all strategies proposed to limit VILI have altered the ventilatory variables associated with a single tidal cycle. Lower tidal volume, lower plateau pressures and higher positive end-expiratory pressure (PEEP) settings have been used to avoid VILI, decrease length of intensive care unit (ICU) stay and curtail the associated mortality rate [3]. Although less well studied, lung injury arising in the course of mechanical ventilation may also relate to non-ventilatory factors such as body position, $PaCO_2$, acid-base state, pulmonary vascular pressure changes, body temperature, concomitant pathologies, and pharmacologic agents. In this chapter, we review a selected subset of these non-ventilatory factors and propose mechanisms for their actions. Our objective is to focus on those amenable to modification at the bedside.

▌ Pathophysiology of VILI

Although VILI is a complex process initiated and propagated through several mechanisms, generally speaking, damage resulting from excessive mechanical stress can be classified into two broad categories: structural and inflammatory. The injury process is initiated by mechanical stress and depends on the magnitude, frequency and cumulative effect of this stimulus. Repetitive over-stretching and cyclic recruitment-derecruitment of collapsed areas that are exposed periodically to high pressure favor injury that disrupts the integrity of the epithelial membrane [4].

Simultaneously, these mechanical forces activate intracellular signaling cascades within epithelial cells. This activation culminates in recruitment of polymorphonuclear leukocytes (PMN), production of pro-inflammatory cytokines, vasodilatation and alveolar edema – collectively a process termed 'biotrauma' [5]. Once formed, alveolar edema has two opposing effects. On one hand, completely flooded alveoli are theoretically subject to lower shearing stresses than atelectatic units, as the gas-liquid interface is eliminated and alveolar dimensions increase. Furthermore, decreased surface tension in partially flooded units would cause capillaries that are fully embedded in the alveolar walls to bulge into the interior, encouraging their rupture. On the other hand, the increased weight of the edematous lung may promote small airway compression and accentuate the tendency for tidal opening and closure to occur [6]. If alveolar units do not have enough time to recover between deleterious cycles (e.g., at a high respiratory rate), the result is disruption of alveolar architecture by apoptosis, capillary-alveolus barrier fracture, consumption of surfactant, increased alveolar edema, collapse of alveolar capillaries, and dilatation of extra-alveolar microvessels. Overt breaks in the blood-gas barrier may arise when the applied mechanical force is extreme. These microscopic breaks, or 'stress fractures', arise very quickly after high pressure ventilatory cycles are initiated and involve both the cellular membranes of individual cells as well as larger tears that traverse intracellular boundaries. The presence of alveolar hemorrhage implies breaks of sufficient size to allow it (Fig. 2).

Because stresses severe enough to disrupt structural collagen are most likely to arise at the junctions of aerated and non-aerated tissue, hemorrhagic edema tends to form preferentially in gravitationally dependent regions. In such zones, inflam-

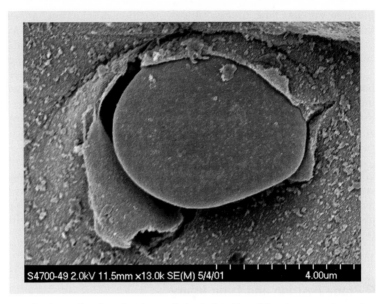

S4700-49 2.0kV 11.5mm ×13.0k SE(M) 5/4/01   4.00um

Fig. 2. Rupture of the alveolar-capillary boundary by ventilation-induced lung injury in an experimental rat

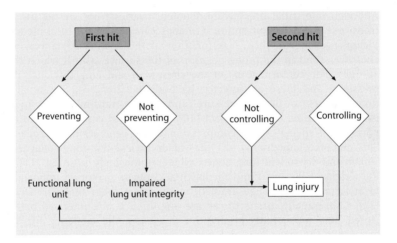

Fig. 3. 'Two Hit' theory of lung injury

mation may be a secondary epiphenomenon to barrier disruption rather than a primary event. The potential for mechanical ventilation to induce a systemic cytokine release and for a protective lung ventilation strategy to attenuate this response, has been well demonstrated in the clinical context [7].

The 'two hit hypothesis' is a plausible but as yet unproven theory proposed to explain the pathogenesis of VILI (Fig. 3). This theory suggests that inflammatory mechano-signaling requires both a supra-physiologic mechanical stress (first hit), as well as one or more 'second hit' co-factors (such as endotoxin or hyperoxia) to promote the signaling process already mentioned [8]. Thus, a mechanical stress that otherwise might be well tolerated culminates in inflammatory injury when paired with another potentially noxious influence. Secondary variables that modulate VILI are viewed to influence the degree of mechanical stress applied to vulnerable structures, the mechano-signaled inflammatory response to overstretching, or both. Although each of the contributing variables shown experimentally to be of importance in VILI can be conceptualized within this framework, we emphasize that a complete mechanistic understanding of VILI remains elusive at this time, and that our presentation schema is more an organizational device rather than a confirmed scientific classification.

Several clinical interventions that are not related to ventilation strategy have genuine potential for manipulation as therapeutic tools for controlling or preventing iatrogenic lung injury. These include prone positioning, acid-base modification, temperature regulation and preconditioning, and modulation of precapillary and postcapillary pulmonary pressures. We will review these topics, with the objective to delineate the potential clinical applications of each.

▌ Prone Position and Lung Injury

The transpulmonary pressure that determines tissue stress is not only a function of plateau pressure but also of the local pressure that surrounds the alveolus. Although interstitial pressure undoubtedly varies from site to site within a given transverse plane, by convention it is approximated by the local pleural pressure [9]. Pleural pressure, in turn, is a function of the relative elastances of the lung and chest wall (and in the prone position of the surface against which the thorax rests, as well). The conformations of the chest wall and lung influence regional pleural pressures, and these are affected by body position. ALI accentuates the gravitational gradient of pleural pressure (and thus of transpulmonary pressure) that exists in the supine healthy subject [10]. Controversy continues as to the relative importance of edema-caused compression in the generation of dependent atelectasis, but computed tomography (CT) has made it clear that lung collapse is most prevalent in the dependent lung zones, whatever the body position [11]. When supine, the weight of the heart and mediastinal contents makes an important contribution to atelectasis, as they are cradled by the lower lobes that partially support them [12]. Conceptually, tissue forces are amplified at the interface between open and closed lung units. Judged solely on this basis, the tendency for VILI should be greatest in the dependent and middle lung zones. In fact, when high plateau pressures are used with insufficient PEEP to keep the high-risk dependent units continually patent, VILI does prevail in the dorsal regions of large anesthetized animals – even in those with initially healthy lungs [13]. Other co-factors, such as secretion retention and microvascular pressure (discussed below) may also contribute to this regional predilection for injury, but these are likely to be of secondary importance.

Although the supine position has traditionally been favored for the care of the critically ill, there are important reasons to question this practice. The great majority of mammals – including our closest primate relatives – orient themselves in the prone position, and healthy humans normally spend only a small fraction of their time supine. Anatomically, the shapes of the lung and the chest wall are more closely matched in the prone position, so that the gravitational gradient of pleural pressure is markedly attenuated. Moreover, the airways drain more effectively in the prone position, and the weight of the heart is borne by the anterior chest wall rather than by the lungs, further reducing the tendency for dependent atelectasis to occur. The resulting reduction in the regional heterogeneity of transpulmonary pressure is likely to account for improved ventilation-perfusion (V/Q) matching in the prone position [14]. These observations apply equally to normal and acutely injured lungs. Better V/Q matching and reduced atelectasis result in improved oxygenation. With regard to VILI, studies conducted in large animals with initially normal or pre-injured lungs demonstrate that ventilatory patterns that result in severe injury produce less damage when the animal is oriented in the prone position [13]. Virtually all of the positional reduction in injury is experienced in the dependent regions. By necessity, information regarding VILI in humans is inferential, as VILI cannot be ethically inflicted nor effectively separated from the underlying ALI/ARDS condition.

Results from randomized clinical trials of prone positioning in ALI and ARDS simultaneously have been disappointing and enlightening [15, 16]. While virtually all observational studies and randomized clinical trials have demonstrated improved oxygenation in the prone position [17], none has shown a consistent survival advantage across all study patients. Unfortunately, neither of the large reported trials has succeeded in recruiting the number of patients targeted by their prospective power analyses [15, 16]. Moreover, if mortality is selected as the primary outcome variable, questions must be raised regarding trial design. In the largest randomized controlled trial yet reported, proning was used for less than one third of each day, patients were studied at varied times after injury onset, and fewer than one half of the targeted number of patients were enrolled [15]. In that landmark Italian trial however, several interesting *post hoc* analyses were informative. Those patients with the most severe disease were statistically more likely to benefit from proning, as were those predisposed to VILI by exposure to very large tidal volumes. It is also of interest that the cohort of patients who experienced improved CO_2 exchange (believed to indicate recruitment) as a result of proning had a reduced mortality rate [18]. Taken together, such data suggest that proning may beneficially impact VILI and mortality in those patients most at risk, especially when recruitment results from the intervention. The relative efficacy of prone positioning in the prevention of mortality would be expected to be a function of the severity and nature of the lung injury (primary vs. secondary), the timing of study entry, the length of the proning period per day, the duration of the proning intervention, the co-morbid conditions, and of other factors. The recently published Spanish trial of prone positioning extended the proning interval closer to 20 hours per day and showed an encouraging, if statistically insignificant, trend toward lower mortality in patients who were proned [16].

▌ CO_2, Acidosis and Lung Injury

Not only does the mechanical stress associated with high pressure ventilatory cycles incite injury, but the association of hyperventilation and hypocapnia with worsened lung injury has been reported. In fact, hypocapnia and hyperventilation may be independent causes of broncopulmonary dysplasia [19]. Hypocapnia appears to mediate parenchymal injury by altering surfactant function and by increasing permeability in airway and parenchymal microvessels [20]. It stands to reason that although the obligate hypoventilation associated with lung protective strategies of ventilation has been termed 'permissive' hypercapnia, hypercapnia itself may be associated with increased survival in ARDS, an association supported by outcome data from a 10-year study [21].

If this association is true, is it hypercapnia or acidosis that is beneficial? Unquestionably, the severity of acidosis predicts an adverse outcome in diverse clinical contexts, including cardiac arrest and sepsis [22]. However, although acidosis occurs commonly in the setting of critical illness and often heralds a poor prognosis, it is likely that the etiology of the underlying condition resulting in the acidosis, rather than the acidosis *per se*, is the key adverse factor. Indeed, acidosis may constitute a protective adaptation in the context of cellular stress, and may confer beneficial effects in the setting of acute organ injury [23].

Intracellular pH is normally lower than extracellular pH, and enzymatic reactions need appropriate pH and temperature for optimal functioning, specifically for ATP generation and protein synthesis. Both PCO_2 and HCO_3 affect the plasma pH, but raised PCO_2 results in rapid inward diffusion of highly soluble carbon dioxide molecules, which quickly lowers intracellular pH. This CO_2-associated alteration of pH occurs more rapidly than is possible by inward migration of the H+ ions resulting from metabolic acidosis or than can be offset by H_2CO_3 retention.

Hypercapnic acidosis alters the activity of polymorphonuclear phagocytes, platelet-activating factor, phospholipase A_2, cell adhesion molecules, cell apoptosis [24], lipid peroxidation, xanthine oxidase, free-radical formation, and superoxide. Simultaneously, hypercapnic acidosis down-regulates lung nitric oxide (NO) production [25] and increases cAMP formation (both having protective potentials in the setting of lung injury) [26]. One likely mechanism underlying these protective actions of hypercapnic acidosis is the attenuated activity of the transcription regulator nuclear factor-kappa beta (NF-κB) [27]. Hypercapnia reduces tissue metabolism, improves surfactant function and prevents nitration of proteins [28]. At the oxygen supply-demand level, it increases local tissue blood flow and causes rightward displacement of the hemoglobin-oxygen disassociation curve, thereby assisting in tissue oxygen and nutrient delivery. Acidosis also decreases sarcoplasmic calcium release, dampens mitochondrial respiration and reduces the activity of enzymes that produce inflammatory metabolic intermediates [21]. These changes favor cellular functioning, control of inflammatory response, improved cardiac function, and maintenance or reactivation of hypoxic pulmonary vasoconstriction, with resultant improvement V/Q matching.

Broccard et al. found that isolated perfused rabbit lungs exposed to high ventilating pressure plus hypercapnia experienced less weight gain and lower protein and hemoglobin concentrations in bronchoalveolar lavage (BAL) fluid than did lungs that underwent high pressure-controlled ventilation and normocapnia. These authors concluded that respiratory acidosis decreased the severity of VILI in this experimental model [29]. Supporting this contention is the work of Sinclair et al., who investigated whether hypercapnic acidosis protects against VILI *in vivo* using anesthetized paralyzed rabbits ventilated in the volume controlled mode. The hypercapnic group showed significantly lower plateau pressures, changes in PaO_2, BAL fluid protein concentration, and injury score than did the normocapnic animals [30].

Laffey et al. investigated whether therapeutic hypercapnia, i.e., the active administration of inspired CO_2, would protect against ALI in an *in vivo* animal model of lung ischemia-reperfusion. They concluded that therapeutic hypercapnia is protective versus ischemia-reperfusion lung injury and proposed that mechanisms of protection may include preservation of lung mechanics, attenuation of pulmonary inflammation and reduction of free radical mediated injury [24].

To return to the question at hand – hypercapnia vs. pH in lung protection – there is increasing evidence that the beneficial effects of hypercapnic acidosis in ALI relate to the acidosis, rather than to the elevated $PaCO_2$ *per se* [31]. Hypercapnia at normal pH caused injury to the alveolar epithelial cell monolayer [32] and decreased surfactant protein A function *in vitro* [33]. In the isolated lung, the protective effect of hypercapnic acidosis in ischemia-reperfusion induced ALI was greatly attenuated if the pH was buffered towards normal. In view of the potential for vascular modulation of VILI, it is of interest that buffering hypercapnic acidosis simultaneously caused significant pulmonary vasodilation [31] (*vide infra*).

Many effects of hypercapnia in models of systemic organ injury appear to be a function of the associated acidosis, as well. The myocardial protective effects of hypercapnic acidosis are also seen with metabolic acidosis, both in *ex vivo* and *in vivo* models. Metabolic acidosis delays the onset of cell death in isolated hepatocytes exposed to anoxia and to chemical hypoxia. Correcting the pH to 7.4 abolished the protective effect and accelerated hepatocyte death [34].

Although limited acidosis has beneficial effects on the intracellular milieu, extreme acidosis may jeopardize adequate function of the cell. In many clinical conditions, a common rationale for buffering the plasma is to ameliorate the haemodynamic consequences of acidosis. In the setting of hypercapnic acidosis, bicarbonate may not be the ideal agent to compensate it, as bicarbonate further increases intracellular CO_2 levels. It has been suggested that the amino alcohol trometamine (THAM) may have a role in these clinical situations, as it does not further increase intracellular CO_2 levels. In addition, the positive effects of hypercapnic acidosis on inflammation may be preserved without reaching dangerous CO_2 levels in the intracellular milieu [35].

In general, these experimental findings demonstrate that hypercapnic acidosis induced by direct administration of CO_2 or permitted by mechanical ventilation strategy is protective in multiple models of ALI and systemic organ injury. These protective effects appear to be a function of the intracellular acidosis rather than the hypercapnia *per se*. Whatever the precise mechanism may be, the potential for un-buffered hypercapnia to attenuate ALI and systemic organ injury is clear.

Nevertheless, the concomitant use of protective ventilatory strategies and permissive hypercapnia needs more clinical study to define their optional use in medical practice. For example, the dose-response relationship of hypercapnia to physiologic response is not well understood in critical illness. Moreover, it is necessary to evaluate the possible utility of therapeutic hypercapnia dissociated from the excessively low tidal volume and frequencies that may promote atelectasis.

▋ Vascular Pressure and Lung Injury

The pulmonary vascular tree can be considered as a series of three segments: arterial, intermediate or middle (which includes alveolar capillaries and contiguous microvessels), and venous. Under normal conditions the arterial and venous segments (which are extra-alveolar) contribute most to overall pulmonary vascular resistance, but the compliant intermediate segment is influenced primarily by alveolar pressures, and as a consequence, it undergoes the greatest change in overall vascular resistance that occurs during ventilation [36].

We have studied the interaction between vascular pressure and alveolar pressure in different animal model experiments, which collectively underscore the potential for deleterious interactions to occur between lung volumes and pulmonary hemodynamics [37–40]. Our initial experiments demonstrated that increased flow and vascular pressure within and upstream from the intermediate segment influenced the severity of VILI resulting from an unchanging adverse pattern of ventilation. Higher pre-capillary pressure dramatically increases the damage resulting from a given ventilatory protocol. In keeping with this concept, Dreyfuss and Saumon found that ventilation with negative pressure caused lung damage more severe that the associated equivalent ventilation by positive pressure, implicating involvement of increased blood flow in ventilation-related damage [41]. Those same investigators provided further support for this hypothesis by showing that rats given dopamine to increase cardiac output suffered increased albumin leak when ventilated with high pressure, and ascribed a major portion of the protective effect of PEEP in the setting of high pressure ventilation to its reduction of pulmonary perfusion [42].

Later work by Broccard and colleagues showed that lowering post-capillary pressure increased the edema and filtration coefficient resulting from a fixed pattern of ventilation and upstream pre-capillary pressure [43]. In other words, vascular pressures as well as the characteristics of the tidal cycle appear to be of fundamental importance to the genesis of VILI. In addition, the minute ventilation, the number of the stress cycles of a potentially damaging character that occur per unit time or their cumulative number, might be important, as well [37–39]. The effects of respiratory frequency and vascular pressures on VILI are not mediated primarily by pulsatile vascular pressure *per se* but rather by a phenomenon related to cyclic

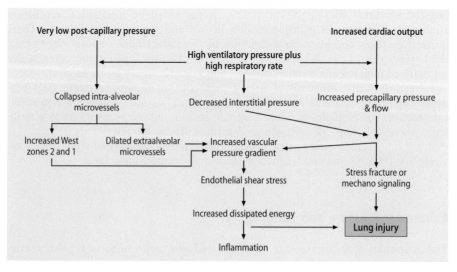

Fig. 4. Hypothetical interaction between airspace and pulmonary vascular pressures in the causation of ventilator-induced lung injury (VILI)

modulation of the vascular microenvironment induced by ventilation [38–40]: cyclic changes in perivascular pressure might be instrumental in the genesis of VILI (Fig. 4).

At first consideration, the fact that lowering post capillary pressure might accentuate the edema resulting from VILI seems paradoxical: in other disease settings reducing capillary pressure often confers benefit on lung functioning. Lower pressure limits exudation of protein-rich fluid, which may inactivate surfactant and further alter membrane permeability by increasing surface tension. Furthermore, edematous lungs tend to collapse under their own weight and to develop dependent atelectasis. When tidal airway pressures are high enough, such compression may lead to cyclic opening and collapse, and amplified shear stress. Such conditions could account for the preferentially dependent distribution of VILI [42]. At the same time, flooding the alveoli of dependent regions can reduce regional mechanical stress by preventing their tidal expansion and collapse. In fact, excessive reduction of capillary pressure may promote vascular derecruitment, alter ventilation-perfusion matching, and contribute to vascular stress because it tends to impose zone 2 conditions during positive pressure ventilation [44]. This extension of zone 2 can amplify the increase in vascular resistance caused by inspiration and augment tidal intramural pressure changes and stress in the vessels located upstream from the narrowed and/or collapsed vessels. Consequently, alveolar collapse occurring in the course of mechanical inflation tends to redistribute flow toward extra-alveolar vessels, thereby increasing their transmural pressure and rate of fluid filtration.

During positive pressure ventilation, the majority of capillaries embedded within the alveolar wall are compressed by the expansion of adjoining alveoli. At the same time, lung expansion decreases interstitial pressure, which increases the transmural pressure of the vessels in the intermediate segment. Raising pre-capillary and/or reducing post-capillary microvascular pressures simultaneously, increases the pressure gradient and energy dissipated across the middle segment of the pulmonary microvasculature. These actions appear to worsen edema and/or accentuate barrier injury when airway mechanical stresses are sufficiently high [38]. On the other hand, cyclic opening and closure of the microvessels may amplify shear forces and stretching of the vascular endothelium (similar to that undergone by alveolar wall), with the potential to initiate inflammation-mediated tissue breakdown. Thus, by promoting alveolar vascular collapse and amplifying extra-alveolar vascular stress, excessive reductions in lung volume and microvascular pressure have the potential to contribute to VILI [37].

If raising pre-capillary microvascular pressure and reducing post-capillary pressure might both amplify VILI, how can pre-capillary microvascular pressure be reduced without compromising systemic organ perfusion or lowering pulmonary post-capillary pressures excessively? Reducing tissue demands for O_2 reduces obligate blood flow through the lung, which in turn deceases both upstream microvascular pressure and the luminal transcapillary pressure gradient. Although more studies are clearly necessary to determine the exact relationship between vascular pressure and lung injury, it would seem prudent to diminish unnecessary demands for ventilation and cardiac output: the direct clinical implication is that conditions of agitation, high fever, pain and work of breathing should be avoided when potentially damaging alveolar pressures are approached.

▌ Temperature Preconditioning and Lung Injury

Maintenance of appropriate thermoregulation is essential for normal cellular functioning. Beyond certain defined physiologic limits, enzymatic functioning may be induced or impaired, distorting normal homeostasis. Extremes of temperature may culminate in protein degradation or overt cellular disruption. It is clear that the pace at which temperature aberrations are accomplished strongly impacts their ultimate physiologic effects. Slowly cooling into the range of tolerable hypothermia slows metabolic processes sufficiently to allow tolerance to certain high-risk surgical procedures. In recent years it has also been demonstrated that hypothermia of modest proportions may improve the prognosis of cardiac arrest [45]. Deliberate 'icing' of recently traumatized tissue reduces edema and limits inflammation. Whereas extreme hypothermia due to environmental exposure may be life threatening to a healthy subject, re-warming must be accomplished slowly to prevent life threatening consequences. Extreme hyperthermia is a genuine emergency that must be reversed as rapidly as possible. In recently published work, several groups of investigators have shown that moderate to extreme hypothermia attenuates the adverse response in models of VILI induced purely by mechanical forces and in models characterized by pre-existing inflammation [46].

Preconditioning is a process whereby cells or tissues exposed to a sub-lethal stimulus are transiently protected from a subsequent noxious stress. When preconditioning is conducted using a stressful stimulus (e.g., high temperatures) applied for a tolerable interval, heat shock proteins (HSP) are elaborated (mainly HSP 72) [47]. These HSP act as molecular chaperones against injury for certain classes of vital intracellular proteins, preventing premature folding and denaturation and allowing normal protein assembly, conformation and interactions to proceed under otherwise adverse environmental conditions. Available data also suggest that HSP 72 has significant anti-apoptotic properties in relation to caspase 3, and that it reduces both the level of tumor necrosis factor (TNF)-α and its cytotoxicity [48]. Thermal preconditioning attenuates VILI-associated decreases in lung compliance, reduces the production of inflammatory cytokines, and increases the amount and percentage of large surfactant aggregates (the active portion form) [49]. Following thermal exposure, full expression of these HSP requires hours to develop. It has been demonstrated that experimental animals that have been pre-stressed by heat exposure are more resistant to the adverse effects of such noxious influences as endotoxin when later exposed to it [50].

Although appropriate heat pre-conditioning may be lung protective, heat exposure occurring simultaneously with high pressure ventilation accentuates rather than attenuates VILI. Presumably, the heat shock class of proteins has not yet been elaborated during simultaneous exposure to heat and mechanical stress, whereas destructive inflammatory enzymes are up-regulated, edema clearance mechanisms are overwhelmed, and/or metabolic demands outstrip the delivery of vital energy substrates. Moderate cooling of experimental animals also appears to afford a VILI-protective effect when the mechanical stress is applied simultaneously with the cooling challenge [46]. Although it has yet to be confirmed in patients, such observations illustrate the potential for thermal manipulation to reduce the risk of VILI. Although clearly of unproven benefit and certainly not advocated for clinical application, preventing hyperthermia when high alveolar pressures are necessary or even inducing mild hypothermia (33–35 °C) may eventually prove viable options to reinforce our treatment to VILI.

Conclusion

VILI is undoubtedly a dynamic and complex process that depends on considerably more than the tidal pressures and PEEP which have received the most investigative attention. Many basic experiments have helped us to better understand the multiple cofactors that modulate its expression and have suggested novel therapeutic options. Closer attention to these non-ventilator variables may offer us a chance to further reduce the iatrogenic morbidity associated with the ventilation of patients with acute respiratory failure.

References

1. Brower RG, Matthay M, Schoenfeld D (2002) Meta-analysis of acute lung injury and acute respiratory distress syndrome trials. Am J Respir Crit Care Med 166:1515–1517
2. The ARDS network (2000) Ventilation with lower tidal volumes as compared with traditional tidal volumes for acute lung injury and the acute respiratory distress syndrome. N Engl J Med 342:1301–1308
3. Amato MB, Barbas CS, Medeiros DM, et al (1998) Effect of a protective-ventilation strategy on mortality in the acute respiratory distress syndrome. N Engl J Med 338:347–354
4. Ricard JD, Dreyfuss D, Saumon G (2003) Ventilator-induced lung injury. Eur Respir J 22:2s–9s
5. Ricard JD, Dreyfuss D (2001) Cytokines during ventilator-induced lung injury: a word ofd caution. Anesth Analg 93:251–252
6. Marttynowicz MA, Minor TA, Walters BJ, Hubmayr RD (1999) Regional expansion of oleic acid-injured lungs. Am J Respir Crit Care Med 160:250–258
7. Ranieri VM, Suter AS, Tortorella C, et al (1999) Effect of mechanical ventilation on inflammatory mediators in patients with acute respiratory distress syndrome: a randomized controlled trial. JAMA 282:54–61
8. Pugin J (2003) Molecular mechanisms of lung cell activation induced by cyclic stretch. Crit Care Med 31:S200–S206
9. Nunn JF (1993) Distribution of pulmonary ventilation and perfusion. In: Nunn JF (ed) Nunn's Applied Respiratory Physiology, 4th Ed. Butterworth-Heinemann, Oxford, pp 156–197
10. Pelosi P, Tubiolo D, Mascheroni D, et al (1998) Effects of the prone position on respiratory mechanics and gas exchange during acute lung injury. Am J Respir Crit. Care Med 157:387–393
11. Gattinoni L, Pelosi P, Crotti S, Valenza F (1995) Effects of positive end-expiratory pressure on regional distribution of tidal volume and recruitment in adult respiratory distress syndrome. Am J Respir Crit Care Med 151:1807–1814
12. Marini JJ, Culver BH, Butler J (1981) Mechanical effect of lung distention with positive pressure on ventricular function. Am Rev Respir Dis 124:382–386
13. Broccard A, Shapiro R, Schmitz L, Adams AB, Nahum A, Marini J (2000) Prone positioning attenuates and redistributes ventilator-induced lung injury in dogs. Crit Care Med 28:295–303
14. Johansson MJ, Wiklund A, Flatebo T, Nicolaysen A, Nicolaysen G, Walther SM (2004) PEEP affects regional redistribution of ventilation differently in prone and supine sheep. Crit Care Med 32:2039–2044
15. Gattinoni L, Tognoni G, Pesenti A, et al (2001) Effect of prone positioning on the survival of patients with acute respiratory failure. N Engl J Med 345:568–573
16. Mancebo J, Rialp G, Fernández R, Gordo F, Albert RK (2003) Prone vs supine position in ARDS patients. Results of a randomized multicenter trial. Am J Respir Crit Care Med 167:A180 (abst)
17. Chatte G, Sab JM, Dubois JM, Sirodot M, Gaussorgues P, Robert D (1997) Prone position in mechanically ventilated patients with severe acute respiratory failure. Am J Respir Crit Care Med 155:473–478

18. Gattinoni L, Vagginelli F, Carlesso E, et al (2003) Prone-Supine Study Group Decrease in PaCO$_2$ with prone position is predictive of improved outcome in acute respiratory distress syndrome. Crit Care Med 31:2727–2733

19. Milberg JA, Davis DR, Steinberg KP, Hudson LD (1995) Improved survival in patients with acute respiratory syndrome. JAMA 273:306–309

20. Tobin MJ (1994) Mechanical ventilation. N Engl J Med 330:1056–1061

21. Laffey J, O'Croinin D, McLoughlin P, Kavanagh B (2004) Permissive hypercapnia. Role in protective lung ventilatory strategies. Intensive Care Med 30:347–356

22. Jorgensen EO, Holm S (1999) The course of circulatory and cerebral recovery after circulatory arrest: influence of prearrest, arrest and postarrest factors. Resuscitation 42:173–182

23. Laffey JG, Kavanagh BP (1999) Carbon dioxide and the critically ill – too little of a good thing? Lancet 354:1283–1286

24. Laffey JG, Tanaka M, Engelberts D, et al (2000) Therapeutic hypercapnia reduces pulmonary and systemic injury following in vivo lung reperfusion. Am J Respir Crit Care Med 162:2287–2294

25. Adding LC, Agvald P, Persson MG, Gustafsson LE (1999) Regulation of pulmonary nitric oxide by carbon dioxide is intrinsic to the lung. Acta Physiol Scand 167:167–174

26. Shibata K, Cregg N, Engelberts D, Takeuchi A, Fedorko L, Kavanagh BP (1998) Hypercapnic acidosis may attenuate acute lung injury by inhibition of endogenous xanthine oxidase. Am J Respir Crit Care Med 158:1578–1584

27. Takeshita K, Suzuki Y, Nishio K, et al (2003) Hypercapnic acidosis attenuates endotoxin-induced nuclear factor KB activation. Am J Respir Cell Mol Biol 29:124–132

28. Holmes JM, Duffner LA, Jappil JC (1994) The effect of raised carbon dioxide on developing rat retinal vasculature exposed to elevated oxygen. Curr Eye Res 13:779–782

29. Broccard A, Hotchkiss J, Vannay Ch, et al (2001) Protective effects of hypercapnic acidosis on ventilator-induced lung injury. Am J Respir Crit Care Med 164:802–806

30. Sinclair S, Kregenow D, Lamn W, Starr I, Chi E, Hlastala M (2002) Hypercapnic acidosis is protective in an in vivo model of ventilator-induced lung injury. Am J Respir Crit Care Med 166:403–408

31. Laffey J, Engelberts D, Kavanach B (2000) Buffering hypercapnic acidosis worsens acute lung injury. Am J Respir Crit Care Med 161:141–146

32. Lang JD Jr, Chumley P, Eiserich JP, et al (2000) Hypercapnia induces injury to alveolar epithelial cells via a nitric oxide-dependent pathway. Am J Physiol Lung Cell Mol Physiol 279:L994–L1002

33. Zhu S, Basiouny KF, Crow JP, Matalon S (2000) Carbon dioxide enhances nitration of surfactant protein A by activated alveolar macrophages. Am J Physiol Lung Cell Mol Physiol 278:L1025–L1031

34. Gores GJ, Nieminen AL, Fleishman KE, Dawson TL, Herman B, Lemasters JJ (1998) Extracellular acidosis delays onset of cell death in ATP-depleted hepatocytes. Am J Physiol 255:C315–C322

35. Weber T, Tschernich H, Sitzwohl C, et al (2000) Tromethamine buffer modifies the depressant effect of permissive hypercapnia on myocardial contractility in patients with acute respiratory distress syndrome. Am J Respir Crit Care Med 162:1361–1365

36. Marini JJ, Hotchkiss J, Broccard A (2003) Bench-tobedside review: Microvascular and airspace linkage in ventilator-induced lung injury. Crit Care 7:435–444

37. Broccard A, Hotchkiss JR, Suzuki S, Olson D, Marini JJ (1999) Effects of mean airway pressure and tidal excursion on lung injury induced by mechanical ventilation in an isolated perfused rabbit lung moodel. Crit Care Med 27:1533–1541

38. Broccard A, Hothchkiss JR, Kuwayama N, et al (1998) Consequences of vascular flow on lung injury induced by mechanical ventilation. Am J Respir Crit Care Med 157:1935–1942

39. Hohtchkiss JR, Blanch LL, Murias G, et al (2000) Effects of decreased respiratory frequency on ventilator induced lung injury. Am J Respir Crit Care Med 161:463–468

40. Hotchkiss JR, Blanch LL, Naviera A, Adams AB, Olson D, Marini JJ (2001) Relative roles of vascular and airspace pressures in ventilator induced lung injury. Crit Care Med 29:1593–1598

41. Dreyfuss D, Saumon G (1998) Ventilator-induced lung injury: lessons from experimental studies. Am J Respir Crit Care Med 157:294–323

42. Dreyfuss D, Saumon G (1993) Role of the tidal volume, FRC, and end-inspiratory volume in the development of pulmonary edema following mechanical ventilation. Am Rev Respir Dis 148:1194–1203
43. Broccard A, Vannay Ch, Feihl F, Schaller M (2002) Impact of low pulmonary vascular pressure on ventilator induced lung injury. Crit Care Med 30:2183–2190
44. West JB (1962) Regional differences in gas exchange in the lung of erect man. J Appl Physiol 17:893–901
45. Bernard SA, Gray TW, Buist MD, et al (2002) Treatment of comatose survivors of out-of-hospital cardiac arrest with induced hypothermia. N Engl J Med 346:557–563
46. Suzuki S, Hotchkiss JR, Toshimichi T, Olson D, Adams AB, Marini JJ (2004) Effect of core body temperature on ventilator-induced lung injury. Crit Care Med 32:144–149
47. McCormick PH, Chen G, Tlerney S, Kelly CJ, Bouchier-Hayes DJ (2003) Clinically relevant thermal preconditioning attenuates ischemia-reperfusion injury. J Surg Res 109:24–30
48. Yoo CG, Lee S, Lee CT (2000) Anti-inflammatory effect of HSP induction. J Immunol 164:5416–5423
49. Ribeiro S, Rhee K, Tremblay L, Veldhuizen R, Lewis J, Slutsky A (2001) Heat stress attenuates ventilator-induced lung dysfunction in an ex vivo rat lung model. Am J Respir Crit Care Med 163:1451–1456
50. Villar J, Ribeiro SP, Mullen JB, Kuliszewski M, Post M, Slutsky AS (1994) Induction of the heat shock response reduces mortality rate and organ damage in a sepsis-induced acute lung injury model. Crit Care Med 22:914–921

Assessment of Alveolar Recruitment: New Approaches

G. K. Wolf and J. H. Arnold

▋ Introduction

As we enter the era of lung protective ventilation, there is emerging evidence that ventilation strategy makes a significant difference in outcome. The mortality rates from acute lung injury (ALI) and acute respiratory distress syndrome (ARDS) vary from 30 to 60%. A low tidal volume strategy of 6 ml/kg compared to 12 ml/kg reduced the mortality from 39.8 to 31.0% in 861 patients with ALI [1]. On the other hand, an inappropriate ventilation strategy may produce ventilator-associated lung injury (VALI), which is histopathologically identical to ALI. In a recent study, 24% of patients who did not have ALI at the onset of ventilation developed ALI after a mean of 2.5 days of mechanical ventilation [2]. About one third of the patients in this study were ventilated with tidal volumes of 12–16 ml/kg. Although other risk factors (blood transfusion, academia, and restrictive lung disease) are implicated, the use of large tidal volumes appeared to be the most significant risk factor for the development of ALI.

Lung protective ventilation not only prevents the progression of lung injury, but also limits further multisystem organ failure (MOF). The injured lung fuels MOF by releasing inflammatory mediators such as interleukin (IL)-6 or tumor necrosis factor (TNF)-a into the systemic circulation. The release of pro-apoptotic factors, translocation of bacteria and peripheral immune suppression will furthermore contribute to MOF. A lung protective ventilation strategy may reduce the release of cytokines; TNF-a, IL-6, and IL-8 were reduced in patients ventilated with a lung protective strategy over a control group in 44 patients [3].

In addition to volutrauma, atelectrauma caused by cyclic opening and closing of alveoli is an important contributor to ALI [4, 5]. Reversal of atelectasis with positive end expiratory pressure (PEEP) has become a priority in the management of ARDS. However, a high PEEP level *per se* does not improve mortality. A recent study using a tidal volume of 6 ml/kg showed no significant difference in mortality between a PEEP of 8.3 cm of water and 13.2 cm of water [6, 7]. Adverse effects of PEEP that counteract beneficial effects include hemodynamic compromise by reducing right ventricular preload and alveolar overdistension by increased plateau pressures.

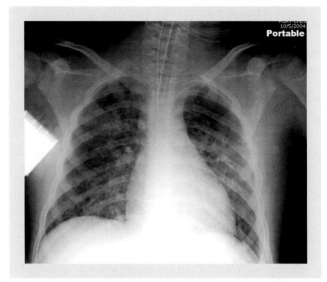

Fig. 1. Chest x-ray of a 12-year-old child with ARDS secondary to sepsis. Findings 24 hours after intubation. The chest x-ray reveals diffuse opacity. (Patient at Children's Hospital, Boston)

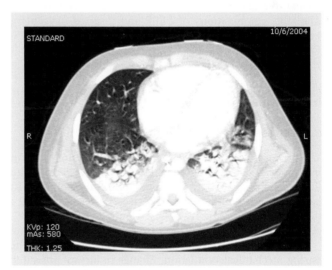

Fig. 2. Chest CT of the same patient as in Fig. 1 on the same day. There is marked alveolar collapse along the gravitational axis in the dorsal, dependent parts of the lung and in the retrocardiac space, not identified by chest x-ray

▌ Chest Radiography

The patient's chest x-ray is routinely used to assess the progression of lung disease. Comparisons between chest computed tomography (CT) and plain chest x-ray in patients with ARDS have clearly shown the low accuracy of frontal bedside x-ray in assessing lung morphology and the distribution of alveolar collapse [8]. Figure 1 shows the chest x-ray of a 16-year-old patient with ARDS secondary to sepsis on day two of mechanical ventilation. The chest x-ray reveals diffuse bilateral homogeneous densities, whereas the chest CT obtained on the same day shows marked abnormality of dependent lung with relative sparing of the anterior lung regions (Fig. 2).

Retrocardiac atelectasis and atelectasis posterior to the diaphragm will not be identified easily by an antero-posterior (AP) chest x-ray but will cause significant impairment in arterial oxygenation. These areas are subject to alveolar collapse in the supine patient due to compression of lung tissue by the heart and abdominal contents.

▌ Arterial Oxygenation

Arterial desaturation as a result of atelectasis is based on the presence of intrapulmonary arterio-venous shunts, which reflects perfusion of non-aerated areas. Alveolar recruitment is associated with improving gas exchange [9, 10]. Suter et al. showed as early as 1975, in 15 patients with acute pulmonary failure, that PEEP improved oxygen transport and decreased physiologic deadspace. They furthermore commented that at optimal PEEP, tidal ventilation occurs on the steep part of the pressure-volume curve during highest compliance [11]. A high correlation between alveolar recruitment and increase in arterial oxygenation was found in a study of 16 patients with ARDS, where recruitment was evaluated with chest CT [12].

In clinical practice, the level of PEEP is usually coupled to the patient's supplemental oxygen requirement, a method that was also used in the ARDSnet trial [1]. Allowable combinations of PEEP and inspired oxygen fraction (FiO_2) in this trial were, for example, FiO_2 0.3/PEEP 5 cmH_2O, FiO_2 0.5/PEEP 8 or 10 cmH_2O and FiO_2 0.8/PEEP 14 cmH_2O.

▌ Assessment of Global Lung Volume

Pressure-volume Curves

The pressure-volume (P/V) curve of the respiratory system has been studied in animal models and in patients with ALI. The P/V curve, characterized by a lower inflection point (LIP) and an upper inflection point (UIP), indicates two potential hazardous areas of ventilation: atelectasis below the LIP and overdistension above the UIP (Fig. 3) [13]. In theory, ventilating in the 'safe zone' between these two points, potentially minimizes atelectrauma and volutrauma.

Dynamic pressure-time curves are generated by application of a constant flow during mechanical ventilation. Change in airway pressure is plotted against time. A straight pressure-time curve indicates constant compliance and minimal stress, a downward concavity inadequate recruitment and an upward concavity overdistension. The shape of the pressure-time curve has been used to identify a lung-protective ventilatory strategy in an animal model of ALI [14].

While it is an important theoretical concept, the application of a static P/V curve at the bedside is limited. A slow inflation maneuver with a positive airway pressure of 40 cm of water over 40 seconds requires sedation and neuromuscular paralysis. Identification of the LIP is potentially difficult and may vary between repeated measurements and different observers.

Imaging the lung in the CT scanner has helped to understand that recruitment occurs along the entire P/V curve. CT images in humans with ALI have convincingly shown that recruitment occurs along the entire P/V curve, well above the LIP

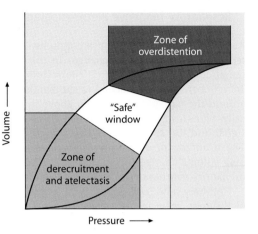

Fig. 3. Ventilating in the 'safe window' during acute lung injury (ALI) is achieved with an adequate PEEP level in combination with low tidal volumes. Note that the 'safe window' is in the area between lower inflection point and upper inflection point. This graph, meant to illustrate high frequency ventilation, applies to conventional ventilation as well. From [13] with permission

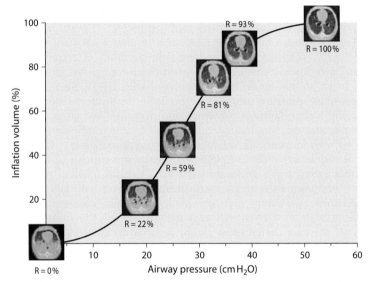

Fig. 4. Recruitment in an experimental ARDS model (canine model). Recruitment occurs along the entire steep part of the pressure-volume curve. R indicates the percentage of atelectasis recruited. At the presumed LIP (second CT image from the left) only 22% of atelectasis is reversed. From [15] with permission

(Fig. 4) [15]. Furthermore, in a canine-model of ARDS, reversal of atelectasis occurred up to airway pressures of 54 cmH$_2$O [16], indicating a large potential for recruitment in dorsal lung areas at airway pressures considered well beyond the 'safe zone'.

Respiratory Inductive Plethysmography

Respiratory inductive plethysmography is a non-invasive respiratory monitoring technique that quantifies changes in the cross-sectional area of the chest wall and the abdominal compartment. The technique uses two elastic bands, which contain Teflon-coated wires attached to the bands in a zigzag form. One is typically placed around the patient's chest, 3 cm above the xyphoid process, and the second is typically placed around the abdomen. Each of these bands produces an independent signal and the sum of these two signals is calibrated against a known gas-volume. The accuracy of respiratory inductive plethysmography in the determination of lung volume changes during the use of conventional ventilation and high frequency oscillatory ventilation (HFOV) has been investigated in a number of animal studies.

Gothberg and colleagues [17] assessed the accuracy of respiratory inductive plethysmography in measuring lung volumes in a newborn animal model. Respiratory inductive plethysmography-derived lung volumes showed a good correlation with injected gas volumes ($r^2 = 0.98$–0.99). P/V curves generated with respiratory inductive plethysmography demonstrated good correlation with the reference method. The authors further reported a change in respiratory inductive plethysmography-derived lung volume after surfactant instillation. This study showed that changes in lung compliance may be detected with respiratory inductive plethysmography during a P/V maneuver and confirmed the accuracy of respiratory inductive plethysmography measurements in the quantification of global lung volumes.

In an animal model of ALI managed with HFOV, Brazelton and colleagues [18] quantified pressure-volume curves using respiratory inductive plethysmography during a super syringe maneuver and demonstrated close correlation with the reference method. Respiratory inductive plethysmography-derived lung volumes correlated with known lung volumes during supersyringe ($r^2 = 0.78$). The authors report that respiratory inductive plethysmography was capable of tracking volume changes and creating a P/V curve during HFOV. Critical opening pressures were identified in 3 of 5 animals during a recruitment maneuver with HFOV. At high mean airway pressures, respiratory inductive plethysmography consistently underestimated lung volumes. Because chest wall expansion is limited, the authors suggested that isovolumic pressure changes may not be detected by respiratory inductive plethysmography [18]. Weber and colleagues used a newborn animal-model to detect lung overdistension during HFOV using respiratory inductive plethysmography [19]. Lung compliance calculated using lung volumes detected by respiratory inductive plethysmography were different before and after induction of lung injury by repetitive saline lavage. This finding demonstrates the potential for respiratory inductive plethysmography to detect a change in lung mechanics during HFOV and the potential to quantify lung volumes non-invasively. Improvements in global lung compliance can be monitored continuously, which may prevent inadvertent lung overdistension produced by delayed weaning of ventilator settings.

Using the same model of lung injury, the authors subsequently described a mathematical prediction tool to optimize mean airway pressure during HFOV using respiratory inductive plethysmography [20]. This model is based on the assumption that the time constant varies significantly depending on the state of lung inflation; different values for effective lung compliance are derived from the specific mean airway pressure. According to this model, the optimal mean airway pressure is indicated by the largest effective compliance. The advantage of this approach is that only relative volume changes are used; therefore, respiratory inductive plethysmography does not have to be accurately calibrated. In the clinical setting, the approach suggested in this study is limited due to the inhomogeneous pattern of alveolar collapse. Average effective compliance includes the compliance of overdistended as well as atelectatic lung tissue.

Respiratory inductive plethysmography has been used in the clinical setting to quantify lung volume changes during suctioning in mechanically ventilated patients in two studies [21, 22]. Maggiore and colleagues [21] compared the loss of lung volume during in-line vs. open suctioning using respiratory inductive plethysmography. Open suctioning caused a greater loss of lung volume than in-line suctioning. Average lung volume loss after disconnection vs. close suctioning was 1466 ml and 531 ml, respectively (p < 0.01). Recruitment maneuvers using the triggering function of the ventilator to deliver 40 cmH2O during endotracheal suctioning prevented the loss of lung volume during suctioning. In a study in the pediatric population, Choong and colleagues came to similar conclusions [22]. These authors further noted that loss of lung volume was related to disconnection from the ventilator rather than to suctioning and was most pronounced in patients with low pulmonary compliance. These two studies show the potential of respiratory inductive plethysmography to contribute to the understanding of derecruitment in the clinical arena.

Although inductive plethysmography offers the potential for non-invasive and continuous assessment of lung volume at the bedside, a number of limitations must be acknowledged. As presently configured, inductive plethysmography allows the quantification of absolute volume change only retrospectively, after appropriate calibration. Finally, it must be acknowledged that even the accurate assessment of lung volume change with a portable, bedside device has its limitations. While many have suggested that the generation of P/V curves at the bedside allows application of lung protective ventilatory strategies and the estimation of the optimal mean airway pressure during mechanical ventilation and HFOV, it is important to emphasize that the information derived from P/V curves is limited. Clearly, the assessment of global lung mechanics does not provide information about changes in regional lung volume or alterations in regional lung behavior.

▌ Assessment of Regional Lung Volumes

Computed Tomography

Twenty years ago first reports of CT in patients during general anesthesia fundamentally changed the understanding of the distribution of atelectasis. Within 5 minutes of induction and muscle relaxation, patients without ALI had developed atelectasis along the gravitational axis, most pronounced in the dorsal lung regions [23]. Gattinoni and colleagues further investigated the inhomogenity of lung disease in patients with ALI using CT [15, 24, 25]. The most important finding is the heterogeneous nature of lung disease during mechanical ventilation: normal to hyperinflated lung is frequently located in nondependent lung areas (ventral in the supine position), ground glass opacification in the middle lung, and consolidation of lung parenchyma in the most dependent lung (dorsal in the supine position). Alveolar collapse is distributed along the gravitational axis as well as the craniocaudal axis. The lung collapses under its own weight, and from mechanical compression of the heart. In a supine patient, pressure from the abdomen accounts for the collapse of the lower lobes, especially dorsal to the diaphragm. In addition, a 'mosaic' distribution of normal and collapsed areas were described in CT, a distribution that does not follow the gravitational or cranio-caudal axis [12].

Positron Emission Tomography Scan

Positron emission tomography (PET) scans have been used to assess the topographical distribution of ventilation and pulmonary blood flow. PET scans, in healthy spontaneously breathing volunteers, have demonstrated a vertical gradient for ventilation and perfusion [26].

In the clinical setting during prone positioning, ventilation-perfusion matching improves primarily by redistribution of ventilation. Recruitment of the previously atelectatic dorsal lung improves ventilation-perfusion matching.

Assessment of ventilation and perfusion during recruitment maneuvers has demonstrated that after a sustained inflation, pulmonary blood flow is diverted to nonaerated regions. Worsening oxygenation after the recruitment maneuver was associated with an increase of intrapulmonary shunt in atelectatic regions. This can be explained by overdistension of nondependent areas resulting in redistribution of pulmonary bloodflow to atelectatic areas. Such changes in pulmonary perfusion persisted for 4–5 min after the recruitment maneuver [27].

Electrical Impedance Tomography

The technical aspects of electrical impedance tomography (EIT) were developed over 20 years ago. Recent interest in this technology has been generated by a number of hardware and software improvements that may allow accurate detection of regional lung volume change. The EIT hardware injects small amounts of electrical current sequentially, using electrodes applied circumferentially to the patient's chest. The receiving electrode calculates the voltage differential and determines the impedance change between the transmitting and receiving electrodes. This creates a tomogram depicting the distribution of tissue electrical properties in a cross sectional image (Fig. 5). A cross sectional image of the lung, comprised of 1024 data points in a 32×32 array, is created using a mathematical algorithm called 'back-projection' [28, 29]. The thickness of this cross-sectional 'slice' of the thorax varies depending on the circumference of the chest and is typically between 15 and 20 cm [30]. It is important to emphasize that no absolute impedance values are generated; rather, impedance changes are generated by referencing all measured voltages to a baseline measurement.

One of the currently available systems is the 'Goe MF II' system that was developed at the University of Göttingen, Germany and is now distributed by Viasys, USA. Other systems used in the past were the Sheffield Mark 1 system and the DAS 01-P system [31, 32]. A comparison study of the three systems showed that the Goe MF II system has the most beneficial signal to noise ratio and allows dynamic measurements at low lung volumes [33].

In current systems, 16 electrodes are applied around the thorax of the patient, although a prototype device that uses 32 electrodes is currently being developed. The scanning rate of the 'Goe MF II' system is between 13 and 44 scans/sec (Hz). This means that the system can generate up to 44 cross-sectional images per second.

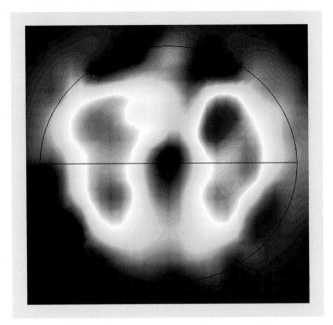

Fig. 5. EIT image of the lung. The orientation is similar to a CT-image. Both lung fields show equal impedance change during spontaneous breathing

The advantage of EIT over respiratory inductive plethysmography is the quantification of regional as well as global changes in lung volume. During offline analysis, a functional impedance image as well as the time course of impedance change vs. time can be displayed. The so-called functional EIT image is a virtual EIT monitor displaying impedance changes within the lung. Standard deviation of impedance change is averaged over 4 seconds in this display. This feature provides the investigator with an almost continuous real-time image of the impedance changes that occur during the ventilatory cycle and are likely directly related to alterations in regional gas volume.

Local impedance change vs. time images can be generated by selecting a specific region of interest within the tomogram. In addition to impedance changes, ventilatory pressures can be recorded simultaneously using a pressure module. Impedance changes can be correlated with airway pressures at a specific time and provide important information about regional changes in lung mechanical behavior in response to alterations in ventilator settings.

The proper interpretation of changes in lung impedance must account for the fact that there are multiple tissues in the thorax and that changes in intrathoracic pressure produce complex interactions between the intrathoracic organs. In general, an increase in aerated lung volume results in a positive impedance change and a decrease in aerated lung volume produces a negative impedance change.

It is essential to recognize that intrathoracic blood volume as well as pulmonary and aortic blood flow influences the EIT signal. Typically, an increase in pulmonary blood volume results in a decrease in relative impedance. Cardiopulmonary interactions during mechanical ventilation influence the EIT signal as follows: a higher mean airway pressure will, to some extent, lower pulmonary blood volume, because blood is displaced due to increasing alveolar pressure. The displacement of blood away from the region of interest will increase measured impedance. This increase in relative impedance change due to displacement of blood volume occurs simultaneously with an increase of impedance change secondary to increasing lung volume. It may be difficult to differentiate between the two effects since they occur at the same time.

In addition, the relative impedance is altered by changes in both right- and left-heart output [34]. The cardiac output-related impedance change is significantly smaller than impedance changes caused by cardiopulmonary interactions. Both physiologic phenomena – alteration of intrathoracic blood volume and blood flow – can be altered by either direct changes in cardiac function or secondarily, by cardiopulmonary interaction during mechanical ventilation.

In an animal model of ALI managed with HFOV, van Genderingen and colleagues assessed regional lung mechanics with EIT [35]. Regional and local impedance change vs. time plots were described during an inflation-deflation maneuver on HFOV. EIT measurements were compared to strain gauge plethysmography and helium dilution. During a pressure volume maneuver using a supersyringe method, the authors reported a regional inhomogenity of lung disease, manifested by different shapes of the P/V curves in dependent (collapsed) and nondependent (recruited) areas. This finding has previously been described by other authors and is related to collapse of alveolar tissue along the gravitational axis [36–38]. During the same P/V maneuver using HFOV, the pressure-impedance curves in dependent and nondependent lung areas were more homogenous. The authors suggested that HFOV has a 'homogenizing effect' and alveolar recruitment is achieved by the opening of 'sticky airways' during HFOV. This finding was not verified by other imaging techniques such as reversal of atelectasis documented by chest CT. This is the first study demonstrating that EIT is capable of tracking lung volume changes during HFOV in an animal model. It also shows the significance of EIT as a functional imaging technique to obtain more insight regarding recruitment phenomena during HFOV.

Frerichs and colleagues compared regional atelectasis using EIT and CT in an animal model of ALI [39]. The animals were ventilated with five different tidal volumes at three different PEEP levels. Local air content was compared with CT and EIT in ventral, middle, and dorsal lung areas on the left and on the right side of the lung. The correlation was strongest in the dependent areas ($r^2 = 0.86$) and acceptable in nondependent areas ($r^2 = 0.66$). The authors attributed the worsening correlation in nondependent areas to movement artifacts during tidal ventilation that increased variability in the lung density measured by CT. These artifacts do not occur during EIT. Time resolution of the EIT scans (13 scans/second) was higher than time resolution of CT scans (3.3 scans/second). The significance of this study is that it confirmed the correlation of impedance changes and volume changes using CT as a reference method in an animal model.

Kunst and colleagues [37] identified regional P/V curves in an animal model with ALI. P/V curves obtained with the supersyringe method were correlated to pressure-impedance curves determined by EIT. The authors were able to show distinct differences in regional pressure-impedance curves by dividing the lung into four different layers. The LIP was 8 cm higher in the most dependent lung compared to the nondependent part of the lung. The authors attributed these differences to increased collapse of atelectasis-prone lung in dorsal areas following the induction of ALI. This study demonstrates the potential for EIT to detect regional alveolar collapse during mechanical ventilation.

A dynamic approach to assess regional recruitment was described in a similar animal model by the same authors. During conventional ventilation, regional impedance changes over time were compared in dependent and nondependent areas [37]. During ALI, impedance changes were decreased in dorsal lung areas, suggesting regional collapse. After a recruitment maneuver, the authors reported improving regional impedance changes in previously collapsed areas. In theory, a ratio of equal impedance changes in dependent and nondependent parts of the lung suggests homogeneous distribution of ventilation to all lung regions. However, this concept has not yet been associated with improved physiologic or pathologic outcomes. Therefore, it remains speculative whether the equalization of impedance changes in all lung areas detected by EIT scans produces optimal lung protection.

The correlation of regional impedance changes in patients with ALI with lung density measurements by CT has been recently verified in a study by Victorino and colleagues [40]. In this study, a slow inflation maneuver was recorded with EIT in 10 intubated and mechanically ventilated adult patients. Subsequently, the same inflation maneuver was performed in the CT scanner. Air content seen on the CT scan was compared to regional impedance changes in the EIT-slice (Fig. 6). Both techniques detected imbalances in ventilation of dependent and nondependent lung areas (upper/lower ratio = 82/18% and 75/25% for EIT and CT). Regional impedance changes on the EIT image showed good correlation ($r^2 = 0.92$) to changes in air content detected by CT. Furthermore, EIT scans showed good reproducibility (SD 4.9%) between repeated measurements on the same patient. It should be noted that CT and EIT images were not obtained simultaneously due to electromagnetic interference of the EIT equipment in the CT scanner. Nevertheless, the authors attempted to minimize this methodological problem by averaging EIT scans obtained prior to and after CT as well as the use of standardized recruitment maneuvers prior to each inflation sequence. This study confirmed that regional impedance changes are closely correlated with regional volume changes identified by CT. This is relevant to

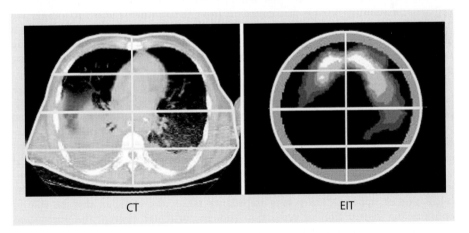

CT   EIT

Fig. 6. Comparison of a CT scan and an electrical impedance tomography (EIT) image during mechanical ventilation of a patient with acute lung injury (ALI). The gray and white areas in the EIT images reflect areas with impedance change (volume changes) and correlate to well inflated areas in the CT scan. There is no impedance change on the EIT scan in the dorsal areas, where atelectasis is present on the CT scan. From [40] with permission

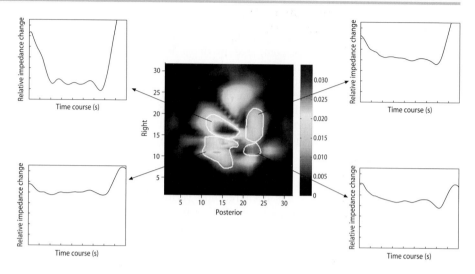

Fig. 7. Derecruitment maneuver in a pediatric patient with ARDS. The gray areas in the EIT image in the middle indicate large impedance change. This corresponds to volume loss in previously well-recruited lung areas during suctioning. The graphs display the magnitude of impedance change over time. Loss of lung volume was most pronounced in the upper right (upper left in the image) lung area

the future use of EIT at the bedside, where ventilation and recruitment strategies could potentially target regional atelectasis identified by the EIT image.

Our group has utilized EIT to detect lung volume changes during a standardized suctioning maneuver in children ventilated with a high frequency oscillatory device (Sensormedics 3100A, Viasys Corp, Yorba Linda, CA). We were able to demonstrate that EIT can be used to detect and quantify regional lung volume changes in the pediatric population during disconnection from the ventilator and suctioning. We have demonstrated considerable regional heterogeneity in volume changes during a derecruitment maneuver. The regional impedance change in four different lung areas during suctioning shows a significant difference in impedance change during derecruitment (Fig. 7).

The experimental data regarding current EIT technology suggest a reliable correlation between global lung volume changes and global impedance changes in multiple animal models. Furthermore, regional impedance changes have demonstrated acceptable correlation with regional changes in lung volume seen on CT during mechanical ventilation. Alveolar recruitment has been demonstrated using EIT by generating regional pressure-impedance curves for different lung areas. In the clinical setting, the most non-compliant area with the highest LIP can be carefully monitored in order to apply adequate airway pressure for recruitment. Furthermore, by calculation of upper to lower lung impedance ratios, the clinician may be able to optimize the distribution of ventilation and, in particular, prevent the overdistension of non-dependent lung during aggressive lung recruitment maneuvers.

▌ Conclusion

As we further delineate the inhomogeneous distribution of lung disease, it is increasingly evident that regional assessment of alveolar recruitment is essential to guide ventilator management of patients with ARDS. Respiratory inductance plethysmography and EIT are two non-invasive monitoring devices that have the potential to be used in the clinical arena. EIT is the only bedside method that offers the potential for repeated, non-invasive measurements of regional lung volume changes. It offers the potential to detect regional atelectasis at the bedside and to alter the ventilation strategy in real time to reverse it. However, the continued evolution of EIT technology is essential. As EIT devices evolve to meet these challenges, it will be important for investigators to standardize the definitions of alveolar recruitment, explore the optimal relationships between regional impedance change ratios, and ultimately to demonstrate the superiority of EIT-guided ventilator management in providing lung protective ventilation.

References

1. The Acute Respiratory Distress Syndrome Network (2000) Ventilation with lower tidal volumes as compared with traditional tidal volumes for acute lung injury and the acute respiratory distress syndrome. N Engl J Med 342:1301–1308
2. Gajic O, Dara SI, Mendez JL, et al (2004) Ventilator-associated lung injury in patients without acute lung injury at the onset of mechanical ventilation. Crit Care Med 32:1817–1824
3. Ranieri VM, Suter PM, Tortorella C, et al (1999) Effect of mechanical ventilation on inflammatory mediators in patients with acute respiratory distress syndrome: a randomized controlled trial. JAMA 282:54–61
4. Chu EK, Whitehead T, Slutsky AS (2004) Effects of cyclic opening and closing at low- and high-volume ventilation on bronchoalveolar lavage cytokines. Crit Care Med 32:168–174
5. Slutsky AS (1999) Lung injury caused by mechanical ventilation. Chest 116:9S–15S
6. Brower RG, Lanken PN, MacIntyre N, et al (2004) Higher versus lower positive end-expiratory pressures in patients with the acute respiratory distress syndrome. N Engl J Med 351:327–336
7. Levy MM (2004) PEEP in ARDS–how much is enough? N Engl J Med 351:389–391
8. Rouby JJ, Puybasset L, Nieszkowska A, Lu Q (2003) Acute respiratory distress syndrome: lessons from computed tomography of the whole lung. Crit Care Med 31:S285–295
9. Maggiore SM, Jonson B, Richard JC, Jaber S, Lemaire F, Brochard L (2001) Alveolar derecruitment at decremental positive end-expiratory pressure levels in acute lung injury: comparison with the lower inflection point, oxygenation, and compliance. Am J Respir Crit Care Med 164:795–801
10. Ranieri VM, Eissa NT, Corbeil C, et al (1991) Effects of positive end-expiratory pressure on alveolar recruitment and gas exchange in patients with the adult respiratory distress syndrome. Am Rev Respir Dis 144:544–551
11. Suter PM, Fairley HB, Isenberg DI (1975) Optimun end-expiratory airway pressure in patients with acute pulmonary failure. N Engl J Med 292:284–289
12. Malbouisson LM, Muller JC, Constantin JM, Lu Q, Puybasset L, Rouby JJ (2001) Computed tomography assessment of positive end-expiratory pressure-induced alveolar recruitment in patients with acute respiratory distress syndrome. Am J Respir Crit Care Med 163:1444–1450
13. Froese AB (1997) High-frequency oscillatory ventilation for adult respiratory distress syndrome: let's get it right this time! Crit Care Med 25:906–908
14. Ranieri VM, Zhang H, Mascia L, et al (2000) Pressure-time curve predicts minimally injurious ventilatory strategy in an isolated rat lung model. Anesthesiology 93:1320–1328
15. Gattinoni L, Caironi P, Pelosi P, Goodman LR (2001) What has computed tomography taught us about the acute respiratory distress syndrome? Am J Respir Crit Care Med 164:1701–1711
16. Pelosi P, Goldner M, McKibben A, et al (2001) Recruitment and derecruitment during acute respiratory failure: an experimental study. Am J Respir Crit Care Med 164:122–130

17. Gothberg S, Parker TA, Griebel J, Abman SM, Kirsella JP (2001) Lung volume recruitment in lambs during high-frequency oscillatory ventilation using respiratory inductive plethysmography. Pediatr Res 49:38–44
18. Brazelton TB 3rd, Watson KF, Murphy M, Al-Khadra E, Thompson JE, Arnold JH (2001) Identification of optimal lung volume during high-frequency oscillatory ventilation using respiratory inductive plethysmography. Crit Care Med 29:2349–2359
19. Weber K, Courtney SE, Pyon KH, Chang GY, Pandit PB, Habib RH (2000) Detecting lung overdistention in newborns treated with high-frequency oscillatory ventilation. J Appl Physiol 89:364–372
20. Habib RH, Pyon KH, Courtney SE (2002) Optimal high-frequency oscillatory ventilation settings by nonlinear lung mechanics analysis. Am J Respir Crit Care Med 166:950–953
21. Maggiore SM, Lellouche F, Pigeot J, et al (2003) Prevention of endotracheal suctioning-induced alveolar derecruitment in acute lung injury. Am J Respir Crit Care Med 167:1215–1224
22. Choong K, Chatrkaw P, Frndova H, Cox PN (2003) Comparison of loss in lung volume with open versus in-line catheter endotracheal suctioning. Pediatr Crit Care Med 4:69–73
23. Brismar B, Hedenstierna G, Lundquist H, Strandberg A, Svensson L, Tokics L (1985) Pulmonary densities during anesthesia with muscular relaxation – a proposal of atelectasis. Anesthesiology 62:422–428
24. Gattinoni L, Presenti A, Torresin A, et al (1986) Adult respiratory distress syndrome profiles by computed tomography. J Thorac Imaging 1:25–30
25. Gattinoni L, D'Andrea L, Pelosi P, Vitale G, Pesenti A, Fumagalli R (1993) Regional effects and mechanism of positive end-expiratory pressure in early adult respiratory distress syndrome. JAMA 269:2122–2127
26. Musch G, Layfield JD, Harris RS, et al (2002) Topographical distribution of pulmonary perfusion and ventilation, assessed by PET in supine and prone humans. J Appl Physiol 93:1841–1851
27. Musch G, Harris RS, Vidal Melo MF, et al (2004) Mechanism by which a sustained inflation can worsen oxygenation in acute lung injury. Anesthesiology 100:323–330
28. Barber DC (1989) A review of image reconstruction techniques for electrical impedance tomography. Med Phys 16:162–169
29. Brown BH (2003) Electrical impedance tomography (EIT): a review. J Med Eng Technol 27:97–108
30. Blue RS, Isaacson D, Newell JC (2000) Real-time three-dimensional electrical impedance imaging. Physiol Meas 21:15–26
31. Frerichs I (2000) Electrical impedance tomography (EIT) in applications related to lung and ventilation: a review of experimental and clinical activities. Physiol Meas 21:R1–21
32. Hahn G, Beer M, Frerichs I, Dudykevych T, Schroder T, Hellige G (2000) A simple method to check the dynamic performance of electrical impedance tomography systems. Physiol Meas 21:53–60
33. Hahn G, Thiel F, Dudykevych T, et al (2001) Quantitative evaluation of the performance of different electrical tomography devices. Biomed Tech (Berl) 46:91–95
34. Smit HJ, Vonk Noordegraaf A, Marcus JT, Boonstra A, de Vries PM, Postmus PE (2004) Determinants of pulmonary perfusion measured by electrical impedance tomography. Eur J Appl Physiol 92:45–49
35. van Genderingen HR, van Vught AJ, Jansen JR (2004) Regional lung volume during high-frequency oscillatory ventilation by electrical impedance tomography. Crit Care Med 32:787–794
36. Arnold JH (2004) Electrical impedance tomography: on the path to the Holy Grail. Crit Care Med 32:894–895
37. Kunst PW, Vazquez de Anda G, Bohm SH, et al (2000) Monitoring of recruitment and derecruitment by electrical impedance tomography in a model of acute lung injury. Crit Care Med 28:3891–3895
38. Kunst PW, de Vries PM, Postmus PE, Bakker J (1999) Evaluation of electrical impedance tomography in the measurement of PEEP-induced changes in lung volume. Chest 115:1102–1106
39. Frerichs I, Hinz J, Herrmann P, et al (2002) Detection of local lung air content by electrical impedance tomography compared with electron beam CT. J Appl Physiol 93:660–666
40. Victorino JA, Borges JB, Okamoto VN, et al (2004) Imbalances in regional lung ventilation: a validation study on electrical impedance tomography. Am J Respir Crit Care Med 169:791–800

Lung Biopsy in Acute Respiratory Distress Syndrome

S. Y. Donati, C. Doddoli, and L. Papazian

▌ Introduction

The etiological diagnosis of pulmonary infiltrations on chest radiography in intensive care unit (ICU) patients remains an everyday problem, especially in cases of acute respiratory distress syndrome (ARDS) where numerous factors can come into play. In terms of survival, Meduri et al. demonstrated the potential benefits of anti-inflammatory treatment instituted in the late stages of ARDS during the fibroproliferative phase [1]. However, the benefits of this approach require differentiation of an infection and the beginning of fibrosis. Current microbiological examinations (tracheal aspiration, protected specimen brush [PSB], bronchoalveolar lavage [BAL]) lack sensitivity and/or specificity for the diagnosis of infection. The unsuitable character of these examinations for the diagnosis of fibrosis, despite the possibility of dosing serum and alveolar biological markers of fibrosis, such as procollagen III, justify performing histologic and microbiologic analysis of lung parenchyma samples obtained by biopsy.

After a discussion of the pathologic lesions found in ARDS, we will attempt to define the indications for lung biopsy in patients with ARDS. We will describe the different sampling techniques used, as well as the treatment and analysis of samples. We will conclude with the clinical consequences of such research and propose an attitude for ICU practice.

▌ ARDS: Histological Aspects

The mechanisms of ARDS development are only partially known despite the fact that they have been studied for over 20 years. These mechanisms differ according to whether the ARDS is primary (direct aggression of the alveoli) or secondary (indirect systemic aggression). Despite these physiopathologic differences, the anatomopathologic abnormalities encountered are quite similar. In fact, during ARDS, there is a succession, or even coexistence, of three phases that can be distinguished histologically.

Early Phase

In the early phase (or exsudative phase), an intraalveolar and interstitial exudate made up of plasmatic proteins, fibrin, and inflammation cells essentially with polynuclear neutrophils and eosinophils, will appear in the first hours and persist for at least one week [2]. During this phase, the alveolar surfactant is altered by a modification in its composition and its functional capacities (alteration of its tensioactive properties). At this stage, there can already be associated morphological lesions of the alveolocapillary barrier with stripping of the endothelial and epithelial basal membrane. Cellular destruction therefore involves the type I epithelial cells (cellular lysis and/or apoptosis) rather than the endothelial cells. The intensity of the epithelial lesions is recognized as an important prognostic factor in ARDS [3]. Macroscopically, the lung has a 'heavy' appearance, edematous or even hemorrhagic, with the section showing a consolidated parenchyma.

Fibro-proliferative Phase

This interstitial and alveolar exudate is then infiltrated by macrophages and fibroblasts. Various activated proteases (elastase, neutrophils, gelatinases) will damage the basal membrane and the extracellular matrix. This so-called organization (or proliferation) phase is characterized by the proliferation of type II pneumocytes, endothelial cells and fibroblasts. The latter have the morphological characteristics of myofibroblasts. Fibroblast proliferation is mediated by signaling molecules (fibronectin, collagen fragments, fibrin, elastin), growth factors and tumor necrosis factor (TNF)-α. Alveolar collapse occurs in the most severely damaged regions with the occasional appearance of real endoalveolar buds. From a macroscopic point of view, the lung has a pale gray color and a smooth surface.

Vascular Lesions. During these first two phases there is increased pulmonary capillary permeability (in part responsible for the exudate) as well as a reduction in the number and the volume of these capillaries [4]. Microthrombi are found with the presence of fibrinoplatelet clusters in the arterioles and capillaries associated with fibrin clots in the pre-acinary and acinary arterioles. At the level of the pulmonary artery, the presence of thrombi appears to be the rule as seen in an autopsy study where this type of lesion was found in 95% of the cases [5]. The vascular structural modification, which can subsequently occur (microcirculatory fibrous occlusion, smooth muscle hypertrophy), thereby contributes to pulmonary arterial hypertension, which is frequently described in ARDS and is associated with poor outcome.

Fibrosis Phase

The proliferation phase can evolve toward fibrosis, a factor of poor outcome [6]. Such fibrosis was found in 40% of the cases in a series of open-lung biopsies performed in 36 patients with ARDS [7]. Fibrosis is formed by an anarchic endoalveolar and septal deposit of type III collagen, then type I, secreted by the fibroblasts. Alveolar and capillary spaces are therefore obstructed, considerably disturbing pulmonary architecture and function. At this stage, the edema has usually disappeared. In addition, there is intraalveolar angiogenesis in response to excessive growth factor production. Macroscopically, the lung has a rough appearance, with a pale and spongiform appearance in sections. Numerous cystic areas and fibrous scars are often observed. Fibrosis can be detected beginning on the fifth day of ARDS. The process most certainly begins earlier given the presence of procollagen III (precursor of collagen synthesis) at elevated levels in the alveolar liquid after 24 hours of evolution [8, 9]. Elevated plasma and alveolar procollagen III levels appear to be predictive markers for ARDS mortality [10, 11]. However, to our knowledge, no study has correlated procollagen levels with the presence of fibrosis confirmed by lung biopsy.

These three phases are, in reality, superimposed in space and time, thereby creating a great heterogeneity of pulmonary lesions in the same patient.

▌ Lung Biopsy Indications in ARDS

There are two essential reasons that move a clinician to perform or prescribe lung parenchyma sampling within the framework of ARDS:
▌ Define an etiology that is potentially curable when less invasive examinations such as BAL have not been conclusive,
▌ Reveal the signs of fibrosis in order to prescribe a possible anti-inflammatory corticoid treatment that could contribute to the chances for survival [1].

Such potentially immunosuppressive corticotherapy is not without risk. In pulmonary infection, microbiologic sampling techniques can lack sensitivity or specificity [12–15], particularly for virus, to contraindicate or delay corticotherapy after beginning an adapted anti-infectious treatment. A series of 36 patients with ARDS who had undergone surgical pulmonary biopsy had cytomegalovirus (CMV) in 50% of the cases [7]. Moreover, biologic analysis of alveolar liquid by dosage of certain markers such as cytokines, alveolar proteins, procollagen III for diagnosis of fibrosis is not yet in current practice.

Lung biopsy could, therefore, be indicated when initial examinations are not conclusive, when ARDS is not evolving favorably after five days (no reduction in Lung Injury Score [LIS] [16]) or earlier if a neoplasic etiology is suspected. The absolute or relative contraindications, hemorrhagic, hemodynamic, or respiratory risks must be taken into account according to the technique under consideration. The risk of transporting a patient to the operating room if the procedure is not possible at the bedside in the ICU must also be evaluated.

▌ Lung Biopsy Techniques

Transparietal Biopsies

Transparietal (percutaneous) biopsy can be performed under fluoroscopy, tomodensitometry, or ultrasound with a specific needle. The major risk of pneumothorax in a ventilated patient makes this technique inadvisable, particularly in ARDS patients. In addition, the yield of this technique in the framework of a diffuse process is very debatable given the small sample size. However, this type of sampling has a place in peripheral radiological opacity exploration, especially in thoracic oncology.

Transbronchial Biopsies

Transbronchial biopsy is performed under bronchial endoscopy (flexible fiberscope or rigid endoscope) directed or not by fluoroscopy. Four to seven biopsies are performed in the same territory to provide for both microbiologic and histologic analyses. This is an attractive technique for pneumologists because it is usually practiced with a flexible fiberscope in awake patients under local anesthesia. A few studies have demonstrated the feasibility and safety of this technique in patients under mechanical ventilation [6, 17, 18]. Simple measures must therefore be taken during this procedure: increase of FiO_2 to 1, discontinuation of positive end-expiratory pressure (PEEP) and rise of maximum pressure alarms. In a recent study of 38 mechanically ventilated patients [19], all with unexplained pulmonary infiltration, BAL and transbronchial biopsy were successively performed. They provided a diagnosis in 74% of the subjects and led to a modification in treatment in 63% of the cases. Transbronchial biopsy alone ensured a diagnosis in 63% of the cases whereas BAL alone provided a diagnosis in 29%. In the subgroup of late-phase ARDS patients (n = 11), the diagnosis was established in 64% of the cases by associating both diagnostic methods: fibroproliferation was found in all of the cases, leading to prescription of corticoids. An examination of the various studies on the subject reveals that transbronchial biopsy provides a diagnosis in an average of 40% of the cases. Nevertheless, the yield of this technique is controversial given the small size of the samples or their low numbers, which sometimes make a quality histological examination difficult [7]. In a study of 116 transbronchial biopsies, Fraire et al. reported a correlation between the number of fragments obtained, the number of alveoli per fragment (more than 20) and the specificity of the histologic results in the diagnosis of infectious pneumonia [20]. A study comparing transbronchial biopsy with open-lung biopsy in 20 patients with chronic pulmonary infiltration demonstrated the superiority of the surgical technique with a diagnosis in 94% of the cases for surgical biopsy and 59% with transbronchial biopsy [21]. However, there are still some arguments in favor of the latter, such as the simplicity of its performance and the possibility to repeat the examination more easily than in the case of surgical biopsy. The risks of this technique in addition to those inherent to bronchial endoscopy are essentially pneumothorax, pneumomediastinum, and hemoptysis. The lateral bronchi of the basal pyramid appear to offer less risk in terms of pneumothorax [22]. In cases of diffuse pulmonary pathology, the American Thoracic Society does not recommend systematic use of fluoroscopy since it did not appear to modify yield or the risks of this procedure in a non-randomized prospective study [23]. The risk of hemoptysis is reduced by ensuring that the coagulation results and platelet count are compatible with the procedure. An old prospective series of 5450 transbronchial biopsies performed in non-ventilated patients reported a mortality rate of 0.25% (13 deaths, including 9 attributable to hemorrhagic complications, the majority with hemostasis problems). This same study showed the need for pneumothorax drainage in 5.5% of the cases [24]. Studies performed in ventilated patients have reported a mean incidence of 12% for pneumothorax (requiring drainage) without persistent bronchopleural fistula [6, 17, 18, 25, 26] and of 11% for moderate bleeding.

Surgical Biopsies

Surgical lung biopsies are performed by video-assisted thoracoscopy or by thoracotomy. With ARDS, only biopsy by thoracotomy (open-lung biopsy) can be performed since it is impossible to do the selective intubation required for surgical thoracoscopy. These open-lung biopsies can be performed at the bedside in the ICU. This technique is of great interest for patients who can only be transported to the operating room with great difficulty given their frequent hemodynamic and respiratory instability.

Technique. Anticoagulants must be stopped, when possible, at least six hours before the biopsy. The surgeon and the intensivist together must choose the side for sampling. The choice is preferably the most pathologic side unless pleural symphysis is suspected or in case of a history of lung resection on the same side. These elements are evaluated from the patient's history, chest x-ray and, if necessary, thoracic CT scan. During the biopsy, FiO_2 is set at 1. The patient is positioned in the supine position. A pad is positioned along the scapula homolateral to the biopsy in order to tilt the patient approximately 15°. The homolateral upper limb is held in abduction with the forearm folded up over the head. A portable monopolar electrocoagulator is essential to complete hemostasis. An anterolateral thoracotomy of approximately 10 cm is performed in the fifth intercostal space. Pleural liquid (serofibrinous effusion is present in two-thirds of the patients) is sampled for cytologic and microbiologic analysis. Extreme care must be taken in handling the pulmonary tissue in order to avoid alveolar rupture. Particular attention is given to hemostasis. A single but broad biopsy is performed in an area that appears to be macroscopically pathologic. It is most often performed at the level of the lingula, from the middle or the lower lobes. The biopsy is performed with mechanical forceps with linear stapling. The ventilator must be temporarily disconnected in order to limit tissue thickness to ensure better aerostasis. The parenchymatous sample is then cut into four parts and each fragment is packaged in a specific manner for histologic, bacteriologic, virologic, and parasito-mycologic analyses. Two drains – an anterior and a posterior – are inserted. The mean duration of the procedure is 30 minutes. Verification by chest X-ray is performed at the end of the procedure.

Monitoring. Monitoring is essentially clinical and radiological. Air leaks are evaluated, blood loss is evaluated daily and the surgical wound is regularly examined for any local complications. Chest X-ray is performed daily until the drains are taken out which is usually done after weaning from the ventilator.

Complications. It appears that no cases of peroperative death directly attributable to the biopsy have been reported in the literature [7, 27–30]. The postoperative complications generally reported are prolonged air leak (15 to 20% of cases) [7, 28, 30]. Evolution, most often spontaneously favorable, can require mobilization of the thoracic drains or placement of a new pleural drain. Other complications such as parenchymatous or pleural infections or hemorrhages are rarely observed [7, 30]. Table 1 summarizes the results concerning the ventilatory conditions and complications encountered in series of surgical pulmonary biopsies [7, 27, 28, 31–34].

Packaging, Preparation and Analysis of the Samples

Packaging of the samples. The transbronchial biopsies must be immediately fixed in formalin 10% or in Bouin liquid. It is unadvisable to fragment this type of biopsy owing to the risk of damaging it and making morphologic analysis impossible. The minimum duration of fixing in formalin is usually short for small samples for which the time of sampling must be noted. Once fixed, the sample is handled conventionally by an anatomopathologic laboratory: dehydration, inclusion in paraffin, and preparation of several histologic sections stained with hematoxylin-eosin. Depending on the conventional morphologic aspect and the clinical context, the analysis can be completed by immunohistochemical study of specific antibodies. On average, the histologic results of a biopsy are available 24 hours after the sampling.

Table 1. Comparison of seven series of surgical biopsies

	n	Place	PEEP	PaO$_2$/FiO$_2$	Complications
Hill [31]	42	ICU	6.5 (0–15)	84 (30–350)	1 bubbling 1 hemothorax 1 infection
Ashbaugh [32]	10	?	10–20	42–74	0
Warner [33]	20	OR	?	?	?
Meduri [27]	7	OR	?	?	?
Canver [28]	27	OR	9±0.8	?	6 bubbling 2 pneumothorax
Meduri [34]	12	OR	?	?	1 bubbling
Papazian [7]	37	ICU (25) OR (12)	5–16	79–304	1 pneumothorax 1 hemothorax

OR: operating room

Table 2. Principal staining used for biopsies

Staining	Principal infectious agents
▍ Gram/Giemsa	Bacteria
▍ Gomori-Grocott	Fungal agents (pneumocystis, aspergillus, histoplasma…)
▍ PAS (Periodic Acid Schiff)	Fungal agents
▍ Ziehl	Mycobacteria

For morphologic analysis of transbronchial biopsy, three whole biopsy fragments are sent directly to the different laboratories (bacteriology, virology and parasito-mycology) in dry sterile jars for staining according to the clinical orientation (Table 2), direct immunofluorescence for legionella and culture on bacteriologic, virologic and mycologic media.

Surgical lung biopsies performed by thoracotomy require, for optimal results, good coordination of the intensivist, the surgeon and the pathologist. In order to avoid contamination, samples for infectious purposes are ideally sent directly from the operating room or the ICU to the microbiology laboratory in dry sterile jars where they are processed like the transbronchial biopsy. Samples for histologic purposes are sent to the anatomopathologic laboratory at a cool temperature in a dry flask with a screwed top and without the addition of a liquid. Samples must therefore be delivered as soon as possible – within a maximum of one hour following the sampling. On reception and according to the clinical context communicated by the intensivist, specific analyses for microbiologic purposes can then be performed on the surgical specimen. Fragments can be frozen in nitrogen for molecular biology study or immunofluorescence or be placed in glutaraldehyde for study by electronic microscopy. The rest of the surgical specimen is fixed in formalin 10%. If the biopsy is small, it is always better to favor conventional morphology and fix the entire sample in formalin. The fixed fragment is processed in a conventional manner in an anatomopathologic laboratory like the transbronchial biopsy.

▮ Clinical Consequences

The clinical consequences of pulmonary biopsy performed within the framework of ARDS can be major. Therapeutic modifications can be prescribed according to the anatomopathologic and/or microbiologic results: corticotherapy in case of fibroproliferation or fibrosis; prescription or modification of anti-infectious treatment, particularly in the framework of a cytomegalovirus or herpes infection [7]. In the same manner, a prognosis can be totally changed by these results: discovery of a potentially curable etiology, diagnosis of primary or secondary lung cancer (carcinomatous lymphangitis essentially in the framework of ARDS), fibrosis, which could benefit from anti-inflammatory treatment, worsening the vital prognosis. The time period before a specific treatment is administered (particularly corticotherapy in case of fibrosis) can be shortened by the carrying out of a rapid analysis before fixing and a more detailed analysis of the principal specimen, with a small fragment immediately taken to an anatomopathologic laboratory. In the same manner, immediate analysis makes it possible to avoid prescription of potentially deleterious corticotherapy if signs of infection, particularly viral, are detected. In a series of 36 patients [7] where prescription of corticotherapy was considered before surgical biopsy, only 40% (15 patients) really had an indication for anti-inflammatory treatment on receipt of the anatomopathologic results owing to the presence of fibroproliferation or fibrosis. Only six patients benefited from such treatment straightaway – the nine others had CMV on biopsy.

▮ Conclusion

We propose a practical attitude to the diagnosis and specific treatment of ARDS, based on lung biopsy. BAL is used to look for etiology and anti-infectious treatment is prescribed if pulmonary infection is suspected. If ARDS persists after 7–10 days of evolution despite an adapted treatment and if the BAL is negative, surgical biopsy is undertaken and followed by specific treatment once the results are known.

References

1. Meduri GU, Headley AS, Golden E, et al (1998) Effect of prolonged methylprednisolone therapy in unresolving acute respiratory distress syndrome: a randomized controlled trial. JAMA 280:159–165
2. Ware LB, Matthay MA (2000) The acute respiratory distress syndrome. N Engl J Med 342:1334–1349
3. Ware LB, Matthay MA (2001) Alveolar fluid clearance is impaired in the majority of patients with acute lung injury and the acute respiratory distress syndrome. Am J Respir Crit Care Med 163:1376–1383
4. Tomashefski J (2000) Pulmonary pathology of acute respiratory distress syndrome. Clin Chest Med 21:435–466
5. Tomashefski J, Davies P, Boggis C, Zapol W, Reid L (1983) The pulmonary vascular lesions of the adult respiratory distress syndrome. Am J Pathol 112:112–126
6. Martin C, Papazian L, Payan MJ, Saux P, Gouin F (1995) Pulmonary fibrosis correlates with outcome in adult respiratory distress syndrome: a study in mechanically ventilated patients. Chest 107:196–200
7. Papazian L, Thomas P, Bregeon F, et al (1998) Open-lung biopsy in patients with acute respiratory distress syndrome. Anesthesiology 88:935–944

8. Marshall RP, Bellingan G, Webb S, et al (2000) Fibroproliferation occurs early in the acute respiratory distress syndrome and impacts on outcome. Am J Respir Crit Care Med 162:1783–1788

9. Chestnutt AN, Matthay MA, Tibayan FA, Clark JG (1997) Early detection of type III procollagen peptide in acute lung injury. Pathogenetic and prognostic significance. Am J Respir Crit Care Med 156:840–845

10. Clark JG, Milberg JA, Steinberg KP, Hudson LD (1995) Type III procollagen peptide in the adult respiratory syndrome. Ann Intern Med 122:17–23

11. Meduri GU, Tolley EA, Chinn A, Stentz F, Postlehwaite A (1998) Procollagen types I and III aminoterminal propeptide levels during acute respiratory distress syndrome and in response to methylprednisolone treatment. Am J Respir Crit Care Med 158:1432–1441

12. Torres A, El-Ebiary M, Padro L, et al (1994) Validation of different techniques for the diagnosis of ventilator-associated pneumonia. Comparison with immediate postmortem pulmonary biopsy. Am J Respir Crit Care Med 149:324–331

13. Marquette CH, Georges H, Wallet F, et al (1993) Diagnostic efficiency of endotracheal aspirates with quantitative bacterial cultures in intubated patients with suspected pneumonia. Am Rev Respir Dis 148:138–144

14. Chastre J, Fagon JY, Bornet-Lesco M (1995) Evaluation of bronchoscopic techniques for the diagnosis of nosocomial pneumonia. Am J Respir Crit Care Med 152:231–240

15. Papazian L, Thomas P, Garbe L, et al (1995) Bronchoscopic or blind bronchial sampling techniques for the diagnosis of ventilator-associated pneumonia. Am J Respir Crit Care Med 152:1982–1991

16. Murray JF, Matthay MA, Luce JM, Flick MR (1988) An expanded definition of the adult respiratory distress syndrome. Am Rev Respir Dis 138:720–723

17. Papin TA, Grum CM, Weg JG (1986) Transbronchial biopsy during mechanical ventilation. Chest 89:168–170

18. Pincus PS, Kallenbach JM, Hurwitz MD, et al (1987) Transbronchial biopsy during mechanical ventilation. Crit Care Med 15:1136–1139

19. Bulpa PA, Dive AM, Mertens L, et al (2003) Combined bronchoalveolar lavage and transbronchial lung biopsy: safety and yield in ventilated patients. Eur Respir J 21:489–494

20. Fraire AE, Cooper SP, Greenberg SD, Rowland LP, Langston C (1992) Transbronchial lung biopsy. Histopathologic and morphometric assessment of diagnostic utility. Chest 102:748–752

21. Burt ME, Flye MW, Webber BL, Path FF, Wesley RA (1981) Prospective evaluation of aspiration needle, cutting needle, transbronchial and open biopsies in chronic infiltrate lung diseases. Ann Thorac Surg 32:146–151

22. Dierkesmann R, Dobbertin I (1998) Different techniques of bronchoscopy. Pulmonary endoscopy and biopsy techniques. Eur Respir Monogr 9:1–21

23. Anders GT, Johnson JE, Bush BA, Matthews JI (1988) Transbronchial biopsy without fluoroscopy. A seven-year survey. Chest 94:557–560

24. Herf SM, Surrat PM, Arora NS (1977) Deaths and complications associated with transbronchial lung biopsy. Am Rev Respir Dis 115:708–711

25. O'Brien JD, Ettinger NA, Shevlin D, Kollef MH (1997) Safety and yield of transbronchial biopsy in mechanically ventilated patients. Crit Care Med 25:440–446

26. Turner JS, Willcox PA, Hayhurst MD, Potgieter PD (1994) Fiberoptic bronchoscopy in the intensive care unit. A prospective study of 147 procedures in 107 patients. Crit Care Med 22:259–264

27. Meduri GU, Belenchia JM, Estes RJ, Wunderink RG, El Torky M, Leeper Kv Jr (1991) Fibroproliferative phase of ARDS. Clinicals findings and effects of steroids. Chest 100:943–952

28. Canver CC, Mentzer RM Jr (1994) The role of open lung biopsy in early and late survival of ventilator-dependent patients with diffuse lung disease. J Cardiovasc Surg 35:151–155

29. McKenna RJ Jr, Mountain CF, Mc Martney MJ (1984) Open lung biopsy in immunocompromised patients. Chest 86:671–674

30. Flabouris A, Myburgh J (1999) The utility of open lung biopsy in patients requiring mechanical ventilation. Chest 115:811–817

31. Hill JD, Ratliff JL, Parrot JC, et al (1976) Pulmonary pathology in acute respiratory insufficiency: lung biopsy as a diagnostic tool. J Thorac Cardiovasc Surg 71:64–71

32. Ashbaugh DG, Maier RV (1985) Idiopathic pulmonary fibrosis in adult respiratory distress syndrome. Diagnosis and treatment. Arch Surg 120:530–535
33. Warner DO, Warner MA, Divertie MB (1988) Open lung biopsy in patients with diffuse pulmonary infiltrates and acute respiratory failure. Am Rev Respir Dis 137:90–94
34. Meduri GU, Chinn AJ, Leeper KV, et al (1994) Corticosteroid rescue treatment of progressive fibroproliferation in late ARDS. Patterns of response and predictors of outcome. Chest 105:1516–1527

Cardiac Crises

The Critically Ill Cardiac Surgery Patient:
How to Avoid Postoperative Catastrophe?

J. Boldt and A. Lehmann

▌ Introduction

The percentage of the population that is greater than 60 years of age will increase dramatically in the next years [1]. With improvements in surgical techniques, extracorporal oxygenation equipment, anesthesiologic management, and postoperative care, patients with advanced age are increasingly referred for cardiac surgery [2]. The extent of cardiac surgery in older patients increases the probability of clinical manifestations of organ dysfunction [3–5]. As elderly patients have a narrower physiological reserve and often suffer from co-existing diseases, they are at an increased risk of perioperative morbidity and mortality; perioperative mortality in the elderly undergoing coronary artery bypass surgery is reported to be 3–7 times higher than in younger patients [6–9].

Cardiopulmonary bypass (CPB) is associated with complex pathophysiological processes that have been compared to the pathophysiologic alterations associated with sepsis or systemic inflammatory response syndrome (SIRS). The non-physiologic perfusion during CPB and the blood contact with the non-endothelial synthetic surfaces of the CPB equipment activates the coagulation cascade, alters the vascular endothelial layer, and promotes the expression of leukocyte adhesion molecules by which post-bypass end-organ damage is mediated [10]. This inflamma-

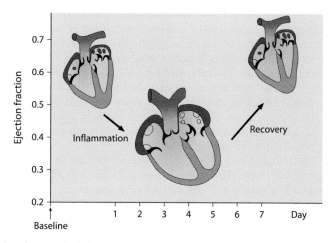

Fig. 1. Changes in myocardial performance by inflammation

tory response may have detrimental consequences for myocardial performance that may be associated with hemodynamic catastrophe and, subsequently, may result in (multiple) organ dysfunction (Fig. 1).

Our knowledge of the cellular and molecular pathophysiology of the development of post-perfusion organ dysfunction has been enlarged in recent years. Several pharmacological manipulations have been aimed at attenuating the negative consequences of CPB. Currently, the area of most intense investigation is drugs that modulate the inflammatory cascade [11, 12]. Approaches focused on manipulating the inflammatory process associated with CPB include the use of aprotinin or corticosteroids, and the specific inhibition of inflammatory mediators (e.g., by monoclonal antibodies).

▌ Prevention of Postoperative Organ Dysfunction by PDE-III Inhibitors?

Use of phosphodiesterase (PDE) III inhibitors may be another promising approach to prevent CPB-related postoperative organ dysfunction. Intracellular cyclic nucleotide levels play an important role in the regulation of several immunological processes. Elevation of intracellular cyclic adenosine monophosphate (cAMP) and/or cyclic guanosine monophosphate (cGMP) concentration by inhibition of PDE is known to modulate the inflammatory response [13]. Moreover, the positive inotropic and vasodilating properties of specific inhibitors of PDE-III result in improved systemic hemodynamics and organ perfusion [14].

To prove the value of PDE-III inhibitors on inflammation and organ function, patients >80 years and scheduled for elective aorto-coronary bypass surgery were studied in a prospective, randomized study [15]. The PDE-III inhibitor enoximone was given prophylactically prior to the start of CPB. Interleukins and soluble adhesion molecules were measured from arterial blood samples, liver function was assessed using the monoethyl-glycinexylidide (MEGX) test and by measuring alpha-glutathione S-transferase (alpha-GST) plasma levels, splanchnic perfusion was assessed by continuous gastric tonometry, and renal function was evaluated by measuring creatinine and alpha-1-microglobulin (alpha-1-MG). Interleukins increased significantly more in the control than in the enoximone-pretreated patients. Soluble adhesion molecules were increased significantly more in the control patients. pHi decreased in the control group, whereas it remained unchanged in the enoximone-treated patients. Liver function was more altered in the control than in the enoximone-pretreated patients: alpha-1-MG increased significantly more in the control than in the enoximone group indicating less tubular damage in the enoximone group. The major result from the study was that pretreatment with the PDE-III inhibitor enoximone in cardiac surgery patients aged >80 years resulted in less postoperative inflammation and improved markers of organ function in comparison to a placebo-treated control group.

Endothelial cell activation commonly occurs in cardiac surgery patients undergoing CPB [16]. Expression of endothelial cell adhesion molecules is believed to play a key role in the inflammatory process in these patients [17]. The non-physiologic perfusion during CPB and the blood contact with the non-endothelial synthetic surfaces of the CPB equipment activate the vascular endothelial layer and promote expression of leukocyte adhesion molecules by which postbypass end organ damage is mediated. Both leukocytes and endothelial cells express particular adhesion molecules that are responsible for the cell-cell interactions. By this cell-cell interplay, trafficking and migration of leukocytes across the vascular endothelial barrier into tissues is induced. Expression of adhesion molecules are upregulated during CPB and some of the soluble adhesion molecules measured in the circulating blood appear to be excellent markers for endothelial damage [18]. An increased expression of L-selectin of more than double baseline values has been reported after CPB [19]. This increase was not reduced by methylprednisolone given at the start of anesthesia. Plasma levels of soluble adhesion molecules were significantly more elevated in untreated controls than in enoximone-pretreated patients. Blease et al. [20] also showed that PDE inhibition inhibited induction of E-selectin expression. The attenuated increase in soluble adhesion molecules by pretreatment with enoximone in elderly patients may indicate preservation of endothelial integrity.

Altered organ function is a common phenomenon after cardiac surgery. Liver function deteriorated significantly less in enoximone-pretreated than in the control patients [15]. Others have also reported that PDE-III inhibitors may have beneficial effects on liver function: use of the PDE-III inhibitor milrinone was shown to enhance indocyanine green (ICG) elimination and lactate metabolism in patients undergoing hepatic resection surgery [21]. Whether this beneficial effect is due to improved (micro-) circulation, attenuation of inflammation or direct effects on hepatic cells is still a matter of discussion.

Several studies have documented altered oxygen delivery to splanchnic organs in cardiac surgery patients and have emphazised the risk that intestinal organs become ischemic during CPB [22]. Deficits in splanchnic blood flow are likely to play an important role in the development of organ dysfunction in critically ill patients. Maintaining hemodynamic stability is no guarantee of an adequate splanchnic perfusion and cannot protect against significant postoperative complications [23]. The PCO_2 gap as a marker of splanchnic perfusion remained almost unchanged in enoximone-pretreated patients but increased significantly in the control group indicating a preserved splanchnic perfusion after CPB by pretreatment with enoximone. Administration of the PDE-III inhibitor milrinone in cardiac surgery intensive care patients was also shown to increase hepatosplanchnic blood flow by approximately 10% [24]. Disturbed renal function has often been reported after cardiac surgery [25]. Elderly patients especially often show reduced renal function and thus appear to be especially prone to develop renal dysfunction postoperatively [26]. In elderly patients, creatinine serum levels were slightly elevated already prior to surgery, but did not increase significantly during the study period. Alpha-1-microglobulin, a more sensitive marker for the early phase of renal failure, was significantly more increased in the non-treated than in the enoximone-pretreated patients, indicating considerable beneficial effects of enoximone on renal function in the elderly cardiac surgery patient [15].

The mechanisms by which the PDE-III inhibitor enoximone may exert its beneficial effects are not completely known. The positive inotropic and vascular relaxant actions of this compound are apparently due to selective inhibitory effects on the cyclic AMP-specific, cyclic GMP-inhibited form of PDE. The inflammatory process is beneficially modulated by this elevation of intracellular cAMP and cGMP, including blockade of the production and release of proinflammatory cytokines (e.g., tumor necrosis factor [TNF]-a, interleukin [IL]-6), attenuated lipopolysaccharide (LPS)-induced leukocyte-endothelial adhesion/emigration, and macromolecular extravasation. Additionally, increased intracellular cAMP concentrations are known to inhibit the secretory function of neutrophils [27]. The increase in microperfusion secondary to PDE-III inhibitors may be of particular benefit in the elderly in the post-bypass period, because microcirculatory deficits are common after CPB and may induce organ dysfunction.

▌ Combination of Beta-blockers and PDE-III Inhibitors

Prevention of perioperative myocardial ischemia represents an important approach to improve postoperative outcome in cardiac surgery patients (Fig. 2). At present, beta-blockers seem to be the most effective regimen to reduce cardiac morbidity and mortality [28, 29]. Acutely administered beta-blockers have been shown to be of benefit in protecting patients from sudden death. The beneficial effects of beta-blocking substances are primarily related to heart rate reduction. Aside from this cardioprotective effects of beta-blockers, this class of compounds may additional possess cellular effects by inhibition of protein kinases. By this mechanism, beta-blockers affect endothelin synthesis, neutrophil chemotaxis, inflammation, nitric oxide (NO) synthesis, and others [30, 31]. In a retrospective database analysis covering approximately 2500 patients undergoing coronary artery bypass graft surgery, perioperative use of β-adrenergic antagonists was associated with a substantial reduction in the incidence of postoperative neurological complications [32]. These results indicate a potential neuroprotective effect of beta-blockers in cardiac surgery patients aside from their myocardial properties.

Beta-blockers are, however, associated with considerable negative inotropic effects. This may limit their use in cardiac surgery patients who are at risk of developing low output failure. β-receptor stimulating substances (e.g., dobutamine, epinephrine) are often needed to treat myocardial pump failure and subsequently prevent low output syndrome. Catecholamines, however, show reduced efficacy in beta-blocked patients and in patients showing 'downregulation' phenomenon. Thus it seems reasonable that a combination of PDE-III induced positive inotropy and β-receptor blockade might offer advantages by producing beneficial hemodynamic ef-

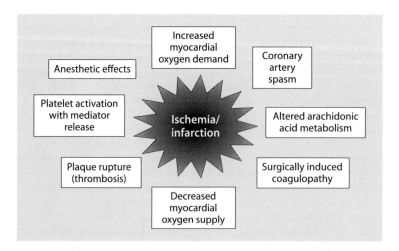

Fig. 2. The importance of perioperative ischemia in cardiac surgery patients

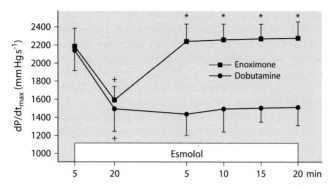

Fig. 3. Influence on myocardial contractility (assessed by measuring dp/dt$_{max}$) of acutely blocking β-receptors by using the ultra-short acting beta-blocker esmolol in patients undergoing cardiac surgery. The depressed myocardial contractility could not be treated by administering the β-receptor agonist dobutamine but by giving the phosphodiesterase (PDE) III inhibitor enoximone (modified from [33])

fects and by compensating each other's limitations in a complementary way [33, 34] (Fig. 3).

In a prospective, randomized, placebo controlled study, the influence of prophylactic use of a combination of i.v. beta-blocker esmolol and PDE-III inhibitor enoximone before CPB on postbypass hemodynamics, inflammation, endothelial and organ function was assessed in elderly cardiac surgery patients [35]. The elderly esmolol+enoximone-treated patients showed less increase in markers of myocardial ischemia (troponin T, creatine kinase (CK)-MB) than the untreated control group. This myocardial protective effect may be attributed only to the use of the beta-blocker, but the PDE-III inhibitor may have contributed to the effects because an increase in (myocardial) blood flow has been shown with these substances.

Not only the heart profited from the use of esmolol + enoximone. Kidney and liver integrity were also preserved from the negative influence of CPB. These beneficial effects on organ function may (mainly) be attributed to the effects of PDE-III inhibitors on perfusion. PDE-III inhibitors increase cardiac output through combined positive inotropic and vasodilative effects ('inodilators'). Because altered microperfusion is an important mechanism for deteriorated organ function in the post-bypass period, maintenance of adequate blood flow by enoximone may be an important maneuver. In several of the untreated control patients, standard β-receptor agonists were used to improve pump function and organ perfusion in the postbypass period. Unmasked peripheral vasoconstrictive response to dobutamine and epinephrine has been reported in patients under beta-blocker therapy resulting in increased systemic vascular resistance (SVR) and decreased cardiac index. This may have contributed to the reduced splanchnic perfusion (higher PCO$_2$ gap), deteriorated kidney integrity (as shown by increased beta-N-acetyl-D-glucosaminidase [NAG] urine concentrations), and liver function (as shown by increased GST-alpha plasma levels) in the untreated control patients. By contrast, use of PDE-III inhibitor in patients treated with a β_1-selective blocker increased stroke volume and decreased heart rate and myocardial oxygen consumption.

The microvasculature is a key battleground for inflammatory processes, with evidence of a central role for the endothelium in modulating inflammation. The endothelium is not only an inert cellular layer, but endothelial cells actively and reactively participate in inflammation and hemostasis [36]. Both leukocytes and endothelial cells express particular adhesion molecules that are responsible for the cell-cell interactions. By this cell-cell interplay, trafficking and migration of leukocytes across the vascular endothelial barrier into tissues is modulated. The release of soluble adhesion molecules into the circulation correlated with the degree of trauma depending on the associated ischemia/reperfusion injury [37]. An increased expression of adhesion molecule L-selectin of more than double the baseline values was seen after CPB [19]. Plasma levels of all measured circulating adhesion molecules were significantly lower in the enoximone + esmolol-treated than in the non-treated control patients indicating less endothelial injury in the treatment group. This may be due either to the reduced inflammatory response, as pro-inflammatory cytokines induce expression and release of adhesion molecules, or due to improved (micro-) circulation that attenuates development of tissue hypoxia.

The timing for preventing postoperative organ dysfunction appears to be essential. Organ protection should start as early as possible preoperatively and should be continued during the entire perioperative period. Thus it seems to be valuable to start administration of esmolol+enoximone immediately after induction of anesthesia, more than 1 hr prior to the start of CPB.

▮ Ca^{++}-agonist Levosimendan: A Novel Approach to Prevent Hemodynamic Catastrophe

The most important cause of death for patients with acute myocardial infarction (AMI) reaching the hospital alive is cardiogenic shock. Moreover, cardiogenic shock complicates 7–10% of all cases of AMI [38]. Drugs given to treat cardiogenic shock in this situation may relieve symptoms (e.g., hemodynamic low output syndrome),

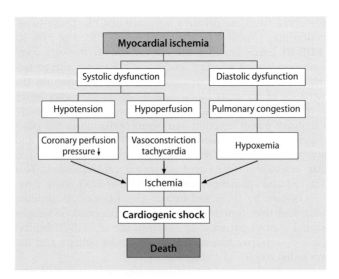

Fig. 4. Myocardial ischemia is directly associated with negative consequences for myocardial function by which low output may be induced resulting in organ perfusion/oxygenation deficits and finally in death

but they cannot treat the cause of ischemic cardiogenic shock. The goals of any pharmacological therapy in (ischemia-based) cardiogenic shock are to treat myocardial ischemia, to restore nutritional blood flow, and to prevent further damage of vital organs (Fig. 4).

Levosimendan is a new positive inotropic drug, belonging to the class of calcium sensitizers. The concept of calcium sensitization hypothesizes that myocardial contractility is increased by drugs directly interacting with contractile proteins [39]. Levosimendan stabilizes the calcium induced conformational change in cardiac troponin C (cTnC) only during systole by binding to the calcium-saturated conformation of cTnC [40]. In contrast to other positive inotropic drugs, levosimendan does not increase intracellular calcium. Therefore, levosimendan exerts its positive inotropic effects by prolonging the effective cross-bridging time [41]. It does not increase the number of actin-myosin crossbridges. Positive inotropy with normal levels of intracellular calcium avoids the undesired side-effects of increased intracellular calcium such as increased oxygen consumption and risk of fatal arrhythmia. The calcium-dependent binding of levosimendan to cTnC has no influence on the affinity of calcium to cTnC resulting in minimal effects on diastole. Besides increasing contractility by acting on cTnC, levosimendan was found to preserve diastolic function [42]. Uncoupling of myocardial calcium metabolism may play an important role in the detrimental effects on ischemic myocardium mediated by excessive NO levels [43].

Levosimendan activates ATP sensitive potassium channels (K_{ATP}-channels) in vascular smooth muscle cells, cardiac myocytes, and in mitochondria. Opening K_{ATP}-channels is an obligatory step of ischemic and pharmacological preconditioning of the human myocardium [44]. Thus aside from its positive inotropic properties, levosimendan has vasodilating effects and anti-ischemic properties by opening K_{ATP}-channels ('inoprotective' substance). At doses simultaneously increasing myocardial contractility, levosimendan has been shown to reduce experimental infarct size [45]. In experimental settings, it increased animals' survival rate and increased the number of rats without any arrhythmia in regional myocardial ischemia [46]. Levosimendan was also found to enhance the contractile function of stunned myocardium in dogs [47].

Based on its positive inotropic and anti-ischemic effects, levosimendan has been proposed for patients with myocardial ischemia simultaneously requiring inotropic support. Consequently, levosimendan is recommended by the guidelines of the European Society of Cardiology [48]. It may also be of value for treating acute worsening of heart failure [49] and for treating acute heart failure after myocardial infarction in the critically ill cardiac surgery patient [50]. In patients with cardiogenic shock of surgical and non-surgical origin and in patients with ischemic cardiogenic shock after cardiac surgery, levosimendan significantly increased cardiac index and decreased elevated SVR [50, 51]. Thus, in patients showing ischemic heart failure and undergoing (acute) cardiac surgery, levosimendan might be of advantage as an inoprotective drug.

Conclusion

The complexity of the pathogenesis of organ dysfunction secondary to cardiac surgery may offer a large number of opportunities for pharmacological interventions to improve post-bypass organ function. Therapy in this situation should not only be focused on improving systemic hemodynamics; improving organ perfusion and tissue perfusion/oxygenation are of similar importance to avoid development of multiple organ dysfunction syndrome. Especially in the elderly and the critically ill cardiac surgery patient, prevention of development of postoperative catastrophe is of greater importance than only treating symptoms of deteriorated post-bypass hemodynamics.

Beta-blockers are widely accepted as the most effective class of drugs to prevent myocardial ischemia. They are, however, associated with some negative side-effects, e.g., depressed myocardial performance with the risk of further deterioration of reduced systemic and regional perfusion. As conventional catecholamines are often ineffective in this situation, PDE-III inhibitors appear to be a promising approach to improve global and local hemodynamics. As they also have some beneficial effects on inflammatory response, early (preventive) use of PDE-III inhibitors combined with beta-blockers may be helpful to avoid post-bypass complications. Whether outcomes will be improved by this approach has to be assessed in large prospective randomized clinical trials. Finally, the calcium channel blocker levosimendan offers another strategy to avoid post-bypass catastrophe especially in the critically ill cardiac surgery patient already showing severe myocardial ischemia preoperatively. "Thanks to the human heart by which we live" (William Wadsworth) – if we always remember this, it will us help to improve postoperative outcome in the cardiac surgery patient.

References

1. Veering BT (1999) Management of anaesthesia in the elderly patients. Curr Opin Anaesthesiol 12:333–336
2. Harris J (1999) Cardiac surgery in the elderly. Heart 82:119–120
3. Christenson JT, Simonet F, Schmuziger M (1999) The influence of age on the outcome of primary coronary artery bypass grafting. J Cardiovasc Surg 40:333–338
4. Wick G, Grubeck-Loebenstein B (1997) The aging immune system: primary and secondary alterations of immune reactivity in the elderly. Exp Gerontol 32:401–413
5. Priebe HJ (2000) The aged cardiovascular risk patient. Br J Anaesth 85:763–778
6. Amano HH, Yoshida S, Takahashi A, Nagano N, Kohmoto T (2000) Coronary artery bypass grafting in the elderly. Chest 117:1262–1270
7. MacDonald P, Johnstone D, Rockwood K (2000) Coronary artery bypass surgery for elderly patients: is our practice based on evidence or faith? CMAJ 162:1005–1006
8. Cook TM, Day CJ (1998) Hospital mortality after urgent and emergency laparatomy in patients aged 65 years and over. Risk and prediction of risk using multiple logistic regression analysis. Br J Anaesth 80:776–781
9. Rady MY (1998) Perioperative determinants of morbidity and mortality in elderly patients undergoing cardiac surgery. Crit Care Med 26:225–235
10. Boyle EM, Pohlman TH, Johnson MC, Verrier ED (1997) Endothelial cell injury in cardiovascular surgery: the systemic inflammatory response. Ann Thorac Surg 63:277–284
11. Royston D (1997) The inflammatory response and extracorporeal circulation. J Cardiothorac Vasc Anesth 11:341–354
12. Miller BE, Levy JH (1997) The inflammatory response to cardiopulmonary bypass. J Cardiothorac Vasc Anesth 11:355–366
13. Németh ZH, Haskó G, Szabó C, Vizi ES (1997) Amrinone and theophylline differentially regulate cytokine and nitric oxide production in endotoxemic mice. Shock 7:371–375
14. Ichioka S, Nakatsuka T, Sato Y, Shibata M, Kamiya A, Harii K (1998) Amrinone, a selective phosphodiesterase III inhibitor, improves microcirculation and flap survival: a comparative study with prostaglandin E. J Surg Res 75:42–48

15. Boldt J, Brosch C, Suttner S, Piper SN, Lehmann A, Werling C (2002) Prophylactic use of the phospodiesterase III inhibitor enoximone in elderly cardiac surgery patients: effect on hemodynamics, inflammation, and markers of organ function. Intensive Care Med 28:1462–1469
16. Hill GE (1998) Cardiopulmonary bypass-induced inflammation: is it important? J Cardiothorac Vasc Anesth 12 (suppl):S21–S25
17. Verrier ED, Morgan EN (1998) Endothelial response to cardiopulmonary bypass surgery. Ann Thorac Surg 66:S17–S19
18. Paret G, Prince T, Keller N, et al (2000) Plasma soluble E-selectin after cardiopulmonary bypass in children: is it a marker of the post- operative care? J Cardiothorac Vasc Anesth 14:433–437
19. Toft P, Christiansen K, Tönnesen E, Noelsen CH, Lillevang S (1998) Changes in adhesion molecule expression and oxidative burst activity of granulocytes and monocytes during open-heart surgery with cardiopulmonary bypass compared with abdominal surgery. Eur J Anaesthesiol 31:283–288
20. Blease K, Burke Gaffney A, Hellewell PG (1998) Modulation of cell adhesion molecule expression and function on human lung microvascular endothelial cells by inhibition of phosphodiesterase 3 and 4. Br J Pharmacol 124:229–237
21. Orii R, Sugawara Y, Hayashida M, et al (2000) Effects of amrinone on ischaemia-reperfusion injury in cirrhotic patients undergoing hepatectomy: a comparative study with prostaglandin E_1. Br J Anaesth 85:389–395
22. Fiddian-Green RG (1990) Gut mucosal ischemia during cardiac surgery. Sem Thorac Cardiovasc Surg 2:389–399
23. Mythen MG, Webb AR (1994) The role of gut mucosal hypoperfusion in the pathogenesis of postoperative organ dysfunction. Intensive Care Med 20:203–209
24. McNicol L, Andersen LW, Liu G, Doolan L, Beak L (1999) Markers of splanchnic perfusion and intestinal translocation of endotoxins during cardiopulmonary bypass: Effects of dopamine and milrinone. J Cardiothorac Vasc Anesth 13:292–298
25. Roques F, Nashef SA, Michel P, et al (1999) Risk factors and outcome in European cardiac surgery: analysis of the EuroSCORE multinational database of 19030 patients. Eur J Cardiothorac Surg 15:816–822
26. Lindeman RD (1992) Changes in renal function with aging: Implications for treatment. Drugs Aging 2:423–431
27. Zurier RB, Weismann G, Hoffstein S, Kammermann S, Thai HH (1974) Mechanisms of lysosomal enzyme release from human leukocytes. Effects of cAMP and cGMP, autonomic agonists, and agents which affect microtubule function. J Clin Invest 53:297–309
28. London MJ (2003) Perioperative beta blockade: Facts and controversies. Ann Cardiac Anaesth 6:117–125
29. Ferguson TB Jr, Coombs LP, Peterson ED; Society of Thoracic Surgeons National Adult Cardiac Surgery Database (2002) Preoperative beta-blocker use and mortality and morbidity following CABG surgery in North America. JAMA 287:2221–2277
30. Wei S, Chow LT, Sanderson JE (2000) Effect of carvedilol in comparison with metoprolol on myocardial collagen postinfarction. J Am Coll Cardiol 36:276–281
31. Port JD, Bristow MR (2001) Altered beta-adrenergic receptor gene regulation and signaling in chronic heart failure. J Mol Cell Cardiol 33:887–905
32. Amory DW, Grigore A, Amory JK, et al (2002) Neuroprotection is associated with beta-adrenergic receptor antagonists during cardiac surgery: evidence from 2575 patients. J Cardiothorac Vasc Anesth 16:270–277
33. Boldt J, Kling D, Zickmann B, Dapper F, Hempelmann G (1990) Haemodynamic effects of the phosphodiesterase inhibitor enoximone in comparison with dobutamine in esmolol-treated cardiac surgery patients. Br J Anaesth 64:611–616
34. Metra M, Nodari S, D'Aloia A, et al (2002) Beta-blocker therapy influences the hemodynamic response to inotropic agents in patients with heart failure: a randomized comparison of dobutamine and enoximone before and after chronic treatment with metoprolol or carvedilol. J Am Coll Cardiol 40:1248–1258

35. Boldt J, Brosch Ch, Lehmann A, Suttner St, Isgro F (2004) The prophylactic use of the beta-blocker esmolol in combination with phosphodiesterase inhibitor III enoximone in the elderly cardiac surgery patient. Anesth Analg 99:1009–1117

36. Galley HF (1999) Cytokine-endothelial cell interaction. Br J Intensive Care 9:147–151

37. Seekamp A, Jochum M, Ziegler M, et al (1998) Cytokines and adhesion molecules in elective and accidental trauma-related ischemia/reperfusion. J Trauma 44:874–882

38. Hochman JS (2003) Cardiogenic shock complicating acute myocardial infarction: expanding the paradigm. Circulation 107:2998–3002

39. Sorsa T, Heikkinen S, Abott MB, et al (2001) Binding of levosimendan, a calcium sensitizer, to cardiac troponin C. J Biol Chem 276:9337–9343

40. Ukkonen H, Saraste M, Akkila J, et al (2000) Myocardial efficiency during levosimendan infusion in congestive heart failure. Clin Pharmacol Ther 68:522–531

41. Remme WJ (1993) Inodilator therapy for heart failure. Early, late, or not at all? Circulation 87 (5 suppl):IV97–IV107

42. Yokoshiki H, Katsube Y, Sunagawa M, Sperelakis N (1997) Levosimendan, a novel CA^{2+} sensitizer, activates the ATP-sensitive K^+ channel in rat ventricular cells. J Pharmacol Exp Ther 283:375–383

43. Webb JG, Lowe AM, Sanborn TA, et al (2003) Percutaneous coronary intervention for cardiogenic shock in the SHOCK trial. The SHOCK investigators. J Am Coll Cardiol 42:1380–1386

44. Jamali IN, Kersten JR, Pagel PS, Hettrick DA, Warltier DC (1997) Intracoronary levosimendan enhances contractile function of stunned myocardium. Anesth Analg 85:23–29

45. Perrault LP, Menasche P (1999) Preconditioning: can nature's shield be raised against surgical ischemic-reperfusion injury? Ann Thorac Surg 68:1988–1994

46. Haikala H, Kaheinen P, Levijoki J, Linden IB (1997) The role of cAMP- and cGMP-dependent protein kinases in the cardiac actions of the new calcium sensitizer, levosimendan. Cardiovasc Res 34:536–546

47. Moiseyev VS, Poder P, Andrejevs N, et al (2002) Safety and efficacy of a novel calcium sensitizer, levosimendan, in patients with left ventricular failure due to an acute myocardial infarction. A randomized, placebo-controlled, double-blind study (RUSSLAN). Eur Heart J 23:1422–1432

48. Hunt SA, Baker DW, Chin MH, et al (2001) ACC/AHA guidelines for the evaluation and management of chronic heart failure in the adult: Executive summary a report of the American College of Cardiology/American Heart Association task force on practice guidelines (committee to revise the 1995 guidelines for the evaluation and management of heart failure). Circulation 104:2996–3007

49. Delle Karth G, Buberl A, Geppert A, et al (2003) Hemodynamic effects of a continuous infusion of levosimendan in critically ill patients with cardiogenic shock requiring catecholamines. Acta Anaesthesiol Scand 47:1251–1256

50. Lehmann A, Lang J, Boldt J, Isgro F, Kiessling AH (2004) Levosimendan in patients with cardiogenic shock undergoing surgical revascularization: a case series. In electronic publication: Med Sci Monit 10:MT89–MT93

51. Lehmann A, Boldt J, Lang J, Isgro F, Blome M (2003) Is levosimendan an inoprotective drug in patients with acute coronary syndrome undergoing surgical revascularization? Anasthesiol Intensivmed Notfallmed Schmerzther 38:577–582

B-Type Natriuretic Peptide to Assess Cardiac Function in the Critically Ill

A.S. McLean and S.J. Huang

▌ Introduction

Brain natriuretic peptide, or B-type natriuretic peptide (BNP), is a member of the natriuretic peptide family, which also includes atrial natriuretic peptide (ANP), C-type natriuretic peptide (CNP), and urodilatin. BNP was first isolated from porcine brain and subsequently found in human brain, heart, and other organs [1, 2]. The atria are the main source of BNP in normal subjects. However, chronic ventricular stress (myocyte stretch), as in heart failure, results in increased ventricular mRNA expression and concentration of the peptides [3, 4].

The BNP gene contains the destabilizing 'TATTTAT' sequence, suggesting a high turnover rate of the BNP mRNA and spontaneous synthesis of BNP, in response to physiological stimuli. BNP gene expression is induced within 1 hour in response to volume and pressure overloading. The gene sequence also implies rapid degradation of the mRNA after the loss of stimuli [5]. The first product synthesized is a 132-amino acid preprohormone, which is then processed into a 108-amino acid precursor protein (proBNP). ProBNP is cleaved into the biologically active 32-amino acid carboxyl-terminal peptide (BNP) and a 76-amino acid amino-terminal (N-terminal) fragment (NT-proBNP) by the endoprotease furin (Fig. 1) [6]. BNP contains a 17-amino acid ring structure, which is common to the natriuretic peptides and is highly conserved in the family. This ring structure is necessary for the binding to its receptors (Fig. 1).

The main physiological stimuli for BNP secretion is volume expansion and pressure overload of the cardiac ventricles [7, 8]. In contrast to ANP, where secretion is effected by exocytosis of storage granules, the secretion of BNP is controlled at the transcription level in response to the stimuli. Once in the active form, BNP binds to type-A NP receptor (NPR-A) [9]. NPR-A is coupled to guanylate cyclase, via a kinase-like moiety, which leads to the formation of the second messenger cyclic guanosine monophosphate (cGMP). A type-C receptor (NPR-C) is also present on cell surfaces but is believed to be responsible for the clearance of the natriuretic peptides (Fig. 2) [10].

▌ Physiology of Heart Failure

The low output state of heart failure leads to the adaptive activation of the renin-angiotensin-aldosterone system (RAAS) and the sympathetic nervous system. Although the activation of both systems provides a short term favorable hemody-

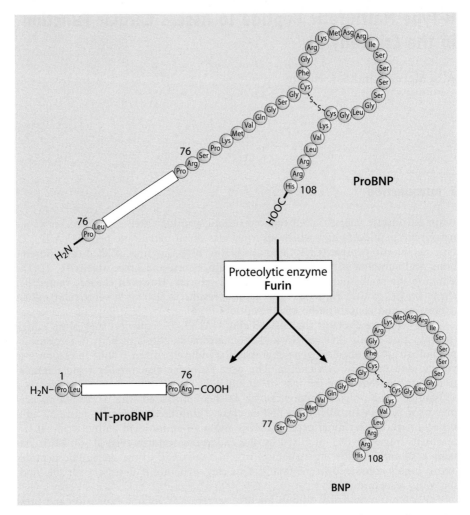

Fig. 1. BNP – structure and relationship. Human BNP is synthesized as a preprohormone of 132 amino acids that is processed to a 108-amino acids precursor (proBNP). ProBNP is subsequently cleaved into the mature biologically active 32-amino acids C-terminal fragment (BNP) and a 76-amino acids fragment (NT-proBNP)

namic response in these patients, unfortunately their activation also promotes the symptoms and progression of the disease. Tachycardia, increased peripheral resistance, and volume overload are common amongst the heart failure population and are partly due to the activation of the RAAS and the sympathetic nervous system. Other deleterious effects include rendering patients refractory to diuretics as a result of angiotensin II-induced increased Na^+ reabsorption, downregulation of cardiac β_1-adrenoceptor which leads to reduced contractility, tachycardia-induced cardiomyopathy, and myocardial remodeling [11–13]. Multiple studies have shown that angiotensin-converting enzyme (ACE) inhibitors and beta-blockers improve clinical outcomes in heart failure patients [14, 15].

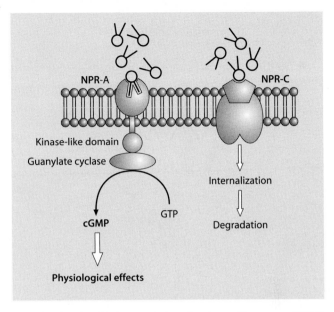

Fig. 2. Signal transduction pathway for BNP. BNP binds to type A natriuretic peptide receptor (NPR-A) and activates the guanylate cyclase which in turn catalyses the conversion of GTP to cyclic GMP (cGMP). BNP clearance is effected by binding to the type C receptor (NPR-C), which leads to internalization and degradation of the peptide. From [30] with permission

▌ Role of BNP in Heart Failure

The end results of the maladaptive responses of the RAAS and the sympathetic nervous system are the increase in preload and afterload, and hence cardiac wall stress. It is now believed that the activation of the natriuretic peptide systems (ANP and BNP) can counter-regulate these maladaptive responses. This is supported by studies that demonstrated that natriuretic peptide antagonism promotes RAAS activation and Na$^+$ retention [16]. An animal model study demonstrated that inhibition of natriuretic peptide degradation improves renal hemodynamic and tubular responses, whereas the administration of a natriuretic peptide receptor antagonist attenuated such responses in mild heart failure [17].

The release of BNP is associated with hemodynamic improvement, including reductions in both preload and systemic vascular resistance (SVR) [18]. This is brought forth mainly by vasodilation and the abilities to decrease renin release, inhibiting endothelin-1 response to angiotensin II, inhibiting sympathetic activity and decreasing aldosterone production [18, 19]. The reduced aldosterone activity promotes natriuresis and diuresis (Fig. 3). The vasodilatory effect on the coronary circulation improves oxygen supply to the myocardium [20].

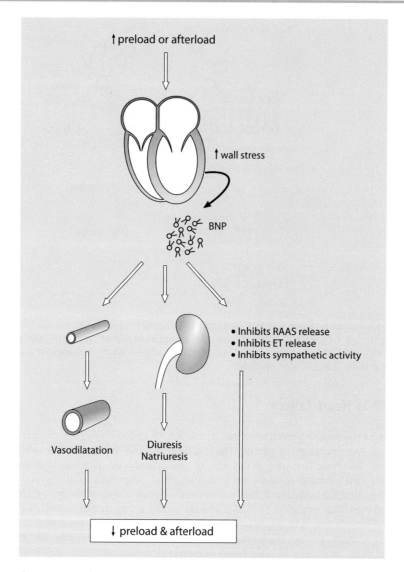

Fig. 3. Actions of BNP. In response to cardiac wall stress, the ventricular myocardium synthesizes and se-
cretes BNP. BNP causes (**a**) vasodilatation; (**b**) promotion of diuresis and natriuresis; and (c) inhibition of
the renin-angiotensin-aldosterone system (RAAS), endothelin-1 (ET) release and the sympathetic system.
As a result, the preload and afterload are reduced

■ Primary Application of BNP – Screening for Cardiac Disease

The use of BNP for the diagnosis of heart failure is well established in the outpatient and in the emergency settings [21, 22]. In the Breathing Not Properly (BNP)
study, conducted in the emergency setting, a plasma BNP cut-off of 100 pg/ml
yielded a sensitivity of 90% and a specificity of 76% in diagnosing heart failure

[23]. BNP levels were found to be proportional to New York Heart Association class, and were significantly more accurate than clinical judgment and traditional diagnostic methods in identifying heart failure patients [24].

In a recent study, approximately 30% of all patients admitted to a general intensive care unit (ICU) were identified as having some form of cardiac dysfunction, either overt or covert [25]. Given the substantial proportion of patients with cardiac dysfunction, early detection or diagnosis is important because timely interventions can be taken to prevent the deterioration of the condition, and possibly provide a better prognosis [26].

When BNP was used as a screening tool in the ICU, the concentration was significantly higher in patients with cardiac dysfunction. A cut-off value of 144 pg/ml offered 92% sensitivity and 86% specificity in predicting the presence of cardiac dysfunction, suggesting a high degree of test accuracy in this clinical setting (the area under the receiver operating characteristic cure [AUC] was 0.96). The negative predictive value achieved was 97% [25]. The high sensitivity and negative predictive value imply that a value less than the cut-off rules out probable cardiac dysfunction.

▌ Factors Affecting BNP Levels

The use of BNP as a screening tool is complicated by the presence of a number of confounding factors (Fig. 4). The most notable confounding factors in the intensive care population are age and gender – BNP level increases with age and is higher in females. Together, these two factors account for almost 30% of the variation in BNP concentrations in the intensive care setting [27]. The cut-offs for males and females are 100 pg/ml and 200 pg/ml (the AUCs were 0.92 and 0.96), respectively. At these cut-offs, the sensitivities and specificities were 87 and 89% for males, and 83 and 85% for females. Therefore, adjusting the normal range for age and gender, rather than using a single cut-off, will be important for optimal test interpretation.

Other factors may also affect BNP levels in the critical care setting, e.g. brain disorders/injury (e.g. subarachnoid hemorrhage) and renal failure. It has been speculated that BNP is released from damaged brain cells in brain disorder patients [28]. However, it is now known that although BNP is expressed in the brain, the level of gene transcripts are at least 1 to 2 orders of magnitude less than the cardiac ventricles making it unlikely that they account for the high circulating BNP concentrations observed [29]. Other studies instead support the notion that BNP is mainly of cardiac origin resulting from brain injury-induced myocardial depression [30].

BNP levels are often elevated in chronic renal failure [31]. Although it is often believed that such an increase is due to decreased renal clearance, supportive evidence is absent. In fact, the lack of correlation between BNP and creatinine in noncardiac intensive care patients strongly suggests that renal function plays a minor role, if any, in elevating plasma BNP levels. Further, the finding that BNP levels are only elevated in renal failure patients with cardiac dysfunction suggests that the elevation is likely to be mediated via the adverse effects of renal dysfunction on the heart [27, 32].

Treatment and management options in the ICU may also have profound effects on BNP levels. For example, BNP and NT-proBNP can be eliminated during hemo-

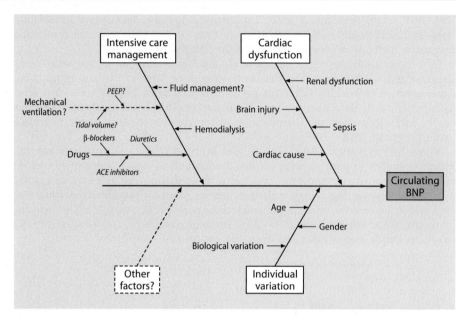

Fig. 4. Cause and effect (fishbone) diagram showing the factors affecting BNP levels in the intensive care population. The main factor that determines BNP levels is cardiac dysfunction, which could be the result of existing cardiac cause, sepsis- or brain injury-induced myocardial depression, and renal dysfunction. Other confounding factors include age, gender, and day-to-day biological variation. Intensive care management and treatment may also play a role in affecting the BNP levels

dialysis [33]. While BNP is cleared by both high- and low-flux membranes, NT-proBNP is cleared to a lesser extent by low flux membranes. Moreover, both BNP and NT-proBNP seem to be released into the circulation during hemodialysis sessions as shown by increasing post-dialysis plasma concentrations despite the demonstrated clearance. Variations in BNP levels can also be affected by drug treatments. While β-adrenoceptor antagonists can increase BNP level, ACE inhibitors and diuretics may reduce it [34, 35].

There are other unproven but potential confounding factors which can affect BNP levels in the critical care setting, two common ones being fluid loading and mechanical ventilation. Intravascular volume expansion resulting from fluid infusion increases the preload, and can theoretically elevate BNP level by increasing the right ventricular wall stress. Similarly, excessive positive end-expiratory pressure (PEEP) can lead to an increase in right ventricular afterload and hence wall stress.

▌ Limitations

BNP is increased in a wide spectrum of cardiac diseases in the intensive care population. These include left ventricular systolic and/or diastolic dysfunction, wall hypertrophy, right ventricular volume or pressure overload, arrhythmias, and valvular lesions [25, 27]. Substantial overlap of plasma BNP concentrations between different classes of cardiac dysfunction has been confirmed in many studies [36–38].

The attempt to use BNP alone to diagnose and differentiate different types of cardiac dysfunction is therefore impossible.

The use of BNP levels in correlating severity of heart disease has also been called into doubt by the recent multicenter REDHOT study, which was conducted in heart failure patients in the emergency setting. In contrast to the previous studies, the REDHOT study failed to show a correlation of BNP levels with the New York Heart Association class. There was also a lack of correlation between the severity of congestive heart failure as perceived by emergency department physicians and that determined by BNP levels [22, 39]. These rather unexpected results prompt more carefully designed studies and interpretation of results.

∎ Recommended Application in the Critical Care Setting

Given the wide range of confounding factors and the limited applications of BNP, BNP measurement is best used as a 'rule-out' test for cardiac dysfunction in the intensive care setting. The measurements should preferably be performed when patients are admitted, prior to further clinical interventions. Since the reference range may vary depending on the assay method and the nature of the control population, it is best to establish the reference range for one's own geographical attribute and use the same assay method all the time. If this is not feasible, a cut-off point of 140 pg/ml is suggested for both genders in the intensive care population. If the BNP is <140 pg/ml, then the presence of cardiac dysfunction is highly unlikely. We, however, highly recommend taking gender difference into account. In this case, cut-offs of 100 pg/ml and 200 pg/ml are recommended for males and females, respectively. If the BNP level is higher than the recommended cut-off, further cardiac assessments should be carried out to confirm the presence of cardiac dysfunction and, if present, to ascertain the type and degree of cardiac dysfunction. It is noteworthy that an increased BNP level is sometimes predictive of future cardiac events. For example, in acute pulmonary embolism, BNP elevation is highly predictive of right ventricular dysfunction [40]. It is important to remember that BNP should not be treated as a standalone diagnostic test. The results must be used and interpreted within the clinical context.

There is always a choice between BNP and NT-proBNP. While the two provide similar sensitivities and specificities in detecting cardiac dysfunction, their plasma half-lives are different. BNP has a half-life of 20 min and NT-proBNP around 2 h [41]. Theoretically, the shorter BNP half-life should render BNP more useful as a guide in monitoring therapy, e.g., reflecting the change in pulmonary capillary wedge pressure every 2 h. The longer half-life for NT-proBNP suggests that meaningful changes can only be observed every 12 h [42]. However, the use of either peptide as a monitoring tool is complicated by the fact that intra-individual biological variations are great, reaching as high as 40% for healthy patients and 24% for stable patients with congestive heart failure. Accordingly, meaningful serial results can only been seen with a change of 129 and 77% (for $p < 0.05$) for these two group of patients, respectively [43]. Given the vigorous hemodynamic management in the ICU, hour-to-hour (or day-to-day) intra-subject variations may even be higher. Further work is needed to determine the actual intra-individual variation in this population.

▌ Conclusion

The use of BNP as a diagnostic tool in the intensive care setting is not as well established as in cardiology or emergency settings. The diverse pathophysiological conditions, presence of confounding factors, and vigorous intensive care management procedures limit the precise interpretation of an elevated BNP in this setting. Based on available knowledge, we recommend that BNP is best used for confirming or ruling out probable cardiac dysfunction in the intensive care setting, where it has clearly been demonstrated to be useful. Other proposed uses of BNP should await further research. BNP measurements should not be used in place of formal cardiac assessments or in isolation from the clinical context. They certainly do not supplant echocardiography, which remains the technique of choice for assessing ventricular function. More research is required to investigate the effects of different management and treatment procedures on BNP levels. In this regard, the ICU provides an unsurpassable environment to study such effects on BNP levels.

References

1. Sudoch T, Kangawa K, Minamino N (1988) A new natriuretic peptide in porcine brain. Nature 332:78–81
2. Saper CB, Hurley KM, Moga MM, et al (1989) Brain natriuretic peptides: Differential localization of a new family of neuropeptides. Neurosci Lett 96:29–34
3. Hystad ME, Geiran OR, Attramadal H, et al (2001) Regional cardiac expression and concentration of natriuretic peptides in patients with severe chronic heart failure. Acta Physiol Scan 171:395–403
4. Luchner A, Stevens TL, Borgeson DD, et al (1998) Differential atrial and ventricular expression of myocardial BNP during evolution of heart failure. Am J Physiol 274:H1684–1689
5. Nakagawa O, Ogawa Y, Itoh H, et al (1995) Rapid transcriptional activation and early mRNA turnover of brain natriuretic peptide in cardiocyte hypertrophy. Evidence for brain natriuretic peptide as an 'emergency' cardiac hormone against ventricular overload. J Clin Invest 96:1280–1287
6. Sawada Y, Suda M, Yokoyama H, et al (1997) Stretch-induced hypertrophic growth of cardiocytes and processing of B-type natriuretic peptide are controlled by proprotein-processing endopretease furin. J Biol Chem 272:20545–20554
7. Yasue H, Yoshimura M, Sumida H, et al (1994) Localisation and mechanism of secretion of B-type natriuretic peptide in comparison with those of A-type natriuretic peptide in normal subjects and patients with heart failure. Circulation 90:195–203
8. Maeda K, Tsutamoto T, Wada A, Hisanaga T, Kinoshita M (1998) Plasma brain natriuretic peptide as a biochemical marker of high left ventricular end-diastolic pressure in pateints with symptomatic left ventricular dysfunction. Am Heart J 135:825–832
9. Suga S, Nakao K, Hosoda K, et al (1992) Receptor selectivity of natriuretic peptide family, ANP, BNP and CNP. Endocrinology 130:229–239
10. Almeida FA, Suzuki M, Scarborough RM, Lewicki JA, Maack T (1989) Clearance function of type C receptor of atrial natriuretic factor in rats. Am J Physiol 256:R469–R475
11. Ikram H, Chan W, Espiner EA, Nicholls MG (1980) Haemodynamic and hormone responses to acute and chronic furosemide therapy in congestive heart failure. Clin Sci 59:443–449
12. Shinbane JS, Wood MA, Jensen N, Ellenbogen KA (1997) Tachycardia-induced cardiomyopathy: a review of animal and clinical studies. J Am Coll Cardiol 29:709–715
13. Tsutamoto T, Wada A, Maeda K, et al (2001) Effect of spironolactone on plasma brain natriuretic peptide and left ventricular modelling in patients with congestive heart failure. J Am Coll Cardiol 37:1228–1233
14. Konstam MA, Kronenberg MW, Rousseau MF, et al (1993) Effects of the angiotensin converting inhibitor enalapril on the long-term progression of left ventricular dilatation in patients with asymptomatic systolic dysfunction. Circulation 88:2277–2283

15. Groenning BA, Nilsson JC, Sondergaard L, Fritz-Hansen T, Larsson HB, Hildebrandt PR (2000) Antiremodeling effects on the left ventricle during beta-blockade with metaprolol in the treatment of chronic heart failure. J Am Coll Cardiol 36:2072–2080
16. Stevens TL, Burnett JC Jr, Kinoshita M, Matsuda Y, Redfield MM (1995) A functional role for endogenous atrial natriuretic peptide in a canine model of early left ventricular dysfunction. J Clin Invest 95:1101–1108
17. Chen HH, Lainchbury JG, Matsuda Y, Harty GJ, Burnett JC Jr (2001) Endogenous natriuretic peptides participate in renal and humoral actions of acute vasopeptidase inhibition in experimental mild heart failure. Hypertension 38:187–191
18. Abraham WT, Lowes BD, Ferguson DA, et al (1998) Systemic haemodynamic, neurohormonal, and renal effects of a steady-state infusion of human brain natriuretic peptide in patients with haemodynamically decompensated heart failure. J Card Fail 4:37–44
19. Brunner-La Rocca HP, Kaye DM, Woods RL, Hastings J, Esler MD (2001) Effects of intravenous brain natriuretic peptide on regional sympathetic activity in patients with chronic heart failure as compared with healthy control subjects. J Am Coll Cardiol 37:1221–1227
20. Okumura K, YasueH, Fujii H, et al (1995) Effects of brain (B-type) natriuretic peptide on coronary artery diameter and coronary hemodynamic variables in humans: comparison with effects on systemic hemodynamic variables. J Am Coll Cardiol 25:342–348
21. Cowie MR, Struthers AD, Wood DA, et al (1997) Value of natriuretic peptides in assessment of patients with possible new heart failure in primary care. Lancet 350:1349–1353
22. Maisel AS, Krishnaswamy P, Nowak RM, et al (2002) Rapid measurement of B-type natriuretic peptide assay in emergency diagnosis of heart failure. N Engl J Med 347:161–167
23. Maisel AS, McCord J, Nowak RM, et al (2003) Bedside B-type natriuretic peptide in the emergency diagnosis of heart failure with reduced or preserved ejection fraction. Results from the Breathing Not Properly Multinational Study. J Am Coll Cardiol 41:2010–2017
24. McCullough PA, Nowak RM, McCord J, et al (2002) B-type natriuretic peptide and clinical judgement in emergency diagnosis of heart failure: analysis from Breathing Not Properly (BNP) Multinational Study. Circulation 106:416–422
25. McLean AS, Tang B, Nalos M, Huang SJ, Stewart DE (2003) Increased B-type natriuretic peptide (BNP) level is a strong predictor for cardiac dysfunction in the intensive care unit patients. Anaesth Intensive Care 31:21–27
26. McLean AS, Huang SJ, Ting I (2004) B-type natriuretic peptide: Is there a place in the critical care setting? Crit Care Shock 7:117–124
27. McLean AS, Huang SJ, Nalos M, Tang B, Stewart DE (2003) The confounding effects of age, gender, serum creatinine, and electrolyte concentrations on plasma B-type natriuretic peptide concentrations in critically ill patients. Crit Care Med 31:2611–2618
28. Berendes E, Van Aken H, Raufhake C, Schmidt C, Assmann G, Walter M (2001) Differential secretion of atrial and brain natriuretic peptide in critically ill patients. Anesth Analg 93:676–682
29. Gerbes AF, Dagnino L, Nguyen T, Nemer M (1994) Transcription of brain natriuretic peptide and atrial natriuretic peptide genes in human tissues. J Clin Endocrinol Metabol 78:1307–1311
30. Espiner EA, Leikis R, Ferch RD, et al (2002) The neuro-cardio-endocrine response to acute subarachnoid haemorrhage. Clin Endocrinol 56:629–635
31. Akiba T, Tachibana K, Togashi K, Hiroe M, Marumo F (1995) Plasma human brain natriuretic peptide in chronic renal failure. Clin Nephrol 44:S61–S64
32. McCullough PA, Sandberg KR (2003) B-type natriuretic peptide and renal disease. Heart Fail Rev 8:355–358
33. Wahl HG, Graf S, Renz H, Fassbinder W (2004) Elimination of the cardiac natriuretic peptides B-type natriuretic peptide (BNP) and N-Terminal proBNP by hemodialysis. Clin Chem 50:1071–1074
34. Luchner A, Burnett JC Jr, Jougasaki M, Hense HW, Riegger GA, Schunkert H (1998) Augmentation of the cardiac natriuretic peptides by beta-receptor antagonism: evidence from a population-based study. J Am Coll Cardiol 32:1839–1844
35. Yoshimura M, Yasue H, Tanaka H, et al (1994) Responses of plasma concentrations of A type natriuretic peptide and B type natriuretic peptide to alacepril, an angiotensin-converting enzyme inhibitor, in patients with congestive heart failure. Br Heart J 72:528–533

36. Luchner A, Burnett JC Jr, Jougasaki M, et al (2000) Evaluation of brain natriuretic peptide as marker of left ventricular dysfunction and hypertrophy in the population. J Hypertens 18:1121–1128
37. Fruhwald FM, Fahrleitner A, Watzinger N, et al (1999) Natriuretic peptides in patients with diastolic dysfunction due to idiopathic dilated cardiomyopathy. Eur Heart J 1415–1423
38. Pfister R, Scholz M, Wielckens K, Erdmann E, Schneider CA (2004) Use of NT-proBNP in routine testing and comparison to BNP. Eur J Heart Failure 6:289–293
39. Maisel A, Hollander JE, Guss D, et al (2004) Primary results of the Rapid Emergency Department Heart Failure Outpatient Trial (REDHOT). J Am Coll Cardiol 44:1328–1333
40. Kruger S, Graf J, Merx MW, et al (2004) Brain natriuretic peptide predicts right heart failure in patients with acute pulmonary embolism. Am Heart J 147:60–65
41. Mair J, Friedl W, Thomas S, Puschendorf B (1999) Natriuretic peptides in assessment of left-ventricular dysfunction. Scan J Clin Lab Invest Suppl 230:132–142
42. McCullough PA, Omland T, Maisel AS (2003) B-type natriuretic peptide: a diagnostic breakthrough for clincians. Rev Cardiovasc Med 4:72–80
43. Wu AHB, Smith AC, Mather JF, et al (2003) Biological variation for NT-pro- and B-type natriuretic peptides and implications for therapeutic monitoring of patients with congestive heart failure. Am J Cardiol 92:428–431

Management of Acute Myocardial Infarction

W. J. Brady, A. Baer, and C. A. Ghaemmaghami

▌ Introduction

Though the recognition of angina pectoris dates to the 18th century, myocardial infarction (MI) was not characterized until the early 20th century. Simultaneous to the identification of MI was the initial introduction and subsequent application of the electrocardiogram (EKG) – the first objective method of the coronary origin of the presentation. During the next 50 years, angina pectoris and MI were further characterized and diagnosed; unfortunately, the management of ischemic heart disease (IHD), however, did not progress as significantly. From this point in medical history to the 1960s, management consisted primarily of pain relief coupled with strict bed rest for prolonged periods and management of resultant congestive heart failure (CHF); acute complications such as cardiogenic shock and sudden cardiac death were invariably fatal events. Subsequently, the introduction and widespread use of cardiopulmonary resuscitation, external defibrillation, and antidysrhythmic agents gave the clinician a powerful tool in the management of sudden cardiac death and other malignant dysrhythmias. Overall management, however, was still aimed at the complications of IHD rather than the syndrome itself.

With the recognition of the thrombotic nature of the acute coronary syndrome (ACS) within the last several decades, the stage was set for the next most significant advance in the management of the more acute forms of IHD, namely acute myocardial infarction (AMI). Early coronary angiography coupled with intra-arterial administration of streptokinase ushered in the era of acute reperfusion therapies, certainly the most significant advance in the recent past. Clinicians were now able not only to treat the acute complications of the illness but also to interrupt, if not halt, the primary process, thereby markedly reducing morbidity and mortality.

▌ Treatment of AMI

Treatment of patients with AMI follows the five basic approaches:
1) increase myocardial oxygen supply
2) decrease the force of myocardial contraction and therefore oxygen demand
3) increase metabolic substrate availability to the myocardium
4) protect injured myocardial cell function by decreasing inflammation or toxic injury, and
5) prevent re-occlusion of the coronary artery.

The initial therapeutic agents which should be considered in the AMI patient include nitroglycerin, morphine, aspirin, heparin, and beta-adrenergic blocking agents. Additional issues may include pain relief and anxiolysis. While these initial medications are administered, the clinician must address the issue of reperfusion therapies, including fibrinolysis and percutaneous coronary intervention. Such reperfusion therapies are a must in the ST segment elevation AMI (STEMI) presentation. In the patient with non-ST segment elevation AMI (NSTEMI), fibrinolysis has not demonstrated benefit while, depending on the clinical status of the individual, coronary angiography with potential percutaneous coronary intervention may be indicated early in the hospital course. In the early phase of management, immediate concerns center on protecting and monitoring of an adequate airway with appropriate gas exchange as well as restoration and maintenance of the circulatory volume.

Nitroglycerin

Nitroglycerin provides significant benefit to ACS patients by reductions in the preload and afterload as well as coronary vasodilation. The most significant positive effect is coronary vasodilation; direct vasodilation of coronary arteries may increase perfusion of ischemic myocardium. The next most significant effect is preload reduction which reduces myocardial oxygen demand. A meta-analysis of various prefibrinolytic studies of intravenous nitroglycerin in AMI patients noted a 35% mortality reduction [1]. In the initial setting, patients with possible ACS and adequate systemic perfusion should receive a sublingual nitroglycerin tablet (0.4 mg). If symptoms are not relieved with two sublingual tablets, the patient should be started on i.v. nitroglycerin. Care must be exercised in patients with bradycardia, hypotension, inferior wall STEMI, and right ventricular infarction when administering nitroglycerin; this caution is advised because a sudden decrease in preload associated with nitroglycerin use can result in profound hypotension. Initial i.v. nitroglycerin infusion rates should start at 10 micrograms/minute with titration to a pain-free state. The clinician should increase the infusion at regular intervals, allowing for a 10% reduction in the mean arterial pressure if normotensive and a 20 to 30% reduction if hypertensive. Maximal benefit is likely achieved at 200 micrograms/minute though certain patients may receive additional benefit at higher infusion rates.

Morphine Sulfate

The use of morphine sulfate for the treatment of ACS has not been extensively evaluated. Morphine sulfate exerts its beneficial effects via several mechanisms, including analgesic, anxiolytic, and vasodilatory properties. Morphine sulfate is a potent analgesic; the relief of pain decreases oxygen consumption and myocardial work. The anxiolytic properties also contribute to reductions in myocardial oxygen demand. Some vasodilatory effects are also noted that can decrease preload to the heart with positive impact on cardiac work and oxygen need. If a patient with possible ACS is unresponsive to nitroglycerin, administration of morphine sulfate should be considered. Standard doses of morphine sulfate are 2 to 5 mg delivered intravenously, repeated every 5 to 30 minutes as necessary. Significant adverse effects include hypotension, respiratory depression, and allergy. Intravenous fluids and naloxone are the primary treatments for hypotension and respiratory depression, respectively. Allergic phenomenon is treated in typical fashion.

Beta-adrenergic Blocking Agents

Beta-adrenergic blocking agents are effective in reducing catecholamine-mediated events in the heart, thereby lowering myocardial oxygen demand. Beta-blockade has been demonstrated to be effective in decreasing mortality for patients with AMI as well as reducing infarct size, ischemic pain, malignant ventricular dysrhythmias, and recurrent infarction. The mortality reduction ranges from 10 to 15%. Beta-adrenergic blocking agents perhaps are most useful in patients with significant sympathetic hyperactivity, manifested by tachycardia and systemic hypertension, although most AMI patients without contraindication will also demonstrate benefit.

Intravenous metoprolol can be given in 5 mg increments by slow infusion over 1 to 2 minutes; the total dose of 15 mg is reached via two consecutive administrations performed at 5-minute intervals. Esmolol is an ultra-short-acting beta-blocker that can be given to patients who potentially will not tolerate beta-adrenergic antagonism, such as patients with mild CHF or a history of bronchospasm. Other agents in this class that may be used include atenolol and propranolol. Contraindications to beta-adrenergic blockade include pulmonary edema, other signs of acute CHF, bronchospasm, atrioventricular block, bradycardia, and hypotension. Despite the potentially beneficial effects of this treatment in the early phase of management in the AMI patient, clinicians appear to use this medication less often than is possible.

Angiotensin-Converting Enzyme Inhibitors

Angiotensin-converting enzyme (ACE) inhibitor agents have been long known to benefit patients with CHF of various causes. It has also been suggested that ACE inhibitors may reduce morbidity and mortality after AMI. In particular, patients treated with ACE inhibitors experience a reduction in cardiovascular mortality, decreased rates of significant CHF development, and fewer recurrent AMIs. These benefits are noted to increase when ACE inhibitors are used in conjunction with other agents such as aspirin and fibrinolytics. The mechanism of action regarding a reduction in recurrent AMI is unknown but may involve a reduction in plaque rupture due to decreased intracoronary shear force.

Captopril, enalipril, lisinopril, or ramipril may be used in this setting. The ultimate doses used should be maximized; care must be exercised with these potent agents such that initial doses should be low and applied cautiously in order to avoid hypotension. Therapy should be initiated early in the post-AMI course, preferably within the first 24 hours. In patients with asymptomatic left ventricular (LV) dysfunction, therapy should be applied for a minimum of 2 to 4 months; in those patients with symptomatic CHF, ACE inhibitors should be administered indefinitely. Contraindications to ACE inhibitor therapy include hypotension; relative contraindications include volume depletion and borderline perfusion. Renal function must be closely monitored during therapy.

Calcium Channel Blocking Agents

The primary benefit of calcium channel blockers appears to be with symptom resolution, similar to the effect of beta-blockade. Unfortunately, these agents may be accompanied by a significant vasodilatory effect resulting in hypotension and therefore the potentiation of the coronary ischemic process. As with beta-blocking agents, calcium channel blockers have substantial negative inotropic effect, further affecting perfusion. AV nodal blockade is also a significant side effect that may be exacerbated in patients previously treated with beta-blockers or with ischemic-related conduction disturbance. In most instances of AMI, calcium channel blocker agents are not recommended.

Aspirin

Aspirin, the standard and perhaps most significant antiplatelet agent, represents the most cost-effective treatment available for patients with AMI. Aspirin should be administered in all patients suspected of AMI who do not have allergy or significant gastrointestinal bleeding; the medication should be given empirically, early in the evaluation/treatment course prior to the return of clinical information. Aspirin irreversibly inhibits platelet function by the acetylation of cyclo-oxygenase. As such, aspirin halts the production of pro-aggregatory thromboxane A2; it also possesses indirect antithrombotic effects *in vitro*. Lastly, aspirin exerts beneficial effect in the vascular endothelium by inactivation of cyclo-oxygenase, thereby reducing the production of anti-aggregatory prostacyclin. The ISIS-2 trial provides the strongest evidence that aspirin independently reduces the mortality of patients with AMI without fibrinolytic therapy (overall 23% reduction) and is synergistic when used with fibrinolytic therapy (42% reduction in mortality) [2]. Standard doses range from 160 to 324 mg given orally; in those patients unable to take medication orally, aspirin may also be given via nasogastric tube or the rectum in suppository form. Minimal side effects are noted, particularly with the 160 mg dose.

Glycoprotein IIb-IIIa Receptor Inhibitors

The glycoprotein IIb-IIIa receptor inhibitors represent a relatively recent addition to the therapeutic armamentarium employed in the AMI patient. This class of medication has provided the clinician with potent antiplatelet therapy; the glycoprotein IIb-IIIa receptor inhibitors, however, have demonstrated clinical utility in only a subset of ACS patients – those undergoing percutaneous coronary intervention. During platelet stimulation, surface receptors are activated, particularly the membrane glycoprotein IIb-IIIa receptors. These receptors represent the final common pathway for platelet activation and ultimate aggregation. Once activated, the glycoprotein IIb-IIIa receptors allow the various circulating factors, von Willebrand factor and fibrinogen, to link into a chain-like arrangement; this linked-chain formation ultimately results in platelet adhesion and clot.

Three agents in this class currently enjoy widespread clinical use, including abciximab, eptifibatide, and tirofiban. Abciximab was the first such glycoprotein receptor inhibitor to have undergone large clinical trials. As a monoclonal antibody specific for the glycoprotein IIb-IIIa receptor, it provides prolonged inhibition of platelet aggregation even after cessation of drug infusion. Numerous trials have demonstrated its effectiveness in AMI patients. Yet only a subset of these patients actually derive benefit from its application – the patient who is managed with percutaneous coronary intervention with or without intracoronary stent. The EPIC (Evaluation of 7E3 for the Prevention of Ischemic Complications) trial [3] investigated the effect of the drug in high-risk unstable angina and AMI patients scheduled for percutaneous coronary intervention, demonstrating a 35% reduction in mortality rate, recurrent MI, and need for unplanned rescue therapies (surgical revascularization, repeat percutaneous coronary intervention, and intra-aortic balloon pump [IABP]) balanced by an increase in hemorrhagic complications. The EPILOG trial [4] further evaluated the effect of abciximab in ACS presentations, including AMI patients, who underwent invasive coronary interventions; these investigators noted a 68% reduction in death or nonfatal AMI in the treatment group with a lower incidence of major bleeding episodes than in the EPIC study. In the GRAPE study, which investigated the use of glycoprotein IIb-IIIa receptor inhibitors in patients scheduled for urgent percutaneous coronary intervention [5], increased rates of TIMI (Thrombolysis in Myocardial Infarction) grade 3 flow were noted in the abciximab group.

Eptifibatide, a synthetic peptide, prevents binding of fibrinogen to the glycoprotein IIb/IIIa receptor; this antagonism blocks platelet aggregation and subsequent thrombus formation. The IMPACT-AMI investigators [6] reported the results in AMI patients receiving fibrinolytic agents and varying doses of eptifibatide (i.e., non-mechanical means of reperfusion); they noted an increase in TIMI grade 3 flow at 90 minutes with similar rates of death, recurrent MI, and the need for revascularization procedures. In the IMPACT-II trial [7], ACS patients bound for percutaneous coronary intervention demonstrated a modest reduction in the rate of revascularization, AMI, or death at 30 days; this modest benefit was lost at six months. Tirofiban is a synthetic, non-peptide, shorter acting glycoprotein IIb-IIIa receptor inhibitors with a similar mechanism of action to eptifibatide. The PRISM [8] and PRISM-PLUS [9] trial investigators did not demonstrate significant benefit in ACS patients with a short-term reduction in ischemic events (PRISM [8]) and benefit limited to angiographic variables (intracoronary thrombus burden, improved perfusion grade, and decreased severity of obstruction) (PRISM-PLUS trial [9]).

Recent work has confirmed the most appropriate use of glycoprotein IIb-IIIa receptor inhibitors in the AMI patient – the patient scheduled for percutaneous coronary intervention with or without intracoronary stenting. The GUSTO IV trial revealed that abciximab did not alter the rate of death or recurrent MI at 1 month in patients with ACS while hemorrhagic complications occurred more often in the active treatment groups [10]. A meta-analysis of glycoprotein IIb-IIIa receptor inhibitor use in ACS patients reinforces this conclusion – that patients who undergo percutaneous coronary intervention benefit markedly from glycoprotein inhibitor administration; other ACS groups do not derive significant benefit from its application [11]. As such, the American College of Cardiology (ACC)/American Heart Association (AHA) has provided the following guidelines [12]:

▌ Class I (evidence and/or general consensus treatment is effective) – glycoprotein IIb-IIIa receptor inhibitors should be given, in addition to acetylsalicylic acid and heparin, to patients in whom percutaneous coronary intervention is planned

▌ Class IIa (conflicting evidence and/or a divergence of opinion regarding effectiveness) – glycoprotein IIb-IIIa receptor inhibitors should be given to patients already receiving heparin, acetylsalicylic acid, and clopidogrel in whom percutaneous coronary intervention is planned, and

▌ Class IIb (efficacy less well established by evidence and/or opinion) – eptifibatide or tirofiban, in addition to acetylsalicylic acid and heparin, may be given to patients without continuing ACS who have no other high-risk features and in whom percutaneous coronary intervention is not planned.

Other Anti-platelet Agents

Ticlopidine inhibits the transformation of the glycoprotein IIb-IIIa receptor into its high-affinity ligand-binding state. This irreversibly inhibits platelet aggregation and lasts for the duration of the life of the platelet. Ticlopidine has non-linear kinetics and, after repeated dosing, reaches a maximal effect after 8 to 11 days of dosage. In patients with unstable angina, a significant reduction in total coronary events is noted; this drug may be considered if aspirin is thought to be inadequate or ineffective. Because of the time delay to the onset of action, ticlopidine's use in the emergency department is limited; it is not suited for use at the onset of AMI and cannot replace aspirin in the acute phase. Furthermore, ticlopidine is associated with a risk of neutropenia and agranulocytosis. It should therefore be reserved for patients who are intolerant of aspirin therapy but need an antiplatelet agent as prophylaxis for AMI. The standard dosage of ticlopidine is 250 mg twice daily taken with food (to lessen gastric intolerance).

Clopidogrel is a ticlopidine analog. Its advantages are a rapid onset of action and an i.v. route of administration. It also prevents the transformation of the glycoprotein IIb-IIIa receptor into its high-affinity state. It also appears to promote formation of platelet cAMP and therefore lowers platelet calcium. While its use in the hospitalized coronary stent population is reasonably well defined, information regarding acute treatment in the emergency department AMI patient is lacking.

Heparin

The heparins have been shown to have a profound synergistic effect with aspirin in preventing death and cardiovascular complications in the AMI patient. The term *heparin* refers not to a single structure but rather to a family of mucopolysaccharide chains of varying length and composition – hence the term *unfractionated* – with pronounced antithrombotic properties. Unfractionated heparin is composed of a mixture of polysaccharide chains with varying molecular weights. Low molecular weight (LMW) heparins constitute approximately one third of the molecular weight of unfractionated heparin and are less heterogeneous in size. At pharmacologic doses, unfractionated heparin binds to antithrombin, forming a complex, which then is able to inactivate factor II (thrombin) and activated factor X, thus preventing the conversion to fibrin and ultimate clot formation. Unfractionated heparin also potentiates the inactivation of factors XIa and IXa via antithrombin; additional anticoagulant effects are mediated via platelet interaction. LMW heparin inhibits the coagulation system in a similar fashion to that of unfractionated heparin with action at varying levels of the cascade, including antithrombin, thrombin, and factor Xa.

The practical advantages of LMW heparin over unfractionated heparin are numerous. LMW heparin inactivates factor Xa, which is resistant to inactivation by unfractionated heparin. LMW heparin has lesser binding characteristics to coagulation factors, resulting in higher bioavailability. LMW heparin has a longer half-life and less individual variability of the anticoagulant response when compared with unfractionated heparin. It has a lower affinity for von Willebrand factor, increased vascular permeability, and a weak effect on platelet function. These differences could explain why LMW heparin produces less bleeding than unfractionated heparin with equivalent or higher antithrombotic effects. The long half-life of LMW heparins and their predictable anticoagulant response to weight-adjusted doses allow once-daily subcutaneous administration without laboratory monitoring. LMW heparins are the agents of choice when heparin is contraindicated by non-availability of activated partial thromboplastin time (aPTT) measurements but the disadvantage is expense. The urgent need for a percutaneous procedure or surgical therapy is a consideration in the application of LMW heparin in that the serum half-life is considerably longer compared to unfractionated heparin; unfractionated heparin, with its shorter half-life, may be a more reasonable alternative in this instance.

The clinical advantages of LMW heparin over unfractionated heparin are less pronounced. In general, it appears that LMW heparin, particularly enoxaparin with its favorable anti-factor Xa/antifactor IIa ratio, offers a short-term benefit in the ACS patient which lessens significantly beyond the first week of treatment. The FRISC trial [13] established that the combination of aspirin, beta-blocker and LMW heparin significantly decreased the rate of nonfatal AMI or death at 1 week with a less pronounced effect at 40 to 150 days coupled with an increased number of minor bleeding episodes. The FRIC study [14] investigated the use of LMW (dalteparin) compared to unfractionated heparin in patients with unstable coronary disease (unstable angina and NSTEMI). The rates of death, recurrent angina, AMI, and the need for revascularization procedures, were similar at 1 week and 45 days. In this study, both forms of heparin provided similar benefit in these ACS patients. In the ESSENCE study [15], a benefit was found with LMW heparin at 30 days; the risk of minor bleeding was higher.

Unfractionated heparin should be administered early in patients with AMI. The initial dose is 80 U/kg by IV bolus, followed by a maintenance infusion of 18 U/kg/ hr. The aPTT should be titrated to 1.5 to 2.5 times control using the maintenance infusion. LMW heparin may be administered in a twice-daily regimen subcutaneously at a dose of 1 mg/kg; doses should be reduced for patients with pronounced renal insufficiency. Contraindications to heparin therapy include active, life-threatening hemorrhage or predisposition to such hemorrhage.

Other Anticoagulants

Hirudin, hirulog, and argatroban are potent antithrombin anticoagulants. Hirudin is an amino acid peptide derived from two sources: leech salivary gland (naturally derived form) and the laboratory (synthetic version). It binds directly with high affinity to thrombin and can inactivate thrombin already bound to fibrin (clot-bound thrombin). Hirudin also inhibits thrombin-induced platelet aggregation. Hirudin has not been associated with drug-induced thrombocytopenia. In the OASIS-2 trial [16], no benefit of hirudin was found over standard therapy in patients with ACS patients; of concern, patients in the hirudin group more often experienced major hemorrhage requiring transfusion. The HIT-4 trial [17] investigated the use of hirudin as an adjunct to fibrinolysis in AMI patients, noting no major difference in rates of death, recurrent acute coronary ischemia, major bleeding, or stroke. Hirulog is a bifunctional 20-amino acid peptide designed on the structure of hirudin. It has similar properties to huridin, but in addition interacts at the catalytic site of thrombin. In the HERO trial [18], AMI patients were treated with streptokinase and aspirin; hirulog appeared to be more effective than heparin in producing early patency in patients treated with aspirin and streptokinase without increasing the risk of adverse outcome including death. Argatroban is an arginine derivative that binds to thrombin with intermediate affinity and is a competitive antagonist inhibiting fibrinogen cleavage and platelet activation by thrombin. Compared with heparin, argatroban is significantly more effective in the prevention of platelet-rich thrombi after vascular injury. The MINT trial [19] demonstrated that argatroban had an effect on reperfusion produced by tissue plasminogen activator in AMI with higher rates of TIMI grade 3 flow at 90 min in the treatment group yet rates of death, recurrent myocardial infarction, cardiogenic shock, and revascularization was not significantly different. These agents demonstrate little to no benefit over standard anticoagulant therapy in the AMI patient.

Reperfusion Therapy

Selected patients suffering from AMI benefit from acute reperfusion therapy. The goal of reperfusion therapy is the restoration of normal flow through the infarct-related epicardial coronary artery. This improvement in blood flow through the coronary artery in turn results in improved myocardial perfusion, limitation of infarct size, reduction of serious morbidity, and improved survival. Pharmacologic and mechanical methods of reperfusion are both effective under specific clinical conditions. Considering both methods, prompt initiation of reperfusion therapy is still the most critical determinant of outcome. The importance of early coronary artery patency was affirmed by the GUSTO investigators in their angiographic substudy when they demonstrated that 90 minute patency predicted rates of survival and preserved LV function that were superior to those of patients not achieving normal coronary flow [20].

Indications for reperfusion therapy are derived from large randomized trials [2, 21, 22] assessing the efficacy of fibrinolytic agents and percutaneous coronary intervention in patients presenting with AMI and who meet specific EKG criteria. These criteria (Table 1) include the onset of symptoms consistent with ACS for less than 12 hours, an absence of contraindications, and an EKG indicating:

▌ ST segment elevation of ≥1 mm in two anatomically contiguous limb leads
▌ ST segment elevation of ≥2 mm in two anatomically contiguous precordial leads, or
▌ new bundle branch block (left and right).

Although not supported by large clinical trials, reperfusion therapy should also be considered in those patients with acute posterior wall and right ventricular (RV) infarctions that are associated with ST segment elevation in the additional EKG leads. Similarly, patients with known left bundle branch block (LBBB) exhibiting certain abnormal ST segment deviations and the appropriate clinical presentation may benefit from rapid reperfusion therapy [23].

Table 1. Indications for reperfusion therapy

▌ Onset of symptoms consistent with cardiac ischemia for less than 12 hours
▌ 12-lead electrocardiogram indicating:
– ST segment elevation of ≥1 mm in two contiguous limb leads;
– ST segment elevation of ≥1mm in two contiguous precordial leads, or
– New bundle branch block (either Left or Right).
▌ Absence of contraindications

Clinical studies of AMI patients undergoing early reperfusion therapy show a strong correlation between time-related myocardial necrosis and reperfusion therapy with respect to resultant left ventricular function and patient survival. In an analysis of all major fibrinolytic AMI trials prior to 1994, the number of lives saved per thousand treated declined from 35 when treated within the first hour of symptom onset to 25 when treated between the second and third hours after symptom onset. The rate of decline in the survival benefit decelerates sharply between the sixth and twelfth hours [24]. In the National Registry of Myocardial Infarction (NRMI) 2 and 3, a comparison of time-to-fibrinolytic agent to survival revealed a significant trend: compared to door-to-therapy times under 30 minutes, the adjusted odds of death increased by 11% and 23% for patients with door-to-therapy times between 61 to 90 minutes and greater than 90 minutes, respectively. Similarly, an increase in the risk of significant LV functional impairment also increased at each 30-minute interval [25–27]. Furthermore, an analysis of NRMI 2 registry data shows that in percutaneous coronary intervention-treated patients, a door-to-balloon time greater than 2 hours was associated with an increased relative risk of mortality compared with individuals managed with percutaneous coronary intervention initiated earlier in the hospital course (odds ratio 1.41) [25]. Per current ACC/AHA guidelines, initiation of fibrinolytic therapy (i.e., door-to-needle time) is recommended within 30 minutes of arrival in the emergency department. In the case of a percutaneous coronary intervention-based strategy, the target is a maximum time of 90 to 120 minutes from emergency department presentation to the time of the first intra-coronary balloon inflation (i.e., door-to-balloon time) [28]. Theoretically, the time from onset of symptoms to the diagnosis of STEMI could be very short in patients sustaining an AMI while hospitalized. This short time to diagnosis when coupled with prompt action could potentially improve outcomes with a reduction in the risks of major complication. Similarly, the clinical impact of a short delay (e.g., 30 mins) to arrange percutaneous coronary intervention may be absorbed because of the very early diagnosis in this patient group. Data on the optimal timing for reperfusion therapy primarily comes from large fibrinolytic trials, so extrapolation to catheter-based strategies may not be entirely applicable. Because there are no large studies investigating the optimal treatment of established inpatients who sustain STEMIs while hospitalized, these issues remain very unclear and call for prudent on-site, individual clinical judgment.

Table 2. Fibrinolytic agents

Chemical Name	Streptokinase	rt-PA	rPA	TNK-tPA
▌Generic name		alteplase	reteplase	tenecteplase
▌Trade name		Activase	Retevase	TNKase
▌Plasminogen activation	indirect	direct	direct	direct
▌Patency at 90 mins				
TIMI grade 3	29–32%	45–63%	60%	66%
TIMI grade 2 or 3	54–60%	73–82%	83%	88%
▌Cost	~ $ 300	$ 2200	$ 2200	$ 2200
▌Antigenic properties	yes	no	no	no

Fibrinolysis

Since the mid-1980s, the use of various fibrinolytic agents in the treatment of AMI has been extensively studied. Currently, there are four commonly used, FDA-approved fibrinolytic agents for treatment of AMI: streptokinase, recombinant tissue plasminogen activator (alteplase, t-PA), reteplase (rPA), and tenecteplase (TNK-tPA) (Table 2). The ISIS-2 trial established the efficacy of streptokinase – and the fibrinolytic concept – by demonstrating a 25% relative reduction in 35-day mortality in comparison to placebo when used in conjunction with aspirin [29]. The subsequent GUSTO trial showed a slight superiority of t-PA over streptokinase in respect to 30-day survival and no significant difference in major bleeding complications [30]. Further investigations of the newer agents, rPA and TNK-tPA, with comparisons to t-PA have shown them to have equivalent survival benefits and comparable risks of major hemorrhage [31–33]. Major hemorrhage is the most common serious complication from fibrinolytic therapy. Contraindications to fibrinolysis are listed in Table 3. The intracranial hemorrhage rate for patients treated in clinical trials with fibrinolytic agents ranges from 0.6 to 1% [34]. Increased risk of intracranial hemorrhage in fibrinolytic-treated patients appears to be most closely related to advancing patient age and the presence of systemic hypertension [35-37]. In the NRMI 2 Registry, the adjusted odds ratios by age group for intracranial hemorrhage after t-PA administration were: 1 for ages less than 65 years, 2.71 for ages 65 to 74 years, and 4.34 for ages greater than 75 years [36]. Other major bleeding generally appears at the sites of vascular puncture, therefore, vascular access to non-compressible sites is contraindicated prior to or during fibrinolysis. The addition of higher dose of unfractionated heparin is associated with increased rates of significant hemorrhage [38].

Table 3. Contraindications to fibrinolysis

Absolute
Any previous history of hemorrhagic stroke
History of stroke within 6 months
Intracranial/intraspinal neoplasm, aneurysm, or AVM
Intracranial/intraspinal surgery within past 2 months
Suspected aortic dissection
Suspected pericarditis
Active bleeding
Known bleeding disorder
Major surgery, trauma, or bleeding within 2 weeks
Relative
Traumatic CPR or CPR > 10 mins
Oral anticoagulant therapy
Hemorrhagic ophthalmologic conditions
Pregnancy or within 1 week postpartum
Active peptic ulcer disease
Uncontrolled hypertension (diastolic blood pressure > 100 mmHg)
Ischemic or embolic stroke > 6 months ago
Significant trauma or major surgery > 2 wks & < 2 months
Subclavian or internal jugular cannulation

Streptokinase is considered to be the first generation of fibrinolytic agents. Streptokinase is a natural product which binds plasminogen and converts it into a plasmin-like agent. This agent in turn converts both circulating and fibrin-bound plasminogen into circulating plasmin. The ensuing systemic lytic state depletes fibrinogen, plasminogen, factors V and VIII [34]. Because of the associated anticoagulation seen with streptokinase, concomitant heparin administration may be of little benefit and can increase the risk of major hemorrhage. Patients can develop antistreptococcal antibodies after administration to streptokinase. This sensitization can cause a serious hypersensitivity reaction, especially on re-exposure.

With t-PA, the second generation of fibrinolytic agents was introduced. t-PA has more specificity to action against fibrin located in clots but can cause a mild general fibrinogen depletion that is less severe than that seen with streptokinase. t-PA has a relatively short half-life of 3 to 8 minutes so it is administered as an infusion rather than a bolus. The so-called 'accelerated' or 'front-loaded' method for administration of t-PA refers to the 90-minute protocol used in the GUSTO trial (Table 4). The third generation of fibrinolytic agents are variants of t-PA that have either been identified as spontaneous human mutations (e.g., reteplase) or specifically engineered to have certain beneficial properties (e.g., tenecteplase). Both reteplase and tenecteplase are recombinant products and nonantigenic. These agents appear to provide greater earlier patency rates of infarct vessels over streptokinase or t-PA [33]. Notably rPA causes fibrinogen depletion greater than that of t-PA but less that

Table 4. Fibrinolytic and heparin dosing guidelines

	Fibrinolytic agent	Heparin
Streptokinase	1.5 million units i.v over 60 minutes	UFH: 12500 unit SC every 12 hours
t-PA (alteplase)	Bolus: 15 mg IV Infuse: 0.75 mg/kg i.v. over 30 min (max. 50 mg) then 0.50 mg/kg i.v. over 60 min (max. 35 mg)	UFH: 60 units/kg bolus (max. 4000 units) then 12 units/kg/hr (max 1000 units/hr) Maintain APTT 50–70 sec
rPA (reteplase)	Double bolus: 10 U IV bolus followed by a second 10 U i.v. bolus in 30 min	UFH: 60 unit/kg bolus (max. 4000 units) then 12 units/kg/hr (max. 1000 units/hr) Maintain APTT 50–70 sec
TNK-tPA (tenecteplase)	Weight-based single i.v. bolus: <60 kg 30 mg 60–69 kg 35 mg 70–79 kg 40 mg 80–89 kg 45 mg ≥90 kg 50 mg	Enoxaparin: 30 mg i.v. then 1 mg/kg SC every 12 hrs – OR – UFH: 60 unit/kg bolus (max. 4000 units) then 12 units/kg/hr (max. 1000 units/hr) Maintain APTT 50–70 sec

UFH: unfractionated heparin; i.v.: intravenously; SC: subcutaneously

than of streptokinase. Contrastingly, tenecteplase has more fibrin specificity and an increased resistance to plasminogen activator inhibitor-1 (PAI-1) [39]. Both tenecteplase and reteplase have longer half-lives than t-PA, allowing for single- and double-bolus administration, respectively.

Despite the higher cost of t-PA over streptokinase, the absolute survival benefit of 1.1% was justified in a formalized cost-effectiveness analysis based on outcomes from the GUSTO trial, revealing a cost per year of life saved of $32,678 [40]. Since the pricing of all second and third generation fibrinolytics are equivalent, the findings related to t-PA should be generalizable to the entire class of new agents.

Ultimately, the selection of fibrinolytic agent is less important than the prompt decision to administer one. The benefits of early administration of a fibrinolytic agent outweigh the differences in survival benefit between any of the individual agents.

Combination Therapies

Multiple combinations of a fibrinolytic agent with anticoagulants, thrombin inhibitors, and/or platelet aggregation inhibitor have been studied in randomized controlled trials [41]. The ASSENT-3 study group reported the superiority of a combined treatment regimen of either tenecteplase plus enoxaparin or reduced-dose tenecteplase plus abciximab over tenecteplase plus unfractionated heparin in terms of efficacy and safety at 30-days (Table 5). Considering the excellent clinical outcomes, the ease of administration (bolus therapy for both agents), and lower comparative cost, the tenecteplase/enoxaprin regimen appears to be the most attractive fibrinolytic option at this time (Table 4 for heparin dosing guidelines) [41].

Table 5. ASSENT-3 results – Combination regimens using tenecteplase (TNK-tPA) for treatment of ST segment elevation acute myocardial infarction [41]

	TNK-tPA (full-dose) +enoxaparin (n = 2040)	TNK-tPA (half-dose) +UFH+abciximab (n = 2017)	TNK-tPA (full-dose) +UFH (n = 2038)	p value
Simple endpoints				
Death at 30 days	5.4%	6.6%	6.0%	0.25
In-hospital reinfarction	2.7%	2.2%	4.2%	0.0009
Refractory ischemia	4.6%	3.2%	6.5%	<0.0001
Intracranial hemorrhage	0.9%	0.9%	0.9%	0.98
Major bleeding (not ICH)	3.0%	4.3%	2.2%	0.0005
Combined endpoints				
Efficacy (death, reinfarct, ischemia)	11.4%	11.1%	15.4%	0.0001
Efficacy + Safety (death, reinfarct, ischemia, ICH, major bleeding)	13.8%	14.2%	17.0%	0.0081

UFH: unfractionated heparin; ICH: intracranial hemorrhage

Percutaneous Coronary Intervention

The strategy of primary percutaneous coronary intervention for AMI has been competing with that of fibrinolytic therapy since the early 1980s. The development of second and third generation fibrinolytic agents has been paralleled by improvements in operator expertise, equipment, and the adjunctive medical strategies used in the setting of percutaneous coronary intervention. A strategy of primary percutaneous coronary intervention results in patency rates in the infarct artery of approximately 90% versus the 50 to 80% patency rates typically seen with fibrinolytic therapy. These differences in patency rates may not translate into improvements in short-term mortality yet they appear to result in fewer subsequent episodes of reinfarction and intractable ischemia [42, 43].

One important conceptual benefit of percutaneous coronary intervention over fibrinolysis is the additive diagnostic value of immediate coronary angiography. Fifteen to twenty percent of patients may have spontaneous reperfusion at the time of catheterization; these patients could be potentially subjected to unnecessary risks of hemorrhage if they received fibrinolytic therapy. The early definition of coronary anatomy can identify patients with indications for early coronary artery bypass graft (CABG) surgery and can aid in the management of patients in the first few days after AMI. Additionally, the infrequent, unexpected angiographic diagnosis of aortic dissection in the setting of EKG ST segment, an absolute contraindication to lytic therapy, can lead to proper surgical management instead of a predictably disastrous outcome.

Multiple small clinical trials have been conducted comparing primary percutaneous coronary intervention with fibrinolysis for STEMI [44]. In a quantitative review of 10 trials comparing primary percutaneous coronary intervention with fibrinolytic therapy conducted prior to 1996, Weaver et al. [44] describe lower rates of 30-day mortality, reinfarction, total stroke rate, and hemorrhagic stroke rate in patients undergoing percutaneous coronary intervention (Table 6). These trials were conducted prior to the advent of routine intracoronary stenting and the adjunctive use of glycoprotein IIb-IIIa receptor inhibitors [43, 45–47]. Subsequent trials comparing percutaneous coronary intervention combined with stents and/or glycoprotein IIb-IIIa receptor inhibitors with percutaneous coronary intervention alone show incremental benefits to the combined approach [48, 49].

The most recent comprehensive investigation of the combined percutaneous coronary intervention-stent-glycoprotein IIb-IIIa receptor inhibitor strategy is the DANAMI-2 trial. [50]. Conducted on a nearly nationwide sample population in Denmark, investigators randomized 1572 patients to receive either percutaneous coro-

Table 6. Comparison of percutaneous coronary intervention with fibrinolytic therapy for ST segment elevation acute myocardial infarction. An analysis of 10 clinical trials before 1996 [44]

	PCI (n = 1290)	Fibrinolytic (n = 1316)	p Value
▌ Mortality at 30-days	4.4%	6.5%	0.02
▌ Death+reinfarction	7.2%	11.9%	<0.01
▌ Total stroke	0.7%	2.0%	0.007
▌ Hemorrhagic stroke	0.1%	1.1%	<0.01

nary intervention or accelerated treatment with alteplase (t-PA). Stents and glyco-protein IIb-IIIa receptor inhibitors were available and used at the discretion of the treating physicians. Significant differences were observed in a composite endpoint of death, reinfarction, or disabling stroke at 30 days between the groups, with rates of 8.5% in the percutaneous coronary intervention group versus 14.2% in the fibri-nolytic group. This study was actually stopped early by its safety board due to the significant benefits seen early in the percutaneous coronary intervention arm.

Reperfusion Therapy – Accessibility and Expertise

Because of the limited availability of percutaneous coronary intervention, fibrinolysis remains the most commonly utilized strategy in eligible STEMI patients [51]. Further complicating the access issue is the question of center expertise. The differ-ences in outcome for patients undergoing percutaneous coronary intervention in high- versus low-volume procedure centers have been well described [52–54]. In an analysis of the NRMI 2 and 3 registries, 30-day mortality rates after AMI were 3.4 vs 6.2% in high-volume versus low-volume percutaneous coronary intervention cen-ters. In fact, there was no significant difference between outcomes in patients treated with primary percutaneous coronary intervention versus fibrinolysis (6.2 vs 5.9%) in low-volume centers [52]. The encouraging results of AIR-PAMI and DA-NAMI-2 trials which included comparisons of fibrinolysis to transport to primary percutaneous coronary intervention centers have led some to advocate the transfer of patients at high risk for mortality or complications to expert centers able to pro-vide primary percutaneous coronary intervention services [50, 53]. This approach may be appropriate when delays can be minimized with proactive system planning and the availability of high quality interfacility transport [54–56].

Current Indication and Contraindications
for Primary Percutaneous Coronary Intervention

The most recent ACC/AHA guidelines advocate primary percutaneous coronary in-tervention as an alternative to fibrinolytic therapy in patients with STEMI "........who can undergo angioplasty of the infarct-related artery within 12 hour of onset of symptoms or greater than 12 hour if symptoms persist, if performed in a timely fashion by persons skilled in the procedure, and supported by experienced person-nel in an appropriate laboratory environment....." (Table 7). These guidelines further recommend primary percutanous coronary intervention in candidates for

Table 7. American College of Cardiology/American Heart Association recommended characteristics of car-diac interventional laboratories eligible to deliver percutaneous coronary intervention for ST segment ele-vation acute myocardial infarction (AMI) [28]

▌Balloon dilatation within 90 ± 30 min of admission and diagnosis of AMI

▌A documented clinical success rate (TIMI grade 2 or 3 flow) in greater than 90% of patients without emergency CABG, stroke, or death

▌Emergency CABG rate less than 5% among all patients undergoing the procedure

▌Actual performance of angioplasty in a high percentage of patients (85% brought to the lab)

▌Mortality rate less than 10%

reperfusion therapy for whom fibrinolytic therapy is contraindicated or who are within the first 18 hours of cardiogenic shock due to STEMI [28].

Patients with intravenous contrast dye allergy may be ineligible for a percutanous coronary intervention-based strategy depending on prior reactions, and careful consideration must be taken in patients with known severe renal dysfunction. Additionally, severe peripheral vascular disease may complicate the arterial access needed for percutanous coronary intervention.

Intra-aortic Balloon Pump

An IABP may be inserted through a sheath in the femoral artery into the descending aorta. It is a long balloon on a catheter that is timed with the cardiac cycle to inflate during diastole and deflate during systole. IABPs increase flow to the coronary arteries and increase cardiac output while decreasing cardiac work. These devices are used to treat refractory angina and cardiogenic shock. Aortic insufficiency can worsen with the use of an IABP. Complications from balloon pumps include embolization and arterial occlusion causing limb ischemia. Patients with IABPs should be systemically heparinized; vascular assessments must be performed regularly. Significant peripheral vascular disease is a relative contraindication to an IABP.

Patient Transfer

Indications for transfer of a patient with AMI to a regional tertiary care facility with angioplasty and cardiovascular surgery capability include patients with fibrinolytic therapy contraindications who may benefit from percutaneous or surgical revascularization, persistent hemodynamic instability, persistent ventricular dysrhythmias, or postinfarction/postreperfusion ischemia. Hospital transfer for percutanous coronary intervention is required in patients with fibrinolytic agent contraindications. The urgent transfer of a fibrinolytic-eligible AMI patient for percutanous coronary intervention to another institution is not recommended until fibrinolytic therapy is initiated unless angioplasty is initiated within approximately 120 minutes of initial diagnosis – this time interval is supported by the medical literature yet individual cases may alter the consideration.

References

1. Yusuf S, Collins R, MacMahon S, et al (1988) Effect of intravenous nitrates on mortality in acute myocardial infarction: an overview of the randomized trials. Lancet I:1088–1092
2. ISIS-2 (Second International Study of Infarct Survival) Collaborative Group (1988) Randomized trial of intravenous streptokinase, oral aspirin, both, or neither amount 17, 187 cases of suspected acute myocardial infarction: ISIS-2. Lancet 2:349–360
3. The EPIC Investigators (1994) Use of a monoclonal antibody directed against the platelet glycoprotein IIb/IIIa receptor in high-risk coronary angioplasty. N Engl J Med 330:956–961
4. The Epilog Investigators (1997) Platelet glycoprotein IIb/IIIa receptor blockade and low-dose heparin during percutaneous coronary revascularization. N Engl J Med 336:1689–1696
5. Lambert F, Zijlstra F, Olsson H, et al (1999) Abciximab in the treatment of acute myocardial infarction eligible for primary percutaneous transluminal coronary angioplasty. J Am Coll Cardiol 33:1528–1532
6. Ohman EM, Kleiman NS, Gacioch G, et al (1997) Combined accelerated tissue-plasminogen activator and platelet glycoprotein IIb/IIIa integrin receptor blockade with Integrilin in

acute myocardial infarction. Results of a randomized, placebo-controlled, dose-ranging trial. IMPACT-AMI Investigators. Circulation 95:846–854

7. The IMPACT-II Investigators (1997) Randomized placebo-controlled trial of effect of eptifibatide on complications of percutaneous coronary intervention: IMPACT II. Integrilin to Minimize Platelet Aggregation and Coronary Thrombosis-II. Lancet 349:1422–1428

8. Platelet Receptor Inhibition in Ischemic Syndrome Management (PRISM) Study Investigators (1998) A comparison of aspirin plus tirofiban with aspirin plus heparin for unstable angina. N Engl J Med 338:1498–1505

9. Zhao XQ, Theroux P, Snapinn SM, Sax FL (1999) Intracoronary thrombus and platelet glycoprotein IIb/IIIa receptor blockade with tirofiban in unstable angina or non-Q-wave myocardial infarction. Angiographic results from the PRISM-PLUS trial (Platelet receptor inhibition for ischemic syndrome management in patients limited by unstable signs and symptoms). PRISM-PLUS Investigators. Circulation 100:1609–1615

10. GUSTO IV-ACS Investigators (2001) Effect of glycoprotein IIb/IIIa receptor blocker abciximab on outcome in patients with acute coronary syndromes without early coronary revascularisation: The GUSTO IV-ACS randomised trial. Lancet 357:1915–1924

11. Boersma E, Harrington RA, Moliterno DJ, et al (2002) Platelet glycoprotein IIb/IIIa inhibitors in acute coronary syndromes: A meta-analysis of all major randomised clinical trials. Lancet 359:189–198

12. Braunwald E, Antman EM, Beasley JW, et al (2002) ACC/AHA guideline update for the management of patients with unstable angina and non-ST-segment elevation myocardial infarction–2002: summary article: a report of the American College of Cardiology/American Heart Association Task Force on Practice Guidelines (Committee on the Management of Patients With Unstable Angina). Circulation 106:1893–1900

13. Wallentin L, Ohlsson J, Swahn E, et al (1996) Low molecular weight heparin during instability in coronary artery disease. Lancet 347:561–568

14. Klein W, Buchwald A, Hillis SE, et al (1997) Comparison of low-molecular-weight heparin with unfractionated heparin acutely and with placebo for 6 weeks in the management of unstable coronary artery disease. Fragmin in unstable coronary artery disease study (FRIC). Circulation 96:61–68

15. Cohen M, Demers C, Gurfinkel EP, et al (1997) A comparison of low-molecular-weight heparin with unfractionated heparin for unstable coronary artery disease. Efficacy and Safety of Subcutaneous Enoxaparin in Non-Q-Wave Coronary Events Study Group. N Engl J Med 337:447–452

16. Organisation to Assess Strategies for Ischemic Syndromes (OASIS-2) Investigators (1999) Effects of recombinant hirudin (lepirudin) compared with heparin on death, myocardial infarction, refractory angina, and revascularisation procedures in patients with acute myocardial ischaemia without ST elevation: a randomised trial. Lancet 353:429–438

17. Neuhaus KL, Molhoek GP, Zeymer U, Tebbe U, Molhoek P, Schroder R (1998) Recombinant hirudin (lepirudin) for the improvement of thrombolysis with streptokinase in patients with acute myocardial infarction: Results of the HIT-4 trial. J Am Coll Cardiol 32:876–881

18. White HD, Aylward PE, Frey MJ, et al (1997) Randomized, double-blind comparison of hirulog versus heparin in patients receiving streptokinase and aspirin for acute myocardial infarction (HERO). Hirulog Early Reperfusion/Occlusion (HERO) Trial Investigators. Circulation 96:2155–2161

19. Jang IK, Brown DF, Giugliano RP, et al (1999) A multicenter, randomized study of argatroban versus heparin as adjunct to tissue plasminogen activator (TPA) in acute myocardial infarction: Myocardial infarction with novastan and TPA (MINT) study. J Am Coll Cardiol 33:1879–1885

20. The GUSTO Angiographic Investigators (1993) The effects of tissue plasminogen activator, streptokinase, or both on coronary-artery patency, ventricular function, and survival after acute myocardial infarction. N Engl J Med 329:1615–1622

21. Gruppo Italiano per lo Studio della Streptochinasi nell'Infarto Miocardico (GISSI) (1986) Effectiveness of intravenous thrombolytic treatment in acute myocardial infarction. Lancet 1:397–402

22. Dundar Y, Hill R, Dickson R, Walley T (2003) Comparative efficacy of thrombolytics in acute myocardial infarction: a systematic review. Q J Med 96:103–113

23. Sgarbossa EB, Pinski SL, Barbagelata A, et al (1996) Electrocardiographic diagnosis of evolving acute myocardial infarction in the presence of left bundle branch block. N Engl J Med 334:481–487

24. Fibrinolytic Therapy Trials (FTT) Collaborative Group (1994) Indications for fibrinolytic therapy in suspected acute myocardial infarction: Collaborative overview of early mortality and major morbidity results from all randomized trials of more than 1000 patients. Lancet 343:311–322

25. Cannon CP, Gibson CM, Lambrew CT, et al (2000) Relationship of symptom-onset-to-balloon time and door-to-balloon time with mortality in patients undergoing angioplasty. JAMA 283:2941–2947

26. Peterson LR, Chandra NC, French WJ, Rogers WJ, Weaver WD, Tiefenbrunn AJ (1999) Reperfusion therapy in patients with acute myocardial infarction and prior coronary artery bypass surgery (National Registry of Myocardial Infarction-2). Am J Cardiol 84:1287–1291

27. Cannon CP, Gibson CM, Lambrew CT, et al (2000) Longer thrombolysis door-to-needle times are associated with increased mortality in acute myocardial infarction: an analysis of 85589 patients in the National Registry of Myocardial Infarction 2 & 3. J Am Coll Cardiol 2000;35 (suppl A):376A (abst)

28. Ryan TJ, Antman EM, Brooks NH, et al (1999) 1999 update: ACC/AHA guidelines for the management of patients with acute myocardial infarction. J Am Coll Cardiol 34:890–911

29. Rosamond WD, Chambless LE, Folsom AR, et al (1998) Trends in the incidence of myocardial infarction and in mortality due to coronary heart disease, 1987 to 1994. N Engl J Med 339:861–867

30. The GUSTO Investigators (1993) An international randomized trial comparing four thrombolytic strategies for acute myocardial infarction. N Engl J Med 329:673–682

31. The GUSTO III Investigators (1997) A comparison of reteplase with alteplase for acute myocardial infarction. N Engl J Med 337:1118–1123

32. Assessment of the safety and efficacy of a new thrombolytic (ASSENT-2) Investigators (1999) Single-bolus tenecteplase compared with frontloaded alteplase in acute myocardial infarction: the ASSENT-2 double blind randomized trial. Lancet 354:716–722

33. Bode C, Smalling RW, Berg G, et al (1996) Randomized comparison of coronary thrombolysis achieved with double-bolus reteplase and front-loaded, accelerated alteplase in patients with acute myocardial infarction. Circulation 94:891–898

34. Ohman EM, Harrington RA, Cannon CP, Agnelli G, Cairns JA, Kennedy JW (2001) Intravenous thrombolysis in acute myocardial infacrtion. Chest 119 (Suppl 1):253S–277S

35. Simoons ML, Maggioni AP, Knaterud G, et al (1993) Individual risk assessment for intracranial hemorrhage during thrombolytic therapy. Lancet 342:1523–1528

36. Angeja BG, Rundle AC, Gurwitz JH, Gore JM, Barron HV (2001) Death or nonfatal stroke in patients with acute myocardial infarction treated with tissue plasminogen activator. Am J Cardiol 87:627–630

37. Barron HV, Rundle AC, Gore JM, Gurwitz JH, Penney J (2000) Intracranial hemorrhage rates and effect of immediate beta-blocker use in patients with acute myocardial infarction treated with tissue plasminogen activator. Am J Cardiol 85:294–298

38. Metz BK White HD, Granger CB, et al (1998) Randomized comparison of direct thrombin inhibition versus heparin in conjunction with fibrinolytic therapy for acute myocardial infarction: Results from the GUSTO-IIb Trial. J Am Coll Cardiol 31:1493–1498

39. Keyt BA, Paoni NF, Refino CJ, et al (1994) A faster acting and more potent form of tissue plasminogen activator. Proc Natl Acad Sci USA 91:3670–3674

40. Mark DB, Hlatky MA, Califf RM, et al (1995) Cost effectiveness of thrombolytic therapy with tissue plasminogen activator as comared with streptokinase for acute myocardial infarction. N Engl J Med 332:1418–1424

41. Assessment of the safety and efficacy of a new thrombolytic regimen (ASSENT)-3 Investigators (2001) Efficacy and safety of tenecteplase in combination with enoxaparin, abciximab, or unfractionated heparin: the ASSENT-3 randomised trial in acute myocardial infarction. Lancet 358:605–613

42. Grines CL, Cox DA, Stone GW, et al (1999) Coronary angioplasty with or without stent implantation for acute myocardial infarction. N Engl J Med 341:1949–1956

43. Grines CL, Browne KF, Marco J, et al (1993) A comparison of immediate angioplasty with thrombolytic therapy for acute myocardial infarction. N Engl J Med 328:673–679
44. Weaver WD, Simes RJ, Betriiu A, et al (1997) Comparison of primary angioplasty and intravenous thrombolytic therapy for acute myocardial infarction: a quantitative review. JAMA 278:2093–2098
45. Ziljstra F, de Boer MJ, Hoorntje J, Reiffers S, Reiber JH, Suryapranata H (1993) A comparison of immediate coronary angioplasty with intravenous streptokinase in acute myocardial infarction. N Engl J Med 328:680–684
46. Gibbons RJ, Holmes DR, Reeder GS, Bailey KR, Hopfenspirger MR, Gersh BJ (1993) Immediate angioplasty compared with the administration of a thrombolytic agent followed by conservative treatment for myocardial infarction. N Engl J Med 328:685–691
47. de Boer MJ, Hoorntje J, Ottervanger JP, Reiffers S, Suryapranata H, Ziljstra F (1994) Immediate coronary angioplasty versus intravenous streptokinase in acute myocardial infarction: left ventricular ejection fraction, hospital mortality and reinfarction. J Am Coll Cardiol 23:1004–1008
48. Zorman S, Zorman D, Noc M (2002) Effects of abciximab pretreatment in patients with acute myocardial infarction undergoing primary angioplasty. Am J Cardiol 90:533–536
49. Suryapranata H, van't Hof A, Hoorntje J, de Boer MJ, Ziljstra F (1998) Randomized comparison of coronary stenting with balloon angioplasty in selected patients with acute myocardial infarction. Circulation 97:2502–2505
50. Andersen HR, Nielsen TT, Rasmussen K, et al (2003) A comparison of coronary angioplasty with fibrinolytic therapy in acute myocardial infarction. N Engl J Med 349:733–742
51. Rogers WJ, Canto JG, Lambrew CT, et al (2000) Temporal trends in the treatment of over 1.5 million patients with myocardial infarction in the U.S. from 1990 through 1999. J Am Coll Cardiol 36:2056–2063
52. Magid DJ, Calogne BN, Rumsfeld JS, et al (2000) Relation between hospital primary angioplasty volume and mortality for patients with acute MI treated with primary angioplasty vs. thrombolytic therapy. JAMA 284:3131–3138
53. McGrath PD, Wennberg DE, Dickens JD, et al (2000) Relation between operator and hospital volume and outcomes following percutaneous coronary interventions in the era of the coronary stent. JAMA 284:3139–3144
54. Canto JG, Every NR, Magid DJ, et al (2000) The volume of primary angioplasty procedures and survival after acute myocardial infarction. N Engl J Med 342:1573–1580
55. Grines CL, Westerhausen, Grines LL, et al (2002) A randomized trial of transfer for primary angioplasty versus on-site thrombolysis in patients with high–risk myocardial infarction. J Am Coll Cardiol 39:1713–1719
56. Dalby M, Montalescot G (2002) Transfer for primary angioplasty: Who and how? Heart 88:570–572

Quantifying Cardiac Dyssynchrony in Man

M. R. Pinsky

▌ Introduction

Presently, cardiac resynchronization therapy has been approved to treat heart failure patients with prolonged QRS. In a large prospective clinical trial, cardiac resynchronization therapy improved long-term outcome and often reversed objective measures of heart failure. The principal behind cardiac resynchronization therapy is that matched left ventricular (LV) or biventricular pacing will restore normal excitation-contraction coupling, improving LV ejection efficiency. However, not all subjects demonstrate benefit from this highly invasive and risky procedure. The mechanism(s) by which cardiac resynchronization therapy improves cardiac performance and induces reverse remodeling is unknown, but dyssynchronous contraction increases myocardial oxygen consumption (MVO_2) and, thus, reduces ejection efficiency. If cardiac resynchronization therapy improves cardiac performance by reversing dyssynchrony, then we should be able to identify pre-operatively those patients whom it would benefit the most and where in the heart optimal pacing should be delivered. Furthermore, we should be able to define the effectiveness of cardiac resynchronization therapy at the time of pacemaker insertion to optimize its placement. To understand this important and rapidly evolving clinical field, one must first define basic concepts of contractility and the determinants of MVO_2. This chapter will focus on the mechanisms by which dyssynchronous LV contraction may impair ejection efficiency and how to quantify it at the bedside.

▌ Relationship between MVO_2 and Ventricular Mechanical Function

Suga and Sagawa demonstrated that LV contractility could be defined by the slope of the LV end-systolic pressure-volume relation [1]. This finding not only allowed one to quantify LV contractility and its changes in patients in response to therapy, disease and time, but also opened up new understandings of the relationship between LV contraction and MVO_2. In that regard, these workers extended their initial pioneering studies on contractility-defining end-systolic pressure-volume relation by incorporating the graphic area inside the LV pressure-volume (P/V) loop (stroke work or SW) plus the end-systolic pressure-volume relation-defined left-sided triangle of potential work (PE) (Fig. 1), called the LV pressure-volume area [2]. They demonstrated that changes in the LV pressure-volume area induce proportional changes in MVO_2. Thus, any process that increases either LV volume or ejection pressure also increases MVO_2, and does so in a predictable fashion. Similarly,

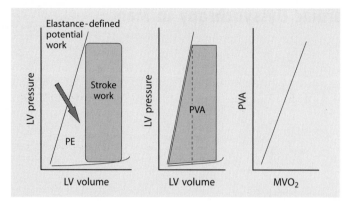

Fig. 1. Relation between left ventricular (LV) pressure-volume relations, end-systolic elastance-defined potential energy (PE), the resultant pressure-volume area (PVA) and myocardial O_2 consumption (MVO_2). From [2] with permission

any process that reduces LV pressure-volume area also reduces MVO_2. Importantly, increasing dyssynchronous LV contractions shifts the LV end-systolic pressure-volume relation to the right (with volume on the x axis). However, the actual impact of this shift on MVO_2 has not been quantified in humans and remains an area of intense interest.

▍ Pacing-induced LV Contraction Asynchrony Causes Cardiac Dilation

Ventricular pacing and abnormally conducted beats increase contraction dyssynchrony. Initially, pacing was thought to have minimal effects on contraction synchrony, because when viewed from the perspective of the whole ventricle, little change could be ascertained when compared to normally conducted beats [3]. However, Badke et al. [4] observed marked regional differences in myocardial contraction when analyzed by multiple dimensions using ultrasonic crystals. Park et al. [5] showed that increasing contraction dyssynchrony, as exemplified by RV and LV pacing in their canine model, did not change the end-systolic pressure-volume relation slope (Ees) but did induce progressive LV dilation proportional to the degree of dyssynchrony (Fig. 2). Any process that results in an increased LV volume for a constant LV ejection pressure and stroke volume (SV) will also increase MVO_2. Subjects with heart failure have a close correlation between conduction delays and contraction dyssynchrony [6]. Thus, the finding that many patients with prolonged QRS heart failure treated with cardiac resynchronization therapy demonstrate a decrease in LV end-diastolic volume (LVEDV) without a change in ejection pressure or SV, suggests that cardiac resynchronization therapy improves ejection effectiveness by reducing contractile dyssynchrony [7, 8]. Although redistribution of local work has been proposed to explain these data [9], reduced mitral regurgitation and metabolism [10] have all been suggested as possible mechanisms by which bi-ventricular pacing improves LV performance in these subjects. Importantly, the observation that some patients with wide QRS cardiomyopathy receive no benefit from

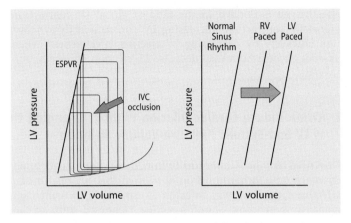

Fig. 2. Effect of increasing dyssynchronous LV contraction by pacing in the left and right ventricles, as assessed by the end-systolic pressure-volume relation (ESPVR) induced by rapid preload reduction via inferior vena caval (IVC) occlusion. From [5] with permission

bi-ventricular pacing, demonstrates that the mechanism by which it improves contractile effectiveness is not understood.

▌ Regional Contraction Dyssynchrony is the most Common Cardiac Contraction Abnormality Seen

Contraction dyssynchrony accounts for much of the observed clinically relevant increase in morbidity from heart disease. Regional myocardial dyssynchrony, characterized by regional wall motion abnormalities (RWMA), is common in patients with both normal [11–14] and abnormal [15–17] cardiac physiology. RWMA are monitored intraoperatively to detect regional myocardial ischemia [18–20]. However, the impact of RWMA on global LV performance has not been quantified. If a quantitative measure of regional myocardial dysfunction could be developed that was easy to use, it would minimize subjective bias in the diagnosis of myocardial ischemia [12], and aid in the evaluation of treatments and titration of therapies used to restore regional myocardial function, including both revascularization and cardiac resynchronization therapy. Later on in this chapter, we shall describe some candidate methods that promise to quantify LV ejection effectiveness.

LV ejection reflects the summed contraction of many cardiac muscle cells whose function is altered by LV volume, arterial impedance, coronary blood flow, and excitation-contraction coupling [14, 20, 21]. LV contraction is normally heterogeneous [13, 22]. The apex and base differ in their onset of contraction and in their response to inotropes [11, 23]; the apex being slightly phase lagged in relation to the base region and somewhat more dynamic. This degree of dyssynchrony is necessary for proper mechanical functioning of the mitral valve apparatus and causes minimal cardiac dilation. However, as LV contraction becomes more asynchronous among cardiac regions, LV ejection effectiveness decreases. LV ejection efficiency is usually defined as the ratio of external work (stroke work) to energy consumed (MVO$_2$). In this chapter, we use a new term, LV ejection effectiveness. LV ejection effectiveness is defined as the ratio of global LV contraction to phase-specific regional LV contraction. Increasing LV contraction dyssynchrony decreases LV ejection efficiency by decreasing LV ejection effectiveness, whereas aortic stenosis or akinetic myocardium may decrease LV ejection efficiency but not LV ejection effectiveness.

∎ RWMA Induce Cardiac Dilation Without Changing the Slope of LV End-Systolic Pressure-Volume Relation

One need not have abnormally conducted beats to develop regional contraction dyssynchrony. Strum and Pinsky showed that regional dyskinesis induced by sub-selective coronary artery infusion of esmolol in an acute canine model induced regional dyssynchrony, caused a similar rightward shifts of the LV end-systolic pressure-volume relation but did not alter Ees (Fig. 3) [24]. Importantly, these changes occurred without changes in QRS morphology. Thus, any form of contraction dyssynchrony (RWMA), whether electrical or mechanical, may cause cardiac dilation decreasing LV ejection efficiency (SW/MVO$_2$). This observation is important, because it demonstrates that contraction dyssynchrony may add to the overall efficiency burden of the myocardium, independent of conduction defects.

Burkhoff et al. [25] demonstrated that although RV pacing altered both the LV pressure/volume area and MVO$_2$, their relationship to each other remained constant. However, they used an isolated heart preparation perfused with a cell free perfusate for their analysis, whereas Baller et al. [26] using intact dogs showed that RV pacing was associated with a higher MVO$_2$ and thus lower LV ejection efficiency than seen with atrial pacing. Thus, in intact animals, increasing dyssynchrony decreased LV contraction efficiency. This is clinically important because:

∎ RWMA are the most common cardiac abnormalities;
∎ pacing for rate control normally increases contraction dyssynchrony;

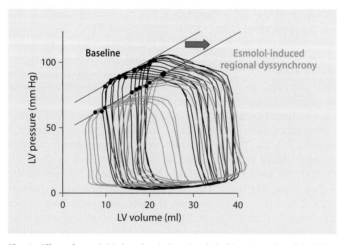

Fig. 3. Effect of esmolol-induced apical regional dyskinesis on the global LV pressure-volume relationship and the end-systolic pressure-volume relationship in an acute canine model. From [24] with permission

▮ patients requiring ventricular pacing usually have impaired ventricular pump function and coronary reserve;

▮ cardiac resynchronization therapy has been approved for the management of wide complex heart failure patients without clear titration end-points for therapy other than measuring developed pressure; and

▮ inotropic agents used in patients with RWMA may improve or impair LV ejection effectiveness, presumably based on their effects on LV ejection synchrony.

The principal hypothesis of this chapter is that changes in LV ejection synchrony reflect a primary determinant of both LV ejection effectiveness and the response of the patient to therapeutic interventions, such as pacing, cardiac resynchronization therapy, and pharmacotherapies.

▮ Hypothetical Relation between Dyssynchrony and MVO$_2$

With contraction dyssynchrony, not all regions of the myocardium reach minimal length or relax at the same time. If a region of the heart reaches minimal volume too late, relative to other regions of the heart, then not only is its contribution to global ejection diminished, the contribution of the remaining contracting elements is also diminished because global end-ejection will be delayed making these normally contracting segments reach end-ejection early. Thus, dyssynchrony decreases

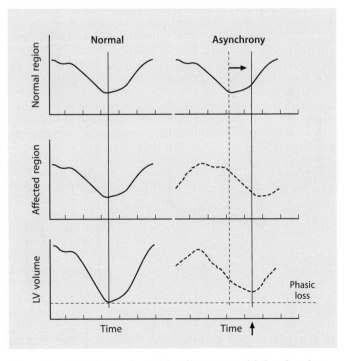

Fig. 4. Schematic representation of the effect of delayed regional end-ejection on global stroke volume

LV ejection efficiency by a greater amount than that predicted by the regional dyssynchrony itself. In Fig. 4, the shortening of the affected region is held constant but is delayed by 60° from the other region. Note that:

▊ regional maximal shortening of affected elements may be unchanged or increased despite a reduced contribution to global end-ejection, and

▊ the contribution of normally contracting elements to global end-ejection will be reduced despite normal contraction synchrony.

Collectively, this impairment can be considered a *'phasic loss'* of ejection stroke volume. As LV ejection dyssynchrony increases, MVO_2 should increase more than predicted from the LV pressure/volume area relation described in Fig. 1 because the LV pressure/volume area will not describe all the mechanical work done by the contracting myocardium. There are two primary theoretical reasons for this assumption:

▊ asynchronously contracting myocardial elements though not completely contributing their contraction to global ejection are still contracting under load and require energy and contribute to MVO_2 and

▊ since global LV wall stress increases as LV volume increases, any process that increases LV volume for a constant ejection pressure and SV must increase MVO_2 for the entire heart.

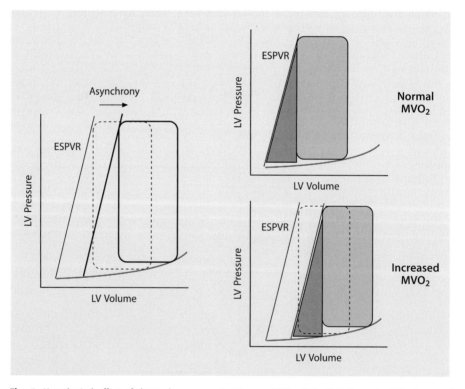

Fig. 5. Hypothetical effect of dyssynchronous contraction on MVO_2. Note that the potentially increased MVO_2 would not be measured using traditional means as described in Figure 1. ESPVR: end-systolic pressure/volume relation

Wiggers initially described the negative impact of ventricular pacing [27]. The greater the distance the excitation wave front has to travel from the pacing site to the His-Purkinje system, the greater will be the degree of dyssynchrony. With pacing this is manifest electrically as a prolonged QRS duration, which has an inverse relation with peak-developed pressure [28]. Usually dyssynchronous contraction occurs because of either conduction abnormalities or regional myocardial contractile pathology. With regional myocardial contractile pathologically, such as during ischemia or stunning, excitation usually proceeds normally but dysfunctional regions contract more slowly. The impact of dyssynchrony on MVO_2 should be predictable from the LV pressure-volume area analyses of Suga et al. [2] (Fig. 5). With normal contraction, MVO_2 is proportional to the SW (light gray area) plus the elastance-defined internal work (dark gray area). With increasing dyssynchrony, LV end-systolic pressure-volume relation is shifted to the right, with volume on the x-axis. Thus, MVO_2 should increase in proportion to the increase in 'area' defined by the parallelogram of the LV end-systolic pressure-volume relation with and without asynchronous contraction (hatched area). As described below, regional phase angle analysis will allow us to define the shift of the LV end-systolic pressure-volume relation, thus defining ejection effectiveness. However, though attractive as a mechanism to define LV efficiency, the validity of this association has not been established.

▌ Pacing in Heart Failure to Improve LV Synchrony

Patients with dilated cardiomyopathy often develop abnormal conduction characterized by left bundle branch block (LBBB) [15]. LBBB contraction patterns induce widespread LV wall motion abnormalities [23]. Blanc et al. showed that LV pacing could improve LV ejection while decreasing LV filling pressure in 23 patients with severe heart failure, although the mechanisms were not defined [29]. Potential mechanisms include not only normalization of ventricular activation sequence, but also increased filling time, decreased mitral regurgitation and optimizing mechanical atrio-ventricular delay [30]. Interestingly, Auricchio and Salo showed that optimization of A-V sequential pacing to the LV or RV site was markedly different amongst patients [31]. Stellbrink et al. [32] reported on the impact of cardiac resynchronization therapy on 6-month LV function in 25 patients. Although LVEDV tended to decrease at 6 months, while LV ejection fraction increased, 4/25 patients deteriorated (non-responders). Non-responders had significantly higher initial LVEDV than responders. No comment was made about dyssynchrony. The potential that cardiac resynchronization therapy can reverse congestive heart failure (CHF) remodeling (referred to as reverse remodeling) is very exciting. Abraham et al. [33] reported on the MIRACLE cardiac resynchronization therapy study in 453 patients with moderate-to-severe symptoms of heart failure associated with an ejection fraction of $\geq 35\%$ and a QRS interval of ≥ 130 msec. Two hundred and twenty-eight patients were randomly assigned to the cardiac resynchronization therapy group. As compared with the control group, 225 patients assigned to cardiac resynchronization therapy experienced an improvement in the distance walked in six minutes (+39 vs. +10 m, p = 0.005), functional class (p < 0.001), quality of life (–18.0 vs. –9.0 points, p = 0.001), time on the treadmill during exercise testing (+81 vs. +19 s, p = 0.001), and ejection fraction (+4.6 percent vs. –0.2 percent, p < 0.001). In addition, fewer cardiac resynchronization therapy patients than control patients required hospitalization (8 vs. 15%) or intravenous medications (7 vs. 15%) for the treatment of heart failure (p < 0.05 for both comparisons). However, improvement was variable, with almost 40% of study patients showing no improvement or worsening function as compared to 60% in the control group. Other small multicenter cardiac resynchronization therapy clinical trials have recently documented similar long-term success rates [34, 35].

Several clinical groups have examined the impact of site of ventricular pacing. Although intra-operative epicardial pacing leads have been used [36], they do not create as uniform an excitation waveform as endocardial pacing [37]. Furthermore, though multisite pacing has been tried [38], LV pacing [39, 40], and specifically LV free wall pacing [41] appears to be best at decreasing dyssynchrony. Importantly, cardiac resynchronization therapy may improve LV ejection synchrony without improving electrical synchrony [42] suggesting that mechanical factors are more important than conduction changes in defining performance. We hypothesize that in these clinical studies, improvement in LV ejection parallels reductions in ejection dyssynchrony. In support of our hypothesis, Kass et al. [7] demonstrated that cardiac resynchronization therapy responders had a reduction in LV end-systolic volume for a constant LVEDV and ejection pressure during LV pacing. No changes in LV diastolic compliance were seen. If cardiac resynchronization therapy improved LV contraction synchrony, then we would expect such a parallel shift in the LV end-systolic volume at a constant ejection pressure.

▌ Regional Phase Angle Analysis defines LV Ejection Effectiveness

While dyssynchrony may delay regional contraction, quantifying its impact by time to peak strain or similar measures in msec does not easily lend itself to mathematical modeling nor is it constant as heart rate varies. We developed a canine model to validate a simplified method to quantify contraction dyssynchrony by measuring both the regional phase angle (a) and SV of each of four regional LV volumes defined by the electrode pair of the conductance catheter aligned along the long axis of the LV lumen [43]. We also measured segmental length changes using sonomicrometer crystals to serve as a gold standard for local dyssynchrony. We induced regional dyskinesis by sub-selective left coronary artery esmolol injection. This allowed us to measure regional ejection effectiveness (proportion of regional SV used in global ejection) and ejection efficiency (proportion of total LV contraction that results in ejection) of involved (apical) and remote regions of the heart during reversible LV dyskinesis. By dividing one cardiac cycle into 360° and assigning global end-ejection as 0°, the amount of early or late contraction of a region can be measured as a phase angle, a, from 0° to ±180°. Assuming that regional volume change during the cardiac cycle approximates a sine wave, then the calculated effective regional SV, that portion of the maximal regional volume change that contributes to global ejection, will equal the product of the maximal regional volume change and cos a. LV ejection efficiency can then be defined as the ratio of the sum of regional maximal SVs to LV SV, or more simply the mean weighted average cos a of all LV regions. Data from one dog for the involved apical regional volume are shown in Figure 6. Note that during esmolol infusion, the dyskinetic segment reaches minimal volume at a post-systolic contraction. Only that portion of the apical contraction that coincided with global end-ejection ejection contributes to LV ejection. The

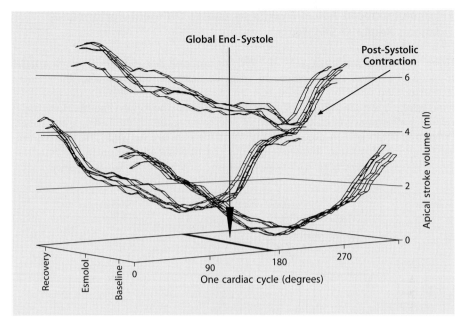

Fig. 6. Effect of esmolol-induced apical regional dyskinesis on the apical LV volume over a cardiac cycle. Five sequential cardiac cycles are shown for one animal during initial baseline conditions, esmolol-induced paresis and then following recovery in an acute canine model. From [43] with permission

remainder of the delayed contraction occurs into a dilating LV. As expected, uninvolved apical and papillary regional phase angles increased 10 to 16% relative to baseline (p < 0.05), whereas apical ultrasonic crystals displayed a 27% increase in the phase angle (p < 0.05). Esmolol increased apical and papillary mean regional systolic time intervals (p < 0.05), but tended to reduce systolic time intervals in the uninvolved basal regions (p = ns). Importantly, esmolol induced no significant change in any regional maximal SV, but induced marked reductions in effective regional SV (Fig. 6). When regional SVs were measured as effective SV, defined as the product of the maximal regional SV and the cosine of its phase angle, apical SV decreased and uninvolved chordal and basal SVs increased (p < 0.05).

Importantly, 1) measures of maximal regional SV alone did not identify this inefficiency because maximal apical contraction was unaltered by esmolol, only its phase relation to global end-ejection was altered (descending arrow, Fig. 6), and 2) referencing apical ejection volume to global end-ejection via the formula regional SV · cos α accurately described the effective regional SV. We can calculate regional effective SV from the product of maximal regional SV and cosine α. Echocardiographic imaging measures only absolute movement, and thus, would be insensitive to phase shifts. We can determine effective regional SV and SW by normalizing each region by its phase angle. Importantly, Kedem et al. [44] found that MVO$_2$ was proportional to the degree of dyssynchrony. The ratio of the sum of all regional effective SVs to global SV equates with ejection efficiency (ratio of an index of MVO$_2$ to cardiac work). Thus, this simple construct has profound applications in the analysis of RWMA physiology, in general, and ventricular pacing, in particular.

▌ Esmolol-induced Apical Dyskinesis Causes Different Performance Among Regional Segments

Using our above model of sub-selective left anterior descending coronary arterial infusion of esmolol (9 mg bolus) in an acute canine model, we also documented that associated with this regional segment contraction delay (Fig. 6), the global LV end-systolic pressure-volume relation was shifted to the right (Fig. 3). However, if cardiac performance is only analyzed in selective regions of the heart, a completely different pattern is seen depending on where the data are derived. The affected apical region's P/V relation demonstrated marked impairment in contractile function,

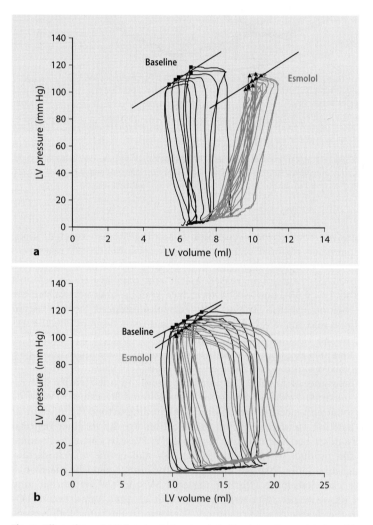

Fig. 7. Effect of esmolol-induced apical regional dyskinesis on the: **a** apical, and **b** remote basal LV pressure-volume relationship and the end-systolic pressure-volume relationship in an acute canine model. From [24] with permission

whereas analysis of an unaffected basal region revealed no alterations in LV performance (Fig. 7) [24]. Note the affected apical regional P/V relation with a rightward shift of the end-systolic pressure-volume relation with volume on the x-axis and collapse of the SW generated. Recall that the effect of this selective regional dysfunction was a parallel shift of the global LV end-systolic pressure-volume relation to the right (Fig. 3). These data collectively demonstrate that both pacing-induced dyssynchrony and regional myocardial contractile dysfunction induce parallel shifts of the LV end-systolic pressure-volume relation to the right and for similar reasons. Thus, a single method of dyssynchrony analysis will quantify LV ejection effectiveness when alterations in LV contraction are induced by either abnormally conducted beats or regional differences in contractility.

▌ Cardiac Resynchronization Therapy and Dyssynchrony Analysis

Animal studies have proven useful in understanding the potential mechanisms of improved LV performance with cardiac resynchronization therapy. Heart failure is a physical state associated with specific pro-inflammatory gene-induced structure modulations in the cardiac myocytes though selective localization of matrix metalloproteinases [45] and early and persistent activation of apoptosis [46], referred to as remodeling. Yin et al. [47] developed myocardial contraction maps using tissue Doppler acceleration imaging in a porcine model, documenting the intramyocardial origin of pacing-induced contraction. Data such as these suggest that uneven strain is a primary inducer of remodeling. Following on that concept, Wyman et al. [48] developed 3-D LV maps of temporal and spatial dynamics of ventricular contraction in a canine model. They demonstrated, using volume strain imaging, that pacing induces marked spatial and temporal differences in myocardial contraction. Potentially, the reverse remodeling seen in cardiac resynchronization therapy responders [49] may be used to rationalize a trial of cardiac resynchronization therapy to subjects with marked contraction dyssynchrony prior to CHF expression.

Several groups have attempted to determine the long-term impact of cardiac resynchronization therapy by acute changes in LV contraction dyssynchrony using tissue Doppler imaging (TDI). Ansalone et al. [50] documented a 52% improvement in overall regional contraction synchrony following cardiac resynchronization therapy in 21 patients but could not identify which patients would improve. If cardiac resynchronization therapy improves LV performance by reducing LV ejection dyssynchrony, then there should be a relation between the degree of dyssynchrony prior to cardiac resynchronization therapy, the improved synchrony with cardiac resynchronization therapy, and LV performance. Hemodynamic improvement following cardiac resynchronization therapy tends to be greatest in those subjects with most asynchronous myocardium at baseline [51], and when the pacing site is centered near the most delayed region of contraction [52]. In one study, longitudinal TDI in 20 long-term cardiac resynchronization therapy survivors suggested that delayed LV basal contraction predicted a good response [53]. Breithardt et al. [54] quantified contraction dyssynchrony grossly by comparing the differences in phase angles between maximal contraction of the septum (Φ_S) and lateral wall (Φ_L) using QRS at $0°$ (referred to as Φ_{LS}), where $\Phi_{LS} = \Phi_L - \Phi_S$. Negative Φ_{LS} values connoted lateral wall contracting early and vice versa. They separated their patients into those with minimal Φ_{LS} (Type 1), positive Φ_{LS} (Type 2) and negative Φ_{LS} (Type 3).

They saw that only Type 2 and 3 patterns were associated with improved performance following cardiac resynchronization therapy. That Φ_{LS} did not predict exactly the degree of subsequent improvement (note 3 Type I subjects without improvement following cardiac resynchronization therapy) may reflect poor pacing site selection to reverse dyssynchrony or inaccurate estimation of dyssynchrony by using entire lateral and septal wall movement to define regional dyssynchrony.

▌ Quantification of Left Ventricular Contraction Dyssynchrony

Dyssynchrony can be analyzed in a number of ways. Echo-contrast imaging has been described in the assessment of regional systolic function [55], but is still in evolution. Similarly, tagged magnetic resonance imaging (MRI) has been traditionally used to assess myocardial movement [48], but does not easily lend itself to clinical practice. Echo color kinesis applies a semi-automated quantitative analysis of digital color-coded data to the acoustic quantification (AQ) algorithm. Although we have used color kinesis and AQ previously, we do not use this method in our analysis because:

▌ AQ and color kinesis examine only endothelial movement and not myocardial movement, and thus are no more specific than the method used by Breithardt et al. [54] described above;

▌ are subject to technical errors due to rotational and movement artifact; and

▌ would require two separate imaging devices.

Fauchier et al. [56] quantified both inter and intraventricular dyssynchrony in patients with idiopathic dilated cardiomyopathies using a Fourier phase analysis of radionuclide angioscintigraphy. They estimated mean LV and RV contraction phase angles along the lines of our phase angle analysis. The greater the dispersion of phase angles among the individual regions of each ventricle, quantified simply by their standard deviation, the higher the 80-month mortality rate. RV dyssynchrony was more predictive of mortality than LV dyssynchrony, presumably because of the greater influence of septal dyssynchrony in RV than LV dynamics. Still, in our proposed model we shall quantify phase dispersion among regions normalized to both tissue mass and amplitude of contraction, thus unifying these variables into a functional dyssynchrony measure.

▌ Tissue Doppler Imaging

TDI is a modification of color flow instrumentation to measure the relatively low velocity of cardiac tissue motion by bypassing the high pass filter and inputting the lower frequency Doppler shift data directly into the autocorrelator. These high amplitude tissue Doppler velocity data are color-coded and superimposed on conventional M-mode and 2-D images in real time. Color images are recorded on a customized computer interfaced directly with the ultrasound system. Major advantages of TDI over color kinesis are the ease of imaging and the strength of the signal. Thus, operator error is minimized and reproducibility of measured tissue velocity is increased.

TDI provides an objective quantitative assessment of global and regional LV function and can be used to quantify dyssynchrony based on the above model [57]. We applied this imaging process in our model of regional dyssynchrony induced by sub-selective intracoronary infusion of esmolol. TDI can measure not only tissue velocity but also transmyocardial velocity gradient. Since the ventricular wall thickens during systole, a transmyocardial velocity gradient develops from the near to the far wall. Although the velocity gradient is linear if transmural contraction is synchronous, it becomes non-uniform with dyssynchrony and regional ischemia. Furthermore, differences in transmyocardial velocity gradients among regions can then be used to quantify global LV contraction dyssynchrony.

TDI to Assess Dyssynchrony

These TDI images were further refined to phase differences among regions of the contracting heart. Using our canine model of RV and LV pacing to induce regional LV dyssynchrony, we saw that RV pacing caused marked septal contraction dyssynchrony, whereas LV pacing induced more long axis dyssynchrony than did RV pacing (Fig. 8). These data demonstrate that regional volume measures and TDI data collected non-invasively can be displayed in a fashion necessary to define both phase angle and amplitude of regional contraction.

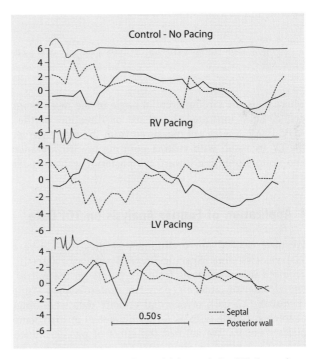

Fig. 8. Effect of sinus rhythm (top), right ventricular (RV) (middle), and left ventricular (LV) (bottom) pacing on tissue Doppler measures of septal and posterior wall velocities during a single cardiac cycle in an acute canine model

Model Development Based on TDI and Fourier Analysis

Wyman et al. [48] estimated an 'activation delay vector' (ADV) by summing a vectorized representation of the mechanical activation time $[t_{act}(c,l)]$ values at each mesh point for a single 2-D plane. Data from their study and our own TDI readouts are presented as both a two-dimensional point and its vector. The magnitudes are equal to $t_{act}(c,l)$, whereas the phases are determined from the spatial locations of the mesh points. Larger ADV values indicate a greater imbalance in contraction from one side of the left ventricle to the other, and smaller ADV values indicate a spatially and temporally balanced contraction. The ADV is calculated by:

$$ADV = \frac{4}{CL} \sum_{l=1}^{L} \left[\sum_{c=1}^{C} t_{act}(c,l) \cdot \frac{r_c}{\| r_c \|} \right] \quad [58] \tag{Eq. 1}$$

where the summations are across all circumferential (C=24) and longitudinal (L=7–9) or base to apex mesh indices. The last term is a unit vector in the direction of the spatial location of $t_{act}(c,l)$. Although the ADV can be calculated as a vector in three-dimensional space, it is reduced to the circumferential plane by using r_c instead of $r_{c,l}$ in the last term of Eq. 1. This is done because the spatio-temporal dyssynchrony observed in the mechanical activation in the longitudinal direction is usually much smaller than in the circumferential direction. Thus, we may use this simplification for our mid-axis measures and analyses. The last term of Eq. 1 is determined by

$$\frac{r_c}{\| r_c \|} = [\cos(\phi_c), \sin(\phi_c)] = \left[\cos\left(2\pi \frac{c}{C}\right), \sin\left(2\pi \frac{c}{C}\right) \right] \quad [59] \tag{Eq. 2}$$

where ϕ_c is the circumferential angle of the mesh point with the circumferential index c. Eq. 2 indicates the phase or direction of the imbalance indicated by the ADV. Phase angles are measured from the reference vector between the septum and the LV free wall with vectors pointing toward the anterior wall considered positive and vectors pointing toward the posterior wall considered negative.

Application of Fourier Analysis on TDI Data

We have carried out preliminary studies to analyze regional dyssynchrony using TDI velocity data. Specifically, TDI velocity data (GE Vingmed Ultrasound) were acquired in apical views from six points on the mitral annular plane: infero-septal, lateral, inferior, anterior, posterior, antero-septal. Using a computer-based software (EchoPak-PC, GE), myocardial velocity data were obtained from a specified region of interest (circle with ~ 6 mm diameter) at high temporal resolution (~ 100 samples/s) (Fig. 9). We studied the effect of pacing-induced dyssynchrony on LV ejection effectiveness in eight open-chested anesthetized dogs. Selective RV free wall pacing creates an asynchronous contraction pattern similar to native LBBB with posterior-inferior and early septal contraction, decreased LV dP/dt and decreased LV developed pressure.

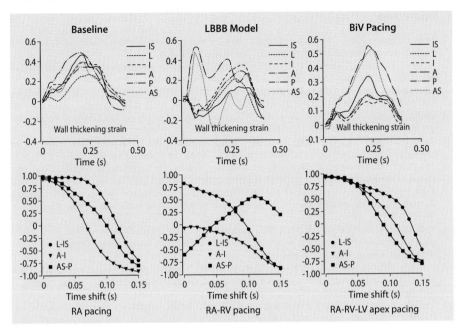

Fig. 9. Top: Six-point tissue Doppler measures of left ventricular (LV) velocity during the cardiac cycle during sinus rhythm (baseline) (left), left bundle branch block (LBBB) model (middle), and biventricular (BiV) pacing (right) for a single cardiac cycle of one animal. Bottom: Cross-correlation of the Fourier analysis power spectrum of opposing regions to define tuning of power. Note that both baseline and BiV pacing restore zero delay power (synchrony) in this acute canine model

Simultaneous apical LV pacing (BiV) reversed the contraction dyssynchrony, restored LV ejection pressure, LV dP/dt and volumes and decreased the variance of regional time to peak strain as compared to RV pacing, creating a contraction pattern similar to sinus pacing. Importantly, the time to end-ejection is not reduced by biventricular pacing, thus conduction abnormalities persisted but were off set by biventricular pacing. Neither biventricular pacing using LV posterior-inferior free wall pacing or LV apical pacing alone caused improved contraction synchrony. Biventricular pacing using either apical or free wall sites decreased the dispersion of regional phase angles, estimated as the standard deviation (SD) of their time to peak strain, from 38 msec with RV pacing to 25 and 23 msec with biventricular pacing free wall and apex, respectively, as compared to 22 msec for sinus beats. However, only apical biventricular pacing increased peak strain while decreasing time to peak strain. Thus, location on the LV free wall and its timing relative to native contraction patterns are key determinants of resynchronization-induced improved LV ejection effectiveness. Moreover, cardiac resynchronization is associated with predictable changes in global LV performance, as characterized by the LV end-systolic pressure-volume relation, developed pressure, and dP/dt.

References

1. Suga H, Sagawa K (1974) Instantaneous pressure-volume relationships and their ratio in the excised supported canine left ventricle. Circ Res 35:117–134
2. Suga H, Hayashi T, Shirahata M (1981) Ventricular systolic pressure-volume area as predictor of cardiac oxygen consumption. Am J Physiol 240:H39–H44.
3. Grover M, Glanz SA (1983) Endocardial pacing affects left ventricular end-diastolic volume and performance in the intact anesthetized dog. Circ Res 53:72–83
4. Badke FR, Boinay P, Covell JW (1980) Effect of ventricular pacing on regional ventricular performance. Am J Physiol 238: H858–H867
5. Park RC, Little WC, O'Rourke RA (1985) Effect of alteration of LV activation sequence on the LV end-systolic pressure-volume relation in closed-chest dogs. Circ Res 57:706–717
6. Toussaint J-F, Lavergne T, Kerrou K, et al (2002) Ventricular coupling of electrical and mechanical dyssynchronization in heart failure patients. Pacing Clin Electrophysiol 25:178–182
7. Kass DA, Chen C-H, Curry C, et al (1999) Improved LV mechanics from acute VDD pacing in patients with dilated cardiomyopathy and ventricular conduction delay. Circulation 99:1567–1573
8. Mulukutta S, Stetten GD, Jacques DC, Gorcsan J (2000) Quantification of left ventricular phase asynchrony in patients with left bundle branch block using tissue Doppler echocardiography. Circulation 102:II-384 (abst)
9. Prinzen FW, Hunter WC, Wymann BT, et al (1999) Mapping of regional myocardial strain and work during ventricular pacing: Experimental study using magnetic imaging tagging. J Am Coll Cardiol 33:1735–1742
10. Delhass T, Arts T, Prinzen FW, Reneman RS (1993) Relation between regional electrical activation time and subepicardial fiber strain in the canine left ventricle. Pflugers Arch 423:78–87
11. Pandian NG, Skorton DJ, Collins SM, Falsetti HL, Burke ER, Kerber RE (1983) Heterogeneity of left ventricular segmental wall thickening and excursion in 2-dimensional echocardiograms of normal human subjects. Am J Cardiol 51:1667–1673
12. Thys DM (1987) The intraoperative assessment of regional myocardial performance: Is the cart before the horse? J Cardiothorac Anesth 1:273–275
13. LeWinter M, Kent R, Kroener J, Carew T, Covell J (1975) Regional differences in myocardial performance in the left ventricle of the dog. Circ Res 37:191–199
14. Haendchen RV, Wyatt HL, Maurer G, et al (1983) Quantification of regional cardiac function by two-dimensional echocardiography I. Patterns of contraction on the normal left ventricle. Circulation 67:1234–1245
15. Xiao HB, Roy C, Gibson DG (1994) Nature of ventricular activation in patients with dilated cardiomyopathy: evidence for bilateral bundle branch block. Br Heart J 72:167–174
16. Bonow RO (1990) Regional left ventricular nonuniformity: effects on left ventricular diastolic function in ischemic heart disease, hypertrophic cardiomyopathy, and the normal heart. Circulation 81:III54–III65
17. Little W, Reeves R, Arciniegas J, Katholi R, Rogers E (1982) Mechanism of abnormal interventricular septal motion during delayed left ventricular activation. Circulation 65:1486–1491
18. Gallagher KP, Matsuzaki M, Koziol JA, Kemper WS, Ross J (1984) Regional myocardial perfusion and wall thickening during ischemia in conscious dogs. Am J Physiol 247:H727–H738
19. Buffington CW, Coyle RJ (1991) Altered load dependence of post-ischemic myocardium. Anesthesiology 75:464–474
20. Miura T, Bhargava V, Guth BD, et al (1993) Increased afterload intensifies asynchronous wall motion and impairs ventricular relaxation. J Appl Physiol 75:389–396
21. Shroff SG, Naegelen D, Clark WA (1990) Relation between left ventricular systolic resistance and ventricular rate processes. Am J Physiol 258:H381–H394
22. Diedericks J, Leone BJ, Fox P (1989) Regional differences in left ventricular wall motion in the anesthetized dog. Anesthesiology 70:82–90
23. Freedman RA, Alderman EL, Sheffield LT, Saporito M, Fisher LD (1987) Bundle branch block in patients with chronic coronary artery disease: angiographic correlates and prognostic significance. J Am Coll Cardiol 10:73–80

24. Strum DP, Pinsky MR (2000) Esmolol-induced regional wall motion abnormalities do not affect regional ventricular elastances Anesth Analg 90:252–261

25. Burkhoff D, Oikawa RY, Sagawa K (1986) Influence of pacing site on canine left ventricular contraction. Am J Physiol 251:H428–H435

26. Baller D, Wolpers HG, Zipfel J, Bretschneider HJ, Hellige G (1988) Comparison of RA, RV apex and AV sequential pacing on MVO$_2$ and cardiac efficiency. Pacing Clin Electrophysiol 11:394–403

27. Wiggers CJ (1925) The muscular reactions of mammalian ventricles to artificial surface stimuli. Am J Physiol 73:346–378

28. Burkhoff D, de Tombe PP, Hunter WC, Kass DA (1991) Contractile strength and mechanical efficiency of left ventricle are enhanced by physiological afterload. Am J Physiol 260:H569–H578

29. Blanc JJ, Etienne Y, Gilard M, et al (1997) Evaluation of different ventricular pacing sites in patients with severe heart failure. Circulation 96:3273–3277

30. Auricchio A, Stellbrink C, Block M, et al (1998) Effect of pacing chamber and atrio-ventricular delay on acute systolic function of paced heart failure patients in PATH-CHF Study. Pacing Clin Electrophysiol 21 (Part II):837 (abst)

31. Auricchio A, Salo RW (1997) Acute hemodynamic improvement by pacing in patients with severe congestive heart failure. Pacing Clin Electrophysiol 20:313–324

32. Stellbrink C, Breithardt O-A, Franke A, et al (2001) Impact of cardiac resynchronization therapy using hemodynamically optimized pacing on left ventricular remodeling in patients with congestive heart failure and ventricular conduction disturbances. J Am Coll Cardiol 38:1957–1965

33. Abraham WT, Fisher WG, Smith AL, et al (2002) Cardiac resynchronization in chronic heart failure. N Engl J Med 346:1845–1853

34. Molhoek SG, Bax JJ, van Erven L, et al (2002) Effectiveness of resynchronization therapy in patients with end-stage heart failure. Am J Cardiol 90:379–383

35. Leclercq GD, Tang AS, Bucknall C, Luttikhuis HO, Kirstein-Pedersen A (2002) Cardiac resynchronization therapy in advanced heart failure: the multicenter InSync clinical study. Eur I Heart Fail 4:311–320

36. Tanaka H, Okishige K, Mizuno T, et al (2002) Temporary and permanent biventricular pacing via left ventricular epicardial leads implanted during primary cardiac surgery. Jpn J Thorac Cardiovas Surg 50:284–289

37. Garrigue S, Jais P, Espil G, et al (2001) Comparison of chronic biventricular acing between epicardial and endocardial left ventricular stimulation using Doppler tissue imaging in patients with heart failure. Am J Cardiol 88:858–862

38. Varma C, O'Callaghan P, Mahon NG, et al (2002) Effect of multisite pacing on ventricular contraction. Heart 87:322–328

39. Touiza A, Etienne Y, Gilard M, Fatemi M, Mansourati J, Blanc JJ (2001) Long-term left ventricular pacing: assessment and comparison with biventricular pacing in patients with congestive heart failure. J Am Coll Cardiol 38:1966–1970

40. Breithardt OA, Stellbrink C, Franke A, et al (2002) Acute effects of cardiac resynchronization therapy on left ventricular Doppler indices in patients with congestive heart failure. Am Heart J 143:34–44

41. Butter C, Auricchio A, Stellbrink C, et al (2001) Effect of resynchronization therapy stimulation site on systolic function of heart failure patients. Circulation 104:3026–3029

42. Leclercq C, Faris O, Tunin R, et al (2002) Systolic improvement and mechanical resynchronization does not require electrical synchrony in the dilated failing heart with left bundle-branch block. Circulation 106:1760–1763

43. Strum DP, Pinsky MR (2000) Modeling of asynchronous myocardial contraction by effective stroke volume analysis. Anesth Analg 90:243–251

44. Kedem J, Lee WW, Weiss HR (1994) An experimental technique for estimating regional myocardial segment work *in vivo*. Ann Biomed Eng 22:58–65

45. Bradham WS, Moe G, Wendt KA, et al (2002) TNF-α and myocardial matrix metalloproteinases in heart failure: relationship to LV remodeling. Am J Physiol 282:H1288–295

46. Moe GW, Naik G, Konig A, Lu X, Feng Q (2002) Early and persistent activation of myocardial apoptosis, bax and caspases: insights into the mechanisms of progression to heart failure. Pathophysiology 8:183–192
47. Yin L, Belohlavek M, Packer DL, Greenleaf SF, Seward JR (2000) Myocardial contraction maps using tissue Doppler acceleration imaging. Chin Med J (Eng) 113:763–768
48. Wyman BY, Hunter WC, Prinzen FW, Faris OP, McVeigh ER (2002) Effects of single- and biventricular pacing on temporal and spatial dynamics of ventricular contraction. Am J Physiol 282:H372–379
49. Yu CM, Chau E, Sanderson JE, et al (2002) Tissue Doppler echocardiographic evidence of reverse remodeling and improved synchrony by simultaneously delaying regional contraction after biventricular pacing therapy in heart failure. Circulation 105:438–445
50. Ansalone G, Giannanontoni P, Ricci R, et al (2001) Doppler myocardial imaging in patients with heart failure receiving biventricular pacing treatment. Am J Heart 142:881–896
51. Sogaard P, Kim WY, Jensen HK, et al (2001) Impact of acute biventricular pacing on left ventricular performance and volumes in patients with severe heart failure. A tissue Doppler and three-dimensional echocardiographic study. Cardiology 95:173–182
52. Ansalone G, Giannantoni P, Ricci R, Trambaiolo P, Fedele F, Santini M (2002) Doppler myocardial imaging to evaluate the effectiveness of pacing sites in patients receiving biventricular pacing. J Am Coll Cardiol 39:489–499
53. Mandarino W, Gorcsan J, Pinsky MR (1998) Assessment of left ventricular contractile state by preload-adjusted maximal power using echocardiographic automated border detection. J Am Coll Cardiol 31:861–868
54. Breithardt OA, Stellbrink C, Kramer A, et al (2002) Echocardiographic quantification of left ventricular asynchrony predicts an acute hemodynamic benefit of cardiac resynchronization therapy. J Am Coll Cardiol 40:536–545
55. Kawaguchi M, Murabayashi T, Fetics BJ, et al (2002) Quantification of basal Dyssynchrony and acute resynchronization from left or biventricular pacing by novel echo-contrast variability imaging. J Am Coll Cardiol 39:2052–2058
56. Fauchier L, Marie O, Casset-Senon D, Babuty D, Cosnay P, Fauchier JP (2002) Interventricular and intraventricular dyssynchrony in idiopathic dilated cardiomyopathy. J Am Coll Cardiol 40:2022–2030
57. Gorcsan JG, Strum DP, Mandarino WA, Gulati VK, Pinsky MR (1997) Quantitative assessment of regional LV contractility by tissue Doppler imaging. Circulation 95:2423–2433
58. Berger DS, Robinson KA, Shroff SG (1996) Wave propagation in the coupled left ventricle-arterial system: implications for aortic pressure. Hypertension 27:1079–1089

Diastolic Heart Failure and Critical Illness

R. Pirracchio and A. Mebazaa

▌ Introduction

Diastolic heart failure is a common entity the frequency of which is widely underestimated. Some data available in the literature suggest that nearly half the patients with congestive heart failure (CHF) have preserved left ventricular (LV) ejection fraction (LVEF > 50%) [1–4]. If CHF is clearly defined as a pathophysiological state in which the heart is unable to pump blood at a rate commensurate with metabolic demand or to do so only from an elevated filling pressure, several guidelines have proposed that the diagnosis of CHF should require objective evidence of LV dysfunction, like an echographic measurement of LVEF [5]. As echographic signs of diastolic heart failure are of poor sensibility and specificity, the use of such criteria in the diagnosis of CHF leads to an underestimation of the frequency of diastolic heart failure. Nevertheless, more than a pathophysiological distinction, differences between systolic and diastolic heart failure are of clinical importance since diastolic heart failure is supposed to be associated with a better long-term survival than CHF [6, 7].

Very limited data are actually available concerning the clinical relevance of diastolic heart failure in the critical care setting. We will try to clarify those situations of critical illness where identifying and treating diastolic heart failure could be of clinical importance.

▌ Definitions and Diagnosis

Similar to systolic heart failure, diastolic heart failure is described as a chronic disease during which some acute decompensations can occur. These acute events can either be *de novo* or appear during the evolution of the CHF.

Chronic Diastolic Heart Failure

Since the early 90s, various guidelines have been published in order to clarify the definition and the diagnosis of diastolic heart failure [7–10]. According to the American College of Cardiology and the American Heart Association, "the diagnosis of diastolic heart failure is generally based on the finding of typical symptoms and signs of heart failure in patients with preserved left ventricular ejection fraction and no valvular abnormalities on echocardiography" [9]. For the Study Group on diastolic heart failure of the European Society of Cardiology, a diagnosis of diastolic heart failure should be made only in case of "evidence of abnormal left ventricular relaxation, diastolic distensibility or diastole stiffness" [7].

Vasan and Levy tried to rationalize the diagnosis with pragmatic criteria which are not yet widely used in the cardiologic literature [8]. They separated three sequential steps for the diagnosis: (1) diagnosis of CHF, (2) preserved systolic LV function (LVEF > 50%), (3) documentation of LV diastolic dysfunction if feasible. Accordingly, the authors proposed to classify subjects suspected of suffering from diastolic heart failure into three groups:

1) 'definite diastolic heart failure', for patients with clinical evidence of CHF, objective evidence of preserved LVEF within 72 hours of the CHF event, and documentation of LV diastolic dysfunction
2) 'probable diastolic heart failure', for patients having clinical evidence of CHF, preserved LVEF without documentation of LV diastolic dysfunction (after exclusion of valvular diseases or core pulmonale)
3) 'possible diastolic heart failure', for patients with clinical evidence of CHF, objective evidence of preserved systolic LV function but not at the time of the CHF event, and no evidence of diastolic LV dysfunction.

A clinical setting typical of diastolic heart failure (Table 1) can upgrade a patient from a 'possible' to a 'probable' diastolic heart failure.

Whether the diagnosis of diastolic heart failure requires some objective evidence of diastolic failure still remains controversial. Zile et al. recently provided a prospective comparison of cardiac catheterization and echocardiography in patients suspected of having diastolic heart failure (CHF symptoms and LVEF > 50%) [11]. The authors concluded that "objective measurement of LV diastolic function serves to confirm rather than establish the diagnosis of diastolic heart failure. The diagnosis of diastolic heart failure can be made without measurement of parameters that reflect LV diastolic function" [12].

Finally, from a clinical point of view, diastolic heart failure can be responsible for symptoms that occur at rest, with less than ordinary physical activity, or with ordinary physical activity. Thus, New York Heart Association classification (NYHA) can be used in diastolic heart failure as well as in systolic heart failure. Of note, the global incidence of diastolic heart failure may be underestimated if paraclinical investigations are only made at rest (see below).

Table 1. Reasons to upgrade diagnosis from possible diastolic heart failure to probable diastolic heart failure [8]

▌Markedly elevated blood pressure (systolic BP > 160 mmHg or a diastolic BP > 100 mmHg) during the episode of heart failure

▌Echocardiographic concentric LV hypertrophy without wall-motion abnormalities

▌A tachyarrhythmia with a shortened diastolic filling period

▌Precipitation of event by the infusion of a small amount of intravenous fluid

▌Clinical improvement in response to therapy directed at the cause of diastolic dysfunction (such as lowering blood pressure, reducing heart rate, or restoring the atrial booster mechanism)

Acute Decompensation of Diastolic Heart Failure

In critical illness, limited data are available in the literature. Diastolic heart failure definition in critical illness is basically the same as in CHF and the diagnosis is also based on the association of heart failure symptoms and a preserved LVEF. The factors that promote fluid overload and precipitate heart failure are similar in diastolic heart failure and systolic heart failure [13].

If we consider acute diastolic heart failure as a pathological situation leading to an impairment in LV diastolic filling, numerous clinical situations could be considered as acute diastolic dysfunction. For example, acute tamponade, acute right heart failure, or acute mitral regurgitation may lead to LV filling abnormalities [14]. Acute settings discussed below are those in which LV diastolic properties are truly impaired. This includes acute exacerbation of chronic diastolic heart failure, hypertensive crisis, severe sepsis, and myocardial ischemia.

▌ Epidemiology

It seems clear that the prevalence and the prognosis of diastolic heart failure are highly dependant on age, gender, and above all the method used to diagnose diastolic heart failure.

Masoudi et al. [15] published in 2003 an epidemiological study in which 19710 patients suffering from heart failure were analyzed. Thirty five percent had preserved LVEF. Among them, 79% were women, whereas only 49 of the 65% suffering from systolic heart failure were women. Patients with diastolic heart failure were 1.5 years older than those with impaired ejection fraction.

Zile and Brutsaert [16] reviewed the data published during the last decade and found that: in patients <50 years, diastolic heart failure represented <15% of the cause of CHF; 50–70 years, the proportion rose to 33%, and >70 years, up to 70% of the CHF were due to diastolic heart failure.

The morbidity from diastolic heart failure remains very high, with a 1-year readmission rate approaching 50%. The morbidity varies according to age and underlying diseases [16, 17]. Data published in the early 90s reported less annual mortality in diastolic heart failure than in systolic heart failure: 5 to 8% in diastolic heart failure versus 10 to 15% in systolic heart failure [18, 19]. More recent studies have reported higher mortality rates. Chen and colleagues [20] analyzed all inhabitants of Olmsted County, Minnesota, between 1996 and 1997 with a new diagnosis of diastolic heart failure. They reported mortality rates as high as 29% at 1 year, 39% at 2 years, and 60% at 3 years. Again, it appears that age and the criteria chosen for the diagnosis of diastolic heart failure can strongly affect the mortality rates.

▌ Pathophysiology of Diastolic Heart Failure

Left Ventricular Pressure/volume Relationship

Systolic, diastolic, and combined heart failure are commonly described using the plotting of LV pressure-volume (P/V) loops.

In case of diastolic dysfunction (Fig. 1), the LV chamber is unable to fill at low left-atrial pressures resulting in abnormalities in the P/V relationship during diastole. The diastolic P/V curve (compliance curve) is displaced upward and to the

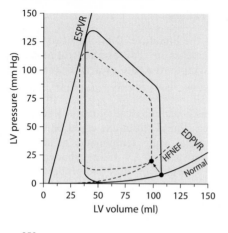

Fig. 1. Modification of the pressure/volume loop in heart failure with normal ejection fraction (HFNEF) also named diastolic heart failure, associating a shift in the end-diastolic pressure-volume relationship (EDPVR) without any change in the end-systolic pressure-volume relationship (ESPVR). From [46] with permission

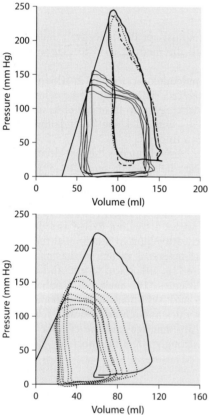

Fig. 2. Pressure/volume (P/V) loops in two patients with diastolic heart failure before (*dashed line*) and after (*dark solid line*) sustained isometric handgrip. From [21] with permission

left. Thus, for a given end-diastolic volume, end-diastolic pressures (also assessed by the pulmonary artery occlusion pressure [PAOP]) are increased. Kawaguchi et al. [21] recently demonstrated that although normal at baseline, P/V loops can be altered during effort. Maneuvers like sustained isometric handgrips can uncover a NYHA stade 2 diastolic heart failure (Fig. 2).

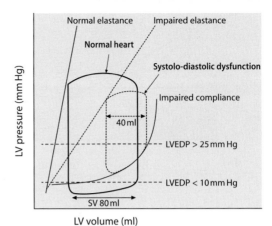

Fig. 3. Left ventricular (LV) pressure/volume loops in combined systolo-diastolic heart failure. LVEDP: left ventricular end-diastolic pressure

In case of systolic dysfunction (Fig. 3), LV contractility is depressed resulting in abnormalities in the P/V relationship during systole. The end-systolic P/V slope (LV systolic elastance slope) is shifted downward and to the right. In addition, the LV end-systolic and end-diastolic volumes are increased. The P/V loop is shifted upward and to the right but remains on the same diastolic P/V curve (LV compliance curve).

Some patients may have combined systolic and diastolic dysfunction (Fig. 3): a modest increase in end-diastolic volume may result in a large increase in end-diastolic pressure if ventricular chamber compliance is markedly altered.

Diastole: New Concepts

According to Zile and Brutsaert [16], diastole can be defined as "the time period during which the myocardium loses its ability to generate force and shorten and returns to an unstressed length and force". Basically, this period represents the part of heart revolution during which the ventricles are filling. Thus diastolic heart failure occurs when the ventricular chamber is unable to accept a volume of blood sufficient to maintain cardiac output at normal diastolic pressures.

The diastole process can be divided into two phases: the first represents LV pressure decline at constant volume, so called isovolumic relaxation; the second is LV chamber filling so called auxotonic relaxation. From a cellular point of view, relaxation is a high energy-consuming process. Release of calcium from troponin C, detachment of the actin-myosin cross-bridge, phosphorylation of phospholamban necessary to activate the ATPase-induced calcium sequestration into the sarcoplasmic reticulum, sodium/calcium exchanger-induced extrusion of calcium from the cytoplasm, and return of the sarcomere to its rest length are all energy consumers.

Zile et al. recently performed a multicenter, prospective study using cardiac catheterization and echocardigraphy to assess the diastolic properties of the left ventricle in 47 patients suffering from diastolic heart failure and 10 normal controls [22]. The authors concluded that diastolic heart failure is characterized by alteration of both LV active relaxation and passive stiffness that could be assessed by the following measures (Fig. 4):

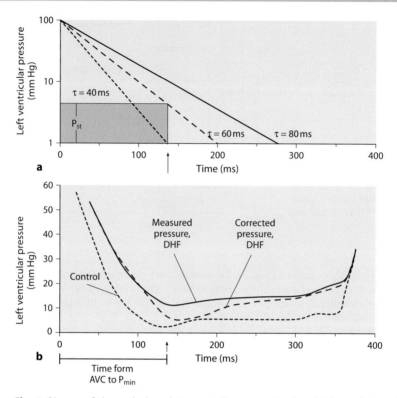

Fig. 4. Diagram of the method used to correct the measured value of left ventricular minimal diastolic pressure for slow relaxation rate. Assuming the physiological concept that active relaxation could be completed after 3.5 τ [47], it is possible to plot the decrease in the left ventricular pressure from the point of aortic valve closure to the theoretical time at which ventricular pressure would approach zero in the absence of filling. By measuring the time from the closure of the aortic valve to Pmin, it is possible to determine the contribution of active relaxation to the left ventricular minimal pressure (Pmin). Thereafter, by subtracting the pressure contribution of slowed relaxation from Pmin, it is possible to obtain a corrected pressure tracing and Pmin, which are used to calculate the corrected passive-stiffness constant. From [22] with permission

▌ τ is the time constant of the isovolumic relaxation
▌ Pmin is the LV minimal pressure after the opening of the mitral valve
▌ PPre-A is the LV pressure just before atrial contraction
▌ EDP is the end-diastolic pressure just after the atrial contraction.

Zile and colleagues [22] showed that in diastolic heart failure, in contrast to normal subjects, relaxation was incomplete at the time of Pmin. Thus, τ was abnormal and Pmin increased with a positive correlation between τ and Pmin. In their study, incomplete relaxation accounted for 7 ± 1 mmHg of the measured Pmin. The authors also reported increased EDP and decreased end diastolic volume (EDV), suggesting increased ventricular stiffness in diastolic heart failure patients. These data suggest that patients with heart failure and preserved ejection fraction have significant abnormalities in both active relaxation and passive stiffness.

Antithesis: More than a Specific Alteration of Diastole?

Some authors recently emphasized that while diastolic parameters are often abnormal in heart failure with normal ejection fraction, they are not necessarily the major component of the dysfunction, nor do they necessarily explain the clinical features. Leite-Moreira et al. remind us that any rise in LV afterload can affect diastole by prolonging relaxation, compromising filling and elevating end-diastolic pressures [23].

Kawaguchi et al. measured LV P/V relations in 10 patients supposedly suffering from diastolic heart failure, 9 asymptomatic normotensive age-matched subjects, 14 asymptomatic normotensive young subjects, and 25 age- and blood-pressure-matched controls [21]. The authors reported a significant increase in both arterial and end-systolic elastance (Ees, Ea) in diastolic heart failure patients and a positive correlation between these two parameters. End-diastolic P/V relations were shifted upward in diastolic heart failure patients but this study clearly emphasizes the fact that end-diastolic P/V relation shift depends on the loading conditions. On the basis of such results, the authors discussed the following hypothesis: diastolic heart failure is essentially due to a combined increase in Ees and Ea. This can influence heart function in several ways: limitation of contractile reserve, high systolic pressure sensitivity to cardiac loading leading to huge hypertensive responses during exertion, increase in myocardial energy consumption, and delay in ventricular chamber relaxation. According to Kawaguchi et al., diastolic dysfunction is present in CHF with normal ejection fractions, but the nature of end-diastolic P/V relations are highly dependent on loading conditions and not merely due to diastolic dysfunction.

▌ Clinical Presentations

Chronic Diastolic Heart Failure

Diastolic heart failure generally occurs in women, in the elderly (50% after 70 years of age), and in those with a history of hypertension. Apart from this, the clinical presentation of diastolic heart failure has no other specificity and the diagnosis is made based on the presence of symptoms of heart failure with preserved systolic function. Table 2 summarizes the prevalence of specific symptoms of CHF in systolic versus diastolic heart failure [16]. The most frequent causes of diastolic heart failure are listed in Table 3 [24].

Diastolic Heart Failure in Acute Situations

Acute Hypertensive Crisis: Ghandi and colleagues [25], recently performed a prospective observational study focusing on echocardiographic profiles at H0, H24 and H72 in patients presenting with acute pulmonary edema and severe arterial hypertension. They wanted to test the hypothesis that such patients suffer from a transient LV systolic dysfunction due to the hypertensive crisis. By contrast to their initial hypothesis, they found that the LVEF and the regional wall motion were similar during the acute episode and after 24 and 72 h of adequate treatment. Moreover 50% of their patients had preserved ejection fraction (LVEF > 50%) and 89% of the patients who had a preserved ejection fraction after treatment also had no sign of

Table 2. Prevalence of specific symptoms and signs in systolic (SHF) *vs* diastolic (DHF) heart failure [16]. Data are expressed as percent of patients in each group presenting with the specified symptom or sign

	DHF (EF > 50%)	SHF (EF < 50%)
Symptoms		
Dyspnea on exertion	85	96
Paroxysmal nocturnal dyspnea	55	50
Orthopnea	60	73
Physical examination		
Jugular venous distension	35	46
Rales	72	70
Displaced apical impulse	50	60
S3	45	65
S4	45	66
Hepatomegaly	15	16
Edema	30	40
Chest radiograph		
Cardiomegaly	90	96
Pulmonary venous hypertension	75	80

EF: ejection fraction

Table 3. Major causes of diastolic heart failure [24]

Myocardial
- Impaired relaxation
  - Epicardial or microvascular ischemia
  - Myocyte hypertrophy
  - Cardiomyopathies
  - Aging
  - Hypothyroidism
- Increased passive stiffness
  - Diffuse fibrosis
  - Post-infarct scarring
  - Myocyte hypertrophy
  - Infiltrative (e.g., amyloidosis, hemochromatosis, Fabry's disease)

Endocardial
- Fibroelastosis
- Mitral or tricuspid stenosis

Epicardial/Pericardia
- Pericardial constriction
- Pericardial tamponade

Coronary microcirculation
- Capillary compression
- Venous engorgement

Other
- Volume overload of the contralateral ventricle
- Extrinsic compression by tumor

systolic dysfunction during the acute episode. Similarly, in patients with an impaired ejection fraction, no differences were found between H0, H24 and H72, suggesting that acute diastolic failure may play a major role also in patients with baseline systolic dysfunction. The pathophysiology of transient diastolic heart failure in hypertensive crisis remains poorly understood but it seems like diastolic heart failure could be uncovered by an acute hypertensive crisis. In case of diastolic heart failure at rest, it is clear that a small increase in LV end-diastolic volume (LVEDV) will lead to a marked elevation in LV end-diastolic pressure (LVEDP). But the explanation is less clear in patients without any diastolic dysfunction at rest. Some authors proposed that hypertensive crisis would lead to a huge increase in coronary perfusion pressure and thus in coronary turgor [26]. Nevertheless, it is unlikely that an increase in coronary blood volume can cause by itself a significant increase in wall thickness.

Myocardial Ischemia: Pennock and colleagues [27] analyzed by echocardiographic and Doppler studies early and late hemodynamic consequences of a circumflex artery ligation in a rabbit model. One hour after the experimental infarct, the rabbits exhibited significant alteration of the LV filling pattern: decrease in E and A waves, A wave reversal velocities, and increase in the mean pulmonary venous systolic-to-diastolic ratio. Three weeks after the coronary ligation, the rabbits still exhibited significant abnormalities in filling pattern. Stugaard and colleagues [28] assessed LV diastolic function in 20 patients during coronary angioplasty and in 8 anesthetized dogs during an experimental coronary occlusion. Diastolic function was explored using a recent Doppler technology, called M-mode Doppler, which allows determination of the time difference between the occurrence of the peak velocity in the apical region and in the mitral tip. The authors reported, in their patients, a significant increase in time difference in comparison with normal values. Coronary artery occlusion in dogs resulted in the same increase in time difference. Moreover, the evolution in time difference was significantly correlated with the variation in time constant of isovolumetric relaxation. Interestingly, the authors tried to investigate whether the changes in filling patterns were associated with ischemic induced tachycardia, increase in intracavitary pressures, or reduction in stroke volume rather than with the ischemic process itself. To answer this question, they performed successively pacing tachycardia, volume loading and caval restriction. None of these procedures significantly altered the time difference.

Sepsis: The role of diastolic dysfunction in septic patients has been questioned since the late 1980s. Stahl et al. showed in 1990 that, in a canine model of hyperdynamic sepsis, myocardial compliance was significantly altered [29]. Jafri et al. published, in the same year, a transmitral Doppler analysis of 13 patients in septic shock, 10 with sepsis without shock, and 33 controls. They reported that, in septic shock as well as in sepsis without shock, the LV filling pattern was significantly altered in comparison with controls [30]. More recently, Poelaert and colleagues [31] characterized systolic and diastolic function in 25 consecutive patients in vasopressor dependant septic shock, using transesophageal echocardiography (TEE) and pulmonary artery catheters. They found that 8 of the 25 patients had no regional wall motion abnormality and a normal LV filling pattern (transmitral E/A wave ratio > 1; pulmonary vein S/D wave ratio > 1); 11 had evidence of abnormal left auricular filling (S/D < 1) but with a preserved systolic function and E/A wave ratio. According to the investigators, transmitral flow in this group could be considered as 'pseudo-normalized'. Finally, 6 of the 25 patients exhibited both systolic and diastolic dysfunction. The authors concluded "cardiac effects of septic shock can be expressed in various degrees, ranging from a normal pattern, through diastolic dysfunction up to both poor LV systolic and diastolic function resulting in combined cardiogenic-septic shock" [31]. It should also be emphasized that impairment of diastolic properties could be an independent predictor of mortality in severe sepsis [32].

▍ Supplementary Investigations

Cardiac Catheterization

The gold standard for the diagnosis of diastolic heart failure is still cardiac catheterization with the assessment of increased ventricular filling pressures at normal chamber volumes and preserved systolic function. With the use of a high-fidelity micromanometer catheter, it is possible to acquire various data including LV pressure, rate of LV pressure decline (dP/dt), and the time constant of isovolumic relaxation (τ).

Diastolic heart failure is characterized by a rise in LVEDP. Zile et al. found a LVEDP above 16 mmHg in 92% of patients with heart failure and normal ejection fraction [12]. Relaxation abnormality is characterized by an increase in the time constant of isovolumic relaxation. In the series of Zile et al., τ was abnormal ($\geq$48 ms) in 79% of the patients.

Chamber stiffness can be assessed by analyzing the diastolic P/V relationship; the stiffness is represented by the slope of the tangent drawn to the curve at any point. Thus, operating stiffness changes throughout filling: lower at the beginning, higher at the end. If LV stiffness increases, the P/V curve is shifted upward and to the left, so that at any point the slope of the tangent becomes steeper.

Echocardiography

Echocardiography provides some fundamental information, such as the normality of LVEF (LVEF > 50%). As demonstrated by Gandhi et al., measurements of ejection fraction even performed several days after an episode of acute exacerbation of CHF correlate with acute measurements [25].

Several echographic criteria have been studied in order to provide a non-invasive assessment of LV diastolic function. The first is the mitral inflow profile. This flow usually has two components: the E wave, which reflects early diastolic filling, and the A wave, which represents the subsequent contribution from atrial systole. These waves are influenced by LV relaxation, LV compliance, and atrial pressure. Normal diastole is characterized by a predominant E wave, showing that most of the LV filling occurs during the early phase of diastole. Mitral inflow abnormalities are of three types:

▍ in mild diastolic dysfunction, relaxation is impaired, and atrial contraction contributes relatively more to ventricular filling: A wave > E wave, with prolonged E wave deceleration time (usually > 240 ms)

▍ in moderate diastolic dysfunction, relaxation is impaired, LV compliance is decreased, and atrial pressure increased: pseudonormal pattern with an E wave again predominant, but the E wave deceleration time is shorter

▌ in severe diastolic dysfunction, LV compliance is extremely low: restrictive pattern with high E wave velocity, usually more than twice the A wave velocity.

Zile et al. reported a lack of sensitivity of the mitral inflow analysis for the diagnosis of diastolic heart failure. In their study [12], the E/A ratio was abnormal in only 48% of the patients presenting signs of CHF with a normal ejection fraction. The E wave deceleration time was found to be more sensitive (abnormal in 64% of the patients).

Pulmonary vein flow can also be measured. There are two waves of pulmonary vein flow, one during systole, the other during diastole. The elevation of the left atrial pressure impairs atrial filling and the pulmonary vein diastolic wave becomes predominant. Nevertheless, pulmonary vein flow abnormalities poorly discriminate systolic and diastolic heart failure.

New, promising modalities like Doppler tissue imaging or color M-mode mitral flow propagation wave need to be validated [33, 34].

Other: Neuroendocrine Profile

B-type natriuretic peptide (BNP) is now recognized as a specific marker of heart failure in patients presenting with acute dyspnea [35]. This peptide also seems to be of interest for the distinction of diastolic heart failure and lung disease in emergency settings. In a study by Maisel et al., when patients with diastolic heart failure were compared with patients without CHF, a BNP value of 100 pg/ml had a sensitivity of 86%, a negative predictive value of 96%, and an accuracy of 75% for detecting abnormal diastolic dysfunction [36]. In this series, patients with diastolic heart failure had significantly lower BNP levels than those with systolic heart failure (413 pg/ml vs 821 pg/ml, $p < 0.001$). Nevertheless, the authors concluded that BNP adds a modest discriminatory value in differentiating diastolic from systolic heart failure.

▌ Treatment

Very few data are currently available concerning the therapeutic strategy for diastolic heart failure. The guidelines are essentially based on pathophysiological concepts and on a small number of prospective clinical trials.

General Treatment

The general treatment of diastolic heart failure has two major goals: to limit the consequences of the cardiac filling abnormalities and to control the factors responsible for the diastolic dysfunction.

Symptom-targeted therapy should focus on the reduction of pulmonary congestion at rest and during exercise. The two ways of reducing pulmonary capillary pressure are to optimize blood volume and to improve LV filling. LV diastolic pressures can be substantially decreased by the reduction in LV diastolic volumes. Indeed, because of the steep diastolic P/V relation, a small decrease in diastolic volume can lead to a great decrease in diastolic pressure. Thus, diuretics to reduce global blood volume and nitrates to decrease central blood volume could be considered as a first step of symptomatic treatment. The second step of symptom-targeted therapy should focus on improving diastolic filling. Therefore, heart rate control should be considered as a major issue. In fact, tachycardia and non-sinus rhythms are poorly tolerated in patients with diastolic heart failure. First, rapid heart rates induce an increase in myocardial oxygen consumption, and a decrease in coronary perfusion time, both promoting myocardial ischemia even in the absence of underlying coronary disease. Second, tachycardia may shorten diastolic time and thus lead to an incomplete filling. Third, recent data suggest that, in diastolic heart failure, relaxation velocity does not increase in response to tachycardia and may even decrease. This may contribute to the elevation of the end diastolic pressures. Furthermore, the loss of sinus rhythm and thus atrial systole is usually poorly tolerated. Beta-blockers, nondihydropyridine calcium-channel blockers like verapamil can be prescribed in order to prevent tachycardia and to improve filling [37, 38]. Finally, it is still not clear whether digitalis may be of interest in the treatment of diastolic heart failure. In the Digitalis Investigation Group trial, the subgroup of patients with normal ejection exhibited fewer symptoms and lower hospitalization rates under digitalis treatment. As long as the pathophysiological interest of digitalis drugs remains unclear in diastolic heart failure, more evidence is needed of their effects before extending their use to these patients.

Specific Treatment

The renin-angiotensin-aldosterone system seems to play a great role in the development of diastolic heart failure and particularly in myocardial remodeling and in fluid retention. Naturally, ACE inhibitors, angiotensin receptor antagonists, and aldosterone antagonists have been proposed in the treatment of diastolic heart failure. A small short-term study performed by Aronow and colleagues focused on the effect of enalapril on diastolic heart failure in elderly patients with prior myocardial infarction [39] and reported a benefit in terms of exercise capacity. The CHARM-preserved study was a multicenter, randomized, double blinded study comparing, in diastolic heart failure, the effects of a selective angiotensin-receptor blocking agent (candesartan) versus a placebo [40]. Between 1999 and 2000, 3023 patients NYHA class II to IV, with a LVEF higher than 40% were enrolled in the study (1514 in the candesartan group, 1509 in the placebo group). After 36 months of follow-up, the authors could only conclude that candesartan significantly reduced the rate of hospitalization. No other differences were observed between the two groups. Losartan, another angiotensin-receptor blocker has been shown to increase exercise tolerance [41].

New agents targeting intracellular calcium homeostasis are currently under evaluation. MCC-135 is one of these drugs, which is supposed to improve calcium reuptake by the sarcoplasmic reticulum. MCC-135 is currently under evaluation in a phase II, double-blind, placebo-controlled study in patients suffering from CHF NYHA II and III and either systolic or diastolic heart failure [42].

Levosimendan is a calcium sensitizer modulating the interaction between troponin and calcium. This inotropic drug has recently been proposed to improve cardiac performance after an acute episode of myocardial ischemia [43]. Twenty-four patients were randomized after percutaneous angioplasty to receive either placebo or levosimendan. In the treated group, LVEDV and the time constant of isovolumic LV pressure fall significantly decreased, indicating an obvious improvement in the diastolic function.

Finally, nitric oxide (NO)-donor effects have also been investigated. Paulus et al. [44] performed intracoronary injections of sodium nitroprusside in normal hearts. The authors showed that NO-donors caused an earlier onset of LV relaxation, a fall in LV minimum and end-diastolic pressures, an increase in LVEDV and a down and rightward displacement of the LV diastolic P/V relation. These results are consistent with a direct NO-induced improvement in diastolic function. Interestingly, the stimulation of endogenous NO release from the coronary endothelium, by intracoronary infusion of a substance P agonist, produced similar results [45].

▌ Conclusion

In summary, diastolic heart failure is a very common pathology, the incidence of which is frequently underestimated. While diastolic heart failure is recognized as the mechanism involved in CHF with a preserved LV function, it seems that diastolic dysfunction can also account for acute heart failure occurring in critical care situations. Hypertensive crisis, sepsis, and myocardial ischemia are frequently associated with acute diastolic heart failure. The diastolic dysfunction can affect either active relaxation, passive stiffness, or both. With a better understanding of cardiomyocyte function, intracellular calcium metabolism impairment appears to be involved frequently in the development of diastolic failure. Symptomatic treatment focuses on the reduction of pulmonary congestion and the improvement of LV filling. Specific treatments are lacking, but encouraging data are emerging concerning the use of renin-angiotensin-aldosterone axis blockers, NO donors, or new agents such as levosimendan.

References

1. Kupari M, Lindroos M, Iivanainen AM, Heikkila J, Tilvis R (1997) Congestive heart failure in old age: prevalence, mechanisms and 4-year prognosis in the Helsinki Ageing Study. J Intern Med 241:387–394
2. Senni M, Tribouilloy CM, Rodeheffer RJ, et al (1998) Congestive heart failure in the community: a study of all incident cases in Olmsted County, Minnesota, in 1991. Circulation 98:2282–2289
3. Mosterd A, Hoes AW, de Bruyne MC, et al (1999) Prevalence of heart failure and left ventricular dysfunction in the general population; The Rotterdam Study. Eur Heart J 20:447–455
4. Vasan RS, Larson MG, Benjamin EJ, Evans JC, Reiss CK, Levy D (1999) Congestive heart failure in subjects with normal versus reduced left ventricular ejection fraction: prevalence and mortality in a population-based cohort. J Am Coll Cardiol 33:1948–1955
5. Remes J, Miettinen H, Reunanen A, Pyorala K (1991) Validity of clinical diagnosis of heart failure in primary health care. Eur Heart J 12:315–321
6. Vasan RS, Benjamin EJ, Levy D (1995) Prevalence, clinical features and prognosis of diastolic heart failure: an epidemiologic perspective. J Am Coll Cardiol 26:1565–1574
7. European Study Group on Diastolic Heart Failure (1998) How to diagnose diastolic heart failure. Eur Heart J 19:990–1003
8. Vasan RS, Levy D (2000) Defining diastolic heart failure: a call for standardized diagnostic criteria. Circulation 101:2118–2121
9. Hunt SA, Baker DW, Chin MH, et al (2001) ACC/AHA guidelines for the evaluation and management of chronic heart failure in the adult: executive summary. A report of the American College of Cardiology/American Heart Association Task Force on Practice Guidelines (Committee to revise the 1995 Guidelines for the Evaluation and Management of Heart Failure). J Am Coll Cardiol 38:2101–2113

10. Remme WJ, Swedberg K (2001) Guidelines for the diagnosis and treatment of chronic heart failure. Eur Heart J 22:1527–1560
11. Zile MR (2003) Diastolic heart failure. Diagnosis, prognosis, treatment. Minerva Cardioangiol 51:131–142
12. Zile MR, Gaasch WH, Carroll JD, et al (2001) Heart failure with a normal ejection fraction: is measurement of diastolic function necessary to make the diagnosis of diastolic heart failure? Circulation 104:779–782
13. Tsuyuki RT, McKelvie RS, Arnold JM, et al (2001) Acute precipitants of congestive heart failure exacerbations. Arch Intern Med 161:2337–2342
14. Pierard LA, Lancellotti P (2004) The role of ischemic mitral regurgitation in the pathogenesis of acute pulmonary edema. N Engl J Med 351:1627–1634
15. Masoudi FA, Havranek EP, Smith G, et al (2003) Gender, age, and heart failure with preserved left ventricular systolic function. J Am Coll Cardiol 41:217–223
16. Zile MR, Brutsaert DL (2002) New concepts in diastolic dysfunction and diastolic heart failure: Part I: diagnosis, prognosis, and measurements of diastolic function. Circulation 105:1387–1393
17. Aurigemma GP, Gaasch WH (2004) Clinical practice. Diastolic heart failure. N Engl J Med 351:1097–1105
18. Setaro JF, Soufer R, Remetz MS, Perlmutter RA, Zaret BL (1992) Long-term outcome in patients with congestive heart failure and intact systolic left ventricular performance. Am J Cardiol 69:1212–1216
19. Judge KW, Pawitan Y, Caldwell J, Gersh BJ, Kennedy JW (1991) Congestive heart failure symptoms in patients with preserved left ventricular systolic function: analysis of the CASS registry. J Am Coll Cardiol 18:377–382
20. Chen HH, Lainchbury JG, Senni M, Bailey KR, Redfield MM (2002) Diastolic heart failure in the community: clinical profile, natural history, therapy, and impact of proposed diagnostic criteria. J Card Fail 8:279–287
21. Kawaguchi M, Hay I, Fetics B, Kass DA (2003) Combined ventricular systolic and arterial stiffening in patients with heart failure and preserved ejection fraction: implications for systolic and diastolic reserve limitations. Circulation 107:714–720
22. Zile MR, Baicu CF, Gaasch WH (2004) Diastolic heart failure – abnormalities in active relaxation and passive stiffness of the left ventricle. N Engl J Med 350:1953–1959
23. Leite-Moreira AF, Correia-Pinto J, Gillebert TC (1999) Afterload induced changes in myocardial relaxation: a mechanism for diastolic dysfunction. Cardiovasc Res 43:344–353
24. Angeja BG, Grossman W (2003) Evaluation and management of diastolic heart failure. Circulation 107:659–663
25. Gandhi SK, Powers JC, Nomeir AM, et al (2001) The pathogenesis of acute pulmonary edema associated with hypertension. N Engl J Med 344:17–22
26. Wexler LF, Grice WN, Huntington M, Plehn JF, Apstein CS (1989) Coronary hypertension and diastolic compliance in isolated rabbit hearts. Hypertension 13:598–606
27. Pennock GD, Yun DD, Agarwal PG, Spooner PH, Goldman S (1997) Echocardiographic changes after myocardial infarction in a model of left ventricular diastolic dysfunction. Am J Physiol 273:H2018–2029
28. Stugaard M, Smiseth OA, Risoe C, Ihlen H (1993) Intraventricular early diastolic filling during acute myocardial ischemia, assessment by multigated color m-mode Doppler echocardiography. Circulation 88:2705–2713
29. Stahl TJ, Alden PB, Ring WS, Madoff RC, Cerra FB (1990) Sepsis-induced diastolic dysfunction in chronic canine peritonitis. Am J Physiol 258:H625–633
30. Jafri SM, Lavine S, Field BE, Bahorozian MT, Carlson RW (1990) Left ventricular diastolic function in sepsis. Crit Care Med 18:709–714
31. Poelaert J, Declerck C, Vogelaers D, Colardyn F, Visser CA (1997) Left ventricular systolic and diastolic function in septic shock. Intensive Care Med 23:553–560
32. Munt B, Jue J, Gin K, Fenwick J, Tweeddale M (1998) Diastolic filling in human severe sepsis: an echocardiographic study. Crit Care Med 26:1829–1833
33. Garcia MJ, Thomas JD, Klein AL (1998) New Doppler echocardiographic applications for the study of diastolic function. J Am Coll Cardiol 32:865–875

34. Nagueh SF, Middleton KJ, Kopelen HA, Zoghbi WA, Quinones MA (1997) Doppler tissue imaging: a noninvasive technique for evaluation of left ventricular relaxation and estimation of filling pressures. J Am Coll Cardiol 30:1527–1533
35. Morrison LK, Harrison A, Krishnaswamy P, Kazanegra R, Clopton P, Maisel A (2002) Utility of a rapid B-natriuretic peptide assay in differentiating congestive heart failure from lung disease in patients presenting with dyspnea. J Am Coll Cardiol 39:202–209
36. Maisel AS, McCord J, Nowak RM, et al (2003) Bedside B-Type natriuretic peptide in the emergency diagnosis of heart failure with reduced or preserved ejection fraction. Results from the Breathing Not Properly Multinational Study. J Am Coll Cardiol 41:2010–2017
37. Aronow WS, Ahn C, Kronzon I (1997) Effect of propranolol versus no propranolol on total mortality plus nonfatal myocardial infarction in older patients with prior myocardial infarction, congestive heart failure, and left ventricular ejection fraction > or = 40% treated with diuretics plus angiotensin-converting enzyme inhibitors. Am J Cardiol 80:207–209
38. Setaro JF, Zaret BL, Schulman DS, Black HR, Soufer R (1990) Usefulness of verapamil for congestive heart failure associated with abnormal left ventricular diastolic filling and normal left ventricular systolic performance. Am J Cardiol 66:981–986
39. Aronow WS, Kronzon I (1993) Effect of enalapril on congestive heart failure treated with diuretics in elderly patients with prior myocardial infarction and normal left ventricular ejection fraction. Am J Cardiol 71:602–604
40. Yusuf S, Pfeffer MA, Swedberg K, et al (2003) Effects of candesartan in patients with chronic heart failure and preserved left-ventricular ejection fraction: the CHARM-Preserved Trial. Lancet 362:777–781
41. Warner JG Jr, Metzger DC, Kitzman DW, Wesley DJ, Little WC (1999) Losartan improves exercise tolerance in patients with diastolic dysfunction and a hypertensive response to exercise. J Am Coll Cardiol 33:1567–1572
42. Zile M, Gaasch W, Little W, et al (2004) A phase II, double-blind, randomized, placebo-controlled, dose comparative study of the efficacy, tolerability, and safety of MCC-135 in subjects with chronic heart failure, NYHA class II/III (MCC-135-GO1 study): rationale and design. J Card Fail 10:193–199
43. Sonntag S, Sundberg S, Lehtonen LA, Kleber FX (2004) The calcium sensitizer levosimendan improves the function of stunned myocardium after percutaneous transluminal coronary angioplasty in acute myocardial ischemia. J Am Coll Cardiol 43:2177–2182
44. Paulus WJ, Vantrimpont PJ, Shah AM (1994) Acute effects of nitric oxide on left ventricular relaxation and diastolic distensibility in humans. Assessment by bicoronary sodium nitroprusside infusion. Circulation 89:2070–2078
45. Paulus WJ, Vantrimpont PJ, Shah AM (1995) Paracrine coronary endothelial control of left ventricular function in humans. Circulation 92:2119–2126
46. Burkhoff D, Maurer MS, Packer M (2003) Heart failure with a normal ejection fraction: is it really a disorder of diastolic function? Circulation 107:656–658
47. Weisfeldt ML, Weiss JL, Frederiksen JT, Yin FC (1980) Quantification of incomplete left ventricular relaxation: relationship to the time constant for isovolumic pressure fall. Eur Heart J (Suppl):119–129

Severe Heart Failure in the ICU

F. Ginsberg and J. E. Parrillo

▌ Introduction

Heart failure is a syndrome caused by abnormal cardiac performance resulting in signs and symptoms related to salt and fluid retention, increased left ventricular (LV) filling pressures, and/or decreased cardiac output. Typical symptoms include dyspnea at rest or with exertion, fatigue, cough, swelling, orthopnea, and paroxysmal nocturnal dyspnea. Physical examination often reveals pulmonary rales, elevated jugular venous pressure (JVP), signs of cardiomegaly, S_3 gallop, hepatic enlargement, and edema. Manifestations of more severe heart failure include marked dyspnea at rest, possibly leading to respiratory failure, cyanosis, cool extremities, and altered mental state. Life expectancy is reduced in patients with heart failure, and death can occur at the end of progressive worsening of the syndrome or can occur suddenly in patients otherwise felt to have been stable.

Heart failure is a very common clinical illness. Five million Americans are affected, females as frequently as males [1]. It is estimated that 1% of the population of Americans over age 65 are affected by heart failure, and 20% of hospital admissions in patients over age 65 are due to heart failure [2]. Five hundred and fifty thousand new cases of heart failure are diagnosed in the United States annually, with a total of nearly one million annual hospital discharges with a primary diagnosis of heart failure [1]. Thus, the treatment of heart failure incurs a very large burden on the US health care system. Epidemiologic data show significant increases in both the incidence and prevalence of heart failure in the US population over the past decade [2], likely influenced by the aging of the population with an increased incidence of hypertension, and improved treatment and survival of patients with ischemic heart disease.

▌ Pathophysiology

Manifestations of heart failure can be thought of as due primarily to LV systolic dysfunction or diastolic dysfunction, although clinically many patients will experience heart failure with both abnormalities. Systolic heart failure results from the inability of the heart to expel blood normally due to depressed LV contraction. Diastolic heart failure is caused by a reduction in LV compliance leading to impaired diastolic filling and higher LV diastolic pressures with resultant increases in pulmonary artery occlusion pressure (PAOP).

Conditions commonly associated with diastolic heart failure, or congestive heart failure (CHF) in the setting of normal systolic function, include hypertension and

a   Ventricular remodeling after acute infarction

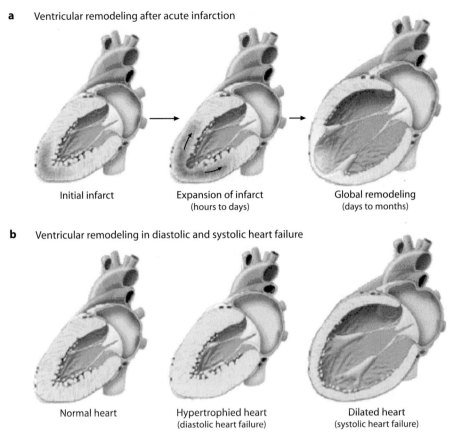

| Initial infarct | Expansion of infarct (hours to days) | Global remodeling (days to months) |

b   Ventricular remodeling in diastolic and systolic heart failure

| Normal heart | Hypertrophied heart (diastolic heart failure) | Dilated heart (systolic heart failure) |

Fig. 1. Ventricular remodeling after infarction (*Panel a*) and in diastolic and systolic heart failure (Panel b). At the time of an acute myocardial infarction — in this case, an apical infarction — there is no clinically significant change in overall ventricular geometry (*Panel a*). Within hours to days, the area of myocardium affected by the infarction begins to expand and become thinner. Within days to months, global remodeling can occur, resulting in overall ventricular dilatation, decreased systolic function, mitral-valve dysfunction, and the formation of an aneurysm. The classic ventricular remodeling that occurs with hypertensive heart disease (*middle of Panel b*) results in a normal-sized left ventricular cavity with thickened ventricular walls (concentric left ventricular hypertrophy) and preserved systolic function. There may be some thickening of the mitral-valve apparatus. In contrast, the classic remodeling that occurs with dilated cardiomyopathy (*right side of Panel b*) results in a globular shape of the heart, a thinning of the left ventricular walls, an overall decrease in systolic function, and distortion of the mitral-valve apparatus, leading to mitral regurgitation. From [2] with permission

LV hypertrophy, and acute coronary ischemia. Diastolic heart failure is common in elderly populations, likely due to progressive diastolic compliance abnormalities seen with aging. Uncommon conditions leading to diastolic heart failure include infiltrative and restrictive cardiomyopathies and chronic constrictive pericarditis (Fig. 1, panel B).

Systolic heart failure, the focus of this chapter, is initiated by conditions leading to damage of LV myocardium. The most common of these conditions are atherosclerotic heart disease with acute myocardial infarction (AMI) and myocardial ischemia; hypertension; dilated cardiomyopathy (i.e., idiopathic, alcoholic, or viral) and valvular heart disease. Chronic myocardial ischemia can result in an entity termed 'hibernating' myocardium. In this setting, chronic severe ischemia leads to dysfunctional but viable myocardium resulting in significant LV contractile dysfunction. Damage to LV myocardium leads to a series of systemic maladaptive responses commonly termed neurohormonal activation [2, 3]. Two major systems involved in neurohormonal activation are the renin-angiotensin system and the sympathetic nervous system.

Activation of the renin-angiotensin system leads to elevated levels of renin, angiotensin II, and aldosterone [3]. These hormones have deleterious consequences on cardiac function. Negative hemodynamic effects include salt and fluid retention, endothelial dysfunction, and vasoconstriction. These agents also contribute to a process known as LV remodeling [2, 3]. In remodeling, the cardiac muscle is affected by myocyte hypertrophy, myocardial interstitial fibrosis, and apoptosis (leading to cell death) with reduced numbers of myocytes. As a result of remodeling, there is progressive LV dilatation, a change in LV geometry, and progressive worsening of LV contractile force. In addition, the change in LV geometry leads often to increasing mitral regurgitation as the size of the mitral annulus increases, and the physical relationship of the mitral valve structures is altered [2, 3] (Fig. 1, panel a).

Sympathetic nervous system activation is, in part, mediated via decreased cardiac output with resultant tachycardia, increased myocyte oxygen consumption, and peripheral vasoconstriction [4]. Renal effects of sympathetic nervous system activation lead to further activation of the renin-angiotensin system. Increased circulating norepinephrine levels also contribute to cardiac myocyte injury and death [4]. Arrhythmias become more common. Thus, a detrimental positive feedback loop is established, causing progressive deterioration in LV structure and performance over time. It is thus clear that systolic heart failure is an illness that progressively worsens over time.

▌ Prognosis

Despite many recent advances in heart failure therapy, the prognosis remains poor. Overall, five-year survival in patients with heart failure is only 50% [3]. If heart failure is diagnosed before age 65, males have an 80% 8-year mortality and females a 70% 8-year mortality. Patients hospitalized for treatment of heart failure have a 25% incidence of re-hospitalization within six months and a 60% 4-year mortality [2].

Recently reported randomized trials of outpatient pharmacologic therapy (reviewed below) reveal annual mortality rates of approximately 10% in patients with Class II–III heart failure and 20–50% annual mortality rates in patients who are Class IV. Studies of treatment in patients with severe heart failure awaiting cardiac transplantation reveal a 1-year mortality of 75% and a 2-year mortality rate of 92% [5]. In chronic heart failure, survival relates most closely to severity of LV dysfunction, severity of associated coronary artery disease and functional class. However, in patients admitted for treatment of decompensated heart failure, short-term prognosis is related most closely to the presence of hypotension, myocardial ischemia, and an altered hemodynamic profile of low cardiac output and high LV end diastolic pressure (LVEDP). The presence of hyponatremia also augurs a poorer prognosis in these patients [6].

Finally, the prognosis for patients who present with heart failure and cardiogenic shock due to AMI is dismal, with 80–90% in-hospital mortality with medical therapy alone. Mortality remains 40–50% even with aggressive supportive therapy and emergency revascularization strategies [7].

Approach to the Patient – Overview

In addition to evaluating specific pharmacologic therapies for patients with heart failure, other potential or aggravating factors must be looked for and corrected when possible (Table 1). Environmental factors such as inadvertent excessive salt and fluid intake or excess alcohol consumption are common. Patient compliance with often complicated regimens of numerous medications must be assessed. Emotional and physical stressors should be corrected when feasible.

Concomitant administration of medications for non-cardiac conditions can have detrimental effects as well. A partial listing includes corticosteroids, which cause fluid retention and aggravate hypertension, and nonsteroidal anti-inflammatory drugs (NSAIDs). NSAIDs also aggravate salt and water retention and can interfere with the beneficial renal effects of ACE-inhibitors and loop diuretics [8]. Metformin

Table 1. Causes of acutely decompensated heart failure

Environmental
▌ Excess salt and fluid intake
▌ Excess alcohol consumption
▌ Medication noncompliance or misunderstanding
▌ Emotional or physical stress

Adverse Medication Effects
▌ Calcium channel blockers
▌ Antiarrhythmics (Types 1A, IC)
▌ Non-steroidal anti-inflammatory drugs (NSAIDs)
▌ Corticosteroids
▌ Metformin, thiazolindinediones (TZDs)
▌ Cancer chemotherapy

Cardiovascular Conditions
▌ Acute ischemia/infarction
▌ Pulmonary embolism
▌ Uncontrolled hypertension
▌ Arrhythmia
▌ Worsening valvular regurgitation
▌ Endocarditis

Extra-Cardiac Illness
▌ Sepsis, infection, hypoxia
▌ Renal failure, urinary obstruction
▌ Thyroid disease
▌ Anemia, blood loss
▌ Obstructive sleep apnea
▌ Bilateral renal artery stenosis

and thiazolindinediones can contribute to water retention and aggravate the symptoms and signs of heart failure. Certain cancer chemotherapies can cause myocardial damage. Cardiac medications such as calcium channel blockers and anti-arrhythmic drugs can also have direct negative effects on LV contractility.

Acute and chronic extra-cardiac conditions may also cause cardiac decompensation. Pulmonary embolus, infectious illnesses and sepsis are common. Anemia, blood loss and thyroid disease need to be assessed and corrected. Renal failure often has similar etiologies to heart failure (e.g., hypertension, vascular disease), and worsening renal function will often aggravate heart failure. Obstructive sleep apnea can also lead to exacerbation of heart failure symptoms and can be effectively treated. Influenza and pneumococcal vaccines should be administered to patients to prevent the cardiac decompensation associated with respiratory infections.

Lastly, coexistent cardiovascular illnesses can aggravate heart failure. Recurrent coronary ischemia should always be suspected, evaluated and corrected with revascularization strategies when appropriate. Uncontrolled hypertension and cardiac arrhythmias (most commonly atrial fibrillation and ventricular arrhythmias) frequently accompany LV dysfunction. Worsening valve regurgitation, endocarditis, and bilateral renal artery stenosis are other examples of conditions which can lead to heart failure exacerbations and which are treatable.

Goals of treatment of heart failure can be assessed as either short-term, to improve acute hemodynamic decompensation in hospitalized patients, or long-term. In patients admitted to the hospital with severe decompensation, short-term goals include improving symptoms by correcting fluid overload and improving hemodynamics with reduction in PAOP, reduction in mean right atrial pressure, and increase in cardiac output. Additional goals include preserving renal function, preventing arrhythmias, and preventing further myocardial necrosis in patients with ischemic and non-ischemic disease. Therapies to prevent or attenuate chronic remodeling and which have been shown to improve long-term prognosis should also be instituted or strengthened while patients are hospitalized.

Long-term goals of therapy include improving symptoms of dyspnea and fatigue and improving exercise tolerance. Therapy should decrease the need for repeated hospitalizations for heart failure exacerbations. Treatments shown to improve life expectancy need to be initiated to decrease the risk of death due to progressive LV failure as well as sudden arrhythmic death.

Pharmacologic treatment of CHF involves combinations of multiple medications. These drugs have been shown to improve symptoms and functional capacity, decrease the need for repeated hospitalization, and improve mortality. Therapies are aimed at improving fluid balance as well as correcting the neurohormonal activation responsible for the progressive decline in LV function. Pharmacologic agents need to be started early in the course of the disease to prevent or attenuate the process of remodeling. For example, these therapies ideally are started in the early phase post-myocardial infarction, or when LV systolic dysfunction is diagnosed even in the absence of clinical symptoms of the heart failure syndrome. Symptomatic abnormal LV function can be seen in 40% of patients post-myocardial infarction as well as in the settings of diabetes mellitus and chronic hypertension.

Specific Pharmacologic Therapies for Treatment of Chronic Heart Failure

Diuretics

Loop diuretics are routinely used in patients with signs or symptoms of fluid retention [1]. Once patients are euvolemic, diuretics are continued to prevent fluid reaccumulation. A flexible dosing schedule, based on daily weights and close telephone contact with a heart failure treatment team member, can be very effective in maintaining a euvolemic state [9].

Furosemide is the most common loop diuretic used. Bumetanide or torsemide are also effective. Torsemide may be helpful in patients with suboptimal responses to furosemide due to its more consistent absorption [3]. Metolazone or a thiazide diuretic can be used in addition to a loop diuretic in patients with more severe heart failure, due to their synergistic effects [3]. Patients must be periodically monitored for side effects of these agents including azotemia, hypokalemia, alkalosis, hyponatremia, and hypomagnesemia.

Beta-blockers

Catecholamine levels are increased in heart failure, and higher levels correlate with worse disease severity [4]. Catecholamines have direct negative effects on the myocardium including induction of myocyte hypertrophy and apoptosis [4]. Clinically, these effects are evident as left ventricular dilatation, increased ischemia, increased peripheral vasoconstriction, and cardiac arrhythmias.

Beta-blockers interfere with catecholamine mediated activation of cardiac β-receptors, thereby attenuating β-receptor mediated increases in heart rate and oxygen consumption and preventing sympathetic nervous system mediated effects on remodeling. In addition, the newer agent, carvedilol, blocks α-receptors, which mediate vasoconstriction and increased cardiac contractility, as well as β-receptors.

Several large trials using beta-blockers in thousands of patients with chronic CHF, or in post-myocardial infarction patients with reduced ejection fractions below 40%, have demonstrated statistically significant and consistent reductions in the need for rehospitalization for heart failure and reductions in mortality. The BHAT study showed a relative 26% reduction in mortality at two years in post-myocardial infarction patients treated with propranolol [10, 11]. The CIBIS II trial using bisoprolol showed a 34% relative risk reduction in hospitalizations and mortality at

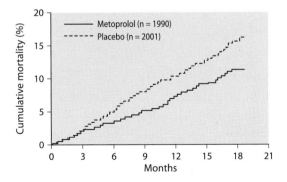

Fig. 2. Results of the MERIT-HF (Metoprolol CR/XL Randomized Intervention Trial in Heart Failure). The addition of metoprolol to conventional therapy was associated with a 34% reduction in the risk of death for any reason (95% confidence interval, 19 to 47% decrease; p < 0.0001). From [4] with permission

16 months of therapy [12], and MERIT-HF showed a relative reduction of 33% in these endpoints at 12 months using metoprolol [13] (Fig. 2). The CAPRICORN trial using the combined alpha- and beta-blocker carvedilol instituted within three weeks of myocardial infarction showed a 23% relative reduction in all cause mortality at two years [14]. More severe heart failure patients, symptomatic classes III and IV were studied in the COPERNICUS trial [15]. Patients with ejection fractions under 25% began therapy with carvedilol in hospital. In 10.4 months, a 35% relative mortality reduction was seen, with improvement in mortality beginning as early as three weeks after therapy initiation (Fig. 3). In these trials, beta-blockers were not discontinued more frequently than placebo for perceived side effects, and there was no increased risk of heart failure exacerbation due to beta-blocker therapy when compared with placebo even in the early phases of drug administration [16]. Several trials with carvedilol have shown an approximate 6% absolute increase in LV ejection fraction after a minimum of two years of therapy [17].

Beta-blockers should be instituted early and titrated up to maximal recommended doses (e.g., metoprolol 200 mg daily or carvedilol 25 mg bid) or maximally

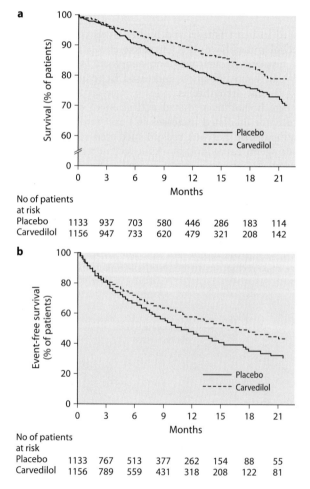

Fig. 3. Results of treatment with carvedilol in chronic heart failure class III and IV patients. From [15] with permission

tolerated doses. These medications should be started in the hospital in post-myo-cardial infarction patients or in patients with heart failure at the earliest possible time regardless of ejection fraction. They should be used in heart failure due to ischemic or nonischemic cardiomyopathy once other therapies have resulted in the patient becoming euvolemic. Beta-blockers should be instituted in 'compensated' patients as well, as these patients have a high likelihood of symptom progression within 12 months. Lastly, this therapy is beneficial as 'add on' treatment to angio-tensin converting enzyme (ACE) inhibitors and diuretics.

ACE Inhibitors

These agents act to decrease the effects of the renin-angiotensin system activation by blocking the conversion of angiotensin I to angiotensin II, thus counteracting the deleterious effects of angiotensin II and aldosterone. Multiple studies have shown benefits of ACE inhibitor therapy in post-myocardial infarction patients as well as patients with cardiomyopathy and heart failure. The SAVE trial with capto-pril involved post-myocardial infarction patients with ejection fractions under 40%. A relative risk reduction of 20% in mortality was noted at 3.5 years [18]. The SOLVD trial, using enalapril in patients with Class II–III heart failure and ejection fractions less than 35%, showed a 10% relative risk reduction in mortality at 3.5 years. Enalapril given to patients less ill, with asymptomatic LV dysfunction and ejection fractions under 35%, showed a reduction in the clinical diagnosis of heart failure and a statistically significant reduction in heart failure hospitalizations at three years [19]. A meta-analysis performed of 32 trials involving 7105 patients with the use of captopril, enalapril, ramipril, quinapril, or lisinopril found that ACE inhibitors reduced the risk of death and hospitalization due to heart failure [20]. Thus, these positive results of ACE inhibitors are felt to be class effects and not specific to any particular agent.

Side effects of these agents include cough, worsening renal function in patients with renal artery stenosis, angioneurotic edema, and hyperkalemia. The dose of ACE inhibitors should be increased as renal function and blood pressure allow. Studies have shown that medium doses of ACE inhibitors when compared to low doses significantly reduce hospitalization rates for heart failure. However, higher doses given routinely do not significantly reduce cardiovascular events further. Further improvement in symptoms and mortality is thus best achieved by adding on beta-blocker therapy rather than by increasing ACE inhibitor doses to even higher levels.

Angiotensin Receptor Blockers

Angiotensin receptor blockers work to counter the effects of angiotensin II at the tissue level by blocking angiotensin II receptors. Multiple studies have shown bene-fits of these medications in patients with heart failure. Large numbers of patients in the reported series have been studied, even more than in the ACE inhibitor trials. Generally in these studies, angiotensin receptor blockers are used as a substi-tute for ACE inhibitors. More recently, they have been evaluated as medications giv-en in combination with ACE inhibitors and beta-blockers.

The RESOLVD trial, using candesartan in heart failure patients with a mean ejection fraction of 27%, showed equivalent mortality rates and similar exercise tol-

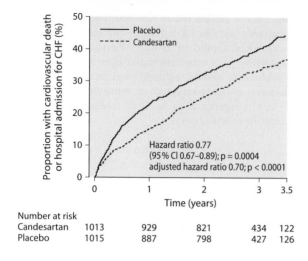

Fig. 4. Kaplan-Meier cumulative event curves for primary outcome in the CHARM trial. From [2] with permission

Number at risk				
Candesartan	1013	929	821	434	122
Placebo	1015	887	798	427	126

erance and functional class to patients treated with enalapril at 3.5 years [21]. ELITE II, a study using losartan compared with captopril in patients with ejection fractions under 40%, showed no difference in mortality or CHF admissions. Losartan was better tolerated because of the lower incidence of problematic cough [22]. ValHeft 2001 showed that valsartan as a substitute for ACE inhibitor therapy was associated with a relative 33% risk reduction in mortality when compared with placebo. A worse mortality for valsartan in patients who were already taking ACE inhibitors and beta-blockers was seen, but the small number of patients in this subgroup made conclusions somewhat suspect [23]. In CHARM, candesartan was prescribed for patients with ejection fractions under 40%. A 17.5 % relative risk reduction in cardiovascular death and CHF admissions was seen when this angiotensin receptor blocker was used as a substitute for ACE inhibitors [24] (Fig. 4), and a 10% relative risk reduction was seen as add on therapy to ACE inhibitors. In this study, significant improvement in outcome and no increased mortality was seen when this angiotensin receptor blocker was used as add on therapy to patients taking both ACE inhibitors and beta-blockers [25], contradicting the results of ValHeft.

In conclusion, angiotensin receptor blockers are a logical and appropriate choice for patients who cannot be maintained on ACE inhibitors because of side effects such as cough. Patients with angioneurotic edema during ACE inhibitor therapy can often be treated with ARBs without developing this complication [26, 27]. Adding angiotensin receptor blocker therapy onto ACE inhibitors and beta-blockers likely achieves a small additional benefit.

Aldosterone Antagonists

These drugs work to counteract the salt and water retention caused by aldosterone. In addition, this hormone is felt to be involved in the progressive myocardial fibrosis that occurs in the remodeling process. In the RALES trial, the aldosterone antagonist spironolactone was given to patients with Class III–IV heart failure with ejections fractions less than 35%. A relative 24% reduction in mortality was seen in treated patients over two years, with reduced cardiovascular death and reduced need for rehospitalization [28]. In the EPHESUS trial, the aldosterone antagonist eplerenone was used in post-myocardial infarction patients who were diabetic or who showed evidence for heart failure with ejection fractions under 40%. Again, an impressive, statistically significant relative risk reduction of 42% for cardiovascular mortality was seen in patients treated with eplerenone in a mean follow up of 16 months [29]. Thus, the use of these agents is effective at improving outcomes in patients with functional Class III–IV heart failure. These medications are contraindicated in patients with renal insufficiency and creatinine levels over 2.5 mg%, or in patients with baseline potassium levels greater than 5.0 mmol/l.

Other Agents

Digoxin works by inhibiting the myocyte sodium/potassium pump, leading to increased intracellular calcium levels and increased inotropy. However, digoxin is a relatively weak inotropic agent. In addition, it has vagotonic effects. The use of digoxin in heart failure has been studied in large numbers of patients. A decreased need for rehospitalizaiton for heart failure was seen with this therapy, but there was no improvement in mortality [30]. Therefore, digoxin is indicated only for patients with symptomatic heart failure [1]. It is also useful in heart failure patients with chronic atrial fibrillation to help control the ventricular rate. Digoxin is not useful in the setting of acute heart failure.

Combination therapy with the vasodilators hydralazine and isosorbide dinitrate was associated with mortality improvement when compared to placebo in one study done in the era prior to the advent of ACE inhibitor or beta-blocker therapy for heart failure [31]. This combination of medications is indicated for patients who unable to tolerate either ACE inhibitors or angiotensin receptor blockers due to the presence of significant renal insufficiency or hyperkalemia [1].

▌ Treatment of Acute/Severe Heart Failure

Patients requiring hospitalization for acute or severe heart failure can be classified into three groups. The first group includes patients presenting in acute heart failure, generally without a history of chronic CHF, who often present in pulmonary edema. Most common etiologies in this group are AMI and acute coronary ischemia. Acute anterior wall infarction can involve a large area of myocardium leading to acute pulmonary edema and low cardiac output. Acute inferior wall myocardial infarction can be associated with right ventricular (RV) infarction with resultant heart failure and low cardiac output. Acute ischemia can cause acutely 'stunned' poorly functioning myocardium without necrosis, which can also result in acute heart failure. Mechanical complications of infarction, such as acute mitral regurgitation due to papillary muscle infarction or ventricular septal rupture also result in acute heart failure.

Relief of coronary ischemia and reperfusion of ischemic/infarcted myocardium is the mainstay of therapy in heart failure due to acute coronary ischemic syndromes or myocardial infarction. Urgent initiation of nitrates for coronary vasodilation (in the absence of hypotension), and anti-thrombotic and antiplatelet therapy is necessary. Parenteral beta-blockers are useful to lower blood pressure and reduce myocardial oxygen demand. However, reperfusion strategies utilizing thrombolytic therapy or urgent coronary angiography and revascularization are usually necessary in addition to medical therapy for optimal outcomes. Urgent cardiac surgery is indicated to repair lesions responsible for acute severe mitral regurgitation or ventricular septal rupture.

The prognosis of patients presenting with cardiogenic shock and LV failure due to AMI remains poor. In addition to vasopressors and inotropic agents (see below), intra-aortic balloon counterpulsation (IABP) is used early to improve the markedly abnormal hemodynamic state. IABP reduces afterload, increases cardiac output, increases coronary perfusion pressure and coronary blood flow without increasing myocardial oxygen demand. However, the use of IABP has only conferred survival benefit in these patients when combined with a strategy of emergency revascularization with percutaneous coronary intervention or coronary artery bypass surgery [7]. IABP is not useful for patients with chronic CHF. It is contraindicated in patients with aortic valve insufficiency or aortic dissection.

Other causes of acute severe heart failure include hypertensive crisis and acute severe valvular regurgitation. The latter syndrome often is due to acute rupture of chordae tendineae in the setting of myxomatous mitral valve degeneration and mitral valve prolapse. Infective endocarditis is another potential etiology. Afterload reduction with intravenous diuretics and parenteral vasodilators is very useful in these conditions. However, urgent cardiac surgery and valve replacement is usually needed for patients with acute valve regurgitation and heart failure.

A second group of patients hospitalized with severe heart failure are those suffering an acute exacerbation in the setting of chronic CHF. Potential causes of heart failure exacerbation are listed earlier in this chapter (Table 1). However, in one study, no specific precipitators were identified in 40% of hospitalized patients [8]. Factors which predict more likely need for hospital treatment include symptoms of heart failure of more than 18 months duration, heart failure due to ischemic heart disease, the presence of atrial fibrillation, lower functional class, and the presence of tachycardia or hypotension [8]. In studies evaluating inpatient medical therapy of CHF, the majority of patients were male, had previous myocardial infarction, were hypertensive and diabetic, and had a mean ejection fraction of 24% [32]. One-third of these patients were in atrial fibrillation.

Lastly, a group of patients are admitted with refractory or end stage heart failure. These patients are very ill and have a very poor prognosis. Cardiac transplantation is a viable option for some of these patients. For the majority, however, therapy is aimed primarily at palliation of symptoms rather than prolongation of life.

▌ Pharmacologic Therapy for Severe Heart Failure

Loop Diuretics

Although no randomized clinical trials exist, the use of furosemide or other loop diuretics is supported by a long history of clinical success [33]. The action of i.v. bolus furosemide begins at 30 minutes and peaks at 1–2 hours. The half-life is six hours, so twice daily dosing is usually required [8]. Patients with chronic heart failure or associated chronic renal insufficiency may exhibit resistance to oral or intravenous bolus furosemide. In these conditions, there is delayed oral absorption and less amount of drug is delivered to the renal tubules, and there is reduced responsiveness to the drug's diuretic effect causing this resistance. Constant delivery of diuretic with i.v. infusions over eight hours has been shown to result in superior diuresis and natriuresis when compared to bolus i.v. administration [34]. A low incidence of ototoxicity side effects was seen. Also, diuretics which act distally in the renal tubule, such as metolazone, or aldosterone blockers such as spironolactone can be added. Hypokalemia and hypomagnesemia are frequent side effects of loop diuretics and can potentiate the occurrence of arrhythmias. Electrolyte levels must be carefully monitored during aggressive diuretic therapy.

These agents often will worsen renal function due to alterations in renal hemodynamics. However, some degree of azotemia often needs to be accepted to obtain adequate relief of dyspnea and edema.

Vasodilators

Nitroglycerin. Intravenous nitroglycerin is an effective venodilator and coronary vasodilator. It is very useful in heart failure due to acute coronary ischemia as it improves coronary blood flow. Intravenous nitroglycerin at doses beginning at 5 µg/min is effective in lowering preload and lowering PAOP, but it reduces afterload less effectively than nitroprusside. A major limitation of the use of intravenous nitroglycerin is the rapid development of tolerance to the drug's effect, often occurring after 24 hours of therapy. Thus having a "nitrate free" period during the daily dosage regimen is often required. Nitrates are often added to chronic heart failure therapy with beta-blockers and ACE inhibitors if blood pressure allows.

Nitroprusside. Intravenous sodium nitroprusside is a powerful venous and arterial dilator. It is a drug of choice in treating hypertension related heart failure and pulmonary edema. A significant reduction of afterload and preload leads to decreased right atrial pressure, decreased systemic vascular resistance (SVR), decreased mean systemic blood pressure, decreased PAOP, and increased cardiac index in patients with heart failure and LV dysfunction. Limitations of nitroprusside use include inducing a coronary 'steal' syndrome in patients with active coronary ischemia [8]. In addition, toxic metabolites can accumulate with more prolonged administration. In patients with significant hepatic dysfunction, thiocyanate levels rise, and in patients with renal dysfunction, cyanide is generated.

Enalaprilat

The ACE inhibitor enalaprilat is an i.v. bolus formulation which can be used in patients with chronic CHF on chronic oral ACE inhibitor therapy who are unable to take oral medications. The maximal action occurs in 1-4 hours after administration, with a six-hour duration of action.

Inotropes, Inodilators, and Vasopressors

Dobutamine. Dobutamine is a potent β_1 agonist. It also has β_2- and α-agonist properties. Its major effect is increased myocardial contractility. It also has venodilator properties. At doses of 2.5–15 µg/kg/min, dobutamine will lower SVR and pulmonary capillary wedge pressure. Dobutamine causes a slight rise in heart rate and will lead to increased cardiac output.

A limitation of dobutamine use is that in patients with heart failure, β-receptors may be chronically downregulated, thus limiting its hemodynamic effects. In addition, dobutamine leads to increased myocardial oxygen demand and oxygen consumption, and this can be detrimental in patients with ischemia. Increases in ventricular arrhythmia have been associated with dobutamine use [35]. In addition, tolerance to dobutamine effects have been demonstrated in patients with infusions lasting over 72 hours, theoretically due to induction of β-receptor down-regulation [36].

Milrinone. Milrinone is an inhibitor of phosphodiesterase, which leads to increased intracellular cyclic AMP and calcium. It is thus an inotropic agent which acts 'downstream' from the receptor. Hemodynamic effects include reduction of mean right atrial pressure, and reduction in pulmonary and systemic vascular resistances. In heart failure, stroke volume and cardiac output are increased with a slight fall in mean systemic arterial pressure [32, 37]. Milrinone acts as a coronary vasodilator, and there is no net increase in myocardial oxygen consumption. Arterial blood pressure and PAOP tend to be lowered more so than with dobutamine, and milrinone's action is more prolonged. There is no tolerance or attenuation of its effects. Milrinone is started as a bolus dose, 50–75 µg/kg, with a maintenance infusion recommended at 0.375–0.75 µg/kg/min. Doses need to be reduced in patients with renal failure.

Dopamine. Dopamine effects include increasing renal blood flow at low doses (1–5 µg/kg/min), increasing myocardial contractility and chronotropy (3–7 µg/kg/min) and vasoconstriction (5–20 µg/kg/min) [38]. Dobutamine is a less useful agent for treatment of heart failure because its effects result in tachycardia, coronary vasoconstriction, increased afterload, and increased oxygen consumption. Dobutamine generally will lead to a greater rise in cardiac output than dopamine. Dopamine can be used when significant hypotension is part of the hemodynamic picture. Although dopamine at low doses is frequently used as add on therapy to inotropic agents in an attempt to increase renal blood flow and augment diuresis, no controlled trials have demonstrated dopamine's usefulness in this setting. No significant benefit of 'renal dose dopamine' has been shown in preventing acute renal failure in high risk patients or in the treatment of established renal failure [36].

Norepinephrine. Norepinephrine is a sympathomimetic agent with strong α-agonist and weak β-agonist effects. In patients with heart failure, norepinephrine's main effect is to raise blood pressure by increasing SVR, with little effect on cardiac output. It will increase myocardial oxygen demand. Its use in the setting of heart failure is restricted to patients with the most severe hypotension unresponsive to dopamine or in patients with complicating illnesses such as sepsis [36, 39].

B-natriuretic Peptide

B-natriuretic peptide (neseritide) is a hormone produced by ventricular and atrial myocytes in response to stretch from chamber dilatation. It is a counter regulatory peptide to the renin-angiotensin hormones, and it causes both venous and arterial dilation, natriuresis, and diuresis. Hemodynamic effects include rapid reduction in PAOP and mean right atrial pressure, exceeding the effects of intravenous nitroglycerin when compared directly [32]. Unlike sympathomimetic drugs, it is not proarrhythmic and does not induce tolerance. It can potentiate the effects of loop diuretics. However, some patients do not respond to neseritide. Significant hypotension may limit its use in some patients [8].

▌ Clinical Considerations in Treatment of Patients with Exacerbations of CHF

Pulmonary Artery Catheterization and Tailoring Therapy to Hemodynamic Measurements

Goals of therapy in treating acute or severe heart failure are similar to treating chronic heart failure, including relieving dyspnea, maximizing improvements in hemodynamic status, and preserving renal function. Therapies should ideally not increase the risk of ischemia, myocyte necrosis and arrhythmia. Treatments should also decrease the need for repeat hospitalization.

Careful serial clinical assessments are useful in guiding pharmacologic therapy. Important signs to note and follow include JVP, the presence of an S_3 gallop, daily weights, pulmonary examination, urine output, and pulse oximetry. Serial chest x-rays, measurements of renal function and electrolytes, electrocardiogram (EKG) signs of ischemia, and natriuretic peptide serum levels can also be useful. However, it is also important to note that findings on physical examination are often insensitive indicators of hemodynamic status. Pulmonary artery catheterization, while controversial as a routine management tool, is often helpful and necessary to determine precise baseline measurements of cardiac output and PAOP as well as to help guide intensive i.v. drug therapy. Although pulmonary artery pressure monitoring has not been shown to improve prognosis in patients with heart failure, significant adverse effects have also not been demonstrated in these patients. When patients present with recurrent or refractory heart failure, renal failure, the syndrome of diminished cardiac output with pulmonary edema, or severe heart failure complicating myocardial infarction, pulmonary artery pressure monitoring is mandated.

Aggressive therapy with parenteral vasodilators and diuretics tailored to an early response in hemodynamic measurements obtained by bedside pulmonary artery catheter (PAC) monitoring has been advocated as an effective method to obtain more rapid and sustained improvement in patients with acute severe heart failure [9, 40]. Specific hemodynamic goals include reducing PAOP to less than 16 mmHg, reducing mean right atrial pressure to less than 8 mmHg, reducing SVR to less than 1200 dynes-sec-cm^{-5}, with improvement of cardiac index to over 2.6 l/min/m^2, and maintaining systolic blood pressure over 80 mmHg. PAOP can be lowered to a normal value of 10–12 mmHg in many patients with significant LV dysfunction without untoward effects [9, 41].

Improvement in hemodynamics has been obtained with aggressive intravenous vasodilator therapy using intravenous nitroprusside, intravenous nitroglycerin, or neseritide. The choice of agents depends on matching the specific hemodynamics and clinical picture of the patient's presentation with the predicted effects of each vasodilator (Table 2) [32, 37, 42, 43].

Consecutive patients with severe heart failure were evaluated and classified according to hemodynamic measurements, PAOP, and cardiac index [44]. Patients were described as 'dry' with an average PAOP of 17 mmHg or 'wet' with an average reading of 29 mmHg. Patients were described as 'warm' with an average cardiac in-

Table 2. A comparison of hemodynamic effects of parenteral vasodilators and inotropic agents

	Nitroprusside	Neseritide	Dobutamine	Milrinone
▌Mechanism of Action	balanced vasodilator	vasodilator, natriuretic	beta-1 stimulator	phospho diesterase inhibitor
▌Heart Rate	--	--	slight ↑	slight ↑
▌Arrhythmia	--	--	+	+
▌Mean RA Pressure	↓	↓	↓	↓↓
▌LVEDP	↓↓	↓↓	↓	↓↓
▌Mean Arterial Pressure	↓	↓	–	↓
▌SVR	↓↓	↓↓	↓↓	↓↓
▌C.I.	↑	↑	↑↑	↑↑
▌dp/dt (inotropy)	--	--	↑↑	↑
▌Hypotension	+	+	--	+
▌Direct Na+ Excretion	--	+	--	--
▌Other considerations:	increased cyanide and thiocyanate levels with prolonged infusion	cannot follow serum BNP level during infusion		more vasodilator response at higher doses

Key: – minimal or no effect, + positive effect, ↑ or ↓ mild increase or decrease, ↑↑ or ↓↓ moderate increase or decrease

dex of 2.1 l/min/m^2, or 'cold' with cardiac index averaging 1.6 l/min/m^2. Thus, patients were divided as either being 'wet/warm', 'wet/cold', 'dry/warm', or 'dry/cold'. Importantly, the severity of symptoms and findings on physical examination did not predict the hemodynamic status [44]. Also, the hemodynamic picture did not predict the response to therapy and survival was similar in all four groups, although the 'dry/warm' patients had slightly better outcomes than the 'wet/cold' patients.

Use of Inotropic Agents

In patients with persistent or problematic hypotension or low cardiac index, treatment with inotropic agents or vasopressors can be added. Dobutamine and milrinone are the most commonly used agents. Again, the choice of agents depends on the specific clinical circumstances. Dobutamine tends to cause a slight rise in heart rate and has little effect on mean arterial pressure (MAP), whereas milrinone often causes low MAP due to more prominent lowering of SVR [42, 43]. Patients who do not respond to dobutamine may have a favorable response to milrinone. Milrinone is being used now more often than dobutamine in view of its more potent vasodilator properties. In addition, its effects are not primarily mediated through β-receptors, which is an important consideration in patients receiving concomitant beta-blocker therapy.

Several studies have compared vasodilator and inotropic therapy or milrinone with placebo. The use of intravenous inotropic therapy in the form of a 48-hour infusion of milrinone has been evaluated for routine therapy in patients admitted with Class III–IV heart failure when inotropic therapy was not felt to be essential [45]. When compared with standard therapy without milrinone, no improvement in symptom relief, hospital length of stay, or re-hospitalization rate within 60 days was demonstrated. In fact, milrinone therapy was associated with an increased risk of hypotension and atrial arrhythmias. Thus, milrinone and other inotropic agents are not recommended for routine use in patients with decompensated heart failure.

Neseritide has been compared to dobutamine in patients with severe heart failure. Neseritide infusion was associated with less tachycardia and ventricular arrhythmia [35]. In another study, there was a trend toward improved survival with neseritide [46], and mortality and re-hospitalization rates at six months were lower with neseritide [47]. In the FIRST study of Class III and IV heart failure patients, a 14-day average dobutamine infusion was associated with an increased risk of morbid events and higher short-term death rates. In patients listed for transplant with baseline systolic blood pressures under 100 mmHg and ejection fractions under 20%, 12 hour per day infusions of dobutamine and nitroprusside given over an average of 20 days were compared, showing better relief of symptoms and increased survival favoring nitroprusside [48]. A study of oral milrinone in Class IV heart failure patients was associated with a 53% increased risk of mortality when compared with placebo [49]. No clinical studies have shown improved short-term or medium term outcomes with inotropic therapy. In fact, the use of inotropic agents has been associated with a worse prognosis for survival [8]. The negative effects of inotropic agents are believed to be related to their property to stimulate sympathetic nervous system activation with increased myocardial oxygen demand, increasing serious cardiac arrhythmias, myocardial ischemia, and further myocyte loss. Stimulation of chronic hibernating myocardium may result in necrosis of tissue. Thus, the use of inotropic agents is not routine and is now restricted to short-term therapy (i.e., less than 72 hours) in patients with severe heart failure and problematic hypotension or critical hypoperfusion. Clinical examples where inotropic agents may be useful include cardiogenic shock due to AMI or RV myocardial infarction (until revascularization can be achieved), in patients awaiting cardiac transplantation, or patients with end stage heart failure (see below).

Conversion to Oral Medications

Once hemodynamics have been improved and are at, or near, goal, oral therapy can be added and parenteral medications weaned [9]. ACE inhibitors are added, or doses maximized in patients already taking this medicine. Nitrates can be added to maintain lower PAOP, if blood pressure allows. Low doses of beta-blockers are added when the patient is determined to be stable and euvolemic. Beta-blocker doses are then titrated up over 6–8 weeks to maximal tolerated doses. The use of milrinone has been suggested as a 'bridge to beta-blocker therapy'. Improvement in hemodynamics seen in the hospital with this strategy can very often be maintained with long-term outpatient oral therapy. A combination of aggressive parenteral therapy, targeted to optimal hemodynamics, followed by conversion to oral therapy utilized in patients referred for listing for cardiac transplantation has resulted in improvement, so that 30% of patients were able to be removed from the transplant listing [9].

Patients with Refractory or End Stage CHF

As patients with heart failure survive longer due to improved medical therapy and improved treatment of ischemic heart disease (IHD), and as the incidence of sudden cardiac death decreases with the more wide-spread use of internal cardioverter defibrillators (see below), the number of patients developing truly end stage or refractory heart failure is expected to increase [50]. Some patients may indeed become 'dependent' on i.v. inotropic infusions because of unacceptable symptomatic hypotension. Current ACC/AHA guidelines for evaluation and management of chronic heart failure indicate that long-term intermittent infusion of a positive inotropic drug as standard therapy for symptomatic systolic dysfunction is contraindicated [1]. However, continuous i.v. infusion of an inotrope can be recommended for palliation of symptoms in patients with refractory end stage heart failure. In this setting, quality of remaining life takes precedence over prolonging life. These patients will have been deemed poor candidates for biventricular pacing, cardiac transplantation, or ventricular assist devices (see below). The decision to use inotropic agents in this circumstance is one that should be carefully individualized.

▌ Myocarditis

Myocarditis, defined as inflammation of heart muscle, is a cause of acute heart failure. Myocarditis can eventually lead to dilated cardiomyopathy with chronic heart failure. A large body of experimental animal data indicates that viral myocarditis resulting in activation of immune mechanisms can result in chronic dilated cardiomyopathy [51]. Some patients with idiopathic dilated cardiomyopathy have biopsy evidence of myocardial inflammation. Thus, many patients diagnosed with idiopathic dilated cardiomyopathy may have had unrecognized myocarditis leading to their chronic heart failure.

Patients with myocarditis can have no or very mild symptoms and the illness can be unrecognized and resolve spontaneously [51]. However, several studies reporting autopsies from younger patients who have experienced unexpected sudden death have shown myocarditis in a significant number of these cases [52]. Another group of patients with myocarditis will develop significant LV dysfunction with the clinical heart failure syndrome. In a minority of cases, myocarditis can present with fulminant heart failure and cardiogenic shock with a high mortality rate [51].

An infectious etiology of myocarditis is common. Viral agents such as enterovirus, adenovirus, and human immunodeficiency virus (HIV) have been implicated as causative agents by serologic data as well as by examination of cardiac cell genomes. The protozoa *Trypanosoma cruzi* is the etiologic agent in Chagas' disease, a form of myocarditis, endemic in Central and South America, that can lead to chronic heart failure. Immune mechanisms are pathogenetic in the myocarditis due to giant cell arteritis, and the myocarditis associated with progressive systemic sclerosis, systemic lupus erythematosis, and polymyositis [52].

Myocarditis is a diagnosis made on clinical grounds and should be suspected in patients who present with new onset heart failure, with or without antecedent flu-like symptoms. Elevated leukocyte count, elevated sedimentation rate, elevated creatinine kinase levels and serum troponin levels and EKG changes suggestive of myocardial ischemia or infarction may be seen, but are often not present. Endomyocardial biopsy has been advocated to aid in the diagnosis of myocarditis. However, the

Dallas criteria, histologic findings of both inflammation and myocyte necrosis in biopsy specimens, have been very insensitive in making the diagnosis and have a high degree of inter-observer variability. In patients suspected of having myocarditis on clinical grounds, only 10–67% of patients have had positive biopsies in reported series [51, 52].

Pharmacologic management of the heart failure due to myocarditis is similar to the management of heart failure from other causes. Diuretics, ACE inhibitors, and beta-blockers are useful. Many patients will experience significant improvement in LV function during the first six months after diagnosis. Patients with acute fulminant heart failure may require intravenous vasodilator and inotropic therapy, and may be candidates for implantation of ventricular assist devices as a bridge to recovery. A number of reported cases of fulminant myocarditis have required mechanical cardiac assistance and then recovered fully to normal ventricular function. Consideration of cardiac transplantation may be necessary for patients who do not improve.

Immunosuppressive therapy for myocarditis has been tried with limited success. Several placebo controlled trials of therapy with prednisone with or without cyclosporine or azathioprine or immune globulin have shown modest improvement in LV ejection fractions with therapy, but without improvement in mortality or rehospitalizations for heart failure [51]. One study defined patients as having heart failure of over six months duration and inappropriate expression of HLA antigens on myocardial biopsy. Therapy with prednisone and azathioprine resulted in significant improvement in LV ejection fraction and clinical functional class at two years, but without differences in mortality, transplantation rate, or rehospitalization rate [53]. Immunosuppressive therapy should be reserved for patients who present with persistent or worsening active immune mediated myocardial damage with ventricular dysfunction.

▌ Arrhythmia Management and Device Therapy

Sudden death, due to presumed sustained ventricular arrhythmia, is a frequent occurrence in heart failure patients, especially in patients with cardiomyopathy due to coronary artery disease. It is estimated that 30% of patients with heart failure and ejection fractions under 30% die suddenly. Prophylactic antiarrhythmic drug therapy aimed at reducing this incidence has been evaluated. In the CAST trial, patients with coronary artery disease, a history of myocardial infarction, and frequent premature ventricular contractions on baseline holter monitoring had an increased mortality when treated with the Class IC antiarrhythmics encainide or flecainide [54], despite good suppression in frequency of arrhythmia on follow up Holter monitoring. This adverse effect on mortality is presumed due to the known potential for these drugs to worsen arrhythmia ('proarrhythmia') in many of these patients. Therefore, type IA and type IC antiarrhythmic drugs should be used with great caution in patients with heart failure and coronary artery disease, when benefits of therapy outweigh potential risks, and when other agents have failed.

Amiodarone was then tried as primary prevention of sudden death, as the proarrhythmic effect of this medication is much less frequent than with type I antiarrhythmics. Six hundred and seventy-five patients with ejection fractions under 40% and heart failure were randomized to treatment with amiodarone or placebo, with no survival difference between the two groups at 45 months [55]. However, there was a trend toward reducing mortality with amiodarone in patients with nonischemic cardiomyopathy. In another study, 1,486 post-myocardial infarction patients with ejection fractions under 40% were randomized to amiodarone or placebo with no difference in mortality at 21 months, although there was a suggestion of a reduction in deaths due to arrhythmia [56]. Unlike the CAST trial, there was no observed increased risk of death with amiodarone. Thus, this medication is considered safe and can be used in heart failure patients with supraventricular arrhythmias.

The use of implanted cardioverter defibrillator therapy was compared to antiarrhythmic drugs as secondary prevention of sudden cardiac death in patients who had been resuscitated from cardiac arrest or who survived ventricular tachycardia associated with syncope. In AVID, 1016 of these patients who also had ejection fractions under 40% were randomized to receive implanted cardioverter defibrillators or antiarrhythmic drugs (over 90% of these patients received amiodarone). There was a statistically improved survival with implanted cardioverter defibrillator therapy at 1, 2, and 3 years of follow up [57]. In two other studies of similar patients, a non-significant reduction in all cause mortality and arrhythmic death was seen with implanted cardioverter defibrillators when compared to amiodarone [58, 59], and increased mortality was seen with propafenone therapy (a Class IC antiarrhythmic) [59]. Taken together, these studies have established implanted cardioverter defibrillators as first line therapy in preference to antiarrhythmic drugs in coronary artery disease/heart failure patients surviving cardiac arrest or surviving an episode of sustained ventricular tachycardia.

The effects of implanted cardioverter defibrillator therapy on mortality have more recently been evaluated as primary prevention of arrhythmic death in patients with coronary heart disease, previous myocardial infarction, and LV dysfunction without symptomatic clinical arrhythmia. In MADIT I, post-myocardial infarction patients with ejection fractions less than 35% and non-sustained ventricular tachycardia on monitoring without symptomatic episodes, were studied with electrophysiologic testing and programmed stimulation. Patients were enrolled in this study if they had inducible ventricular tachycardia not suppressed with antiarrhythmic therapy. At two years of follow up, total mortality was significantly reduced from 39% in the medically treated group (standard medical therapy with or without amiodarone) to 15% in the implanted cardioverter defibrillator group [60]. In the MUSTT study, a similar cohort of patients showed an improvement in mortality from 55% in patients treated with medication to 24% in patients treated with implanted cardioverter defibrillators at five years [61]. Lastly, in MADIT II, the patient population was extended to include patients with a history of myocardial infarction and ejection fraction of less than 30%. Importantly, in this study, neither ventricular arrhythmias seen on cardiac monitoring nor electrophysiologic study was necessary for inclusion. A statistically significant improvement in total mortality was seen in patients treated with implanted cardioverter defibrillators from 19.8 to 14.2% at four years [62]. It should be noted that Class IV heart failure patients were not included in any of these studies (Fig. 5).

Thus, the approved use of implanted cardioverter defibrillator therapy for prevention of sudden cardiac death has been extended as prophylactic primary prevention therapy in patients with ischemic cardiomyopathy and inducible ventricular tachycardia on electrophysiologic study, and in patients with low ejection fractions (less than 30%) and prolonged QRS duration on EKG without any electrophysiologic testing criteria. Approved indications for implanted cardioverter defibrillator

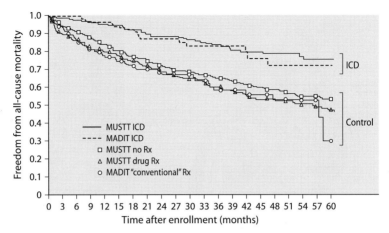

Fig. 5. Kaplan-Meier survival curves for all-cause mortality in MUSTT and MADIT. From [70] with permission

therapy as primary prevention of sudden arrhythmic cardiac death will likely be extended in the future to a broader patient population with heart failure. The usefulness of implanted cardioverter defibrillator therapy in the treatment of patients with non-ischemic cardiomyopathy however is still uncertain.

▌ Resynchronization Therapy

In many patients with heart failure, the contraction of the intraventricular septum and LV free wall lacks normal coordination, and is termed dyssynchronous. This often coexists with conduction system disease in the His-Purkinje system, with marked QRS prolongation seen on EKG [63]. In fact, left bundle branch block (LBBB) pattern with long QRS duration is associated with an increase in all cause mortality in heart failure patients. Pacemaker therapies have been developed to correct this LV dyssynchrony, involving timed pacing of both left and right ventricles. This is termed biventricular pacing or resynchronization therapy. Standard dual chamber transvenous leads are placed in the right atrium (in the absence of chronic atrial fibrillation) and right ventricle. The LV free wall is paced via an electrode passed through the coronary sinus into an epicardial lateral cardiac vein. Alternatively, an epicardial LV lead can be placed via thoracoscopy. The pacemaker is programmed to coordinate timing of atrial stimulation with ventricular stimulation, and septal stimulation via the right ventricle with left ventricular lateral wall stimulation [63] (Fig. 6).

In the MIRACLE trial, 453 patients with ejection fractions under 35% and Class III–IV heart failure and QRS duration greater than 130 msec were treated with resynchronization therapy or standard medical therapy. At six months of follow up, biventricular pacing patients showed a statistically significant improvement in six minute walking distance, quality of life score, and New York Heart Association functional class, with fewer hospitalizations for recurrent heart failure [63]. No significant mortality improvement was noted in this relatively short follow up. There was an 8% rate of unsuccessful LV lead placement, and a 1.2% incidence of serious

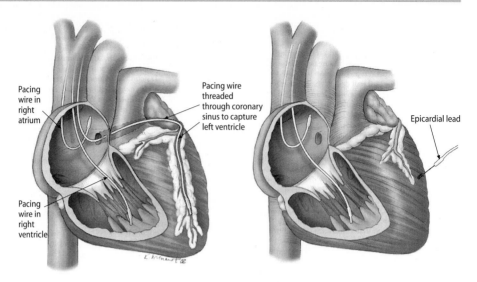

Fig. 6. Schematic to show placement of pacing wires in biventricular pacing (left panel). Lack of coronary sinus venous branch necessitates epicardial placement of third lead via minimally invasive surgical procedure (right panel)

complications of implantation of the pacemaker device, including coronary sinus dissection or perforation. A meta analysis of three major resynchronization trials concluded that a statistically significant 51% reduction in death from progressive heart failure was associated with chronic resynchronization therapy in 1634 patients [64].

▌ Combination Devices

Most recently, devices containing biventricular pacing and implanted cardioverter defibrillator therapy have been evaluated in patients with heart failure. These devices are used to attempt to decrease morbidity and mortality associated with progressive heart failure as well as decrease mortality associated with sudden serious ventricular arrhythmia. Initial reports indicate biventricular pacing does not interfere with appropriate implanted cardioverter defibrillator detection and termination of ventricular arrhythmias [65]. The COMPANION trial enrolled 1634 patients with ejection fractions under 35%, Class III and IV heart failure, and QRS duration greater than 120 msec and normal sinus rhythm with PR interval greater than 150 msec [66]. These patients were randomized to receive medical therapy alone versus medical therapy combined with biventricular pacing and medical therapy combined with biventricular pacing and implanted cardioverter defibrillator therapy. In these three groups, 16-month mortality was significantly improved from 19 to 15% with biventricular pacing alone, and further to 11% with combined resynchronization and implanted cardioverter defibrillator therapy. A 20% relative improvement in all cause mortality plus all cause hospitalization was also noted in both treatment groups [66].

Thus, it can be seen that newer combination biventricular pacemaker/defibrillator therapy will have an important role in providing both symptomatic as well as life extending benefits in patients with heart failure.

Ventricular Assist Devices

It is estimated that approximately 60 000 patients annually are affected with end-stage heart failure and could benefit from cardiac transplantation. However, the pool of donor hearts is currently only approximately 3000 per year and is not increasing. In addition, a mortality rate of 30% has been reported in patients listed for and awaiting heart transplantation [36]. Thus, there is a role for mechanical ventricular assist devices as treatment for patients with the most severe heart failure. These devices are mechanical pumps which take over the function of the failing ventricle. They provide normal hemodynamics, cardiac output, and flow to vital organs [67]. Ventricular assist devices can thus be used as a 'bridge' to transplantation or to recovery of LV function. Their use has also been advocated as chronic, stand-alone 'destination' therapy.

Ventricular assist devices are most often used as univentricular devices, but have been biventricular in 10–20% of cases. With improved technology, pumps have been made smaller. They are inserted via a mid-line sternotomy, with the inflow conduit inserted at the LV apex. The outflow conduit is inserted in the ascending aorta. The pump is small enough to be implanted in the abdominal wall and is connected to an external power pack via a driveline through the skin. The power pack is small enough to be wearable, so patients have freedom of movement and can participate in rehabilitation efforts. Current devices have textured blood contacting surfaces so anticoagulation therapy is not required [68] (Figs. 7 and 8).

Patients selected for LV assist devices have end-stage heart failure with persistent hypotension or cardiogenic shock. Life expectancy for these patients is estimated to be less than four months [67]. Contraindications for placing these devices include irreversible end-organ damage, severe chronic obstructive pulmonary disease (COPD), need for hemodialysis, or uncorrected coagulopathy. Immediate complications of device placement include bleeding, air embolization, end-organ failure, and LV failure. The latter is often due to severe pulmonary hypertension, which can be treated with inhaled nitric oxide administration. Longer term complications include sepsis, thromboembolic complications, and device failure.

In patients awaiting transplantation, LV assist devices are associated with a 91% rate of improvement with recovery to hospital discharge, and a 74% rate of survival to transplantation. As destination therapy, patients have survived with these devices for over two years. There have been case reports of significant improvement in LV function during LV assist device therapy, such that the LV assist device was removed after a period of 160–790 days, with long-term survival thereafter without the need for transplantation [69]. Thus, some left ventricles with end stage systolic dysfunction may actually show significant improvement in function and improvement in histologic abnormalities after long-term unloading by ventriclar assista devices [69].

The REMATCH trial compared LV assist devices as destination therapy with standard medical therapy in 129 patients with Class IV heart failure, ejection fractions less than 25%, and initial dependence on intravenous inotropic therapy [5].

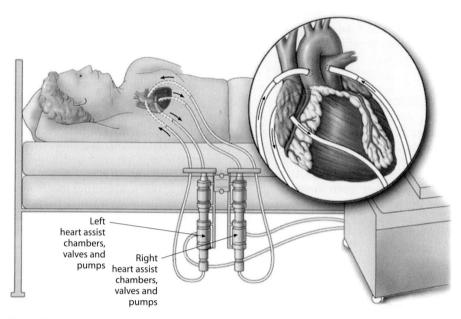

Fig. 7. Biventricular assist device. Blood is removed from the right atrium and injected into the pulmonary artery. Blood is removed from the left atrium and injected into the aorta. The Abiomed biventricular assist device has the ability to completely substitute for left and right heart function

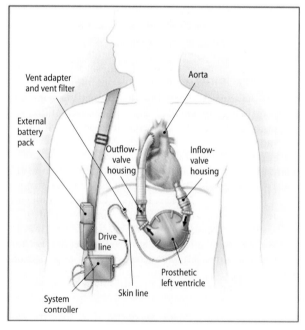

Fig. 8. Components of the left ventricular assist device. Modified from [5] with permission

This study showed improved survival and measured quality of life in patients treated with the LV assist device. Survival at one year was 52% with the LV assist device as compared with 25% with medical therapy, and two-year survival was 23% compared with 8% respectively. However, there was a significant 35% complication rate at two years with LV assist device therapy, most often due to infection, bleeding, and device malfunction. Causes of death in these patients were most often sepsis and device failure, not heart failure.

With refinements in design and technological improvements, long-term mechanical support of the failing left ventricle may be feasible for indefinite periods of time, especially if the incidence of infectious and thromboembolic complications can be reduced. Progress towards making these devices smaller and totally implantable will advance treatments toward the goal of a reliable artificial heart.

References

1. Hunt S, Baker D, Chin M, et al (2001) ACC/AHA Guidelines for the evaluation and management of chronic heart failure in the adult: Executive Summary. Circulation 104:2996–3007
2. Jessup M, Brozena S (2003) Heart failure. N Engl J Med 348:2007–2018
3. Wu A, Cody R (2003) Medical and surgical treatment of chronic heart failure. Curr Probl Cardiol 28:225–260
4. Packer M (2001) Current role of beta-adrenergic blockers in the management of chronic heart failure. Am J Med 110:81S–84S
5. Rose E, Gelijns A, Moskowitz A, et al (2001) Long-term use of a left ventricular assist device for end-stage heart failure. N Engl J Med 345:1435–1443
6. Chin M, Goldman L (1996) Correlates of major complications or death in patients admitted to the hospital with congestive heart failure. Arch Intern Med 156:1814–1820
7. Hochman J, Sleeper L, Webb J, et al (1999) Early revascularization in acute myocardial infarction complicated by cardiogenic shock. SHOCK Investigators. Should we emergently revascularize occluded coronaries for cardiogenic shock. N Engl J Med 341:625–634
8. Jain P, Massie B, Gattis W, et al (2003) Current medical treatment for the exacerbation of chronic heart failure resulting in hospitalization. Am Heart J 145:S3–S17
9. Steimle A, Stevenson L, Chelimsky-Fallick C, et al (1997) Sustained hemodynamic efficacy of therapy tailored to reduce filling pressures in survivors with advanced heart failure. Circulation 96:1165–1172
10. BHAT Trial Research Group (1982) A randomized trial of propranolol in patients with acute myocardial infarction. I. Mortality results. JAMA 747:1707–1714
11. BHAT Trial Research Group (1983) A randomized trial of propranolol in patients with acute myocardial infarction. II. Morbidity results. JAMA 250:2814–2819
12. CIBIS II Investigators (1999) The Cardiac Insufficiency Bisoprolol Study II: A randomized trial. Lancet 353:9–13
13. The MERIT-HF Study Group (2000) Effects of controlled release metoprolol on total mortality, hospitalizations and well-being in patients with heart failure. JAMA 283:1295–1302
14. The CAPRICORN Investigators (2001) Effect of carvedilol on outcome after myocardial infarction in patients with left ventricular dysfunction: The CAPRICORN Randomized Trial. Lancet 357:1385–1390
15. Packer M, Coats A, Fowler M, et al (2001) Effect of carvedilol on survival in severe chronic heart failure. N Engl J Med 344:1651–1658
16. Krum H, Roecker E, Mohacsi P, et al (2003) Effects on initiating carvedilol in patients with severe chronic heart failure. Results from the COPERNICUS Study. JAMA 289:712–718
17. Bristow M, Gilbert E, Abraham W, et al (1996) Carvedilol produces dose related improvements in left ventricular function and survival in subjects with chronic heart failure. Circulation 94:2807–2816
18. Pfeffer M, Braunwald E, Moye L, et al (1992) Effect of captopril on mortality and morbidity in patients with left ventricular dysfunction after myocardial infarction. N Engl J Med 327:669–677

19. The SOLVD Investigators (1992) Effect of enalapril on mortality and the development of heart failure in asymptomatic patients with reduced left ventricular ejection fractions. N Engl J Med 327:685–691

20. Garg R, Yusuf S (1995) Overview of randomized trials of angiotensin converting enzyme inhibitors on mortality and morbidity in patients with heart failure. JAMA 273:1450–1456

21. The RESOLVD Pilot Study Investigators (1999) Comparison of candesartan, enalapril, and their combination in congestive heart failure. Circulation 100:1056–1064

22. Pitt B, Poole-Wilson P, Segal R, et al (2000) Effect of losartan compared with captopril on mortality in patients with symptomatic heart failure: Randomized trial – The Losartan Heart Failure Survival Study (ELITE II). Lancet 355:1582–1587

23. Cohn J, Tognoni G (2001) A randomized trial of the angiotensin receptor blocker valsartan in chronic heart failure. N Engl J Med 345:1667–1675

24. Granger C, McMurray J, Yusuf S, et al (2003) Effects of candesartan patients with chronic heart failure and reduced left ventricular systolic function intolerant to angiotensin-converting enzyme inhibitors. The CHARM Alternate Trial. Lancet 362:772–776

25. McMurray J, Ostergren J, Swedberg K, et al (2003) Effects of candesartan in patients with chronic heart failure and reduced left ventricular systolic function taking angiotensin-converting enzyme inhibitors. The CHARM – Added Trial. Lancet 362:759–766

26. Manohair P, Pina I (2003) Therapeutic role of angiotensin II receptor blockers in the treatment of heart failure. Mayo Clinic Proc 78:334–338

27. Sharma D, Buyse M, Pitt B, et al (2000) Meta-Analysis of observed mortality data from all controlled double–blind multiple dose studies of losartan in heart failure. Am J Cardiol 85:187–192

28. Pitt B, Zannad F, Remme W, et al (1999) The effect of spironolactone on morbidity and mortality in patients with severe heart failure. N Engl J Med 341:709–717

29. Pitt B, Remme W, Zannad F, et al (2003) Eplerenone, a selective aldosterone blocker, in patients with left ventricular dysfunction after myocardial infarction. N Engl J Med 348:1309–1321

30. The Digitalis Investigation Group (1997) The effect of digoxin on mortality and morbidity in patients with heart failure. N Engl J Med 336:525–533

31. Cohn J, Archibald D, Ziesche S, et al (1986) Effect of vasodilator therapy on mortality in chronic congestive heart failure. Results of a Veteran's Administration Cooperative Study. N Engl J Med 314:1547–1552

32. Publication Committee for the VMAC Investigators (2002) Intravenous nesiritide versus nitroglycerin for treatment of decompensated congestive heart failure: A randomized controlled trial. JAMA 287:1531–1540

33. Poole-Wilson P (2002) Treatment of acute heart failure: Out with the old, in with the new. JAMA 287:1578–1580

34. Dormans T, Van-Meyel, J, Gerlag, P, et al (1996) Diuretic efficacy of high dose furosemide in severe heart failure: bolus injection versus continuous infusion. J Am Coll Cardiol 28:376–382.

35. Burger A, Horton D, LeGemtel T, et al (2002) Effect of neseritide (B-type natriuretic peptide) and dobutamine on ventricular arrhythmias in the treatment of patients with acutely decompensated congestive heart failure: The PRECEDENT Study. Am Heart J 144:1102–1108

36. Chattergee K, DeMarco T (2003) Role of nonglycosidic inotropic agents: Indications, ethics, and limitations. Med Clin N Am 87:391–418

37. Colucci W, Elkayam U, Horton D, et al (2002) Intravenous nesiritide, a natriuetic in the treatment of decompensated congestive heart failure. N Engl J Med 343:246–253

38. Leier C, Binkley P (1998) Parenteral inotropic support for advanced congestive heart failure. Prog Cardiovasc Dis 41:207–224

39. Stevenson L (2003) Clinical use of inotropic therapy for heart failure: Looking backward or forward? Part I: Inotropic infusions during hospitalization. Circulation 108:367–372

40. Stevenson L (1999) Tailored therapy for hemodynamic goals for advanced heart failure. Eur J Heart Fail 1:251–257

41. Stevenson L, Tillisch J (1986) Maintenance of cardiac output with normal filling pressures in patients with dilated heart failure. Circulation 74:1303–1308

42. Colucci W, Wright R, Jaski B, et al (1986) Milrinone and dobutamine in severe heart failure: Differing hemodynamic effects and individual patient responsiveness. Circulation 73:175–183

43. Jaski B, Fifer M, Wright R, et al (1985) Positive inotropic and vasodilator actions of milrinone in patients with severe congestive heart failure. J Clin Invest 75:643–649

44. Shah M, Hasselblad V, Stinnett S, et al (2001) Hemodynamic profiles of advanced heart failure: Association with clinical characteristics and long-term outcomes. J Card Fail 7:105–113

45. Cuffe M, Califf R, Adams K, et al (2002) Short-term intravenous milrinone for acute exacerbation of chronic heart failure: A randomized control trial. JAMA 287:1541–1547

46. Abraham W, Adams K, Fonarow G, et al (2003) Comparison of in-hospital mortality in patients treated with neseritide versus other parenteral vasoactive medications for acutely decompensated heart failure: An analysis from a large prospective registry database. J Card Fail 2003; 9:S81 (abst)

47. Silver M, Horton D, Ghali J, et al (2002) Effect of neseritide versus dobutamine on short-term outcomes in the treatment of patients with acute decompensated heart failure. J Am Coll Cardiol 39:798–803

48. O'Connor C, Gattis W, Uretsky B, et al (1999) Continuous intravenous dobutamine is associated with an increased risk of death in patients with advanced heart failure: Insights from the Flolan International Randomized Survival Trial (FIRST). Am Heart J 138:78–86

49. Packer M, Carver JR, Rodeheffer RJ, et al (1991) Effect of oral milrinone on mortality in severe chronic heart failure. The PROMISE Study Research Group. N Engl J Med 325:1468–1475

50. Stevenson L (2003) Clinical use of inotropic therapy for heart failure: Looking backward or forward? Part II: Chronic inotropic therapy. Circulation 108:492–497

51. Feldman A, McNamara D (2000) Myocarditis. N Engl J Med 19:1388–1398

52. Parrillo J (2001) Inflammatory cardiomyopathy (myocarditis) which patients should be treated with anti-inflammatory therapy. Circulation 104:4–6

53. Wojnicz R, Nowalany-Kozielska E, Wojciechowska C, et al (2001) Randomized, placebo-controlled study for immunosuppressive treatment of inflammatory dilated cardiomyopathy: two-year follow-up results. Circulation 104:39–45

54. The Cardiac Arrhythmia Suppression Trial Investigators (1989) Preliminary Report: Effect of encainide and flecainide on mortality in a randomized trial of arrhythmia suppression after myocardial infarction. N Engl J Med 321:406–412

55. Singh S, Fletcher R, Fisher S, et al (1995) Amiodarone in patients with congestive heart failure and asymptomatic ventricular arrhythmia. N Engl J Med 333:77–82

56. Julian D, Camm A, Frangin G, et al (1997) Randomized trial of effect of amiodarone on mortality in patients with left ventricular dysfunction after recent myocardial infarction: EMIAT. Lancet 349:667–674

57. The AVID Investigators (1997) A comparison of antiarrhythmic drug therapy with implantable defibrillators in patients resuscitated from near-fatal ventricular arrhythmias. N Engl J Med 337:1576–1583

58. Connolly S, Gent M, Roberts R, et al (2000) Canadian Implantable Defibrillator Study (CIDS): A randomized trial of the implantable cardioverter defibrillator against amiodarone. Circulation 101:1297–1302

59. Kuck K, Cappato R, Siebels J, et al (2000) Randomized comparison of antiarrhythmic drug therapy with implantable defibrillators in patients resuscitated from cardiac arrest: The Cardiac Arrest Study Hamburg (CASH). Circulation 102:748–754

60. MADIT Investigators (1995) Improved survival with an implanted defibrillator in patients with coronary disease at high risk for ventricular arrhythmia. N Engl J Med 335:1933–1940

61. Buxton A, Lee, K, Fisher J, et al (1999) A randomized study of the prevention of sudden death in patients with coronary artery disease. N Engl J Med 341:1882–1890

62. MADIT II Investigators (2001) Prophylactic implantation of a defibrillator in patients with myocardial infarction and reduced ejection fraction. N Engl J Med 346:877–883

63. Abraham W, Fisher W, Smith A, et al (2002) Cardiac resynchronization in chronic heart failure. N Engl J Med 346:1845–1853

64. Bradley D, Bradley E, Baughman K, et al (2003) Cardiac resynchronization and death from progressive heart failure. A meta analysis of randomized control trials. JAMA 289:730–740

65. Young J, Abraham W, Smith A, et al (2003) Combined cardiac resynchronization and implantable cardioversion defibrillation in advanced chronic heart failure. The MIRACLE ICD Trial. JAMA 289:2685–2694
66. Salukhe T, Francis D, Sutton R (2003) Comparison of medical therapy, pacing and defibrillation in heart failure (COMPANION) trial terminated early; combined biventricular pacemaker-defibrillators reduce all cause mortality and hospitalization. Int J Cardiol 87:119–120
67. Goldstein G, Oz M, Rose E (1998) Medical progress: Implantable left ventricular assist devices. N Engl J Med 339:1522–1533
68. Nemeh H, Smedira N (2003) Mechanical treatment of heart failure: The growing role of LVADs and artificial hearts. Cleve Clin J Med 70:223–234
69. Muller J, Wallukat G, Weng Y, et al (1997) Weaning from mechanical cardiac support in patients with idiopathic dilated cardiomyopathy. Circulation 96:542–549
70. Prystowsky E (2000) Screening and therapy for patients with nonsustained ventricular tachycardia. Am J Cardiol 86 (Suppl):34k–39k

Weaning-induced Cardiac Dysfunction

B. Lamia, X. Monnet, and J. L. Teboul

▌ Introduction

Mechanical ventilation can be beneficial for the cardiovascular system in patients suffering from left heart failure [1]. In this regard, mechanical ventilation is used routinely as a therapy for acute heart failure even using a non-invasive mode [2]. Conversely, the cardiovascular consequences of abrupt transfer from mechanical ventilation to spontaneous breathing could be responsible for weaning failure in patients with left-side heart failure. Accordingly, cardiogenic pulmonary edema and/ or myocardial ischemia have been reported to occur abruptly during weaning from mechanical ventilation in patients with preexisting cardiac disease [3–7].

▌ Consequences of the Transfer from Mechanical Ventilation to Spontaneous Breathing on the Cardiovascular System

The two major consequences of transferring a patient from mechanical ventilation to spontaneous breathing are:
▌ the increase in respiratory muscle activity, which results in increased work of breathing and in decreased intrathoracic pressure, and
▌ the increase in sympathetic tone.

Increase in Work of Breathing

As a result of respiratory muscle activity, spontaneous breathing causes an increase in global oxygen demand [8, 9]. This results in increases in cardiac work and myocardial oxygen demand that can lead to myocardial ischemia in patients with coronary artery disease. In addition, the increased oxygen demand of the respiratory muscles may lead to blood flow redistribution towards the respiratory muscles with subsequent risks of hypoperfusion of critical organs [10–14].

Negative Intrathoracic Pressure

During weaning from mechanical ventilation, intrathoracic pressure becomes negative [3]. This leads to an increase in the systemic venous return pressure gradient and a decrease in the left ventricular (LV) ejection pressure gradient [1, 15]. The increase in systemic venous return pressure gradient can be responsible for an increase in central blood volume [16] with subsequent risks of pulmonary edema formation. During spontaneous inspiration, the pressure surrounding the left ventricle decreases while the pressure surrounding the extrathoracic arterial compartment remains constant. Consequently, the left ventricle must generate a higher pressure – i.e., transmural pressure – before blood can leave the thorax. This condition is sensed by the left ventricle as an increased afterload [1].

Increase in Sympathetic Tone

The emotional stress due to the abrupt disconnection from the ventilator in patients ventilated for a long time can result in a dramatic adrenergic response. Lemaire et al. [3] measured a two-fold increase in epinephrine and norepinephrine blood levels during weaning of patients with chronic obstructive pulmonary disease (COPD). Acute development of marked hypoxemia and hypercapnia may also contribute to this catecholamine release, which can play a role in the induction of LV dysfunction through several mechanisms. Adrenergic discharge is responsible for:
▌ the increase in systemic arterial pressure and thus in LV afterload, and
▌ the increase in myocardial oxygen demand (tachycardia and increased systolic wall stress) that is potentially deleterious in the setting of coronary artery disease.

▌ Main Cardiovascular Causes of Weaning Failure

Myocardial Ischemia

Mechanisms. In a patient with preexisting coronary artery disease, weaning from mechanical ventilation has potential to induce some degree of myocardial ischemia through several mechanisms:
▌ Myocardial oxygen demand might be potentially increased:
  - As mentioned earlier, the increased work of breathing results in an increased myocardial oxygen demand.
  - As we shall discuss later, the potential increase in LV afterload during weaning-induced loaded inspiration may lead to increased systolic LV wall stress and hence myocardial oxygen demand.
  - The excessive catecholamine release associated with difficult weaning [3, 17] may also result in increased myocardial oxygen demand related to tachycardia.
▌ Myocardial oxygen delivery might be reduced because of the following mechanisms:
  - Weaning-induced hypoxemia that can be secondary to 1) worsening of ventilation/perfusion ratios heterogeneity, as described during weaning from mechanical ventilation in patients with COPD [18], 2) onset of weaning-induced pulmonary edema as described below, and 3) decrease in PvO_2 related to excessive increase in global oxygen demand [19]. The decreased PaO_2 combined with respiratory acidosis may lead to low values of SaO_2, which may significantly lower the amount of oxygen delivered to the myocardium.
  - Decrease in diastolic arterial pressure related to the decrease in intrathoracic pressure during inspiration that may be significant in patients with marked inspiratory efforts due to difficult weaning. As diastolic arterial pressure is the inflow pressure to coronary perfusion, a decrease in coronary blood flow

could subsequently occur. In addition, tachycardia induced by excessive cate-cholamine release in difficult weaning is able to shorten the coronary perfu-sion time by reducing the duration of diastole.

Clinical Correlates. Evidence of development of myocardial ischemia during weaning in patients with preexisting coronary artery disease has been shown in numerous stud-ies. In a series of 12 patients ventilated for acute myocardial infarction (AMI) and pul-monary edema, Rasanen et al. [20] observed five cases of myocardial ischemia during the switch from mechanical ventilation to spontaneous breathing. Lemaire et al. [3] have suggested that weaning-induced LV dysfunction can play a role in preventing successful weaning in patients with COPD and preexisting LV disease. They observed, in 15 patients who were recovering from acute cardiopulmonary decompensation, that weaning was associated with segmental wall motion abnormalities, suggesting the on-set of myocardial ischemia [3]. To evaluate the possibility that myocardial ischemia may occur during weaning, Hurford et al. [4] performed Thallium 201 myocardial scintigraphy in 15 ventilator-dependent patients able to breathe spontaneously and comfortably for at least 10 minutes. During spontaneous breathing, eight out of 15 pa-tients exhibited decreased myocardial Thallium uptake at redistribution on delayed images indicating decreased myocardial perfusion during spontaneous ventilation [4]. Chatila et al. [6] examined the rate of occurrence of ST segment abnormalities during weaning in a population of 93 patients (49 had known coronary artery dis-ease). Only 6% of the patients exhibited ST segment abnormalities during the weaning period. This occurrence was associated with the highest rate of weaning failure [20]. Similar results were found by the same group of investigators in 83 patients suffering from coronary artery disease [6].

A case of ischemic LV failure and ischemic mitral insufficiency during weaning from mechanical ventilation was recently reported [21]. Transluminal angioplasty made weaning possible. This suggests that acute ischemic mitral insufficiency may contribute to cardiac failure during weaning and that angioplasty can allow suc-cessful weaning [21].

▌ Cardiogenic Pulmonary Edema

A marked increase in pulmonary artery occlusion pressure (PAOP) has been ob-served during weaning in patients with pre-existing left heart disease [3, 19, 22]. Several mechanisms may explain this abnormality:

Increase in LV Afterload

Effects of Negative Intrathoracic Pressure. As pointed out earlier, a marked decrease in intrathoracic pressure during inspiratory efforts should result in an increased LV afterload [1]. This effect is likely to play a role in the development of acute LV dys-function that may occur in association with acute exacerbation of COPD [23]. In this regard, increased aortic transmural pressures consistent with increased LV afterload were measured during a Mueller maneuver in normal volunteers [24] and in cardiac surgery patients [15].

In a series of patients with COPD and without pre-existing LV disease, a weaning-induced increase in LV afterload was suggested by a decrease in LV ejection fraction during the transfer from mechanical ventilation to spontaneous breathing [25].

Influence of increased sympathetic tone. Independent of any change in intrathoracic pressure an increase in LV afterload may occur during weaning because of the systemic hypertension related to marked catecholamine discharge [3, 26].

Increase in LV Preload

The fall in intrathoracic pressure during spontaneous inspiration is responsible for the widening of the systemic venous return pressure gradient owing to the decrease in right atrial pressure while the peripheral venous pressure remains unchanged relative to the atmospheric pressure. The resulting increase in right ventricular (RV) preload leads to increased RV stroke volume, pulmonary venous return, and LV preload, provided that the right ventricle is preload dependent. This necessarily

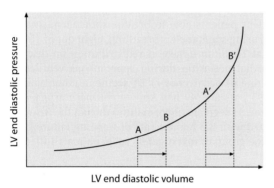

Fig. 1. Left ventricular (LV) end-diastolic pressure/LV end-diastolic volume relationship. Note that the relationship is curvilinear, such that when LV end-diastolic volume increases during weaning, the increase in LV end-diastolic pressure is low if the LV volume is previously normal (from A to B) while the increase in pressure is marked when the LV volume is previously high (from A' to B')

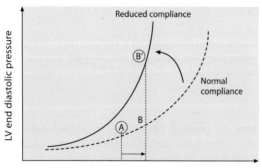

Fig. 2. Left ventricular (LV) end-diastolic pressure/LV end-diastolic volume relationship in normal and reduced LV compliance. Note that when LV end-diastolic volume increases during weaning, the increase in LV end-diastolic pressure remains low if the LV volume and compliance are previously normal (from A to B). By contrast, when the compliance of the left ventricle is either previously low or decreased by the weaning process *per se*, the increase in LV volume induced by weaning results in a marked increase in LV end-diastolic pressure (from A to B')

induces an increase in LV filling pressures, particularly in the case of preexisting cardiac disease. Indeed, in the presence of a dilated cardiomyopathy, a further increase in LV end-diastolic volume will result in a marked increase in LV filling pressure (Fig. 1). In the presence of a reduced LV ventricular compliance, the increase in LV end-diastolic volume induced by weaning will result in a marked increase in LV filling pressure (Fig. 2). These mechanisms probably explain in part, the rise in PAOP observed during weaning in patients with pre-existing cardiac disease, in whom an increase in LV end-diastolic volume was actually measured during weaning from ventilation [3].

Decrease in LV Compliance

The transfer from mechanical ventilation to spontaneous breathing can reduce LV compliance and induce an increase in PAOP provided that the pulmonary venous return is maintained or increased. This phenomenon may result either from the onset of myocardial ischemia or from biventricular interdependence. This mechanism can occur during weaning especially when RV impedance increases secondary to an increase in pulmonary artery pressure [25]. The latter phenomenon may occur as a consequence of:

▌ weaning-related worsening of hypoxemia,
▌ weaning-related respiratory acidosis,
▌ weaning-induced increase in PAOP,
▌ weaning-induced alveolar vessel compression related to dynamic pulmonary hyperinflation created by tachypnea.

The resulting increase in RV afterload associated with the simultaneous increase in systemic venous return and RV filling may lead to a marked enlargement of the right ventricle during the transfer from mechanical ventilation to spontaneous breathing. This may decrease the ability of the left ventricle to fill during diastole and hence may result in a marked increase in PAOP. This phenomenon is likely to occur in patients with pre-existing RV disease and has been considered as responsible for weaning-induced pulmonary edema in COPD patients [3].

In summary, numerous mechanisms can contribute to increase PAOP during the transfer from mechanical ventilation to spontaneous breathing. However, in the absence of left heart disease, the increase in PAOP is limited [9, 27]. By contrast, marked increases in PAOP have been reported to occur in patients suffering from left heart disease who failed to wean because of the onset of cardiogenic pulmonary edema [3, 19, 22].

▌ Diagnosis of the Cardiac Origin of the Weaning Failure

The diagnosis of weaning-induced cardiac dysfunction can be evoked in high-risk patients (COPD and chronic left heart disease) after discarding the classical causes of weaning failure. To establish such a diagnosis, it is useful to perform a weaning trial over a one-hour period of spontaneous breathing either using a T-piece or pressure support with low levels of insufflation pressure (7–10 cm H_2O). Detection of weaning-induced myocardial ischemia can be made with ST segment monitoring [5–7] although this method may suffer from a lack of sensitivity [28]. Detection of weaning-induced pulmonary edema may require pulmonary artery catheterization showing a significant increase in PAOP during the weaning test [3, 19]. The decrease in mixed venous oxygen saturation (SvO_2) during the trial may also detect weaning failure from a cardiovascular origin [19]. Whether monitoring of central venous oxygen saturation ($ScvO_2$) [29] could also be useful remains undetermined. The PiCCO system, by showing an increase in extravascular lung water (EVLW) during weaning, could be helpful for detecting weaning-induced pulmonary edema. However, its clinical utility for that purpose remains to be established.

▌ Treatment of Weaning-induced Cardiac Dysfunction

The treatment must be logically adjusted according to the mechanism that is most likely to have occurred. This requires an individual pathophysiological analysis. Diuretics can be considered when excessive increase in LV preload is assumed to be the predominant mechanism [3]. Treatment by nitrates seems a logical consideration when weaning-induced pulmonary edema is presumed to be related to a marked increase in LV preload and/or occurrence of myocardial ischemia. Vasodilators could be considered when augmentation of LV afterload is presumed to be the predominant mechanism. In this regard, phosphodiesterase inhibitors were demonstrated to allow successful weaning in patients with weaning-induced pulmonary edema [22, 30].

▌ Conclusion

Weaning-induced cardiac dysfunction may occur in some patients suffering from left heart disease, in particular when associated with airway obstruction and/or right heart disease. Among the numerous pathophysiological mechanisms, myocardial ischemia and increase in LV afterload must be underlined. Detecting such phenomena may allow successful weaning after applying the most appropriate treatment.

References

1. Pinsky MR (1989) Effects of changing intrathoracic pressure in the normal and failing heart. In: Scharf SM, Casidy SS (eds) Heart-lung Interactions in Health and Disease. Marcel Dekker, New York, pp 839–876
2. International consensus conferences in intensive care medicine: Noninvasive positive pressure ventilation in acute respiratory failure (2001) Am J Respir Crit Care Med 163:283–291
3. Lemaire F, Teboul JL, Cinotti L, et al (1988) Acute left ventricular dysfunction during unsuccessful weaning from mechanical ventilation. Anesthesiology 69:171–179
4. Hurford WE, Lynch KE, Strauss RN, Lowenstein E, Zapol WM (1991) Myocardial perfusion as assessed by thallium-201 scintigraphy during the discontinuation of mechanical ventilation in ventilator-dependent patients. Anesthesiology 74:1007–1016
5. Hurford WE, Favorito F (1995) Association of myocardial ischemia with failure to wean from mechanical ventilation. Crit Care Med 23:1475–1480
6. Chatila W, Ani S, Cuaglianone D, Jacob B, Amoateng-Adjepong Y, Manthous CA (1996) Cardiac ischemia during weaning from mechanical ventilation. Chest 109:577–583
7. Srivastava S, Chatila W, Amoateng-Adjepong Y, et al (1999) Myocardial ischemia and weaning failure in patients with coronary artery disease: an update. Crit Care Med 27:2109–2112
8. Field S, Kelly SM, Macklem PT (1982) The oxygen cost of breathing in patients with cardiorespiratory disease. Am Rev Respir Dis 126:9–13

9. De Backer D, Haddad PE, Preiser JC, Vincent JL (2000) Hemodynamic responses to successful weaning from mechanical ventilation after cardiovascular surgery. Intensive Care Med 26:1201–1206

10. Viires N, Sillye G, Aubier M, Rassidakis A, Roussos C (1983) Regional blood flow distribution in dog during induced hypotension and low cardiac output. Spontaneous breathing versus artificial ventilation. J Clin Invest 72:935–947

11. Mohsenifar Z, Hay A, Hay J, Lewis MI, Koerner SK (1983) Gastric intramural pH as a predictor of success or failure in weaning patients from mechanical ventilation. Ann Intern Med 119:794–798

12. Bocquillon N, Mathieu D, Neviere R, Lefebvre N, Marechal X, Wattel F (1999) Gastric mucosal pH and blood flow during weaning from mechanical ventilation in patients with chronic obstructive pulmonary disease. Am J Respir Crit Care Med 160:1555–1561

13. Uusaro A, Chittock DR, Russell JA, et al (2000) Stress test and gastric-arterial PCO_2 measurement improve prediction of successful extubation. Crit Care Med 28:2313–2319

14. Hurtado FJ, Beron M, Oliviera W, et al (2001) Gastric intramucosal pH and intraluminal PCO_2 during weaning from mechanical ventilation. Crit Care Med 29:70–76

15. Buda AJ, Pinsky MR, Ingels NB, Daughters GT, Stinson EB, Alderman EL (1979) Effect of intrathoracic pressure on left ventricular performance. N Engl J Med 301:453–459

16. Schmidt H, Rohr D, Bauer H, Bohrer H, Motsch J, Martin E (1997) Changes in intrathoracic fluid volumes during weaning from mechanical ventilation in patients after coronary artery bypass grafting. J Crit Care 12:22–27

17. Oh TE, Bhatt S, Lin ES, Hutchinson RC, Low JM (1991) Plasma catecholamines and oxygen consumption during weaning from mechanical ventilation. Intensive Care Med 17:199–203

18. Torres A, Reyes A, Roca J, Wagner PD, Rodriguez-Roisin R (1989) Ventilation-perfusion mismatching in chronic obstructive pulmonary disease during ventilator weaning. Am Rev Respir Dis 140:1246–1250

19. Jubran A, Mathru M, Dries D, Tobin MJ (1998) Continuous recordings of mixed venous oxygen saturation during weaning from mechanical ventilation and the ramifications thereof. Am J Respir Crit Care Med 158:1763–1769

20. Rasanen J, Nikki P, Heikkila J, et al (1984) Acute myocardial infarction complicated by respiratory failure. The effects of mechanical ventilation. Chest 85:21–28

21. Demoule A, Lefort Y, Lopes ME, Lemaire F (2004) Successful weaning from mechanical ventilation after coronary angioplasty. Br J Anaesth 93:295–297

22. Paulus S, Lehot JJ, Bastien O, Piriou V, George M, Estanove S (1994) Enoximone and acute left ventricular failure during weaning from mechanical ventilation after cardiac surgery. Crit Care Med 22:74–80

23. Teboul JL, Lemaire F (1996) Left ventricular function during acute respiratory failure of chronic obstructive pulmonary disease. In: Derenne JP, Whitelaw WA, Similowski T (eds) Acute respiratory failure in chronic obstructive pulmonary disease. Marcel Dekker, New York, pp 429–51

24. Scharf SM, Brown R, Tow DE, Parisi AF (1979) Cardiac effects of increased lung volume and decreased pleural pressure in man. J Appl Physiol 47:257–262

25. Richard C, Teboul JL, Archambaud F, Hebert JL, Michaut P, Auzepy P (1994) Left ventricular function during weaning of patients with chronic obstructive pulmonary disease. Intensive Care Med 20:181–186

26. Dryden CM, Smith DC, McLintic AJ, Pace NA (1993) The effect of preoperative beta-blocker therapy on cardiovascular responses to weaning from mechanical ventilation and extubation after coronary artery bypass grafting. J Cardiothorac Vasc Anesth 7:547–550

27. Teboul JL, Abrouk F, Lemaire F (1988) Right ventricular function in COPD patients during weaning from mechanical ventilation. Intensive Care Med 14:483–485

28. Martinez EA, Kim LJ, Faraday N, et al (2003) Sensitivity of routine intensive care unit surveillance for detecting myocardial ischemia. Crit Care Med 31:2302–2308

29. Reinhart K, Kuhn HJ, Hartog C, Bredle DL (2004) Continuous central venous and pulmonary artery oxygen saturation monitoring in the critically ill. Intensive Care Med 30:1572–1578

30. Valtier B, Teboul JL, Lemaire F (1990) Left ventricular dysfunction while weaning from mechanical ventilation. Contribution of enoximone. Arch Mal Coeur Vaiss 83:83–86

Circulatory Shock

Resuscitation from Circulatory Shock: An Approach Based on Oxygen-derived Parameters

B. Vallet, E. Wiel, and G. Lebuffe

▌ Introduction

Resuscitation from 'circulatory shock' requires an emergency and global approach, which is supposed to be based on limited clinical features for establishing diagnosis and probabilistic therapy. The efficacy of this initial therapeutic strategy then becomes part of the diagnostic approach: if the chosen therapy is successful, it confirms the diagnosis retrospectively. This initial diagnostic approach is essentially based on physician knowledge of global hemodynamics and oxygen-derived parameters. It can be helped by rapidly available oxygen-derived biologic markers.

Circulatory failure results in a decrease in oxygen delivery (DO_2) associated with a decrease in cellular partial pressure of oxygen (PO_2). When a critical PO_2 value is reached, oxidative phosphorylation is limited and leads to a shift from aerobic to anaerobic metabolism. The result is a rise in cell and blood lactate concentration, associated with a decrease in adenosine triphosphate (ATP) synthesis. Adenosine diphosphate (ADP) and hydrogen ion accumulate and together with raised serum lactate lead to metabolic lactic acidosis. This state is called 'dysoxia' and can be accepted as a definition for 'shock', a state in which inadequate tissue oxygenation produces cellular injury. Shock often, but not only, results from circulatory failure and decreased DO_2.

▌ Understanding the Underlying Pathophysiology of Global Flow and DO_2

Addressing the Global Adequacy of Tissue Oxygenation

Adequacy of tissue oxygenation is defined by an adapted oxygen supply (or DO_2) to oxygen demand [1]. Oxygen demand varies according to tissue type and according to time. Although oxygen demand cannot be measured or calculated, oxygen uptake or consumption (VO_2) and DO_2 can both be quantified; they are linked by a simple relationship:

$$VO_2 = DO_2 \times O_2ER$$

where O_2ER represents oxygen extraction ratio (O_2ER in %; VO_2 and DO_2 in ml O_2/kg/min). DO_2 represents the total flow of oxygen in the arterial blood and is given as the product of cardiac output by arterial oxygen content (CaO_2):

$$DO_2 = \text{cardiac output} \times CaO_2$$

with CaO_2 being the product of hemoglobin (Hb, g/100 ml), arterial oxygen saturation (SaO_2, %) and Hb oxygen capacity (1.39 ml O_2/g Hb):

$$CaO_2 = Hb \times SaO_2 \times 1.39$$

Under physiological control, oxygen demand equals VO_2 (≈ 2.4 ml O_2/kg/min for a DO_2 of 12 ml O_2/kg/min, which corresponds to a 20% O_2ER). The rate of oxygen delivered by blood is physiologically larger than the rate of VO_2: DO_2 is adapted to oxygen demand. When oxygen demand increases (as during exercise for example), DO_2 has to adapt and increase.

During circulatory shock and/or severe hypoxemia, as DO_2 declines secondary to a decrease in cardiac output and/or a decrease in CaO_2, VO_2 can be maintained by a compensatory increase in O_2ER, VO_2 and DO_2 therefore remaining independent. But as DO_2 falls further, a critical point (DO_2crit) is reached; O_2ER can no longer compensate for this fall in DO_2 and, at this critical level, VO_2 becomes DO_2-dependent (Fig. 1). At this DO_2crit (4 ml/kg/min), for a VO_2 about 2.4 ml/kg/min, O_2ER reaches its critical point (O_2ERcrit) of 60%. When VO_2 is higher, DO_2crit is higher as well. Increase in O_2 extraction occurs via two fundamental adaptive mechanisms [2]:

- Redistribution of blood flow among organs via an increase in sympathetic adrenergic tone and central vascular contraction (this is responsible for a decreased perfusion in organs with low O_2ER, such as the skin and splanchnic area, and a maintained perfusion in organs with high O_2ER [heart and brain]);
- Capillary recruitment within organs responsible for peripheral vasodilation (opposite to central vasoconstriction).

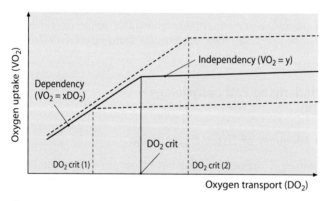

Fig. 1. O_2 uptake (VO_2)-to-O_2 supply (DO_2) relationship. When VO_2 is supply independent ("independency") following the relation $VO_2 = y$, whole body O_2 needs are met. When VO_2 becomes DO_2 dependent ("dependency") according to the relation $VO_2 = x\, DO_2$, VO_2 starts to be linearly dependent on DO_2 at the critical DO_2 value ("DO_2crit"), which corresponds to "dysoxia" (insufficient ATP synthesis as related to needs) and shock state. DO_2crit is influenced by global organism oxygen needs: when VO_2 is decreased (rest, sedation, hypothermia...), the DO_2crit is decreased as well [lower dotted line; DO_2crit(1)]; conversely, increased VO_2 (increased muscle activity, awakening, hyperthermia, sepsis...) is associated with increased DO_2crit [upper dotted line; DO_2crit(2)]

Using Mixed Venous Oxygen Saturation to Assess Adequacy of Global Tissue Oxygenation

In the clinical setting, mixed venous O_2 saturation (SvO_2) can be used for assessing whole body VO_2-to-DO_2 relationships. Indeed, according to the Fick equation, tissue VO_2 is proportional to cardiac output:

$$VO_2 = \text{cardiac output} \times (CaO_2 - CvO_2)$$

where CvO_2 is mixed venous blood oxygen content. To some extent, $VO_2 \approx$ cardiac output $\times (SaO_2-SvO_2) \times Hb \times 1.39$ and $SvO_2 \approx SaO_2-VO_2 /(\text{cardiac output} \times Hb \times 1.39)$.

Four situations can be responsible for a decrease in SvO_2: hypoxemia (decrease in SaO_2), an increase in VO_2, a fall in cardiac output, and/or a decrease in Hb. At DO_2crit, SvO_2 is about 40% (SvO_2crit) with an O_2ER of 60% and a SaO_2 of 100%. This SvO_2crit has been identified in humans [3]. It is important to emphasize that for the same decrease in CaO_2 (induced by either a decrease in Hb or SaO_2), the decrease in SvO_2 will be more pronounced if cardiac output cannot adapt. Hence, SvO_2 represents adequacy of global cardiac output to CaO_2 decrease. A 40% SvO_2 can be taken as an imbalance between arterial blood oxygen supply and tissue oxygen demand with evident risk of dysoxia. In the clinical setting, a decrease in SvO_2 of 5% from its normal value (77 to 65%) is representative of a significant fall in DO_2 and/or an increase in oxygen demand (Fig. 2). If initial probabilistic treatment (fluid resuscitation and/or low dose inotropes, and/or red blood cell transfusion) does not restore SvO_2 to a minimal 65%, Hb, SaO_2, and cardiac output should then be individually measured in order to introduce the appropriate treatment.

Assessing Global Flow

Global flow is dependent on preload, myocardial contractility, afterload, and heart rate. Regional flow distribution is not homogeneous and is dependent on central and peripheral vascular tone, which ultimately results in the composite systemic

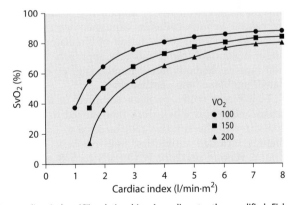

Fig. 2. Venous O_2 saturation (SvO_2)-to-cardiac index (CI) relationship. According to the modified Fick equation, the relationship SvO_2/CI is curvilinear. Consequently, when oxygen uptake (VO_2) is constant, CI variations lead to large variations in SvO_2 when the initial CI value is low. In contrast, when initial CI values are already high, CI variations do not influence SvO_2 very much. These relationships are modified when CI variations are associated with large modifications in VO_2

vascular resistances (SVR). As an oversimplification, mean arterial pressure (MAP) can be estimated as the product of flow by SVR. When flow decreases, MAP remains stable when SVR increases; this corresponds to increased sympathetic adrenergic tone and central vascular contraction in low O_2ER organs and preserved peripheral vasodilation in high O_2ER organs. Overall, O_2ER increases and SvO_2 decreases.

Minimal data exist to guide selection of the threshold for blood pressure maintenance. Arbitrary values of a systolic blood pressure (SBP) of 90 mmHg or a MAP of 60–65 mmHg have traditionally been chosen. MAP is a better reflection of arterial pressure-head, but in the presence of an arterial line, SBP is likely to be a more accurate pressure measurement and is typically used [4].

Observation of an inappropriate tissue perfusion (raised blood lactate level, metabolic acidosis, $SvO_2 < 40\%$, decreased urinary flow...) and its persistence despite probabilistic therapy (fluid, low dose inotropes, red cells) should lead to optimizing flow according to the Frank-Starling curve. This can be assessed by invasive and non-invasive investigative procedures (see later).

During circulatory shock, when O_2ER crit is reached, VO_2-to-DO_2 dependency with a rise in blood lactate levels implies oxygen debt. Several authors have reported that oxygen debt is related to the likelihood of multiple organ failure (MOF) and mortality in postoperative or polytrauma patients [5, 6]. Patients who survived MOF have been shown to have higher cardiac index, lower SVR, higher VO_2, and higher SvO_2 than non-survivors [7, 8]. Rixen and Siegel [6] demonstrated that the degree of tissue oxygen debt is related to an enhanced inflammatory response, associated with an increased risk of acute respiratory distress syndrome (ARDS), and higher mortality rates.

Recent research has emphasized the potential interest of central venous oxygen saturation ($ScvO_2$) for detecting global oxygenation impairment [6]. Experimental studies reported that changes in SvO_2 and $ScvO_2$ closely reflect circulatory disturbances during periods of hypoxia, hemorrhage and subsequent resuscitation. Fluctuations in these two parameters correlated well although absolute values differed [9, 10]. Finally, observational data found $ScvO_2$ to be a useful parameter in detecting occult tissue hypoperfusion in both sepsis and cardiac failure [11, 12]. An important feature with $ScvO_2$ monitoring is that $ScvO_2$ can be continuously provided by central venous catheters equipped with optic fibers (PreSep®, Edwards Lifesciences). In initial resuscitation of circulatory shock, insertion of a central venous line is a standard, rapid and easy approach, much easier than any other invasive or non-invasive hemodynamic monitoring, especially in patients who are not yet sedated, intubated, and ventilated.

In a recent study, patients admitted to the emergency department with severe sepsis and septic shock were randomized to standard therapy (n = 133) or to early goal-directed therapy (n = 130) targeted to achieve a $ScvO_2$ of >70% [13]. Standard therapy included antibiotics, fluid resuscitation and vasoactive drugs to achieve a central venous pressure (CVP) between 8 and 12 mmHg, MAP >65 mmHg, and urine output >0.5 ml/kg/h. The patients in the early goal-directed therapy group, in addition to the same previous goals, had to reach an $ScvO_2$ of >70% by optimizing fluid administration, hematocrit to >30%, and/or prescription of inotrope (dobutamine to <20 µkg/min). Initial $ScvO_2$ in both groups was quite low (49 ± 12%), reminding us that severe sepsis is a hypodynamic shock before any fluid resuscitation has started. This study demonstrated a significant reduction in hospital mortality: 30.5% in the early goal-directed therapy group compared with 46.5% in the standard therapy (p=0.009). An important point in this study is that 99.2% of patients receiving early goal-directed therapy achieved their hemodynamic goals within the first 6 hours compared with 86% of those receiving standard therapy. From the 1st to the 72nd hour, the total fluid loading was not different between the two groups ($\approx 13\,400$ ml); in contrast, from the 1st to the 7th hour the amount of fluid received was significantly larger in the early goal-directed therapy patients (≈ 5000 ml vs 3500 ml). In the follow-up period between the 7th and the 72nd hour, in patients receiving early goal-directed therapy, mean $ScvO_2$ was higher ($70.6 \pm 10.7\%$ vs $65.3 \pm 11.4\%$; p=0.02), mean arterial pH was higher (7.40 ± 0.12 vs 7.36 ± 0.12; p=0.02), and lactate plasma levels were lower (3.0 ± 4.4 mmol/l vs 3.9 ± 4.4 mmol/l; p=0.02), as was base excess (2.0 ± 6.6 mmol/l vs 5.1 ± 6.7 mmol/l; p=0.02). MOF score was significantly altered in patients receiving standard therapy when compared to early goal-directed therapy patients. This is the first study demonstrating that early identification of patients with sepsis, associated with early initiation of goal-directed therapy in order to achieve adequate tissue oxygenation by DO_2 ($ScvO_2$ monitoring), significantly improves mortality rates [13].

▌ Deciding the Diagnostic and Treatment Strategy (Fig. 3)

Strategy relies, therefore, on shock definition (dysoxia) and it starts with an early and rapid estimation of oxygen deficit, rapidly followed by an early probabilistic treatment. The response to this early probabilistic treatment (modification in lactate, ar-

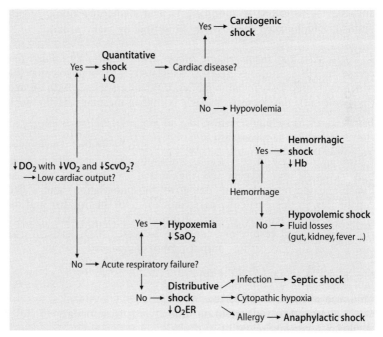

Fig. 3. How to interpret a shock state at the initial stages. DO_2: oxygen supply; VO_2: oxygen uptake; $ScvO_2$: central venous oxygen saturation; SaO_2: arterial oxygen saturation; Q: cardiac output; Hb: hemoglobin; O_2ER: oxygen extraction ratio

terial pH, $ScvO_2$ or SvO_2) then suggests which type of complementary investigation to carry out (echocardiography, esophageal Doppler, scan...) and the type of monitoring to install (invasive systolic arterial blood pressure variations, Swan-Ganz catheter...), which will help then to refine the diagnosis and optimize treatment.

Diagnosing the Type of Shock

Quantitative shock (decreased DO_2)

▌ *Decreased flow (hypovolemic, cardiogenic shock).* Decrease in flow can be related to either decrease in circulatory volume (absolute or relative hypovolemia) or to a failure of the cardiac pump.

Hypovolemia is 'absolute' after severe hydration defect, plasma or blood losses; it can be 'relative' when fluid administration is insufficient to compensate a loss in vascular tone in the context of sepsis or anaphylaxis (or use of large doses of sedative drugs). In that context, there is an inadequacy between the content (volume) and the vascular capacity, and abnormal sympathetic tone is associated with an altered capillary recruitment. Relative hypovolemia is therefore often associated with altered redistribution of flow among and within organs. It is important to notice that shock can result from a mixture of quantitative and distributive features, and a mixture of absolute and relative hypovolemia.

Cardiac failure can result from either myogenic injury (infectious, viral or ischemic disease), or an 'obstacle' to ventricular ejection (increased right ventricle [RV] afterload, increased vascular pulmonary resistance, increased left ventricle [LV] afterload, increased SVR), and/or a lack of ventricular filling (decreased RV or LV preload, valvulopathy, decrease in filling time by tachycardia).

▌ *Decreased CaO_2 (hemorrhagic shock, acute respiratory failure, poisoning).* A decrease in Hb is not necessarily associated with hypovolemia (hemodilution in which decreased DO_2 remains modest). When associated with an acute hemorrhage (hypovolemia), the decrease in DO_2 is higher inasmuch as the decrease in flow is larger.

Hemoglobin capacity to carry oxygen can also be limited. During carbon monoxide poisoning, decrease in DO_2 results from a loading competition on Hb between carbon monoxide and oxygen, and 'maximized' by abnormal oxygen utilization (carbon monoxide interacts with oxidative phosphorylation) and a decrease in O_2ER capabilities. In this particular case, shock is both quantitative and distributive.

In case of an acute respiratory disorder (altered gas exchange or abnormal central or peripheral respiratory control), decreased SaO_2 leads to a decreased CaO_2 and DO_2 as soon as cardiac output cannot compensate.

Distributive shock (decreased O_2ER)

This type of shock is linked to:

▌ An altered flow redistribution among organs secondary to inflammation, anaphylaxis, or abusive use of sedation

▌ A decrease in capillary recruitment secondary to altered vascular reactivity, increased intravascular coagulation, increased blood cell adhesion, and/or endothelial edema

▌ An abnormal mitochondrial function (mitochondrial injury or dysfunction) such as described in the so-called 'cytopathic hypoxia' [14].

Distributive shock often coexists with hypovolemic and/or cardiogenic shock.

Deciding when to Admit the Patient to the Intensive Care Unit (ICU)

Admission to the ICU is needed when hemodynamic instability is present and requires use of inotropes (inoconstrictors or inodilators); this occurs when shock does not respond to initial therapy (fluid administration, low dose inotropes, red cell infusion), requires ventilatory support (with a non-invasive interface or after intubation), necessitates hemofiltration (severe electrolyte disorder, fluid overflow, poisoning), and more generally when invasive procedures become necessary (invasive blood pressure monitoring). A patient becomes eligible for an ICU bed at the time at which failure of one or more organ develops.

Choosing the Appropriate Monitoring

The discussion of monitoring type does not have any meaning until the cardiorespiratory emergency has been treated. The minimal monitoring device consists of an electrocardiogram, pulse oximeter, and rapid arterial pressure recordings (every five minutes and at the best continuous and invasive). A central venous catheter allows measurement of CVP, which often cannot help much in deciding on fluid administration (it is indicative at least when it remains < 5–8 mmHg), but which facilitates infusion of drugs, crystalloids or colloids. The central venous line allows also for monitoring and/or sampling of $ScvO_2$ (a surrogate for mixed SvO_2) if the catheter is not equipped with optic fibers. Central venous catheters are easier, should be cheaper and less iatrogenic to use than Swan-Ganz catheters.

A Swan-Ganz catheter (at best with continuous cardiac output and SvO_2 monitoring) and/or any non-invasive flow assessment (transesophageal echo, esophageal Doppler) is recommended when optimized cardiac output is doubtful according to the Frank-Starling curve. This requires that some preliminary cardiorespiratory stability has been obtained. In that context, fluid administration should be continued (the heart is preload-dependent) until cardiac output does not increase any more (becomes preload-independent); when cardiac output is not sufficient to satisfy MAP, urine output, and/or when SvO_2 remains low, and/or when lactate concentration remains elevated, an inotrope should be given. Cardiac echography must be conducted in the context of congestive heart failure (CHF) and/or myocardial ischemia to diagnose ventricle or valve dysfunction. In the sedated, intubated and ventilated patient, recordings of systolic pressure variation (SPV) and/or pulse pressure variation (ΔPP) can be helpful; the heart remains preload-dependent until SPV is smaller than 10 mmHg and/or ΔPP is less than 10% [15]. Arrhythmia unfortunately precludes this type of evaluation.

Iterative blood gas analysis (another approach justifying insertion of an arterial line), metabolic acidosis and lactate concentration evaluation, assess global tissue oxygenation, thus complementing $ScvO_2$ or SvO_2 information.

▌ Therapeutic Principles: Symptomatic and Etiologic Treatments

Symptomatic Treatment

Emergency therapeutic principles of care need to be decided at the time the initial diagnostic strategy is considered. Supplemental oxygen and ventilatory support must be given in response to acute respiratory failure (primary respiratory failure: acute lung injury [ALI], mechanics failure...; secondary: respiratory distress) either through a face mask, or through a chest tube. Acute circulatory failure is treated by initial fluid loading in absence of LV failure (see below). If decreased global contractility is present, inotropic support with either dobutamine or dopamine should be considered. In case of anaphylactic shock, intravenous epinephrine must be given to treat allergy-induced vasodilation.

Fluid loading is the first step in treatment [16]. The first goal is to optimize LV preload in order to improve DO_2 by increasing cardiac output [17]. There is however an associated risk of interstitial edema, in particular pulmonary edema. Unless the patient has ALI, fluid loading aims at maximizing flow [17] according to the Frank-Starling relationship, decreased lung gas exchange being detected by a decrease in SaO_2 (or by a decrease in its surrogate, pulse oximetry).

Swan-Ganz derived pulmonary artery occlusion pressure (PAOP) has long been the most widely used static clinical variable for guiding fluid infusion. In septic shock, it is accepted that maximal cardiac output is obtained for values of PAOP between 12 and 15 mmHg [17]. In order to better estimate LV preload, LV end-diastolic surface has been proposed. In fact, in the sedated, intubated and ventilated patient, ventilatory-induced SPV predicts increased systolic ejection volume to fluid loading much better than PAOP [18].

Synthetic colloids are first line agents. They may induce less pulmonary edema than crystalloids, especially in septic shock. Crystalloids are recommended as first line agents during anaphylactic shock. Normalization of hemoglobin concentration by red blood cell transfusion is not required. However, a hemoglobin concentration between 8 and 10 g/dL [17] might be useful in patients with severe sepsis and/or coronary disease and/or decreased cardiac contractility. In those latter cases decreased hemoglobin concentration is not compensated for by increased cardiac output, and DO_2crit is reached more rapidly.

Catecholamines help in restoring perfusion pressure and insuring cardiac output in order to allow sufficient DO_2; this should allow regional flow distribution and improved O_2ER. All catecholamines are inotropes; they can be distinguished into:

▌ inodilators, when they combine inotrope properties and vasodilation (low dose dopamine, any dose of dobutamine or dopexamine);

▌ inoconstrictors, when they combine inotrope properties and vasoconstricting effects (high dose dopamine, any dose of epinephrine or norepinephrine).

Inodilators increase flow; inoconstrictors increase perfusion pressure. Due to variable individual sensitivity to catecholamines, dose titration is heavily recommended [17]. More potent vasopressors such as vasopressin and its derivatives are now being tested [19]. It is important to emphasize that a rise in blood pressure may not be a surrogate for clinical benefit. Indeed, in a large placebo-controlled clinical trial, administration of the nonselective nitric oxide (NO) inhibitor, N^G-methyl-L-arginine, in septic shock produced both significant increases in blood pressure and significant increases in mortality [20].

In septic shock, one study demonstrated that increasing MAP from 65 to 85 mmHg was associated with no difference in organ perfusion variables [21]. Because increasing blood pressure through vasoconstriction may be associated with a decrease in flow, a trade-off may exist between increased blood pressure and decreased cardiac index that will vary based on the choice of vasopressor or combined inotrope/vasopressor [4].

Other Therapeutic Principles

The importance of correction of metabolic acidosis, and the use of intravenous bicarbonate for shock-induced anion gap acidosis, has been emphasized too much in the past. Indeed, clinical studies, including one randomized, prospective trial, failed to show any hemodynamic benefit from bicarbonate therapy either to increase cardiac output or to decrease vasopressor requirements, regardless of the degree of acidemia. Cardiac function does not appear to be decreased for arterial pH values higher than 7. Bicarbonate infusion, apart from in renal or digestive losses, is therefore not recommended, unless the patient requires hemodialysis or hemodiafiltration for hyperkalemia [22].

In septic shock, stress-dose (low dose) steroid therapy (hydrocortisone 300 mg/day) needs to be considered, especially if the decrease in blood pressure requires high/increasing concentrations of vasopressors, once antibiotics are adapted and/or the infectious site is controlled [23]. Intravenous hydrocortisone is administered after the serum cortisol level has been assessed (before and after corticotropin stimulation test). The duration for treatment is 5 days minimum when a positive clinical response is present. Beyond 72 hours, absence of any hemodynamic improvement suggests that the hydrocortisone treatment is futile.

The place of high-volume hemofiltration in the treatment of septic shock remains to be defined.

Although, not oriented toward better circulatory efficacy, a number of treatments are essential in the treatment of septic shock [16]. Infectious source control and its eradication are primordial. Empiric or probabilistic antibiotics need to be directed against Gram-negative microorganisms, but also to potentially resistant ones. This justifies double or triple antibiotherapy, which theoretically offers the following advantages: activity spectrum widening, antibacterial synergy, increased bactericidal speed, and decreased risk for emergent resistant germs.

▌ Prognosis

The main prognostic factors for circulatory shock lie in the number of organ failures present on admission, delay starting treatment, and the response to symptomatic treatment; in case of septic shock, control of the infectious source and its sensitivity to medical and surgical treatment are essential. Early goal-directed therapy certainly determines the severity of MOF and prognosis, as clearly demonstrated by the recent trial from Rivers et al. [13].

References

1. Vallet B, Tavernier B, Lund N (2000) Assessment of tissue oxygenation in the critically ill. Eur J Anaesth 17:1–10
2. Vallet B (1998) Vascular reactivity and tissue oxygenation. Intensive Care Med 24:3–11
3. Ronco JJ, Fenwick JC, Tweeddale MG, et al (1993) Identification of the critical oxygen delivery for anaerobic metabolism in critically ill septic and nonseptic humans. JAMA 270:1724–1730
4. Dellinger RP (2003) Cardiovascular management of septic shock. Crit Care Med 31:946–955
5. Shoemaker WC, Appel PL, Kram HB (1988) Tissue oxygen debt as a determinant of lethal and nonlethal postoperative organ failure. Crit Care Med 16:1117–1120
6. Rixen D, Siegel JH (2000) Metabolic correlates of oxygen debt predict posttrauma early acute respiratory distress syndrome and the related cytokine response. J Trauma 49:392–403
7. Shoemaker WC, Appel PL, Kram HB, et al (1993) Hemodynamic and oxygen transport monitoring to titrate therapy in septic shock. New Horiz 1:145–159
8. Rady MY, Rivers EP, Martin GB, et al (1999) Continuous central venous oximetry and shock index in the emergency department: use in the evaluation of clinical shock. Am J Emerg Med 10:538–541
9. Reinhart K, Kuhn HJ, Hartog C, Bredle DL (2004) Continuous central venous and pulmonary artery oxygen saturation monitoring in the critically ill. Intensive Care Med 30:1572–1578
10. Scalea TM, Holman M, Fuortes M, et al (1988) Central venous blood oxygen saturation: an early, accurate measurement of volume during hemorrhage. J Trauma 28:725–732
11. Ander DS, Jaggi M, Rivers E, et al (1998) Undetected cardiogenic shock in patients with congestive heart failure presenting to the emergency department. Am J Cardiol 82:888–891
12. Rady MY, Rivers EP, Nowak RM (1996) Resuscitation of the critically ill in the ED: responses of blood pressure, heart rate, shock index, central venous oxygen saturation, and lactate. Am J Emerg Med 14:218–225
13. Rivers E, Nguyen B, Havstad S, et al (2001) Early goal-directed therapy in the treatment of severe sepsis and septic shock. N Engl J Med 345:1368–1377
14. Fink MP (2002) Bench-to-bedside review: cytopathic hypoxia. Crit Care 6:491–499
15. Michard F, Boussat S, Chemla D, et al (2000) Relation between respiratory changes in arterial pulse pressure and fluid responsiveness in septic patients with acute circulatory failure. Am J Respir Crit Care Med 162:134–138
16. Dellinger RP, Carlet JM, Masur H, et al (2004) Surviving Sepsis Campaign guidelines for management of severe sepsis and septic shock. Intensive Care Med 30:536–555
17. Task force of the American College of Critical Care Medicine, Society of Critical Care Medicine (1999) Practice parameters for hemodynamic support of sepsis in adult patients in sepsis. Crit Care Med 127:639–660
18. Tavernier B, Makhotine O, Lebuffe G, et al (1998) Systolic pressure variation as a guide to fluid therapy in patients with sepsis-induced hypotension. Anesthesiology 89:1313–1321
19. Dünser MW, Mayr AJ, Ulmer H, et al (2003) Arginine vasopressin in advanced vasodilatory shock. A prospective, randomized, controlled study. Circulation 107:2313–2319
20. Lopez A, Lorente JA, Steingrub J, et al (2004) Multiple-center, randomized, placebo-controlled, double-blind study of the nitric oxide synthase inhibitor 546C88: effect on survival in patients with septic shock. Crit Care Med 32:21–30
21. LeDoux D, Astiz ME, Carpati CM, et al (2000) Effects of perfusion pressure on tissue perfusion in septic shock. Crit Care Med 28:2729–2732
22. Forsythe SM, Schmidt GA (2000) Sodium bicarbonate for the treatment of lactic acidosis. Chest 117:260–267
23. Annane D, Sebille V, Charpentier C, et al (2002) Effect of treatment with low doses of hydrocortisone and fludrocortisone on mortality in patients with septic shock. JAMA 288:862–871

Is there a Place for Epinephrine in the Management of Septic Shock?

B. Levy, S. Gibot, and P.E. Bollaert

▌ Introduction

In contrast to norepinephrine-dobutamine, epinephrine, when used in septic shock, increases lactate level together with a slightly enhanced lactate/pyruvate (L/P) ratio, decreases global splanchnic flow, and elevates tonometric mucosal PCO_2 gap (tonometer PCO_2, $PaCO_2$), a surrogate marker of gastric mucosal metabolism and/or perfusion.

Based on these observations, The Task Force of the American College of Critical Care Medicine and the Society of Critical Care Medicine recommends the use of epinephrine only in patients who fail to respond to traditional therapies [1]. Nevertheless, invasive arterial and pulmonary artery monitoring, although essential to the rational management of septic shock, may take time to establish. Fluid therapy and vasoactive therapy may be immediately required in order to maintain acceptable blood pressure levels. In this setting, there is good reason to choose a broad-spectrum catecholamine such as epinephrine or dopamine rather than a pure α-adrenergic agonist which can cause substantial reductions in cardiac output, or a pure β-agonist such as dobutamine which can exacerbate vasodilation and hypotension through its β_2-adrenergic action [2].

The aim of this chapter is to provide an alternative point of view regarding the somewhat dark side of epinephrine and to moderate the interpretation of pharmacological data.

▌ Epinephrine Effects in Volunteers [3–4]

Hemodynamic Effects of Epinephrine in Volunteers

In volunteers, epinephrine increases heart rate (HR) as well as mean arterial pressure (MAP) due mainly to a rise in systolic blood pressure. Conversely, diastolic blood pressure falls, irrespective of the dosage. Vasodilatation occurs in the calf vascular bed while blood flow in skin capillaries and arteriovenous anastomoses decreases. Concentration-dependent increases in stroke volume and cardiac output occur without any changes in end-diastolic volume, along with decreases in vascular resistances of the systemic circulation, calf, and adipose tissue. Coronary blood flow, blood flow to skeletal muscles, as well as hepatic blood flow increase while splanchnic vascular resistances decrease. However, renal blood flow decreases with an increase in the filtration fraction.

Metabolic Effects of Epinephrine in Volunteers

In healthy volunteers, epinephrine induces hyperglycemia and hyperlactatemia. Since insulin secretion is suppressed by α-adrenergic stimulation, plasma concentrations of insulin remain low. Hyperglycemia is induced by an increase in glucose production caused by an increase in hepatic glycogenolysis and an increase in gluconeogenesis. There is also a marked increase in oxygen consumption (VO_2). In skeletal muscle, epinephrine increases glycolysis and glycogenolysis inducing an upsurge in lactate. Muscular lactate serves as a substrate for hepatic neoglucogenesis (Cori Cycle). Epinephrine also increases lipolysis and decreases muscular proteolysis.

▌ Epinephrine Effects in Septic Shock

Epinephrine is Effective in Restoring Global Hemodynamics

In patients unresponsive to volume expansion or other catecholamine infusions, epinephrine can increase MAP, primarily by increasing cardiac index and stroke volume together with more modest increases in systemic vascular resistance (SVR) and HR. This is an important advantage, especially in patients with altered cardiac function. The effects of epinephrine in hyperdynamic or normodynamic septic shock are highly predictable correlating an increase in MAP with an increase in cardiac index [5]. Using epinephrine as a first line agent, Moran et al. reported a linear relationship between epinephrine dosage and HR, MAP, cardiac index, left ventricular stroke work index (LVSWI), and oxygen delivery and consumption [6]. Despite an increase in oxygen consumption, no adverse cardiac side effects have been described in septic shock. Electrocardiographic (EKG) changes indicating ischemia or arrhythmias have not been reported in septic patients. In patients with right ventricular failure, epinephrine increases right ventricular function by improving contractility [7]. Considering global hemodynamics, epinephrine is more effective than dopamine and is just as efficient as norepinephrine [8].

Summary: In septic shock, epinephrine increases arterial pressure and cardiac index.

Epinephrine Increases Lactate Concentration

In human septic shock, epinephrine increases lactate levels without any increase in L/P ratio when the latter is normalized to pH. This rise in lactate is transient, however, since levels return to baseline values after 12 hours [8]. Epinephrine infusion is associated with an increase in lactate concentration not only in septic conditions but also under fully aerobic conditions such as in healthy volunteers at rest and during exercise. In a model of endotoxic shock, we demonstrated that the infusion of epinephrine was associated with a significant increase in lactate without any change in L/P ratio. Moreover, epinephrine use was not associated with a decrease in tissue ATP [9], hence demonstrating that epinephrine-induced hyperlactatemia is probably related to direct effects of epinephrine on carbohydrate metabolism and not to cellular hypoxia. Indeed, elevated blood lactate concentrations during shock states are often viewed as evidence of tissue hypoxia, with lactate levels being proportional to the defect in oxidative metabolism [10]. However, many tissues generate pyruvate and lactate under aerobic conditions (so-called aerobic glycolysis) in a process linking glycolytic ATP supply to activity of membrane ion pumps such as Na^+,K^+-ATPase [10]. Stimulation of aerobic glycolysis, i.e., glycolysis not attributable to oxygen deficiency or glycogenolysis, occurs not only in resting, well-oxygenated skeletal muscles but also during experimental hemorrhagic shock and experimental sepsis, and is closely linked to stimulation of active sarcolemmal Na^+,K^+-ATPase transport under epinephrine stimulation. Epinephrine stimulates the release of lactate from skeletal muscle through stimulation of Na^+, K^+ adenosine triphosphatase for oxidation purposes or gluconeogenesis (Cori cycle). Thus, increased lactate production is the result of aerobic glycolysis rather than the result of anaerobic glycolysis. Although this is an adenosine 5'-triphosphate (ATP)-consuming process, the source of energy in the liver ultimately comes from fatty acids. Hence, lactate provides glycolytic ATP to several peripheral cells, this ATP derived from energy-producing lipid oxidation.

Summary: Epinephrine transiently increases lactate concentration through an increase in aerobic glycolysis.

Epinephrine Increases PCO$_2$ Gap

In a clinical setting of dopamine-resistant septic shock, we compared the effects of norepinephrine-dobutamine versus epinephrine alone on gastric tonometry using saline tonometry [8]. Despite similar increases in arterial pressure and oxygen delivery in both groups, PCO_2 gap increased in epinephrine-treated patients. This increase was transient however as both groups had the same normal PCO_2 gap after 24 hours (Fig. 1). Moreover, the amplitude of PCO_2 gap increase was moderate and consistently below 18 mmHg [11]. This suggests one of two possibilities [12]:

▌ that epinephrine increases splanchnic oxygen utilization and CO_2 production through a thermogenic effect especially if gastric blood flow does not increase to the same extent, inducing a mismatch between splanchnic oxygen delivery and splanchnic oxygen consumption;

▌ a second hypothesis would be that epinephrine decreases mucosal blood flow with a decrease in CO_2 efflux, the net result being an increase in PCO_2 gap.

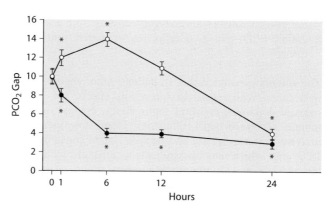

Fig. 1. Evolution of PCO$_2$ gap (tonometer PCO$_2$–arterial PCO$_2$) during infusion of epinephrine (*open circles*) or norepinephrine-dobutamine (*closed circles*) * $p < 0.01$ versus baseline. (From [8] with permission)

The latter hypothesis is not sustained however by Duranteau et al. [13] who demonstrated, using laser Doppler flow, that epinephrine induces higher gastric mucosal blood flow than norepinephrine and dopamine without significant change in PCO_2 gap. Moreover, De Backer et al. [14] did not observe any variation in PCO_2 gap during epinephrine infusion using air tonometry. Conversely, also using air tonometry, we have frequently observed (personal data) a decrease in PCO_2 gap in the early phase of septic shock when using epinephrine as a first line agent. It is our hypothesis that the improvement in arterial pressure and oxygen delivery induced by epinephrine in severely hypotensive patients may offset the putative deleterious effects on mucosal oxygenation.

Summary: Epinephrine inconsistently increases PCO_2 gap in septic shock.

Epinephrine Decreases Splanchnic Blood Flow and Increases the SvO_2-ShO_2 Gradient

Epinephrine decreases splanchnic blood flow, with transient increases in arterial, splanchnic, and hepatic venous lactate concentrations. The reduction in splanchnic blood flow has been associated with a decrease in oxygen delivery and a reduction in oxygen consumption [15]. These effects may be due to a reduction in splanchnic oxygen delivery to a level that impairs nutrient blood flow, likely resulting in a reduction in global tissue oxygenation, but may be potentially reversed by the concomitant administration of dobutamine. The addition of dobutamine to epinephrine-treated patients has been shown to improve gastric mucosal perfusion, as assessed by improvements in intramucosal pH (pHi), arterial lactate concentration, and PCO_2 gap [16]. It is not clear whether a transient decrease in hepatosplanchnic blood flow in septic shock is deleterious. The mucosa and the submucosa are known to receive most of splanchnic blood flow. Indocyanine green (ICG) clearance explores both splanchnic blood flow and liver function. De Backer et al. [14] compared epinephrine, norepinephrine, and dopamine titrated for the same MAP, using three different tools to evaluate splanchnic perfusion and splanchnic metabolism. Splanchnic perfusion was assessed by the following means:

▌ ICG clearance as a reflection of global hepatosplanchnic blood flow;
▌ hepatic venous oxygen saturation (ShO_2) and the gradient of mixed venous oxygen saturation (SvO_2) and ShO_2 as a reflection of the balance between splanchnic oxygen delivery and oxygen consumption; and
▌ gastric PCO_2 gap as a reflection of gastric mucosa perfusion/metabolism adequacy.

The authors concluded that in patients who responded to dopamine, no differences were found with regard to splanchnic effects. On the other hand, in nine of ten cases of dopamine-resistant septic shock, epinephrine when associated with dobutamine, decreased hepatosplanchnic blood flow, increased SvO_2-ShO_2 gradient, and increased arterial lactate and hepatic lactate consumption without any net effect on PCO_2 gap, which may also indicate a constant blood flow in the mucosa. Moreover, the absence of variation in PCO_2 gap argues against a deleterious effect of epinephrine on splanchnic circulation since the gut mucosa is probably the area of the body most sensitive to a decrease in blood flow. In various animal models, a decrease in splanchnic blood flow is associated with an increase in PCO_2 gap. The more likely explanation is that the energetic cost of metabolic processes induced by epinephrine such as neoglucogenesis and lactate consumption decreases the ability of the liver to metabolize ICG. Nevertheless, metabolizing ICG is not a natural process. Because epinephrine does not decrease liver lactate consumption, liver energy equilibrium is likely to remain stable.

On the other hand, in patients with septic shock, at doses that induced the same MAP, Seguin et al. [17] demonstrated that epinephrine did not modify ICG clearance and enhanced gastric mucosal blood flow more than the combination of dobutamine at 5 μg/kg per minute and norepinephrine.

Moreover, the effects of epinephrine may be different according to the studied area. Duranteau et al. [13], using laser Doppler flow, demonstrated that epinephrine induced higher gastric mucosal blood flow than norepinephrine without any significant changes in pHi. Thus, it is likely that despite a relative decrease in splanchnic blood flow in the epinephrine-treated patient, the gut mucosa receives sufficient blood flow to meet its metabolic needs. In fact, epinephrine exerts both sides of its β-2 properties: a redistribution of blood flow from the splanchnic bed to the muscular bed, and a redistribution of splanchnic flow towards the mucosa.

Summary: In dopamine resistant septic shock, epinephrine inconsistently decreases global splanchnic blood flow. The clinical significance of this is as yet unknown.

▌ Limitation of Splanchnic Blood Flow Estimation

The clarification of the role of epinephrine in septic patients is somewhat limited by the few techniques currently available to estimate splanchnic tissue oxygenation, in addition to each of these techniques having its own limitations. The ICG method used by De Backer et al. and other teams for splanchnic blood flow determination actually measures liver venous blood flow, which fails to distinguish supply from the portal vein and the hepatic artery. Consequently, changes in distribution of blood flow between the muscularis and the mucosa of the gut are not detectable by this method. Tonometric measurement raises the same types of concern because it only represents flow conditions in the gastric region. It has been shown, at least in an animal model, that changes in blood flow to the various organs in the splanchnic region are quite variable following induction of sepsis. An increase in SvO_2-ShO_2 gradient signifies that the splanchnic area consumes more oxygen than the rest of the body. It does not mean that the splanchnic area is hypoxic.

▌ Other Properties of Epinephrine

Epinephrine decreases kalemia. This characteristic is of importance in patients with shock and hyperkalemia. We have observed dramatic increases in potassium levels after switching epinephrine for norepinephrine. The hemodynamic effects of epinephrine (MAP and cardiac index increase) were obtained without the adjunction of dobutamine conversely to norepinephrine. This may prove to be important from a practical standpoint in situations such as transportation.

▮ Does the Choice of Catecholamine Influence Patient Evolution and Prognosis?

Currently, there is no prospective randomized clinical study indicating that one catecholamine is superior to the other during septic shock. A recent meta-analysis by the Cochrane group [18] failed to demonstrate any difference between tested vasopressors. Furthermore, no study has demonstrated a relationship between improvement in PCO_2 gap or ICG clearance after pharmacological intervention and an improvement in prognosis. Thus, all current data regarding the splanchnic effects of catecholamine should be considered as pharmacological investigations of a vasoactive agent evaluated by a particular monitoring device. The discrepancy observed between all of these measurements further highlights the absence of clinical relevance.

▮ Catecholamine Use is not only Limited to Specialized ICUs

The initial choice of catecholamine in the ICU is relatively well standardized, at least for hyperkinetic septic shock. Hemodynamic evaluation is easy and accessible (even if the type of monitoring remains debatable) with the choice of catecholamine based on rational evaluation. This is not the case for many situations in other clinical settings. For example, catecholamines are used on the ward, during transportation, in the emergency room, and even in the patient's home. Physicians are often young and/or with little experience in ICU treatment. Diagnosis is not always straightforward and in some cases it may be difficult to distinguish between cardiogenic, hypovolemic or septic shock. In these particular circumstances, it seems more appropriate to use a catecholamine with predictable effects such as epinephrine rather than a strong vasoconstrictor such as norepinephrine.

▮ Conclusion

Two opposite points of view are proposed. First, why should we use epinephrine, a drug with such potentially negative effects, when there are other alternatives in the treatment of septic patients On the other hand, epinephrine is commonly used worldwide, and reported morbidity and mortality rates are no different from those observed with other vasopressors. A French study comparing epinephrine and norepinephrine-dobutamine is currently in progress and may help us to decide whether Dr. Jekyll or Mr. Hyde represents the true nature of epinephrine in the treatment of septic shock [19].

References

1. Hollenberg SM, Ahrens TS, Annane D, et al (2004) Practice parameters for hemodynamic support of sepsis in adult patients: 2004 update. Crit Care Med 32:1928–1948
2. Rudis MI, Basha MA, Zarowitz BJ (1996) Is it time to reposition vasopressors and inotropes in sepsis? Crit Care Med 24:525–537
3. Bearn AG, Billing B, Sherlock S (1951) The effect of adrenaline and noradrenaline on hepatic blood flow and splanchnic carbohydrate metabolism in man. J Physiol 115:430–441

4. Ensinger H, Weichel T, Lindner KH, Grunert A, Georgieff M (1995) Are the effects of nor-adrenaline, adrenaline and dopamine infusions on VO2 and metabolism transient? Intensive Care Med 21:50–56
5. Wilson W, Lipman J, Scribante J, et al (1992) Septic shock: does adrenaline have a role as a first-line inotropic agent? Anaesth Intensive Care 20:470–474
6. Moran JL, O'Fathartaigh MS, Peisach AR, Chapman MJ, Leppard P (1993) Epinephrine as an inotropic agent in septic shock: a dose-profile analysis. Crit Care Med 21:70–77
7. Le Tulzo Y, Seguin P, Gacouin A, et al (1997) Effects of epinephrine on right ventricular function in patients with severe septic shock and right ventricular failure: a preliminary descriptive study. Intensive Care Med 23:664–670
8. Levy B, Bollaert PE, Charpentier C, et al (1997) Comparison of norepinephrine and dobutamine to epinephrine for hemodynamics, lactate metabolism, and gastric tonometric variables in septic shock: a prospective, randomized study. Intensive Care Med 23:282–287
9. Levy B, Mansart A, Bollaert PE, Franck P, Mallie JP (2003) Effects of epinephrine and norepinephrine on hemodynamics, oxidative metabolism, and organ energetics in endotoxemic rats. Intensive Care Med 29:292–300
10. James JH, Luchette FA, McCarter FD, Fischer JE (1999) Lactate is an unreliable indicator of tissue hypoxia in injury or sepsis. Lancet 354:505–508
11. Levy B, Gawalkiewicz P, Vallet B, Briancon S, Nace L, Bollaert PE (2003) Gastric capnometry with air-automated tonometry predicts outcome in critically ill patients. Crit Care Med 31:474–480
12. Chapman MV, Mythen MG, Webb AR, Vincent JL (2000) Report from the meeting: Gastrointestinal Tonometry: State of the Art. 22nd–23rd May 1998, London, UK. Intensive Care Med 26:613–622
13. Duranteau J, Sitbon P, Teboul JL, et al (1999) Effects of epinephrine, norepinephrine, or the combination of norepinephrine and dobutamine on gastric mucosa in septic shock. Crit Care Med 27:893–900
14. De Backer D, Creteur J, Silva E, Vincent JL (2003) Effects of dopamine, norepinephrine, and epinephrine on the splanchnic circulation in septic shock: which is best? Crit Care Med 31:1659–1667
15. Meier-Hellmann A, Reinhart K, Bredle DL, Specht M, Spies CD, Hannemann L (1997) Epinephrine impairs splanchnic perfusion in septic shock. Crit Care Med 25:399–404
16. Levy B, Bollaert PE, Lucchelli JP, Sadoune LO, Nace L, Larcan A (1997) Dobutamine improves the adequacy of gastric mucosal perfusion in epinephrine-treated septic shock. Crit Care Med 25:1649–1654
17. Seguin P, Bellissant E, Le Tulzo Y, et al (2002) Effects of epinephrine compared with the combination of dobutamine and norepinephrine on gastric perfusion in septic shock. Clin Pharmacol Ther 71:381–388
18. Mullner M, Urbanek B, Havel C, Losert H, Waechter F, Gamper G (2004) Vasopressors for shock. Cochrane Database Syst Rev CD003709
19. Levy B (2003) Epinephrine in septic shock: Dr. Jekyll or Mr. Hyde? Crit Care Med 31:1866–1867

Resuscitation

New Options for Pharmacological Management of Cardiac Resuscitation

M. H. Weil, W. Tang, and S. Sun

▌ Introduction

Cardiovascular disease continues to be the leading cause of death in the Western world [1]. In the United States, approximately one half of the 2 million deaths each year are due to cardiovascular disease. Of these deaths, approximately one-third or 350,000 occur suddenly and outside of the hospital. Thus, each minute, one person is the victim of 'sudden (cardiac) death' in the United States, and almost one half of the victims are under 65 years of age [2]. The huge human and economic costs are equivalent to the fatal crash of two 747 aircraft each day and are therefore self-evident [3].

Though the initial success of cardiopulmonary resuscitation (CPR) is approximately 39% (range 13 to 59%), a majority of victims die within 72 hours, primarily due to heart failure and/or recurrent ventricular fibrillation (VF). CPR itself therefore yields a functional survival rate of only 1.4 to 5% [4–7].

A major commitment of our group has been on myocardial function after successful resuscitation from cardiac arrest. After resuscitation following an interval of 3 min or more of untreated cardiac arrest, 'post-resuscitation myocardial dysfunction' is observed. Our group first identified this phenomenon in rats and subsequently in pigs [8, 9]. The same phenomenon, namely, profound but reversible myocardial failure after resuscitation from cardiac arrest, has been documented in human victims [5, 6].

The magnitude of the problem of post resuscitation myocardial dysfunction and its often fatal outcome has been further documented in multicenter studies on human victims. In the Brain Resuscitation Clinical Trial I [10], 262 victims were successfully resuscitated. Approximately 70% died within the first 72 hours after hospital admission. During the first 8 hours after resuscitation, 45% of patients manifested arterial hypotension, 26% supraventricular and ventricular arrhythmias, and 25% recurrent cardiac arrest as a primary event. In the Brain Resuscitation Clinical Trial II [4], 516 patients were resuscitated and 62% of the patients died within the first week. During the first 24 hours, 65% of the resuscitated patients had systemic hypotension.

In studies on high-dose epinephrine in 6 emergency centers that enrolled 1280 victims of out-of-hospital cardiac arrests, 32% of patients were initially resuscitated [5]. Though 10% of these patients died prior to admission to the hospital, 43% of the remaining victims died during the first 72 hours. Arterial hypotension and fatal ventricular arrhythmias were also identified as predominant causes. Only 4.5% of victims were discharged alive from the hospital. In a second multicenter study on high dose epinephrine, 650 victims of cardiac arrest were enrolled. Spontaneous circulation was initially restored in 21% of the victims. However, a majority of patients died within the first 48 hours after hospital admission and only 4% were discharged alive from the hospitals [6]. We view the reversible global myocardial injury following successful CPR as akin to myocardial stunning following reversible regional myocardial ischemic injury in settings of coronary artery occlusion. This may explain, at least in part, the high fatality rate due to ventricular arrhythmias and contractile failure within the initial 72 hours after successful resuscitation from cardiac arrest.

▌ Myocardial Oxygen Consumption and Metabolism During Cardiac Arrest

Unlike most other tissues, the myocardium predominately utilizes fatty acids as an energy source. Approximately 70% of the energy which provides for myocardial contraction is derived from oxidation of fatty acids. The resting coronary blood flow in the human averages about 225 ml/min, which is approximately 0.8 ml/g/min of heart muscle. During the resting state, the ATP content is approximately 20 µmol/g dry weight and the myocardial oxygen consumption is 5 mmol/hr/g dry weight. The heart regenerates its entire ATP pool every 5 seconds [11]. Therefore the energy reserve of the myocardium is very small under physiological conditions.

During global myocardial ischemia following cardiac arrest, fatty acid oxidation ceases. Cardiac function is now dependent on anaerobic glycolysis. This emergency pathway provides only about 5% of the energy normally produced by oxidation of glucose. Consequently, the energy requirements of the fibrillating heart rapidly exceed availability. All residual ATP is hydrolyzed and anaerobically generated lactate accounts for excesses of protons and specifically H^+ [12]. The excesses of H^+ are buffered by intracellular bicarbonate such that myocardial PCO_2 is strikingly increased. In initial studies on myocardial tissue PCO_2 in our Institute, the CO_2 tension increased from 45 to more than 350 mmHg and coronary venous lactate increased from 0.8 to more than 12 mmol/l during 7 min of untreated VF [13]. Pharmacological interventions, which either prevent rapid increases or produce rapid reductions of myocardial metabolism, would minimize ischemic injury and prevent or minimize post resuscitation myocardial dysfunction. These actions would be characterized by lesser increases in myocardial PCO_2 and H^+ and delayed fall of myocardial PO_2 [14, 15]. Our group is uniquely postured to use tissue PCO_2 and PO_2 measurements since we have pioneered this technology. Hypothermia has recently been demonstrated to improve neurological outcomes and post resuscitation survival [16].

Box 1. Suggested further related references for pharmacology in CPR

Becker LB, Ostrander MP, Barrett J, Kondos GT (1991) CPR Chicago: outcome of cardiopulmonary resuscitation in a large metropolitan area – where are the survivors? Ann Emerg Med 20:355–361

Bernard SA, Gray TW, Buist MD, et al (2002) Treatment of comatose survivors of out-of-hospital cardiac arrest with induced hypothermia. N Engl J Med 346:549–556

Brown CG, Werman HA (1990) Adrenergic agonists during cardiopulmonary resuscitation. Resuscitation 19:1–16

Bruce DS, Bailey EC, Setran DP, et al (1996) Circannual variations in bear plasma albumin and its opioid-like effects on guinea pig ileum. Pharmacol Biochem Behav 53:885–889

Chen CL, Chen L, Fallon JT, et al (1996) Functional and structural alterations with 24-hour myocardial hibernation and recovery after reperfusion. A pig model of myocardial hibernation. Circulation 94:507–516

Chien S, Maley R, Oeltgen PR, et al (1997) Canine lung transplantation after more than 24 hours of normothermic preservation. J Heart Lung Transplant 16:340–351

Haikala H, Kaivola J, Nissinen E, Wall P, Levijoki J, Lindén I-B (1995) Cardiac troponin C as a target protein for a novel calcium sensitizing drug, levosimendan. J Mol Cell Cardiol 27:1859–1866

Heusch G, Rose J, Skyschally A, Post H, Schulz R (1996) Calcium responsiveness in regional myocardial short-term hibernation and stunning in the in situ porcine heart: inotropic responses to postextrasystolic potentiation and intracoronary calcium. Circulation 93:1556–1566

Jennings RB, Hawkins HK, Lowe JE, Hill ML, Klotman S, Reimer KA (1978) Relation between high energy phosphate and lethal injury in myocardial ischemia in the dog. Am J Pathol 92:187–214

Link RE, Desai K, Hein L, et al (1996) Cardiovascular regulation in mice lacking α_2-adrenergic receptor subtypes b and c. Science (Wash DC) 273:803–805

Lomasney JW, Cotecchia S, Leftkowitz RJ, Caron MG (1991) Molecular biology of α-adrenergic receptors: implications for receptor classification and for structure-function relationships. Biochim Biophys Acta 1095:127–139

Maldonado FA, Weil MH, Tang W, et al (1993) Myocardial hypercarbic acidosis reduces cardiac resuscitability. Anesthesiology 78:343–352

McPherson BC, Yao Z (2001) Signal transduction of opioid-induced cardioprotection in ischemia-reperfusion. Anesthesiology 94:1082–1088

Oeltgen PR, Welborn JR, Nichols PA, Spurrier WA, Bruce DS, Su TP (1987) Opioids and hibernation. ii. Effects of kappa opioid u69593 on induction of hibernation in summer-active ground squirrels by "hibernation induction trigger" (HIT). Life Sci 41:2115–2120

Oeltgen PR, Horton ND, Bolling SF, Su TP (1996) Extended lung preservation with the use of hibernation trigger factors. Ann Thorac Surg 61:1488–1493

Pollesello P, Ovaska M, Kaivola J, et al (1994) Binding of a new Ca^{2+}-sensitizer, levosimendan, to recombinant human cardiac troponin C. J Biol Chem 269:28584–28590

Sorsa T, Heikkinen S, Abbott MB, et al (2001) Binding of levosimendan, a calcium sensitizer, to cardiac troponin C. J Biol Chem 276:9337–9343

Yokoshiki H, Katsube Y, Sunagawa M, Sperelakis N (1997) Levosimendan, a novel Ca^{2+} sensitizer, activates the glibenclamide-sensitive K^+ channel in rat arterial myocytes. Eur J Pharmacol 333:249–259

Yu LC, Cai YP (1993) Effects of opioid receptors antagonist administration to suprachiasmatic nucleus on hibernation of ground squirrels Citellus dauricus. Comparative Biochem Physiol – C: Comparative Pharmacol Toxicol 104(2):249–252

▌ Current Vasopressor Agents Increase the Severity of Myocardial Ischemia During CPR

The primary goal of the initial pharmacological intervention during CPR is to increase coronary perfusion pressure by increasing peripheral vascular resistance. Optimally, an adrenergic drug would maximize arterial blood flow to the coronary and cerebral circuits by increasing arterial pressure during chest compression. These benefits would be likely to accrue primarily from α-adrenergic agonists. Epinephrine is a powerful agonist of α_1-, β_2-, β_1- and α_2-adrenergic receptors. It has been the preferred adrenergic agent for the treatment of human cardiac arrest for more than 40 years. There is unequivocal evidence that its efficacy is due to its α-adrenergic vasopressor effects. Yet, adverse effects include the β- and α_1-adrenergic effects of epinephrine which increase both inotropic and chronotropic actions on the heart. As a result, these actions provoke disproportionate increases in myocardial oxygen consumption, especially during VF. Accordingly, it increases the demand of the globally ischemic myocardium for oxygen during cardiac arrest [17]. If the heart is resuscitated, greater ischemic injury accounts for greater post resuscitation myocardial dysfunction [5, 6].

Epinephrine increases myocardial lactate concentration and decreases myocardial ATP content even though coronary blood flow may be doubled [18]. Epinephrine also increases the severity of post resuscitation myocardial dysfunction and decreases post resuscitation survival when compared with epinephrine combined with the β_1-blocking agent, esmolol [17]. Epinephrine increases the incidence of ventricular arrhythmias, ventricular tachycardia (VT) and (recurrent) VF. These ventricular arrhythmias were significantly decreased after β-adrenergic blockade. Epinephrine also produces pulmonary ventilation/perfusion defects and therefore increases pulmonary arteriovenous admixture with decreases in arterial oxygen tension and increases in arterial CO_2 tension with decreases in end-tidal PCO_2 [19].

In the most recent guidelines for CPR [1], a non-adrenergic vasopressor agent, vasopressin, is recommended as an alternative for epinephrine. Unfortunately, the long half-life of the agent produces persistent arterial vasoconstriction following successful resuscitation. This is associated with even more severe post-resuscitation myocardial dysfunction than epinephrine in the early hours after restoration of spontaneous circulation [20]. In pigs, post-resuscitation systemic vascular resistance (SVR) of the vasopressin group is two-fold greater than that of the epinephrine group. This explains the significantly lower cardiac output and reduced myocardial contractility in the first 4 hours following successful resuscitation under experimental conditions. A recent study failed to document survival benefit for vasopressin during CPR [21].

With the recognized limitations of epinephrine for the management of cardiac resuscitation, including the adverse β- and to a lesser extent α_1-adrenergic effects together with the potential limitations of vasopressin, our group has focused on more selective adrenergic agonists. This prompted our trials with selective α_2-adrenoceptor agonists. Three subtypes of α_2-receptors are now identified, namely α_{2A}, α_{2B}, and α_{2C}. Alpha$_{2A}$-agonists like clonidine, acting centrally on the medulla, mediate a tonic sympatho-inhibitory effect accounting for reductions in arterial blood pressure, myocardial contractility, and heart rate. This contrasts with α_{2B} peripheral vasoconstrictor actions. Alpha$_{2B}$ subtype receptors, which are less abundant in brain tissue, provoke a predominant peripheral vasoconstrictor response [22]. A third receptor, namely a_{2C}, has a predominant central nervous system effect like a_{2A}, but its cardiovascular actions are not as yet well defined [23].

Since a_2-adrenoceptor agonists have centrally acting vasodilator effects and peripherally acting vasoconstrictor effects, it is only the peripheral action that is of moment in the initial management of cardiac arrest. We therefore sought a selective a_2-agonist, which does not gain entry into the brain. It is in this context that we demonstrated that one selective a_2-agonist, a-methylnorepinephrine (aMNE), is as effective as epinephrine for initial cardiac resuscitation but without the a_1- or β-effects by which myocardial oxygen consumption is increased. Accordingly, adverse effects on post-resuscitation myocardial function and survival are avoided [24]. In addition, there is evidence that a_2-adrenergic agonists increase endothelial nitric oxide (NO) production which mitigates endogenous a-adrenergic vasoconstrictor effects on coronary arteries and thereby potentially improves coronary blood flow [25].

When we compared aMNE to epinephrine in a rat model of cardiac arrest and resuscitation, aMNE significantly improved the likelihood of initial resuscitation, post-resuscitation myocardial function and survival. The incidence of post-resuscitation ventricular arrhythmias was strikingly reduced [24]. We then compared the effects of aMNE on post-resuscitation myocardial function with vasopressin. We again demonstrated that myocardial function was significantly better in animals treated with aMNE [26]. Based on these preliminary studies, we recognize that the selective a_2-adrenergic agonist has the following advantages for CPR: (1) the oxygen requirements of the fibrillating heart are not increased and therefore the severity of myocardial ischemic injury is lessened; (2) post synaptic a_2-adrenergic receptors do not desensitize during systemic ischemia in contrast to a_1-adrenergic receptors, allowing for more persistent vasoconstriction; (3) increases in endothelial NO production in the coronary circuit after a_2 stimulation favor improved coronary blood flow.

▌ Myocardial Hibernation Produced by Opioid Receptor Activation as an Option for Minimizing Ischemic Injury

Hibernation is a seasonal state in black bears, woodchucks, and ground squirrels. The metabolic change is triggered by climatic conditions. Hibernation is associated with striking increases in endogenous opiate concentration in serum [27]. The transition from wakeful to somnolent states is traced to opiate agonists acting on receptors in the brain [28]. Systemic temperature is significantly reduced. This is associated with a dramatic reduction in myocardial oxygen consumption and energy production. Accordingly, hibernating animals consume less than 10% of systemic oxygen when contrasted with the pre-hibernating state [29]. It is to this extent that the term 'hibernation' has made its way into medical settings in which there is a reduction in myocardial metabolic rate and therefore oxygen demand when the temperature is normal. It is in this physiological setting that marked reductions in perfusion and oxygen delivery to the heart do not produce myocardial ischemic injury. Accordingly, we have addressed the concept of opioid-mediated 'hibernation' in settings of cardiac arrest and resuscitation.

Three unique classes of opioid receptors have been identified in the central nervous system. These are designated δ, κ, and μ. Moreover, subtypes have more recently been identified for each class of receptor. Each receptor group has a discrete pharmacological profile [30]. Hibernation appears to be mediated predominantly by the δ-class of receptors, and more specifically δ_1 and δ_2 receptors [31, 32].

Experimental observations support the concept of myocardial hibernation. In isolated saline-perfused rat hearts, a 40% reduction in coronary perfusion was followed by a 30% decrease in left ventricular systolic pressure, dP/dt, and oxygen consumption. This reduced perfusion was adequate for sustaining myocardial metabolism such that there was no evidence of myocardial ischemia with lactate production [33]. When a coronary artery was partially occluded in pigs, lactate extraction was reduced. The coronary venous effluent had increased concentrations of H^+ and CO_2. Yet, both acidosis and hypercarbia gradually returned to control values during the subsequent 180 min of reduced coronary blood flow [34]. Metabolic adjustments to reduced coronary blood flow were also confirmed by Arai et al. [35], Chen et al. [36], and Heusch [37]. The evidence is persuasive that significant reductions in coronary blood flow prompt a protective mechanism by which there is a downregulation of regional oxygen consumption in the myocardium such that the myocardium is protected against ischemic injury while systemic temperature is kept normal. This downregulation of regional oxygen consumption after coronary occlusion has recently been explained by activation of the δ-opiate receptors [31].

In a recent study on isolated perfused rabbit hearts, Benedict et al. [31] administered opiates as a pharmacological option akin to that of myocardial hibernation. Post-ischemic myocardial mechanical function was significantly improved in hearts pretreated with the δ-opiate agonists, beprenorphrine and pentazocine. Histologically, the hearts treated with the δ-opiate agonists maintained ultrastructural integrity when compared with untreated controls. The evidence supported the concept that myocardial hibernation is mediated by δ-opiate receptors.

There are distinctive roles of δ_1- and δ_2-opioid receptor activation for myocardial protection. In a rat model of regional myocardial ischemia, Fryer et al. [38] demonstrated that after 30 min of coronary artery occlusion and 2 hours reperfusion, the infarct size was significantly reduced from 60% to 37% in animals treated with the δ-opioid receptor agonist, DADLE. Interestingly, this protective effect was completely abolished by a selective δ_1- but not a δ_2-opioid receptor antagonist. In both rat and rabbit isolated heart preparations, Kato and Foex [39] and Bolling et al. [40] independently demonstrated that activation of δ_1-opioid receptor reduced infarct size but did not improve post-ischemic myocardial function. However, a selective δ_2-antagonist completely abolished the improved post-ischemic myocardial mechanical function that followed opioid activation. These studies, together with our preliminary studies pinpointed the potential role of δ-opioid receptor agonists for myocardial protection during global myocardial ischemia of cardiac arrest and resuscitation.

∎ The Potential Role of Myocardial Calcium Sensitizers for the Treatment of Post-resuscitation Myocardial Dysfunction

Though post-resuscitation myocardial dysfunction is associated with poor outcomes following cardiac arrest, there are currently no optimal strategies for restoring post-resuscitation myocardial function following resuscitation from cardiac arrest. In a porcine model of cardiac arrest and resuscitation, Dr. Kern and his colleagues demonstrated that high dose dobutamine but not intra-aortic balloon counterpulsation restored myocardial systolic and diastolic functions after prolonged cardiac arrest [41, 42]. The duration of survival, however, was not addressed. In addition, activation of β-adrenergic receptors by dobutamine following successful resuscitation increases heart rate and myocardial oxygen consumption, and may further increase myocardial injury even though coronary perfusion may have been restored.

Because of these limitations in treatment, our group has investigated the effects of levosimendan on post-resuscitation myocardial dysfunction and duration of survival. Levosimendan, a myocardial calcium sensitizer, restored post-resuscitation myocardial function through two different mechanisms. The predominant mechanism of action is traced to calcium sensitization of the contractile proteins in myocardium. This effect is obtained by calcium-dependent binding of the drug to cardiac troponin C. Due to the calcium dependency, levosimendan does not impair relaxation as is the case with β-adrenergic agonists. For the same reason, its positive inotropic effect is associated with little chronotropic effect. Secondly, levosimendan opens up K-ATP channels, both in vascular and in cardiac muscle. As demonstrated by others and us it has both afterload reduction and anti-ischemic effects [43].

Cardiac muscle contraction is controlled by the calcium-induced change in troponin C. Levosimendan binds selectively to calcium saturated cardiac troponin C. This binding stabilizes the conformation of troponin C, which triggers contraction. Most importantly, levosimendan does not affect myosin ATPase activity [44]. Its positive inotropic effect is therefore not associated with increased crossbridge cycling rate and coincident increases in myocardial oxygen consumption [45].

The positive inotropic and lusitropic effects have been demonstrated in isolated blood perfused normal and failing canine hearts [46], in isolated perfused guinea pig hearts [47], and in ventricular muscle strips obtained from human hearts with end-stage heart failure [45]. In addition, levosimendan produced only a small increase in the automaticity of the sino-atrial node, the A-V junctional area and the Purkinje fibers of the rabbit hearts. Its inotropic effect is therefore not accompanied by electrical instability and alterations of rhythmicity.

In a dog model of regional myocardial ischemia, levosimendan significantly improved both systolic and diastolic myocardial functions without significant changes in heart rate, left ventricular diastolic pressure, and oxygen consumption [48]. Similar results were also observed in preliminary studies in human patients (Kleber F et al. personal communication) and by our group in a rat and a pig model of global myocardial ischemia. The anti-ischemic effect of levosimendan was also demonstrated recently in a dog model of regional myocardial ischemia. A 50% reduction of infarct size followed administration of levosimendan [49].

▌ Benefits of Adrenergic Blocking Agents

The potential beneficial effects of activating the α_2- and blocking the β-adrenergic receptors, either exogenously or endogenously during CPR, were initially investigated in a rat model of cardiac arrest and resuscitation. Seven groups of Sprague-Dawley rats were randomized to receive:

▌ epinephrine combined with the selective α_1-blocking agent, prazocine, and non-selective β-blocking agent, propranolol;
▌ epinephrine combined with non-selective β-blocking agent, propranolol;
▌ epinephrine combined with selective α_1-blocking agent, prazocine;
▌ epinephrine combined with selective α_2-blocking agent, yohimbine;
▌ saline placebo combined with non-selective β-blocking agent, propranolol;
▌ saline placebo combined with selective α_1-blocking agent, prazocine; and
▌ saline placebo combined with selective α_2-blocking agent, yohimbine.

The blocking agents were administered 15 min prior to inducing VF. VF remained untreated for 4 min. CPR, including mechanical ventilation and precordial compression, was initiated after 4 min of untreated VF and continued for 8 min. Either epinephrine or saline placebo was administered at 2 min after start of CPR. CPR was continued for an additional 6 min followed by a 2-J DC electrical shock. If VF was not reversed, a second 2-J DC shock was delivered. Each animal was restored to spontaneous circulation. Myocardial function was impaired significantly in all animals following successful resuscitation. However, the severity of post-resuscitation myocardial dysfunction was significantly reduced in animals pre-treated with β- and/or α_1-adrenergic blocking agents. This was associated with a significantly increased duration of post resuscitation survival. All animals pre-treated with both β- and α_1-adrenergic blocking agents survived for more than 72 hours.

We then investigated the beneficial effects of an α_2-agonist in our porcine model of CPR. Three groups of 5 male domestic pigs weighing 37 ± 3 kg were investigated. VF was untreated for 7 min prior to start of precordial compression, mechanical ventilation, and attempted defibrillation. Animals were randomized to receive central venous injections of equipressor doses of:

▌ epinephrine;
▌ epinephrine in which both α_1- and β-adrenergic effects were blocked by prior administration of prazosin and propranolol; and
▌ vasopressin during CPR.

All but one animal was successfully resuscitated. After α_1- and β-adrenergic blockade, epinephrine produced significantly better cardiac output and fractional area change, together with lesser increases in troponin-I. Post-resuscitation neurological function was also improved after α_1- and β-block in comparison with both unblocked epinephrine and vasopressin. We therefore demonstrated in two animal models that combined α_1- and β-adrenergic blockade, leaving relatively selective α_2-vasopressor agonist effects, resulted in improved post-resuscitation cardiac and neurological recovery and prolongation of survival.

▌ Conclusion

There are presently no pharmacological interventions for management of cardiac arrest that are of proven clinical benefit for ultimate survival. Epinephrine in conventional doses increases initial success of resuscitation but there is persuasive evidence that it compromises post-resuscitation survival. To the contrary, there is increasing evidence that it is the selective α_2-agonist action that has the dual advantage of improving initial resuscitation and yet minimizing the post resuscitation adverse effect of β- and α_1-adrenergic agonists. There has been increasing experimental evidence over more than two decades that the administration of β-adrenergic blocking agents prior to or during CPR may itself be beneficial. The rationale is to minimize adrenergically primed increases in tissue ischemia and especially myocardial ischemia. The anticipated benefits of vasopressin for survival have not been realized and we suspect adverse effects of the increased afterload induced by its prolonged action.

The effort to minimize tissue ischemia during the low or no flow interval prompted research into 'hibernation' beginning with myocardial preservation. This led to investigations of opioid receptor agonists. It is a promising but not as yet well explored option for reducing the severity of tissue injury during the hypoxia of the no flow or low flow state.

Finally, the initial laboratory and clinical findings with levosimendan have been encouraging. It is likely to emerge as a major inotrope with the advantage that it does not increase myocardial oxygen demand and therefore avoids any additional ischemic injury.

References

1. American Heart Association (2000) Guidelines 2000 for Cardiopulmonary resuscitation and emergency cardiovascular care. Circulation 102:I-1–I-380
2. American Heart Association (1992) Heart and Stroke Facts. AHA, Dallas
3. Weil MH, Becker L, Budinger T, et al (2001) Workshop Executive Summary report: post-resuscitative and initial utility in life saving efforts (PULSE). Circulation 103:1182–1184
4. Brain Resuscitation Clinical Trial II Study Group (1991) A randomized clinical study of a calcium-entry blocker (lidoflazine) in the treatment of comatose survivors of cardiac arrest. N Engl J Med 324:1125–1231
5. Brown CG, Martin DR, Pepe PE (1992) A comparison of standard-dose and high-dose epinephrine in cardiac arrest outside the hospital. N Engl J Med 327:1051–1055
6. Stiell IG, Herbert PC, Weitzman BN (1992) High-dose epinephrine in adult cardiac arrest. N Engl J Med 327:1045–1050
7. Lombardi G, Gallagher J, Gennis P (1994) Outcome of out-of-hospital cardiac arrest in New York City: the Pre-hospital Arrest Survival Evaluation (PHASE) study. JAMA 271:678–683
8. Tang W, Weil MH, Sun SJ, Gazmuri RJ, Bisera J, Rackow EC (1993) Progressive myocardial dysfunction after cardiac resuscitation. Crit Care Med 21:1046–1050
9. Gazmuri RJ, Weil MH, Bisera J, Tang W, Fukui M, McKee D (1996) Myocardial dysfunction after successful resuscitation from cardiac arrest. Crit Care Med 24:992–1000
10. Brain Resuscitation Clinical Trial I Study Group (1986) A randomized clinical study of thiopental loading in comatose survivors of cardiac arrest. N Engl J Med 314:397–403
11. Depre C, Taegtmeyer H (2000) Metabolic aspects of programmed cell survival and cell death in the heart. Cardiovasc Res 45:538–548.
12. Katz AM, Reuter H (1979) Cellular calcium and myocardial cell death. Am J Cardiol 44:188–190
13. Kette F, Weil MH, Gazmuri RJ, Bisera J, Rackow EC (1993) Intramyocardial hypercarbic acidosis during cardiac arrest and resuscitation. Crit Care Med 21:901–906
14. Weil MH, Tang W (1997) Cardiopulmonary resuscitation: A promise as yet largely unfulfilled. Disease-A-Month 43:429–504
15. Tang W, Weil MH, Sun SJ, Pernat A, Mason E (2000) Ischemic preconditioning improves post resuscitation myocardial dysfunction: the role of KATP channel activation. Am J Physiol 279:H1609–H1615
16. Hypothermia after Cardiac Arrest Study Group (2002) Mild therapeutic hypothermia to improve the neurologic outcome after cardiac arrest. N Engl J Med 346:549–556
17. Tang W, Weil MH, Sun S, Noc M, Yang L, Gazmuri RJ (1995) Epinephrine increases the severity of postresuscitation myocardial dysfunction. Circulation 92:3089–3093
18. Ditchey RV, Lindenfeld JA (1988) Failure of epinephrine to improve the balance between oxygen supply and demand during closed-chest resuscitation in dogs. Circulation 78:382–389
19. Tang W, Weil MH, Gazmuri RJ, Sun S, Duggal C, Bisera J (1991) Pulmonary ventilation/perfusion defects induced by epinephrine during cardiopulmonary resuscitation. Circulation 84:2101–2107
20. Prengel AW, Lindner KH, Keller A, Lurie KG (1996) Cardiovascular function during the post-resuscitation phase after cardiac arrest in pigs: A comparison of epinephrine versus vasopressin. Crit Care Med 24:2014–2019
21. Wenzel V, Krismer AC, Arntz HR, Sitter H, Stadlbauer KH, Lindner KH (2004) A comparison of vasopressin and epinephrine for out-of-hospital cardiopulmonary resuscitation. N Engl J Med 350:105–113

22. Kable JW, Murrin LC, Bylund DB (2000) In vivo gene modification elucidates subtype-specific function of a_2-adrenergic receptors. J Pharmacol Exper Ther 293(1):1
23. Gavras I, Gavras H (2001) Role of alpha$_2$-adrenergic receptors in hypertension. Am J Hypertens 14:171S–177S
24. Sun S, Weil MH, Tang W, Kamohara T, Klouche K (2001) Alpha-methylnorepinephrine, a selective alpha$_2$-adrenergic agonist for cardiac resuscitation. J Am Coll Cardiol 37:951–956
25. Ishibashi Y, Duncker DJ, Bache RJ (1997) Endogenous nitric oxide masks alpha$_2$-adrenergic coronary vasoconstriction during exercise in the ischemic heart. Circ Res 80:196
26. Klouche K, Weil MH, Tang W, Povoas H, Kamohara T, Bisera J (2002) A selective a-adrenergic agonist for cardiac resuscitation. J Lab Clin Med 140:27–34
27. Bruce DS, Bailey EC, Crane SK, Oeltgen PR, Horton ND, Harlow HJ (1997) Hibernation-induction trigger. I. Opioid-like effects of prairie dog plasma albumin on induced contractility of guinea pig ileum. Pharmacol Biochem Behav 58:621–625
28. Bourhim N, Elkebbaj MS, Ouafik L, Chautard TH, Giraud P, Oliver C (1993) Opioid binding sites in jerboa (Jaculus orientalis) brain: a biochemical comparative study in the awake-active and induced hibernating states. Comparative Biochem Physiol – B: Comparative Biochem 104:607–615
29. Wang LCH (1997) Energetic and field aspects of mammalian torpor in the Richardson's ground squirrel. In: Wang LCH, Hudson JW (eds) Strategies in Cold: Natural Torpidity and Thermogenesis. Academic Press, New York, pp 109–145
30. Clark JA, Liu L, Price M, Hersh B, Edelson M, Pasternak GW (1989) Kappa opiate receptor multiplicity: evidence for two U50,488-sensitive kappa 1 subtypes and a novel kappa 3 subtype. J Pharmacol Exp Ther 251:461–468
31. Benedict PE, Benedict MB, Su TP, Bolling SF (1999) Opiate drugs and delta-receptor-mediated myocardial protection. Circulation 100:357–360
32. Sigg DC, Coles JA, Jr., Oeltgen PR, Iaizzo PA (2002) Role of delta-opioid receptor agonists on infarct size reduction in swine. Am J Physiol Heart Circ Physiol 282:H1953–H1960
33. Keller AM, Cannon PJ, Wolny AC (1991) Effect of graded reductions of coronary pressure and flow on myocardial metabolism and performance: a model of "hibernating" myocardium. J Am Coll Cardiol 17:1661–1670
34. Fedele FA, Gewirtz H, Capone RJ, Sharaf B, Most AS (1988) Metabolic response to prolonged reduction of myocardial blood flow distal to a severe coronary artery stenosis. Circulation 78:729–735
35. Arai AE, Pantely GA, Anselone CG, Bristow, Bristow JD (1991) Active downregulation of myocardial energy requirements during prolonged moderate ischemia in swine. Circ Res 69:1458–1469
36. Chen CL, Ma L, Dyckman W, et al (1997) Left ventricular remodeling in myocardial hibernation. Circulation 96 (Suppl II): II46–II50
37. Heusch G (1998) Hibernation myocardium. Physiol Rev 78:1055–1085
38. Fryer RM, Wang Y, Hsu AK, Gross G (2001) Essential activation of PKC-d in opioid-initiated cardioprotection. Am J Physiol 280:H1346–H1353
39. Kato R, Foex P (2000) Fentanyl reduces infarction but not stunning via d-opioid receptors and protein kinase C in rats. Br J Anaesth 84:608–614
40. Bolling SF, Badhwar V, Schwartz CF, Oeltgen PR, Kilgore K, Su TP (2001) Opioids confer myocardial tolerance to ischemia: Interaction of delta opioid agonists and antagonists. J Thorac Cardiovasc Surg 122:476–481
41. Kern KB, Hilwig RW, Berg RA, et al (1997) Postresuscitation left ventricular systolic and diastolic dysfunction. Treatment with dobutamine. Circulation 95:2611–2613
42. Tennyson H, Kern KB, Hilwig RW, Berg RA, Ewy GA (2002) Treatment of post resuscitation myocardial dysfunction: aortic counterpulsation versus dobutamine. Resuscitation 54:69–75
43. Kopustinskiene DM, Pollesello P, Saris NEL (2001) Levosimendan is a mitochondrial KATP channel opener. Eur J Pharmacol 428:311–314
44. Haikala H, Levijoki J, Linden I-B (1995) Troponin C-mediated calcium sensitization by levosimendan accelerates the proportional development of isometric tension. J Mol Cell Cardiol 27:2155–2165

45. Hasenfuss G, Pieske B, Castell M, Kretschman B, Maier L, Hanjörg J (1998) Influence of the novel inotropic agent levosimendan on isometric tension and calcium cycling in failing human myocardium Circulation 98:2142–2147
46. Todaka K, Wang J, Yi GH, et al (1996) Effects of levosimendan on myocardial contractility and oxygen consumption. J Pharmacol Exp Ther 279:120–127
47. Haikala H, Kaheinen P, Levijoki J, Linden I-B (1997) The role of cAMP- and cGMP-dependent protein kinases in the cardiac actions of the new calcium sensitizer, levosimendan. Cardiovasc Res 34:536–546
48. Jamali IN, KerstenJR, Pagel PS, Hettrick DA, Warltier DC (1997) Intracoronary levosimendan enhances contractile function of stunned myocardium. Anesth Analg 85:23–29
49. Kersten JR, Montgomery MW, Pagel PS, Warltier DC (2000) Levosimendan, a new positive inotropic drug, decreases myocardial infarct size via activation of KATP channels. Anesth Analg 90:5–11

Cardiopulmonary Resuscitation (CPR) Instructions Provided by Emergency Medical Dispatchers

J. G. Wigginton, L. P. Roppolo, and P. E. Pepe

▌ Introduction

In the circumstance of out-of-hospital sudden cardiac death, basic cardiopulmonary resuscitation (CPR) will improve the patient's chance of surviving neurologically intact, particularly when provided immediately by witnessing bystanders [1–5]. Unfortunately, the frequency of bystander CPR remains low in most communities and, as a result, this shortcoming has become one of the major limiting steps in terms of improving outcomes following out-of-hospital sudden cardiac death [1, 6].

With the evolution of sophisticated dispatch programs for emergency medical services (EMS) systems in the 1970 and 80s, many communities developed a mechanism to provide medical care instructions over the telephone to bystanders at an emergency scene prior to arrival of professional responders [7–10]. In most venues, those so-called "pre-arrival instructions" included protocols to provide CPR directives over the telephone while awaiting the arrival of emergency responders [8–12]. Therefore, it has become an expectation, even by the public, that emergency medical dispatch (EMD) personnel receiving calls at public safety answering points (e.g., 911 telephone centers in the United States, 999 in Australia, and 113 in parts of Europe) will be trained to provide CPR pre-arrival instructions whenever applicable [12–14]. Such pre-arrival instructions have increased the frequency of bystander CPR and are believed to improve survival chances by increasing the number of persons receiving CPR and by facilitating earlier intervention [11, 13, 15].

Although based on most of the same science and subsequent standardized protocols originally developed for bystander CPR [15], it has become clear that dispatch CPR pre-arrival instructions need to be somewhat different considering the non-visual, logistical and unique emotional aspects of gaining accurate, instantaneous telephone assessments of the situation in critical emergencies [16, 17]. Also, expeditious and unemotional compliance with multiple directives (moving the unresponsive patient onto a hard surface, opening an airway, providing rescue breathing and chest compressions) can be extremely difficult, especially when (undemonstrated) instructions are provided, for the first time, over the telephone, to a frightened person in a stressful situation [16–20]. Therefore, the routine provision of medical pre-arrival instructions as a special methodology has been recognized as an essential link in the 'chain of survival' and an international standard of care [15–17].

In examining various techniques recommended to improve effectiveness of 'dispatch life support', the evidence suggests the intuitive concept that on-scene rescuers function better with fewer sequential steps [16–20]. In the past, dispatch CPR instructions had included the traditional 'A-B-C' techniques taught in CPR classes,

Table 1. Sample recommendations regarding dispatcher-assisted CPR instructions provided by emergency medical dispatch (EMD) personnel to bystanders at the scene of a presumed cardiac arrest. (Adapted from the 2003 recommendations of the *National Academies of Emergency Dispatch*)

- To avoid confusion, rescuers stating they have been trained in CPR (and who are not requesting CPR assistance) should be instructed to provide those techniques they have learned
- Otherwise, EMD personnel should provide chest compressions-only CPR Instructions in the immediate few minutes after a sudden collapse. Such chest compressions-only instructions also should be given to individuals declining to perform rescue breathing or those unsure of techniques to perform
- Though dependent on the local EMS system, rescue breaths can be provided by the untrained rescuer after approximately 4 minutes of chest compressions – or about 400 consecutive compressions. Specifically, two rescue breaths can be given and, subsequently, every minute thereafter. This 100:2 compression to ventilation ratio can be continued until the arrival of professional responders
- Dispatchers should provide current standardized for rescue breathing in their CPR instructions for child and adult cases involving probable respiratory and trauma etiologies
- Dispatcher CPR protocols should account for EMS system features and receive quality oversight and expert medical direction

namely *airway* maintenance, rescue *breathing*, and *circulation*-inducing chest compressions. However, researchers are now finding certain problems with ventilation during CPR. Although some concern exists that would-be rescuers do not perform CPR because they have fear of communicable diseases, more importantly there are also evolving physiological concerns [20–23]. For example, frequent interruption of chest compressions to provide rescue breaths will counteract against the maintenance of coronary perfusion pressure, the key determinant of resuscitation [22, 23].

More to the point, some investigators have now considered the deletion of the rescue breathing component of CPR, especially in the first few minutes after out-of-hospital sudden cardiac death. In addition to maintaining coronary perfusion pressure, another basis for deferring rescuer-assisted breathing is the recognition that some degree of ventilation breathing can occur without it, at least for a while. For example, because of rapid chest recoil during the release phase of chest compressions, some air movement can take place [24, 25]. Also, in many cases, spontaneous respirations (so-called 'agonal' breaths), also transpire [25–27]. In fact, these gasping respirations tend to occur in those most likely to survive [26, 27]. In certain animal models, these sources of ventilation can maintain adequate oxygenation and carbon dioxide clearance for several minutes [25, 27–30].

Recognizing these issues, in the late 1990s, the American Heart Association (AHA) and other members of the International Liaison Committee on Resuscitation (ILCOR) called for a re-appraisal of rescue breathing and also formal studies of traditional procedures. The AHA allowed for 'compressions-only' CPR instructions [6, 15] in cases where persosn declined to perform mouth-to-mouth or in the case of dispatcher pre-arrival instructions in whoich the caller did not know how to perform CPR. More recently, a working group for the Council of Standards of the National Academies of Emergency Dispatch was asked to develop an EMD CPR protocol that provides for 'chest compressions' only instructions (Table 1). In the following discussion, we review the rationale for these modifications and hopefully inspire targets for future research efforts.

∎ The Unique Physiology of Cardiac Arrest and CPR Conditions

Most cases of out-of-hospital sudden cardiac death are due to primary cardiac processes, generally ventricular fibrillation (VF) leading to sudden, unexpected collapse [1]. While VF and other sudden cardiac arrest processes rapidly lead to global ischemia, they are usually not caused by it. For example, at the onset of VF, the bloodstream and most body tissues, including much of the heart itself, are well-oxygenated. Furthermore, basic CPR provides only limited forward blood flow and oxygen is not rapidly circulated or consumed. Therefore, arterial oxygen saturations may persist for several minutes following the onset of VF onset [25, 30]. Also, during CPR conditions, there is little need to attempt to eliminate CO_2, regardless of the cause of the cardiac arrest [25]. During manual chest compressions, cardiac output and pulmonary blood flow are dramatically diminished from normal circulatory conditions. Even when compressions are started immediately, there is pronounced reduction in tissue oxygen delivery [25, 31]. In such severe shock states, a significant reduction in total body CO_2 production ensues as well as a pursuant reduction in the need to eliminate it [25, 31]. Metabolism of residual tissue oxygen may continue (or even accelerate) in certain organs such as the brain and heart during the immediate first few minutes following sudden circulatory arrest. However, this consumption of oxygen eventually wanes. Although this transient persistence of oxygen consumption can lead to a concomitant surplus of CO_2 in those specific tissues, return blood flow to the lungs (to eliminate that CO_2) still is severely compromised despite optimal performance of chest compressions [25]. Due to increased blood flow, rescuers can increase end-tidal CO_2 production somewhat with stronger and persistent chest compressions, but this amplification is hardly enough to 'normalize' ventilatory needs [25, 32]. Until strong spontaneous circulation is returned, substantially less ventilation is needed in most cases, particularly when using current CPR techniques [25, 32].

It needs to be recognized that certain out-of-hospital CPR cases result from cardiac arrest caused by hypoxemic etiologies such as drowning, choking, or respiratory failure. However, these cases constitute a relatively small percentage of the situations for which dispatchers must provide CPR pre-arrival instructions. Circumstantially, these cases are also easier to discern: an unresponsive child being pulled from water, a chronic lung disease patient with several hours of worsening dyspnea, or a person at dinner turning cyanotic and grasping their throat before their collapse [15]. Therefore, a major target of this discussion is the out-of-hospital sudden cardiac death case without evidence of other pre-disposing respiratory circumstances. Regardless of the etiology, however, less ventilation (CO_2 removal) will be needed in very low flow states.

Although ventilatory demands to remove CO_2 generally will remain low prior to the return of spontaneous circulation, blood oxygen saturation still requires the maintenance of the inflation (or re-inflation) of certain dependent lung zones that are subject to alveolar closure [25, 33]. Particularly with vigorous chest compressions, lung deflation, and thus red cell de-saturation, eventually becomes an important issue [24, 33]. The central question is to determine the point at which assisted lung inflation is going to be required.

As mentioned previously, there are other potential sources of oxygenation and ventilation during cardiac arrest and the performance of CPR. In addition to some air being forcefully expelled from the thorax during the compression phase of chest compressions, it is passively inhaled during the elastic recoil of the chest wall, assuming an open airway [25]. Also, in VF and most other cases of out-of-hospital sudden cardiac death, the brainstem and respiratory apparatus usually remain oxygenated until the sudden cessation of circulation. Therefore, gasping commonly occurs in that early phase of sudden cardiac arrest and is associated with a better outcome, possibly reflecting lesser/shorter ischemic insult to the brain [26, 27]. Considering that it occurs most often when bystanders witness the collapse from out-of-hospital sudden cardiac death, gasping may be preserved for longer periods of time with early, effective CPR, because of the maintenance of improved oxygenation of the central nervous system and respiratory musculature [26, 27].

Although gasping eventually deteriorates due to the less than optimal perfusion of the brain and respiratory muscles during CPR, they may still provide relatively effective respirations during the first few minutes after a sudden cardiac arrest [6, 26, 27]. In fact, the unique mechanics of gasping may actually improve the effectiveness of CPR. Especially in their early phases, gasping breaths can generate a larger and stronger respiratory effort than a normal resting breath, creating better oxygenation (more lung units recruited), more CO_2 removal (larger tidal volume and more alveolar ventilation per breath), and even more blood flow due to enhanced cardiac preload [27]. Specifically, these stronger inspiratory efforts enhance negative intrathoracic pressures during inspiration, thus significantly enhancing venous return to the heart [27].

▌ The Importance of Not Interrupting Chest Compressions

Adequate restoration of coronary artery perfusion is the single most important determinant of successful resuscitation. While standard CPR can help to restore coronary perfusion, recent data indicate that it may take many seconds (e.g., 10–15 seconds) to build up a pressure head during chest compressions and, more importantly, that interruption causes that pressure head to suddenly fall off, dramatically, and almost immediately [23, 24, 34, 35]. While recognizing the more optimal conditions of the animal laboratory, left ventricular myocardial blood flows in swine receiving chest compressions-only CPR have the potential to be nearly as high as the pre-arrest baseline [23]. Yet with frequent interruptions, such blood flows may never be achieved or only sustained for a few seconds each minute. Therefore, there is significant concern about the frequent interruption of chest compressions to perform what may be a relatively unnecessary action (ventilation) in the immediate minutes following sudden cardiac arrest [6, 23, 24].

So can ventilatory interruption be avoided altogether? Several experimental models have explicitly demonstrated that animals can maintain adequate ventilation (removal of CO_2), even as long as twelve minutes, with continuous chest compressions-only following VF-induced arrest [22, 23, 30, 32, 34]. Animal models also demonstrate that adequate oxygenation (red cell saturation) can be maintained, at least for several minutes with chest compressions-only after sudden cardiac arrest [25, 30], a period of time that would correspond to the dispatch phase of cardiac arrest in rapid response EMS systems.

A recent clinical trial indeed supports the notion that such ventilatory assistance may not be needed during CPR, at least in those first few minutes after a sudden cardiac arrest [12]. In this clinical trial from the Seattle 911 dispatch office, there was an impressive trend toward improved survival (14.7 versus 10.4%) when chest compressions-only CPR instructions from dispatchers were compared to standard

ABC instructions [12]. Recognizing the average 911 call to scene arrival interval was 4 to 5 minutes, the main explanations for these impressive results most likely stem from the findings that: 1) the compressions-only CPR instructions were easier to complete (more patient compliance and success); 2) the bystanders began the chest compressions much earlier; and 3) the chest compressions were not interrupted, or presumably interrupted less often [12].

This particular concern, interruption of chest compressions, is more likely to be exaggerated when CPR instructions are given over the phone for the first time to an individual without prior CPR training. Dispatchers attempting to give traditional CPR instructions over the phone for the first time not only spend significant amounts of time addressing the movement of the patient onto the floor and then positioning the head and neck, but also, to give a breath, they must explain pinching the nose and how to deliver the initial breaths. As shown in the Seattle trial, CPR instructions with chest compressions-only can be provided more quickly and these all-important chest compressions can be begun, on average, about a minute and a half earlier than when instructions for standard CPR are provided [12]. More importantly, using current standards for CPR [15], once chest compressions are begun, it seems that they are continually interrupted to provide intermittent rescue breathing. Some studies have shown that recommended rates of compressions (e.g., 100 per minute) are rarely achieved [32]. The more frequently compressions are interrupted (i.e. 5:1 versus 15:2 compression:ventilation ratios), the less apt is the rescuer to achieve and sustain reasonable coronary perfusion [22, 23]. Considering that it may take 10 seconds (or more) to restore the same level of pressure head, the average amount of coronary perfusion over a minute is dramatically diminished, even with 15:2 ratios, re-enforcing the concept that chest compressions should be interrupted as infrequently as possible, particularly in the first few minutes after a sudden VF arrest. Intuitively, this would be further exaggerated in the setting of dispatchers providing CPR per-arrival instructions over the telephone to the novice rescuer. Ideal CPR is, more than likely, not being performed and the time to deliver a breath is likely to be more protracted.

▌ Limitations to Compressions-Only CPR

While the idea of compressions-only CPR seems increasingly attractive, beyond several minutes of cardiac arrest (perhaps more than four or five minutes), or with pharmacological paralysis (blocked gasping), some form of ventilatory support also becomes increasingly necessary, particularly to maintain lung inflation and red cell saturation [6, 25]. In asphyxial arrest, assisted ventilation is theoretically more of a priority because the arrest is presumably secondary to significant and progressive interval of hypoxemia and tissue hypoxia [36]. Likewise, there is concern that certain patients may not be able to gasp or have the ability to overcome an occluded (relaxed) airway. In many of the experiments cited, the animals had 'pre-intact' airways because of pre-arrest placement of endotracheal tubes. In the actual clinical situation, the patient's agonal respiratory efforts may have to overcome a relaxed, occluded airway to gasp. Also, before many of the experimental data supporting compressions are extrapolated to humans, it should be noted that animals may also gasp more than humans and perhaps, in part, because they receive more optimal compressions in the laboratory setting [6, 27]. Furthermore, even with the promising clinical trial results from the Seattle dispatch office [12], that particular EMS system had unique features, including very rapid response intervals, and, therefore, the results may not be applicable to other venues with longer EMS response times.

Nevertheless, one animal study compared six minutes of standard CPR (including assisted ventilation with a patent airway) to chest compressions-only CPR with a totally occluded airway. This study found no difference in 24-hour survival between the two groups [37]. While arterial blood gases predictably were not as good with the occluded airway, hemodynamic parameters remained significantly better with compressions-only, suggesting that, despite poorer saturation, overall oxygen delivery to the tissues may be matched by the improved flows [6, 27]. While this study was not a true model of hypoxic etiology because VF was induced initially and then the endotracheal tube was clamped, it did demonstrate that chest compressions-only CPR can be effective for the first few minutes, even if there is no ventilation in an arrest of cardiac origin.

Assimilating the Experimental and Clinical Information

Assimilating the information discussed previously, in experimental models of sudden death (i.e., VF-induced versus those of respiratory origin), animals may tolerate several minutes (four to five minutes) of chest compressions-only CPR in terms of their respiratory status, particularly when there are gasping respirations. Eventually, some degree of support needs to begin to maintain red cell saturation (lung inflation). However, removal of CO_2 appears to be maintained for even longer periods of time without assisted rescue breaths. One might then conclude that, in cases of sudden cessation of circulation, chest compressions-only CPR may be adequate for several minutes. Rescue breaths may then be needed to generate an adequate lung inflation for red cell saturation, but the frequency of those breaths should still remain low [33].

Recent animal studies support this conclusion. Comparing different chest compression-ventilation ratios, a group of swine receiving compressions-only CPR for 4 minutes followed by a compression-ventilation ratio of 100:2 (for more than ten minutes) achieved better neurological outcomes than those receiving more frequent breaths (15:2 ratio) for the entire CPR phase [38]. Not surprisingly, both of these groups had better outcomes than those receiving no assisted breaths at all over the 10-minute CPR period [38].

Still, some investigators would argue that, once ventilations are begun, current standards of 15:2 compression to ventilation ratios are still superior than lower ratios. In recent animal studies, 15:2 ratios appeared to be superior to 50:2 in terms of tissue oxygen delivery to the brain [39]. However, the experiments were conducted with mechanical devices that provided only 2 to 3 second pauses for ventilation and the authors cautioned that the data should not be immediately extrapolated to lay bystanders. Therefore, less frequent breaths may be recommended for less than ideal CPR.

Several clinical investigations still support the survival advantages of bystander CPR using both ventilation and chest compressions over so-called 'incomplete CPR', when defined as either compressions alone or ventilatory assistance alone [3–5]. However, when just examining chest compressions alone, the differences were not as striking [3–5]. If just chest compressions were performed, the reported quality of the CPR was generally very good in close to half of the cases and, among these cases, there were relatively better outcomes in terms of long term survival (15 versus 12%) when compared to cases involving combined ventilations and compressions in general [3]. Also, in many of the cases, the bystander-performed CPR may not have begun until after the first few minutes following the arrest and was then continued well beyond that early phase. In other words, the bulk of the data support the compressions-only approach at the dispatch office, at least in EMS systems with rapid response and especially in cases of sudden witnessed collapse [12].

There still remains concern that those with toxic overdose, respiratory depression, witnessed choking, hanging or strangulation, drowning, smoke inhalation, allergic reactions, severe trauma, and prolonged arrest interval would benefit more from earlier assisted breathing [40]. These conditions presumably lead to secondary cardiac arrest from evolving hypoxemia and hypoxia, making them less likely to be gasping adequately at the time of cardiac arrest. Nevertheless, even if assisted breathing were to start earlier, the compression to ventilation ratio might still be higher (e.g., 30:2 or 50:2), at least for adults. Likewise, children would be considered candidates for earlier ventilation because respiratory failure and shock are presumably the most common causes of out-of-hospital cardiopulmonary arrest in children [41]. Nevertheless, while recommended ventilation to compression ratios for children would likely remain higher than ratios for adults, experimental modeling and evolving research still point out a need for modification of future pediatric guidelines as well [35].

▌ Other Advantages of Compression-Only CPR

In addition to concerns about interrupting chest compressions and thus severely compromising coronary perfusion, pauses to provide mouth-to-mouth ventilation may actually be detrimental for other reasons. First of all, the expired gas delivered by a rescuer contains much higher levels of CO_2 and reciprocally lower levels of oxygen than ambient air [6, 42]. Therefore, rescue breaths are slightly more hypoxic and hypercarbic than gasping breaths and chest compression-induced ventilation [6, 42, 43]. Also, when no endotracheal tube is in place, assisted ventilation may not only lead to inadequate alveolar ventilation, but also to increased gastric insufflation and the secondary risk of aspiration of gastric contents [6, 43, 44]. Proper rescue breathing is also more difficult to perform than chest compressions alone and it may be aesthetically unpleasant for many would-be rescuers [6, 12]. Bystanders at cardiac arrest scenes are also more likely to perform it if they feel free to do compressions only [6, 20, 21].

Above all, continuous, uninterrupted, compressions-only CPR may prolong gasping and, in turn, prolong better perfusion. Because gasping is believed to provide better gas exchange (oxygenation and CO_2 clearance) and enhanced venous return [26, 27], its prolongation may, as a result, also delay rapid cardiovascular deterioration because it promotes better oxygenation and blood flow. Following cardiac arrest, there is diminishing oxygenation to the peripheral vascular musculature resulting in peripheral vascular relaxation and declining aortic pressure and subsequent worsening perfusion of the coronary arteries [45]. Intermittent positive pressure rescue breaths may not only inhibit venous return and be less effective breaths in terms of gas exchange, but they may also diminish blood flow to the brainstem and respiratory apparatus because of repeated and protracted interruptions of blood flow. Therefore, rescue breathing may lead to a more rapid deterioration of both gasping and, in turn, diminished flow and oxygenation. Therefore, paradoxically, by not breathing for the gasping patient, one may prolong better oxygenation, better ventilation, and longer periods of more adequate perfusion during CPR. Continuous chest compressions may, thus, have other indirect effects that go beyond simple out thrusts of blood from the thorax in that they may actually result in better and more prolonged respiratory functions.

▌ Timing and Frequency of Rescue Breaths in Pre-Arrival Instructions

Use of a very low frequency of rescue breaths seems to be a major departure from current CPR standards that recommend 15:2 compressions to ventilations for adults and 5:1 for children [15]. At the same time, the introduction of some breathing after several minutes of cardiac arrest, even at a 100:2 ratio, may be considered a more 'conservative' approach than the current recommendations. Dispatchers are already advised to use and continue with chest compressions-only pre-arrival instructions for the untrained rescuer. One could easily argue that dispatchers should continue with pre-arrival instructions with chest compressions only until rescuers arrive to avoid confusion and interruption of chest compressions. However, there is also an issue of rescuer fatigue with constant compressions over several minutes [46, 47]. Furthermore, although compression-ventilation ratios of 50:2 may be optimal in terms of some experimental modeling [35], concerns about pauses for ventilation are probably exaggerated in the circumstance of dispatch pre-arrival instructions.

▌ Conclusion

In summarizing a recommendation for dispatchers, the available evidence indicates that the best strategy would be to provide chest compressions alone for the first four or five minutes following a sudden witnessed cardiac arrest. Then one might provide some degree of lung inflation, but at a rate much less frequently than currently recommended, perhaps only once or twice a minute [35, 38]. Although it may not provide the best respiratory support for some patients who do not gasp immediately (or adequately) after their cardiac arrest, it probably captures the majority of persons likely to survive [4, 26, 27]. More importantly, the best available experimental and clinical evidence indicates that it appears to improve their overall chances of surviving neurologically intact [12, 38].

References

1. Cummins RO, Ornato JP, Thies WH, Pepe PE (1991) Improving survival from sudden cardiac arrest: the "chain of survival" concept. Circulation 83:1832–1847
2. Martens PR, Mullie A, Buylaert W, Calle P, van Hoeyweghen R (1992) Early prediction of non-survival for patients suffering cardiac arrest – a word of caution. The Belgian Cerebral Resuscitation Study Group. Intensive Care Med 18:11–14
3. Bossaert L, Van Hoeyweghen R and the Cerebral Resuscitation Group (1989) Bystander cardiopulmonary resuscitation (CPR) in out-of-hospital cardiac arrest. Resuscitation 17 (Suppl):55–69
4. Van Hoeyweghen RJ, Bossaert LL Mullie A, et al (1993) Quality and efficiency of bystander CPR. Resuscitation 26:47–52

5. Holmberg M, Holmberg S, Herlitz J for the Swedish Cardiac Arrest Registry (2001) Factors modifying the effect of bystander cardiopulmonary resuscitation on survival in out-of-hospital cardiac arrest patients in Sweden. Eur Heart J 22:511–519

6. Becker LB, Berg RA, Pepe PE, et al (1997) A reappraisal of mouth-to-mouth ventilation during bystander-initiated cardiopulmonary resuscitation. Circulation 96:2102–2112

7. Zachariah BS, Pepe PE (1995) The development of emergency medical dispatch in the USA: a historical perspective Eur J Emerg Med 2:109–112

8. Clawson JJ (1981) Dispatch priority training: strengthening the weak link. JEMS 6:32–36

9. Clawson JJ (1990) Dispatch life support: establishing standards that work JEMS 15:80–86

10. Clawson JJ (1986) Telephone treatment protocols: reach out and help someone JEMS 11:43–44

11. Rea TD, Eisenberg MS, Culley LL, Becker L (2001) Dispatcher-assisted cardiopulmonary resuscitation and survival in cardiac arrest. Circulation 104:2513–2516

12. Hallstrom A, Cobb L, Johnson E, Copass M (2000) Cardiopulmonary resuscitation by chest compression alone or with mouth-to-mouth ventilation. N Engl J Med 342:1546–1553

13. National Association of Emergency Physicians Position Paper (1989) Emergency Medical Dispatching. Prehosp Disaster Med 4:163–166

14. Billittier AJ, Lerner EB, Tucker W, Lee J (2000) The lay public's expectations of pre-arrival instructions when dialing 9-1-1. Prehosp Emerg Care 4:234–237

15. American Heart Association (2000) Guidelines 2000 for cardiopulmonary resuscitation and emergency cardiovascular care: International consensus on science. Circulation 102 (Suppl 8): I43–I44

16. Clawson JJ (1986) The hysterical threshold: gaining control of the emergency caller. JEMS 11:40–41

17. Dorph E, Wik L, Steen PA (2003) Dispatcher-assisted cardiopulmonary resuscitation. An evaluation of efficacy amongst elderly. Resuscitation 56:265–273

18. Handley JA, Handley AJ (1998) Four-step CPR – improving skill retention. Resuscitation 36:3–8

19. American College of Emergency Physicians (1988) Guidelines for Emergency Medical Services Systems. Ann Emerg Med 17:742–745

20. Locke CJ, Berg RA, Sanders AB, et al (1995) Bystander cardiopulmonary resuscitation: Concerns about mouth-to-mouth contact. Arch Intern Med 155:938–943

21. Ornato JP, Hallagan LF, McMahan SB, Peeples EH, Rostafinski AG (1990) Attitudes of BCLS instructors about mouth-to-mouth resuscitation during the AIDS epidemic. Ann Emerg Med 19:151–156

22. Berg RA, Sanders AB, Kern KB, et al (2001) Adverse hemodynamic effects of interrupting chest compressions for rescue breathing during cardiopulmonary resuscitation for ventricular fibrillation cardiac arrest. Circulation 104:2465–2470

23. Kern KB, Hilwig RW, Berg RA, Sanders AB, Ewy GA (2002) Importance of continuous chest compressions during cardiopulmonary resuscitation: improved outcome during a simulated single lay-rescuer scenario. Circulation 105:645–649

24. Idris AH, Banner MJ, Wenzel V, et al (1994) Ventilation caused by external chest compression is unable to sustain effective gas exchange during CPR: a comparison with mechanical ventilation. Resuscitation 28:143–150

25. Idris AH, Florete O Jr, Melker RJ, Chandra NC (1996) The physiology of ventilation, oxygenation, and carbon dioxide elimination during cardiac arrest. In: Paradis NA, Halperin HR, Nowak RM, (eds) Cardiac Arrest: The Science And Practice Of Resuscitation Medicine. Williams & Wilkins, Baltimore, pp 391–392

26. Clark JJ, Larsen MP, Culley LL, Graves JR, Eisenberg MS (1992) Incidence of agonal respirations in sudden cardiac arrest. Ann Emerg Med 21:1464–1467

27. Yang L, Weil MH, Noc M, Tang W, Turner T, Gazmuri RJ (1994) Spontaneous gasping increases the ability to resuscitate during experimental cardiopulmonary resuscitation. Crit Care Med 22:879–883

28. Berg RA, Kern KB, Hilwig RW, et al (1997) Assisted ventilation does not improve outcome in a porcine model of single-rescuer bystander cardiopulmonary resuscitation. Circulation 95:1635–1641

29. Noc M, Weil MH, Tang W, Turner T, Fukui M (1995) Mechanical ventilation may not be essential for initial cardiopulmonary resuscitation. Chest 108:821–827
30. Chandra NC, Gruben KG, Tsitlik JE, et al (1994) Observations of ventilation during resuscitation in a canine model. Circulation 90:3070–3075
31. Pepe PE, Culver BH (1985) Independently measured oxygen consumption during reduction of oxygen delivery by positive end-expiratory pressure. Am Rev Respir Dis 132:788–792
32. Milander MM, Hiscok PS, Sanders AB, Kern KB, Berg RA, Ewy GA (1995) Chest compression and ventilation rates during cardiopulmonary resuscitation: the effects of audible tone guidance. Acad Emerg Med 2:708–713
33. Pepe PE (2001) Acute respiratory insufficiency. In: Harwood-Nuss AL, Linden CH, Lutten RC, Shepherd SM, Wolfson AB (eds) The Clinical Practice Of Emergency Medicine, 3rd edn. Lippincott-Raven Publishers, Philadelphia, pp. 657–663
34. Kern KB (2000) Cardiopulmonary resuscitation without ventilation. Crit Care Med 28: N186–189
35. Babbs CF, Nadkarni V (2004) Optimizing chest compression to rescue ventilation ratios during one-rescuer CPR by professionals and laypersons: children are not just little adults. Resuscitation 61:173–181
36. Berg RA (2000) Role of mouth-to-mouth rescue breathing in bystander cardiopulmonary resuscitation for asphyxial cardiac arrest. Crit Care Med 28:N193–195
37. Kern KB, Hilwig RW, Berg RA, Ewy GA (1998) Efficacy of chest compression-only BLS CPR in the presence of an occluded airway. Resuscitation 39:179–188
38. Sanders AB, Kern KB, Berg RA, Hilwig RW, Heidenrich J, Ewy GA (2002) Survival and neurologic outcome after cardiopulmonary resuscitation with four different chest compression-ventilation ratios. Ann Emerg Med 40:553–662
39. Dorph E, Wik L, Stromme TA, Eriksen M, Steen PA (2003) Quality of CPR with three different ventilation:compression ratios. Resuscitation 58:193–201
40. Dorph E, Wik L, Stromme TA, Eriksen M, Steen PA (2004) Oxygen delivery and return of spontaneous circulation with ventilation:compression ratio 2:30 versus chest compressions only CPR in pigs. Resuscitation 60:309–318
41. Sirbaugh PE, Pepe PE, Shook JE, et al (1999) A prospective, population-based study of the demographics, epidemiology, management, and outcome of out-of-hospital pediatric cardiopulmonary arrest. Ann Emerg Med 33:174–184
42. Wenzel V, Idris AH, Banner MJ, Fuerst RS, Tucker KJ (1994) The composition of gas given by mouth-to-mouth ventilation during CPR. Chest 106:1806–1810
43. Rottenberg EM, Dzwonczyk R, Reilley TE, Malone M (1994) Use of supplemental oxygen during bystander-initiated CPR. Ann Emerg Med 23:1027–1031
44. Lawes EG, Baskett PJ (1987) Pulmonary aspiration during unsuccessful cardiopulmonary resuscitation. Intensive Care Med 13:379–382
45. Lee SK, Vaaganes P, Safar P, Stezoski SW, Scanlon M (1989) Effect of cardiac arrest time on cortical cerebral blood flow during subsequent standard external cardiopulmonary resuscitation in rabbits. Resuscitation 17:105–117
46. Ashton A, McCluskey A, Gwinnutt CL, Keenan AM (2002) Effect of rescuer fatigue on performance of continuous external chest compressions over 3 minutes. Resuscitation 55:151–155
47. Ochoa JF, Ramalle-Gomara E, Lisa V, Saralegui I (1998) The effect of rescuer fatigue on the quality of chest compressions. Resuscitation 37:149–152

Thrombolytic Therapy
During Cardiopulmonary Resuscitation

F. Spöhr and B. W. Böttiger

▌ Introduction

Thrombolytic therapy is a causal, effective and well-established treatment for acute myocardial infarction (AMI) and massive pulmonary embolism [1, 2]. Because of the fear of severe bleeding complications, however, thrombolysis has been widely withheld in patients with cardiac arrest who require cardiopulmonary resuscitation (CPR) [3–5]. It has been estimated that AMI or pulmonary embolism are the underlying diseases in more than 50–70% of patients suffering from cardiac arrest and requiring CPR [6, 7]. Since the prognosis of patients suffering from cardiac arrest is very poor, and few specific therapeutic options have been shown to improve survival in these patients [8, 9], new therapeutic approaches to improve the outcome of patients with cardiac arrest are most intriguing. Increasing clinical experience and data from recent studies have suggested that thrombolysis during CPR can significantly improve hemodynamic stabilization and even microcirculatory reperfusion which may be most important for the neurological outcome of surviving patients [10]. Yet the major drawback to using thrombolytics during or shortly after CPR has been the potential risk of severe bleeding.

This chapter focuses on recently available experimental and clinical data on the efficacy of thrombolysis during CPR. In addition, safety aspects will be addressed.

▌ Mechanisms of Action of Thrombolysis During CPR

There are two different mechanisms contributing to the effect of thrombolytic therapy during CPR. First, thrombolytic agents act specifically at the site of coronary thrombosis or pulmonary emboli when used during CPR. Therefore, they treat a condition that contributes to 50–70% of cardiac arrests [6, 7]. If pulmonary embolism is the cause of cardiac arrest, chest compressions may amplify the effect of thrombolysis, because thrombolytic drugs can act more effectively on blood clots that have been mechanically fragmented [11]. In addition, experimental and clinical studies suggest a second mechanism of action that may be of particular importance. After cardiac arrest, microcirculatory reperfusion failure is common and represents one of the most important causes for cerebral dysfunction. This phenomenon is also referred to as the 'no-reflow' phenomenon. It prolongs cerebral ischemia and affects outcome after cardiac arrest [12, 13]. Although the underlying pathophysiology has not been conclusively elucidated, leukocyte-endothelial interactions and coagulation activation have been shown to contribute to the microcirculatory perfusion failure [14, 15]. In a clinical study with patients after cardiac arrest, a marked activation of blood coagulation was reported which was not counterbalanced by an appropriate activation of endogenous fibrinolysis [16]. Thrombolytic treatment may cause a reduction of the 'no-reflow' phenomenon, as shown by experimental data in cats [14]. Thus, under experimental conditions, thrombolytic drugs may improve microcirculatory reperfusion substantially and, therefore, contribute to an improved neurological outcome. Even after prolonged resuscitation, both the direct actions of thrombolytics on coronary thrombosis or pulmonary emboli and the effect of thrombolytics on microcirculatory reperfusion may contribute to the exceptionally good neurological performance of patients reported by different authors [17–19].

Clinical Data on Thrombolysis During CPR

The first report on thrombolysis during CPR in a patient presenting with acute pulmonary embolism was published 30 years ago [20]. Since then, many case reports and case series have followed, most of them demonstrating an exceptional success rate even after prolonged CPR and failure to restore a spontaneous circulation by regular treatment. These case reports and case series have been reviewed before [11, 21]. Although the unusual success suggested by these anecdotal reports may be, in part, attributed to a selection bias in publication, outcome data were regarded as exceptionally high [18]. In addition, several clinical studies on thrombolysis during CPR both in- and out-of-hospital have been performed.

In-hospital Studies

The first prospective study of 20 patients with massive pulmonary embolism undergoing CPR was presented by Köhle et al. [22]. After pulmonary angiography, streptokinase was administered locally. Return of spontaneous circulation was achieved in 11 patients (55%). In another prospective study, Gramann and colleagues treated 28 patients suffering from AMI with thrombolytics during resuscitation. Nine patients could be stabilized primarily, but only three patients were long-term survivors [23]. Kürkciyan et al. retrospectively compared a group of 21 patients presenting with cardiac arrest after massive pulmonary embolism who were given a bolus dose of recombinant tissue plasminogen activator (alteplase, rt-PA) during CPR with a group of 21 patients receiving standard treatment for cardiac arrest after massive pulmonary embolism. The number of patients with return of spontaneous circulation was significantly higher in the thrombolysis group compared to the non-thrombolyis group (17 vs. 9), while the number of survivors was not significantly different in both groups (2 vs. 1) [24]. In a prospective study including 30 patients with prehospital (83%) and in-hospital (17%) cardiac arrest, thrombolysis using tenecteplase was performed after failure of conventional resuscitation efforts. Of these patients, 30% had return of spontaneous circulation, 17% were admitted to the intensive care unit (ICU), 10% survived 24 hours and 7% of these patients were finally discharged from hospital [25]. Recently, a prospective, randomized, double-blind, placebo-controlled pilot study with patients who were resuscitated in-hospital after an out-of-hospital cardiac arrest was performed. In this study, 35 patients received tenecteplase or placebo as the first drug given during CPR. There were no differences in survival between the tenecte-

Table 1. Thrombolysis during CPR: In-hospital studies

Reference	Study type	Underlying disease	Number of patients	Thrombolytic agent	CPR-related bleeding	Number of survivors
Köhle 1984 [22]	Prospective	PE	20	SK	–	11
Scholz 1990 [43]	Retrospective	PE	9	SK/UK/rt-PA	Pectoral/sternal hemorrhage, liver laceration	5
Gramann 1991 [23]	Prospective	AMI	28	SK/rt-PA	Pericardial/ sternal hemorrhage (4)	3
Scholz 1992 [44]	Retrospective	AMI	6	SK/UK/rt-PA	–	3
Kurkciyan 2000 [24]	Retrospective	PE	21	rt-PA	2 liver ruptures, mediastinal bleeding	2
Kleiner 2003 [25]	Prospective	n.r.	30	TNK	–	2
Fatovich 2004 [26]	Randomized, placebo-controlled	n.r.	19	TNK	–	1
Total			**133**		**9 (6.7%)**	**27 (20.3%)**

AMI: myocardial infarction, CPR: cardiopulmonary resuscitation, n.r.: not reported, PE: pulmonary embolism, rt-PA: recombinant tissue plasminogen activator (alteplase), SK: streptokinase, TNK: tenecteplase, UK: urokinase

plase and placebo group at hospital discharge, although patients treated with tenecteplase more often achieved return of spontaneous circulation compared to the control group [26]. However, due to funding difficulties, the study was not powered to show a significant difference in outcome.

In conclusion, in-hospital clinical studies suggest an improved rate of return of spontaneous circulation in patients with cardiac arrest due to AMI or massive pulmonary embolism. In addition, they report a markedly improved long-term survival (20.3%, see Table 1) compared to patients receiving standard treatment in hospital (approx. 15% survivors [27, 28]).

Out-of-hospital Studies

Four studies on out-of-hospital thrombolysis with a total of 299 patients have been published (Table 2). Patients with out-of-hospital CPR are known to have a very poor prognosis. It has been estimated that only about 5% of patients who suffer from out-of-hospital cardiac arrest survive without severe neurological impairment [18], and conventional CPR is not successful in the majority of cases [29]. Klefisch and colleagues performed 'rescue thrombolysis' in 34 patients with suspected AMI or massive pulmonary embolism during CPR. Five patients presenting with ventricular fibrillation refractory to conventional treatment of cardiac arrest survived,

Table 2. Thrombolysis during CPR: Out-of-hospital studies

Reference	Study type	Number of patients	Thrombolytic agent	CPR-related bleeding	Number of survivors
Klefisch 1995 [30]	Prospective	34	SK	hemothorax	5
Bottiger 2001 [19]	Prospective, controlled	40	rt-PA	–	6
Lederer 2001 [31]	Retrospective, controlled	108	rt-PA	2 pericardial tamponades, 1 hemothorax	27
Abu-Laban 2002 [42]	Prospective, randomized, controlled	117	rt-PA	1 pulmonary hemorrhage, 1 major hemorrhage (not clearly specified)	1
Total		**299**		**6 (2.0%)**	**39 (13.0%)**

CPR: cardiopulmonary resuscitation, rt-PA: recombinant tissue plasminogen activator (alteplase), SK: streptokinase

three of them without neurological impairment [30]. In a prospective study that was performed in our department, 40 patients with out-of-hospital cardiac arrest received thrombolytic treatment with rt-PA during CPR after resuscitation had been unsuccessful for more than 15 minutes. Six patients (15%) were discharged from the hospital alive, five of them without severe neurological impairment [19]. These results were confirmed by a retrospective chart review of 108 out-of-hospital patients receiving rt-PA during CPR. Fifty-two patients (48.1%) survived the first 24 hours, 27 patients (27%) survived to discharge. This was a significant improvement in outcome compared to a matched pairs control group who were treated for cardiac arrest without thrombolysis (15.4% survivors) [31]. A randomized, double-blind, placebo-controlled trial on out-of-hospital thrombolysis during cardiac arrest did not reveal beneficial effects of thrombolytic treatment with rt-PA on survival. However, most of the patients in that study presented with pulseless electrical activity of the heart, and in more than one third of patients there was no witnessed collapse. The outcome of the control group, which received standard treatment (CPR without thrombolysis), was 0%, and therefore, was poorer than in any other study on cardiac arrest ever published. Because of these methodological drawbacks, the study has been widely criticized [32].

In conclusion, data from the first studies on thrombolysis during CPR after out-of-hospital cardiac arrest suggest a beneficial effect of this treatment on outcome and potentially even on neurological performance of survivors.

▌ Safety of Thrombolysis during and after CPR

The risks of thrombolytic therapy in general have been classified into five major categories: intracranial hemorrhage, systemic hemorrhage, immunologic complications, hypotension, and reperfusion injury [33]. Arterial hypotension and allergic reactions can usually be treated effectively in the setting of resuscitation, since the use of vasopressors is a standard treatment in cardiac arrest. A reperfusion injury may be caused by toxic metabolites from dying tissue and by clogging of the microcirculatory vessels due to aggregation of white blood cells [33]. Thus, severe hemorrhage represents the major safety concern in thrombolysis during or shortly after CPR. To estimate the risk caused by the combination of CPR and thrombolysis, it is important to classify bleeding complications, because both thrombolysis and CPR can cause significant bleeding complications even if they are not combined [34].

Hemorrhagic complications are not unusual after CPR without thrombolysis. Among CPR-related bleeding, hemorrhages of the great vessels, the heart, the lung, and abdominal bleeding are most common [29, 35]. From several retrospective and prospective autopsy studies [29, 36, 37], hemorrhagic complications may be estimated to occur in more than 15% of all patients after CPR [34]. On the other hand, thrombolysis itself clearly increases the bleeding risk. A meta-analysis of nine large randomized trials on thrombolysis for treatment of AMI revealed an incidence of 1.1% of major bleeding, defined as bleeding that required transfusion or was life-threatening, within the first 35 days after thrombolysis, compared to an incidence of 0.4% in the control group. In addition, the risk of intracranial bleeding after thrombolysis for AMI was 0.8% compared to 0.1% in the control group without thrombolysis [38]. After thrombolysis for massive pulmonary embolism, the incidence of intracranial bleeding may be up to 1.9%, one third being fatal [39]. Therefore, the risk for severe bleeding events in patients with AMI or pulmonary embolus who are administered thrombolytics even without CPR can be estimated to be between 1.9 and 3.0% as compared to 0.5% in patients not receiving thrombolytics [34]. The major question is if CPR-related bleeding occurs more frequently or is aggravated by thrombolysis.

In studies on thrombolysis shortly *after* CPR, very few bleeding complications related to CPR have been reported [34]. In a subgroup analysis of the Spanish multi-center registry on thrombolysis after CPR (ARIAM – analysis of delay in AMI), two hemorrhagic strokes (not CPR-related) and two not clearly specified hematomas that required transfusion occurred in 303 patients treated by CPR after AMI, 67 of whom had received thrombolysis after CPR. None of these bleeding events was fatal [40]. In a study on 132 patients receiving thrombolysis for treatment of AMI after out-of-hospital CPR, Kurkciyan and colleagues found 13 hemorrhagic complications. Two of these were most probably related to CPR, but the others (cerebral, gastrointestinal bleeding, bleeding from puncture sites) were not causally related to CPR. Interestingly, of seven bleeding complications in the control group (133 patients receiving CPR without thrombolysis), six were probably CPR-related (thoracic, liver, myocardial bleeding) [41]. In summary, the incidence of CPR-related bleeding complications in currently available retrospective studies on thrombolysis after CPR was 1.2%. Therefore, these studies do not suggest a relevant increase in hemorrhagic complications compared to CPR without thrombolysis.

The incidence of CPR-related bleeding complications reported by several clinical in-hospital studies on thrombolysis *during* CPR was significantly higher than that reported in studies on thrombolysis *after* CPR. Seven studies including 133 patients showed CPR-related bleeding complications in nine cases (6.7%). However, this incidence does not exceed the incidence of hemorrhagic complications of about 15% resulting from CPR without thrombolysis that has been suggested in the studies mentioned above. Gramann et al. reported 28 cases of AMI with cardiac arrest refractory to standard CPR treatment. Thrombolysis was used during CPR as an *ultima ratio*. Nine patients could be primarily stabilized, four of them showing mainly thoracic bleeding complications. One of these hemorrhages (pericardial bleeding) led to a fatal outcome [23]. No other fatal bleedings related to CPR have been reported in any of the in-hospital studies.

According to Table 2, the overall incidence of severe bleeding incidents related to CPR that was reported from the four out-of-hospital studies on thrombolysis during CPR was 2.0%. Klefisch et al. reported the successful resuscitation of five out of 34 patients presenting with cardiac arrest refractory to advanced cardiac life support who were administered thrombolytics during CPR. One patient showed a hemothorax after prolonged resuscitation (75 min) [30]. In their retrospective study with 108 patients, Lederer and colleagues reported six severe bleeding incidents in a subgroup of 45 non-surviving patients. Three of these were directly related to CPR (Table 2). However, in the corresponding control group without thrombolysis, the incidence of severe bleeding events was not significantly different [31]. The recent study by Abu-Laban et al. reported a pulmonary hemorrhage in the sole surviving patient, and one more major hemorrhage which was not clearly specified [42]. In summary, the overall incidence for CPR-related bleeding complications of 2.0% in 299 patients after out-of-hospital thrombolysis *during* CPR suggests that thrombolysis during out-of-hospital resuscitation is not likely to contribute to an increased bleeding risk.

▌ Outlook

In order to assess the efficacy and safety of prehospital thrombolytic therapy in cardiac arrest of presumed cardiac origin, a large randomized, double-blind, placebo-controlled trial has been recently started (http://www.erc.edu/index.php/newsitem/en/nid=146). The Thrombolysis in Cardiac Arrest Study (TROICA) is designed to randomize approximately 1000 patients with prehospital cardiac arrest of presumed cardiac origin either to receive a weight-adjusted dose of tenecteplase or placebo during CPR. The primary endpoint of the study is the 30-day survival rate, additional endpoints include the neurological performance of surviving patients and the incidence of bleeding complications. Results of the study are expected for the end of 2005.

▌ Conclusion

From clinical studies, there is increasing evidence that thrombolytic therapy during CPR can contribute to stabilization in patients with cardiac arrest caused by AMI or massive pulmonary embolism. Direct action of thrombolytics on coronary thrombosis or pulmonary emboli as well as beneficial effects of thrombolytics on the microcirculatory perfusion appear to be two major mechanisms of action that may explain the exceptionally good outcome data. Although thrombolysis is clearly associated with a higher incidence of bleeding events, currently available data suggest that these potential risks probably do not outweigh the benefits that are associated with thrombolysis in the setting of cardiac arrest. Currently, the efficacy and safety of this promising treatment is being assessed in a large, randomized, placebo-controlled multicenter trial.

References

1. Bode C, Nordt TK, Runge MS (1994) Thrombolytic therapy in acute myocardial infarction-selected recent developments. Ann Hematol 69:S35–40
2. Arcasoy SM, Kreit JW (1999) Thrombolytic therapy of pulmonary embolism: a comprehensive review of current evidence. Chest 115:1695–1707
3. Curzen N, Haque R, Timmis A (1998) Applications of thrombolytic therapy. Intensive Care Med 24:756–768
4. Ryan TJ, Antman EM, Brooks NH, et al (1999) 1999 update: ACC/AHA guidelines for the management of patients with acute myocardial infarction: executive summary and recommendations: a report of the american college of cardiology/American Heart Association Task Force on Practice Guidelines (Committee on Management of Acute Myocardial Infarction). Circulation 100:1016–1030
5. The Task Force on the Management of Acute Myocardial Infarction of the European Society of Cardiology (1996) Acute myocardial infarction: pre-hospital and in-hospital management. Eur Heart J 17:43–63
6. Silfvast T (1991) Cause of death in unsuccessful prehospital resuscitation. J Intern Med 229:331–335
7. Spaulding CM, Joly LM, Rosenberg A, et al (1997) Immediate coronary angiography in survivors of out-of-hospital cardiac arrest. N Engl J Med 336:1629–1633
8. Kudenchuk PJ, Cobb LA, Copass MK, et al (1999) Amiodarone for resuscitation after out-of-hospital cardiac arrest due to ventricular fibrillation. N Engl J Med 341:871–878
9. The HACA Group (2002) Mild therapeutic hypothermia to improve the neurologic outcome after cardiac arrest. N Engl J Med 346:549–556
10. Bottiger BW, Spohr F (2003) The risk of thrombolysis in association with cardiopulmonary resuscitation: no reason to withhold this causal and effective therapy. J Intern Med 253:99–101
11. Padosch SA, Motsch J, Bottiger BW (2002) Thrombolysis during cardiopulmonary resuscitation. Anaesthesist 51:516–532
12. Hossmann KA (1993) Ischemia-mediated neuronal injury. Resuscitation 26:225–235
13. Safar P, Stezoski W, Nemoto EM (1976) Amelioration of brain damage after 12 minutes' cardiac arrest in dogs. Arch Neurol 33:91–95
14. Fischer M, Bottiger BW, Popov-Cenic S, Hossmann KA (1996) Thrombolysis using plasminogen activator and heparin reduces cerebral no-reflow after resuscitation from cardiac arrest: an experimental study in the cat. Intensive Care Med 22:1214–1223
15. Bottiger BW (1997) Thrombolysis during cardiopulmonary resuscitation. Fibrinolysis (Suppl 2):93–100
16. Bottiger BW, Motsch J, Bohrer H, et al (1995) Activation of blood coagulation after cardiac arrest is not balanced adequately by activation of endogenous fibrinolysis. Circulation 92:2572–2578
17. Bottiger BW, Bohrer H, Bach A, Motsch J, Martin E (1994) Bolus injection of thrombolytic agents during cardiopulmonary resuscitation for massive pulmonary embolism. Resuscitation 28:45–54
18. Newman DH, Greenwald I, Callaway CW (2000) Cardiac arrest and the role of thrombolytic agents. Ann Emerg Med 35:472–480
19. Bottiger BW, Bode C, Kern S, et al (2001) Efficacy and safety of thrombolytic therapy after initially unsuccessful cardiopulmonary resuscitation: a prospective clinical trial. Lancet 357:1583–1585
20. Renkes-Hegendörfer U, Herrmann K (1974) Successful treatment of a case of fulminant massive pulmonary embolism with streptokinase. Anaesthesist 23:500–501
21. Bottiger BW, Martin E (2001) Thrombolytic therapy during cardiopulmonary resuscitation and the role of coagulation activation after cardiac arrest. Curr Opin Crit Care 7:176–183
22. Kohle W, Pindur G, Stauch M, Rasche H (1984) Hochdosierte Streptokinasetherapie bei fulminanter Lungenarterienembolie. Anaesthesist 33:469
23. Gramann J, Lange-Braun P, Bodemann T, Hochrein H (1991) Der Einsatz von Thrombolytika in der Reanimation als Ultima ratio zur Überwindung des Herztodes. Intensiv- und Notfallbehandlung 16:134–137

24. Kurkciyan I, Meron G, Sterz F, et al (2000) Pulmonary embolism as a cause of cardiac arrest: presentation and outcome. Arch Intern Med 160:1529–1535
25. Kleiner DM, Ferguson KL, King K, Bozeman WP (2003) Empiric tenecteplase use in cardiac arrest refractory to standard advanced cardiac life support interventions. Circulation 108 (Suppl IV):318–319
26. Fatovich DM, Dobb GJ, Clugston RA (2004) A pilot randomised trial of thrombolysis in cardiac arrest (The TICA trial). Resuscitation 61:309–313
27. Bedell SE, Delbanco TL, Cook EF, Epstein FH (1983) Survival after cardiopulmonary resuscitation in the hospital. N Engl J Med 309:569–576
28. Ballew KA, Philbrick JT, Caven DE, Schorling JB (1994) Predictors of survival following in-hospital cardiopulmonary resuscitation. A moving target. Arch Intern Med 154:2426–2432
29. Bedell SE, Fulton EJ (1986) Unexpected findings and complications at autopsy after cardiopulmonary resuscitation (CPR). Arch Intern Med 146:1725–1728
30. Klefisch F, Gareis R, Störk T, Möckel M, Danne O (1995) Präklinische ultima-ratio Thrombolyse bei therapierefraktärer kardiopulmonaler Reanimation. Intensivmedizin 32:155–162
31. Lederer W, Lichtenberger C, Pechlaner C, Kroesen G, Baubin M (2001) Recombinant tissue plasminogen activator during cardiopulmonary resuscitation in 108 patients with out-of-hospital cardiac arrest. Resuscitation 50:71–76
32. Bottiger BW, Padosch SA, Wenzel V, et al (2002) Tissue plasminogen activator in cardiac arrest with pulseless electrical activity. N Engl J Med 17:1281–1282
33. Califf RM, Fortin DF, Tenaglia AN, Sane DC (1992) Clinical risks of thrombolytic therapy. Am J Cardiol 69:12A–20A
34. Spohr F, and Bottiger BW (2003) Safety of thrombolysis during cardiopulmonary resuscitation. Drug Saf 26:367–379
35. Nagel EL, Fine EG, Krischer JP, Davis JH (1981) Complications of CPR. Crit Care Med 9:424
36. Powner DJ, Holcombe PA, Mello LA (1984) Cardiopulmonary resuscitation-related injuries. Crit Care Med 12:54–55
37. Krischer JP, Fine EG, Davis JH, Nagel EL (1987) Complications of cardiac resuscitation. Chest 92:287–291
38. Fibrinolytic Therapy Trialists' (FTT) Collaborative Group (1994) Indications for fibrinolytic therapy in suspected acute myocardial infarction: collaborative overview of early mortality and major morbidity results from all randomised trials of more than 1000 patients. Lancet 343:311–322
39. Kanter DS, Mikkola KM, Patel SR, Parker JA, Goldhaber SZ (1997) Thrombolytic therapy for pulmonary embolism. Frequency of intracranial hemorrhage and associated risk factors. Chest 111:1241–1245
40. Ruiz-Bailén M, Aguayo de Hoyos E, Serrano-Córcoles MC, Díaz-Castellanos MA, Ramos-Cuadra JA, Reina-Toral A (2001) Efficacy of thrombolysis in patients with acute myocardial infarction requiring cardiopulmonary resuscitation. Intensive Care Med 27:1050–1057
41. Kurkciyan I, Meron G, Sterz F, et al (2003) Major bleeding complications after cardiopulmonary resuscitation: impact of thrombolytic treatment. J Intern Med 253:128–135
42. Abu-Laban RB, Christenson JM, Innes GD, et al (2002) Tissue plasminogen activator in cardiac arrest with pulseless electrical activity. N Engl J Med 346:1522–1528
43. Scholz KH, Hilmer T, Schuster S, Wojcik J, Kreuzer H, Tebbe U (1990) Thrombolysis in resuscitated patients with pulmonary embolism. Dtsch Med Wochenschr 115:930–935
44. Scholz KH, Tebbe U, Herrmann C, et al (1992) Frequency of complications of cardiopulmonary resuscitation after thrombolysis during acute myocardial infarction. Am J Cardiol 69:724–728

Suspended Animation for Delayed Resuscitation

X. Wu, T. Drabek, and P. M. Kochanek

Introduction

Since its appearance in the utopian novel *Looking Backward* by the American author Edward Bellamy in 1888, "Suspended Animation" remained a hypothetical technical term in science fiction for nearly a century. In 1984, Dr. Peter Safar, the father of modern cardiopulmonary resuscitation (CPR), and Dr. Ronald Bellamy, a US Army surgeon, redefined suspended animation and consolidated the concept with sound scientific rationales and potential practical values in medicine [1]. By the end of the last century, a series of experiments, mostly conducted in the Safar Center for Resuscitation Research at the University of Pittsburgh, showed that suspended animation is feasible in a large animal model of cardiopulmonary arrest, and that suspended animation might ultimately be feasible in a clinical setting [1]. To appreciate the scientific concept of suspended animation, a brief review of current resuscitation of traumatic cardiopulmonary arrest is helpful.

The Challenge of Traumatic Cardiopulmonary Arrest in Resuscitation

In the civilian setting, 50% of deaths due to trauma occur at the accident scene, with another 30% occurring within a few hours of injury [2]. In the military setting, a similar picture of rapid deterioration has been reported. For example, the majority of the US soldiers killed in action in Vietnam without brain trauma had penetrating truncal injuries and exsanguinated to cardiopulmonary arrest within minutes [1]. These injuries were often surgically repairable. Unfortunately, for a large portion of the acute mortality from rapid exsanguination cardiopulmonary arrest in both civilian and military settings, no effective methods have been established to reliably improve survival. The technical obstacles are formidable. Shortening rescue and transport time barely impact the irreversible deterioration of the brain that occurs 5 min after cardiopulmonary arrest. The need for surgical repair in these patients is also obvious, but not feasible in the setting of exsanguination cardiopulmonary arrest. Finally, conventional CPR is generally futile in these cases because of a volume-depleted and trauma-disrupted circulatory system. More aggressive treatments with thoracotomy and aortic cross clamping have also not improved the poor outcome in these patients [3]. The grim prognosis has led the National Association of EMS Physician Standard and Clinical Practice Committee and the American College of Surgeons Committee on Trauma to publish guidelines for termination of resuscitation in pre-hospital traumatic cardiopulmonary arrest. If patients with either blunt or penetrating trauma are found apneic, pulseless, and without pupillary reflexes, or spontaneous movement, termination of resuscitation efforts is recommended [4]. In the military setting, resuscitation efforts are generally stopped if a patient fails to respond to 1 l of hetastarch [5].

Few studies have tried to address this problem. One group proposed the use of intra-aortic balloon catheter to stop bleeding beyond the descending aorta and infuse blood or other solutions into the aorta above the balloon to avoid ischemic injuries in the heart and the brain [6]. This approach is similar to thoracotomy and aortic cross-clamping, but less invasive. However, outcome studies of this technique are lacking. This chapter focuses on a unique resuscitation concept, which is called suspended animation for delayed resuscitation that we have been developing over the past 20 years.

▌ The Concept of Suspended Animation

Facing the challenge of traumatic cardiopulmonary arrest, Drs. Safar and Bellamy jointly created the concept of suspended animation in 1984. Instead of futilely trying to restart the circulation in the setting of exsanguination cardiopulmonary arrest, preservation was proposed as the initial intervention to buy time for transport and surgical repair. After the anatomic defect in the circulation is repaired, cardiopulmonary bypass (CPB) is initiated as part of a delayed resuscitation.

▌ Development of Suspended Animation Experimental Models

Different from profound hypothermic cardiopulmonary arrest in neurological and cardiovascular surgery, a clinically-relevant suspended animation model should have these two key features: 1) the pre-existence of insults at normal or near normal body temperatures, including trauma, hemorrhage, and cardiopulmonary arrest; and 2) a trauma-disrupted circulatory system that makes fluid replacement and chest compression futile. Any technology that relies on intact circulatory system, such as CPB, cannot be relied upon for induction of hypothermia in some cases. Because of its complexities, a step-by-step approach has been taken in the establishment of suspended animation models.

1980s: Feasibility of Organism Preservation after Hemorrhagic Shock

In the late 1980s, Tisherman et al. conducted a ground-breaking series of suspended animation experiments in dogs. The pre-existing insults were 30 or 60 min of hemorrhagic shock at a mean arterial pressure (MAP) of 30 or 40 mmHg. Hypothermic preservation was induced by closed-chest CPB with hemodilution using crystalloids. At the end, delayed resuscitation was performed with CPB. Profound cerebral hypothermia ($< 10\,^\circ$C) induced at the beginning of a 60–120 min exsanguination cardiopulmonary arrest improved neurologic outcome, vs deep hypothermia ($15\,^\circ$C) [7, 8–10]. This series established the premise for the suspended animation concept by showing that the pre-existing hemorrhagic shock did not obviate the potential efficacy of hypothermic preservation.

1999–2002 Clinically Relevant Suspended Animation Model – without Trauma

The second series, again carried out in dogs, took one step closer towards the ideal suspended animation model in that:
1) suspended animation was initiated after cardiopulmonary arrest, assuming that most victims would have cardiopulmonary arrest when approached by paramedics, and that people would be more willing to initiate suspended animation after rather than before cardiopulmonary arrest;
2) 2–5 min of cardiopulmonary arrest was allowed to elapse, assuming the time that was required for vascular cannulation; and
3) one-way flush was used, assuming the existence of the disrupted circulatory system that does not allow CPB to function properly.

The solutions were administered into the aortic arch using a balloon catheter, and drained out from the right atrium via an external jugular catheter.

Typically, the suspended animation model that was developed has three phases:
1) a hemorrhage and cardiopulmonary arrest phase: 5 min of rapid exsanguination followed by 2–5 min cardiopulmonary arrest;
2) a suspended animation phase: up to 3 h of preservation; and
3) a delayed resuscitation phase: initiated with 2 h of CPB for re-warming and return of spontaneous circulation, followed by up to 96 h of intensive care.

The final outcome is assessed at 72 or 96 h based on evaluation of Overall Performance Category (OPC, 1–5) and neurologic deficit score (NDS). A histological deficit score (HDS) was also developed which quantifies neuronal damage in 19 brain regions.

2002–2003: Clinically-relevant Suspended Animation Model – with Trauma

The success of suspended animation in non-trauma models prompted us to explore whether suspended animation would work in the setting of experimental trauma with a superimposed exsanguination cardiopulmonary arrest. Nozari et al. added trauma in the form of a thoracotomy, laparotomy, and splenic transection into the above suspended animation model in dogs [11]. Splenectomy was performed during the arrest that followed. As expected, coagulopathy due to hemodilution, hypothermia, and ischemia were greatly worsened by trauma, even with use of fresh donor blood during resuscitation. Nevertheless, 60 min of cardiopulmonary arrest plus severe trauma could be reversed to intact survival in about 50% of the dogs. In the rest, multiple organ failure (MOF) occurred, and evaluation of neurologic function was not possible. Histology revealed that there was almost no brain injury in any of the dogs. In subsequent studies, based on studies in clinical sepsis and MOF showing efficacy of plasma exchange in decreasing the microangiopathy, Nozari et al. reported that plasma exchange not only decreased the MOF seen after trauma and suspended animation, but also had improved neurologic outcomes after 2 h of exsanguination cardiopulmonary arrest [12].

▌ Therapeutic Windows for Suspended Animation

Two studies have been conducted to explore how much the pre-existing duration of cardiopulmonary arrest or hemorrhagic shock limit the efficacy of suspended animation. In a 30 min cardiopulmonary arrest model, initiation of 2 °C normal saline flush was delayed by 2, 5 or 8 min from the onset of cardiopulmonary arrest. All dogs received 100 ml/kg normal saline flushed into the thoracic aorta via a balloon catheter over 4 min. Delays in flush did not change the efficacy of brain cooling. When cooling was delayed by 2 or 5 min, all 12 dogs regained consciousness after resuscitation. In contrast, those with 8 min delay remained comatose and severely disabled [13]. This suggests that the time window for the onset of the flush is between 5 and 8 min for suspended animation to be successful after cardiopulmonary arrest.

All of the initial work with suspended animation used a paradigm in which exsanguination cardiopulmonary arrest was rapidly induced – over 5 min. This was done to model the rapid exsanguination that was observed in the battlefield in lethal combat casualties from gunshot wounds. However, not all exsanguination cardiopulmonary arrest occurs rapidly. Thus, it was not clear if suspended animation would be effective if induced in the setting of an exsanguination cardiopulmonary arrest that had developed over a much longer period of hemorrhagic shock such as 1–2 h or more. To answer this question, dogs were gradually but continuously hemorrhaged until cardiopulmonary arrest, using a paradigm that resulted in cardiopulmonary arrest at between 1.5 and 2.5 h after the onset of hemorrhage. Before cardiopulmonary arrest, about 60 to 90% of the estimated total blood volume was removed (Wu et al.; unpublished data). Upon cardiopulmonary arrest, the arterial blood gases revealed the following mean values for key physiological parameters including

- ▌ pH ~7.0,
- ▌ base excess ~– 15 mmol/l,
- ▌ lactate ~15 mmol/l, and
- ▌ K^+~7.0 mmol/l.

After 2 min of cardiopulmonary arrest, either conventional CPR or suspended animation was initiated. Conventional CPR included chest compression, pressure-controlled ventilation, and vigorous volume replacement. In contrast, suspended animation was rapidly induced with flush of 20 l of ice-cold saline via a femoral artery, and maintained for a period of 60 min. We found that while all dogs treated with CPR died before 16 h, all but one dog treated with suspended animation survived to >72 h. Surprisingly, to produce intact neurological outcome in this paradigm, it was necessary to follow suspended animation with a 36 h period of mild hypothermia (34 °C). Thus, prolonged hemorrhagic shock prior to exsanguination cardiopulmonary arrest should not preclude the possibility of survival with intact neurological outcome after suspended animation treatment.

▌ The Development of Hypothermic Approaches for Suspended Animation

Hypothermia so far is the most reliable and potent approach for preservation during cardiopulmonary arrest. Behringer et al. conducted a series of experiments that systemically explored specific details of the optimal hypothermic approach [14–17].

Table 1. Studies of hypothermic approaches

CA time	Flush solution			Achieved/target Tty*	Outcome
	Volume	Approach	Avg. Efficiency (C/ml)		
15 min	25 ml/kg (24 °C)	Intra-aortic balloon catheter		36 a	
20 min	25 ml/kg (24 °C)	Intra-aortic balloon catheter		35.7 a	62 (8–67) (n=6)
20 min	25 ml/kg (4 °C)	Intra-aortic balloon catheter	0.16	34 a	5 (0–49) (n=6)
30 min	25 ml/kg (4 °C)	Intra-aortic balloon catheter		34 a	69 (54–100) (n=6)
30 min	100 ml/kg (4 °C)	Intra-aortic balloon catheter	0.10	28 a	4 (0–18) (n=7)
60 min	~159 ml/kg (4 °C)	Intra-aortic balloon catheter		20 t	13 (0–27) (n=6)
60 min	~306 ml/kg (4 °C)	Intra-aortic balloon catheter	0.08	15 t	0 (0–3) (n=5)
60 min	~469 ml/kg (4 °C)	Intra-aortic balloon catheter		10 t	0 (0–0) (n=3)
90 min	~578 ml/kg (4 °C)	Intra-aortic balloon catheter	0.048	10 t	0 (0–0) (n=6)
120 min	~666 ml/kg (4 °C)	Femoral artery catheter	0.046	7 a	10 (0–39) (n=4)

CA: cardiopulmonary arrest; *: a=achieved; t=targeted; Tty: tympanic membrane temperature

As shown in Table 1, a linear relationship exists between brain temperature and effective preservation durations ($r=0.97$) in suspended animation. To achieve 20-min preservation, cooling to brain temperature of 34 °C is needed; for 30 min, 28 °C is needed; for 60 min, 15 °C appears sufficient; while for 90 min, ≤10 °C is needed. The efficacy of ice-cold saline for cooling, however, decreased dramatically as the brain temperature decreased. During a temperature reduction from 37 to 15 °C, 1 ml/kg ice-cold saline reduced brain temperature by ~0.16 °C; from 15 to 10 °C, however, the same amount of cold fluid reduced brain temperature by only ~0.018 °C/ml/kg – a reduction in cooling efficiency by a factor of nearly ten. When the tympanic membrane temperature was reduced to 7 °C, the effective preservation time appeared to be 2–3 h, but the requirement of large amount of fluid to achieve this temperature in our paradigm limits its application on the field.

Alam et al. [18] studied the impact of rate of cooling on outcome in a model of large blood vessel laceration in pigs. Thirty min after vascular injury, cooling with CPB was initiated to achieve a pharyngeal temperature of 10 °C at an averaged speed of 0.5, 0.9, and 1.35 °C/min. The cardiopulmonary arrest lasted for 60 min, followed by re-warming and delayed resuscitation. Six weeks later, the survival rates were 37.5%, 62.5%, and 87.5% respectively, supporting the notion that the most rapid cooling rate is maximally efficacious. However, it is unclear if cooling at an even faster rate (>2 °C/min) would further improve outcome. We found one-way flush with ice-cold saline was faster in cooling than CPB. At ~1.2 l/min with one-way flush, the cooling rate (to achieve a temperature of 10 °C) was about 2.5 °C/min [17]. Surprisingly, cooling with CPB (recirculation), although slower, appeared to yield better neurological outcome [19]. Although there were other factors that may be responsible for the differences in outcomes, some transplantation researchers believe flush solutions that are administered at very low temperatures can be detrimental for organ preservation [20, 21]. The optimal cooling rate for induction of hypothermic suspended animation remains to be determined.

The rate of re-warming from profound hypothermic suspended animation also influences outcome. Using CPB, Alam et al. induced 10 °C hypothermic cardiopulmonary arrest in their pig vascular injury model [22]. When pigs were re-warmed at the maximal rate that was technically achievable (~0.52–0.8 °C/min depending on core temperatures), the 6 week survival rate was only 30%, in contrast to 90% survival with somewhat slower re-warming at 0.5 °C/min. Surprisingly, substantially slower re-warming at 0.25 °C/min also produced poor outcome (6 week survival rate 50%). We have not set a target re-warming rate. Instead, the CPB water bath is set at a temperature that is 5 °C higher than the core blood temperatures. In ~45–60 min the dogs were re-warmed to 34 °C from 10 °C. This approach results in an average rate of re-warming of ~0.4–0.53 °C/min, which fortuitously has produced good outcome and appears to agree with the work discussed above [22].

Maintenance of mild hypothermia during the delayed resuscitation phase also appears to be a crucial adjunct for suspended animation. Empirically, mild hypothermia at 34 °C was kept for 12 h after CPB and satisfactory outcomes can be achieved with this approach for exsanguination cardiopulmonary arrest that occurs rapidly. As discussed above, longer periods of mild hypothermia are needed when prolonged hemorrhagic shock precedes exsanguination cardiopulmonary arrest. In this setting, shorter (12 h) periods of mild hypothermia were insufficient and resulted in delayed neurological deterioration with seizures after re-warming. When hypothermia was extended from 12 to 36 h, there were no seizures and intact neurological outcome could be achieved even after an exsanguination cardiopulmonary arrest that was preceded by over 2 h of hemorrhagic shock and profound acidosis at the time of suspended animation induction (Wu et al., unpublished data).

The Exploration of Pharmacological Approaches

The successful development of pharmacological adjuncts to suspended animation could have dramatic benefits on the potential clinical application of this therapy. Drugs can be easily delivered into the circulation – in contrast to the large fluid volumes needed to cool to levels of profound hypothermia (an aortic flush of ~500 ml/kg in dogs). If a pharmacological agent could completely supplant the need to cool, it would similarly eliminate the need to rapidly cannulate the aorta to administer a flush solution for suspended animation induction.

To this end, we tested the effects of 14 different pharmacological approaches in our suspended animation paradigm (Table 2). The model used was 20 min of exsanguination cardiopulmonary arrest with a potentially portable volume of flush solution (25 ml/kg) at ambient temperature, which achieved only mild cerebral hypothermia. In controls, saline flush started at 2 min of cardiopulmonary arrest produced survival, but with brain damage. In groups of 3 to 6 experiments per drug,

Table 2. Exploration of pharmacological approaches for suspended animation

	OPC 1	OPC 2	OPC 3	OPC 4	NDS (%)	HDS
Control	1/15	3/15	6/15	4/15	40 (18–63)	98 (58–136)
1. Energy metabolism						
▌Adenosine			2/2		50, 43	116, 120
▌Thiopental	2/8		2/8	4/8	52 (22–57)	60 (52–138)
▌Thiop/Phenytoin	1/7		2/7	4/7	55 (38–59)	76 (48–132)
▌Fructose BiPhosphate			2/5	3/5	55 (39–63)	96 (76–102)
2. Membrane stability						
▌MK801			2/5	3/5	50 (33-55)	80 (41–109)
▌YM872			1/3	2/3	43, 55, 63	78, 98, 72
▌Nimodipine			1/2	1/2	33, 66	86, 90
▌Diltiazem			1/2	1/2	47, 64	134, 100
▌Lidocaine			2/3	1/3	27, 48, 52	54, 118, 74
▌Insulin/Glucose	1/4		2/4	1/4	1, 32, 48, 51	NA
3. Protein-kinase inhibitor						
▌W7 *			1/2	1/2	66, 48	108, 98
4. Apoptosis inhibitor						
▌Cycloheximide			3/3		50, 39, 42	92, 72, 70
5. Antioxidant						
▌Tempo	5/8	3/8			9 (3–48)	58 (35–78)
6. Mitochondria protection						
▌Cyclosporine A			1/2	1/2	41, 71	NA

*: W7 = N-(6-amino-hexyl)-5-chloro-1-naphthalenesulphonamide; NDS: neurologic deficit score; OPC: overall performance category; HDS histologic deficit score

various doses were flushed into the aortic arch via an intra-aortic balloon catheter, and in some experiments, additional therapy was given during reperfusion with CPB. The drugs tested were categorized into one (or more) of the following mechanistic strategies:

▌ delaying energy failure,
▌ protecting cell membrane integrity,
▌ preventing structural degradation,
▌ regulating protein synthesis,
▌ preventing re-oxygenation injuries, and
▌ preserving mitochondria.

Remarkably, none of the 14 drugs yielded a breakthrough effect. The brain penetrating antioxidant tempol, however, appeared to produce some benefit [23]. Tempol is available and inexpensive and penetrates the blood-brain barrier, but it is not approved by the US Food and Drug Administration. All 8 dogs that received 150–300 mg/kg of tempol via the aortic arch flush, beginning at 2 min after cardiopulmonary arrest, were normal or near normal, whereas none of the 8 control dogs achieved consciousness. However, histological damage was not mitigated by tempol [23].

The goal of this series was to screen for a breakthrough drug. Clearly, no single pharmacological agent was effective, and we concluded that the efficacy of drugs paled in comparison to hypothermia. However, synergistic effects of drugs with hypothermia are likely, and should be explored in future studies. In addition, we did not carry out studies examining brain pharmacodynamics – and it is thus unclear if each agent was able to penetrate the blood-brain barrier and target the specific mechanism and produce its desired biochemical or molecular effect. Further studies in this regard are needed.

The Exploration of Novel Preservation Solutions

In the history of organ preservation for transplantation, preservation solutions have played a key role. However, in our pilot experiments, various solutions seemed to offer only marginal effects. In a 30 min cardiopulmonary arrest model, we found that neither 5–25% albumin nor Unisol (Organ Recovery Systems Inc., Pittsburgh, PA) improved outcome. In contrast, a combination of polynitroxylated albumin (Synzyme, Irving, CA) and tempol significantly reduced NDS and HDS compared to Unisol [24]. In one study using a 120 min cardiopulmonary arrest model, we evaluated a provocative approach put forth by Taylor et al. [25] using a solution with an intracellular composition to fill the vasculature after the flush (Unisol-I [Intracellular]) and followed this with an extracellular based solution (Unisol-E [Extracellular]) to initiate delayed resuscitation. This approach achieved conscious survival in 5 out of 6 dogs, while normal saline was less successful [14]. In a recirculation study of suspended animation, that was originally designed to reduce fluid requirement, a better outcome with recirculation of diluted blood but without gas-exchange was found over the one-way flush [19]. This observation fuels the speculation that certain components in the blood may be beneficial. As there was no fresh oxygen supply, oxygen carrying capacity of hemoglobin did not produce the observed effects.

In the field of cardiac surgery, Aoki et al. found that intermittent flush of University of Wisconsin solution via the carotid artery over 2 h of a profound hypothermic (15 °C) cardiopulmonary arrest in piglets improved recovery of cerebral blood flow and ATP during early reperfusion, compare to the saline flush group [26]. In an outcome study that followed, however, the piglets that received 50 ml/kg University of Wisconsin solution flushed via the carotid artery, exhibited similar OPC and NDS on day 5, but actually had worse histological deficit versus controls that did no receive any flush during cardiopulmonary arrest [27]. Robbins et al. found that oxygenated 'cerebroplegia' solution, which contained 2.5% glucose, 12.5% mannitol, 22 mEq sodium bicarbonate, 25 mEq/l lidocaine, 0.5 µg/l nitroglycerin, and 5 mg/l calcium chloride, flushed intermittently via the carotid artery during hypothermic cardiopulmonary arrest substantially delayed brain energy depletion [28]. More recently, Taylor et al. [25] developed an asanguinous solution for whole-body perfusion during profound hypothermic cardiopulmonary arrest. The choices of the components for the solution were literature-based, and satisfactory outcome after 3 h cardiopulmonary arrest was achieved. However, it is not clear if the solution has any specific brain preservation effects, since the main problems seen in the controls but absent in the treatment group were cardiac or peripheral nerve injury and/or dysfunction [25].

▌ Devices

Although we believe that suspended animation can be implemented in trauma centers using currently available surgical devices, to induce suspended animation in the field requires the development of a number of related technologies. Most important is the need for the safe and timely cannulation of the aorta by paramedics – who generally lack surgical expertise. For this, Yaffe et al. have been developing a "smart catheter" – an ultrasound-guided approach with a self-sealing catheter that might allow paramedics to percutaneously insert an aortic catheter in the field [29]. Prototypes are also under development for portable cooling and pumping in the field.

▌ Mechanistic Studies

Studies in Large Animals

The most vulnerable organ during prolonged cardiopulmonary arrest, with or without hypothermia, is the brain. When the whole body was cooled to $\sim 10\,^\circ$C for preservation of up to 3 h of cardiopulmonary arrest, lethal extra-cerebral organ injuries were rare using our delayed resuscitation protocol. The mechanisms of brain injury in suspended animation and reperfusion are likely multifactorial. Even when the brain temperature was reduced to $8\,^\circ$C, oxygen consumption remains at $\sim 11\%$ of baseline [30], and ATP and creatine phosphate in the brain were shown to be depleted in 60–90 min during deep hypothermia (12–15 $^\circ$C) [28]. Given that 2 min of normothermic cardiopulmonary arrest precedes the induction of hypothermia in a suspended animation model, energy depletion would occur sooner and may play a major role in the brain injury in our suspended animation model. Release of excitatory amino acids and production of nitric oxide (NO) contribute to neuronal injury during profound hypothermic cardiopulmonary arrest [31].

Proteomic Approaches in Suspended Animation

An initial study in our center focused on the degradation of brain proteins during a prolonged hypothermic or normothermic circulatory arrest. We noted that 30 min of complete ischemia at either 37 or 10 $^\circ$C results in minimal protein degradations as assessed with 1 D and 2 D gel electrophoresis [32]. Future studies will evaluate the effect of reperfusion on protein degradation. In the 1960s, in seminal studies in the field of prolonged hypothermic preservation, White et al. [33] preserved the dog brain at 2 $^\circ$C for hours to days. Remarkably, he used on isolated dog head preparation. After recirculation and re-warming, electroencephalogram (EEG) signals, pupil light reflex and rhythmic gasping were seen in the heads that were preserved for 4 h. However, this electrophysiological activity eventually disappeared as reperfusion at 34 $^\circ$C went beyond 6 h [33]. Incredibly, thus, in 1966, White's finding was consistent with the contemporary concept of 'reperfusion injury' as a key mechanism of damage in brain ischemia.

A Rat Model of Suspended Animation

We chose a dog model for these suspended animation experiments to maximize clinical relevance. However, certain limitations are pertinent to that model. First, there are few molecular tools available for dogs. That limits the evaluation of impact of therapies on the cellular and molecular mechanisms of secondary injury. Understanding molecular mechanisms of ischemia-reperfusion injury, and the impact of suspended animation on these cascades, would allow us to define specific targets for future interventions, and to assess markers of reversibility. Second, the cost and labor-intensiveness of the suspended animation experiment in dogs poses an obstacle to rapid screening of drugs and preservation solutions that would seem promising.

Based on these limitations, we have recently launched a project to develop a rat model of suspended animation to address these drawbacks. The cornerstone of the successful establishment of the model was development of a miniaturized CPB machine that would be effective in rats, because CPB is essential to delayed resuscitation after prolonged periods of suspended animation.

In the past, there were many attempts to develop CPB for small animals [34]; the first one being used in cats as early as in 1937. Over the past sixty years, tremendous improvements have been achieved. Both pulsatile and non-pulsatile models of CPB have been described and tested on various large animals – dogs, cows, sheep, pigs and rabbits. In many studies, perfusion of isolated organs was evaluated, while only a few studies actually implemented CPB in small animals. Often, open-chest cannulation was used, which prevented long-term survival. A limited number of papers reported successful separation of the study animal from CPB. Recently, several centers have reported successful establishment of CPB in rats [35]. Unfortunately, many of these reports are still published only in abstract form.

The absence of a commercially available CPB machine for rodents remains another limiting factor. The static priming volume required in even the smallest pediatric oxygenators approximates 40 ml, which is nearly twice the total blood volume of a rat. Donor blood for the circuit prime is still necessary, even for the custom-made devices that are now available, with priming volumes less than 10 ml. Transfusion of whole blood between rats does not appear to be an important problem with regard to blood compatibility; however, subtle transfusion-related injury may remain underappreciated.

Grocott and co-workers have reported that CPB *per se* causes neurologic and neurocognitive impairment in rats – even in the absence of cardiopulmonary arrest [36, 37]. CPB has also been shown to trigger mesenteric endothelial dysfunction [38], and acute lung injury (ALI) [39] as part of the systemic inflammatory response syndrome. Mechanical ventilation itself leads to endothelial damage, especially superimposed upon ischemia-reperfusion injury [40]. These findings are in accordance with the well-recognized effects of CPB seen in humans. The leading cause of the neurologic injury associated with CPB use in man – microembolism – has not been studied in rats. Current research by investigators using these new CPB devices in rats is focused on the effect of CPB on the brain [41] and is targeting approaches to ameliorate the systemic inflammation [42–44].

As discussed, a proteomic approach was used to assess protein degradation after suspended animation using decapitation to produce global ischemia. Those studies focused solely on the effect of intra-ischemic protein degradation during prolonged global cerebral ischemia with and without hypothermia. The model used precluded the possibility of reperfusion. Remarkably, no major changes in the rat brain proteome were noted after normothermic or hypothermic ischemia – even with durations as long as 30 min [45].

Reperfusion is likely to result in protein degradation via either calcium- or oxidation-mediated pathways. We also anticipate that reperfusion will produce degradation of lipids. Both protein and lipid degradation may have a critical influence on the final outcome. To be able to address these pathways requires substantial molecular tools. Such tools are not available for use with tissue from dogs. In contrast, panoply of molecular tools is available for use with rat tissue. Thus, the ability to develop a rat model of suspended animation was essential to allowing us to pursue these important questions, and is a current area of focus in our laboratory.

In our model, resuscitation from suspended animation was first attempted using miniaturized CPB with small priming volume [46]. In pilot experiments, designed to mirror dog studies, we hypothesized that 30 min of suspended animation would be achievable in rats, and that Plasma-Lyte A would be a more favorable flush solution than normal saline. In our initial studies, hemorrhagic shock was induced with rapid exsanguination (12.5 ml) over 5 min, followed by KCl-induced cardiopulmonary arrest. After 2 min of no-flow, cooling was initiated with ice-cold flush and surface cooling. A target temperature of 10 °C was chosen. After 30 min of suspended animation, reperfusion and re-warming were achieved via CPB over 60 min. Four out of seven rats survived to 24 h at both groups. Favorable outcome (OPC 1) with minimal neurologic impairment on clinical assessment were achieved in both groups, with better results in Plasma-Lyte A group (4/7 rats) vs normal saline group (2/7 rats). Important to the potential future use of this model, microscopic alterations within the brain sections were minimal in the long-term survivors in these studies. Surprisingly, despite normal brain pathology, some extracerebral injury was noted on microscopic examination. Rats cooled with normal saline flush showed more severe heart, lung and kidney injury than those cooled with Plasma-Lyte A.

To our knowledge, this is one of the first descriptions of the successful use of CPB in a rat model that includes cardiopulmonary arrest, and certainly the first study of the successful resuscitation of a rat *after* prolonged cardiopulmonary arrest with deep or profound hypothermia. In our suspended animation studies, the cardiopulmonary arrest is induced before the induction of hypothermia. It is well recognized that it is much more challenging to successfully preserve or resuscitate an organism with hypothermia or any other strategy after the onset of a cardiopulmonary arrest than it is to protect with hypothermia before the insult. All of our studies with suspended animation have tackled the latter more challenging insult. Thus, it appears that suspended animation is achievable in rats and can produce intact neurological outcome and normal brain histopathology. We are currently characterizing this model and pushing the 30 min limit that was achieved in our initial work.

Future studies focused at better organ preservation are underway in many centers. Diverse drugs such as phosphodiesterase (PDE)-4 inhibitor [47], xenon or other volatile anesthetics [48], P-selectin [42], and glutamine [44] have yielded favorable results in terms of ameliorating CPB-induced injury or ischemic injury, respectively. Other promising drugs including delta-opioid agonists or hibernation-induction triggers are emerging on the horizon. Knowledge of the molecular and cellular derangements will help target future therapies.

Successful establishment of this technically demanding model will allow the use of molecular tools to study the effects of suspended animation or deep hypothermia circulatory arrest and reperfusion on neuronal death and organ injury. This will have relevance to cardiac surgery and organ preservation. The ideal recipe for the suspended animation-inducing flush solution remains to be determined. The optimal composition of this 'magic potion' will, hopefully, be determined based on scientific evidence from our molecular studies, but may also require serendipity. Hemodynamic management must also be optimized during reperfusion, to maximize outcome.

▌ Other Possible Applications of Suspended Animation and the Futuristic Perspective of Suspended Animation

In a broad sense, suspended animation can be viewed as a strategy that bridges an organism over an insult that is otherwise incompatible with life. Besides traumatic cardiopulmonary arrest, other potential targets for suspended animation might include refractory normovolemic cardiopulmonary arrest, cardiac or neurosurgical procedures that are impossible without extremely prolonged periods of circulatory arrest, consequences of chemical or biological warfare, and potentially other applications. When the milieu is improved by plasma exchange, administration of antidotes or the anatomic structure is corrected by surgery, delayed resuscitation can be started.

▌ Conclusion

Suspended animation is a novel concept created to resuscitate traumatic cardiopulmonary arrest. We have proven its feasibility in a series of large animal experiments using clinically-relevant suspended animation models. The effectiveness of the hypothermic approach has been repeatedly demonstrated, and the maturity of the techniques prompts us to plan suspended animation clinical trials with currently available devices in trauma centers in the setting of otherwise lethal exsanguination cardiopulmonary arrest (Fig. 1). To make suspended animation eventually

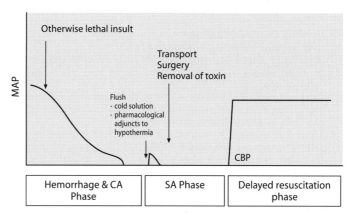

Fig. 1. Potential clinical scenario for application of suspended animation with (SA) delayed resuscitation as developed by investigators at the Safar Center for Resuscitation Research. See text for details. CA: cardiopulmonary arrest; SA: suspended animation; CPB: cardiopulmonary bypass; MAP: mean arterial pressure

a technique for field resuscitation, further, bold developments of cannulation and cooling techniques are also required. The exploration of pharmacologic approaches, however, needs more efforts to develop effective brain oriented preservation cocktails with drugs or solutions. Mechanistic studies using 2D proteomics and lipidomics may unveil the complex ischemic and reperfusion pathophysiology, and shed light into the area of pharmacological intervention.

We have taken the first steps toward moving the concept of suspended animation from science fiction to reality – through rigorous scientific investigation. Further research into suspended animation may lead to a substantial improvement in the resuscitation of trauma-induced cardiopulmonary arrest for the first time in the past decades, benefit cardiovascular and neurological surgeries that need brain preservation techniques, and provide novel insight into the limits of viability of the brain and the entire organism during prolonged cardiopulmonary arrest.

Acknowledgements. This work was supported by the United States Army Medical Research and Materiel Command, Ft. Detrick, Maryland (DAMD 17-01-2-0038). We thank Drs. Samuel Tisherman, Larry Jenkins, Mandeep Chadha, and Mr. William Stezoski for their critical roles on this project. We also thank the technical support team for their work on these studies and the many prior fellows who have contributed enormously to this work. We thank Dr. Lyn Yaffe for key consultative input, and COL Dean Calcagni and Mr. Robert Read of the US Army Telemedicine and Advanced Technology Research Center for their enthusiastic support. This chapter is dedicated to the late Dr. Peter Safar who passed away on August 3, 2003.

References

1. Bellamy R, Safar P, Tisherman SA, et al (1996) Suspended animation for delayed resuscitation. Crit Care Med 24 (Suppl 2):S24–S47
2. Trunkey D (1991) Initial treatment of patients with extensive trauma. N Engl J Med 324:1259–1263
3. Rhee PM, Acosta J, Bridgeman A, Wang D, Jordan M, Rich N (2000) Survival after emergency department thoracotomy: review of published data from the past 25 years. J Am Coll Surg 190:288–298
4. Hopson LR, Hirsh E, Delgado J, et al (2003) Guidelines for withholding or termination of resuscitation in prehospital traumatic cardiopulmonary arrest. J Am Coll Surg 196:475–481
5. Holcomb JB (2003) Fluid resuscitation in modern combat casualty care: lessons learned from Somalia. J Trauma 54 (Suppl 5):S46–S51
6. Manning JE, Katz LM, Pearce LB, et al (2001) Selective aortic arch perfusion with hemoglobin-based oxygen carrier-201 for resuscitation from exsanguinating cardiac arrest in swine. Crit Care Med 29:2067–2074
7. Capone A, Safar P, Radovsky A, Wang YF, Peitzman A, Tisherman SA (1996) Complete recovery after normothermic hemorrhagic shock and profound hypothermic circulatory arrest of 60 min in dogs. J Trauma 40:388–395
8. Tisherman SA, Safar P, Radovsky A, et al (1991) Profound hypothermia (less than 10 degrees C) compared with deep hypothermia (15 degrees C) improves neurologic outcome in dogs after two hours' circulatory arrest induced to enable resuscitative surgery. J Trauma 31:1051–1061
9. Tisherman SA, Safar P, Radovsky A, et al (1990) Deep hypothermic circulatory arrest induced during hemorrhagic shock in dogs: preliminary systemic and cerebral metabolism studies. Curr Surg 47:327–330
10. Tisherman SA, Safar P, Radovsky A, Peitzman A, Sterz F, Kuboyama K (1990) Therapeutic deep hypothermic circulatory arrest in dogs: a resuscitation modality for hemorrhagic shock with 'irreparable' injury. J Trauma 30:836–847

11. Nozari A, Safar P, Wu X, et al (2004) Suspended animation can allow survival without brain damage after traumatic exsanguination cardiac arrest of 60 min in dogs. J Trauma 57:1266–1275

12. Nozari A, Safar P, Tisherman S, et al (2004) Suspended animation and plasma exchange enables full neurologic recovery from lethal traumatic exsanguination, even after 2 h period of no-flow. Crit Care Med (Suppl):A9–36 (abst)

13. Behringer W, Safar P, Wu X, Kentner R, Radovsky A, Tisherman SA (2001) Delayed intra-ischemic aortic cold flush for preservation during prolonged cardiac arrest in dogs. Crit Care Med 29 (Suppl):A17–52 (abst)

14. Behringer W, Safar P, Nozari A, Wu X, Kentner R, Tisherman SA (2004) Intact survival of 120 min cardiac arrest at 10 degree C in Dogs. Cerebral preservation by cold aortic flush. Crit Care Med 29 (Suppl):A71–225 (abst)

15. Behringer W, Prueckner S, Kentner R, et al (2000) Rapid hypothermic aortic flush can achieve survival without brain damage after 30 minutes cardiac arrest in dogs. Anesthesiology 93:1491–1499

16. Behringer W, Prueckner S, Safar P, et al (2000) Rapid induction of mild cerebral hypothermia by cold aortic flush achieves normal recovery in a dog outcome model with 20-minute exsanguination cardiac arrest. Acad Emerg Med 7:1341–1348

17. Behringer W, Safar P, Wu X, et al (2003) Survival without brain damage after clinical death of 60–120 min in dogs using suspended animation by profound hypothermia. Crit Care Med 31:1523–1531

18. Alam HB, Chen Z, Honma K, et al (2004) The rate of induction of hypothermic arrest determines the outcome in a swine model of lethal hemorrhage. Trauma 57:961–969

29. Nozari A, Safar P, Stezoski W, et al (2004) Suspended animation for 90 min cardiac arrest in dogs with small volume arterial flush and veno-arterial extracorporeal cooling. Crit Care Med 31(Suppl):A9–35 (abst)

20. Albes JM, Fischer F, Bando T, Heinemann MK, Scheule A, Wahlers T (1997) Influence of the perfusate temperature on lung preservation: is there an optimum? Eur Surg Res 29:5–11

21. Solberg S, Larsen T, Jorgensen L, Sorlie D (1987) Cold induced endothelial cell detachment in human saphenous vein grafts. J Cardiovasc Surg (Torino) 28:571–575

22. Alam HB, Rhee P, Honma K, et al (2005) The rate of rewarming from profound hypothermic arrest influences the outcome in a swine model of lethal hemorrhage. J Trauma (in press)

23. Behringer W, Safar P, Kentner R, et al (2002) Antioxidant Tempol enhances hypothermic cerebral preservation during prolonged cardiac arrest in dogs. J Cereb Blood Flow Metab 22:105–117

24. Behringer W, Safar P, Kentner R, et al (2004) Novel solutions for intra-ischemic aortic cold flush for preservation during 30 min cardia arrest in dogs. Crit Care Med 29 (Suppl):A71 (abst)

25. Taylor MJ, Bailes JE, Elrifai AM, et al (1995) A new solution for life without blood. Asanguineous low-flow perfusion of a whole-body perfusate during 3 h of cardiac arrest and profound hypothermia. Circulation 91:431–444

26. Aoki M, Jonas RA, Nomura F, et al (1994) Effects of cerebroplegic solutions during hypothermic circulatory arrest and short-term recovery. J Thorac Cardiovasc Surg 108:291–301

27. Forbess JM, Ibla JC, Lidov HG, et al (1995) University of Wisconsin cerebroplegia in a piglet survival model of circulatory arrest. Ann Thorac Surg 60 (Suppl 6):S494–S500

28. Robbins RC, Balaban RS, Swain JA (1990) Intermittent hypothermic asanguineous cerebral perfusion (cerebroplegia) protects the brain during prolonged circulatory arrest. A phosphorus 31 nuclear magnetic resonance study. J Thorac Cardiovasc Surg 99:878–884

29. Yaffe L, Abbott D, Schulte B (2004) Smart aortic arch catheter: moving suspended animation from the laboratory to the field. Crit Care Med 32 (Suppl 2):S51–S55

30. Ehrlich MP, McCullough JN, Zhang N, et al (2002) Effect of hypothermia on cerebral blood flow and metabolism in the pig. Ann Thorac Surg 73:191–197

31. Tseng EE, Brock MV, Lange MS, et al (1998) Monosialoganglioside GM1 inhibits neurotoxicity after hypothermic circulatory arrest. Surgery 124:298–306

32. Chadha M, Kochanek PM, Safar P, Jenkins L (2002) Proteomic changes in rat brain after 30 min of complete cerebral ischemia with hypothermia treatment. Crit Care Med 30 (Suppl): A24 (abst)
33. White RJ, Albin MS, Verdura J, Locke GE (1966) Prolonged whole-brain refrigeration with electrical and metabolic recovery. Nature 209:1320–1322
34. Ballaux PK, Gourlay T, Ratnatunga CP, Taylor KM (1999) A literature review of cardiopulmonary bypass models for rats. Perfusion 14:411–417
35. Gourlay T, Ballaux PK, Draper ER, Taylor KM (2002) Early experience with a new technique and technology designed for the study of pulsatile cardiopulmonary bypass in the rat. Perfusion 17:191–198
36. Mackensen GB, Sato Y, Nellgard B, et al (2001) Cardiopulmonary bypass induces neurologic and neurocognitive dysfunction in the rat. Anesthesiology 95:1485–1491
37. Grocott HP, Mackensen GB, Newman MF, Warner DS (2001) Neurological injury during cardiopulmonary bypass in the rat. Perfusion 16:75–81
38. Doguet F, Litzler PY, Tamion F, et al (2004) Changes in mesenteric vascular reactivity and inflammatory response after cardiopulmonary bypass in a rat model. Ann Thorac Surg 77:2130–2137
39. Senra DF, Katz M, Passerotti GH, et al (2001) A rat model of acute lung injury induced by cardiopulmonary bypass. Shock 16:223–226
40. Sasaki S, Takigami K, Shiiya N, Yasuda K (1996) Partial cardiopulmonary bypass in rats for evaluating ischemia-reperfusion injury. ASAIO J 42:1027–1030
41. Hindman BJ, Moore SA, Cutkomp J, et al (2001) Brain expression of inducible cyclooxygenase 2 messenger RNA in rats undergoing cardiopulmonary bypass. Anesthesiology 95:1380–1388
42. Hayashi Y, Sawa Y, Nishimura M, et al (2000) P-selectin participates in cardiopulmonary bypass-induced inflammatory response in association with nitric oxide and peroxynitrite production. J Thorac Cardiovasc Surg 120:558–565
43. Hayashi Y, Sawa Y, Fukuyama N, Nakazawa H, Matsuda H (2002) Preoperative glutamine administration induces heat-shock protein 70 expression and attenuates cardiopulmonary bypass-induced inflammatory response by regulating nitric oxide synthase activity. Circulation 106:2601–2607
44. Hayashi Y, Sawa Y, Fukuyama N, Nakazawa H, Matsuda H (2001) Inducible nitric oxide production is an adaptation to cardiopulmonary bypass-induced inflammatory response. Ann Thorac Surg 72:149–155
45. Fountoulakis M, Hardmeier R, Hoger H, Lubec G (2001) Postmortem changes in the level of brain proteins. Exp Neurol 167:86–94
46. Houston RJ, de Lange F, Kalkman CJ (1904) A new miniature fiber oxygenator for small animal cardiopulmonary bypass. Adv Exp Med Biol 540:313–316
47. Hamamoto M, Suga M, Nakatani T, et al (2004) Phosphodiesterase type 4 inhibitor prevents acute lung injury induced by cardiopulmonary bypass in a rat model. Eur J Cardiothorac Surg 25:833–838
48. Ma D, Yang H, Lynch J, Franks NP, Maze M, Grocott HP (2003) Xenon attenuates cardiopulmonary bypass-induced neurologic and neurocognitive dysfunction in the rat. Anesthesiology 98:690–698

Intraabdominal Pressure

The Abdominal Compartment Syndrome in the Critically Ill Patient

T. Standl and A. Gottschalk

▌ Introduction

Within the last decade the abdominal compartment syndrome (ACS) has gained increasing interest in intensive care medicine. Although the term 'abdominal compartment syndrome' was established by Kron et al. [1] in patients after surgery of the abdominal aorta, the syndrome has now emerged as a significant problem in many intensive care patients. Several recently published studies demonstrate that the ACS represents a relevant and critical clinical condition which is still underestimated with respect to its incidence and severity [2–4]. Although the negative influence of an increased intraabdominal pressure (IAP) on the respiratory system was described nearly one century ago, the pathophysiology of the ACS has not been understood adequately in the past [5]. However, the widespread use of laparoscopic surgery and the increasing scientific and clinical interest in the pathophysiology of the capnoperitoneum has focused the attention of anesthesiologists and intensivists towards the ACS which previously has often been called an 'epiphenomenon'. Knowledge of the ACS, which can result in rapid development of multiple organ failure (MOF), is crucial to provide timely and adequate treatment, thus decreasing the incidence of MOF [6–9].

▌ Characteristics of the ACS

The term 'compartment' generally describes a closed space with limited compliance where an increase in volume results in an increase of the pressure within this space, e.g., increase in the intracranial pressure (ICP) in patients with intracranial bleeding or edema. Although the relatively elastic abdominal wall and diaphragm allow limited expansion of the abdomen, the intraabdominal space meets the criteria for the possible development of a compartment syndrome. The increase in IAP first leads to a reduction in the venous flow and with further increasing IAP to a decreased arterial perfusion resulting in impairment of organ function. The ACS is now understood to be a combination of respiratory, cardiovascular, splanchnic, renal, and intracranial disturbances resulting from an acute and more or less rapid increase in IAP [10].

The normal IAP was thought to be atmospheric or even subatmospheric, but recent studies have demonstrated a mean value of 6.5 mmHg, which can increase with body mass index [11] and sagittal abdominal diameter [12]. Mechanical ventilation produces a positive IAP which is close to the endexpiratory pressure. Values up to

10 mmHg are considered as normal in ventilated patients. Intraabdominal hypertension (IAH) is assessed according to escalating values for IAP as grade I: 10–15 mmHg; grade II: 16–25 mmHg; grade III: 26–35 mmHg and grade IV: >35 mmHg [13].

Balogh et al. recently defined the ACS as the combination of:

▌ IAP greater than 25 mmHg;

▌ progressive organ dysfunction (urinary output <0.5 ml/kg/h or PaO_2/FiO_2 >150 or peak airway pressure >45 cmH_2O or cardiac index <3 l/min/m^2 despite resuscitation); and

▌ improved organ function after decompression [2].

The ACS can be subdivided into primary and secondary ACS. Primary ACS is caused by diseases such as pancreatitis, intraabdominal aneurysms and malignancies, ascites, or by blunt abdominal or pelvic trauma. Ongoing intraabdominal bleeding due to failed nonoperative management of abdominal organ injuries is the main reason for this situation (Fig. 1) [14]. Secondary ACS is a result of massive volume resuscitation in severe hemorrhagic shock and because of reperfusion injury after surgical aneurysm repair or a complication of damage control laparotomy. In these patients the abdominal content is mainly increased by bowel edema and probably ascites. Additionally, secondary ACS can be caused by intraabdominal 'packing' (Fig. 2) or forced primary closure of the abdominal wall after acute surgical interventions in patients with enormous hernias, ileus, or peritonitis [15].

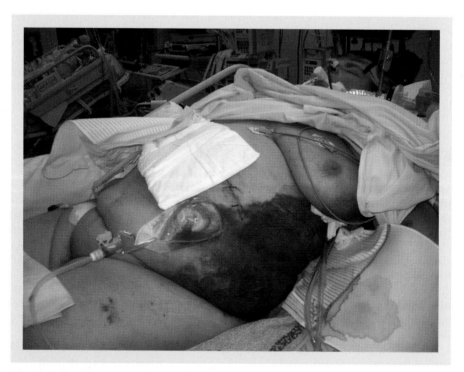

Fig. 1. 68-year-old obese woman after deceleration trauma causing multiple rib fractures and hematothorax on the left side and secondary rupture of the spleen

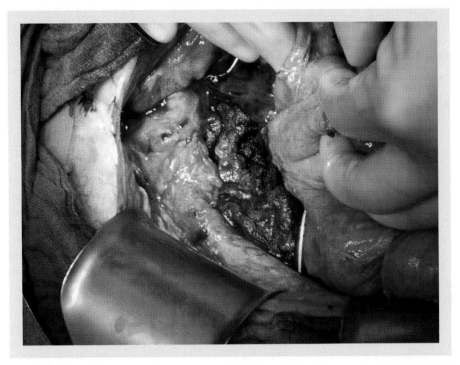

Fig. 2. Abdominal packing because of intrabdominal bleeding which could not be terminated by surgical intervention

Incidence of ACS

It still is difficult to estimate the incidence of ACS in intensive care patients. A main problem is that incidence often has been estimated retrospectively and has included inconsistent definitions of ACS. Additionally heterogenic patient populations, non-standardized diagnosis and therapy, and lack of adequate statistical analyses, such as multivariate analyses of the data, result in difficult estimations of the risk for the development of the ACS.

Of 188 patients with multiple injury undergoing a standardized "goal-orientated resuscitation", 6% developed primary and 8% secondary ACS [8]. In another study, including 311 trauma patients with abdominal or pelvic trauma, the incidence of primary ACS was 5.5% [14]. In a retrospective analysis of 377 patients, primary ACS was the reason for surgical intervention including installation of a laparostoma in 16% of the patients [16]. In a recently published multicenter prospective 1-day-point prevalence epidemiological study in 13 intensive care units (ICUs) in six countries, Malbrain et al. enrolled 97 patients [17]. The prevalence of IAH was 50.5% (defined as IAP > 12 mmHg) and 8.2% had ACS (defined as IAP > 20 mmHg). The only risk factor significantly associated with IAH was the body mass index, while massive fluid resuscitation, renal and coagulation impairment were at the limit of significance. Other predictors for IAH under discussion consist of increased blood lactate levels, mesh closure, abdominal trauma, high crystalloid volume and low systemic blood pressure in surgical and trauma patients, and an increase in the net fluid balance, plateau airway pressure and CO_2 gap [8, 9, 18]. However, independent of the incidence of ACS which varies between different studies, the mortality rate of ACS remains between 29 and 100% [2].

Diagnosis and Monitoring of Increased Intraabdominal Pressure

Clinical examination in intensive care patients only has a limited importance in the diagnosis of ACS. IAP can be measured directly by laparoscopy or by a less invasive indirect technique. The most widely used, but non-continuous technique described by Kron and modified by others is the measurement of the urinary bladder pressure using a transurethral catheter [1]. This technique is easy to perform and shows a good correlation with IAP [19]. However, previous bladder surgery, bladder tumors, neurogenic bladder disorders, and abdominal packing with restricted motion of the bladder wall may result in incorrect, mainly artificially high, values. Other methods of IAP recording include intermittent transgastric IAP measurement via nasogastric tubes, a semi-continuous technique using an esophageal balloon catheter placed in the stomach, or a continuously measuring fully automated gastric air-pouch system [20]. Other techniques use manometry with probes inserted in the inferior vena cava, in the rectum, or in the uterus.

The technique of the urinary bladder pressure measurement requires a urinary catheter with a T-piece allowing continuous sterile access. The patient has to be placed in the supine position. After the bladder is completely emptied the catheter is clamped distal of the T-piece and 50 ml saline is infused into the bladder. In cases where a conventional urinary catheter is in situ, a needle or venous cannula can be inserted into the aspiration port of the urinary catheter and attached to the pressure transducer. The level of the pubic symphysis is used as zero for the preceding calibration.

Malbrain et al. recently reviewed different IAP measurement techniques and concluded that there is no gold standard of IAP measurement, since all the different techniques are difficult to compare [20]. However, the urinary bladder pressure measurement can be used as an estimate for IAP and as a screening method to identify patients at risk. Additionally the authors pointed out that for (multicenter) study purposes, surgical patients, trauma patients, patients at higher risk for IAH, it is preferable to switch to a continuous method for IAP monitoring via the stomach to focus therapy on optimizing IAP. On the background of increasing economical pressure in the health system and especially the costs explosion of intensive care medicine every method of measurement of the IAP has to be evaluated with respect to cost and effectiveness.

Effects of Intraabdominal Hypertension

The increase in IAP results in different pathophysiological changes in vital organs. Short duration increases in IAP, which occur during coughing or Valsalva's maneuver, are not clinically relevant. Nevertheless, continuously and rapidly increasing IAP affects regional blood flow and impairs tissue perfusion significantly. Harmful effects can be expected within hours in the following organ systems:

Cardiovascular System

Increased IAP impairs venous return due to compression of the retroperitoneal veins and due to a direct mechanical restriction of the inferior vena cava, especially at the step in the diaphragm (threshold between the abdominal and thoracic cavity) [4]. Simultaneously the systemic vascular resistance (SVR) increases, causing an increase in the left ventricular afterload. The increased intrathoracic pressure, which is the result of an upward movement of the diaphragm, increases right ventricular afterload and can lead to right ventricular failure and dilatation with impaired left ventricular filling due to displacement of the ventricular septum [21]. High values of central venous pressure (CVP) and pulmonary artery occlusion pressure (PAOP) are artificially induced by the high IAP and do not reflect the volume status [3, 21, 22].

Clinically, patients show a high heart rate to maintain the cardiac output with a reduced stroke volume. A critical hypovolemia in combination with tachycardia and increased SVR can be deleterious, especially in patients with cardiac disease. Aggressive volume substitution in trauma patients performed with crystalloids to improve the oxygen supply to supranormal values $(DO_2 > 600 \text{ ml/min/m}^2)$ caused an increased number of patients with ACS [9]. Therefore, adequate volume substitution in hypovolemic patients should be monitored carefully, e.g., by measurement of the extravascular lung water (EVLW) or repeated transesophageal echocardiography (TEE).

Respiratory System

Impairment of respiratory function is mainly caused by the increased IAP resulting in an upward movement of the diaphragm. The thoracic compliance decreases and an increased pressure is required to ventilate these patients. Additionally, the upward movement of the diaphragm causes compression atelectases in the basal areas of the lung with an increase in the ventilation/perfusion mismatch resulting in a higher shunt fraction with deteriorated oxygenation [3, 22]. The hypoxic pulmonary vasoconstriction is associated with a higher right ventricular stress, since pulmonary arterial pressure increases. In ventilated patients, a significantly higher airway pressure is necessary to maintain sufficient gas exchange including the risk of barotrauma. Moreover, atelectases are a risk factor for the development of bronchopulmonary infections. In animal models, ACS caused intense pulmonary inflammatory infiltration [6].

Intestine and Bowel

The increase in IAP results in impaired perfusion of the stomach, duodenum, jejunum, ileum, and colon. The pathophysiolocigal background is a reduced portal venous flow and a reduced chylus flow via the thoracic duct as well as a reduced arterial flow in the mesenteric arteries. Additionally, cardiac output is often decreased. In severe cases, tissue ischemia can result with alteration of the mucosal barrier and increased bacterial translocation leading to an activation of proinflammatory cytokines (interleukin [IL]-1, IL-6, IL-8, tumor necrosis factor [TNF]-a) and eicosanoids [23]. According to experiments in rats and swine with peritonitis the increase in IAP enhances the incidence of septicemia and endotoxemia [24, 25]. The impaired intestinal immune system in ACS is believed to play an important role in MOF.

Liver

IAP increase reduces hepatic perfusion, since the arterial blood flow in the hepatic artery, as well as the portal venous flow, is reduced [26]. Due to the impaired hepatic microcirculation, paracentral necroses can be detected histologically. An IAP of only 14 mmHg was associated with a significantly increased impairment in liver parenchymal function. The release of endotoxin from the gut further worsens liver function [27]. Clinical signs of impaired liver function can be detected by an increase in the liver enzymes and lactate concentration after 18–24 hours. Ongoing damage of the liver parenchyma is detected with increased bilirubin concentration and alkaline phosphatase activity.

Renal Function

The pathogenesis of renal dysfunction during ACS is complex and multifactorial. IAP of 15–20 mmHg results in oliguria, whereas a pressure of more than 30 mmHg induces anuria [3, 28, 29]. Due to the abdominal pressure and the decreased cardiac output, the venous and arterial blood flows of the kidneys are reduced. With the reduced blood flow in the kidneys, the glomerular filtration rate (GFR) which is mediated by secretion of renin and angiotensin and aldosterone-mediated water reabsorption is also reduced [30, 31]. The compression of the ureters has been implicated also as a contributing factor in the development of renal impairment. However, inserting catheters into both ureters had no favorable effects on diuresis in these patients [10].

Brain

The potential impairment of cerebral function in patients with ACS is often underestimated, although nearly 50% of the patients with severe abdominal trauma additionally have severe head and brain injury [32]. The main reason for the increase in the ICP is the increased intra-thoracic pressure as a result of the upward movement of the diaphragm in patients with ACS. The increased intra-thoracic pressure impairs the venous return from the brain. The increased ICP consequently reduces cerebral blood flow [33, 34]. Especially in patients with severe cerebral trauma, an increase in ICP can have deleterious consequences and must be continuously monitored by invasive probes.

▌ Management of ACS in the ICU

Early identification of patients at risk for ACS is the most important issue with respect to the prognosis of these patients [8, 15]. However, active detection of ACS is not a common practice in many ICUs. On the other hand, clinical examination alone is not sensitive enough to detect an increased IAP, especially in the early stages [35]. Therefore, the detection of independent predictors is of high importance. Hypothermia, a low hemoglobin concentration, and a high base excess in trauma patients have been identified as independent predictors for primary ACS

[8]. Patients with ACS show a higher fluid balance within the first 24 h of admission and higher peak airway pressures [36]. Patients with ACS (n = 44) remained longer in the ICU and in the hospital and showed a higher mortality in comparison to the control group (67 vs. 0%). With respect to secondary ACS it has been shown that the use of a high volume of crystalloids as well as increasing renal insufficiency worsens the prognosis [9, 15]. Based on several case reports and retrospective as well as prospective studies, it has been demonstrated that, in patients with primary ACS, the first 6–12 hrs play the most important role with respect to the dynamics of IAP increase and the further prognosis [8]. When the primary ACS was not detected until 24 h after admission to the hospital more patients developed a severe ACS and showed a higher mortality. Therefore, the decision for fast surgical decompression of the abdomen as the therapy of choice is mainly influenced by the progression of the IAP and the progression of organ dysfunction. Irrespective of the temporary recovery after the decompression surgery and the initial restoration of respiratory, cardiovascular, and renal function, mortality in these patients remains high due to the impaired organ function and imminent MOF [15]. Only improved cardiac index, reduced base excess, and recovered renal function were associated with an improved outcome in patients with ACS after decompression surgery [8]. In a small study with only 14 patients suffering from secondary ACS, decompression surgery lowered the ventilatory pressure and the urinary bladder pressure and resulted in an increase in the arterial pressure and diuresis [37].

Depending on the intraabdominal findings during decompression surgery, the abdomen may not be closed. In the majority of patients, open abdomen treatment has to be performed. The management of the open abdomen in the ICU includes treatment of specially associated risks like desiccation due to a large surface area for fluid loss. Additionally the open abdomen exposes the viscera to trauma and is a route for infection. The simplest method is to place wet abdominal packs soaked in saline over the bowel to prevent desiccation followed by watertight dressing. A synthetic net (e.g., vicryl) can be placed onto the gut and fixed at the edge of the abdominal wall thus preventing herniation of the small intestine (Fig. 3). The risk of abdominal hernias after open abdomen treatment can probably be prevented by using a vacuum assisted closure of the abdomen. Studies demonstrate that wound healing with the use of a vacuum treatment results in a complete closure of the fascia in 80% of patients [38].

The treatment of patients with ACS depends on the dynamics of the IAP. In patients with an IAP < 20 mmHg all treatment possibilities should be considered which are able to minimize the intraabdominal volume. In patients with terminal liver insufficiency and consecutive development of ascites, drainage of the ascites can result in improved hemodynamics and diuresis. Patients with capillary leak syndrome and consecutive interstitial volume shift with edema of the mucosa may profit from an increase in the colloid oncotic pressure using synthetic colloids as well as from the administration of mineralocorticoids. Additionally, negative fluid balance has been established as part of the treatment of ACS as long as the patient's cardiovascular status is stable enough.

Septic patients profit from an increase in the cardiac output with associated improvement in intestinal perfusion by using dobutamine in a small up to a medium dosage after volume substitution [39]. In patients with persistent hypotension the application of norepinephrine is mandatory.

Ventilation of patients with ACS should be performed with low tidal volumes (5–7 ml/kg with respect to standard body weight) and with an optimized ventila-

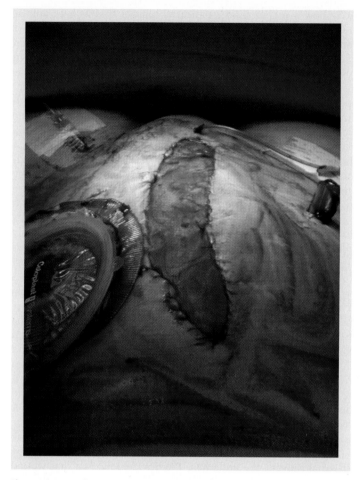

Fig. 3. Patient after ACS with adaptation of the abdominal wall with a synthetic net and temporary colostomy

tion therapy (BiPAP mode with adjusted positive end-expiratory pressure [PEEP] levels and a periodical alveolar recruitment). This ventilation therapy takes the pathological gas exchange into account and provides the development of secondary lung injury [40].

▌ Conclusion

The ACS is still an underestimated and life threatening disorder in intensive care patients. The ACS is caused by a rapidly increasing IAP of more than 25 mmHg, which results in organ dysfunction with possible progressive MOF and fatal outcome. In patients at risk of IAH, repeated measurement of the IAP using urinary bladder pressure measurement should be performed. Because the clinical examination is not very sensitive, all predictors and parameters of organ dysfunction must be registered thoroughly and continuously. The decision to perform prompt abdominal decompression and open abdominal treatment can reduce the functional MOF which is associated with a high incidence of lethal outcome.

References

1. Kron IL, Harman PK, Nolan SP (1984) The measurement of intra-abdominal pressure as a criterion for abdominal re-exploration. Ann Surg 199:28–30
2. Balogh Z, McKinley BA, Cox CS Jr, et al (2003) Abdominal compartment syndrome: the cause or effect of postinjury multiple organ failure. Shock 20:483–492
3. Cullen DJ, Coyle JP, Teplick R, Long MC (1989) Cardiovascular, pulmonary, and renal effects of massively increased intra-abdominal pressure in critically ill patients. Crit Care Med 17:118–121
4. Raeburn CD, Moore EE, Biffl WL, et al (2001) The abdominal compartment syndrome is a morbid complication of postinjury damage control surgery. Am J Surg 182:542–546
5. Emerson H (1911) Intra-abdominal pressures. Arch Intern Med 7:754–784
6. Rezende-Neto JB, Moore EE, Melo de Andrade MV, et al (2002) Systemic inflammatory response secondary to abdominal compartment syndrome: stage for multiple organ failure. J Trauma 53:1121–1128
7. Oda J, Ivatury RR, Blocher CR, Malhotra AJ, Sugerman HJ (2002) Amplified cytokine response and lung injury by sequential hemorrhagic shock and abdominal compartment syndrome in a laboratory model of ischemia-reperfusion. J Trauma 52:625–631
8. Balogh Z, McKinley BA, Holcomb JB, et al (2003) Both primary and secondary abdominal compartment syndrome can be predicted early and are harbingers of multiple organ failure. J Trauma 54:848–859
9. Balogh Z, McKinley BA, Cocanour CS, et al (2003) Supranormal trauma resuscitation causes more cases of abdominal compartment syndrome. Arch Surg 138:637–642
10. Saggi BH, Sugerman HJ, Ivatury RR, Bloomfield GL (1998) Abdominal compartment syndrome. J Trauma 45:597–609
11. Sanchez NC, Tenofsky PL, Dort JM, Shen LY, Helmer SD, Smith RS (2001) What is normal intra-abdominal pressure? Am Surg 67:243–248
12. Sugerman H, Windsor A, Bessos M, Wolfe L (1997) Intra-abdominal pressure, sagittal abdominal diameter and obesity comorbidity. J Intern Med 241:71–79
13. Meldrum DR, Moore FA, Moore EE, et al (1995) Barney resident research award. Cardiopulmonary hazards of perihepatic packing for major liver injuries. Am J Surg 170:537–540
14. Ertel W, Oberholzer A, Platz A, Stocker R, Trentz O (2000) Incidence and clinical pattern of the abdominal compartment syndrome after "damage-control" laparotomy in 311 patients with severe abdominal and/or pelvic trauma. Crit Care Med 28:1747–1753
15. Balogh Z, McKinley BA, Cocanour CS, et al (2002) Secondary abdominal compartment syndrome is an elusive early complication of traumatic shock resuscitation. Am J Surg 184: 538–543
16. Tons C, Schachtrupp A, Rau M, Mumme T, Schumpelick V (2000) Abdominal compartment syndrome: prevention and treatment. Chirurg 71:918–926
17. Malbrain ML, Chiumello D, Pelosi P, et al (2004) Prevalence of intra-abdominal hypertension in critically ill patients: a multicentre epidemiological study. Intensive Care Med 30:822–829
18. Ivatury RR, Porter JM, Simon RJ, Islam S, John R, Stahl WM (1998) Intra-abdominal hypertension after life-threatening penetrating abdominal trauma: prophylaxis, incidence, and clinical relevance to gastric mucosal pH and abdominal compartment syndrome. J Trauma 44:1016–1021
19. Yol S, Kartal A, Tavli S, Tatkan Y (1998) Is urinary bladder pressure a sensitive indicator of intra-abdominal pressure? Endoscopy 30:778–780
20. Malbrain ML (2004) Different techniques to measure intra-abdominal pressure (IAP): time for a critical re-appraisal. Intensive Care Med 30:357–371

21. Robotham JL, Wise RA, Bromberger-Barnea B (1985) Effects of changes in abdominal pressure on left ventricular performance and regional blood flow. Crit Care Med 13:803–809
22. Ridings PC, Bloomfield GL, Blocher CR, Sugerman HJ (1995) Cardiopulmonary effects of raised intra-abdominal pressure before and after intravascular volume expansion. J Trauma 39:1071–1075
23. Sugerman HJ, Bloomfield GL, Saggi BW (1999) Multisystem organ failure secondary to increased intraabdominal pressure. Infection 27:61–66
24. Diebel LN, Dulchavsky SA, Brown WJ (1997) Splanchnic ischemia and bacterial translocation in the abdominal compartment syndrome. J Trauma 43:852–855
25. Bloomfield G, Saggi B, Blocher C, Sugerman H (1999) Physiologic effects of externally applied continuous negative abdominal pressure for intra-abdominal hypertension. J Trauma 46:1009–1014
26. Diebel LN, Wilson RF, Dulchavsky SA, Saxe J (1992) Effect of increased intra-abdominal pressure on hepatic arterial, portal venous, and hepatic microcirculatory blood flow. J Trauma 33:279–282
27. Toens C, Schachtrupp A, Hoer J, Junge K, Klosterhalfen B, Schumpelick V (2002) A porcine model of the abdominal compartment syndrome. Shock 18:316–321
28. Harman PK, Kron IL, McLachlan HD, Freedlender AE, Nolan SP (1982) Elevated intra-abdominal pressure and renal function. Ann Surg 196:594–597
29. Sugrue M, Buist MD, Hourihan F, Deane S, Bauman A, Hillman K (1995) Prospective study of intra-abdominal hypertension and renal function after laparotomy. Br J Surg 82:235–238
30. Bloomfield GL, Blocher CR, Fakhry IF, Sica DA, Sugerman HJ (1997) Elevated intra-abdominal pressure increases plasma renin activity and aldosterone levels. J Trauma 42:997–1004
31. Tal R, Lask DM, Keslin J, Livne PM (2004) Abdominal compartment syndrome: urological aspects. BJU Int 93:474–477
32. Gennarelli TA, Champion HR, Sacco WJ, Copes WS, Alves WM (1989) Mortality of patients with head injury and extracranial injury treated in trauma centers. J Trauma 29:1193–1201
33. Bloomfield GL, Ridings PC, Blocher CR, Marmarou A, Sugerman HJ (1997) A proposed relationship between increased intra-abdominal, intrathoracic, and intracranial pressure. Crit Care Med 25:496–503
34. Bloomfield GL, Ridings PC, Blocher CR, Marmarou A, Sugerman HJ (1996) Effects of increased intra-abdominal pressure upon intracranial and cerebral perfusion pressure before and after volume expansion. J Trauma 40:936–941
35. Kirkpatrick AW, Brenneman FD, McLean RF, Rapanos T, Boulanger BR (2000) Is clinical examination an accurate indicator of raised intra-abdominal pressure in critically injured patients? Can J Surg 43:207–211
36. McNelis J, Marini CP, Jurkiewicz A, et al (2002) Predictive factors associated with the development of abdominal compartment syndrome in the surgical intensive care unit. Arch Surg 137:133–136
37. Biffl WL, Moore EE, Burch JM, Offner PJ, Franciose RJ, Johnson JL (2001) Secondary abdominal compartment syndrome is a highly lethal event. Am J Surg 182:645–648
38. Suliburk JW, Ware DN, Balogh Z, et al (2003) Vacuum-assisted wound closure achieves early fascial closure of open abdomens after severe trauma. J Trauma 55:1155–1160
39. Meier-Hellmann A (2003) Standards in the diagnosis and treatment of sepsis. Anasthesiol Intensivmed Notfallmed Schmerzther 38:107–133
40. Rimensberger PC, Cox PN, Frndova H, Bryan AC (1999) The open lung during small tidal volume ventilation: concepts of recruitment and "optimal" positive end-expiratory pressure. Crit Care Med 27:1946–1952

Non-invasive Modulation of Intraabdominal Pressure

F. Valenza and L. Gattinoni

▋ Introduction

The well-known effects of intraabdominal pressure (IAP) in critically ill patients are increasingly recognized by physicians [1–7]. At high levels of IAP, surgical decompression is an accepted treatment [1, 4, 8], while somewhere in between 12 and 25 mmHg the detrimental consequences of intraabdominal hypertension (IAH) are present but surgical decompression is not recommended. Patients with these values of IAP represent the great majority of those labeled as having IAH, however there is no definite treatment modality for these patients, except for supportive therapy for failing organs.

During the investigation of the effects of IAH in a pig model we have recently shown that an increased IAP may have profound effects on the lung during the course of oleic-induced lung injury. In fact, the amount of edema dramatically increased once IAP increased during lung injury as opposed to abdomen inflation in normal conditions (i.e., without lung injury) [9]. The observation led us to the hypothesis that the application of a negative pressure around the abdomen could be beneficial during IAH.

To investigate the potential benefits of non-invasive abdominal decompression, we first explored the feasibility of application of continuous negative extra-abdominal pressure (NEXAP) in critically ill patients [10]. The results obtained left us with some open questions that we tried to answer with new animal studies [11]. In this brief chapter, we will summarize some of the results we and others have obtained with the use of non-invasive decompression of the abdomen, trying to walk the reader through what we think are the light and shadows of this potential treatment modality.

Saggi et al. [12] and Bloomfield et al. [13] found in animal models that negative pressure around the abdomen significantly decreased IAP. However, to generate negative pressure around the abdomen they used a "… large poncho connected to a vacuum into which the entire animal was placed" [13]. This is somewhat difficult and impractical to obtain in humans. Moreover, the entire body is subjected to negative pressure, a condition much different from the application of negative pressure to the abdomen alone. To overcome this problem we decided to use a rigid shell around the abdomen to generate NEXAP. This shell was originally designed to apply negative pressure around the thorax (Life Care – Nev 100, Respironics). To fit the shell over the abdomen, it is rotated by 180°. In this way NEXAP was applied on the abdomen of 30 consecutive patients, in a random order, at a pressure equal to IAP (NEXAP0), 5 cmH$_2$O (NEXAP-5) or 10 cmH$_2$O (NEXAP-10) more negative than NEXAP0. The results are shown in Figure 1. The figure clearly indicates that

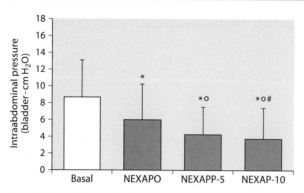

Fig. 1. Effects of the application of a continuous negative extra-abdominal pressure (NEXAP) on intra-abdominal pressure (IAP). ANOVA, * $p < 0.05$ vs Basal; °$p < 0.05$ vs NEXAP0; # $p < 0.05$ vs NEXAP-5

NEXAP does in fact reduce IAP, as assessed by bladder pressure. IAP decreased from 8.7 ± 4.3 mmHg to 6.0 ± 4.2 (Basal vs NEXAP0, $p < 0.001$). Changes were greater when more negative pressure was applied ($p < 0.001$). Average decrease of IAP with NEXAP-10 was 4.5 ± 2.9 mmHg (maximum decrease 11 mmHg).

The application of NEXAP was well tolerated by patients and there were no major side effects. At the end of the protocol, there was mild but reversible erythema on the skin of the abdomen where the shell was applied. Awake patients suffered some degree of discomfort at higher levels of NEXAP, but only one patient was clearly uncomfortable. However, at NEXAP levels equal to baseline IAP (NEXAP0), all patients were comfortable.

These results showed the feasibility of NEXAP in critically ill patients and are similar to those reported by Sugerman and colleagues who used negative pressure to treat headache in awake obese patients affected by pseudotumor cerebri. Patients were intermittently treated several hours a day without major complaints or adverse effects [14].

One of the greatest fears we initially had was related to hemodynamic compromise during NEXAP application. Interestingly, even if we selected patients without major instability, NEXAP did not cause any severe impairment of cardiovascular function: mean arterial pressure (MAP) did not change; when measured, cardiac output was not affected by NEXAP. However, even if patients were stable during NEXAP, central venous pressure (CVP) decreased and heart rate (HR) slightly increased when CVP changes were greater (NEXAP-10), as from a compensatory response to a pre-load decrease.

These results were in line with data previously shown in animal models [12, 13]. However, the changes of pleural pressure occurring with IAH necessitate the use of transmural measurements when dealing with pressure indicators of pre-load such as CVP ($CVP_{tm} = CVP$-Pleural pressure), which were not measured in our human study. Therefore, we were not really able to discriminate a possible artefact of measurement from a possible blood shift out of the thoracic cage secondary to NEXAP. This possible effect of NEXAP is potentially relevant in a critically ill patient, particularly in a scenario in which the volume status/distribution may be altered.

To answer the 'blood shift' question, we moved to the animal laboratory and measured CVP (as in the previous human study). However, we also used volume indicators of pre-load, as these are more valuable methods in this context [15], free

Table 1. Effects of NEXAP on cardiovascular function. Measurements were taken before NEXAP was applied (Pre), immediately after the transition to NEXAP (NEXAP1), after 15 min of NEXAP (NEXAP2), and after NEXAP was lifted (Post)

	Pre	NEXAP1	NEXAP2	Post
GEDV (mL)	289 ± 38	257 ± 44^a	254 ± 38^a	$291 \pm 31^{b,c}$
ITBV (mL)	358 ± 47	318 ± 54^a	314 ± 47^a	$361 \pm 38^{b,c}$
EVLW (mL/kg)	10.9 ± 2.4	9.8 ± 1.4	10.2 ± 1.5	10.6 ± 1.5
CO (mL/min)	2.9 ± 0.5	2.4 ± 0.5^a	2.3 ± 0.6^a	2.7 ± 0.6^c
HR (bpm)	119 ± 12	125 ± 28	122 ± 22	112 ± 15
SV (mL)	25.6 ± 2.8	18.1 ± 8.3^a	20.6 ± 4.6^a	24.2 ± 4.5
AP (mmHg)	105 ± 15	92 ± 17^a	91 ± 18^a	$100 \pm 14^{b,c}$
CVP$_{exp}$ (mmHg)	6.4 ± 1.6	4.0 ± 1.8^a	$4.6 \pm 1.7^{a,b}$	$7.0 \pm 1.6^{a,b,c}$

GEDV: global end-diastolic volume; ITBV: intra-thoracic blood volume; EVLW: extra-vascular lung water; CO: cardiac output; HR: heart rate; AP: arterial blood pressure; CVP$_{exp}$: end-expiratory central venous pressure

ANOVA for repeated measures

[a] $p < 0.05$ vs Pre; [b] $p < 0.05$ vs NEXAP1; [c] $p < 0.05$ vs NEXAP2

from any interference derived from changes in pleural pressures. We measured, as indexes of pre-load, intrathoracic blood volumes (PiCCO system – Pulsion, Medical System AG, Munich, Germany). The results are shown in Table 1. These data, also confirmed by the measurement of pulmonary vein diameter by means of echocardiography in a subset of animals, prove that NEXAP causes a blood shift from the thoracic compartment (pre-load effect). This effect is similar, even if contrary, to that observed during extra-thoracic negative pressure [16–19].

Interestingly, this is possibly the effect that generates the effect of abdominal decompression in the setting of experimental IAH [12, 13] or in the setting of pseudotumor cerebri [14]. Notably, these effects may be deleterious in the absence of IAH when cerebral perfusion pressure (CPP) is borderline.

NEXAP application in humans was also associated with slightly higher airway pressure and lower respiratory system compliance. When looking at the data, the following question rose: is the effect of NEXAP on respiratory mechanics beneficial or detrimental? To answer this question we started from the model described in Figure 2, that we applied to our experimental protocol by measuring single variables. An example of the acute effects of NEXAP on the measured variables is shown in Figure 3.

As one can see from Table 2, the application of NEXAP caused a drop in gastric pressure (Pga) and esophageal pressure (Pes), while end-expiratory airway pressure (PEEP) was similar. Therefore, lung volume (i.e., Ptp=Paw-Pes) increased during NEXAP, as we measured directly in three pigs with the closed helium dilution technique (Fig. 4).

The rise in airway pressure observed may thus be explained by a similar tidal volume over-imposed on a greater lung volume generated by NEXAP. In fact, pressure/volume (P/V) curve analysis showed that cord compliance (considering volume changes equals to individual tidal volumes) decreased from 22.8 ± 5.3 ml/cmH$_2$O to 18.0 ± 5.0 ($p < 0.05$) when NEXAP was applied. However, when we considered the

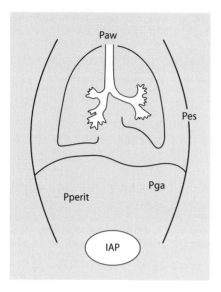

Fig. 2. The figure describes the variables taken into account to explore the cardio-respiratory effect of NEXAP. Paw: airway pressure; Pes: esophageal pressure, used as an estimate of pleural pressure; Pga: gastric pressure; Pperit: peritoneal pressure, directly measured; IAP: bladder pressure

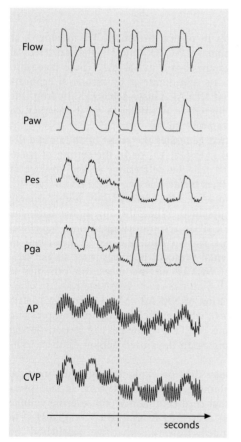

Fig. 3. Example of the acute effects of NEXAP. Flow: air flow during controlled mechanical ventilation; Paw: airway pressure; Pes: esophageal pressure; Pga: gastric pressure; AP: arterial blood pressure; CVP: central venous pressure

Table 2. Effects of NEXAP on respiratory function. Measurements were taken before NEXAP was applied (Pre), immediately after the transition to NEXAP (NEXAP1), after 15 min of NEXAP (NEXAP2), and after NEXAP was lifted (Post)

	Pre	NEXAP1	NEXAP2	Post
▊ **Flow** (L/min)	0.314 ± 0.077	0.311 ± 0.078	0.314 ± 0.093	0.323 ± 0.102
▊ **Vt** (mL/kg)	11.28 ± 1.14	10.89 ± 0.92	11.31 ± 1.17	11.94 ± 1.39^{b}
▊ **RR** (bpm)	19 ± 5	20 ± 5	20 ± 5	19 ± 5
▊ **Paw** (cmH$_2$O)	16.0 ± 3.5	20.2 ± 4.4^{a}	$18.3 \pm 3.2^{a,b}$	$15.3 \pm 2.0^{b,c}$
▊ **PEEP** (cmH$_2$O)	5.7 ± 1.1	5.8 ± 0.9	5.8 ± 0.8	5.7 ± 0.9
▊ **Pes$_{exp}$** (mmHg)	5.4 ± 1.9	4.1 ± 2.0^{a}	4.2 ± 2.1^{a}	$5.4 \pm 1.7^{b,c}$
▊ **Pga$_{exp}$** (mmHg)	6.1 ± 1.7	4.3 ± 2.5	4.1 ± 2.4	$6.9 \pm 1.8^{b,c}$

Vt: tidal volume; RR: respiratory rate: Paw: plateau airway pressure; PEEP: positive end-expiratory pressure; Pes$_{exp}$: end-expiratory esophageal pressure; Pga$_{exp}$: end-expiratory gastric pressure

ANOVA for repeated measures

[a] $p < 0.05$ vs Pre; [b] $p < 0.05$ vs NEXAP1; [c] $p < 0.05$ vs NEXAP2

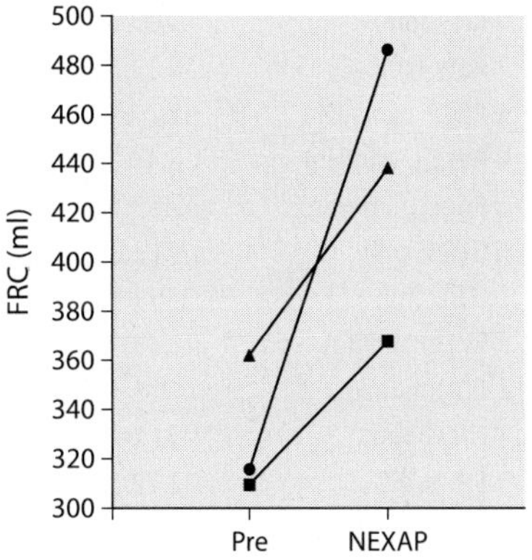

Fig. 4. The figure shows individual data for three animals whose lung volumes were measured by means of helium dilution technique before (Pre) and after (NEXAP) the application of negative extra-abdominal pressure

increase in lung volume induced by NEXAP from pleural pressure drop, assuming unchanged characteristics of the lung (wet-to-dry weight [W/D] ratio at the end of the experiment was within normal range: 5.4 ± 0.5), the decrease in cord compliance was no longer apparent (23.7 ± 8.6 ml/cmH$_2$O, $p = $ n.s. vs basal).

However, the increase in lung volume is not the only explanation. The higher chest wall elastance may contribute to the rise in airway pressure as chest wall elastance increases when IAP was normal. The increase may be due to the stiffer diaphragm, pulled downwards by NEXAP, or to the shell used to apply NEXAP. In fact, at least in one case, shell positioning on the abdomen, before NEXAP application, was associated with a small increase of pleural pressure.

Additionally, during NEXAP application, rib cage and/or xifoid are partly squeezed. This is clearly shown in Figure 5 with the recordings from a human subject whose thorax and abdomen were bent with a Respitrace during NEXAP application. This device allows the assessment of the relative movements of the chest wall (xifoid in this case) and the abdomen. One can clearly see that rib cage vol-

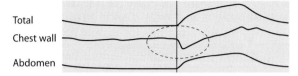

Fig. 5. An example of the effects of NEXAP application is shown. Traces described the partitioning of volume changes obtained by means of RespiTrace. Total volume (Total) rose when NEXAP was applied. Chest wall immediately decreased, to subsequently rise, while abdomen volume increased. This describes the 'squeezing' effect of NEXAP described in the text

Table 3. Effects of NEXAP on cardio-respiratory function during intra-abdominal hypertension obtained by means of helium insufflation (peritoneal pressure of 24.7 ± 5.5 mmHg). Measurements were taken before NEXAP was applied (Pre), immediately after the transition to NEXAP (NEXAP1), after 15 min of NEXAP (NEXAP2), and after NEXAP was lifted (Post)

	Pre	NEXAP1	NEXAP2	Post
▌**Flow** (l/min)	0.293 ± 0.095	0.293 ± 0.091	0.296 ± 0.095	0.298 ± 0.094
▌**Vt** (ml/kg)	9.85 ± 1.42	9.81 ± 1.29	10.15 ± 1.31	10.13 ± 1.21
▌**RR** (bpm)	20 ± 5	20 ± 5	20 ± 5	20 ± 5
▌**Paw** (cmH$_2$O)	30.2 ± 5.2^{d}	29.7 ± 5.1	29.0 ± 4.5	28.6 ± 4.9^{a}
▌**PEEP** (cmH$_2$O)	5.2 ± 0.8	5.4 ± 0.6	5.4 ± 0.8	5.3 ± 0.8
▌**Pes$_{exp}$** (mmHg)	5.4 ± 1.2	5.5 ± 1.2	5.1 ± 1.3	5.2 ± 1.4
▌**Pga$_{exp}$** (mmHg)	12.6 ± 6.9^{d}	11.7 ± 6.4	10.9 ± 6.2	12.9 ± 5.6
▌**GEDV** (ml)	271 ± 36	264 ± 41	258 ± 27	272 ± 36
▌**ITBV** (ml)	336 ± 45	329 ± 52	319 ± 34	337 ± 45
▌**EVLW** (ml/kg)	11.3 ± 1.6	11.0 ± 1.8	10.3 ± 1.2	11.0 ± 1.7
▌**CO** (mL/min)	2.7 ± 0.7	2.5 ± 0.5	2.5 ± 0.5	2.7 ± 0.5
▌**HR** (bpm)	121 ± 28	123 ± 25	118 ± 22	126 ± 14
▌**SV** (ml)	22.3 ± 3.6	21.2 ± 4.7	21.6 ± 3.9	21.3 ± 4.1
▌**AP** (mmHg)	105 ± 14	105 ± 15	102 ± 16	101 ± 16
▌**CVP$_{exp}$** (mmHg)	6.7 ± 2.1	6.8 ± 2.1	6.8 ± 2.1	6.8 ± 2.1

Vt: tidal volume; RR: respiratory rate; Paw: plateau airway pressure; PEEP: positive end-expiratory pressure; Pes$_{exp}$: end-expiratory esophageal pressure; Pga$_{exp}$: end-expiratory gastric pressure; GEDV: global end-diastolic volume; ITBV: intra-thoracic blood volume; EVLW: extra-vascular lung volume; CO: cardiac output; HR: heart rate; AP: arterial blood pressure; CVP$_{exp}$: end-expiratory central venous pressure

ANOVA for repeated measures

[a] $p < 0.05$ vs Pre; [b] $p < 0.05$ vs NEXAP1; [c] $p < 0.05$ vs NEXAP2; [d] $p < 0.05$ vs basal condition

ume decreases immediately after the application of NEXAP, just before the abdomen and the xifoid are pulled up. Therefore, although the net effect of NEXAP is an increase in lung volume, the shell partially squeezes the thorax, possibly contributing to the discomfort of the awake patients. The shell might possibly be better designed, in order to overcome this problem.

The potential of NEXAP is mostly in the above-mentioned 'gray zone' of IAH. However, it is important to know the different effects of NEXAP at different levels of IAP. On a first analysis of human data, it looked as though there was no major different in response between sub-groups of patients. In fact, the difference between basal IAP and IAP at NEXAP0 was not correlated with basal IAP as assessed by linear regression ($R^2 = 0.08$, p = 0.115) or by ANOVA considering basal IAP quartiles as groups (p = 0.163). Moreover, changes were not different when patients were stratified according to sedation and paralysis (p = 0.964), controlled versus assisted ventilator mode (p = 0.849), presence of vasoactive drugs (p = 0.142) or body mass index (p = 0.226, considering median BMI as a cut-off). However, the number of patients was not sufficient to perform sub-analyses confidently and some groups were characterized by a low-normal IAP.

To overcome these limitations we investigated the use of NEXAP in animal experiments with or without IAH induced by means of helium insufflation into the peritoneal space (target pressure: 25 mmHg). Data on the effects of NEXAP during IAH are shown in Table 3. When we performed ANOVA for repeated measure taking into consideration the effects of IAH, NEXAP and the interaction of the two, we found that NEXAP significantly modified several variables during basal condition, but, despite average values followed the same trend during IAH, changes were not statistically different. This observation was similar to that reported by Saggi [12]. It was not due to gas compression, as, in one animal in which the abdomen was inflated with water instead of helium, we obtained results similar to those obtained with gas insufflation.

Interestingly, the effect of NEXAP during IAH became evident when more negative pressure was applied. In fact, effective negative pressure (the true distending abdominal pressure, calculated as the difference between negative pressure and IAP was linearly correlated with percent changes of intra-thoracic blood volume (ITBV, $R^2 = 0.648$, p < 0.001) and CVP ($R^2 = 0.522$, p < 0.05); the greater the effective NEXAP, the greater the drop.

On the contrary, the behavior of respiratory mechanics was different before and after IAH was induced. In fact, NEXAP improved chest wall elastance during IAH, as shown in Figure 6.

The decrease in chest wall elastance may be very valuable in the setting of IAH in the ICU setting. In fact, IAH interferes with respiratory function. Even a minor improvement in respiratory function in a patient mechanically ventilated would be desirable, even if it does not necessarily translate into better oxygenation. With this perspective, it is important to note that the effects of IAP on pleural pressure are not univocal [2, 3, 9, 11, 20, 21]. In fact, we have shown that the rise in pleural

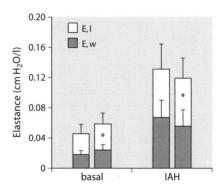

Fig. 6. Figure shows the effects of NEXAP on respiratory mechanics before (basal) and during intra-abdominal hypertension (IAH). Left columns represent values measured before NEXAP application, while right columns are those obtained during NEXAP. Elastance is partitioned into lung (E, l) and chest wall (E, w) components. * p < 0.05 pre before vs NEXAP

(esophageal) pressure may be influenced by the method used to measure pressures (i.e, end-expiratory esophageal pressure as opposed to mean esophageal pressure). Changes in pressure occurring during tidal ventilation (the so called ΔPes) increase with increasing levels of IAP, thus influencing *per se* mean pleural pressures, while lung mechanics and PEEP levels influence end-expiratory esophageal pressure [22]. Therefore, method of measurement, respiratory mechanics and ventilatory settings need to be taken into account when dealing with the improperly called 'transmission of IAP to pleural pressure'.

▌ Clinical Perspectives

As detailed above, the use of negative extra-abdominal pressure is a fascinating tool with a great potential for non-invasive decompression of IAH. In this chapter we have tried to walk the reader through our attempt to learn as much as possible of NEXAP and its possible use. There is much work still to do before NEXAP translates into clinical practice, if ever. In fact, understanding the underlying mechanisms and learning how to use this tool is mandatory.

However, there are more questions we need to answer, particularly whether NEXAP improves organ function when used in patients with IAH in the 'gray zone' of IAP between 12 and 25 mmHg. We are still a long way from the answer, but are on our way.

References

1. Bailey J, Shapiro MJ (2000) Abdominal compartment syndrome. Crit Care 4:23–29
2. Barnes GE, Laine GA, Giam PY, Smith EE, Granger HJ (1985) Cardiovascular responses to elevation of intra-abdominal hydrostatic pressure. Am J Physiol 248:R208–R213
3. Mutoh T, Lamm WJ, Embree LJ, Hildebrandt J, Albert RK (1991) Abdominal distension alters regional pleural pressures and chest wall mechanics in pigs in vivo. J Appl Physiol 70:2611–2618
4. Cullen DJ, Coyle JP, Teplick R, Long MC (1989) Cardiovascular, pulmonary, and renal effects of massively increased intra-abdominal pressure in critically ill patients. Crit Care Med 17:118–121
5. Malbrain ML (1999) Abdominal pressure in the critically ill: measurement and clinical relevance. Intensive Care Med 25:1453–1458
6. Pelosi P, Aspersi M, Chiumello D, et al (2002) Measuring intra abdominal pressure in the intensive care setting. Intensivmedizin und Notfallmedizin 39:509–519
7. Malbrain ML, Chiumello D, Pelosi P, et al (2004) Prevalence of intra-abdominal hypertension in critically ill patients: a multicentre epidemiological study. Intensive Care Med 30:822–829
8. Balogh Z, McKinley BA, Holcomb JB, et al (2003) Both primary and secondary abdominal compartment syndrome can be predicted early and are harbingers of multiple organ failure. J Trauma 54:848–859
9. Quintel M, Pelosi P, Caironi P, et al (2004) An increase of abdominal pressure increases pulmonary edema in oleic acid-induced lung injury. Am J Respir Crit Care Med 169:534–541
10. Valenza F, Bottino N, Canavesi K, et al (2003) Intra-abdominal pressure may be decreased non-invasively by continuous negative extra-abdominal pressure (NEXAP). Intensive Care Med 29:2063–2067
11. Valenza F, Irace M, Guglielmi M, et al (2004) Effects of continuous negative extra-abdominal pressure on cardiorespiratory function during abdominal hypertension: an experimental study. Intensive Care Med Oct 26 (Epub ahead of print)

12. Saggi BH, Bloomfield GL, Sugerman HJ, et al (1999) Treatment of intracranial hypertension using nonsurgical abdominal decompression. J Trauma 46:646–651
13. Bloomfield GL, Saggi BH, Blocher C, Sugerman HJ (1999) Physiologic effects of externally applied continuous negative abdominal pressure for intra-abdominal hypertension. J Trauma 46:1009–1014
14. Sugerman HJ, Felton III WL 3rd, Sismanis A, et al (2001) Continuous negative abdominal pressure device for to treat pseudotumor cerebri. Int J Obes Relat Metab Disord 25:486–490
15. Cheatham ML, Safcsak K, Block EF, Nelson LD (1999) Preload assessment in patients with an open abdomen. J Trauma 46:16–22
16. Borelli M, Benini A, Denkewitz T, Acciaro C, Foti G, Pesenti A (1998) Effects of continuous negative extrathoracic pressure versus positive end-expiratory pressure in acute lung injury patients. Crit Care Med 26:1025–1031
17. Adams J, Osiovich H, Goldberg R, Suguihara C, Bancalari E (1992) Hemodynamic effects of continuous negative extrathoracic pressure and continuous positive airway pressure in piglets with normal lungs. Biol Neonate 62:69–75
18. Pierce J, Jenkins I, Noyes J, Samuels M, Southall D (1995) The successful use of continuous negative extrathoracic pressure in a child with Glenn shunt and respiratory failure. Intensive Care Med 21:766–768
19. Torelli L, Zoccali G, Casarin M, Dalla Zuanna F, Lieta E, Conti G (1995) Comparative evaluation of the haemodynamic effects of continuous negative external pressure (CNEP) and positive end-expiratory pressure (PEEP) in mechanically ventilated trauma patients. Intensive Care Med 21:67–70
20. Ivankovich AD, Miletich DJ, Albrecht RF, Heyman HJ, Bonnet RF (1975) Cardiovascular effects of intraperitoneal insufflation with carbon dioxide and nitrous oxide in the dog. Anesthesiology 42:281–287
21. Ridings PC, Bloomfield GL, Blocher CR, Sugerman HJ (1995) Cardiopulmonary effects of raised intra-abdominal pressure before and after intravascular volume expansion. J Trauma 39:1071–1075
22. Valenza F, Porro GA, Tedesco C, et al (2004) Effects of PEEP on esophageal pressure during intra-abdominal hypertension. Intensive Care Med 30:S430 (abst)

Severe Infections

Rational Use of Antibiotics in the ICU: Optimum Efficacy for the Lowest Costs

A. R. H. van Zanten and K. H. Polderman

▌ Introduction

Critically ill patients treated in the intensive care unit (ICU) for severe infections need to be treated quickly and effectively to improve the chances of a favorable outcome. Early recognition and diagnosis of infections and prompt initiation of antimicrobial treatment have long been recognized as fundamental principles of therapy. In daily practice, the attending physician/intensivist needs to take a number of key aspects of antimicrobial therapy into account. The probability of success in treating bacterial infections depends on factors such as the condition of the patient, the etiology of the infection and the appropriateness of antimicrobial therapy. Selection of antimicrobial drugs is often based on *in vitro* susceptibility of causative pathogens to specific antibiotics, although usually initial treatment is started empirically, based on knowledge of pathogens commonly involved in infections of particular organs in a specific location. The interactions between antibiotics, causative pathogens and host defenses in immunocompetent or immunocompromised patients is highly complex [1]; many ICU patients should be regarded as having (temporarily) diminished immune functions, due to factors such as downregulation of immune function following severe infections [2], administration of drugs such as corticosteroids, underlying chronic diseases, impairment or interruption of local defense systems (e.g., endotracheal intubation and mechanical ventilation) and various other factors.

The administration of antibiotics should therefore be carefully targeted at the proven or suspected causative pathogen(s), using a strategy that takes pharmacokinetics and pharmacodynamics for the applied antibiotic into consideration to increase efficacy and reduce the risk of antimicrobial resistance. In addition, in times of tight budgets and increased workload, economic aspects of drug therapies should also be taken into account.

▌ Does Appropriateness of Initial Antibiotic Therapy Matter?

The early initiation of appropriate antibiotic therapy seems to be a logical approach, to facilitate high bacterial killing rates and to enhance the resolution of infectious complications. On the other hand, the effect of appropriate antibiotics is part of an overall treatment strategy, and cannot be viewed separately from other therapeutic interventions that may affect outcome, such as early goal-directed fluid resuscitation, intensive insulin therapy and many other interventions [3]. With the increasing incidence of antimicrobial drug resistance an increased likelihood of inappropriate antimicrobial therapy over the past few years might have been expected to occur; however, this is far from clear. Metlay and Singer failed to observe a link between inappropriateness of initial antibiotic therapy and outcome in a large study in patients with lower respiratory tract infections, such as community-acquired pneumonia (CAP) and acute exacerbations of chronic bronchitis [4].

In recent years, several groups have addressed the question of whether inappropriate initial antibiotic treatment can lead to adverse outcome. Studies have been performed in various patient groups, including the critically ill. Outcome in patients who received appropriate antibiotic treatment (i.e., where the causative microorganism was susceptible to the drug on *in vitro* testing [3]) were compared to patients in whom antibiotic therapy was inappropriate. The results of some of these studies will be briefly discussed.

Zaidi and associates performed a prospective case control study in 113 ICU patients treated for nosocomial infections. On multivariate analysis and corrected for predicted mortality based on APACHE II scores the authors observed an independent correlation of inappropriate antibiotic treatment with higher mortality (Odds ratio [OR] 70, $p < 0.0001$) [6]. In contrast, Zaragoza et al. found no correlation between appropriateness of initial antibiotic choice in a series of critically ill patients with bloodstream infections. A possible reason for this is the fact that the incidence of relatively low virulent microorganisms such as coagulase-negative staphylococci was higher in patients with inappropriate treatment compared to those with appropriate treatment [7]. In a much larger prospective study in 494 ICU patients with bloodstream infections, Ibrahim et al. [8] found a higher hospital mortality rate in patients receiving inappropriate compared to appropriate antimicrobial treatment (62% vs. 28%, $p < 0.001$). Multiple logistic regression analysis identified inappropriate antibiotics as an independent predictor of hospital mortality, with an odds ratio of 6.9 [5.1–9.2]. The most commonly involved causative pathogens in cases of inadequate antimicrobial treatment were vancomycin-resistant enterococci, *Candida species,* oxacillin-resistant *Staphylococcus aureus,* coagulase-negative staphylococci, and *Pseudomonas aeruginosa* [8]. This illustrates that the inappropriateness of initial antimicrobial therapy will depend to a substantial degree on the prevalence of resistant pathogens in specific settings.

To evaluate the relationship between inappropriate antimicrobial treatment of infections (both community-acquired and nosocomial infections) and hospital mortality for patients requiring ICU admission, Kollef and coworkers performed a prospective study in 2000 consecutive ICU patients, of whom 655 patients (25.8%) had either community-acquired or developed nosocomial infections. In this group they evaluated inappropriate antimicrobial treatment. They observed inadequate antimicrobial therapy most frequently in patients with nosocomial infections, which occurred most frequently following treatment for community-acquired infections (45%). Thirty-four percent of patients had nosocomial infections alone (34%) and 17% had community-acquired infections alone (17%). Main risk factors for inappropriateness of antimicrobial therapy were prior administration of antibiotics (OR 3.4 [2.9–4.2]) and bloodstream infections (OR 1.9 [1.5–2.3]). The infection-related mortality rate was 42% in patients receiving inappropriate antimicrobial treatment, compared to 18% in patients receiving appropriate antibiotic treatment. Inappropriate antimicrobial treatment was found to be the most significant independent determinant of hospital mortality in this study, with an odds ratio of 4.27 [3.4–5.4] [9].

On balance, the administration of the right antibiotics in the treatment of both community-acquired and nosocomial infections in critically ill patients appears to be a major determinant of outcome. In addition to this, clinicians treating patients with severe infections in the ICU should be aware that the presence of specific pathogens may independently affect outcome. For example, in bloodstream infections with *P. aeruginosa,* hospital mortality rates are higher than when *S. aureus* is the cause, even when antibiotic treatment for *Pseudomonas* is appropriate [10]. Experimental studies in bacterial Gram-negative sepsis have shown that appropriate antibiotics alone cannot always prevent adverse outcome including death [11]. Thus although appropriate antibiotic treatment is of paramount importance, many other factors can also affect outcome.

▌ Does the Timing of Appropriate Antibiotic Administration Matter?

Selection of the initial antibiotic treatment is often made empirically. The appropriateness of the initial choice can be evaluated when Gram-stains and/or culture results with information on susceptibility of the causative pathogen(s) become available. This information can lead to changes in antibiotic regimen; if the initial therapy was inadequate the delay (during which the infection was either not treated with effective antibiotics, or suboptimally treated with partly susceptible micro-organisms) may affect outcome.

Several studies have addressed the issue of timing of appropriate antibiotic therapy. In CAP, delayed administration of antibiotics has been linked to increased hospital mortality [12, 13]. The difference reached statistical significance at 8 hours in a study by Meehan and coworkers, implying that administering appropriate antibiotics within 8 h of hospital arrival was associated with improved survival [14]. Similarly, Houck and associates recently reported in a study in 13771 elderly non-ICU patients that patients admitted to a hospital for CAP who received appropriate antibiotics within 4 hours of admission had lower in-hospital mortality compared to patients in whom antibiotics were initiated later (6.8% vs. 7.4%; [OR 0.85 (0.74–0.98)]) [15].

In patients suffering from *Klebsiella pneumoniae* meningitis, timing of appropriate antimicrobial therapy, guided by conscious level but not by the duration of symptoms, was a major determinant of survival and neurological outcome. Based on these findings the authors recommend giving the first dose of an appropriate antibiotic before consciousness decreases to Glasgow Coma Scale (GCS) scores of 7 points or less [16].

In another retrospective cohort study in 269 patients with community-acquired bacterial meningitis microbiologically proven by lumbar puncture performed within 24 hours after presentation, a delay in therapy after arrival at the emergency department was associated with adverse outcome if the patient's clinical situation had advanced to the highest stage of prognostic severity before the initial antibiotic dose was given [17]. In yet another recent cohort study in 109 adult patients with culture-proven community-acquired bacterial meningitis, the timing of appropriate antimicrobial therapy (defined by level of consciousness), was a major determinant of survival and neurological outcome. The authors concluded that the first dose of an appropriate antibiotic should be administered before a patient's consciousness deteriorates to a GCS score ≤10 [18].

Several authors have addressed delays in initiation of appropriate antibiotics in ventilator-associated pneumonia (VAP). Luna et al. and Ibrahim et al. found a trend toward lower mortality if antimicrobial treatment was commenced early in the course of pneumonia; patients with severe VAP in whom antibiotic treatment was initiated after >48 hours after diagnosis were more likely to die than those in whom therapy was started within 48 h after diagnosis [19, 20]. Similarly, Iregui and co-workers reported an odds ratio of 7.7 [4.5–13.1] for mortality if initiation of appropriate antimicrobials in VAP was delayed beyond 24 hours compared to the group receiving timely adequate therapy [21]. These data suggest that it may be important to initiate appropriate therapy early on, in order to increase the likelihood of favorable outcome and reduce morbidity in patients with severe infections.

However, in a recent study, Clec'h and coworkers were unable to demonstrate a strong correlation between timing of adequate antibiotics in VAP in a prospective study of 142 ICU patients. Surprisingly, in a subgroup analysis of patients with lower severity of disease an association with higher mortality and inadequate therapy was found [22]. These findings are difficult to interpret and in sharp contrast with previous findings; the effects of inappropriate therapy on outcome was more profound in more severely ill patient groups such as was demonstrated in the group of meningitis patients in which the effect of inadequate therapy was more deleterious if consciousness level was lower indicating more severe illness and poorer prognosis as well as in patients with bloodstream infections.

In conclusion, the available data suggest that not just the appropriateness of antibiotic treatment but also the speed of initiation of this treatment is a major determinant for outcome in critically ill patients. Earlier initiation of therapy may thus help us to significantly improve outcome; conversely, a prolonged delay may lead to marked reductions in favorable outcome.

▌ Potential Strategies to Reduce Inappropriate Antimicrobial Treatment

Various risk factors that may contribute to inappropriate antimicrobial treatment have been identified. These include recent exposure to antibiotics, use of broad-spectrum antibiotics, prolonged length of stay, prolonged mechanical ventilation, and presence of invasive devices [5]. Several interventions can be used to decrease the risk of inappropriate choice of antibiotics. These include measures such as the use of antibiotic practice guidelines, consulting an infectious disease specialist or microbiologist, and implementing more rapid methods of microbiological identification. Furthermore, intensivists should be familiar with the pathogens most frequently involved in community-acquired and nosocomial infections encountered in their ICU. Initiation of (empirical) antibiotic treatment based on this knowledge as well as individual patient characteristics will increase the likelihood of initiating the right therapy. In many cases this will require initial treatment with broad-spectrum antibiotics, which can be changed when the culture results are known.

Vogtlander et al. studied procedural changes that could improve the chance of timely administration of antibiotics. They were able to reduce the mean time from the initial order to administration of the first dose in different type wards from 2.7 to 1.7 hours in potentially severe cases (p = 0.003) [23].

❚ Pharmacokinetic and Pharmacodynamic Principles in the ICU

Apart from the impact on outcome, inadequate antimicrobial treatment is an important factor in the emergence of antibiotic resistance. Inadequate dosing of antibiotics may play an important role in the emergence of resistance in the ICU [24]. Pharmacokinetic and pharmacodynamic properties of antibiotics should be taken into account to gain insight into the effects of antibiotic treatment in the critically ill.

Pharmacokinetics is the study of the processes of absorption, distribution, metabolism, and excretion of drugs by the body. Pharmacokinetics describes the time course of the drug and its metabolites in the body. In other words: What does the body do to the drug?

After oral ingestion a drug has to be separated from the vehicle, absorbed from the gastric or intestinal mucosa, and then distributed to the body. The percentage of available drug compared to the ingested dose is usually described as the bioavailability of the drug. Total serum drug levels may vary due to differences in the calculated volume of distribution (Vd). Vd is determined by protein binding, blood flow, membrane penetration, and tissue solubility. In critically ill patients the bioavailability of drugs may vary significantly, due to alterations in gastric emptying, environmental pH, and interactions with other enteral substances including continuous enteral nutrition. Therefore, as a rule, the intravenous route of administration is preferable in these patients. When variations in bioavailability are excluded by intravenous administration, three major pharmacokinetic variables remain: Volume of distribution, clearance, and half-life.

During the hyperdynamic states of stress and sepsis half-life may be reduced and Vd expanded. Commonly used dosing regimens of antibiotics may therefore be inadequate in critically ill patients. Subtherapeutic antibiotic concentrations in these patients may account for treatment failures and may lead to the emergence of bacterial resistance [25].

The field of pharmacodynamics addresses the biochemical and physiologic effects of drugs and their mechanisms of action; or more specifically, the reactions between drugs and living organisms, including the responses of the body to pharmacological, biochemical, physiological, and therapeutic actions and effects. In other words, what does the drug do to the body?

In order to increase the chances of a successful treatment, pharmacodynamic principles should be applied. The pharmacokinetic profile of a specific antibiotic and the susceptibility of the target pathogen should determine the required dosage. *In vitro* antimicrobial susceptibility provides information regarding the appropriateness of the selected antibiotic; however, this does not take into account differences in antimicrobial exposure *in vivo*, due to variations in pharmacokinetics and the dosage regimens used.

Recent studies have provided more information on pharmacodynamic principles and the relationship between antimicrobial concentration and bactericidal effect [26, 27]. This information may help to initiate the optimal dosing strategy for specific antibiotics in various clinical settings.

Successful eradication of bacteria results from the antibiotic's microbiological properties and the pharmacokinetic profiles; both of these are important, drug selection should be based on both microbiology and pharmacokinetic/pharmacodynamic parameters.

Pharmacodynamic Properties of Commonly used Antibiotics in the ICU

The pharmacodynamic interaction between antibiotic and pathogen differs between various classes of antibiotics. The bactericidal activity of the different classes of antibiotics can be either time or concentration dependent; it can also be linked to the persistence of drug effects after serum levels have fallen below the minimum inhibitory concentration (MIC) for the target pathogen. This is known as the post-antibiotic effect. Pharmacodynamic parameters are shown in Figure 1.

For aminoglycosides, bacterial killing is determined mainly by the maximum serum concentrations (Cmax) relative to the MIC (Cmax:MIC ratio $\geq$10). This has been shown to correlate closely with improvements in the rate and extent of clinical response [28, 29]. Based on these observations and on the pharmacodynamic properties of aminoglycosides, which have a marked post-antibiotic effect, a once daily administration has been recommended to maximize efficacy while minimizing the potential for drug accumulation and toxicity [30]

In contrast, for fluoroquinolones the pharmacodynamic parameter linked to optimal clinical and microbiological outcome is the area under the concentration–time curve (AUC) relative to the MIC (AUC:MIC ratio) [31, 32]. In patients with nosocomial pneumonia treated with ciprofloxacin, achieving AUC:MIC ratios >125 resulted in clinical and microbiological cure rates above 80%. More recently, Ambrose and colleagues found that for levofloxacin or gatifloxacin, the attainment of AUC:MIC ratios >34 in CAP resulted in improved probabilities of microbiological eradication of *Streptococcus pneumoniae* (AUC:MIC $\geq$34 = 100% eradication; AUC:MIC < 34 = 64% eradication) [33].

For β-lactam antibiotics the bactericidal effect is related to the time during which drug concentrations exceed the MIC of the antibiotic (T>MIC). Optimum β-lactam antibiotic exposure has been shown to improve both microbiological cure rates and the clinical response [34-36].

The optimum level of exposure differs within the class of β-lactam antibiotics: T>MIC of 60–70% for penicillins, 50-70% for cephalosporins and 40–50% for carbapenems [37].

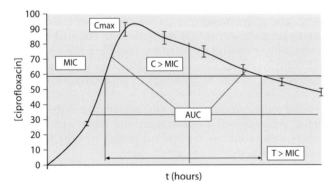

Fig. 1. Concentration-time curve of ciprofloxacin after single intravenous dose. MIC: Minimal Inhibitory Concentration; AUC: Area under the curve (surface area below concentration curve); Cmax: Maximum concentration; T>MIC: time concentration exceeds MIC; C> MIC: concentration above MIC

In order to optimize the $T > MIC$, either higher or more frequent doses can be used. Also, the administration time of the β-lactam antibiotic can be extended from 30 minutes up to several hours, or the daily dose continuously infused over 24 hours. Either of these strategies can further enhance the favorable pharmacodynamic profile of these agents [38].

By applying pharmacodynamic principles, intensivists can make better use of antibiotics, maximize microbiological eradication and improve clinical outcomes.

▌ Clinical Application of Pharmacokinetic/Pharmacodynamic Principles

Although it has been suggested that continuous infusion of β-lactam antibiotics such as cephalosporins may be superior to intermittent (bolus) administration from a pharmacokinetic viewpoint, studies of clinical efficacy in patients with severe infections are scarce [4]. We recently compared pharmacokinetic and pharmacodynamic profiles, antibiotic resistance, and clinical efficacy of continuous vs. intermittent administration of cefotaxime in patients with obstructive pulmonary disease and respiratory tract infections. Although clinical cure rates were comparable in our relatively small group of 93 hospitalized patients, continuous administration of cefotaxime 2 gram after a loading dose of 1 gram led to significantly greater proportions of concentrations $> MIC$ and $> 5 \times MIC$ compared to intermittent dosing (1 gram tid). Continuous administration thus seems preferable from a pharmacodynamic and microbiological perspective. In addition there may be advantages in cost-effectiveness with at least the same clinical efficacy (unpublished data). In an ongoing study in ICU patients the number of unexpectedly low drug levels with increased likelihood of concentrations below MIC for more than 30–50% of the dosing interval was more common in both groups compared to patients in the general ward. This highlights the importance of the large variations in pharmacokinetics in the critically ill.

A theoretical objection against continuous infusion might be that drug equilibration can take more time when compared to intermittent (bolus) administration. In severe infections this delay of onset of antibacterial activity can be relevant. However, this problem can be easily circumvented by administration of an initial loading dose prior to continuous infusion.

Based on these findings we recommend continuous administration of cefotaxime (and perhaps other β-lactam antibiotics) as the preferred mode of administration.

We also evaluated the pharmacokinetics of the fluoroquinolone antibiotic ciprofloxacin in a separate study. We assessed the ratio of AUC to MIC following administration of 400 mg i.v. twice daily, a commonly used dose. It has been determined that an AUC to MIC ratio of 125 for the causative microorganism best predicts efficacy [33] (Fig. 2). We evaluated whether AUCs exceeded MIC values ranging from 0.125 to 2.0 mg/l by at least 125 times and/or whether peak concentration $> 10 \times$ MIC (Cmax/MIC > 10) were reached. These targets were reached with sufficient frequency only when the causative pathogens had MICs < 0.25. Because many bacteria in the critical care setting may exceed this threshold we recommend increasing the standard dosage to at least 1200 mg per day if infections with one of these microorganisms are suspected, or if treatment is given empirically in critically ill patients. This can be achieved either by increasing the doses (to 600 mg bid) or by increasing the dosing frequency (400 mg tid).

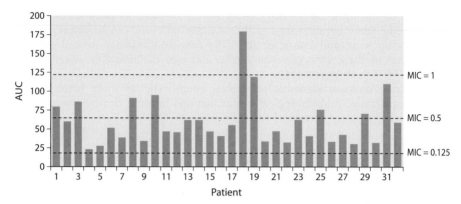

Fig. 2. Area under the curve (AUC$_{1-24}$) in mg*24h/l of ciprofloxacin concentrations over 24 hours in 32 individual critically ill patients treated with ciprofloxacin 400 mg bid i.v. and AUC/MIC > 125 for different theoretical MIC levels of 0.125, 0.5 and 1.0

For aminoglycosides the importance of therapeutic drug monitoring to enhance efficacy and avoid toxicity has been previously demonstrated in the literature [28, 29].

In conclusion, individual treatment strategies combining patient characteristics, bacterial susceptibility, knowledge of pharmacokinetics and therapeutic drug monitoring of antibiotics may help improve microbiological and clinical outcome and decrease the risk of antimicrobial drug resistance in critically ill patients.

∎ Cost Considerations

Although it seems rational to assume that optimizing antibiotic strategies and avoiding inappropriate use of antibiotics in the ICU will also lead to favorable pharmacoeconomic effects, data from the literature are scarce and sometimes confusing. One way to address this issue is to analyze the impact of infections with antibiotic-resistant organisms on morbidity, mortality, and cost. In a review on this subject, Niedermann remarked that many of the available studies were confounded by methodological problems. For example, data on methicillin-resistant *S. aureus* (MRSA) and vancomycin-resistant enterococcus were inconsistent with regard to effects on mortality. However, more firm conclusions could be drawn regarding increased length of stay and higher costs [39]. Infections in patients caused by antibiotic-resistant bacteria led to prolonged length of stay and incurred higher costs compared to patients treated for infections with antibiotic susceptible pathogens.

Furthermore, the institution of an infectious disease consulting service to evaluate and improve antibiotic prescription patterns in various general wards has been shown to substantially reduce the costs for antibiotics without interfering with the quality of care [40].

Another approach is to implement guidelines to restrict the use of certain antimicrobial agents, by means of special order forms and sequential prospective audits of prescriptions. Although inappropriate antibiotic usage may persist for some drugs despite restrictions in access, implementation of such guidelines resulted in a marked reduction in overall antimicrobial costs [41]. Moreover, to optimize antibiotic use it is necessary to be aware of the most commonly cultured pathogens locally and their susceptibility patterns, so that empirical therapy will have a high likelihood of being effective [39].

Other measures to reduce costs, maintain efficacy and reduce the possibility for emergence of resistance include limiting the duration of antibiotic therapy, streamlining antibiotics after culture results have become available and switching antibiotics from the intravenous route to the enteral route where possible.

Additional cost-reducing strategies include negotiation of lower prices for acquiring antibiotics. Antibiotic guidelines and hospital prescription guidelines are often based not just on efficacy data but also take pharmacoeconomic aspects into account. However, it should be realized that drug acquisition costs alone do not determine the overall costs of treatment. Other factors such as nursing workload, necessity for therapeutic monitoring and side effects may significantly influence these costs. For example, in a cost-effectiveness study comparing continuous and intermittent use of five different antibiotics for pneumonia or intraabdominal infections we observed that antibiotic treatment was associated with significant hidden costs mostly determined by the mode of administration [42]. We found that the cheapest drug to buy was one of the most expensive to use. Regarding the method of administration, when all cost drivers were taken into account the cheapest method of administering intravenous antibiotics, perhaps unexpectedly, was through use of a continuous syringe pump [42]. These costs were 3.23 ($ 3.88) per dose, while direct intravenous administration as a bolus cost 11.69 ($ 14.03) per dose. This difference was due in large part to the fact that direct intravenous administration requires more time expenditure by relatively highly trained (and paid) certified nurses or physicians. Moreover, the procedure often requires slow infusion of the antibiotic, which also implies a greater expenditure of time [42]. This example demonstrates that other factors than the drug price alone should be taken into account when assessing total treatment costs, and that continuous administration (apart from its pharmacological advantages) may also be more cost-effective. In this regard, an additional factor that should be considered is that various studies in different settings have shown that increased staff workload is associated with adverse outcome, increased complication rates, increased length of stay, and even with higher mortality [43-46]. If the amount of time spent on administering drugs could be reduced, this would allow health care workers to devote more time to other aspects of patient care, which in itself might lead to improvements in outcome.

∎ Conclusion

For critically ill patients with infectious complications, immediate and adequate institution of antimicrobial therapy appears to be a major determinant of outcome. Several strategies to reduce inadequacy of antibiotic therapy may be implemented, including the use of antibiotic practice guidelines, consultation of experts in microbiology and infectious diseases, quick microbiological detection procedures, and optimizing knowledge of commonly occurring pathogens and related antibiotic susceptibility profiles in one's own ICU.

Antibiotic therapy choices based on integrated information of pharmacokinetics and pharmacodynamics of commonly used antibiotics and frequently encountered pathogens in the ICU may further increase the efficacy of antimicrobial treatment. An individual approach may be necessary as pharmacokinetics in critically ill patients can vary significantly.

When using β-lactam antibiotics, continuous administration can improve pharmacodynamics and reduce costs and workload. When using fluoroquinolones, the risk of underdosing should be taken into account, and when treating microorganisms with relatively low susceptibility, dosages of 1200 mg/day may be required in critically ill patients.

Optimal antibiotic strategies do not necessarily mean more expensive therapies. Rational application of intravenous antibiotic therapy in the ICU can simultaneously improve efficacy, reduce the risk of antibiotic resistance, and also reduce costs and workload. Awareness of these issues and proper application of guidelines as well as pharmacodynamic principles can help us to improve our usage of currently available treatments.

References

1. Bergogne-Berezin E (1997) Interactions among antibiotics, bacteria and the human immune system: the clinical relevance of in vitro testing. J Chemother Suppl 1:109–115
2. Oberholzer A, Oberholzer C, Moldawer LL (2001) Sepsis syndromes: understanding the role of innate and acquired immunity. Shock 16:83–96
3. Polderman KH, Girbes ARJ (2004) Drug intervention trials in sepsis: divergent results. Lancet 363:1721–1723
4. Metlay JP, Singer DE (2002) Outcomes in lower respiratory tract infections and the impact of antimicrobial drug resistance. Clin Microbiol Infect 8 (Suppl 2):1–11
5. Kollef MH (2000) Inadequate antimicrobial treatment: an important determinant of outcome for hospitalized patients. Clin Infect Dis 31 (Suppl 4):S131–S138
6. Zaidi M, Sifuentes-Osornio J, Rolon AL, et al (2002) Inadequate therapy and antibiotic resistance. Risk factors for mortality in the intensive care unit. Arch Med Res 33:290–294
7. Zaragoza R, Artero A, Camarena JJ, et al (2003) The influence of inadequate empirical antimicrobial treatment on patients with bloodstream infections in an intensive care unit. Clin Microbiol Infect 9:412–418
8. Ibrahim EH, Sherman G, Ward S, et al (2000) The influence of inadequate antimicrobial treatment of bloodstream infections on patient outcomes in the ICU setting. Chest 118:146–155
9. Kollef MH, Sherman G, Ward S, Fraser VJ (1999) Inadequate antimicrobial treatment of infections: a risk factor for hospital mortality among critically ill patients. Chest 115:462–474
10. Osmon S, Ward S, Fraser VJ, Kollef MH (2004) Hospital mortality for patients with bacteremia due to Staphylococcus aureus or Pseudomonas aeruginosa. Chest 125:607–616
11. Greisman SE, DuBuy JB, Woodward CL (1979) Experimental gram-negative bacterial sepsis: prevention of mortality not preventable by antibiotics alone. Infect Immun 25:538–557
12. McGarvey RN, Harper JJ (1993) Pneumonia mortality reduction and quality improvement in a community hospital. QRB Qual Rev Bull 19:124–130
13. Dean NC, Silver MP, Bateman KA, et al (2001) Decreased mortality after implementation of a treatment guideline for community-acquired pneumonia. Am J Med 110:451–457
14. Meehan, MP, Fine, MJ, Krumbolz, HM, et al (1997) Quality of care, process and outcomes in elderly patients with pneumonia. JAMA 278:2080–2085
15. Houck PM, Bratzler DW, Nsa W, et al (2004) Timing of antibiotic administration and outcomes for Medicare patients hospitalized with community-acquired pneumonia. Arch Intern Med 164:637–644
16. Fang CT, Chen YC, Chang SC (2000) Klebsiella pneumoniae meningitis: timing of antimicrobial therapy and prognosis. QJM 93:45–53
17. Aronin SI, Peduzzi P, Quagliarello VJ (1998) Community-acquired bacterial meningitis: risk stratification for adverse clinical outcome and effect of antibiotic timing. Ann Intern Med 129:862–869

18. Lu CH, Huang CR, Chang WN, et al (2002) Community-acquired bacterial meningitis in adults: the epidemiology, timing of appropriate antimicrobial therapy, and prognostic factors. Clin Neurol Neurosurg 104:352–358

19. Luna, CM, Vujacich, P, Niederman, MS, et al (1997) Impact of BAL data on the therapy and outcome of ventilator-associated pneumonia. Chest 111:676–685

20. Ibrahim, EH, Sherman, G, Ward, S, Fraser VJ, Kollef MH (2000) The influence of inadequate antimicrobial treatment of bloodstream infections on patient outcomes in the ICU Chest 118:146–155

21. Iregui M, Ward S, Sherman G, Fraser VJ, Kollef MH (2002) Clinical importance of delays in the initiation of appropriate antibiotic treatment for ventilator-associated pneumonia. Chest 122:262–268

22. Clec'h C, Timsit JF, De Lassence A, et al (2004) Efficacy of adequate early antibiotic therapy in ventilator-associated pneumonia: influence of disease severity. Intensive Care Med 30:1327–1333

23. Vogtlander NP, Van Kasteren ME, Natsch S, et al (2004) Improving the process of antibiotic therapy in daily practice: interventions to optimize timing, dosage adjustment to renal function, and switch therapy. Arch Intern Med 164:1206–1212

24. MacGowan AP (2001) Role of pharmacokinetics and pharmacodynamics: does the dose matter? Clin Infect Dis 33 (Suppl 3):S238–S239

25. Fry DE (1996) The importance of antibiotic pharmacokinetics in critical illness. Am J Surg 172:20S–25S

26. Nicolau DP, Quintiliani R, Nightingale CH (1995) Antibiotic kinetics and dynamics for the clinician. Med Clin North Am 79:477–495

27. Craig WA (1998) Pharmacokinetic/pharmacodynamic parameters: rationale for antibacterial dosing of mice and men. Clin Infect Dis 26:1–10

28. Moore RD, Lietman PS, Smith CR (1987) Clinical response to aminoglycoside therapy: importance of the ratio of peak concentration to minimal inhibitory concentration. J Infect Dis 155:93–99

29. Kashuba AD, Nafziger AN, Drusano GL, et al (1999) Optimizing aminoglycoside therapy for nosocomial pneumonia caused by Gram-negative bacteria. Antimicrob Agents Chemother 43:623–629

30. Nicolau DP, Freeman CD, Belliveau PP, et al (1995) Experience with a once-daily aminoglycoside program administered to 2184 adult patients. Antimicrob Agents Chemother 39:650–655

31. Forrest A, Nix DE, Ballow CH, et al (1993) Pharmacodynamics of intravenous ciprofloxacin in seriously ill patients. Antimicrob Agents Chemother 37:1073–1081

32. Drusano G, Labro MT, Cars O, et al (1998) Pharmacokinetics and pharmacodynamics of fluoroquinolones. Clin Microbiol Infect 4 (Suppl 2):S27–S41

33. Ambrose PG, Grasela DM, Grasela TH, et al (2001) Pharmacodynamics of fluoroquinolones against Streptococcus pneumoniae in patients with community-acquired respiratory tract infections. Antimicrob Agents Chemother 45:2793–2797

34. Craig WA, Andes D (1996) Pharmacokinetics and pharmacodynamics of antibiotics in otitis media. Pediatr Infect Dis J 15:255–259

35. Schentagg JJ, Smith IL, Swanson DJ, et al (1984) Role for individualization with cefmenoxime. Am J Med 77:43–50

36. Grant EM, Kuti JL, Nicolau DP, et al (2002) Clinical efficacy and pharmacoeconomics of a continuous-infusion piperacillin–tazobactam program in a large community teaching hospital. Pharmacotherapy 22:471–483

37. Craig WA (2002) The role of pharmacodynamics in effective treatment of community-acquired pathogens. Advanced Studies in Medicine 2:126–134

38. Drusano GL, Craig WA (1997) Relevance of pharmacokinetics and pharmacodynamics in the selection of antibiotics for respiratory tract infections. J Chemother 9 (Suppl 3):38–44

39. Niederman MS (2001) Impact of antibiotic resistance on clinical outcomes and the cost of care. Crit Care Med 29 (Suppl 4):N114–120

40. Lemmen SW, Becker G, Frank U, Daschner FD (2001) Influence of an infectious disease consulting service on quality and costs of antibiotic prescriptions in a university hospital. Scand J Infect Dis 33:219–221

41. Thuong M, Shortgen F, Zazempa V, et al (2000) Appropriate use of restricted antimicrobial agents in hospitals: the importance of empirical therapy and assisted re-evaluation. J Antimicrob Chemother 46:501–508

42. Van Zanten AR, Engelfriet PM, Van Dillen K (2003) Importance of nondrug costs of intravenous antibiotic therapy. Crit Care 7:R184–R190

43. Heyland DK, Rocker GM, Dodek PM, et al (2002) Family satisfaction with care in the intensive care unit: results of a multiple center study. Crit Care Med 30:1413–1418

44. Tarnow-Mordi WO, Hau C, Warden A, Shearer AJ (2000) Hospital mortality in relation to staff workload: a 4-year study in an adult intensive-care unit. Lancet 356:185–189

45. Tucker J, UK Neonatal Staffing Study Group (2002) Patient volume, staffing, and workload in relation to risk-adjusted outcomes in a random stratified sample of UK neonatal intensive care units: a prospective evaluation. Lancet 359:99–107

46. Thorens JB, Kaelin RM, Jolliet P, Chevrolet JC (1995) Influence of the quality of nursing on the duration of weaning from mechanical ventilation in patients with chronic obstructive pulmonary disease. Crit Care Med 23:1807–1815

Pharmacokinetics of Antibiotics During Continuous Renal Replacement Therapy

W. A. Krueger, T. H. Schroeder, and M. Hansen

▌ Introduction

At first glance, dosing of antibotics in patients receiving renal replacement therapy does not seem a complicated issue. For most drugs, well-defined dosage recommendations are available for patients with impaired renal function, including terminal renal failure. Furthermore, it is usually well known whether these drugs may be removed by dialysis. Finally, one may roughly estimate a creatinine clearance of approx. 20 ml/min accomplished by the renal replacement therapy. Thus, dosage recommendations can either be looked up in various lists available in textbooks or on the web for patients receiving renal replacement therapy, or the drugs may be given according to the roughly estimated values for creatinine clearances. So what is the problem? Indeed, many recommendations for patients suffering from acute renal failure are derived from calculations. The dosage recommendations are then given in analogy to patients suffering from chronic renal failure and reduced creatinine clearance.

A closer look at the situation in critically ill patients reveals that the pharmacokinetics of drugs may be complex and sometimes unforeseeable. Very often, the functions of organs other than the kidneys are compromised as well, and in such conditions it is hardly possible to assess their elimination function that might otherwise compensate for the impaired renal drug excretion [1]. Also, there may be interactions of several drugs given concomitantly and conditions may change frequently in individual patients. Finally, there are substantial differences between different types of renal replacement therapies. These differences may relate to the treatment modalities, such as dialysis versus hemofiltration, the filters, their sizes and changing intervals, and – most importantly – the filtrate and dialysis flow rates. There is a strong rationale for using high filtrate flow rates of 35 ml/kg/min, which can improve outcome of patients with acute renal failure [2]. Of course, we do not want to offset the beneficial effects of intensified renal replacement therapy by enhanced elimination of antbiotics used for treatment of septic patients.

At the beginning of this chapter, an outline will be presented on general principles of pharmacotherapy during continuous renal replacement therapy (CRRT). Some general considerations will already answer a number of questions about necessity and extent of dosage adjustment. Of course, this article does not obviate the need for having access to lists for dosage recommendations during renal replacement therapy, but it is easier to understand and memorize such recommendations, once the basic principles are clear. The choice of antibiotics discussed later is based on didactical considerations, as they show the applicability as well as limitations of calculations of the creatinine clearances of renal replacement therapies. Hence, a more detailed understanding of the subject will hopefully contribute to both optimizing antimicrobial therapy and improving patient safety.

▌ General Principles of Pharmacotherapy During Renal Replacement Therapy

The initial dose (loading dose) of an antibiotic is given for rapid achievement of antimicrobially active levels in the blood and at the sites of infection. The loading dose is therefore identical for patients with or without renal failure. One of the few exceptions to this rule pertains bolus administration of aminoglycosides, which will be discussed in more detail later in the chapter.

Two factors must then be considered in order to decide about the timing and amount of subsequent doses. First, one must look up whether dosage reductions are necessary for patients suffering from chronic anuric renal failure (this will be the case for most antibiotics). Additionally, one must consider replacement of the amount of drug removed by the renal replacement therapy (substitution dose).

It is a general rule that drugs that are eliminated by the kidneys are also eliminated by renal replacement therapy – at least, when the renal elimination is mainly based on glomerular filtration [3]. A substitution dose is considered necessary when the clearance achieved by the renal replacement therapy amounts to more than 20–25% of the total body clearance of the drug [4]. This is true for most cephalosporins and penicillins. If the extracorporeal clearance is lower, the dosages recommended for anuric patients are appropriate and no extra dose for the renal replacement therapy is necessary.

Drugs that are almost exclusively eliminated by non-renal pathways can be administered at their usual dosages in isolated renal failure – whether or not renal replacement therapy is used (e.g., moxifloxacin [5]). This rule has theoretical limitations if metabolites are formed that would normally be eliminated by the kidneys, since such metabolites may accumulate and possibly cause hazardous side effects. Unfortunately, data for pharmacokinetics of metabolites during renal replacement therapy are very sparse. This means that the potentially adverse effects of drug breakdown products are not adequately represented in the recommendations.

▌ Principles of Drug Elimination by Renal Replacement Therapy

During dialysis, solutes are removed by diffusion from the blood into the countercurrently flowing dialysis fluid and the coefficients of diffusion depend on the molecular weights. Therefore, small molecules such as potassium are dialyzed very effectively. Vancomycin in contrast is one of the largest drug molecules (approx. 1400 daltons), which means that the extent of removal is comparatively lower during dialysis [6].

During hemofiltration, solutes are removed by convective transport. The driving force is a hydrostatic pressure gradient, which filters plasma water and all solutes along with it. Thus, the elimination of soluble substances is independent of the molecule size, as long as it is below cut-off threshold of the filter membrane. Since the cut-off values of common hemofilter materials (polysulphone, polyamide,

AN69^{TM}) range between 10000 and 30000 daltons, virtually all drugs can be filtered, as long as they are not protein-bound.

Hemodiafiltration combines diffusive and convective elimination principles. Other mechanisms of drug elimination, such as adsorption to the hemofilter or electrostatic interactions with filter membrane materials can usually be neglected (aminoglycosides are a possible exception, as outlined below).

Factors Influencing Drug Elimination

Some pharmacological properties as well as certain characteristics of renal replacement therapies may allow an estimate of the elimination of drugs (Table 1).

Protein Binding and Sieving Coefficient

The sieving coefficient describes the fraction of drug that is eliminated from the plasma into the filtrate. The easiest way to calculate the sieving coefficient is to divide the filtrate concentration by the plasma concentration from samples simultaneously obtained during the elimination phase of the drug. Alternatively, the ratio of the respective AUC-values, which are the areas under the concentration-time curves of the drug in filtrate and in plasma may be calculated [7]. When the sieving coefficient equals 1, the drug passes freely from the blood into the filtrate and is not retained by the hemofilter.

As may be expected, there is an inverse correlation between the sieving coefficient and protein binding. Sieving coefficient values close to 0 are found for highly protein bound drugs such as oxacillin, which means that these drugs are retained together with the proteins and cannot be eliminated by renal replacement therapies [8]. Thus, in cases of high protein binding, no substitution dose is required for the renal replacement therapy and the dose recommended for anuric patients is appropriate. A more theoretical exception is reduced protein binding, e.g., by competitive inhibition by other highly protein bound drugs, high bilirubin levels, changes in pH, or in severe protein deficiency.

Based on theoretical considerations, 1.0 is the maximum value for the sieving coefficient, since higher values suggest active elimination [3]. Rarely, values above 1.0 have been reported, which supposedly are caused by electrostatic interactions of

Table 1. Factors influencing drug elimination during CRRT

	Predictable factors	Variable factors
Drug	Volume of distribution Sieving coefficient	Protein binding (interaction with bilirubin, other drugs, pH-changes)
Filter	Material (cut-off, binding) Surface area of membrane	Partial clotting Protein precipitation at membrane
Modality	Filtrate/dialysate flow rate (Pre-versus post dilution) (blood flow through hemofilter)	Vascular access (recirculation of blood at catheter, clotting of catheter) Interruptions of renal replacement therapy due to diagnostic procedures/ technical failure

charged drugs with the filter materials or with protein precipitates at the filters, so that the elimination is increased for reasons of electroneutrality.

Clearance

Since the sieving coefficient is a drug-specific constant value, the hemofiltration clearance can be calculated by multiplying the sieving coefficient by the filtrate flow rate. Similarly, the clearance of hemodialysis can be calculated. In analogy, the saturation coefficient is determined by dividing the concentration of the drug in the dialysate by the plasma concentration, and the clearance can be derived by multiplication with the dialysate flow rate. However, different from the sieving coefficient, the saturation coefficient is constant only within certain limits. With high dialysate flow rates, the contact time may be too short for complete passage of the drug into the countercurrent flowing dialysate, which means that the saturation coefficient becomes smaller under such conditions. This is especially true for filters with small surfaces, where the contact times are shorter [9]. The maximum elimination is reached once the flow becomes higher than the countercurrent blood flow.

Volume of Distribution

High extracorporeal drug clearances do not necessarily mean that substitution doses are necessary. More importantly, the volume of distribution of the drug has to be considered. The volume of distribution is a virtual value that does not correspond to an anatomical space and it can reach much larger values than the total body volume. It is calculated by dividing the dose of the drug by the plasma concentration of the drug. For a better understanding of the impact of the volume of distribution and clearance on the amount of elimination, one can imagine the volume of distribution being a large barrel and the clearance being the flow of beer through the tap of the barrel. For a large barrel, a substitution dose (buy a new barrel) will be necessary less frequently than for a small barrel, even when the flow through the tap stays the same. A clinical example is azithromycin with a volume of distribution of 25 times the body weight, which results in more than 1000 liters in adults and is due to intracellular trapping of the drug [10]. Thus, the clearance only describes the amount of plasma volume becoming devoid of the substance, whereas volume of distribution determines the fraction of a drug residing in the compartment that is amenable to the extracorporeal clearance.

Even though the volume of distribution for drugs may be substantially different in intensive care unit (ICU) patients compared to healthy volunteers, this is not readily foreseeable in individual cases [11–13]. Betalactam-antibiotics (i.e., penicillins, cephalosporins, carbapenems, monobactams), aminoglycosides, and the macrolide antibiotic, roxithromycin, have volumes of distribution of approx. 20 liters, which means that there is a relevant degree of extracorporeal clearance, as long as these drugs are not protein-bound. In contrast, most macrolides and fluoroquinolones have volumes of distribution of 100 liters or more [10, 14], which means that only small amounts of these drugs are removed by the renal replacement therapy.

Drug-specific Examples

Imipenem-cilastatin

Imipenem is a carbapenem antibiotic, which is mainly eliminated by glomerular filtration and tubular secretion, but is also metabolized by renal dehydropeptidase-I (DHP-1) located in tubular epithelial cells [15]. The metabolites are nephrotoxic, as they accumulate in the epithelial cells. Therefore, imipenem is not available as a single substance for clinical use and is always administered together with cilastatin, which inhibits the DHP-1 and thereby prevents nephrotoxicity. While the two substances have similar elimination characteristics in individuals without renal impairment, cilastatin accumulates relative to imipenem in anuric patients. Hemofiltration eliminates both drugs, but there is still a relative accumulation of cilastatin over imipenem [16–19]. Several authors have recommended a reduced dosage of 2×500 mg of imipenem in its fixed combination with cilastatin during veno-venous hemofiltration [19–21] and during continuous hemodialysis [22]. However, most of these studies were done when filtrate flow rates of 1–1.5 l/h were the standard and it is unclear whether these dosages will be enough for patients being treated with high filtrate flow rates. Furthermore, it has repeatedly been reported that the clearance of imipenem is higher in patients with acute renal failure compared to patients with chronic renal failure. The reasons for the difference in clearances are not known, but could possibly be due to residual activity of the DHP-1 in acute renal failure. Therefore, some authors recommend higher dosages for patients with acute renal failure during treatment with veno-venous hemofiltration (2×1000 mg) [18, 21]. Such doses also seem more appropriate for filtrate flow rates of approx. 3 l/h, which have been shown to improve patient outcome [2].

Meropenem

Meropenem is also a carbapenem antibiotic, but it is almost exclusively eliminated by the kidneys [23] and it is not metabolized by human renal DHP-1 [24]. No difference in clearance has been reported for acute and chronic renal failure [25]. Similar to other beta-lactams, such as cephalosporins, penicillins, and monobactams, the optimal bacteriocidal effect is achieved, as long as the plasma levels stay above the minimal inhibitory concentration (MIC) of the pathogens [26, 27]. But, different to other beta-lactams, carbapenems exert postantibiotic effects against Gram-positive and Gram-negative bacteria [28–30], which means that regrowth does not immediately occur once the plasma levels fall below the MIC of the bacteria. Therefore, it is considered sufficient when the levels exceed the MIC for approximately 30% of the dosage interval (Krueger et al., unpublished data) [31].

During continuous hemodiafiltration with a flow rate of 1600 ml/h (Fig. 1), the plasma levels following 1 g of meropenem b.i.d. exceeded the MIC of intermediately susceptible microorganisms (breakpoint: 8 mg/l [32]) throughout the dosage interval [33]. When 500 mg were given every 12 h during hemofiltration, the levels were still sufficient in all patients for the treatment of infections caused by susceptible bacteria (i.e., MIC < 4 mg/l), but not all patients had plasma levels above the MIC of intermediately susceptible bacteria for more than 30% of the dosage interval (Fig. 2) [34]. No relevant differences were found with respect to the elimination characteristics for meropenem during hemodiafiltration and hemofiltration. Binding of meropenem to commonly used filter materials could be excluded by *in vitro*

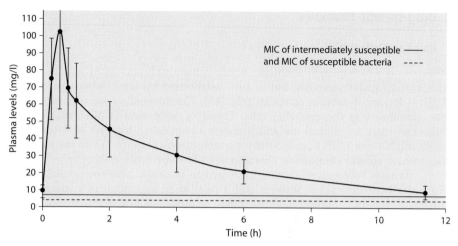

Fig. 1. Levels of meropenem in plasma (means and standard deviations) in eight critically ill patients treated by continuous veno-venous hemodiafiltration. A dose of 1000 mg of meropenem was administered as an i.v. infusion over 30 min. MIC: minimal inhibitory concentration. Adapted from [33] with permission

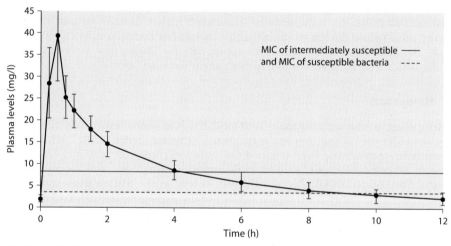

Fig. 2. Levels of meropenem in plasma (means and standard deviations) in eight critically ill patients treated by continuous veno-venous hemofiltration. A dose of 500 mg of meropenem was administered as an i.v. infusion over 30 min. MIC: minimal inhibitory concentration. Adapted from [34] with permission

experiments (polysulphone, polyamide, AN69™ [9]. In conclusion, for both types of renal replacement therapy, 2×500 mg of meropenem is adequate for the treatment of infections caused by bacteria that are susceptible to meropenem and 2×1000 mg in cases of intermediate susceptibility, or in cases where the MICs of the infecting organisms are not known. The higher dosage might also be adequate when renal replacement therapies with filtrate or dialysate flows markedly above 1.5 l/h are used.

Piperacillin-tazobactam

Piperacillin is an acylamino-penicillin, and approximately 60–70% of the dose is eliminated by the kidneys. During continuous veno-venous hemofiltration 2×4000 mg instead of the usual 3×4000 mg has been recommended, but the filtrate flow was relatively low in that study (approximately 800 ml/h) [35]. The spectrum of activity of piperacillin can be extended by combination with an inhibitor of beta-lactamases, which otherwise cleave the antibiotic. In its fixed combination, 4000 mg of piperacillin and 500 mg of the beta-lactamase-inhibitor, tazobactam, show similar kinetics in subjects without renal impairment, but the influence of the different volumes of distribution on the elimination becomes obvious during hemo-filtration. The hemofiltration clearance of tazobactam was higher than the clearance of piperacillin, but the former accumulates due to its higher volume of distribution, when regular doses are given (3×4000/500 mg). Since piperacillin is available as a single substance, some authors recommend the intermittent administration of the antibiotic without the beta-lactamase-inhibitor [36], whereas others use the fixed combination at its regular dose of 3×4000/500 mg [37].

Ciprofloxacin

Approximately 70% of an intravenous dose of the fluoroquinolone antibiotic, cipro-floxacin, is eliminated by the kidneys, 12% is metabolized, and 15% is eliminated with feces due to transintestinal secretion, mainly accomplished by small intestinal epithelial cells [5]. In healthy volunteers and patients with normal renal function, the fecal level of ciprofloxacin after intravenous administration is dose-dependent and up to 800 μg per gram of feces have been found [38, 39]. In renal failure, up to 50% of an intravenous dose is eliminated by transintestinal secretion, but this rela-tive increase only partially compensates decreased renal excretion and the half-life is doubled to approximately 8 hours [40]. In such patients, half of the regular dose of ciprofloxacin has been recommended. The volume of distribution of ciprofloxa-cin is approximately 100 liters, which means that renal replacement therapies con-tribute much less to the elimination, compared to the before mentioned examples of betalactam antibiotics. Therefore, a daily dose of 400 mg has been recommended in patients treated with CRRT [41]. The pharmacokinetics of the 3 (or even 4?) me-tabolites of ciprofloxacin have not been studied during renal replacement therapy.

Aminoglycosides

In contrast to the beta-lactams, the bacteriocidal activity of aminoglycosides is con-centration-dependent [42]. The ratio of peak levels to the MIC correlates with ther-apeutic success [43, 44] and, furthermore, aminoglycosides exert postantibiotic ef-fects, which prevent immediate bacterial regrowth when the drug levels fall below the MICs [42]. Moreover, an interval with low levels even decreases the toxicity [45]. It has, therefore, become clinical practice to administer the total daily dose of aminoglycosides as a bolus over 60 min. Such bolus administration provides plas-ma levels for gentamicin or tobramycin above 20 mg/l, while the trough levels should be kept below 1 mg/l for prevention of renal toxicity and possibly also for prevention of ototoxicity [45]. However, once-daily dosing of aminoglycosides is contraindicated when the creatinine-clearance is below 40 ml/min, since prolonged high levels are likely to increase toxicity [46]. Aminoglycosides should be avoided as much as possible in patients suffering from acute renal failure. If there are no alternatives, a third of the daily dose should be administered at the beginning of aminoglycoside therapy. It is not possible to give general recommendations for subsequent doses, and frequent measurements of the plasma levels are strongly advocated to avoid toxic side effects. Often, a reduction by 50% is necessary on the second day and plasma levels are to be monitored meticulously [3].

Due to its negative charge, an AN69^{TM}-hemofilter with an effective surface area of 1 m^2 can bind approximately 20 mg of tobramycin [47, 48]. Thus, elimination by binding to the membrane is usually not clinically relevant, but needs to be kept in mind when the hemofilter is changed several times a day.

Vancomycin

More than 90% of the glycopeptide, vancomycin, is eliminated by the kidneys, and therefore the regular half-life of 6–8 hours is prolonged to more than 200 hours in terminal renal failure. Since the molecule is very large (approximately 1400 dalton), it was only negligibly eliminated by dialysis with old cuprophane membranes, which have cut-off values of approximately 500 dalton but are not used any more today. With modern high-flux membranes (e.g., polysulphone), the plasma levels fall considerably during dialysis. However, a rebound of plasma levels can be observed a few hours after dialysis, which is due to redistribution, so that therapeutic levels may persist despite the initial fall during dialysis [49]. In contrast, vancomycin is eliminated much more readily by CRRT with high-flux membranes. No general dosage recommendation can be given, and the decision must be based on measurements of the plasma levels [50–52].

Linezolid

Approximately 30% of the dose of linezolid, which is an oxazolidinone antibiotic, is renally excreted and 50% is eliminated as metabolites. The regular dose of 2×600 mg also applies for patients with renal impairment. The protein binding is approximately 30% and the volume of distribution is 40–50 liters in an adult person [53]. Elimination of linezolid by renal replacement therapy has been shown by an *in vitro* extracorporeal circuit model [54], but no dosage adjustment is necessary in patients with renal failure treated with renal replacement therapy [55].

▋ Conclusion

The loading dose of an antibiotic is independent of the renal function. The amount and interval of subsequent doses depend on the extent of extrarenal and extracorporeal elimination. Drugs that are exclusively eliminated by non-renal pathways can be given at their regular doses and the extent of extracorporeal elimination is usually not relevant. Accumulation of drug metabolites in patients with renal impairment treated with renal replacement therapy deserves further attention, but there is still a lack of data in this field. Drugs with narrow therapeutic margins – such as aminoglycosides – should not be used or should be closely monitored by measurement of plasma levels.

The extracorporeal clearance by renal replacement therapy can be calculated by multiplying the filtrate flow with the sieving coefficient, and the latter inversely correlates with protein binding. However, the volume of distribution is even more important in determining whether a substitution dose for the extracorporeal drug clearance is necessary. Beta-lactam antibiotics (penicillins, cephalosporins, carbapenems) have volumes of distribution of approximately 20 liters in an adult person and most beta-lactams have relatively low protein binding. This means that the amount of extracorporeal clearance is relevant, especially in renal replacement therapy with high flow rates. Fluoroquinolones and most macrolides have much higher volumes of distribution and, therefore, the amount of drug removed by renal replacement therapies is relatively low and does not necessitate an extra dose.

References

1. Schroeder TH, Hansen M, Dinkelacker K, et al (2005) Influence of underlying disease on the outcome of critically ill patients with acute renal failure Eur J Anaesthesiol 21 (in press)
2. Ronco C, Bellomo R, Homel P, et al (2000) Effects of different doses in continuous veno-venous haemofiltration on outcomes of acute renal failure: a prospective randomised trial. Lancet 356:26–30
3. Cotterill S (1995) Antimicrobial prescribing in patients on haemofiltration. J Antimicrob Chemother 36:773–780
4. Olbricht CJ (1992) Pharmakotherapie bei kontinuierlicher Hämofiltration CAVH/CVVH. Intensivmed 29:4–8
5. Fuhrmann V, Schenk P, Jaeger W, Ahmed S, Thalhammer F (2004) Pharmacokinetics of moxifloxacin in patients undergoing continuous venovenous haemodiafiltration J Antimicrob Chemother 54:780–784
6. Davies JG, Kingswood JC, Sharpstone P, Street MK (1995) Drug removal in continuous haemofiltration and haemodialysis. Br J Hosp Med 54:524–528
7. Reetze-Bonorden P, Böhler J, Keller E (1993) Drug dosage in patients during continuous renal replacement therapy. Clin Pharmacokinet 24:362–379
8. Golper TA (1985) Continuous arteriovenous hemofiltration in acute renal failure. Am J Kidney Dis 6:373–386
9. Schroeder TH, Krueger WA, Hansen M, Hoffmann E, Dieterich HJ, Unertl K (1999) Elimination of meropenem by continuous hemo(dia)filtration: an *in vitro* one-compartment model. Int J Artif Organs 22:307–312
10. Sörgel F, Kinzig M, Naber KG (1993) Macrolides. In: Bryskier A, Butzler JP, Neu HC (eds) Chemistry, Pharmacology and Clinical Uses. Arnette Blackwell, Paris, France, pp 421–435
11. Lugo G, Castañeda-Hernández G (1997) Relationship between hemodynamic and vital support measures and pharmacokinetic variability of amikacin in critically ill patients with sepsis. Crit Care Med 25:806–811
12. Niemiec PW, Allo MD, Miller CF (1987) Effect of altered volume of distribution on aminoglycoside levels in patients in surgical intensive care. Arch Surg 122:207–212
13. van Dalen R, Vree TB (1990) Pharmacokinetics of antibiotics in critically ill patients. Intensive Care Med 16:235–238
14. Sörgel F, Kinzig M (1993) Pharmacokinetics of gyrase inhibitors, part 1: basic chemistry and gastrointestinal disposition. Am J Med 94 (Suppl 3A):44S–55S
15. Birnbaum J, Kahan FM, Kropp H, McDonald JS (1985) Carbapenems, a new class of antibiotics. Discovery and development of imipenem/cilastatin. Am J Med 78 (Suppl 6A):3–21
16. Keller E, Fecht H, Böhler J, Schollmeyer P (1989) Single-dose kinetics of imipenem/cilastatin during continuous arteriovenous haemofiltration in intensive care patients. Nephrol Dial Transplant 4:640–645
17. Przechera M, Bengel D, Risler T (1991) Pharmacokinetics of imipenem/cilastatin during continuous arteriovenous hemofiltration. Contrib Nephrol 93:131–134

18. Tegeder I, Bremer F, Oelkers R, et al (1997) Pharmacokinetics of imipenem-cilastatin in critically ill patients undergoing continuous venovenous hemofiltration. Antimicrob Agents Chemother 41:2640–2645
19. Vos MC, Vincent HH, Yzerman EPF (1992) Clearance of imipenem/cilastatin in acute renal failure patients treated by continuous hemodiafiltration (CAVHD). Intensive Care Med 18:282–285
20. Alarabi AA, Cars O, Danielson BG, Salmonson T, Wikström B (1990) Pharmacokinetics of intravenous imipenem/cilastatin during intermittent haemofiltration. J Antimicrob Chemother 26:91–98
21. Mueller BA, Scarim SK, Macias WL (1993) Comparison of imipenem pharmacokinetics in patients with acute or chronic renal failure treated with continuous hemofiltration. Am J Kidney Dis 21:172–179
22. Hashimoto S, Honda M, Yamaguchi M, Sekimoto M, Tanaka Y (1997) Pharmacokinetics of imipenem and cilastatin during continuous hemodialysis in patients who are critically ill. ASAIO J 43:84–88
23. Bax RP, Bastain W, Featherstone A, Wilkinson DM, Hutchison M, Haworth SJ (1989) The pharmacokinetics of meropenem in volunteers. J Antimicrob Chemother 24 (Suppl A):311–320
24. Fukasawa M, Sumita Y, Harabe ET, et al (1992) Stability of meropenem and the effect of 1-β-methyl substitution on its stability in the presence of renal dehydropeptidase I. Antimicrob Agents Chemother 36:1577–1579
25. Tegeder I, Neumann F, Bremer F, Brune K, Lötsch J, Geisslinger G (1999) Pharmacokinetics of meropenem in critically ill patients with acute renal failure undergoing continuous venovenous hemofiltration. Clin Pharmacol Ther 65:50–57
26. Craig WA (1995) Interrelationship between pharmacokinetics and pharmacodynamics in determining dosage regimens for broad spectrum cephalosporins. Diag Microbiol Infect Dis 22:89–96
27. Vogelman B, Gudmundsson S, Leggett J, Turnidge J, Ebert S, Craig WA (1988) Correlation of antimicrobial pharmacokinetic parameters with therapeutic efficacy in an animal model. J Infect Dis 158:831–847
28. Bustamante CI, Drusano GL, Tatem BA, Standiford HC (1984) Postantibiotic effect of imipenem on *Pseudomonas aeruginosa*. Antimicrob Agents Chemother 26:678–682
29. Munckhof WJ, Olden D, Turnidge JD (1997) The postantibiotic effect of imipenem: relationship with drug concentration, duration of exposure, and MIC. Antimicrob Agents Chemother 41:1735–1737
30. Nadler HL, Pitkin DH, Sheikh W (1989) The postantibiotic effect of meropenem and imipenem on selected bacteria. J Antimicrob Chemother 24 (Suppl A):225–231
31. Drusano GL, Hutchison M (1995) The pharmacokinetics of meropenem. Scand J Infect Dis Suppl 96:11–16
32. National Committee for Clinical Laboratory Standards (1998) Performance standards for antimicrobial susceptibility testing. Eighth informational supplement. NCCLS, Wayne 18:12
33. Krueger WA, Schroeder TH, Hutchison M, et al (1998) Pharmacokinetics of meropenem in critically ill patients with acute renal failure treated by continuous hemodiafiltration. Antimicrob Agents Chemother 42:2421–2424
34. Krueger WA, Neeser G, Schuster H, et al (2003) Correlation of meropenem plasma levels with pharmacodynamic requirements in critically ill patients receiving continuous venovenous hemofiltration. Chemother 49:280–286
35. Capellier G, Cornette C, Boillot A, et al (1998) Removal of piperacillin in critically ill patients undergoing venovenous hemofiltration. Crit Care Med 26:88–91
36. van der Werf TS, Mulder POM, Zijlstra JG, Uges DRA, Stegeman CA (1997) Pharmacokinetics of piperacillin and tazobactam in critically ill patients with renal failure, treated with continuous veno-venous hemofiltration (CVVH). Intensive Care Med 23:873–877
37. Valtonen M, Tiula E, Takkunen O, Backman JT, Neuvonen PJ (2001) Elimination of the piperacillin/tazobactam combination during continuous venovenous haemofiltration and haemodiafiltration in patients with acute renal failure. J Antimicrob Chemother 48:881–885

38. Krueger WA, Ruckdeschel G, Unertl K (1997) Influence of intravenously administered cipro-floxacin on aerobic intestinal microflora and fecal drug levels when administered simulta-neously with sucralfate. Antimicrob Agents Chemother 41:1725–17230

39. Krueger WA, Ruckdeschel G, Unertl K (1999) Elimination of fecal *Enterobacteriaceae* by in-travenous ciprofloxacin is not inhibited by concomitant sucralfate – a microbiological and pharmacokinetic study in patients. Infection 27:335–340

40. Rohwedder RW, Bergan T, Thorsteinsson SB, Scholl H (1990) Transintestinal elimination of ciprofloxacin. Diag Microbiol Infect Dis 13:127–133

41. Malone RS, Fish DN, Abraham E, Teitelbaum I (2001) Pharmacokinetics of levofloxacin and ciprofloxacin during continuous renal replacement therapy in critically ill patients. Anti-microb Agents Chemother 45:2949–2954

42. Craig WA (1998) Pharmacokinetic/pharmacodynamic parameters: rationale for antibacterial dosing in mice and men. Clin Infect Dis 26:1–12

43. Kashuba AD, Nafziger AN, Drusano GL, Bertino JS (1999) Optimizing aminoglycoside therapy for nosocomial pneumonia caused by Gram-negative bacteria. Antimicrob Agents Chemother 43:623–629

44. Moore RD, Smith CR, Lietman PS (1984) Association of aminoglycoside plasma levels with therapeutic outcome in Gram-negative pneumonia. Am J Med 77:657–662

45. Beaucaire C (2000) Does once-daily dosing prevent nephrotoxicity in all aminoglycosides equally? Clin Microbiol Infect 6:357–362

46. Hatala R, Dinh T, Cook DJ (1996) Once-daily aminoglycoside dosing in immunocompetent adults: a meta-analysis. Ann Intern Med 124:717–725

47. Cigarran-Guldris S, Brier ME, Golper TA (1991) Tobramycin clearance during simulated continuous arteriovenous hemodialysis. Contrib Nephrol 93:120–123

48. Kronfol NO, Lau AH, Barakat MM (1987) Aminoglycoside binding to polyacrylonitril hemo-filter membranes during continuous hemofiltration. Trans Am Soc Artif Intern Organs 33:300–303

49. Böhler J, Reetze-Bonorden P, Keller E, Kramer A, Schollmeyer PJ (1992) Rebound of plasma vancomycin levels after haemodialysis with highly permeable membranes. Eur J Clin Phar-macol 42:635–640

50. Boereboom FTJ, Ververs FFT, Blankestijn PJ, Savelkoul TJF, van Dijk A (1999) Vancomycin clearance during continuous venovenous haemofiltration in critically ill patients. Intensive Care Med 25:1100–1104

51. Foote EF, Dreitlein WB, Steward CA, Kapoian T, Walker JA, Sherman RA (1998) Pharmaco-kinetics of vancomycin when administered during high flux hemodialysis Clin Nephrol 50:51–55

52. Uchino S, Cole L, Morimatsu H, Goldsmith D, Bellomo R (2002) Clearance of vancomycin during high-volume haemofiltration: impact of pre-dilution. Intensive Care Med 28:1664–1667

53. Krueger WA, Unertl KE (2002) Neue Therapieoption für Intensivpatienten mit Infektionen durch Gram-positive Bakterien – Überblick über Linezolid. Anästhesiol Intensivmed Not-fallmed Schmerzther 37:199–204

54. Schroeder TH, Hansen M, Stephan M, Hoffmann E, Unertl K, Krueger WA (2004) Elimina-tion of linezolid by an in vitro extracorporeal circuit model. Int J Artif Org 27:473–479

55. Brier ME, Stalker DJ, Aronow DR, Batts DH, Ryan KK, O'Grady NP, Hopkins NK, Jungblut GL (2003) Pharmacokinetics of linezolid in subjects with renal dysfunction. Antimicrob Agents Chemother 47:2775–2780

Impact of Methicillin Resistance on the Outcome of Severe *Staphylococcus aureus* Infections

A. Combes, C.-E. Luyt, and J.-L. Trouillet

▌ Introduction

Methicillin-resistant *Staphylococcus aureus* (MRSA) was first described in 1961 [1]. Since then, it has emerged as a major cause of nosocomial infections worldwide, with more than 50% of *S. aureus* strains isolated in intensive care units (ICUs) being MRSA [2]. Predisposing factors for MRSA infections include severe underlying condition, prolonged hospital stay, previous antibiotic treatment, and nasal MRSA carriage [3–5]. Despite continuous efforts to control MRSA transmission in the hospital, especially in ICUs, MRSA infections remain a major worldwide concern and the true impact of MRSA on morbidity and mortality remains highly controversial. While some papers [3, 6–12], including a recent meta-analysis of *S. aureus* bacteremia [13], found higher mortality rates for MRSA compared to methicillin-susceptible *S. aureus* (MSSA) infections, many studies failed to identify a relationship between MRSA and mortality [14–23]. These results may reflect the endpoints chosen (crude versus infection-related mortality), major differences in patient populations, preexisting comorbidities, severity of *S. aureus* infection at the time of its diagnosis, sites of these infections and, above all, high rates of inappropriate empiric antibiotic regimens prescribed for MRSA infections. This chapter will first review the factors that might affect outcomes of patients suffering from severe *Staphylococcus aureus* infections. Second, we will discuss the results of studies focusing on the impact of methicillin resistance on the outcome of *S. aureus* bacteremia, surgical wound infections and ventilator-associated pneumonia (VAP).

▌ Factors Related to Increased Crude Mortality for Severe *Staphylococcus aureus* Infections

In most studies published to date, crude hospital or ICU mortality was significantly higher for patients suffering from MRSA vs. MSSA infection. This increase in mortality could relate to the bacteria itself (enhanced virulence for MRSA strains), to host factors (patients characteristics may differ between groups), or to the antimicrobial treatment administered to MRSA patients (Table 1). These variables need to be carefully controlled when comparing outcomes of MSSA and MRSA infections. This can be accomplished by selecting homogeneous groups of patients (for example patients receiving appropriate initial antimicrobial treatment), by matching case and control patients or by including unmatched variables in a multivariate analysis.

Table 1. Factors potentially related to unfavorable outcome for severe methicillin-resistant *Staphylococcus aureus* infections

Factor	Level of evidence
Increased fitness of MRSA strains	0
Host related factors	
▌ Older age	+
▌ Comorbidities	+
▌ Increased disease severity	+
Factors related to antimicrobial treatments	
▌ Suboptimal action of vancomycin	+
▌ Insufficient trough plasma vancomycin level	+
▌ High rates of inappropriate empiric antibiotic treatment	++

Effect of Methicillin Resistance on Bacterial Fitness

To date, no studies have demonstrated a correlation between increased bacterial fitness and nosocomial MRSA strains. Studies of experimental infection in mice and guinea pigs have shown MRSA and MSSA strains to be equally virulent [24, 25]. In several *in vitro* studies, MRSA and MSSA strains have been shown to possess similar virulence factors, adherence properties and bacteriological pathogenicity [24, 26, 27]. Specifically, Laurent et al [28] demonstrated that MSSA and MRSA isolates had similar generation times and Duckworth and Jordens [29] even found significantly less attachment of MRSA to cells and fibronectin compared with MSSA strains. However, recently recognized community–acquired MRSA strains may display significantly higher virulence, which may in part be explained by the activity of the Panton-Valentine leukocidin [30, 31].

Host-related Factors

An important issue when comparing the impact of antimicrobial resistance on outcomes is the appropriate adjustment for differences in epidemiological and clinical characteristics between patients with resistant and susceptible infections. Specifically, age, comorbidities, hospital length of stay before infection onset, and disease severity before and at infection onset are important variables that can independently result in adverse outcomes of resistant infections. Indeed, it has been demonstrated that MRSA-infected patients are older, more frequently suffer from diabetes, peripheral vascular disease, or advanced renal failure, have experienced prolonged antibiotic exposure and extended length of stay in the hospital before infection onset, and also present signs of more severe disease at infection onset.

Various methods have been proposed to adjust for illness severity. Disease severity and organ dysfunction scores are commonly used for patients hospitalized in ICUs. Additionally, an important issue for the accurate assessment of the impact of resistant organisms on infection outcomes is the timing of the assessment of illness severity. The presence of infection may strongly influence disease severity and may represent an intermediate variable in the chain of events between the infection and the outcome [32]. Studies that adjust for disease severity when the infection is patent may underestimate the magnitude of the effect that resistance has on outcomes [32].

Pre-morbid state is frequently evaluated using the McCabe and Jackson scoring system [33], but it is subjectively based on the judgement of the individual reviewing the patient record. The Charlson comorbidity scoring system [34], which evaluates the number of comorbidities before hospital admission, may be a more valuable tool.

Factors Related to Antimicrobial Treatments

One possible explanation for the higher morbidity and mortality associated with MRSA infections advanced in some studies could be the suboptimal antimicrobial action of vancomycin. It has been suggested that vancomycin may be less rapidly bactericidal than semi-synthetic penicillin for the treatment of severe S. aureus infections, such as endocarditis [35, 36]. Moreover, the penetration of vancomycin into lung tissue [37] and pulmonary lining fluid [38] has been reported to be relatively low (blood-to-tissue ratio: 3:1–6:1) and linearly correlated to the plasma concentration.

Insufficient trough plasma vancomycin levels may also explain worse outcomes for MRSA infections. In a previous study by our group, only trough plasma vancomycin levels of 15–20 μg/ml were associated with pulmonary lining fluid concentration exceeding the drug's minimal inhibitory concentrations (MIC) for most Gram-positive cocci [38]. In another study, Rodman et al. [39] screened for appropriateness of initial dosing based on available dosing nomograms of all intravenous vancomycin orders over a 3-month period in a community and teaching hospital. Of the 48 patients who received intravenous vancomycin, only 19 (39.6%) were given initial doses that achieved the desired serum concentration. In this study, older patients were at higher risk for overdosing, whereas younger patients were more likely to be underdosed.

New antibiotic classes broadly active against Gram-positive bacteria, such as linezolid, may offer attractive alternative options for treating MRSA VAP. Linezolid, the first commercially available member of the oxazolidinone class, showed excellent lung penetration, with the epithelial lining fluid concentration exceeding that of blood [40]. Indeed, in their recent retrospective analysis of 2 double-blind studies of patients with MRSA pneumonia, Wunderink et al. [41] demonstrated that linezolid was associated with significantly better survival and clinical cure rate than vancomycin. However, linezolid and vancomycin showed similar cure rates in a randomized open-label trial of MRSA infections, 25% of which were pneumonia [42]. Therefore, additional trials are warranted before linezolid becomes the standard treatment for MRSA infections.

Finally, one of the major confounders in studying MRSA and MSSA pathogenicity might be higher rates of inappropriate empiric antimicrobial treatments prescribed to MRSA patients, which ranged from 8 to 55% in previous studies [9, 14, 16, 17, 43]. Pertinently, this factor was independently associated with hospital mortality in the largest investigation of S. aureus bacteremia [16]. Inappropriate empiric antimicrobial treatment was also found to be the most important independent determinant of hospital mortality among critically ill patients in a study on various infections, for which inappropriate antibiotics had been initially administered to 60% of the patients in the MRSA group vs. 9% of those in the MSSA group [44].

▌ Clinical Studies of Severe *S. aureus* Infections

S. aureus Bacteremia

Previous studies comparing outcomes in MSSA and MRSA bacteremia revealed some conflicting data. Most studies did not find a higher mortality rate among patients with bacteremia involving MRSA [14–20, 22, 23]. Other investigators found significantly higher fatality rates in patients with MRSA bacteremia [8–10, 12, 13]. Probably the most powerful study concerning clinical outcomes in patients with MSSA and MRSA bacteremia was performed by Soriano et al. [16]. These authors compared 225 episodes of MRSA bacteremia with 683 episodes of MSSA bacteremia. In this cohort study, patients with MRSA bacteremia were older and sicker and had, as a consequence, a higher intrinsic mortality rate. Methicillin resistance was associated with shock, a variable recognized to be an independent predictor of mortality. The authors also composed 163 matched pairs of patients with MSSA and MRSA bacteremia on the basis of preexisting comorbidities, prognosis of underlying disease, and length of hospitalization prior to the bacteremia. Despite this matching procedure, there were still more comorbidity factors and a higher rate of shock and related mortality in the MRSA group. In a logistic regression analysis, methicillin resistance was not independently associated with shock and mortality.

Recently Cosgrove et al. [13] performed a meta-analysis to summarize the impact of methicillin-resistance on mortality in *S. aureus* bacteremia. The analysis included 31 studies and a total of 3963 patients with *S. aureus* bacteremia: 2603 patients (65.7%) had MSSA bacteremia and 1360 patients (34.3%) had MRSA bacteremia. Twenty-four studies (77.4%) found no significant difference in the mortality rates for MRSA and MSSA bacteremia, 7 studies (22.6%) found significantly higher mortality rates associated with MRSA bacteremia, and no studies found significantly lower mortality rates associated with MRSA bacteremia. When the results were pooled with a random-effects model, a significant increase in mortality associated with MRSA bacteremia was found (OR, 1.93; 95% CI, 1.54–2.42). However, significant heterogeneity was detected among the study results, suggesting that the included studies were not estimating a single common effect of the impact of methicillin resistance on mortality. Additionally, the authors acknowledged that most of these studies did not include detailed information on the adequacy of the initial antibiotic therapy prescribed for MRSA bacteremia and, as already mentioned above, inadequate antimicrobial therapy for MRSA bacteremia was independently associated with hospital mortality in the largest investigation of *S. aureus* bacteremia [16].

S. aureus Surgical Site Infections

Surgical site infection complicates 2%–5% of all surgery in the United States, with *S. aureus* being the most common cause of the disease [2]. They result in a total of 300 000–500 000 infections each year [2] and are associated with increased morbidity rates, mortality rates, and costs (they are responsible for additional annual hospital charges of >$1.6 billion in the United States alone [45]). It also should be noted that poststernotomy mediastinitis carries the most dreadful prognosis of all surgical site infections. Few studies to date have evaluated the impact of methicillin resistance on the outcomes of surgical site infections. The authors of one study reported an increase in length of hospital stay but no increase in the mortality rate among surgical patients infected with MRSA compared with patients infected with MSSA [46]. Engemann et al. [12] also reported data from 286 patients with surgical site infections (mostly following cardiothoracic and orthopedic procedures). Patients infected with MRSA had a greater 90-day mortality rate (odds ratio, 3.4; 95% confidence interval, 1.5–7.2), greater duration of hospitalization after infection and increased hospital charges than did patients infected with MSSA. Unfortunately, this study did not control for the type of antimicrobial treatments used for both groups of patients.

Data on the impact of methicillin resistance on the outcome of poststernotomy mediastinitis are also very few. In the study by Engemann et al. [12], 68% of the patients who died with MRSA vs. 64% of the patients who died with MSSA (p = 0.80) surgical site infections had mediastinitis. However, Mekontso-Dessap et al. [7] demonstrated, on a limited number of patients (15 patients with mediastinitis due to MRSA and 26 patients with mediatinitis due to MSSA), an increased risk for mortality and treatment failure and longer duration of hospitalization for the MRSA group.

More recently, our group retrospectively analyzed 145 patients with MSSA and 73 patients with MRSA mediastinitis treated with closed drainage with Redon catheters [47]. Importantly, initial empiric antibiotic therapy was appropriate for every patient included in the study. Patients with MRSA mediastinitis were older, had higher disease-severity scores at ICU admission and had longer incubation times. Factors associated with ICU death identified by multivariate analysis were age ≥65 years, incubation time ≤15 days, bacteremia, higher APACHE II score and mechanical ventilation ≥2 days after surgical debridement, but not methicillin resistance. Kaplan-Meier estimates of the cumulative probabilities of ICU survival as a function of the numbers of days after mediastinal debridement did not differ significantly for the two groups (Fig. 1). Additionally, durations of mechanical ventilation and Redon drainage were similar for both groups (only the time to mediastinal effluent sterilization remained longer for MRSA patients). We concluded from

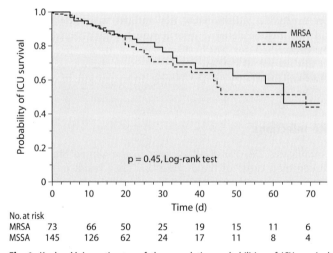

Fig. 1. Kaplan-Meier estimates of the cumulative probabilities of ICU survival for 73 MRSA and 165 MSSA mediastinitis patients for whom initial empiric therapy was always appropriate [47]

these data that methicillin resistance did not significantly affect ICU mortality of patients with poststernotomy mediastinitis benefiting from optimal treatments.

S. aureus Ventilator-associated Pneumonia

The outcomes of ventilator-associated *S. aureus* pneumonia have also rarely been addressed. According to an investigation of an outbreak of nosocomial pneumonia due to gentamicin–methicillin-resistant *S. aureus*, survival rates were comparable for the 17 MRSA- and the 12 MSSA-infected patients [48]. In contrast, Rello et al. [6], comparing 38 MSSA- and 11 MRSA-VAP episodes, demonstrated that unadjusted mortality attributed to pneumonia was 20 times higher for MRSA patients. More recently, Gonzalez et al. [43] studied 32 cases of MRSA and 54 cases of MSSA bacteremic VAP; again mortality did not differ significantly between groups. Notably, more than 25% of the patients in that study did not receive appropriate antibiotic treatment [43]; unfortunately, this information was not provided in the two other papers [6, 48].

To better estimate the true impact of methicillin resistance on mortality, our group recently reported on a large series of patients with *S. aureus* VAP, for whom the initial antibiotic therapy was always appropriate [49]. A retrospective cohort of 97 patients with MSSA and 74 patients with MRSA VAP was analyzed. As expected, patients with MRSA VAP were older, had higher disease-severity scores and had been on mechanical ventilation longer at VAP onset. Factors associated with 28-day death retained by multivariate logistic regression analysis were patient age and the number of organs failing at VAP diagnosis, but not methicillin resistance (Table 2). Additionally, the percentages of infection relapse or superinfection did not differ significantly between the two patient groups. We concluded from this study that after controlling for clinical and physiologic heterogeneity between groups, methicillin resistance did not significantly affect 28-day mortality of patients with *S. aureus* VAP receiving appropriate antibiotics.

Table 2. Factors associated with 28-day mortality according to multivariate logistic regression analysis on a cohort of 97 patients with MSSA and 74 patients with MRSA ventilator-associated pneumonia (VAP) [49]

Factor	Multivariate Analysis	
	OR (95% CI)	p Value
▌ Age	1.05 (1.02-1.08)	0.0009
▌ Day 1 ODIN score	1.90 (1.31-2.78)	0.0007
▌ Methicillin resistance	1.72 (0.73-4.05)	0.22*

OR: odds ratio; CI: confidence interval; Day 1: day on which bronchoscopy for VAP diagnosis was performed; ODIN = Organ Dysfunctions and/or Infection.

* Methicillin resistance was forced into the final multivariate model.

▌ Conclusion

Since methicillin resistance has become a worldwide concern, the debate whether MRSA infections are associated with higher mortality than MSSA infections has been ongoing. Because there is little evidence of MRSA strains being more virulent, differences in outcome may principally relate to patient characteristics before or at the time of infection onset and to the effect of antimicrobial treatment. Indeed, patients infected with MRSA tend to be older, sicker, and more debilitated. In contrast to patients with MSSA infections, they frequently have a history of prior antibiotic use and a longer time of hospitalization. These variables need to be carefully controlled when comparing outcomes of MSSA and MRSA infections. Additionally, high rates of inappropriate empiric antimicrobial treatment might be one of the most important independent determinants of outcome for MRSA-infected patients. In two large series of severe *S. aureus* infections (poststernotmy mediastinitis and VAP), we recently demonstrated that methicillin resistance does not significantly affect ICU mortality of patients receiving appropriate initial empiric antibiotic therapy. Identification of patients with risk factors favoring MRSA infection such as severe underlying condition, a history of multiple hospitalizations or prior antibiotic use should prompt the initiation of an empiric antibiotic regimen including vancomycin (or linezolid in selected cases), which can usually be deescalated 48 to 72 hours later when the results of microbiological sample cultures become available.

References

1. Jevons MP (1961) Celbin-resistant staphylococci. BMJ 1:124–125
2. National Nosocomial Infections Surveillance (NNIS) System Report (2003) Data summary from January 1992 through June 2003, issued August 2003. Am J Infect Control 31:481–498
3. Romero-Vivas J, Rubio M, Fernandez C, Picazo JJ (1995) Mortality associated with nosocomial bacteremia due to methicillin-resistant *Staphylococcus aureus*. Clin Infect Dis 21:1417–1423
4. Pujol M, Pena C, Pallares R, et al (1996) Nosocomial *Staphylococcus aureus* bacteremia among nasal carriers of methicillin-resistant and methicillin-susceptible strains. Am J Med 100:509–516
5. Steinberg JP, Clark CC, Hackman BO (1996) Nosocomial and community-acquired *Staphylococcus aureus* bacteremias from 1980 to 1993: impact of intravascular devices and methicillin resistance. Clin Infect Dis 23:255–259
6. Rello J, Torres A, Ricart M, et al (1994) Ventilator-associated pneumonia by *Staphylococcus aureus*. Comparison of methicillin-resistant and methicillin-sensitive episodes. Am J Respir Crit Care Med 150:1545–1549
7. Mekontso-Dessap A, Kirsch M, Brun-Buisson C, Loisance D (2001) Poststernotomy mediastinitis due to *Staphylococcus aureus*: comparison of methicillin-resistant and methicillin-susceptible cases. Clin Infect Dis 32:877–883
8. Blot SI, Vandewoude KH, Hoste EA, Colardyn FA (2002) Outcome and attributable mortality in critically ill patients with bacteremia involving methicillin-susceptible and methicillin-resistant *Staphylococcus aureus*. Arch Intern Med 162:2229–2235
9. Talon D, Woronoff-Lemsi MC, Limat S, et al (2002) The impact of resistance to methicillin in *Staphylococcus aureus* bacteremia on mortality. Eur J Intern Med 13:31–36
10. Conterno LO, Wey SB, Castelo A (1998) Risk factors for mortality in *Staphylococcus aureus* bacteremia. Infect Control Hosp Epidemiol 19:32–37
11. Ibelings MM, Bruining HA (1998) Methicillin-resistant *Staphylococcus aureus*: acquisition and risk of death in patients in the intensive care unit. Eur J Surg 164:411–418
12. Engemann JJ, Carmeli Y, Cosgrove SE, et al (2003) Adverse clinical and economic outcomes attributable to methicillin resistance among patients with *Staphylococcus aureus* surgical site infection. Clin Infect Dis 36:592–598

13. Cosgrove SE, Sakoulas G, Perencevich EN, Schwaber MJ, Karchmer AW, Carmeli Y (2003) Comparison of mortality associated with methicillin-resistant and methicillin-susceptible *Staphylococcus aureus* bacteremia: a meta-analysis. Clin Infect Dis 36:53–59

14. Harbarth S, Rutschmann O, Sudre P, Pittet D (1998) Impact of methicillin resistance on the outcome of patients with bacteremia caused by *Staphylococcus aureus*. Arch Intern Med 158:182–189

15. Tumbarello M, De Gaetano Donati K, Tacconelli E, et al (2002) Risk factors and predictors of mortality of methicillin-resistant *Staphylococcus aureus* (MRSA) bacteraemia in HIV-infected patients. J Antimicrob Chemother 50:375–382

16. Soriano A, Martinez JA, Mensa J, et al (2000) Pathogenic significance of methicillin resistance for patients with *Staphylococcus aureus* bacteremia. Clin Infect Dis 30:368–373

17. Roghmann MC (2000) Predicting methicillin resistance and the effect of inadequate empiric therapy on survival in patients with *Staphylococcus aureus* bacteremia. Arch Intern Med 160:1001–1004

18. Mylotte JM, Tayara A (2000) *Staphylococcus aureus* bacteremia: predictors of 30-day mortality in a large cohort. Clin Infect Dis 31:1170–1174

19. Hershow RC, Khayr WF, Smith NL (1992) A comparison of clinical virulence of nosocomially acquired methicillin-resistant and methicillin-sensitive *Staphylococcus aureus* infections in a university hospital. Infect Control Hosp Epidemiol 13:587–593

20. Mylotte JM, Aeschlimann JR, Rotella DL (1996) *Staphylococcus aureus* bacteremia: factors predicting hospital mortality. Infect Control Hosp Epidemiol 17:165–168

21. Marty L, Flahault A, Suarez B, Caillon J, Hill C, Andremont A (1993) Resistance to methicillin and virulence of *Staphylococcus aureus* strains in bacteriemic cancer patients. Intensive Care Med 19:285–289

22. French GL, Cheng AF, Ling JM, Mo P, Donnan S (1990) Hong Kong strains of methicillin-resistant and methicillin-sensitive *Staphylococcus aureus* have similar virulence. J Hosp Infect 15:117–125

23. Selvey LA, Whitby M, Johnson B (2000) Nosocomial methicillin-resistant *Staphylococcus aureus* bacteremia: is it any worse than nosocomial methicillin-sensitive *Staphylococcus aureus* bacteremia? Infect Control Hosp Epidemiol 21:645–648

24. Hewitt JH, Sanderson PJ (1974) The effect of methicillin on skin lesions in guinea-pigs caused by methicillin-sensitive and methicillin-resistant *Staphylococcus aureus*. J Med Microbiol 7:223–235

25. Peacock JE, Jr., Moorman DR, Wenzel RP, Mandell GL (1981) Methicillin-resistant Staphylococcus aureus: microbiologic characteristics, antimicrobial susceptibilities, and assessment of virulence of an epidemic strain. J Infect Dis 144:575–582

26. Aathithan S, Dybowski R, French GL (2001) Highly epidemic strains of methicillin-resistant Staphylococcus aureus not distinguished by capsule formation, protein A content or adherence to HEp-2 cells. Eur J Clin Microbiol Infect Dis 20:27–32

27. Schmitz FJ, MacKenzie CR, Geisel R, et al (1997) Enterotoxin and toxic shock syndrome toxin-1 production of methicillin resistant and methicillin sensitive *Staphylococcus aureus* strains. Eur J Epidemiol 13:699–708

28. Laurent F, Lelievre H, Cornu M, et al (2001) Fitness and competitive growth advantage of new gentamicin-susceptible MRSA clones spreading in French hospitals. J Antimicrob Chemother 47:277–283

29. Duckworth GJ, Jordens JZ (1990) Adherence and survival properties of an epidemic methicillin-resistant strain of Staphylococcus aureus compared with those of methicillin-sensitive strains. J Med Microbiol 32:195–200

30. Ellis MW, Hospenthal DR, Dooley DP, Gray PJ, Murray CK (2004) Natural history of community-acquired methicillin-resistant Staphylococcus aureus colonization and infection in soldiers. Clin Infect Dis 39:971–979

31. Okuma K, Iwakawa K, Turnidge JD, et al (2002) Dissemination of new methicillin-resistant Staphylococcus aureus clones in the community. J Clin Microbiol 40:4289–4294

32. Cosgrove SE, Carmeli Y (2003) The impact of antimicrobial resistance on health and economic outcomes. Clin Infect Dis 36:1433–1437

33. McCabe WR, Jackson GG (1962) Gram-negative bacteremia. Arch Intern Med 110:847–864

34. Charlson ME, Pompei P, Ales KL, MacKenzie CR (1987) A new method of classifying prognostic comorbidity in longitudinal studies: development and validation. J Chronic Dis 40: 373–383
35. Levine DP, Fromm BS, Reddy BR (1991) Slow response to vancomycin or vancomycin plus rifampin in methicillin-resistant *Staphylococcus aureus* endocarditis. Ann Intern Med 115: 674–680
36. Small PM, Chambers HF (1990) Vancomycin for *Staphylococcus aureus* endocarditis in intravenous drug users. Antimicrob Agents Chemother 34:1227–1231
37. Cruciani M, Gatti G, Lazzarini L, et al (1996) Penetration of vancomycin into human lung tissue. J Antimicrob Chemother 38:865–869
38. Lamer C, de Beco V, Soler P, et al (1993) Analysis of vancomycin entry into pulmonary lining fluid by bronchoalveolar lavage in critically ill patients. Antimicrob Agents Chemother 37:281–286
39. Rodman DP, McKnight JT, Rogers T, Robbins M (1994) The appropriateness of initial vancomycin dosing. J Fam Pract 38:473–477
40. Conte JE, Jr., Golden JA, Kipps J, Zurlinden E (2002) Intrapulmonary pharmacokinetics of linezolid. Antimicrob Agents Chemother 46:1475–1480
41. Wunderink RG, Rello J, Cammarata SK, Croos-Dabrera RV, Kollef MH (2003) Linezolid vs vancomycin: analysis of two double-blind studies of patients with methicillin-resistant *Staphylococcus aureus* nosocomial pneumonia. Chest 124:1789–1797
42. Stevens DL, Herr D, Lampiris H, Hunt JL, Batts DH, Hafkin B (2002) Linezolid versus vancomycin for the treatment of methicillin-resistant *Staphylococcus aureus* infections. Clin Infect Dis 34:1481–1490
43. Gonzalez C, Rubio M, Romero-Vivas J, Gonzalez M, Picazo JJ (1999) Bacteremic pneumonia due to *Staphylococcus aureus*: a comparison of disease caused by methicillin-resistant and methicillin-susceptible organisms. Clin Infect Dis 29:1171–1177
44. Kollef MH, Sherman G, Ward S, Fraser VJ (1999) Inadequate antimicrobial treatment of infections: a risk factor for hospital mortality among critically ill patients. Chest 115:462–474
45. Martone WJ, Nichols RL (2001) Recognition, prevention, surveillance, and management of surgical site infections: introduction to the problem and symposium overview. Clin Infect Dis 33 (Suppl 2):S67–68
46. Gleason TG, Crabtree TD, Pelletier SJ, et al (1999) Prediction of poorer prognosis by infection with antibiotic-resistant gram-positive cocci than by infection with antibiotic-sensitive strains. Arch Surg 134:1033–1040
47. Combes A, Trouillet JL, Joly-Guillou ML, Chastre J, Gibert C (2004) The impact of methicillin resistance on the outcome of poststernotomy mediastinitis due to Staphylococcus aureus. Clin Infect Dis 38:822–829
48. Lentino JR, Hennein H, Krause S, et al (1985) A comparison of pneumonia caused by gentamicin, methicillin-resistant and gentamicin, methicillin-sensitive *Staphylococcus aureus*: epidemiologic and clinical studies. Infect Control 6:267–272
49. Combes A, Luyt CE, Fagon JY, et al (2004) Impact of methicillin resistance on outcome of Staphylococcus aureus ventilator-associated pneumonia. Am J Respir Crit Care Med 170: 786–792

Clostridium difficile-associated Disease

S. Buyse, E. Azoulay, and B. Schlemmer

▌ Introduction

Since the first description of *Clostridium difficile* in 1935 by Hall and O'Toole [1], the incidence of infection with this organism has increased throughout the world in lockstep with the increasing use of broad-spectrum antibiotics. The clinical and financial burden of *C. difficile*-associated disease is of concern [2]. In this chapter, we will discuss the epidemiology, microbiology, clinical manifestations, and outcome of *C. difficile*-associated disease, with special attention to severe forms and to their management in the intensive care unit (ICU).

▌ Microbiology

C. difficile (Fig. 1) is a Gram-positive, spore-forming, anaerobic bacillus that is widely distributed in the environment. Toxinogenic *C. difficile* strains cause disease, whereas non-toxinogenic strains are harmless members of the commensal flora. Toxin production differs across strains and can be influenced by nutrient availability or other environmental factors [3]. The two toxins identified to date, toxin A (or enterotoxin) and toxin B (or cytotoxin), differ regarding their structure, receptor, and mechanism of pathogenic effects. Many *C. difficile* strains produce both toxins, and only 2% produce toxin B but not toxin A [4]. Both toxins are encoded by a pathogenicity locus. Transcription and translation products are huge single-chain peptides with molecular masses of 308 kDa for toxin A and 270 kDa for toxin B [4]. Each toxin has three functional domains. The toxins share 50% amino acid homology and exhibit similar primary structures. The main target of the pathogenic effects of toxins A and B is the colonocyte.

▌ Epidemiology

C. difficile has been recovered in fecal samples from 2 to 4% of healthy occidental adults and 15% of healthy Japanese adults [5]. The carriage rate in healthy adults ranges from 1 to 4% [6]. Most carriers have non-toxinogenic (i.e., non-pathogenic) strains. The rate of *C. difficile* acquisition varies across populations and according to antibiotic exposure. Moreover, 40 to 80% of children younger than 6 months are asymptomatic carriers [5]. Toxins are detectable in fecal samples from a small minority of these infants; the absence of pathogenic effects may be ascribable to inges-

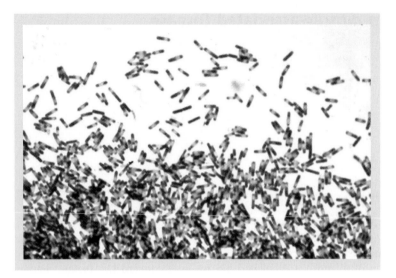

Fig. 1. *Clostridium difficile* (optic microscopy X 1000) (F. Barbut)

tion of IgG anti-toxin A contained in the colostrum or to absence of the toxin A receptor on the colonocyte border in newborns [7]. Although asymptomatic carriers may act as a potential transmission reservoir, they should not receive treatment, as Johnson et al. have shown delayed clearance of the organism after vancomycin administration to healthy carriers followed by an increased risk of recurrent carriage [8]. In hospital wards, environmental contamination with *C. difficile* spores has been demonstrated at 34 to 58% of tested sites, even after detergent-based cleaning [9]. *C. difficile*-associated disease is the most common gastrointestinal nosocomial infection in hospitalized patients older than 60 years of age [9–11]. The diagnosis rests on identification of toxin A and/or toxin B in the feces of a patient with acute diarrhea.

▌ Contamination and Transmission

C. difficile can be found in neonates, healthy adults, or patients with *C. difficile*-associated diarrhea. Transmission is thought to occur via the oro-fecal route [9] and may take place from patient to patient or from healthcare workers to patients. Strain-typing studies during hospital outbreaks suggested transmission via the hands of healthcare workers [9, 10]. Thus, the main reservoirs in hospitals are patients with *C. difficile*-associated disease and asymptomatic carriers of the organism. *C. difficile* can also be transmitted via the environment [10]; vegetative spores usually die after exposure to ambient air, but spores produced under optimal conditions may survive and remain toxinogenic for several months in air, serving as an effective means of dissemination. Patients with severe diarrhea heavily contaminate their immediate environment [11]. McFarland [10] found environmental contamination in 49% of rooms of patients with *C. difficile*-associated diarrhea as compared to only 29% of rooms of patients with asymptomatic *C. difficile* carriage.

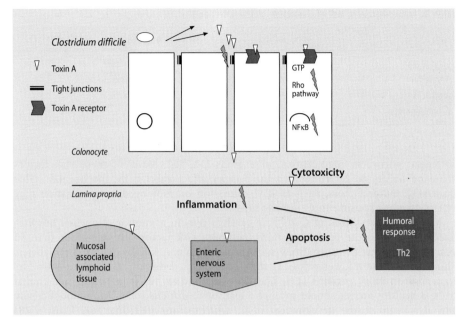

Fig. 2. Effects of toxinogenic *Clostridium difficile* on the intestinal epithelium

Furthermore, contamination was noted in 8% of rooms of patients without *C. difficile*, indicating that cleaning procedures between patients failed to consistently eliminate the organism [10].

▌ Risk Factors

To date, all antibiotics except intravenous aminoglycosides have been incriminated in the development of *C. difficile*-associated disease [9]. The risk varies across antibiotics, however, being highest with broad-spectrum agents such as penicillins (alone or combined with a β-lactamase inhibitor), cephalosporins, and clindamycin (Table 1). Broad-spectrum antibiotics cause major changes in the intestinal flora, particularly when given orally [9]. Thus, the relative risk of *C. difficile*-associated colitis has been estimated at 40 for cephalosporin and 70 for lincosamide [7]. Use of multiple antibiotics or prolonged treatment increases the risk [11]. Wistrom et al. reported that the risk of *C. difficile*-associated disease was significantly greater in patients given antibiotics for more than three consecutive days than in those treated for shorter periods [12]. *C. difficile*-associated disease can be induced by antibiotics to which the organism is susceptible *in vitro* (Table 1), perhaps in part because *C. difficile* overgrowth from persistent spores may occur at a faster rate than restoration of the normal colonic flora.

Other independent risk factors for *C. difficile*-associated disease identified by multivariate analyses of data from case-control studies include current hospitalization [13]; age older than 65 years with a severe underlying illness; non-surgical gastrointestinal procedures (e.g., insertion of a nasogastric tube); and use of stool

Table 1. Antibiotic-related risk of *Clostridium difficile* infection [13]

High risk	Medium risk	Low risk
Clindamycin	Fluoroquinolones	Metronidazole
Ampicillin	Co-trimoxazole	Vancomycin
Amoxicillin	Macrolides	Rifampin
Cephalosporins	Tetracyclines	

softeners, anti-ulcer medications, or enemas [14, 15]. Many of these risk factors share an ability to interfere with the barrier effect exerted by the normal stable flora [11]. Other factors, such as ICU admission or prolonged hospitalization may reflect greater exposure to *C. difficile* [13].

More than two-thirds of *C. difficile* carriers remain asymptomatic when hospitalized [16, 17]; in the remaining third, common risk factors are age older than 60 years and serious co-morbidities such as heart failure, kidney failure, or diabetes. Shim et al. found a lower risk of *C. difficile*-associated disease in asymptomatic carriers than in naive patients [13]. Therefore, acute diarrhea in a patient not known to be a healthy carrier should prompt a test for *C. difficile* toxin. Immunodeficiency can also promote the development of *C. difficile*-associated diarrhea. Thus, a 48-fold increase in the risk of acute *C. difficile*-associated diarrhea was found in patients with low serum IgGs against toxin A [18]. Similarly, the risk of relapse was greater in patients with low serum levels of IgG and IgM antibodies to toxin A. Finally, fecal stasis, enteral nutrition via a nasogastric tube, and anti-acid treatment were associated with an increased risk of *C. difficile*-associated disease. These data suggest that the best preventive strategy may be preservation of normal gut flora, gut motility, and gastric secretion.

ICU patients are often exposed to multiple risk factors for *C. difficile*-associated disease, including broad-spectrum antibiotics, enteral nutrition via a nasogastric tube, and immunodepression. The relative risk of *C. difficile*-associated disease in ICU patients has not yet been determined. Nevertheless, available data point to a major role for this organism in acute diarrhea developing in the ICU.

Pathophysiology

C. difficile-associated diarrhea typically develops when the normal colonic flora is disrupted by antimicrobial therapy, as this impairs resistance to colonization by *C. difficile*. Thus, if *C. difficile* is present in the lumen, it can proliferate and produce toxin A or B, or both. Toxins A and B are the most extensively studied determinants of *C. difficile* virulence. They cause cell death by disrupting the actin cytoskeleton, inducing the production of inflammatory mediators, and disrupting the epithelial tight junction proteins [7, 9]. The *C. difficile* receptor for toxin A is a glycopeptide that has not been identified in human neonates [19]. Most of the toxinogenic strains produce both toxin A and toxin B. Their mechanisms of action are similar: they undergo endocytosis by the cell, alter the actin cytoskeleton, and result in cell death [20, 21] (Fig. 1). They also induce the production of tumor necrosis factor (TNF)-α and pro-inflammatory interleukins (IL), which contribute to the associated inflammatory response and pseudomembrane formation [22]. Toxin A causes necrosis, increased intestinal permeability, and inhibition of protein synthesis. Toxin A also affects phospholipase A2 and therefore prostaglandin and leukotriene production [23]. It damages the villus tips and brush border membranes, an effect that can lead to complete erosion of the mucosa. Viscous, bloody fluid is produced in response to the tissue damage [24]. Toxins A and B have synergistic effects. The prosecretory effect of toxin A is due to increased intestinal secretion of chloride [20]. Both toxins inactivate low-molecular-weight proteins of the Rho family via glycosylation. GTPase inactivation is a key mechanism of cytotoxicity that involves changes in intracellular signaling. *In vivo*, toxin A exerts indirect toxic effects by inducing the secretion of eicosanoids [25]. Production of chemokines, most notably IL-8, induces an influx of inflammatory cells [26]. Pseudomembranous colitis can be induced by either toxin, but toxin B is 1000 times more cytotoxic than toxin A [7, 9]. The enteric nervous system may play a role in the response to toxin A [16]; according to this hypothesis, the pathogenic effect is related to transepithelial signals sent toward neuro-immune cells when toxin A binds to the mucosal border. Non-toxinogenic strains seem devoid of pathogenic effects. However, variations in virulence have been demonstrated across toxinogenic strains and serotypes [7]. Virulent strains with a toxin A-negative/toxin B-positive phenotype have been identified, indicating that toxin A is not indispensable to the pathogenic effect.

▌ Clinical Presentation

C. difficile has been isolated from stool cultures in over 95% of patients with pseudomembranous colitis and in 15–25% of those with antibiotic-associated diarrhea. Clinical presentations of *C. difficile* infection range from mild diarrhea to life-threatening pseudomembranous colitis with megacolon and possible perforation [27, 28]. Depending on the severity of the colitis, manifestations may include abdominal pain with or without a fever, electrolyte disturbances, hypoalbuminemia, and paralytic ileus. When pancolitis develops, there is a risk of toxic megacolon, perforation and secondary endotoxin shock [7, 25]. Diarrhea typically starts within a few days of antibiotic therapy initiation; *C. difficile* infection is rare in patients who have never received antibiotics. The feces usually have a characteristic foul odor; in the absence of pseudomembranous colitis, they are bloody in less than 5% of cases.

More than 90% of *C. difficile* infections occur after or during antibiotic treatment. Antibiotics disrupt the normal colonic flora, allowing *C. difficile* from endogenous or exogenous sources to proliferate in the colon. If the strain is toxinogenic, toxins A and B are usually produced simultaneously, causing fluid secretion, inflammation, and mucosal damage. Symptoms range from mild diarrhea to severe pseudomembranous colitis. The reasons for this variability in clinical expression remain unclear but probably involve both host-related factors and virulence factors such as adhesion or secretion of hydrolytic enzymes [25, 29].

Pseudomembranous colitis can occur without diarrhea, and fulminant forms requiring emergency surgery have been reported [25, 29, 30]. Most patients with pseudomembranous colitis have high-grade fever, tachycardia, severe abdominal pain, and organ failure. Ascitis and intraperitoneal extravasation may be present. Colonoscopy should be performed with caution; this investigation is contraindicated in patients with evidence of perforation. Typical pseudomembranes may be visible in the rectum or colon. However, absence of visible membranes does not rule out the diagnosis, as the sensitivity of endoscopy is poor. Although histology can be helpful [31], endoscopy is not imperative for the diagnosis of *C. difficile* infection [32]. Rather, patients with suspected *C. difficile*-associated disease should undergo stool tests for *C. difficile*.

Pseudomembranous colitis is an uncommon presentation of *C. difficile* infection [33]. Severe disease is rare and systemic manifestations extremely unusual. However, pancreatic, splenic, or intraperitoneal abscesses have been reported [34]. Moreover, a few cases of reactive oligoarthritis within 2 weeks after *C. difficile* infection have been described [35].

Although antimicrobial treatment is usually effective, relapses have occurred in 10% of patients after standard treatment [33]. Among patients with relapsing disease, 40% experience more than one relapse [9, 36]. The only known factor predicting repeated relapses after conventional treatment is the number of previous episodes of *C. difficile*-associated disease [36, 37].

▌ Laboratory Diagnosis

C. difficile is now recognized as the major infectious cause of hospital-acquired diarrhea in industrialized countries. This fact has led a number of hospital microbiology laboratories to look for *C. difficile* (but not other enteropathogens such as *Salmonella* or *Shigella*) in all fecal samples from patients hospitalized for longer than 3 days.

Antibiotics can cause diarrhea by mechanisms independent from *C. difficile*, and many other conditions or drugs are associated with diarrhea. Therefore, microbiological tests are required for the diagnosis of *C. difficile* infection. There are two main techniques, namely, culturing and toxin assays [30]. Culturing requires up to 5 days and fails to distinguish *C. difficile*-associated disease from presence of nontoxinogenic strains or asymptomatic carriage of toxinogenic strains. Few laboratories still perform routine stool cultures for *C. difficile*. However, culturing must be performed when typing is needed to collect epidemiological data on strains in a ward or hospital. *C. difficile* colonies are easily recognized based on their typical morphology when observed under a binocular microscope. The characteristic horse manure odor also assists in identifying the organism.

Assays for one or both *C. difficile* toxins are the laboratory techniques of choice for diagnosing *C. difficile*-associated disease [10]. Although toxin assays are advocated by many authors as the routine diagnostic test of choice, culturing should be performed also to obtain optimal results. Toxin detection is best achieved by the cytotoxin cell-culture assay with confirmation by anti-toxin neutralization. Only liquid stools should be accepted, except in epidemiological investigations. Because cytotoxic activity is lost rapidly, only fresh specimens should be processed; if tests cannot be performed rapidly, specimens should be kept at a temperature no greater than 4 °C. A filtrate of a feces suspension is injected into a cell culture. Presence of toxin results in disruption of the cell cytoskeleton, which manifests as cell rounding in many cell lines. The effect is due mainly to toxin B, which is 1000 times more cytotoxic than toxin A [23]. Most of the cell lines commonly used in clinical microbiology laboratories can serve for fecal cytotoxin detection, including Vero, Hep2,

Table 2. Proposed scheme for the bacteriological diagnosis of *C. difficile*-associated disease (CDAD)

Culture	Fecal Toxin	Conclusion
+	+	CDAD
–	+	Probable CDAD
+	–	Carriage of a non toxinogenic strain or CDAD (damaged toxin)
–	–	No CDAD

fibroblasts, CHO, and HeLa cells. Immunoassay kits (primarily ELISAs) for toxin detection are widely available and simple to use but lack sensitivity [23].

Molecular methods for diagnosing *C. difficile*-associated disease have not been as extensively studied as those for other infectious diseases. This is probably due to the relatively satisfactory results obtained with conventional methods, as described above, and to the well-known interferences between fecal specimens and amplification procedures. Several polymerase chain reaction techniques for amplifying part of the toxin A gene have been tested. However, these expensive approaches seem to have few advantages over the conventional laboratory testing [26].

An algorithm for the routine laboratory diagnosis of *C. difficile*-associated disease can be suggested. Culturing and toxin detection should be performed on all fecal specimens (Table 2). When both tests are negative, *C. difficile*-associated disease is ruled out. A positive finding from both tests indicates *C. difficile*-associated disease requiring treatment and infection-control measures. When the culture is positive but the toxin test is negative, a direct immunoenzymetric assay should be done on several colonies picked directly from the culture plate; this toxin test requires only 30 minutes. If the result is negative, treatment for *C. difficile*-associated disease is not required. If it is positive, *C. difficile*-associated disease is very likely and both antibiotics and infection-control measures are in order. In the tiny minority of patients who have a negative culture but a positive cytotoxin test, a second specimen is usually obtained for a repeat culture with a CCFA including taurocholate medium; the result is usually positive, indicating a need for treatment.

▌ Treatment

The treatment of *C. difficile* infection has changed little in recent years, and there are few proven therapeutic options. If at all possible, the precipitating antibiotics should be stopped [33]. Specific antibiotic therapy is indicated in patients with systemic illness and evidence of colonic inflammation, pseudomembranous colitis, or persistent symptoms despite discontinuation of the precipitating antibiotics. In practice, most patients are started on either vancomycin or metronidazole when the infection is diagnosed and before the precipitating antibiotics are stopped; the latter can be replaced by lower risk agents (Table 1), although this approach is of unproven benefit and is often impossible in critically ill patients. Anti-diarrheal agents should be avoided because they reduce the clearance of pathogenic organisms [38].

The first-line treatment of *C. difficile* infection relies on oral metronidazole for 10 days (400 or 500 mg tid), except in pregnant or breast-feeding women. Alternatively, vancomycin (125 mg qds) can be given for 7–10 days. No statistically significant differences in overall response rates or recurrence rates have been found between these two antibiotics [7, 37]. Mean symptom duration was shorter with vancomycin than with metronidazole. However, vancomycin is far more expensive, and most hospitals now use metronidazole as their first-line agent to reduce selection of glycopeptide-resistant enterococci, which is increased by widespread use of vancomycin [37]. Either antibiotic can be administered via the nasogastric route if it cannot be tolerated orally [7]. The two antibiotics should be given in combination when intravenous administration is required, as the colonic concentration of each agent is unpredictable with this route.

Symptomatic recurrences following treatment of *C. difficile* infection are common and their management is challenging. The first step consists in determining whether the second episode is a relapse (re-emergence of the same strain) or a recurrence (re-infection with a different strain). The common practice of switching from metronidazole to vancomycin or *vice versa* in patients with symptomatic recurrences is illogical, and there is little justification for using experimental treatments in this situation. In practice, the first recurrence should be treated with oral metronidazole, and a relapse should lead to substitution of metronidazole for vancomycin. About one fourth of symptom-free patients continue to excrete *C. difficile* in their faeces, and consequently stool cultures should not be performed after treatment in symptom-free patients. Effective infection-control measures should be implemented, including use of gloves by healthcare workers and surface decontamination with hypochlorite solutions. Relapses should prompt investigations for other conditions, such as ischemic colitis or inflammatory colitis related to *C. difficile* infection. In patients with severe presentations, such as toxic megacolon, vancomycin should be given in a dosage of 500 mg qds through a nasogastric tube to ensure that luminal vancomycin levels are optimal [37].

▌ Alternative Treatments

There has been increasing interest in biological and immunological approaches to the treatment of *C. difficile*-associated disease. Biotherapy seeks to restore the commensal gut flora. Probiotics are live microorganisms that can prevent or treat diseases when taken orally. The yeast *Saccharomyces boulardii*, in particular, has been extensively studied and is commercially available as a freeze-dried preparation. Several placebo-controlled, double-blind trials have evaluated the ability of *S. boulardii* to prevent or treat antibiotic-associated diarrhoea via production of a protease that degrades toxins A and B [39, 40]. Concern has been voiced that administering live microorganisms may carry risks, particularly in frail elderly patients with inflammation of the gut mucosa. Cases of fungemia have been reported in immunocompromised patients following administration of *S. boulardii*, and fungemia has also occurred in an immunocompetent patient given a commercial preparation of *S. boulardii*, demonstrating the potential virulence of this yeast in humans [40]. To date, there is no proof that *S. boulardii* is beneficial in patients with *C. difficile*-associated diarrhea. *S. boulardii* administration is recommended to prevent antibiotic-associated diarrhea and may be useful in patients with recurrent *C. difficile* infections [40]. However, *S. boulardii* is not an appropriate treatment in patients with typical *C. difficile*-associated disease.

In several small series of patients, biological agents have been used to treat or to prevent antibiotic-associated diarrhea including *Lactobacillus acidophilus* [41]. *Lactobacillus GG* therapy has produced conflicting results in patients with acute diarrhea [41, 42] and has not been shown to be capable of restoring the normal gut flora.

Rectal biotherapy and rectal infusion of feces have been suggested as a means of circumventing the gastric-acid mediated degradation of antibiotics used to treat recurrent *C. difficile*-associated disease [43–45]. *In vitro* studies suggest that rectal infusion of feces from healthy individuals may stop the proliferation of toxinogenic *C. difficile* strains [5].

There is also continued interest in the potential role of vaccines and immunotherapy in the treatment of *C. difficile* infection. There have been several reports of patients with *C. difficile*-associated disease refractory to standard antimicrobial therapy who responded to intravenous immunoglobulins. Bovine colostrum contains high levels of IgG immunoglobulins, and a marked increase in specific IgGs can occur following immunization with *C. difficile* toxoids. Bovine immunoglobulin concentrate has been reported to inhibit the cytotoxic and enterotoxic effects of *C. difficile* toxin [46, 47]. However, concern about bovine spongiform encephalopathy is a major obstacle to the use of such preparations in humans. Vaccines for preventing *C. difficile* infection in the elderly are under study and may radically change current treatment strategies.

Some authors recommend sequential antimicrobial treatment in refractory forms of *C. difficile*-associated disease. Tedesco et al. designed the "pulse scheme" [48], which consists of standard metronidazole therapy for 10 days followed by a therapeutic window allowing proliferation of vegetative strains then by another 10-day metronidazole pulse. Only 3% of *C. difficile* strains have an intermediate response to metronidazole therapy [49]. A group working in Spain recently identified a *C. difficile* strain with intermediate susceptibility to vancomycin [50].

▌ Prognosis

The epidemiology of community-acquired *C. difficile*-associated disease has been described, although not extensively studied, and suggests that the incidence and morbidity of *C. difficile*-associated disease may be far less in the community than in hospitals [51]. Mortality also seems lower with the community-acquired variant, although this may reflect selection bias, as patients with severe community-acquired disease may be admitted and therefore possibly included among hospital-acquired cases [51]. Age older than 70 years, co-morbidities, and recurrent *C. difficile*-associated diarrhea are significant risk factors for severe disease and adverse outcomes in patients admitted for *C. difficile*-associated disease [51]. Patients with significant co-morbidities or advanced age may be unable to mount an effective response to *C. difficile* infection. A high index of suspicion should be maintained in patients with these risk factors to ensure that effective treatment is given early [51, 52]. Little is known about predictors of adverse outcomes in patients with fulminant *C. difficile*-associated disease managed in the ICU, but co-morbidity is well known to indicate a poor prognosis [52–54].

Mortality associated with *C. difficile* infections was estimated by Olson et al. in a retrospective study of 908 patients with *C. difficile* infections [55]: six patients died with active pseudomembranous colitis as the main cause of death. In another study, mortality ranged from 35 to 50% in patients requiring colectomy for toxic mega-colon or colonic perforation [52].

▌ Prevention

The key to controlling *C. difficile*-associated disease is the exercise of good judg-ment when using antimicrobial agents [34]. Although awareness of *C. difficile* infec-tion and its link with antibiotic use seems high, continuous feedback to prescribing physicians may be needed to prevent a further increase in the incidence of this dis-ease. Also, patient-to-patient transmission occurs readily, and spores play a major role in cross-infection because they can survive several months in the environment. Hygienic measures such as regular hand washing with sporicidal iodine-based hand-rub solutions (e.g., povidone) are essential to the prevention of *C. difficile* dissemination in hospitals [16, 56]. It is important to note that hydro-alcoholic products usually fail to destroy *C. difficile* spores since they have no sporicidal or detergent properties [56]. Inappropriate use of environmental cleaning agents may promote spore persistence, thereby increasing the risk of infection. Isolation is also essential to prevent environmental contamination, which is an important factor in the spread of *C. difficile* [56]. As soon as *C. difficile* is suspected or identified, full enteric precautions must be implemented and maintained until at least 48 h after the diarrhea resolves. Therefore, patients should be isolated and cohort-nursed for as long as they are contaminated. Disinfection of surfaces in the patient's environ-ment with products containing hypochlorite or aldehyde has been found highly effective in reducing environmental contamination and should be performed daily [10]. Control measures include stringent antibiotic policies; a high index of suspi-cion for *C. difficile* infection; prompt diagnosis, isolation, and treatment of infected patients; and implementation of enteric precautions. Surveillance should be insti-tuted to ensure early detection of outbreaks.

▌ Conclusion

C. difficile is an anaerobic, Gram-positive, spore-forming bacillus that can produce two toxins responsible for pseudomembranous colitis and post-antibiotic diarrhea. Non-toxinogenic strains are not pathogenic. Diarrhea and colonic lesions are caused by toxins A and/or B, whose detection in fecal samples is essential to the di-agnosis. Complications of *C. difficile*-associated disease can be serious. Therefore, detection tests for toxins A and B should be done at the slightest doubt in hospita-lized patients with acute diarrhea after antibiotic therapy. Current treatments for *C. difficile* infection rely on oral metronidazole and other antibiotics. Effective control of *C. difficile* in the hospital requires both restricted use of antibiotics and preven-tion of environmental seeding and bacterial spread. *C. difficile* strains are widely distributed in the hospital, both as a cause and as a result of nosocomial diarrhea. The clinical and financial burden of *C. difficile*-associated disease warrants cam-paigns to promote preventive efforts and research into new treatment options in-cluding immunotherapy and toxin-binding agents.

References

1. Hall JC, O'Toole E (1935) Intestinal flora in new-born infants with a description of a new pathogenic anaerobe, Bacillus difficilis. Am J Dis Child 49:390–402
2. Wilcox MH, Cunniffe JG, Trundle C, Redpath C (1996) Financial burden of hospital acquired Clostridium difficile infection. J Hosp Infect 34:23–30
3. Ward PB, Young GP (1997) Dynamics of Clostridium difficile infection. Control using diet. Adv Exp Med Biol 412:63–75
4. Kato H, Kato N, Watanabe K, et al (1998) Identification of toxin A-negative, toxin B-positive Clostridium difficile by PCR. J Clin Microbiol 36:2178–2182
5. Rolfe RD (1988) Asymptomatic intestinal colonization by Clostridium difficile. In: Rolfe RD, Finegold SM (eds) Clostridium Difficile. Its Role in Intestinal Disease. Academic Press Inc, London, pp 201–225
6. Wongwanish S, Pongpech P, Dhiraoutra C, et al (2001) Characteristics of Clostridium difficile strains isolated from asymptomatic individuals and from diarrheal patients. Clin Microbiol Infect 7:438–441
7. Marteau P, Sobhani I, Beretta O, et al (1991) Physiopathologie des infections intestinales dues á Clostridium difficile. Rôle de l'écosystème colique. Gastroenterol Clin Biol 15:322–329
8. Johnson S, Hofmann SR, Bettin KM (1992) Treatment of asymptomatic C. Difficile carriers with vancomycine or metronidazole. Ann Intern Med 117:297–302
9. Barlett JG (1998) Pseudomembranous enterocolitis and antibiotic-associated colitis. In: Sleisenger MH, Fordtran JS (eds) Gastrointestinal Disease, 6th edition. Saunders, Philadelphia, pp 1633–1647
10. McFarland LV (1991) The epidemiology of Clostridium difficile infections. Gastroenterol Int 4:82–85
11. Bignardi GE (1998) Risk factors for Clostridium difficile infection. J Hosp Infect 40:1–15
12. Wistrom J, Norrby SR, Myhre EB, et al (2001) Frequency of antibiotic associated diarrhea in 2462 antibiotic-treated hospitalized patients: a prospective study. J Antimicrob Chemother 47:43–50
13. Shim JK, Johnson S, Samore MH, et al (1998) Primary symptomless colonisation by Clostridium difficile and decreased risk of subsequent diarrhea. Lancet 351:633–636
14. Bliss DZ, Johnson S, Savik K, Clabots CR, Willard K, Gerding DN (1998) Acquisition of Clostridium difficile and Clostridum difficile associated diarrhea in hospitalized patients receiving tube feeding. Ann Intern Med 129:1012–1019
15. Cunningham R, Dale B, Undy B, Gaunt N (2003) Proton pump inhibitors as a risk factor for Clostridium difficile. J Hosp Infect 54:243–245
16. McFarland LV, Mulligan ME, Kwok RYY, et al (1989) Nosocomial acquisition of Clostridium difficile infection. N Engl J Med 320:204–210
17. Mc Farland LV, Surawicz CM, Greenberg RN, et al (1994) A randomized placebo-controlled trial of Saccharomyces boulaardii in combination with standard antibiotics for Clostridium difficile. JAMA 271:1913–1918
18. Kyne L, Warny M, Qamar A, Kelly CP (2000) Asymptomatic carriage of Clostridium difficile and serum levels of Ig G antibody against toxin A. N Engl J Med 342:390–397
19. Krivan HC, Clark GF, Smith DF (1986) Cell surface binding site for Clostridium difficile enterotoxin: evidence for a glycoconjugate containing the sequence Gal3 Gal1-4GlcNac. Infect Immun 53:573–581
20. Moore R, Pothoulakis C, LaMont JT (1990) Clostridium difficile toxin A increases intestinal permeability and induces Cl-secretion. Am J Physiol 259:G165–172
21. Hecht G, Pothoulakis C, LaMont JT, Madara JL (1988) Clostridium difficile toxin A perturbs cytoskeletal structure and tight junction permeability of cultured human intestinal epithelial monolayers. J Clin Invest 82:1516–1524
22. Just I (1998) Clostridium difficile. In: Rampal P, Boquet P (eds) Recent Advances In the Pathogenesis of Gastrointestinal Bacterial Infections. John Libbey Eurotext, Paris, pp 135–142

23. Chaves-Olarte E, Weidmann M, von Eichel-Streiber C, et al (1997) Toxins A and B from Clostridium difficile differ with respect to enzymatic potencies, cellular substrate specificities and surface binding to cultured cells. J Clin Invest 100:1734–1741

24. Souza MLHP, Melo-Filho AA, Rocha MFG, et al (1997) The involvment of macrophage-derived tumor-necrosis factor and lipooxygenase products on the neutrophil recruitment induced by Clostridium difficile toxin B. Immunology 91:281–288

25. Just I, Wilm M, Selzer J, et al (1995) The enterotoxin from Clostridium difficile monoglycosylates the Rho proteins. J Biol Chem 270:13932–13936

26. Branka JE, Vallette G, Jarry A, et al (1997) Early functional effects of Clostridium difficile toxin A on human colonocytes. Gastroenterology 112:1887–1894

27. Marteau P (1996) Clostridium difficile: clinical spectrum with emphasis on atypical clinical presentations. In: Rambaud JC, LaMont JT (eds) Updates on Clostridium difficile. Springer, Paris, pp 6–14

28. Mogg GAG, Keighley MRB, Burdon DW, et al (1979) Antibiotic-associated colitis. A review of 66 cases. Br J Surg 66:738–742

29. Triadafilopoulos G, Hallstone AE (1991) Acute abdomen as the first presentation of pseudomembranous colitis. Gastroenterology 101:685–691

30. Barbut F, Corthier G, Charpak Y, et al (1996) Prevalence and pathogenicity of Clostridium difficile in hospitalized patients. Arch Intern Med 156:1449–1454

31. Lavergne A, Galian A (1990) Clostridium difficile et anatomie pathologique. In: Rambaud JC, Ducluzeau R (eds) Clostridium Difficile et Pathologie Intestinale. Springer, Paris

32. Tedesco FJ (1979) Antibiotic-associated pseudomembranous colitis with negative proctosigmoioscopic examination. Gastroenterology 77:225–227

33. Talbot RW, Walker RC, Beart RW (1986) Changing epidemiology, diagnosis, and treatment of Clostridium difficile toxin associated colitis. Br J Surg 73:457–460

34. Wolf LE, Gorbach SL, Granowitz EV, et al (1998) Extraintestinal Clostridium difficile 10 years experience at a tertiary care hospital. Mayo Clin Proc 73:934–937

35. Putterman C, Rubinow A (1993) Reactive arthritis associated with Clostridium difficile pseudomembranous colitis. Semin Arthr Rheum 22:420–426

36. Fekety R, Mc Farland LV, Surawicz CM, et al (1997) Recurrent Clostridium difficile diarrhea: characteristics of and risk factors for patients enrolled in a prospective, randomized, double-blinded trial. Clin Infect Dis 24:324–333

37. Wenisch C, Parschalk B, Hasenhundl M, Hirsch AM, Graninger W (1996) Comparison of vancomycin, teicoplanin, metronidazole, and fusidic acid for the treatment of Clostridium difficile-associated diarrhea. Clin Infect Dis 22:813–818

38. Church JM, Fazio VW (1986) A role for colonic stasis in the pathogenesis of disease related to Clostridium difficile. Dis Colon Rectum 29:804–809

39. Castagliuolo I, Riegler MF, Valenick K, et al (1999) Saccharomyces boulardii protease inhibits the effects of Clostridium difficile toxins A and B in human colonic mucosa. Infect Immun 67:302–307

40. Pothoulakis C, Kelly CP, Joshi MA, et al (1993) Saccharomyces boulardii inhibits Clostridium difficile toxin A binding and enterotoxicity in rat ileum. Gastroenterology 104:1108–1115

41. Biller JA, Katz AJ, Flores AF, et al (1995) Treatment of recurrent Clostridium difficile colitis by Lactobacillus GG. J Pediatr Gastroenterol Nutr 21:224–226

42. Beck C, Necheles H (1961) Beneficial effects of the administration of Lactobacillus acidophilus in diarrheal and other intestinal disorders. Am J Gastroenterol 35:522–530

43. Elmer GW, Surawicz CM, McFarland LV (1996) Biotherapeutic agents. A neglected modality for the treatment and prevention of selected intestinal and vaginal infections. JAMA 275:870–876

44. Borriello SP (1990) The influence of the normal gut flora on Clostridium difficile colonisation of the gut. Ann Med 22:61–67

45. Boriello S, Barclay FE (1986) An in vitro model of colonisation resistance to Clostridium difficile infection. J Med Microbiol 21:299–309

46. Sakedo J, Kaeres S, Pothoulaks C (1997) Intravenous immunoglobulin therapy for severe Clostridium difficile colitis. Gut 41:366–370

47. Beales P (2002) Intra-venous immunoglobulin for recurrent Clostridium difficile diarrhea. Gut 51:455–458
48. Tedesco FJ, Gordon D, Fortson WC (1985) Approach to patients with multiple relapse of antibiotic associated pseudomembranous colitis. Am J Gastroenterol 80:867–868
49. Barbut F, Decre F, Burghoffer B, et al (1999) Antimicrobial susceptibilities and serogroups of clinical strains of Clostridium difficile isolated in France in 1991 and 1997. Antimicrob Agents Chemother 43:2607–2611
50. Pelaez T, Alcala L, Alonso R, et al (2002) Reassessment of Clostridium difficile susceptibility to metronidazole and vancomycin. Antimicrob Agents Chemother 46:1647–1650
51. Andrews C (2003) Clostridium difficile-associated diarrhea: Predictors of severity in patients presenting to the emergency departement. Can J Gastroenterol 17:369–373
52. Marts BC, Longo WE, Vernava AM 3rd, Kennedy DJ, Daniel GL, Jones I (1994) Patterns and prognosis of Clostridium difficile colitis. Dis Col Rectum 16:837–845
53. Siemann M, Koch-Dorfler M, Rabenhorst G (2000) Clostridium difficile-associated disease. The clinical course of 18 fatal cases. Intensive Care Med 26:416–421
54. Miller MA (2002) Morbidity, mortality, and healthcare burden of nosocomial Clostridium difficile-associated diarrhea in Canadian hospitals. Infect Control Epidemiol 23:137–140
55. Olson MM, Shanholtzer CJ, Lee JT Jr, Gerding DN (1994) Ten years of prospective Clostridium difficile-associated disease surveillance and treatment at the Minneapolis VA Medical Center, 1982–1991. Infect Control Hosp Epidemiol 15:371–381
56. Wilcox MH, Fawley WN (2000) Hospital disinfectants and spore formation by Clostridium difficile. Lancet 356:1324–1325

Sepsis and MOF: Basic Mechanisms

The TREMS: A Multifaceted Family of Immunoreceptors

S. Gibot and B. Levy

▌ Introduction

Stimulatory immunoreceptors have a central role in allowing the recognition of foreign antigens or pathogens by the immune system [1]. Typical examples of immunoreceptors are the B cell receptor and the T cell receptor, structures used by B and T cells to discriminate between self and non-self. Stimulatory immunoreceptors are composed of ligand-binding sites and associated transmembrane adaptor proteins. The cytoplasmic domain of adaptor proteins contains an immunoreceptor tyrosine-based activation motif (ITAM) with the consensus sequence $YxxL/Ix_{6-8}YxxL/I$ (x representing any amino acid). Among these ITAM-containing adaptor proteins are CD3ζ, FcRγ and DAP12 (DNA activating protein 12, also called KARAP) [1]. Several immunoglobulin (Ig)-like activating receptors have been character-

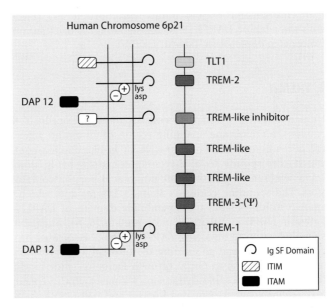

Fig. 1. The *trem* cluster on human chromosome 6. On the left, TREMs are characterized with their adaptor proteins: DAP12 for TREM-1 and -2; unknown adaptors for the other TREMs. Human TREM-3 is a pseudogene. On the right, the *trem* cluster on human chromosome 6 (murine counterpart on chromosome 17). *TREM* genes are closely linked to the MHC II region on the same chromosome

Table 1. Summary of the human TREMs

TREMs	Expression pattern	Regulation	Function
▌ TREM-1	Neutrophils Monocytes CD14^{high} Macrophages	Bacterial and fungal products	Amplification of inflammatory responses
▌ TREM-1sv	Monocytes Lung and liver macrophages	Cell wall fraction of *Mycobacterium bovis* BCG	Unknown
▌ TLT-1	Platelets Megakaryocytes	Platelet activation	Granule constriction and dispersal
▌ TREM-2	Immature dendritic cells Microglia osteoclasts	GM-CSF IL-4	Maturation of dendritic cells, microglia, oligodendrocytes and osteoclasts

IL: interleukin; GM-CSF: granulocyte/macrophage-colony stimulating factor

ized including paired Ig receptors [2], NKp44 [3], and the SHPS-1 family [4]. Recently, a new family of receptors expressed on myeloid cells, distantly related to NKp44, has been described: the Triggering Receptor Expressed on Myeloid cells (TREM) family [5, 6]. The TREM isoforms share low sequence homology to each other and to other IgSF members and are characterized by having only one Ig-like domain. Five *trem* genes have been identified with four encoding putative functional type I transmembrane glycoproteins [7]. The *trem* genes are clustered on human chromosome 6 (and mouse chromosome 17) (Fig. 1). All TREMs associate with the adaptor DAP12 [5–8] for signaling. A brief summary of the human TREM isoforms is depicted in Table 1.

▌ TREM-1

Human TREM-1 (hTREM-1) consists of an extracellular region of 194 amino acid residues, a membrane spanning region of 29 amino acids and a short cytoplasmic tail of 5 amino acids. The extracellular Ig-like domain contains the motif DxGxYxC, which corresponds to a V-type Ig-domain. The Ig domain is connected to the transmembrane region by a 60 amino acid portion containing three *N*-glycosylation sites. The spanning region contains a Lys residue, which forms a salt-bridge with an Asp residue of the transmembrane domain of DAP12, allowing the association between TREM-1 and its adaptor protein [5, 9]. Engagement of TREMs triggers a signaling pathway involving ZAP70 (ζ-chain-associated protein 70) and SYK (spleen tyrosine kinase) and an ensuing recruitment and tyrosine phosphorylation of adaptor molecules such as GRB2 (growth factor receptor binding protein 2), the activation of PI3K (phosphatidylinositol 3-kinase), PLC-γ (phospholipase C-γ), ERK-1,-2 (extracellular-signal-regulated kinase) and p38 MAPK (p38 mitogen-associated protein kinase) [10, 11]. The activation of these pathways ultimately leads to a mobilization of intracellular calcium, a rearrangement of the actin cytoskeleton and activation of transcriptional factors (Fig. 2). Of note, although crystallographic analyses [12, 13] can predict TREM-1 recognition by using antibody-equivalent complemen-

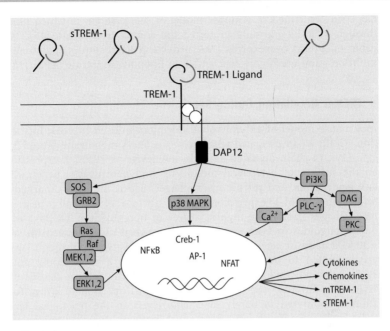

Fig. 2. TREM-1 signaling pathway

tary determining region (CDR) loops (such as TCRs, CD8 and CTLA-4), its natural ligand has yet to be determined.

TREM-1 as an Amplifier of the Inflammatory Response

TREM-1 is expressed by neutrophils, macrophages and mature monocytes (CD14[high]) [5]. Its expression by effector cells is dramatically increased in skin, biological fluids and tissues infected by Gram-positive or Gram-negative bacteria, as well as fungi [14, 15]. By contrast, TREM-1 is not upregulated in samples from patients with non-infectious inflammatory disorders such as psoriasis, ulcerative colitis, or vasculitis caused by immune complexes [15]. In mice, the engagement of TREM-1 with agonist monoclonal antibodies has been shown to stimulate the production of proinflammatory cytokines and chemokines [5, 16] such as interleukin (IL)-8, monocyte chemoattractant protein (MCP)-1, MCP-3 and macrophage inhibitory factor (MIP)-1α, along with rapid neutrophil degranulation and oxidative burst [17]. The activation of TREM-1 in the presence of Toll-like receptor (TLR)2 or TLR4 ligands amplifies the production of proinflammatory cytokines (tumor necrosis factor [TNF]-α, IL-1β, granulocyte-macrophage colony stimulating factor [GM-CSF]); together with the inhibition of IL-10 release [16]. In addition, the activation of these TLRs upregulates TREM-1 expression [5]. Thus, TREM-1 and TLRs appear to cooperate in producing an inflammatory response. Expression of TREM-1 could be under the control of nuclear factor-B (NF-κB) (activated by the TLRs) whereby engagement of TREM-1 plausibly leads to the activation of several transcription complexes which synergize with NF-κB to mount the transcription of proinflammatory genes [10]. The role of TREM-1 as an amplifier of the inflammatory response has been confirmed in a mouse model of septic shock in which blocking signaling through TREM-1 partially protected the animal from death [15]. Moreover, transgenic mice that overexpress DAP12 develop leukocytosis, pulmonary macrophage infiltrates, and are highly susceptible to lipopolysaccharide (LPS) [18].

TREM-1 Regulation During Sepsis

In a mouse model of polymicrobial infection induced by cecal ligation and perforation (CLP), we investigated whether sepsis alters membrane-bound TREM-1 expression [19]. In sham-operated animals, low levels of TREM-1 expression were present on the surface of peripheral monocytes and neutrophils, peritoneal macrophages and neutrophils, and splenic macrophages. Sepsis induced a marked increase (3- to 5-fold) in TREM-1 expression on the surface of all cell-types, with peritoneal macrophages having the highest degree of upregulation. TREM-1 was undetectable on lymphocytes in both groups of mice. Sepsis also induced the appearance of a ~ 30 kDa band in peritoneal lavage fluid samples which, through Western blot analysis, revealed to be specifically recognized by a monoclonal antibody directed against the extracellular domain of TREM-1. The release of this soluble form of TREM-1 (sTREM-1) was markedly increased in peritoneal lavage fluid from septic animals compared to barely detectable levels in the peritoneal lavage fluid from sham-operated animals. In septic shock patients, flow cytometry analysis demonstrated the same patterns with a marked TREM-1 overexpression compared to control patients, with a progressive decline during the recovery phase of the disease. Knapp et al. determined the regulation of TREM-1 upon intravenous LPS challenge in healthy humans [20]. Granulocyte TREM-1 expression was high at baseline and immediately downregulated following LPS administration along with an increase in sTREM-1. Monocytes displayed a progressive upregulation of TREM-1 after LPS administration [20]. Using a symmetrical approach, Passini et al. demonstrated that peripheral neutrophils from septic patients expressed high levels of TREM-1 ligand on the cell surface with a progressive decrease during the recovery period [21]. Interestingly, TREM-1 ligand expression was not detected on neutrophils from patients with non-infectious SIRS (systemic inflammatory response syndrome). Taken together, these data demonstrate that, during sepsis, membrane-bound TREM-1 expression is strongly induced on neutrophils and monocytes/macrophages, along with the release of its soluble form, mainly at the focus of infection. Moreover, considering that both cell-surface and soluble TREM-1 are upregulated during sepsis, it could well offer interesting perspectives in the diagnosis of infection.

TREM-1 in the Diagnosis of Infection

The specific involvement of TREM-1 solely in cases of infection, led us to investigate the diagnostic value of plasma sTREM-1 assay in distinguishing sepsis from severe systemic non-infectious inflammation among newly admitted critically ill patients with suspected infection [22]. Baseline plasma levels of C-reactive protein (CRP), procalcitonin (PCT), and sTREM-1 were higher among septic patients than in subjects with SIRS only. Plasma sTREM-1 level appeared to be the most helpful parameter in differentiating patients with sepsis from those with SIRS. Median plasma sTREM-1 levels at admission were 0 ng/mL (range, 0 to 144 ng/ml) in non-infected patients and 149 ng/ml (range, 30 to 428 ng/ml) in patients with sepsis (p<0.001). Plasma sTREM-1 levels yielded the highest discriminative value with an area under the ROC curve (AUC) of 0.97 followed by PCT (AUC, 0.85) and CRP (AUC, 0.77). At a cut-off level of 60 ng/ml, sTREM-1 was associated with a sensitivity of 96% and a specificity of 89% in differentiating patients with SIRS from those with sepsis or septic shock.

The diagnostic value of sTREM-1 in the context of a more localized infectious process, pneumonia, has also been investigated in a series of 148 consecutive mechanically ventilated patients [23]. sTREM-1 levels were higher in bronchoalveolar lavage (BAL) fluid originating from community-acquired and ventilator-associated pneumonia patients than from non-pneumonia patients but did not differ significantly between community-acquired and ventilator-associated pneumonia patients. BAL fluid levels of TNF-α and IL-1β exhibited the same trend but with a large overlap of values. The presence of sTREM-1 in BAL fluid was associated with a positive likelihood ratio of 10.38. The area under the ROC curve was 0.93 when using sTREM-1 to differentiate pneumonia from non pneumonia. A cut-off value of 5 pg/ml for sTREM-1 had a sensitivity of 98% and a specificity of 90%. Richeldi et al. studied the level of TREM-1 expression in BAL specimens from patients with community-acquired pneumonia, tuberculosis (an intra-cellular infection unable to induce TREM-1 upregulation *in vitro*), and interstitial lung diseases, the latter used as a model of non-infectious inflammatory disease of the lung [24]. TREM-1 expression was significantly increased in lung neutrophils and in lung macrophages of patients with pneumonia (n=7; 387.9±61.4 MFI [mean fluorescence intensity] and 660.5±18.3 MFI respectively) compared to patients with pulmonary tuberculosis (n=7; 59.2±13.1 MFI and 80.6±291.2 MFI), and patients with interstitial lung diseases (n=10; 91.8±23.3 MFI and 123.9±22.8 MFI).

Hence, sTREM-1 may constitute a reliable marker of infection particularly in plasma during sepsis and BAL fluid in cases of pneumonia. It remains to be determined, however, whether sTREM-1 could be useful in other infectious conditions, such as infected ascites or meningitis. The true clinical value of sTREM-1 assessment may be in allowing the clinician to withhold empiric antibiotics for cases where sTREM-1 levels are low, thus eliminating unnecessary antibiotic exposure for the patient.

TREM-1 Pathway as a Therapeutic Target

Bouchon et al. demonstrated that TREM-1 blockade by the use of a fusion protein containing murine TREM-1 extracellular domain and the human immunoglobulin-G (IgG1) Fc portion (mTREM-1/IgG1) protected mice against LPS-induced shock, as well as against microbial sepsis caused by live *Escherichia coli* or CLP [15]. We designed a synthetic peptide (LP17) mimicking a portion of the extracellular domain of TREM-1 and examined its action both *in vitro* and in a model of endotoxemia in mice [25]. LP17 reduced, in a concentration-dependent manner, TNF-α and IL-1β production from monocytes cultured with LPS. Mice treated with a single dose of LP17 60 min before administration of a lethal dose (LD$_{100}$) of LPS were protected from death in a dose-dependent manner. Delayed treatment with LP17 still conferred significant protection against a LD$_{100}$ of LPS. Compared to controls, LP17 reduced cytokines levels by 30%. Similar results were obtained in a model of polymicrobial sepsis model induced by CLP. Modulation of TREM-1 signaling reduces, although not completely, cytokine production and protects septic animals from hyper-responsiveness and death.

▌ TREM-1 Splice Variant

A product containing a 193-base deletion was identified by Gingras et al. as a splice variant of TREM-1 both in $CD14^+$ monocytes, lung, and liver [26]. If translated, this alternative splice variant (TREM-1sv) would encode a 150 amino acid-protein with a molecular mass of 17.5 kDa. The first 136 amino acids of TREM-1sv are identical to the first 136 amino acids of TREM-1 whereas the last 14 amino acids differ completely. Although the hydrophobic signal peptide and the V-type Ig-like domain are conserved, three N-glycosylation sites are lacking. Secretion of TREM-1sv receptor lacking the transmembrane domain could act as a downregulator by competing for the natural ligand of the full-length TREM-1. Nevertheless, the existence of the TREM-1sv remains to be proven. Moreover, this splice variant has been shown to be exclusively overexpressed upon stimulation with the cell wall fraction of *Mycobacterium bovis* BCG but not with LPS [27].

▌ TREM-like Transcript (TLT)-1

Analysis of the murine *trem* cluster revealed a putative regulatory receptor, immediately telomeric to *trem-2*, named TLT-1 by Washington et al. [28]. This cDNA encodes a single open reading frame predicting a 322 amino acid protein containing a single V-type Ig domain. The cytoplasmic region of TLT-1 contains an immunoreceptor tyrosine-based inhibitory motif (ITIM), implying the ability to mediate inhibition through the recruitment of SH-2 domain-containing protein tyrosine phosphatases. In fact, TLT-1 is exclusively expressed in platelets and megakaryocytes and its expression is strongly upregulated upon platelet activation [29, 30]. TLT-1 regulates granule construction or dispersal and thus does not function to inhibit members of the TREM family but rather plays a role in mediating vascular homeostasis and regulating coagulation at sites of injury. TLT-1 is the second ITIM-bearing receptor to be identified in platelets after platelet endothelial cell adhesion molecule (PECAM)-1.

▌ TREM-2

Human TREM-2 was first shown to be expressed by immature monocyte-derived dendritic cells [8]. Ligation of TREM-2 with an agonist monoclonal antibody on immature dendritic cells induced incomplete maturation. As dendritic cell activation influences the degree of expansion of naïve T-cells and the differentiation of helper T-cells, TREM-2 may regulate T-cell responses by activating antigen-presenting cells. Aside from its expression by dendritic cells, TREM-2 has also been detected in the brain [31], microglia [32], and osteoclasts. Humans deficient in TREM-2 develop degenerative brain abnormality and bone cysts in a rare disease known as 'Nasu-Hakola' disease (or polycystic lipomembranous osteodysplasia with sclerosing leukoencephalopathy: PLOSL), a clinical presentation similar to humans lacking DAP12 [33]. Thus, present data indicate that the TREM-2/DAP12 pathway directs the differentiation of myeloid precursors towards dendritic cells, osteoclasts [34], microglia, and oligodendrocytes. It has recently been demonstrated that mouse TREM-2 could bind to both Gram-positive and Gram-negative bacteria as well as to astrocytoma cell lines. TREM-2 binding is inhibited by purified anionic bacterial products, suggesting that TREM-2 receptors likely bind both bacteria and astrocytes via a charge-dependent interaction [35]. Therefore, pattern recognition of anionic ligands by TREM-2 may extend both to pathogens and to self antigens.

■ Other TREM Members

TREM-3 has been detected in murine macrophages and at low levels in T-cells [7]. Transcripts for TREM-3 are upregulated by LPS and downregulated by interferon (IFN)-γ. Analysis of the mouse genome reveals that the *trem-3* gene lies adjacent to the *trem-1* gene and is in close proximity to a number of other single Ig domain receptors, including *trem-2*. In humans, however, TREM-3 is a pseudogene. Other TREM family members, predicted from the genome analysis, have not yet been characterized.

■ Conclusion

TREMs constitute a family of immunoreceptors involved in myeloid cell maturation and activation, amplification of the inflammatory response triggered by the TLRs, platelet and coagulation homeostasis, as well as maintenance of the normal architecture of brain and bone. Although data on this exciting receptor family are rapidly growing, several crucial questions remain unanswered: what are the ligands associated with TREMs? Is TREM-1 a suitable therapeutic target during sepsis? Are *trem*-1 knockout mice resistant to sepsis? Is there a link between *trem*-2 mutations and demyelinizing diseases such as multiple sclerosis? A better knowledge of TREM biology is the key to answering many of these questions.

References

1. Diefenbach A, Raulet DH (2003) Innate immune recognition by stimulatory immunoreceptors. Curr Opin Immunol 15:37–44
2. Kubagawa H, Burrows PD, Cooper MD (1997) A novel pair of immunoglobulin-like receptors expressed by B cells and myeloid cells. Proc Natl Acad Sci USA 94:5261–5266
3. Cantoni C, Bottino C, Vitale M, et al (1999) NKp44, a triggering receptor involved in tumor cell lysis by activated human natural killer cells, is a novel member of the immunoglobulin superfamily. J Exp Med 189:787–796
4. Dietrich J, Cella M, Seiffert M, Buhring HJ, Colonna M (2000) Cutting edge: signal-regulatory protein 1 is a DAP12-associated activating receptor expressed on myeloid cells. J Immunol 164:9–12
5. Bouchon A, Dietrich J, Colonna M (2000) Cutting edge: inflammatory responses can be triggered by TREM-1, a novel receptor expressed on neutrophils and monocytes. J Immunol 164:4991–4995
6. Daws MR, Lanier LL, Seaman WE, Ryan JC (2001) Cloning and characterization of a novel mouse myeloid DAP12-associated receptor family. Eur J Immunol 31:743–791
7. Chung DH, Seaman WE, Daws MR (2002) Characterization of TREM-3, an activating receptor on mouse macrophages: definition of a family of single Ig domain receptors on mouse chromosome 17. Eur J Immunol 32:59–66
8. Bouchon A, Hernandez-Munain C, Cella M, Colonna M (2001) A DAP12-mediated pathway regulates expression of CC chemokine receptor 7 and maturation of human dendritic cells. J Exp Med 194:1111–1122

9. Lanier LL, Bakker AB (2000) The ITAM-bearing transmembrane adaptor DAP12 in lymphoid and myeloid cell function. Immunol Today 21:611–614
10. Colonna M (2003) TREMs in the immune system and beyond. Nature Rev Immunol 3:1–9
11. McVicar DW, Taylor LS, Gosselin P, et al (1998) DAP12-mediated signal transduction in natural killer cells. A dominant role for the Syk protein-tyrosine kinase. J Biol Chem 273:32934–32942
12. Radaev S, Kattah M, Rostro B, et al (2004) Crystal structure of the human myeloid cell activating receptor TREM-1. Structure 11:1527–1535
13. Kelker MS, Foss TR, Peti W, et al (2004) Crystal structure of human triggering receptor expressed on myeloid cells 1 (TREM-1) at 1.47 Å. J Mol Biol 342:1237–1248
14. Colonna M, Fachetti F (2003) TREM-1: a new player in acute inflammatory responses. J Infect Dis 187 (suppl 2):S397–S401
15. Bouchon A, Fachetti F, Weigand MA, et al (2001) TREM-1 amplifies inflammation and is a crucial mediator of septic shock. Nature 410:1103–1107
16. Bleharski JR, Kiessler V, Buonsanti C, et al (2003) A role for triggering receptor expressed on myeloid cells-1 in host defense during the early-induced and adaptive phases of the immune response. J Immunol 170:3812–3818
17. Radsak MP, Salih HR, Rammensee HG, et al (2004) Triggering receptor expressed on myeloid cells-1 in neutrophil inflammatory responses: differential regulation of activation and survival. J Immunol 172:4956–4963
18. Lucas M, Lucas M, Daniel L, et al (2002) Massive inflammatory syndrome and lymphocytic immunodeficiency in KARAP/DAP12-transgenic mice. Eur J Immunol 32:2653–2663
19. Gibot S, Kolopp-Sarda MN, Bene MC, et al (2004) Régulation d'expression de TREM-1 au cours du sepsis expérimental. Réanimation 13 (suppl 1):180 (abst)
20. Knapp S, Gibot S, de Vos A, et al (2004) Cutting edge: expression patterns of surface and soluble triggering receptor expressed on myeloid cells-1 in human endotoxemia. J Immunol 173:7131–7134
21. Passini N, Mariani M, Biffi M, et al (2004) Expression of TREM-1 ligand on neutrophils provides a potential diagnostic tool in sepsis. Shock 21 (suppl 1):418
22. Gibot S, Kolopp-Sarda MN, Bene MC, et al (2004) Plasma level of a triggering receptor expressed on myeloid cells-1: Its diagnostic accuracy in patients with suspected sepsis. Ann Intern Med 141:9–15
23. Gibot S, Cravoisy A, Levy B, et al (2004) Soluble triggering receptor expressed on myeloid cells and the diagnosis of pneumonia. N Engl J Med 350:451–458
24. Richeldi L, Mariani M, Losi M, et al (2004) Triggering receptor expressed on myeloid cells: role in the diagnosis of lung infections. Eur Respir J 24:247–250
25. Gibot S, Kolopp-Sarda MN, Bene MC, et al (2004) A soluble form of the triggering receptor expressed on myeloid cells-1 modulates the inflammatory response in murine sepsis. J Exp Med 200:1419–1426
26. Gingras MC, Lapillonne H, Margolin JF (2002) TREM-1, MDL-1, and DAP12 expression is associated with a mature stage of myeloid development. Mol Immunol 38:817–824
27. Begun NA, Ishii K, Kurita-Taniguchi M (2004) Mycobacterium bovis BCG cell wall-specific differentially expressed genes identified by differential display and cDNA substraction in human macrophages. Infect Immun 12:937–948
28. Washington AV, Quigley L, McVicar DW (2002) Initial characterization of TREM-like transcript (TLT)-1: a putative inhibitory receptor within the TREM cluster. Triggering receptors expressed on myeloid cells. Blood 100:3822–3824
29. Barrow AD, Astoul E, Floto A, et al (2004) Cutting edge: TREM-like transcript, a platelet immunoreceptor tyrosine-based inhibition motif encoding costimulatory immunoreceptor that enhances, rather than inhibits, calcium signalling via SHP-2. J Immunol 172:5838–5842
30. Washington AV, Schubert RL, Quigley L, et al (2004) TREM family member, TLT-1, is found exclusively in the α-granules of megakaryocytes and platelets. Blood 104:1042–1047
31. Paloneva J, Manninen T, Christman G, et al (2002) Mutations in two genes encoding different subunits of a receptor signaling complex result in an identical disease phenotype. Am J Hum Genet 71:656–662

32. Schmid CD, Sautkulis LN, Danielson PE, et al (2002) Heterogeneous expression of the trig-gering receptor expressed on myeloid cells-2 on adult murine microglia. J Neurochem 83:1309–1320
33. Kaifu T, Nakahara J, Inui M, et al (2003) Osteopetrosis and thalamic hypomyelinosis with synaptic degeneration in DAP12-deficient mice. J Clin Invest 111:323–332
34. Cella M, Buonsanti C, Strader C, Kondo T, Salmaggi A, Colonna M (2003) Impaired differ-entiation of osteoclasts in TREM-2-deficient individuals. J Exp Med 198:645–651
35. Daws MR, Sullam PM, Niemi EC, Chen TT, Tchao NK, Seaman WE (2003) Pattern recogni-tion by TREM-2: binding of anionic ligands. J Immunol 171:594–599

Role of Mannose-Binding Lectin in Host Defense

A. N. Tacx, M. H. L. Hart, and A. B. J. Groeneveld

▌ Introduction

Mannose-binding lectin, also called mannan-binding lectin (MBL), is an important acute phase plasma protein and component of the innate, non-specific immune defense system [1–3]. Before specific antibodies can efficiently defend the human body against invading microorganisms, the non-specific response is the first line of defense and the complement system plays an important role herein. Indeed, MBL is able to help complement activation. We will briefly review the biochemistry, function and genetic aspects of MBL, as well as the role of MBL in disease and therapeutic possibilities in MBL deficiency.

▌ The Biochemistry of MBL

MBL is a plasma glycoprotein, also called a collectin. Collectins are proteins containing a collagenous region and a carbohydrate-binding lectin part. MBL contains four domains: a short, cysteine-rich N-terminal region, essential for effective oligomerization; the collagen-like domain; a short alpha-helical neck region; and the large C-terminal C-type carbohydrate recognition domain. The collagen structure is responsible for the tail of the MBL molecule, and together with the three-headed cluster of lectin domains, it forms the basic universal collectin structure [1–3]. MBL interacts with several proteases to activate the lectin pathway of complement: MBL-associated serine proteases (MASP) -1 and -2. The MBL-MASP complex requires calcium for binding to a carbohydrate ligand of a microorganism [1]. MBL is mainly synthesized by hepatocytes. The serum concentration of MBL depends on age and the presence of an acute phase reaction. Interindividual variations in MBL levels are largely caused by genetic factors.

▌ Function of MBL

In recent years, it has become firmly established that MBL plays an important role in the innate immune defense system [1–3]. Several functions of the MBL pathway have been described, including activation of the complement system, promotion of (complement-independent) opsonophagocytosis and modulation of inflammation and apoptosis [4–6]. The MBL pathway is, together with the classical (antibody-mediated) and the alternative (antibody-independent) pathways, another, probably evolutionary 'older' and antibody-independent, route of complement activation [7, 8].

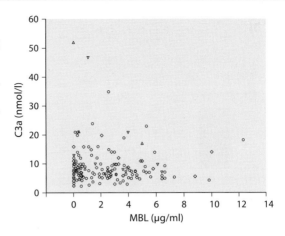

Fig. 1. Relation between MBL levels and activated complement product 3a (C3a) in 177 adult medical (hospitalized) patients with fever, without positive microbiological cultures (circles), with local positive culture (diamonds), with bacteremia only (triangles) and with positive local and blood cultures (inverted triangels). It is shown that even febrile patients with microbial infection and low MBL levels can activate complement. From [13] with permission

When bound to carbohydrate ligands of microbial surfaces, complexes of MBL/ MASP-1 and MBL/MASP-2 become activated [4]. Then, MBL/MASP-2, expressing enzymatic activity identical to C1q esterase, results in sequential cleavage of C2 and C4 [6, 9, 10]. The C4b fragment also binds to the microbial surface and interacts with C2. This complex expresses C3 convertase activity and cleaves C3 in a similar manner to the C3 convertases of both the classical and alternative pathways of complement activation. The MBL/MASP-1 complex is responsible for direct cleavage of C3 [10, 11]. The role of MBL in *in vivo* complement activation remains ill defined, however [12, 13] (Fig. 1). In febrile adult patients hospitalized in medical wards, we could not establish an association between circulating C3a levels as a marker of complement activation, and circulating MBL, even in those patients deficient of MBL and having severe microbial infection and bacteremia [13]. MBL may enhance opsonophagocytosis of microorganisms, either directly or via deposition of complement components activated via the lectin pathway [1, 4, 6]. MBL may modulate cytokine release by monocytes [6]. Other data suggest the presence of an MBL receptor on the surface of polymorphonuclear leukocytes, implying MBL-dependent cell-mediated cytotoxicity [1]. MBL is also a mediator of non-inflammatory clearance of immune complexes and injured/dying cells [5, 8]. It can bind to apoptotic cells and initiate uptake by macrophages [5, 6]. Accumulation of apoptotic cells following MBL deficiency is one of the explanations of systemic autoimmunity, for example in systemic lupus erythematosus (SLE) [8].

▌ Genetics of MBL

The MBL gene is located on the long arm of chromosome 10 and consists of a promotor gene and four exons coding for the protein. The promotor gene resembles that of an acute phase protein. MBL 2 gene mutation usually occurs in exon 1, coding for the cysteine-rich N-terminal domain of the protein. The mutations are located in codon 52, 54 or 57 and are all inherited in an autosomal dominant manner. In case of a codon 52 mutation (D variant), cysteine is replaced by arginine, a codon 54 mutation (B variant) results from replacement of glycine by aspartate and in case of a codon 57 mutation (C variant), glycine is replaced by glutamate. Muta-

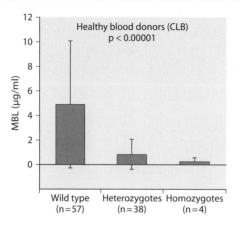

Fig. 2. Distribution (mean ± SD) of mannan-binding lectin (MBL) plasma levels among 99 healthy blood donors at the Central Laboratory for Blood Transfusion Services in Amsterdam, with normal genotypes (wild type), with heterozygous codon 52 or 54 mutations and with homozygous or double heterozygous mutations. Codon 57 mutations did not occur in this sample of healthy Dutch blood donation volunteers

tion is associated with a non-functional rather than an absent protein [6, 14]. The normal or wild-type is called the A variant. The B variant is most commonly responsible for low MBL concentrations in Europeans, occurring in about 25% of individuals [15, 16] (Fig. 2). The C variant is common in African individuals, in whom it reaches frequencies of 50–60% [6, 15]. Mutations in the promotor region of the gene have also been described and are also relevant in terms of functional MBL levels [1, 3, 16]. Heterozygotes may have severe reductions in plasma MBL (about 1/8 of normal levels), depending on the type of the heterozygous mutation, while MBL is usually hardly detectable in homozygotes (Fig. 2). Hence, mild MBL deficiencies are relatively common in most (Caucasian) populations, while severe deficiency affects about 15% of the Caucasian population. In contrast, the prevalence of (genotypic and phenotypic) MBL deficiency is much higher in African populations. This suggests that MBL deficiency may convey some benefit in Africa, for instance by limiting the susceptibility for disease by intracellular microorganisms, such as leishmaniasis and tuberculosis [17].

▌ Detection and Quantification

Normal plasma concentrations of MBL vary between 1000–5500 ng/ml. A MBL plasma-concentration indicative of deficiency is hard to define, since the overlap in MBL levels in patients with different genetic backgrounds is large and methods of determination widely differ among studies. Values below the lower limit of detection of about 200 ng/ml are certainly, and those below 500–800 ng/ml are often, indicative of (heterozygous) MBL deficiency [1, 3, 13, 16, 18–22]. The antigenic level and functional activity of MBL can be measured using techniques such as the radioimmunoassay, the enzyme-linked immunosorbent assay, and complement-dependent erythrocyte hemolysis, mannan binding and complement deposition tests [2, 13, 23–26]. DNA typing methods utilize polymerase chain reaction amplifications for genetic evaluation [2, 16, 18, 19, 21, 22, 27]. The advantage of genotyping over protein measurements is that the genotype is not influenced by the disease process, whereas serum MBL protein, being an acute phase protein, may be influenced by the disease itself. One the other hand, the disadvantage of genotyping is that it cannot prove the relationship between MBL concentration and disease [2].

▌ The MBL Pathway and Disease

MBL or MASP-2 deficiency increases the susceptibility to infectious diseases, often associated with other (humoral) immunodeficiencies, but there are also associations between MBL deficiency and non-infectious diseases including auto-immune diseases, malignancies, atherosclerosis and coronary artery disease [1, 9, 17–19, 22, 28–37].

In animal and (adult) clinical studies, a relation between MBL deficiency and increased infectious disease susceptibility and severity has been described [28, 31, 38, 39]. However, not all studies show a dominant role of the MBL-pathway of complement activation in the defense against microorganisms, and deficiency of MBL may be a cofactor rather than an independent risk factor for infection [13, 30, 40, 41]. MBL deficiency, either genotypic or phenotypic, may predispose to severe infections in adults treated with chemotherapy and after stem cell transplantation, but this association has been refuted by other authors [27, 32, 41]. In contrast, several pediatric studies show that mutations in the MBL gene and resultant MBL deficiency are risk factors for recurrent infections, for example infections of the respiratory system, whether or not associated with cystic fibrosis or other immune defects [3, 20, 29]. Homozygous mutations may be associated with more severe infections than heterozygous mutations [29]. In children with malignancy, (genotypic and phenotypic) MBL deficiency may prolong the duration of febrile, chemotherapy-induced neutropenic episodes [18].

For bacterial, viral, and fungal infections, increased susceptibility and more severe courses are observed in patients with MBL deficiency [1, 3, 36, 42]. *Staphylococcus aureus, Neisseria meningitides,* and beta-hemolytic group A streptococci exhibit strong MBL binding, and infections with these microorganisms in particular may be severe and fatal in humans with (genotypic or phenotypic) MBL deficiency [2–4, 31, 36, 38, 43]. *Streptococcus pneumoniae* less avidly binds MBL, and, indeed, MBL deficiency as a risk factor for invasion by this microorganism has been refuted by other authors [33, 43, 44]. Some reports showed that (homozygous and not heterozygous) MBL deficiency predisposed to *S. pneumoniae* infection [33], while other investigators did not observe such association for *S. pneumoniae* bacteremia in unselected adult patients [44]. The role of MBL in viral infections, for example human immunodeficiency virus (HIV) and hepatitis B/C, is also controversial. MBL deficiency may enhance susceptibility to viral infections, but may or may not affect the course of HIV infections [1, 3, 36].

Candida and aspergillus species also strongly bind to MBL, making the lectin pathway of complement activation an important defense mechanism [36, 42, 43]. A clear role for MBL in the defense against parasitic infections such as malaria has not yet been established [3, 36, 45]. Low levels of MBL can be protective against intracellular microorganisms that use MBL and complement activation for invading cells, including mycobacterial and leishmania species. For *Mycobacterium tuberculosis,* an intracellular microorganism, some studies suggest a protective effect of the B allele of the MBL gene in African-American individuals, but not in other ethnicities [17, 36].

Several reports show evidence of an increased frequency of mutant MBL genes and low plasma MBL concentrations in SLE, but not in rheumatoid arthritis, while low MBL levels may be associated with more severe disease in rheumatoid arthritis [1, 3, 34]. Also, autoantibodies against MBL have been detected in SLE, which adversely affect the functional activity of MBL [34]. Increased risks for vascular complications have been described for certain MBL genotypes in studies on coronary artery disease and type 1 diabetes [22, 35]. Genotypes associated with diminished levels of MBL were predictive of atherosclerosis and coronary artery disease [35], while high levels of MBL seemed to predispose to diabetic cardiovascular complications and nephropathy, possibly due to an enhanced vascular wall inflammation [22]. Inhibition of MBL by antibodies reduces postischemic myocardial reperfusion injury in rats, via an anti-inflammatory response [46].

▮ MBL and Intensive Care

Given the potential association between MBL deficiency and the occurrence (and course and severity) of bacterial infections, there is increasing awareness that MBL deficiency and associated genetic polymorphisms may play a role in nosocomial infections and sepsis in the critically ill. In critically patients with systemic inflammatory response syndrome (SIRS), for instance, (genotypic and phenotypic) MBL deficiency is associated with an increased risk of sepsis, shock and fatality [3, 19, 28, 47]. Variant MBL alleles and MBL deficiency may be associated with more severe inflammatory response to microbial infections than normal genetics and levels, at least in critically ill children [21]. Intensive insulin therapy administered to critically ill patients, may exert an antiinflammatory effect and may thereby counteract the potential adverse effects of low MBL levels [47]. This may be one of the mechanisms by which intensive insulin therapy lowers the incidence and sequelae of bacteremic sepsis and increases survival during critical illness. Indeed, high MBL levels, indicating an acute phase response, were associated with an elevated mortality risk and insulin treatment attenuated the rise in MBL levels [47]. Finally, MBL-mediated complement activation is, at least in part, associated with the inflammatory response after ischemia/reperfusion associated with thoracoabdominal aneurysm repair [48].

▮ Replacement Therapy

The increasing knowledge and understanding of MBL-mediated complement activation leads to new therapeutic strategies involving interference in uncontrolled or insufficient immune defense systems. Because the MBL pathway is an activator of inflammation, studies searching for MBL pathway inhibitors such as C_1 inhibitor and α_2-macroglobulin could lead to therapeutic options in uncontrolled inflammatory (noninfectious) processes [1, 12, 46, 49, 50]. Blockade of the lectin pathway with inhibitory monoclonal antibodies may protect the heart from ischemia-reperfusion injury by reducing tissue inflammation [8, 46]. With MBL genetic mutations conferring the most widespread immune deficiency, investigators are searching for MBL substitutes. Treatment with plasma-derived MBL and recombinant MBL as MBL substitutes is under investigation, with the aim to enforce the host defense to overcome (repeated) microbial infections, particularly when caused by cancer chemotherapy, or modulate the course of autoimmune disease [2, 6, 49–51]. Future therapy with MBL substitutes or inhibitors will have to be based on prospective clinical trials showing a benefit of immune boosting or suppression, respectively.

▌ Conclusion

In the last decades, it has become clear that MBL and the lectin pathway of complement activation play a key role in the innate immune defense system. Also, the
clinical relevance of MBL deficiency and MBL polymorphisms have been elucidated. We now know that MBL deficiency is one of the commonest immune deficiencies in humans, occurring in about 25% and that, despite uncertainties and
controversies in the literature, MBL deficiency most likely increases susceptibility
to infection, particularly in children or when immune function is suppressed by
other primary or secondary defects.

References

1. Petersen SV, Thiel S, Jensenius JC (2001) The mannan-binding lectin pathway of complement activation: biology and disease association. Mol Immunol 38:133–149
2. Kilpatrick DC (2002) Mannan-binding lectin and its role in innate immunity. Transfusion
   Med 12:335–351
3. Kilpatrick DC (2002) Mannan-binding lectin: clinical significance and applications. Biochim
   Biophys Acta 1572:401–413
4. Jack DL, Turner MW (2003) Anti-microbial activities of mannose-binding lectin. Biochem
   Soc Trans 31:753–757
5. Nauta AJ, Raaschou-Jensen N, Roos A, et al (2003) Mannose binding lectin engagement
   with late apoptotic and necrotic cells. Eur J Immunol 33:2853–2863
6. Turner MW (2003) The role of mannose-binding lectin in health and disease. Mol Immunol
   40:423–429
7. Fugita T, Endo Y, Masaru N (2004) Primitive complement system-recognition and activation. Mol Immunol 41:103–111
8. Saevarsdottir S, Vikingsdottir T, Valdimarsson H (2004) The potential role of mannan-binding lectin in the clearance of self-components including immune complexes. Scand J Immunol 60:23–29
9. Stengaard-Pedersen K, Thiel S, Gadjeva M, et al (2003) Inherited deficiency of mannan-
   binding lectin-associated serine protease 2. N Engl J Med 349:554–560
10. Chen R, Wallis R (2004) Two mechanisms for mannose-binding protein modulation of the
    activity of its serine proteases. J Biol Chem 25:26058–26065
11. Thiel S, Petersen SV, Vorup-Jensen T, et al (2000) Interaction of C1q and mannan-binding
    lectin (MBL) with C1r, C1s, MBL-associated proteases 1 and 2, and the MBL-associated pro-
    tein MAp19. J Immunol 165:878–887
12. Gulati S, Sastry K, Jensenius JC, Rice PA, Ram A (2002) Regulation of the mannan-binding
    lectin pathway of complement on Neisseria gonorrhoeae by C1-inhibitor and alpha2-macro-
    globulin. J Immunol 168:4078–4086
13. Tacx AN, Groeneveld ABJ, Hart MH, Aarden LA, Hack CE (2003) Mannan binding lectin in
    febrile adults: no correlation with microbial infection and complement activation. J Clin
    Pathol 56:956–959
14. Terai I, Kobayashi K, Matsushita M, Miyakawa H, Mafune N, Kikuta H (2003) Relationship
    between gene polymorphisms of mannose-binding lectin (MBL) and two molecular forms
    of MBL. Eur J Immunol 33:2755–2763
15. Lipscombe RJ, Sumiya M, Hill AVS, et al (1992) High frequencies in African and non-Afri-
    can populations of independent mutations in the mannose binding protein gene. Hum Mol
    Genet 9:709–715
16. Minchinton RM, Dean MM, Clark TR, Heatley S, Mullighan CG (2002) Analysis of the rela-
    tionship between mannose-binding lectin (MBL) genotype, MBL: levels and fucntion in an
    Australian blood donor population. Scand J Immunol 56:630–641
17. El Sahly HM, Reich RA, Dou SJ, Musser JM, Graviss EA (2004) The effect of mannose bind-
    ing lectin gene polymorphisms on susceptibility to tuberculosis in different ethnic groups.
    Scand J Infect Dis 36:106–108

18. Neth O, Hann I, Turner MW, Klein NJ (2001) Deficiency of mannose-binding lectin and burden of infection in children with malignancy: a prospective study. Lancet 358:614-618

19. Garred P, Strom JJ, Quist L, Taaning E, Madsen HO (2003) Association of mannose-binding lectin polymorphisms with sepsis and fatal outcome, in patients with systemic inflammatory response syndrome. J Infect Dis 188:1394-1403

20. Cedzynski M, Szemraj J, Swierzko AS, et al (2004) Mannan-binding lectin insufficiency in children with recurrent infections of the respiratory system. Clin Exp Immunol 136:304-311

21. Fidler KJ, Wilson P, Davies JC, Turner MW, Peters MJ, Klein NJ (2004) Increased incidence and severity of the systemic inflammatory response syndrome in patients deficient in mannose-binding lectin. Intensive Care Med 30:1438-1445

22. Hansen TK, Tarnow L, Thiel S, et al (2004) Association between mannose-binding lectin and vascular complications in type 1 diabetes. Diabetes 53:1570-1576

23. Dumestre-Perard C, Ponard D, Arlaud GJ, Monnier N, Sim, RB, Colomb MG (2002) Evaluation and clinical interest of mannan binding lectin function in human plasma. Mol Immunol 39:465-473

24. Petersen SV, Thiel S, Jensen L, Steffensen R, Jensenius JC (2001) An assay for the mannan-binding lectin pathway of complement activation. J Immunol Meth 257:107-116

25. Kuipers S, Aerts PC, Sjoholm AG, Harmsen T, Van Dijk H (2002) A hemolytic assay for the estimation of functional mannose-binding lectin levels in human serum. J Immunol Meth 268:149-157

26. Roos A, Bouwman LH, Munoz J, et al (2003) Functional characterization of the lectin pathway of complement in human serum. Mol Immunol 39:655-668

27. Mullighan CG, Heatley S, Doherty K, et al (2002) Mannose-binding lectin gene polymorphisms are associated with major infection following allogeneic hemopoietic stem cell transplantation. Blood 99:3524-3529

28. Summerfield JA, Ryder S, Sumiya M, et al (1995) Mannose binding protein gene mutations associated with unusual and severe infections in adults. Lancet 345:886-889

29. Summerfield JA, Sumiya M, Levin M, Turner MW (1997) Association of mutations in mannose binding protein gene with childhood infection in consecutive hospital series. BMJ 314:1229-1232

30. Mullighan CG, Marshall SE, Welsh KI (2000) Mannose binding lectin polymorphisms are associated with early age of disease onset and autoimmunity in common variable immunodeficiency. Scand J Immunol 51:111-122

31. Hibberd ML, Summerfield JA, Levin M (2001) Variation in the mannose binding (MBL) gene and susceptibility to sepsis. Sepsis 4:201-207

32. Peterslund NA, Koch C, Jensenius JC, Thiel S (2001) Association between deficiency of mannose-binding lectin and severe infections after chemotherapy. Lancet 38:637-638

33. Roy S, Knox K, Segal S, et al (2002) MBL genotype and risk of invasive pneumococcal disease: a case-control study. Lancet 359:1569-1573

34. Seelen MA, Trouw LA, Van der Hoorn JWA, et al (2003) Autoantibodies against mannose-binding lectin in systemic lupus erythematosus. Clin Exp Immunol 134:335-343

35. Best LG, Davidson M, North KE, et al (2004) Prospective analysis of mannose-binding lectin genotypes and coronary artery disease in American Indians. Circulation 109:471-475

36. Eisen DP, Minchinton RM (2003) Impact of mannose-binding lectin on susceptibility to infectious diseases. Clin Infect Dis 37:1496-1505

37. Gomi K, Tokue Y, Kobayashi T, et al (2004) Mannose-binding lectin gene polymorphism is a modulating factor in repeated respiratory infections. Chest 126:95-99

38. Shi L, Takahashi K, Dundee J, et al (2004) Mannose-binding lectin-deficient mice are susceptible to infection with staphylococcus aureus. J Exp Med 199:1379-1390

39. Windbichler M, Echtenacher B, Hehlgans T, Jensenius JC, Schwaeble W, Mannel DN (2004) Involvement of the lectin pathway of complement activation in antimicrobial immune defense during experimental septic peritonitis. Infect Immun 9:5247-5252

40. Aittoniemi J, Rintala E, Miettinen A, Soppi E (1997) Serum mannan-binding lectin (MBL) in patients with infection: clinical and laboratory correlates. APMIS 105:617-622

41. Bergmann OJ, Christiansen M, Laursen I, et al (2003) Low levels of mannose-binding lectin do not affect occurrence of severe infections or duration of fever in acute myeloid leukaemia during remission inudction. Eur J Haematol 70:91-97

42. Ip WK, Lau YL (2004) Role of mannose-binding lectin in the innate defense against candida albicans: enhancement of complement activation, but lack of opsonic function, in phagocytosis by human dendritic cells. J Infect Dis 190:632–640
43. Neth O, Jack DL, Dodds A, Holzel H, Klein NJ, Turner MW (2000) Mannose-binding lectin binds to a range of clinically relevant microorganisms and promotes complement deposition. Infect Immun 68:688–693
44. Kronborg G, Weis N, Madsen HO, et al (2002) Variant mannose-binding lectin alleles are not associated with susceptibility to or outcome of invasive pneumococcal infection in randomly include patients. J Infect Dis 185:1517–1520
45. Garred P, Nielsen MA, Kurtzhaks JAL, et al (2003) Mannose-binding lectin is a disease modifier in clinical malaria and may function as opsonin for *Plasmodium falciparum*-infected erythrocytes. Infect Immun 71:5245–5253
46. Jordan JE, Montalto MC, Stahl GL (2001) Inhibition of mannose-binding lectin reduces postischemic myocardial reperfusion injury. Circulation 104:1413–1418
47. Hansen TK, Thiel S, Wouters PJ, Christiansen JS, Van den Berghe G (2003) Intensive insulin therapy exerts anti-inflammatory effects in critically ill patients and counteracts the adverse effect of low mannose-binding lectin levels. J Clin Endocrinol Metab 88:1082–1088
48. Fiane AE, Videm V, Lingaas PS, et al (2003) Mechanism of complement activation and its role in the inflammatory response after thoracoabdominal aortic aneurysm repair. Circulation 108:849–856
49. Petersen SV, Thiel S, Jensen L, Vorup-Jensen T, Koch C, Jensenius JC (2000) Control of the classical and the MBL pathway of complement activation. Mol Immunol 37:803–811
50. Summerfield JA (2003) Clinical potential of mannose-binding lectin-replacement therapy. Biochem Soc Trans 31:770–773
51. Valdimarsson H, Stefansson M, Vikingsdottir T, et al (1998) Reconstitution of opsonizing activity by infusion of mannan-binding lectin to MBL-deficient humans. Scand J Immunol 48:116–123

Mitochondrial Dysfunction in Sepsis

J. M. Handy

▌ Introduction

While the essence of cellular metabolism and respiration are considered to be essential knowledge in medical education, there are few postgraduate specialties that require this information to be omnipresent during the day-to-day duties of the clinician. Convincing evidence exists to suggest that early improvement of oxygen delivery (DO_2) to the tissues can improve survival in patients with sepsis [1] and with this in mind, it is not hard to imagine the effects that abnormal cellular oxygen utilization could throw into the equation. Recent advances in the scientific literature highlight the need for fluency in the understanding of cellular respiration in order that one can comprehend the pathophysiology in sepsis and the potential for future therapies. The aim of this chapter is to reiterate the physiology of cellular respiration, in particular the role of the tricarboxylic acid (TCA) and electron transport pathways, and then review the recent literature in an attempt to explain where these pathways become dysfunctional during sepsis and why variation may have occurred in clinical studies of improving DO_2 in critically ill patients [1–3].

▌ Cellular Energetics

Before considering the intricacies of oxidative phosphorylation, it is worth contemplating the more fundamental aspects of energy dynamics within systems. The first law of thermodynamics states that, during the course of a chemical reaction in a closed system, energy can neither be created nor destroyed but can be converted from one form to another. The second law of thermodynamics states that in a closed system the total amount of usable energy (termed the Gibbs free energy or δG) is always decreased. In other words, a chemical reaction will only take place spontaneously if the reaction proceeds in the direction that results in a net decrease in the δG. Take the example:

$$A + B \leftrightarrow C$$

If the free energy (δG) of the forward reaction is positive, the reaction will not take place spontaneously and energy will be required to form C from A and B. It is an 'uphill' process and is said to be 'endergonic'. If however the δG is negative then the reaction of A with B to form C is an energetically 'downhill' process and will occur spontaneously. Such a reaction is 'exergonic'.

The clinical relevance of the above is that no enzyme or chemical reaction in the body can take place unless the δG for that reaction is negative (if it is zero, the reaction will remain in equilibrium). In order to make a reaction with a positive δG occur spontaneously it must be 'coupled' to another reaction where the δG is negative such that the sum of their free energies (δG_{tot}) is negative. This coupling can occur in several ways, the most common of which is for both the reactions to take place on the same enzyme. Given that so many of the reactions in the body are energy dependant (endergonic) there is a constant requirement for a highly exergonic reaction to which they can be coupled in order to give a negative δG_{tot} and hence allow the overall reaction to proceed spontaneously. This highly exergonic reaction is provided in the hydrolysis of ATP, where:

$$ATP^{4-} + H_2O \rightarrow ADP^{3-} + HPO_4^{2-} + H^+$$

This process has a δG of –30.5 kJ and therefore occurs spontaneously.

An example of an endergonic reaction is the formation of glycerol-3-phosphate from glycerol:

$$glycerol + HPO_4^{2-} \rightarrow (glycerol\text{-}3\text{-}phosphate)^{2-} + H_2O$$

This has a δG of +9.2 kJ and thus will not occur spontaneously. However if the two reactions are coupled we get the following reaction:

$$glycerol + ATP^{4-} \rightarrow (glycerol\text{-}3\text{-}phosphate)^{2-} + ADP^{3-} + H^+$$

This combined reaction has a δG_{tot} of –30.5 kJ + 9.2 kJ = –21.3 kJ and thus will now proceed spontaneously.

It is obvious from the above why ATP has become the 'universal currency' that can be coupled with energy dependent processes. Hence, ATP depletion rapidly results in these processes coming to a halt. Over the past decade there has been increased interest in the effects of sepsis on the production of ATP and cellular respiration. Increasing evidence is coming to light to suggest that these are impaired in septic patients and in order to understand the pathways that are affected it is necessary to revise the basic physiology of cellular ATP production.

■ ATP Production from Glucose

To make ATP, energy must be absorbed in the form of food, and must subsequently be released and packaged in a usable form. The simplest pathway to follow in order to analyze this process is the formation of ATP from carbohydrates, in particular glucose.

Glucose contains 15.7 kJ/g of free energy and therefore if 1 mole undergoes complete oxidation it will release 2826 kJ, which if collected could be used for energy-dependent cell functions. If this process were to occur in one step (e.g., combustion) this energy would be released in the form of heat and none would be stored. The challenge for the body therefore is to oxidize the glucose in a manner that allows the free energy to be released in a step-wise fashion so that it can be collected and utilized elsewhere. The breakdown of glucose into carbon dioxide (CO_2) occurs in two steps: glycolysis and the citric-acid cycle. These two pathways are used to recycle molecules of two important reducing agents, NADH and FADH$_2$, which donate electrons to the electron transport chain with the resultant production of ATP. They are the key elements that transfer energy from the pathways involved in the breakdown of glucose to that involved in the production of ATP.

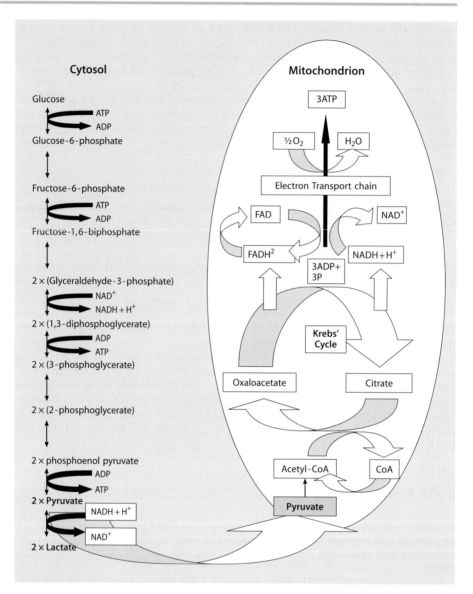

Fig. 1. Aerobic metabolism of glucose. FAD and FADH$_2$=oxidized and reduced Flavin cofactors respectively; CoA=coenzyme A

The process of glycolysis is shown on the left hand side of Figure 1 with the interplay with the TCA cycle (Krebs' cycle) shown on the right hand side. It can be seen that glycolysis utilizes two molecules of ATP and produces four for every glucose molecule metabolized, with a net production of two ATP and two NADH. Here the ATP is formed by a process called 'substrate level phosphorylation' where the energy required to phosphorylate ADP is acquired by direct linkage to the chemical reactions:

1,3-diphosphoglycerate → 3-phosphoglycerate

and:

Phosphoenol pyruvate → pyruvate

These reactions result in the formation of ATP whereas the others in the pathway do not because they are exergonic and contain a δG greater than that required by the endergonic production of ATP from ADP. Indeed this must be a common factor in all reactions involved in the production of ATP.

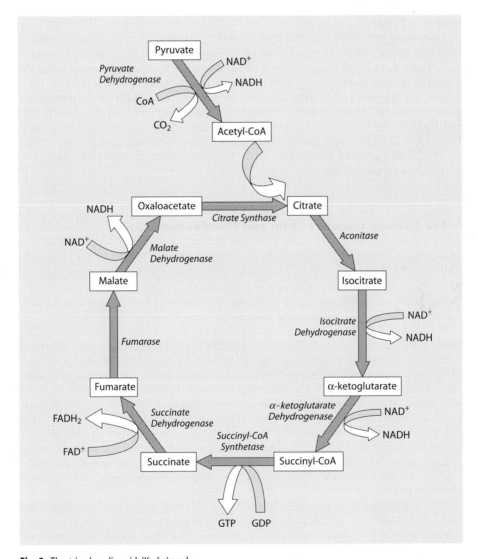

Fig. 2. The tricarboxylic acid (Krebs) cycle

The two pyruvate and two NADH produced by glycolysis subsequently enter the mitochondrion, the former by facilitated diffusion. The fate of the NADH will be discussed later. The pyruvate, meanwhile, is combined with coenzyme A to form acetyl-CoA. The catalyst for this reaction is pyruvate dehydrogenase and is an important enzyme that may be inactivated in sepsis [4]. The resultant acetyl-CoA combines with oxaloacetate to form citrate and so enters the Krebs' cycle depicted in Figure 2. A number of steps in this cycle release free energy that is stored in the reducing agents NADH and $FADH_2$. In addition a molecule of GTP is produced for every cycle. This can be considered as equivalent to ATP in terms of the δG stored in its 'high energy' phosphate bonds. Thus each 'turn' of the Krebs' cycle produces $4NADH + FADH_2 + GTP$. As two molecules of pyruvate enter the cycle for every glucose undergoing glycolysis, the net product is therefore twice this, i.e., $8NADH + 2FADH_2 + 2GTP$.

Combining glycolysis and the Krebs' cycle it is apparent that the equivalent of only four molecules of ATP are produced from the complete oxidation of glucose to CO_2. These have a net energy content of 122 kJ (4×30.5 kJ), which would make the efficiency of the reaction only 4.5% if all the other energy was lost in heat (122/2826 kJ). Fortunately this latter situation is not the case. Much of the energy released is stored in the reduction-oxidation (redox) potential of the NADH and $FADH_2$. It is the release of this energy via the electron transport chain by what is termed the chemiosmotic theory that results in the metabolism of glucose having an overall efficiency of nearly 45%. Thus the importance of these reducing agents cannot be overemphasized.

▌ The Electron Transport Chain and Chemiosmotic Theory

The ability to couple the redox potential of the NADH and $FADH_2$ to the phosphorylation of ADP to form ATP is a stroke of evolutionary genius, the mechanism for which has only recently been adequately elucidated. The essence of the process lies in the ability of the former agents to donate electrons and for the sake of simplicity NADH will be used as the example though the same principles apply to $FADH_2$.

If a chemical element exists in a state that is far from its electrochemical equilibrium, it will have a tendency to achieve equilibrium by gaining or losing electrons. Thus it has an electrical potential that can be termed reduction potential if the element has a propensity to lose electrons. As within a battery, the movement of electrons occurs from areas of low electrical potential (reduction potential) to those with higher electrical potential and in doing so energy is released. They will move in the direction that results in the greatest change in electrical potential and this is the principle behind the one-way movement of electrons through the electron transport chain thus creating an electrical current. The structure of both the mitochondrion and the complexes within the electron transport chain are crucial to the coupling of the redox and phosphorylation reactions in what is termed 'oxidative phosphorylation'.

The mitochondrial membranes are the crucial areas where this coupling takes place. There are two membranes, a convoluted inner membrane, which is largely impermeable and an outer permeable membrane. The inner membrane contains a number of proton channels, pumps, and complexes that are together referred to as the electron transport chain (Fig. 3). Importantly, evidence exists to suggest that a

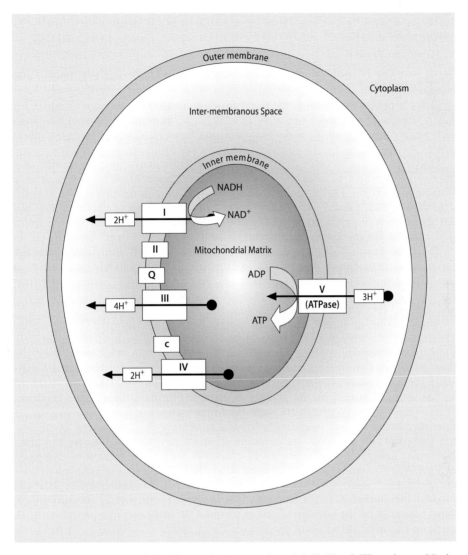

Fig. 3. The electron transport chain. Diagram showing complexes I, II, III, IV and ATP synthetase (V), the mobile electron carriers Coenzyme Q and Cytochrome c, and hydrogen ion movement (solid arrows)

number of these areas within the electron transport chain become dysfunctional in sepsis. All the components of the electron transport chain pathway are proteins with the exception of the NADH and succinate (which are soluble in the mitochondrial matrix) and coenzyme Q (CoQ), the latter of which acts as a mobile carrier of electrons between the primary dehydrogenases and cytochrome b. The electron transport proteins are clustered together to form complexes I, II, III, and IV. Complex I is composed of NADH dehydrogenase, non-heme-iron proteins, and a cofactor and is responsible for transferring electrons from NADH to CoQ. The electrical energy contained within this transfer is referred to as δE and is related to the free energy of the reaction by the Nernst equation:

$$\delta G = -n \cdot F \cdot \delta E$$

where n is the number of electrons involved in the reaction and F is the Faraday constant.

Thus it can be established that the transfer of an electron through Complex I is highly exergonic and results in a δG of –79kJ. This is more than enough to form ATP when coupled with the endergonic reaction between ADP and inorganic phosphate.

Electron transfer through Complex-II, or succinate dehydrogenase, results in a δG of –10 kJ, which is insufficient to drive the synthesis of ATP. Of note it is at Complex-II that the $FADH_2$ donates its electrons and it is for this reason that the oxidation of one molecule of $FADH_2$ results in the formation of only two ATP versus the three ATP produced by NADH due to the latter entering the electron transport chain at the more exergonic Complex-I stage.

The hydrophobic CoQ is reduced by Complexes-I and II and diffuses through the membrane to donate its electrons to Complex-III. The principle components of this latter complex are the heme-proteins, cytochromes b and $c1$, and a non-heme-protein. The iron within the heme-proteins alternates between the oxidized (Fe^{3+}) and reduced (Fe^{2+}) forms as electrons pass within the complex.

After passing through Complex-III, the electrons are transferred by the mobile cytochrome c to Complex-IV. This complex is also known as 'cytochrome oxidase' as it donates its electrons to the ultimate acceptor, oxygen. The reduced oxygen then combines with hydrogen ions to produce water. Complex-IV contains, amongst other proteins, the heme-proteins cytochromes a and $a3$.

The energy released by the passage of electrons through the electron transport chain is used to pump protons through the inner membrane from the matrix to the inter-membrane space. Complexes I, III, and IV achieve this task acting as the proton pumps. Thus a proton concentration gradient is established across the inner membrane and the potential energy so created is termed the 'proton-motive force' or PMF. The movement of these protons down their concentration gradient releases energy that is used by the ATP synthetase (Complex-V) to phosphorylate ADP and produce the desired ATP. The Complex-V is composed of F_1 and F_0 subunits which, when triggered by the passage of protons, bind ADP and inorganic phosphate at its catalytic site with the resultant product, ATP.

Thus from the above complicated pathway, it can be seen that transfer of electrons from NADH via the electron transport chain results in the production of three ATP and those from $FADH_2$ produce two ATP. Thus the eight NADH, two $FADH_2$ and two GTP produced as a result of two pyruvate entering the Krebs' cycle give the equivalent of 30 ATP once they have entered into oxidative phosphorylation. Glycolysis yields two ATP and two NADH equivalent to eight ATP once oxidative phosphorylation has take place and thus the overall oxidation of glucose to water and carbon dioxide yields 38 ATP with an efficiency of nearly 45%, largely as a result of the redox reactions taking place within the chemiosmotic machinery.

❚ Mitochondrial Dysfunction in Sepsis

The delivery of oxygen to tissues in a state of sepsis has commanded a great deal of attention over the past two decades, and yet evidence to support techniques that enhance such delivery has been inconsistent, if not contradictory [1–3]. This reflects the complexity of the pathophysiology underlying cellular and organ dysfunction in sepsis. Over time, however, a number of authors have highlighted the possibility that cellular utilization of oxygen is impaired in sepsis and subsequently a number of studies have produced evidence to support this [5–14]. This phenomenon has not been replicated consistently though [15, 16] suggesting once again that a complex interplay of factors exists in producing the organ dysfunction that we see clinically.

In tissue that exhibits oxygen consumption at a greater rate than it is being delivered, under normal physiological conditions one would expect to see an increase in the extraction ration for oxygen entering and leaving the cells. Thus the distribution of tissue PO_2 should move to the left showing more values nearer zero. However, this has not consistently been found to be the case. Whole body and regional oxygen extraction have been shown to decrease or remain static in a number of studies using animal models of sepsis [5–7] though this phenomenon has not been replicated in human models [15]. In one animal study [7], a group of pigs were infused with *Escherichia coli* lipopolysaccharide (LPS) and were resuscitated once the subsequent septic response ensued. Distal ileal mucosa was analyzed for pH, blood flow and PO_2, and compared with a control group. The surprising finding was that although mucosal blood flow was similar between the two groups, acidosis developed in the septic group in the presence of increased PO_2. Thus, ongoing ATP hydrolysis in the presence of reduced oxygen extraction ratio was observed, inferring that cellular oxygen utilization was dysfunctional.

Subsequent studies have aimed to analyze where the defect in oxygen utilization may lie and whether or not this can be reversed. While considering these studies it is worth referring back to the previously described metabolic pathways involved in ATP production. It is generally accepted that nitric oxide (NO) is upregulated in sepsis [17] and that inducible NO synthase (iNOS) can appear in a number of organs and tissues in animal models of sepsis [18, 19]. A number of studies have highlighted NO and iNOS as contributing to cellular dysoxia [10, 13, 20]. Indeed inhibition of iNOS by the use of aminoguanidine has been shown to restore cellular oxygen utilization to normal values in endotoxemic rats [9, 10]. In conditions of raised NO levels, NO has been shown to inhibit Complex I and the cytochrome a,a_3 portion of Complex IV [13, 21], thus preventing electron transfer to molecular oxygen and thus inhibiting the electron transport chain. This inhibition is associated with a decrease in reduced glutathione concentrations and while *in vitro* data suggest that this state can be reversed by the addition of exogenous glutathione [21], this was not the case when studied in humans [13]. The transfer of electrons along the electron transport chain may be disrupted by competition between oxygen and NO for binding sites on mitochondrial electron transport chain complexes [22]. Of interest, Levy et al. [11] showed that although the inhibition of cytochrome oxidase was competitive early in the septic phase, this became non-competitive by 48 hours. Such observations may explain the variation seen in clinical trials aiming to optimize DO_2 to tissues in septic patients depending on the time period at which interventions were initiated [1, 3]. While NO seems a likely culprit in causing cellular dysoxia, it is the formation of peroxynitrite from the reaction between NO and reduced oxygen that has more potential for toxicity. Peroxynitrite has been shown to inhibit electron transport chain complexes I, II, and V [23], and the enzyme aconitase that converts citrate into isocitrate in the Krebs' cycle [24].

Another possible mechanism for cell dysfunction is the over expression of poly-(adenosine 5′-diphosphate-ribose) synthetase (PARS) in sepsis. This nuclear enzyme is activated in the presence of DNA single-strand breakages, when it triggers the metabolically inefficient transfer of ADP-ribose to nuclear proteins. This results in the rapid depletion of NAD and ATP leading to cell injury and death [25]. It has been shown that PARS production increases in sepsis as a result of increased DNA single-strand breakage caused by reactive oxygen radicals and peroxynitrite. Inhibitors of PARS have been shown to be protective against cell damage in free-radical mediated cell injury [25] and in sepsis [8, 14]. Lastly, as mentioned previously, increased inactivation of the enzyme pyruvate dehydrogenase may occur in sepsis as a result of an increase in pyruvate dehydrogenase kinase levels [4]. This results in reduced conversion of pyruvate to acetyl-CoA and subsequent 'starvation' of substrate for the Krebs' cycle.

▌ Conclusion

The disruption of cellular oxidation utilization may play an important role in causing organ dysfunction in sepsis. Evidence suggests that the pathways involved may include decreased acetyl-CoA formation from pyruvate, inhibitory effects of NO and peroxynitrite on electron transfer complexes, peroxynitrite inhibition of aconitase, and the over production of PARS resulting in NAD depletion. Of particular interest is that the dynamics of such interference appears to change during the time-course of the septic insult, which may explain the inconsistencies seen in the results from clinical trials aiming to improve DO_2 to tissues in critically ill patients. At present, manipulating these disrupting influences has shown variable results with no clinically useful drugs or techniques materializing. However, in the future this situation may be reversed as our knowledge of the pathophysiology behind sepsis and cellular dysoxia improves. It may yet be that a detailed understanding of cellular respiration proves to be an important factor in improving survival in patients with sepsis.

References

1. Rivers E, Nguyen B, Havstad S, et al (2001) Early goal-directed therapy in the treatment of severe sepsis and septic shock. N Engl J Med 345:1368–1377
2. Shoemaker WC, Appel PL, Kram HB, et al (1988) Prospective trial of supranormal values of survivors as therapeutic goals in high-risk surgical patients. Chest 94:1176–1186
3. Hayes MA, Timmins AC, Yau EHS, Palazzo M, Hinds CJ, Watson D (1994) Elevation of systemic oxygen delivery in the treatment of critically ill patients. N Engl J Med 330:1717–1722
4. Vary TC, Siegel JH, Nakatani T, Sato T, Aoyama H (1986) Effect of sepsis on activity of pyruvate dehydrogenase complex in skeletal muscle and liver. Am J Physiol 250:E634–E640
5. Schumacker PT, Kazaglis J, Connolly HV, et al (1995) Systemic and gut O_2 extraction during endotoxaemia: Role of nitric oxide synthesis. Am J Respir Crit Care Med 151:107–115
6. Astiz M, Rackow EC, Weil MH, Schumer W (1988) Early impairment of oxidative metabolism and energy production in severe sepsis. Circ Shock 26:311–320
7. Vandermeer TJ, Wang H, Fink M (1995) Endotoxaemia causes ileal mucosal acidosis in the absence of mucosal hypoxia in a normodynamic porcine model of septic shock. Crit Care Med 23:1217–1226

8. Goldfarb Rd, Marton A, Szabo E, et al (2002) Protective effect of a novel, potent inhibitor of poly(adenosine 5'-diphosphate-ribose) synthetase in a porcine model of severe bacterial sepsis. Crit Care Med 30:974–980

9. King CJ, Tytgat S, Delude RL, Fink M (1999) Ileal mucosal oxygen consumption is decreased in endotoxemic rats but is restored toward normal by treatment with aminoguanidine. Crit Care Med 27:2518–2525

10. Unno N, Wang H, Menconi MJ, et al (1997) Inhibition of inducible nitric oxide synthase ameliorates endotoxin-induced gut mucosal barrier dysfunction in rats. Gastroenterology 113:1246–1257

11. Levy RJ, Vijayasarathy C, Raj NR, Avadhani NG, Deutschman CS (2004) Competitive and non-competitive inhibition of myocardial cytochrome c oxidase in sepsis. Shock 21:110–114

12. Chen HW, Hsu C, Lu TS, Wang SJ, Yang RC (2003) Heat shock pre-treatment prevents cardiac mitochondrial dysfunction during sepsis. Shock 20:274–279

13. Brealey D, Brand M, Hargreaves I, et al (2002) Association between mitochondrial dysfunction and severity and outcome of septic shock. Lancet 360:219–223

14. Jagtap P, Soriano FG, Virag L, et al (2002) Novel phenanthridinone inhibitors of poly(adenosine 5-diphosphate-ribose) synthetase: Potent cytoprotective and antishock agents. Crit Care Med 30:1071–1082

15. Ronco J, Fenwick J, Tweeddale M, et al (1993) Identification of the critical oxygen delivery for anaerobic metabolism in critically ill septic and non-septic humans. JAMA 270:1724–1730

16. Sair M, Etherington PJ, Winlove CP, Evans T (2001) Tissue oxygenation and perfusion in patients with systemic sepsis. Crit Care Med 29:1343–1350

17. Evans T, Carpenter A, Kinderman H, Cohen J (1993) Evidence of increased nitric oxide production in patients with the sepsis syndrome. Circ Shock 41:77–81

18. Chamulitrat W, Skrepnik NV, Spitzer JJ (1996) Endotoxin-induced oxidative stress in the rat small intestine: role of nitric oxide. Shock 5:217–222

19. Chamulitrat W, Skrepnik NV, Spitzer JJ (1996) Nitrosyl complex formation during endotoxin-induced injury in the rat small intestine. Shock 5:59–65

20. Clementi E, Brown GC, Feelisch M, Moncada S (1998) Persistent inhibition of cell respiration by nitric oxide: crucial role of S-nitrosylation of mitochondrial complex I and protective action of glutathione. Proc Natl Acad Sci USA 95:7631–7636

21. Cassina A, Radi R (1996) Differential inhibitory action of nitric oxide and peroxynitrite on mitochondrial electron transport. Arch Biochem Biophys 328:309–316

22. Giuffre A, Sarti P, D'Itri E, et al (2000) On the mechanism of inhibition of cytochrome c oxidase by nitric oxide. J Biol Chem 271: 33404–33408

23. Radi R, Rodriguez M, Castro L, Telleri R (1994) Inhibition of mitochondrial electron transport by peroxynitrite. Arch Bioch Biophys 308:96–102

24. Castro L, Rodriguez M, Radi R (1994) Aconitase is readily inactivated by peroxynitrite, but not its precursor, nitric oxide. J Biol Chem 269:29409–29415

25. Szabo C (1996) DNA strand breakage and activation of poly-ADP ribosyltransferase: A cytotoxic pathway triggered by peroxynitrite. Free Radic Biol Med 21:855–869

Localized Coagulation Activation and Fibrin Deposition in Critically Ill Patients

M. Levi, G. Choi, and M. J. Schultz

▌ Introduction

Most critically ill patients have an activated coagulation system. This activation of coagulation is measurable with highly sensitive assays for molecular markers of activated coagulation proteases, their activation peptides, or protease-protease-inhibitor complexes [1]. In many patients, this activation may go undetected although in the majority of them some abnormality in routine coagulation tests, such as a drop in platelet count or a minor prolongation of global coagulation tests may occur. Most clinicians do not regard these abnormalities as very relevant. In more severe forms of coagulation activation, however, it is now clear that the ensuing formation of intravascular fibrin may contribute to the pathogenesis of multiple organ failure (MOF), in particular in patients with a systemic inflammatory response, for example due to severe infection or trauma [2]. Indeed, in the majority of patients with disseminated intravascular coagulation (DIC), fibrin thrombi can be found in many organs (Table 1) [3].

The pathogenesis of the systemic activation of coagulation and microvascular fibrin formation has become more clear in recent years [4]. The trigger for the activation of the coagulation system is mediated by several pro-inflammatory cytokines, expressed and released by mononuclear cells and endothelial cells. Thrombin generation proceeds via the (extrinsic) tissue factor/factor VIIa route and simultaneously occurring depression of inhibitory mechanisms, such as antithrombin III and the protein C and S system. Also, impaired fibrin degradation, due to high cir-

Table 1. Organ involvement by (micro)thrombi in patients with disseminated intravascular coagulation [3]

Organ	Mean percentage of patients with (micro)thrombi at autopsy
▌ Kidney	70.4
▌ Lung	70.0
▌ Brain	41.1
▌ Heart	40.4
▌ Liver	39.6
▌ Spleen	39.6
▌ Adrenals	37.1
▌ Pancreas	24.1
▌ Gut	20.7

culating levels of plasminogen activator inhibitor (PAI)-1, contributes to enhanced intravascular fibrin deposition.

▌Systemic Versus Localized Responses

Although the mechanisms mentioned above have been demonstrated to occur *in vivo* as a general response upon pro-inflammatory stimuli, it is likely that marked differences in the procoagulant response, as well as the underlying pathogenetic pathway, may exist between cells and tissues [5]. This may be caused by differences in cell-specific gene expression, environmental factors, and organ specific differences. First, localization of coagulation activity may relate to a cell specific gene expression. For example, inflammatory mediators enhance PAI-1 gene expression in a complex and tissue-specific way [6]. Recent studies have demonstrated that the von Willebrand factor promotor contains cell-specific elements, and similar response elements may be involved in protein synthesis in cells in general [7]. Second, the tissue environment may determine whether specific gene transcription occurs [8]. It is not completely clear why specific sites and organs are at greater risk of developing microvascular thrombosis and also local differences in the consequences of (micro)thrombosis are still poorly understood. Environmental factors underlying the inflammatory response are thought to play a role in this differential coagulative response as well. In mice with disturbances in the plasminogen-plasmin system subjected to hypoxia, the formation of fibrin is induced and is particularly evident in the lungs [9]. In contrast, these same mice respond to endotoxemia with fibrin deposition in the microvasculature of the kidney in particular. Similarly, mice with a functional thrombomodulin deficiency had a marked increase in pulmonary fibrin deposition after hypoxic challenge [10]. In addition, when mice with a functional defect in the thrombomodulin gene were challenged with endotoxin in sublethal amounts, fibrin formation was apparent in the lungs, but not in any other organ studied. In the latter model, fibrin was only temporarily present, and had disappeared after 24 hours [11]. These models illustrate the assumption that fibrin formation is a localized phenomenon, rather than a generalized process.

Lastly, various organ systems may markedly differ in their endothelial cell response towards inflammation and injury. In general, endothelial cells play a central role in the coagulation response upon systemic inflammation [12]. The endothelium plays a central role in all major pathways involved in the pathogenesis of hemostatic derangement during severe inflammation. Endothelial cells appear to be directly involved in the initiation and regulation of thrombin generation and the inhibition of fibrin removal. Endothelial cells may express tissue factor, which is the main initiator of coagulation. In addition, physiological anticoagulant pathways, such as antithrombin, the protein C system, or tissue factor pathway inhibitor (TFPI), are mostly located on endothelial cells and endothelial cell dysfunction is directly related to impaired regulation of coagulation. Also, endothelial cells are the main storage site of plasminogen activators and inhibitors and can acutely release these factors, thereby importantly mediating fibrinolytic activity or inhibition. Pro-inflammatory cytokines are crucial in mediating these effects on endothelial cells, which themselves may also express cytokines, thereby amplifying the coagulative response [13]. Although not completely clear, various organs may differ in all these endothelial cell-related factors influencing local coagulation activation and fibrin deposition.

Organ Specific Responses by Endothelial Cells

In their excellent overview, Rosenberg and Aird postulate that endothelial cells integrate different extracellular signals and cellular responses in different regions of the vascular bed [7]. Various exogenous stimuli, such as shear stress, inflammatory mediators, and growth factors, exert their action on endothelial cells and the response of the endothelial cells to transduce the signal may vary between various tissues and even from endothelial cell to endothelial cell within a tissue. As a result, the pro- or anticoagulant response of endothelial cells may differ between organs. Experiments in mice with a targeted deletion of the anticoagulant part of the thrombomodulin gene show abundant fibrin formation in lungs, heart, and spleen [14]. Mice with homozygous deficiencies of plasminogen activators form clots in liver, heart, and lungs, but not in brain or kidneys [15]. PAI deficient mice have fibrin deposition predominantly in kidneys [6]. Rosenberg and Aird state that various mechanisms play a role in the individual response of endothelial cells [7]. Cell-to-cell communication may have important effects, as evidenced by the fact that PAI-1 expression in endothelial cells is upregulated if the culture is incubated with medium from aorta or umbilical vein cell culture but, in contrast, is downregulated by addition of conditioned medium from vascular smooth muscle cells [16, 17]. In addition, cell signaling pathways may vary between endothelial cell subtypes. For example, hemodynamic changes may have opposite reactions in nitric oxide (NO) mRNA expression in endothelial cells from the aorta or from the pulmonary artery [18]. Another example is provided by the experiment showing that endothelial cells from renal and cerebrovascular vessels have decreased prostacyclin production and more apoptosis when exposed to plasma of patients with thrombocytopenic thrombotic purpura, whereas endothelial cells derived from lungs and liver do not respond to this same stimulus [19]. Lastly, also at the level of transcription a differential phenotype of endothelial cells between various organs can be demonstrated. Coagulation proteins, such as von Willebrand factor, have been shown to respond to various promoters by expressing this factor in different tissues, for example exclusively in heart and skeletal muscle or in brain [8]. All these various mechanisms render the endothelial cells with an extreme capacity for differential response to various stimuli in different organs and for integrating multiple extracellular signals within one organ.

Coagulation Activation and the Kidney

Coagulation is important in two groups of renal disorders in man. In one group, the kidney is the major site of disease and localized thrombosis and fibrin formation is superimposed on demonstrable immunological and or endothelial damage. These disorders will not be discussed here. In the second group, renal lesions associated with fibrin formation are involved as a consequence of systemic intravascular coagulation or DIC [20]. In the latter group, acute renal failure is the usual associated renal presentation, occurring in the course of sepsis, major surgery, severe trauma, hypovolemic and cardiogenic shock. The pathogenesis of acute renal failure in these conditions is caused by hypoperfusion resulting in ischemia-reperfusion injury. The decrease in oxygen saturation and hormonal dysregulation causes acute tubular necrosis [21]. In septic shock it has been suggested that microthrombi contribute to acute renal failure [22, 23]. The older literature strongly suggests that intravascular coagulation causes immediate changes that are detrimental to renal function. Electron microscope studies have shown that coagulation causes mesangial swelling and an increase in vacuoles, organelle free ribosomes, and mitochondria [24]. These changes were associated with phagocytosis of fibrin and secretion of basement membrane like material. The glomerular lesions occurring in the course of DIC may resemble those seen in acute glomerulonephritis, with platelets and fibrin deposits intraluminally, swollen endothelium, subendothelial deposits of fibrin cleavage fragments, and cellular proliferative effects. When these processes continue, complete occlusion of glomerular capillaries and hyalinization of glomeruli may follow [20]. The pathophysiology of renal failure in shock is also thought to be influenced by vasoactive substances, and renal damage was markedly reduced by adrenergic blockade in a model of hemorrhagic shock or endotoxin shock [25]. Catecholamine infusion in experimental animals causes shock and DIC. Heparin reduces the effects of catecholamine-induced shock and endotoxin related complications in animal models. It thus appears that the combination of hypoperfusion related ischemia-reperfusion injury and vasoactive reactions are of major influence on the occurrence of acute renal failur in shock. The finding of fibrin deposits suggests that DIC contributes to organ damage, and the observed improvement under heparin treatment supports this concept. The trigger to thrombosis is probably locally induced by the ischemia-reperfusion responses of hypoxia inducible factor (HIF) mediated tissue factor expression [26]. In addition, systemic stimuli such as endotoxin cause cytokine mediated upregulation of tissue factor mRNA in the kidney, while local fibrinolytic defense mechanisms are also activated (urokinase-type plasminogen activator [uPA] and tissue-type plasminogen activator [t-PA], without concurrent upregulation of PAI-1). Furthermore, experimental studies have demonstrated that specific blockade of the factor VII-tissue factor complex reduced fibrin in the kidney [27]. Infusion of hirudin caused a dose dependent decrease in mortality, and also reduced the amount of fibrin deposition in the kidney. An important role of the protein C system in preventing glomerular thrombosis may be inferred from the abundant presence of thrombomodulin expression on endothelial cells in the glomerulus [28]. In inflammatory glomerular disease, such as acute membranoproliferative or lupus glomerulonephritis, an increase in thrombomodulin expression has been implicated [29]. In contrast, in ischemia-reperfusion injury in kidneys, thrombomodulin has been markedly downregulated. Administration of soluble thrombomodulin to rats with renal ischemia-reperfusion injury prevented massive glomerular thrombosis and kidney dysfunction [30]. In another experimental study of renal ischemia and reperfusion, administration of activated protein C (APC) prevented histological changes and the decrease in renal blood flow, and preserved kidney function, whereas treatment with active site-blocked factor Xa, heparin and inactivated protein C were less effective [31]. It therefore appears that inhibition of coagulation also reduces the amount of fibrin in the kidney. This may imply an improvement in renal function, however, there have been no controlled trials in which the beneficial effect of anticoagulant treatment in patients with DIC and acute renal failure was investigated.

▌ Coagulation Activation and the Lung

The lungs are amongst the most frequently affected organs during severe infection and sepsis [32, 33]. Lung injury in this situation is characterized by increased permeability of the alveolar-capillary membrane, diffuse alveolar damage, and the accumulation of pulmonary edema, containing a high concentration of proteases and other proteins. Pathological examination of the injured lung demonstrates epithelial cell injury represented by extensive necrosis of pneumocytes, swelling of endothelial cells with the widening of intercellular junctions, and the formation of hyaline membranes, for an important part composed of fibrin in alveolar ducts and airspaces. At later stages, massive infiltration of neutrophils and other inflammatory cells will occur and fibrin thrombi can be seen in the alveolar capillaries and smaller pulmonary arteries [34]. The abundant presence of intravascular and extravascular fibrin appears to be a specific hallmark of acute lung injury (ALI) following sepsis and is much more outspoken than the fibrin deposition in other organs. Based on this observation, many authors have hypothesized that fibrin deposition plays an important role in the pathogenesis of ALI in sepsis, a concept that is further supported by large clinical studies in patients with sepsis demonstrating the association between lung injury and coagulation abnormalities [35]. Furthermore, the extensive local fibrin deposition may suggest that local activation of coagulation or perturbation of local physiological regulatory systems could be involved in this. Interestingly, it has been shown that effective blocking of the coagulopathy in experimental sepsis attenuates lung injury and local inflammatory activity, which may point at pivotal cross-talk between the (local) mechanisms of coagulation and inflammation [36, 37].

In bronchoalveolar (BAL) fluid from patients with acute respiratory distress syndrome (ARDS), it has been demonstrated that there is activation of coagulation and inhibition of fibrinolysis [38–40]. Almost immediately after the onset of ARDS, an increased but transient procoagulant activity can be detected in BAL fluid. At the same time, fibrinolytic activity is strongly inhibited, and is kept at a low level up to 14 days. Experimental and clinical studies have shown that fibrin deposition is due to tissue factor-mediated thrombin generation and suppressed fibrinolysis [41]. The most important determinants of these local disturbances are tissue factor and PAI-1; high levels of soluble tissue factor can be measured in BAL fluid from patients with ARDS, while increased production of PAI-1 is the most consistent finding reported as being related to suppressed fibrinolytic activity. Recently, lower levels of pulmonary protein C levels were correlated with a higher degree of lung injury and worse outcome in patients with ALI [42].

Similar to ALI and ARDS, pneumonia is characterized by a shift in the alveolar haemostatic balance. In BAL fluid from patients with severe pneumonia a markedly increased procoagulant activity was detected. Concordantly, fibrinolytic activity was depressed in BAL fluid, related to high concentrations of PAI-1 in the lungs. Patients at risk of ventilator-associated pneumonia show similar changes in pulmonary fibrin turnover [43]. Similarly, in mechanically ventilated patients who developed pneumonia, an increase in coagulation products was detected in lung lavage fluids. Interestingly, the diagnosis of pneumonia was preceded by a strong increase in PAI-1 levels in the lungs, with a resulting decrease in fibrinolytic activity. Similar to the inflammatory responses in patients with unilateral pneumonia patients, there is overt activation of coagulation, and depressed fibrinolytic activity due to PAI-1 upregulation [44]. Recently it has been demonstrated that the protein C system is also suppressed at the site of infection, contributing to the procoagulant effects of pulmonary infection [44].

Coagulation Activation and the Intestinal Tract

Acute intestinal ischemia and reperfusion may result in impaired intestinal structure and function, in experimental models characterized by intestinal cell swelling and protein leakage and impaired intestinal absorptive capacity. In addition, intra- and extravascular fibrin deposits may be present, due to activation of mesenteric coagulation and inhibition of fibrinolysis [45]. Upon 20 to 40 minutes occlusion of the superior mesenteric artery and subsequent reperfusion, portal vein plasma levels of thrombin-antithrombin levels increased, indicating local thrombin generation. This increase in portal coagulation activity is associated with a marked fall in protein C activity levels. Simultaneously, markers for fibrinolysis in portal plasma showed a complete inhibition, due to an increase in levels of PAI-1. This activation of coagulation upon ischemia-reperfusion could be almost completely blocked by systemic administration of APC, whereas heparin and antithrombin were less effective (Schoots et al., unpublished data). Interestingly, amelioration of ischemia-reperfusion-induced intestinal intra- and extravascular fibrin deposition by administration of APC caused a significant improvement in intestinal function.

Coagulation Activation and the Liver

The liver is the major site of synthesis of almost all coagulation factors. In addition, Kupffer cells of the liver are most important bacterial scavengers, neutralize bacterial products, and pro-inflammatory cytokines. Impaired synthesis of the physiological anticoagulant proteins antithrombin and protein C, and low levels of free protein S due to acute phase upregulation of C4b-binding protein (the carrier of protein S) are well known consequences of impaired liver function [46]. However, failure of the coagulation system is not only a consequence of liver failure but may also contribute to the pathogenesis of liver failure in systemic inflammatory states. Under these circumstances endothelial cells of the liver show a marked upregulation of tissue factor, leading to local thrombin generation and fibrinogen to fibrin conversion [47]. A marked cross-talk between coagulation and inflammation is also strongly present in liver tissue, as protease activated receptors (PARs) are abundantly present and activated coagulation proteases may not only lead to fibrin formation but also to increased inflammation, and in case of liver tissue, ultimately to tissue fibrosis [48]. Indeed, it has been shown that anticoagulant treatment can prevent ischemia-reperfusion injury in an experimental model in rat livers [49].

Conclusion

The response of the coagulation system upon systemic inflammation may vary considerably between cells, tissues, and organs. This may explain, in part, the variable clinical presentation of MOF in patients with a systemic inflammatory response upon sepsis or trauma. Many coagulation pathways in various organs may act according to parallel routes but marked differences exist in the emphasis of a specific mechanism in a specific organ system. Detailed knowledge on the site specific activation and regulation of coagulation may provide more insight into better management strategies in case of specific organ failures in the setting of a systemic inflammatory response.

References

1. Bauer KA, Rosenberg RD (1987) The pathophysiology of the prethrombotic state in humans: insights gained from studies using markers of hemostatic system activation. Blood 70:343–350
2. Levi M, ten Cate H (1999) Disseminated intravascular coagulation. N Engl J Med 341:586–592
3. Marder VJ, Feinstein D, Francis C, et al (1994) Consumptive thrombohemorrhagic disorders. In: Colman RW, Hirsh J, Marder VJ, et al (eds) Hemostasis and Thrombosis. Basic Principles and Clinical Practice. JB Lippincott Company, Philadelphia, pp 1023–1056
4. Levi M (2004) Current understanding of disseminated intravascular coagulation. Br J Haematol 124:567–576
5. Aird WC (2001) Vascular bed-specific hemostasis: role of endothelium in sepsis pathogenesis. Crit Care Med 29:S28–S34
6. Sawdey MS, Loskutoff DJ (1991) Regulation of murine type 1 plasminogen activator inhibitor gene expression in vivo. Tissue specificity and induction by lipopolysaccharide, tumor necrosis factor-alpha, and transforming growth factor-beta. J Clin Invest 88:1346–1353
7. Rosenberg RD, Aird WC (1999) Vascular-bed–specific hemostasis and hypercoagulable states. N Engl J Med 340:1555–1564
8. Aird WC, Edelberg JM, Weiler-Guettler H, Simmons WW, Smith TW, Rosenberg RD (1997) Vascular bed-specific expression of an endothelial cell gene is programmed by the tissue microenvironment. J Cell Biol 138:1117–1124
9. Yamamoto K, Loskutoff DJ (1996) Fibrin deposition in tissues from endotoxin-treated mice correlates with decreases in the expression of urokinase-type but not tissue-type plasminogen activator. J Clin Invest 97:2440–2451
10. Healy AM, Hancock WW, Christie PD, Rayburn HB, Rosenberg RD (1998) Intravascular coagulation activation in a murine model of thrombomodulin deficiency: effects of lesion size, age, and hypoxia on fibrin deposition. Blood 92:4188–4197
11. ten Cate H (2000) Pathophysiology of disseminated intravascular coagulation in sepsis. Crit Care Med 28 (Suppl 9):S9–S11
12. Levi M, van Der PT, Buller HR (2004) Bidirectional relation between inflammation and coagulation. Circulation 109:2698–2704
13. Levi M, van der Poll T, ten Cate H, van Deventer SJ (1997) The cytokine-mediated imbalance between coagulant and anticoagulant mechanisms in sepsis and endotoxaemia. Eur J Clin Invest 27:3–9
14. Weiler H, Lindner V, Kerlin B, et al (2001) Characterization of a mouse model for thrombomodulin deficiency. Arterioscler Thromb Vasc Biol. 21:1531–1537
15. Pinsky DJ, Liao H, Lawson CA, et al (1998) Coordinated induction of plasminogen activator inhibitor-1 (PAI-1) and inhibition of plasminogen activator gene expression by hypoxia promotes pulmonary vascular fibrin deposition. J Clin Invest 102:919–928
16. Christ G, Seiffert D, Hufnagl P, Gessl A, Wojta J, Binder BR (1993) Type 1 plasminogen activator inhibitor synthesis of endothelial cells is downregulated by smooth muscle cells. Blood 81:1277–1283
17. Gallicchio M, Argyriou S, Ianches G, et al (1994) Stimulation of PAI-1 expression in endothelial cells by cultured vascular smooth muscle cells. Arterioscler Thromb 14:815–823
18. Everett AD, Le Cras TD, Xue C, Johns RA (1998) eNOS expression is not altered in pulmonary vascular remodeling due to increased pulmonary blood flow. Am J Physiol 274:L1058–L1065
19. Mitra D, Jaffe EA, Weksler B, Hajjar KA, Soderland C, Laurence J (1997) Thrombotic thrombocytopenic purpura and sporadic hemolytic-uremic syndrome plasmas induce apoptosis in restricted lineages of human microvascular endothelial cells. Blood 89:1224–1234

20. Kincaid-Smith P (1972) Coagulation and renal disease. Kidney Int 2:183–190
21. Conlon PJ, Kovalik E, Schwab SJ (1995) Percutaneous renal biopsy of ventilated intensive care unit patients. Clin Nephrol 43:309–311
22. Davenport A (1997) The coagulation system in the critically ill patient with acute renal failure and the effect of an extracorporeal circuit. Am J Kidney Dis 30:S20–S27
23. Kanfer A (1992) Glomerular coagulation system in renal diseases. Ren Fail 14:407–412
24. Vassali P, Simon G, Rouiller C (1963) Electron microscopic study of glomerular lesions resulting from intravascular fibrin formation. Am J Pathol 43:579–617
25. Grandchamp A, Ayer G, Truniger B (1971) Pathogenesis of redistribution of intrarenal blood flow in haemorrhagic hypotension. Eur J Clin Invest 1:271–276
26. O'Rourke JF, Pugh CW, Bartlett SM, Ratcliffe PJ (1996) Identification of hypoxically inducible mRNAs in HeLa cells using differential-display PCR. Role of hypoxia-inducible factor-1. Eur J Biochem 241:403–410
27. Yamazaki M, Asakura H, Aoshima K, et al (1994) Effects of DX-9065a, an orally active, newly synthesized and specific inhibitor of factor Xa, against experimental disseminated intravascular coagulation in rats. Thromb Haemost 72:392–396
28. Terada Y, Eguchi Y, Nosaka S, Toba T, Nakamura T, Shimizu Y (2003) Capillary endothelial thrombomodulin expression and fibrin deposition in rats with continuous and bolus lipopolysaccharide administration. Lab Invest 83:1165–1173
29. Mizutani M, Yuzawa Y, Maruyama I, Sakamoto N, Matsuo S (1993) Glomerular localization of thrombomodulin in human glomerulonephritis. Lab Invest 69:193–202
30. Ikeguchi H, Maruyama S, Morita Y, et al (2002) Effects of human soluble thrombomodulin on experimental glomerulonephritis. Kidney Int 61:490–501
31. Mizutani A, Okajima K, Uchiba M, Noguchi T (2000) Activated protein C reduces ischemia/reperfusion-induced renal injury in rats by inhibiting leukocyte activation. Blood 95:3781–3787
32. Idell S (1994) Extravascular coagulation and fibrin deposition in acute lung injury. New Horiz 2:566–574
33. Martin GS, Bernard GR (2001) Airway and lung in sepsis. Intensive Care Med 27(Suppl 1): S63–S79
34. Bellingan GJ (2002) The pulmonary physician in critical care * 6: The pathogenesis of ALI/ARDS. Thorax 57:540–546
35. Welty-Wolf KE, Carraway MS, Ortel TL, Piantadosi CA (2002) Coagulation and inflammation in acute lung injury. Thromb Haemost 88:17–25
36. Miller DL, Welty-Wolf K, Carraway MS, et al (2002) Extrinsic coagulation blockade attenuates lung injury and proinflammatory cytokine release after intratracheal lipopolysaccharide. Am J Respir Cell Mol Biol 26:650–658
37. Welty-Wolf KE, Carraway MS, Miller DL, et al (2001) Coagulation blockade prevents sepsis-induced respiratory and renal failure in baboons. Am J Respir Crit Care Med 164:1988–1996
38. Bertozzi P, Astedt B, Zenzius L, et al (1990) Depressed bronchoalveolar urokinase activity in patients with adult respiratory distress syndrome. N Engl J Med 322:890–897
39. Idell S (1994) Extravascular coagulation and fibrin deposition in acute lung injury. New Horiz 2:566–574
40. Fuchs-Buder T, de Moerloose P, Ricou B, et al (1996) Time course of procoagulant activity and D dimer in bronchoalveolar fluid of patients at risk for or with acute respiratory distress syndrome. Am J Respir Crit Care Med 153:163–167
41. Levi M, van der Poll T, ten Cate H, et al (1998) Differential effects of anti-cytokine treatment on bronchoalveolar hemostasis in endotoxemic chimpanzees. Am J Respir Crit Care Med 158:92–98
42. Ware LB, Fang X, Matthay MA (2003) Protein C and thrombomodulin in human acute lung injury. Am J Physiol Lung Cell Mol Physiol 285:L514–L521
43. Schultz MJ, Millo J, Levi M, et al (2004) Local activation of coagulation and inhibition of fibrinolysis in the lung during ventilator associated pneumonia. Thorax 59:130–135
44. Choi G, Schultz MJ, van Till JW, et al (2004) Disturbed alveolar fibrin turnover during pneumonia is restricted to the site of infection. Eur Respir J 24:786–789
45. Schoots IG, Levi M, Roossink EH, Bijlsma PB, Van Gulik TM (2003) Local intravascular coagulation and fibrin deposition on intestinal ischemia-reperfusion in rats. Surgery 133:411–419

46. Dhainaut JF, Marin N, Mignon A, Vinsonneau C (2001) Hepatic response to sepsis: interaction between coagulation and inflammatory processes. Crit Care Med 29:S42–S47
47. Kobayashi Y, Yoshimura N, Yamagishi H, Oka T (1998) Role of tissue factor in ischemic reperfusion injury: (I). Tissue factor levels of liver tissue and serum after hepatic injury in rats. Transplant Proc 30:3726–3727
48. Chambers RC, Laurent GJ (2002) Coagulation cascade proteases and tissue fibrosis. Biochem Soc Trans 30:194–200
49. Hisama N, Yamaguchi Y, Okajima K, et al (1996) Anticoagulant pretreatment attenuates production of cytokine-induced neutrophil chemoattractant following ischemia-reperfusion of rat liver. Dig Dis Sci 41:1481–1486

The Central and Autonomic Nervous Systems: Essential Regulators of the Immune Response

D. J. van Westerloo, I. A. J. Giebelen, and T. van der Poll

"The brain is the last and grandest biological frontier, the most complex thing we have yet discovered in our universe. The brain boggles the mind."
James D. Watson (*from Discovering the Brain*, National Academy Press, 1992)

▌ Introduction

Of all the organs in our body, the brain is the most versatile and poses the greatest mystery. It contains hundreds of billions of cells interlinked through trillions of connections which generate our thoughts, houses our 'soul', makes us sense, feel, and move through the somatic and sensory nervous system, and orchestrates essential life functions through the autonomic nervous system. The brain consists of extensively connected subsystems, such as the brain stem, limbic system, hypothalamus, and cerebral cortex and many others which are all directly or indirectly connected to sensory (afferent) and effector (efferent) pathways reaching virtually any location in the body. The autonomic nervous system relays input on all vital processes in the body to the brain and controls our heart rate, respiratory rate, blood pressure, gut motility, body temperature, and virtually any essential involuntary process. One could say that in any vital process that takes place there is 'always a brain attached'. Although it is widely accepted that virtually any vital process is supervised and controlled by the central nervous system (CNS), our innate immune response has long been regarded as a totally peripheral system regulated by the interaction of immune competent cells with pathogens and with each other. In this chapter, we will review data that suggest that communication between the immune, nervous, and endocrine systems is in fact an essential homeostatic system that regulates the innate immune response. First we will discuss the classic regulation of innate immunity and the physiological anatomy of the autonomic nervous system; second we will discuss new insights in immune to brain and brain to immune communication and finally focus on the cholinergic anti-inflammatory pathway and the important physiological insights and therapeutic opportunities that arise from the concept that activation of innate immunity is, at least in part, regulated in the CNS.

Classic Regulation of Innate Immunity: the Balance Between Pro- and Anti-Inflammation

Inflammation is a physiologic response of the host to either invasion of micro organisms or local injury. The innate immune system is the first line of defense against invading pathogens. Invading pathogens activate the cells of the innate immune system by a variety of, pathogen class specific, stimuli [1]. As a result of these triggers immune competent cells are activated to release a plethora of pro-inflammatory soluble mediators, such as cytokines (e.g., tumor necrosis factor [TNF]-α, interleukin [IL]-1) and chemokines (e.g., IL-8) [2]. The goal of this inflammatory reaction is to restrain and localize the infection to the infected compartment of the body and ultimately clear the pathogen and remove the injury.

However, the release of all these mediators can be detrimental to the host [3]. Inflammatory reactions must be fine-tuned and regulated in a precise manner since exaggerated inflammation may lead to tissue damage and morbidity. Indeed, in recent years many common diseases have been recognized as 'inflammatory conditions', including atherosclerosis, ischemia reperfusion injury, rheumatoid arthritis, inflammatory bowel disease and fulminant sepsis [2, 4]. In these diseases, there is an induction of the innate immune system, and activation and migration of neutrophils and the cytokine network. To keep the potentially detrimental effects of the pro-inflammatory system in check an anti-inflammatory cytokine system (e.g. IL-10, IL-4) counterbalances the pro-inflammatory systems. In health and disease, the balance between pro- and anti-inflammatory systems is essential to maintain a delicate homeostasis which ensures an adequate host defense with minimal collateral damage due to over aggressive responses of the innate immune system. On the basis of this concept, new therapies have been developed in recent years. Elimination of TNF-α by monoclonal antibodies restores the inflammatory balance and effectively treats 'pro-inflammatory diseases' such as Crohn's disease and rheumatoid arthritis [5].

Physiological Anatomy of the Autonomic Nervous System

The autonomic nervous system provides constant and extremely rapid control of visceral functions, such as arterial pressure, gastrointestinal motility and secretion, urinary bladder emptying, sweating, body temperature, and many other activities of which some are totally and others partially controlled by the autonomic nervous system. The autonomic nervous system consists of sensory neurons and motor neurons that run between the CNS (especially the hypothalamus and medulla oblongata) and internal organs. It differs from the sensory-somatic system in using two groups of motor neurons to stimulate the effectors instead of one. Preganglionic neurons arise in the CNS and run into a ganglion where they synapse with a postganglionic neuron that runs all the way into the effector region. The autonomic nervous system has two subdivisions that usually act reciprocally of each other: the sympathetic and the parasympathetic nervous system.

The motor neurons of the sympathetic nervous system arise in the spinal cord and pass into two large chains of perivertrebral ganglia. Here the preganglionic neuron can synapse directly with a postganglionic neuron, travel up or down the chain to synapse in a ganglion at another level with postganglionic neurons or travel up or downward and terminate in one of the prevertebral ganglia. Either way, from the ganglion the postganglionic fibers travel all the way to their destination in the various organs where norepinephrine is released by the postganglionic neuron. One exception is the sympathetic innervation of the adrenal medulla. Here, preganglionic fibers travel all the way to the medulla without synapsing and end directly on neuronal cells that secrete epinephrine and norepinephrine into the blood stream. The release of norepinephrine results in stimulation of the heartbeat, a rise in blood pressure, dilatation of the bronchi, a shunt of blood away from non-vital organs, and an inhibition of bladder and gastrointestinal peristalsis. Activation of the sympathetic nervous system results in generalized responses since preganglionic neurons usually synapse with many postganglionic neurons and also because the release of epinephrine by the adrenal medulla ensures that even body sites that are not reached by postganglionic sympathetic neurons will be drenched with epinephrine. In short, stimulation of the sympathetic branch of the autonomic nervous system prepares the body for emergency: usually referred to as 'fight or flight' reactions.

About 75% of parasympathetic nerves fibers arise from the tenth cranial nerves, the vagus nerves. Other sympathetic innervation comes from cranial nerves III, VII, and IX and from the second and third sacral spinal nerves. The two vagus nerves originate in the medulla oblongata and wander all the way through the cervical area (where one vagus nerve travels right and the other left of the trachea) and the thoracic and abdominal regions of the body. At several locations both vagus nerves meet and share fibers with each other. The vagus nerve supplies parasympathetic innervation to the heart, the lungs, the esophagus, the small intestine, the proximal half of the colon, the liver, the pancreas, the ureters, and the spleen. Just as the sympathetic nervous system, the vagus nerve has both preganglionic and postganglionic neurons. However, the preganglionic fibers travel uninterrupted to their destination and synapse with postganglionic fibers inside the target organ where short postganglionic fibers spread throughout the organ. Parasympathetic stimulation causes slowing of the heartbeat, lowering of blood pressure, and activation of gastrointestinal peristalsis. In short, parasympathetic innervation returns the body to its resting state after it has been activated by the sympathetic nervous system.

Sympathetic and parasympathetic neurons all secrete one of the two synaptic neurotransmitters, acetylcholine (cholinergic neurons) or norepinephrine (adrenergic neurons). All preganglionic neurons, as well as the postganglionic neurons of the parasympathetic division, are cholinergic whereas (except for sweat glands) postganglionic sympathetic neurons are adrenergic. Before acetylcholine or norepinephrine can exert effects on the target organ they need to bind to specific receptors. Usually binding of a neurotransmitter to a receptor results in either a change in cellular membrane permeability or in the alteration of intracellular enzymes, such as in the case of norepinephrine binding where cyclic AMP (cAMP) is formed in response to receptor binding [6]. Acetylcholine activates two different receptors, muscarinic and nicotinic acetylcholine receptors. Muscarinic receptors are found in all effector cells stimulated by postganglionic neurons whereas nicotinic receptors are found in the synapses between pre and postganglionic neurons. Adrenergic receptors can be divided into α- and β-receptors. Stimulation of α- and β-receptors sometimes has contrary effects on target organs, implicating that the effects of epinephrine and norepinephrine on organs is dependent on the type of receptors present in the particular organ.

▌ Interactions between the CNS and the Immune System

The CNS and the immune system have several important features in common. Both systems are designed to constantly survey the body for danger and mount an appropriate response to these threats. In contrast to classical thinking, these two systems act together in orchestrating the immune response in response to infection or injury. Stimulation or ablation of several regions of the brain can alter immune responses; secondly, inflammatory processes can alter the firing rate of CNS neurons. Thus, there is a cross talk between inflammatory cells and the CNS that can go towards as well as away from an inflamed site of the body.

Immune to Brain Communication

The CNS receives sensory input from the immune system through both humoral and neural routes (Fig. 1). IL-1β, TNF-α, and other immunologically active mediators, can signal the brain in circumscript areas [7]. These so called circumventricular organs include specific sites in the hypothalamus as well as the dorsal vagal complex (DVC) [8]. The DVC consists of the nucleus tractus solitarius (NTS), the dorsal motor nucleus of the vagus (DMN), and the area postrema (Fig. 1) [9]. The DMN is the major site of origin of efferent vagal neurons whereas the main portion of vagal sensory input is received by neurons in the NTS. The area postrema, which lacks a tight blood-brain barrier, is an important circumventricular organ and site for humoral immune-to-brain communication [7]. In fact, reversible inactivation of the DVC completely blocks endotoxin-induced behavioral changes and expression of c-FOS (neuronal activation marker) in forebrain regions of endotoxemic animals [8]. Exactly how cytokines are able to cross the blood brain barrier at these sites and activate the CNS is a matter of debate. Some studies suggest there is active transport of cytokines across the blood brain barrier [6]. Others implicate receptors for cytokines and for bacterial fragments that are constitutively expressed in cells within circumventricular organs and upregulated during inflammation [7]. Binding of cytokines to these receptors induces responses including changes in electrical activity of neurons, induction of transcription factors leading to modifications in gene expression during inflammation, and to a localized release of secondary signal molecules which are able to cross the blood brain barrier [7].

Neural pathways, predominantly the vagus nerve, also signal the brain for danger (Fig. 1) [10]. Cytokines and bacterial products such as endotoxin stimulate afferent neural fibers in the vagus nerve that are processed in the brain and result in the initiation of an acute phase response, induction of fever and upregulation of IL-1β in the brain [10–12].

Fig. 1. Immune to brain communication. The brain receives information from the immune system by humoral as well as neural pathways. Cytokines elicit signaling in the afferent vagus nerve which reach the nucleus tractus solitarius (NTS). From here, projections lead via the area postrema (AP) to the hypothalamus and subsequently the pituitary gland , and also to the dorsal motor nucleus (DMN) of the vagus nerve and the rostro ventrolateral medulla (RVM). All these nuclei are involved in generating responses of the brain back to the immune system (see Fig. 2). Via the humoral route, cytokines can signal through circumventricular organs such as the AP

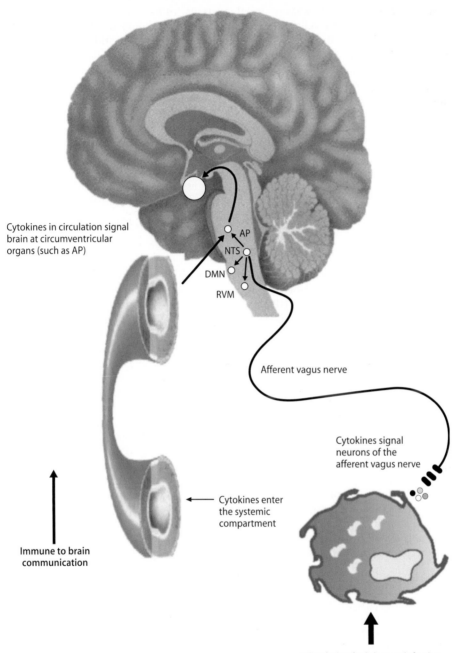

Cytokines in circulation signal
brain at circumventricular
organs (such as AP)

AP

NTS

DMN

RVM

Afferent vagus nerve

Cytokines signal
neurons of the
afferent vagus nerve

Cytokines enter
the systemic
compartment

Immune to brain
communication

Stimulation by injury or infection

Immunogenic stimuli activate vagal afferents either directly by cytokines re-leased by inflammatory cells at the site of infection or injury or indirectly through chemoreceptive cells located in vagal paraganglia [13]. After stimulation by cyto-kines, vagal afferent fibers transmit signals to the DVC [13, 14] where most sensory information is relayed to the NTS.

Whether humoral or neural pathways are essential in relaying information on the presence of inflammation to the brain is largely dependent on the magnitude of the inflammatory response. In experimental studies, it has been shown that when the level of inflammation is low, such as when a low dose of endotoxin is injected intraperitoneally, vagotomy inhibits the stimulation of the hypothalamus-pituitary-adrenal (HPA) axis and the induction of IL-1 in the brain [10, 11] whereas high doses of endotoxin induce responses by the brain independent of the vagus nerve [15, 16]. This implies that neural pathways are essential in the relay of localized in-flammation whereas information about severe systemic inflammation reaches the brain predominantly through humoral pathways.

Brain to Immune Communication

Neuro-endocrine Pathways. When notified of ongoing inflammation, either by humoral or neural pathways as described above, the brain exerts strong anti-inflammatory ef-fects through activation of the HPA axis (Fig. 2). Information received via the afferent vagus in the NTS is relayed to the hypothalamus, which may induce release of a-me-lanocyte stimulating hormone (a-MSH) and corticotropin releasing hormone (CRH). CRH induces adrenocorticotropin hormone (ACTH) release by the pituitary gland and activates a neural-endocrine anti-inflammatory pathway [11, 13, 17]. Upon ACTH stimulation, cortisol is released by the adrenal medulla. Cortisol inhibits pro-inflam-matory gene expression by immune cells by binding to an intracellular receptor with subsequent suppression of nuclear factor kappa B (NF-κB) activity as well as activa-tion of transcription of anti-inflammatory genes [18].

Hard Wired Connections. The CNS and the immune system are directly linked through the autonomic nervous system (Fig. 2). Direct contact between postgan-glionic neurons of the autonomic nervous system and immune cells, either with immune cells in lymphoid organs or with residential or migrated immune cells lo-cated in an inflamed area, provides a direct hard wired link for the CNS to modu-late inflammatory responses *in vivo*. Lymphoid organs are innervated by the para-sympathetic nervous system as well as the sympathetic nervous system [19]. Furthermore, lymphocytes, granulocytes and macrophages have been shown to car-

————————————————————————————➤

Fig. 2. Brain to immune communication. Brain to immune pathways are activated by signals reaching the brain though the systemic compartment and the vagus nerve. The brain responds by activating a neuro-endocrine pathway through the release of adrenocorticotropin releasing hormone (ACTH), which activates cortisol release by the adrenal medulla as well as a-melanocyte stimulating hormone (a-MSH). Cortisol inhibits immune cells through intracellular receptors, a-MSH through the MC4 receptor. Also, vagal efferent activity is activated through the dorsal motor nucleus (DMN), which results in the release of ace-tylcholine (Ach) at vagal post synaptic neurons, inhibiting immune cells through the nicotinic acetylcho-line $a7$ receptor. Furthermore the sympathetic nervous system (SNS) is activated and epinephrine (EN) is released by the adrenal cortex and norepinephrine (NE) at postsynaptic SNS neurons. Both epinephrine and norepinephrine inhibit immune cells through β-receptors

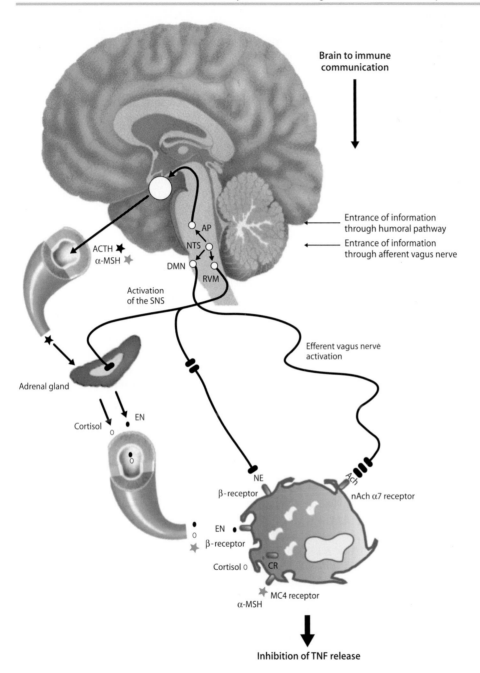

ry receptors for acetylcholine [20, 21] as well as norepinephrine [22] but also for various other substances released by neurones such as vasoactive intestinal peptide (VIP) [23], a-MSH [24] and leptin [24].

Sympathetic Nervous System: Stimulation of Beta Receptors on Immune Cells

The autonomic nervous system is activated upon detection of inflammation either directly or via activation of the NTS through the afferent vagus nerve. With regard to the sympathetic nervous system, there are connections of the NTS with nuclei, such as the rostro ventrolateral medulla (RVM), that activate the sympathetic nervous system (Fig. 2) [25]. Activation of preganglionic neurons of the sympathetic nervous system induces the release of epinephrine by the adrenal medulla into the bloodstream, converting a neural pathway into an endocrine anti-inflammatory pathway, since in response to catecholamines monocytes release less pro inflammatory mediators and are stimulated to produce IL-10 [6, 22, 26, 27]. The major importance of this pathway is shown by experiments where the infusion of β-agonists in humans and animals reduces inflammation during experimental endotoxemia whereas β-receptor antagonists stimulate pro-inflammatory responses [22]. The importance of the sympathetic nervous system in inhibiting the immune response is illustrated by several elegant experiments. In a mouse model of stroke, the hypothesis that a stroke-induced immunodeficiency increased the susceptibility to bacterial infections was tested. Indeed, mice developed spontaneous pneumonia within three days after the induction of stroke. Administration of the β-adrenoreceptor antagonist propranolol drastically reduced the incidence of pneumonia, the defect in lymphocyte activation, and mortality after stroke [27]. This suggests that immunosuppression during stroke is actually catecholamine-mediated. Furthermore, norepinephrine is released by postganglionic neurons which directly affects nearby immune cells through β receptors (Fig. 2).

Parasympathetic Nervous System: the Cholinergic Anti-inflammatory Pathway

Upon activation of the NTS, projections to the area postrema stimulate the HPA axis and projections to the RVM activate the sympathetic nervous system (Fig. 3). However, direct connections between the NTS and the DMN ensure that when signals reach the NTS vagal efferent activity is stimulated as well (Fig. 3). Release of acetylcholine by postganglionic neurons of the vagus nerve inhibits the release of pro-inflammatory cytokines by immune cells (Fig. 3).

In vitro studies have shown that immune cells are susceptible to acetylcholine. When macrophages are exposed to acetylcholine, the principle parasympathetic neurotransmitter, these cells are effectively deactivated [20]. This acetylcholine-induced deactivation is characterized by a dose-dependent reduction in the release of a series of pro-inflammatory cytokines, including TNF-a, IL-1β, IL-6, and IL-18, by macrophages stimulated with endotoxin [20]. Acetylcholine acts through two types of receptors: muscarinic and nicotinic. In addition to the brain and "wire-innervated" peripheral structures, these acetylcholine receptor subtypes are also ex-

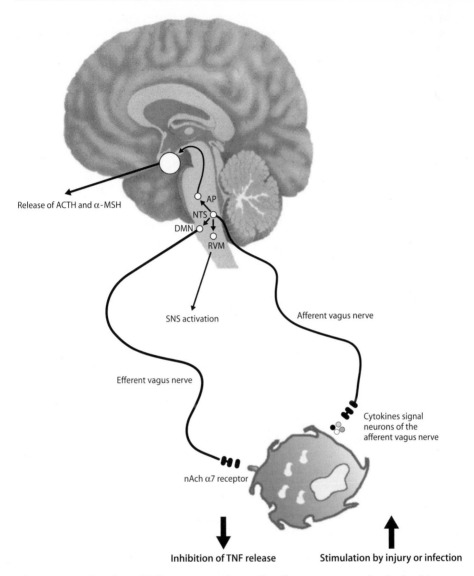

Fig. 3. The cholinergic anti-inflammatory pathway. The afferent vagus nerve is stimulated by cytokines. Information is relayed to nucleus tractus solitarius (NTS). From here, projections lead to the area postrema (AP); this nucleus connects to the hypothalamus which activates the HPA axis. Second, projections to the rostro ventrolateral medulla (RVM) activate the sympathetic nervous system and epinephrine (EN) is released by the adrenal cortex and norepinephrine (NE) at postsynaptic SNS neurons. Finally, through the dorsal motor nucleus (DMN) vagal efferent activity is activated through the dorsal motor nucleus (DMN), which results in the release of acetylcholine (Ach) at vagal post synaptic neurons, inhibiting immune cells through the nicotinic acetylcholine α7 receptor

pressed by immune cells [17, 21, 28-30]. Evidence indicates that the anti-inflammatory effects of acetylcholine are mediated by nicotinic acetylcholine receptors, and in particular by the $a7$ subunit of the nicotinic acetylcholine receptor [21]. *In vitro* studies have shown that acetylcholine and nicotine inhibit endotoxin-induced pro-inflammatory cytokine release by macrophages; this acetylcholine effect can be prevented by nicotine receptor antagonists, and macrophages deficient for the $a7$ subunit of the nicotinic acetylcholine receptor cannot be inhibited with regard to cytokine release by acetylcholine or nicotine [20, 21]. *In vivo* studies in endotoxemia and other models of inflammation have shown that macrophages are directly influenced by vagus nerve derived acetylcholine, suggesting that the vagus nerve provides a hard wired anti-inflammatory pathway called the "cholinergic anti-inflammatory pathway" (Fig. 3) [28]. In these studies, electrical stimulation of the efferent vagus nerve inhibits TNF release induced by injection of endotoxin into rats and mice and prevents shock; however, electrical stimulation of the vagus nerve in mice deficient for the $a7$ subunit of the nicotinic acetylcholine receptor does not result in reduced cytokine release upon endotoxin administration [20]. Besides inflammation induced by endotoxin, the cholinergic anti-inflammatory pathway can also inhibit other types of inflammation *in vivo*. Direct stimulation of the vagus nerve diminished shock and pro-inflammatory cytokine synthesis in liver and heart obtained from animals subjected to ischemia-reperfusion injury induced by transient aortic occlusion [31]. Furthermore, in hypovolemic hemorrhagic shock in rats, stimulation of the vagus nerve increased survival time, reverted hypotension, blunted NF-κB activity in the liver, and reduced TNF levels [32]. Localized inflammation is also affected by the cholinergic anti-inflammatory pathway, as shown in experimental murine arthritis induced by carrageenan where vagus nerve stimulation inhibited the inflammatory response and suppressed the development of paw swelling [33]. In, as of yet unpublished, studies by our group we have shown that the severity of experimental pancreatitis is dependent on nicotinic acetylcholine receptors and the vagus nerve and that the cholinergic anti-inflammatory pathway regulates host defense and the inflammatory response during experimental Gram-negative sepsis. Another line of evidence comes from studies in which vagus nerve activity was stimulated centrally. CNI-1493, a tetravalent guanylhydrazone, has been shown to induce efferent vagus nerve firing when injected intracerebroventrically [33]. CNI-1493 significantly suppressed carrageenan-induced paw edema, even in doses at least 6-logs lower than those required for a systemic effect. Bilateral cervical vagotomy or atropine blockade abrogated the anti-inflammatory effects of CNI-1493 indicating that the intact vagus nerve is required for CNI-1493 activity. Taken together, activation of efferent vagus nerve activity provides the CNS with a fast and powerful anti-inflammatory pathway that is mediated by the release of acetylcholine by postganglionic vagal neurons, which inhibits the release of pro-inflammatory mediators by immune cells in the area of inflammation.

▌ Therapeutic Implications

We have reviewed data that show that the CNS and the immune system are actually two tightly linked systems. The CNS is informed about ongoing inflammation by humoral and neural networks and responds in a reflex like manner by the release of hormones and through activation of the autonomic nervous system. This 'inflammatory reflex' is a powerful, endogenous system designed to restrain the potential detrimental effects of excessive inflammatory responses to the body. The identification of these links between the CNS and the nervous system provides an opportunity to study new therapeutic approaches for diseases in which unrestrained inflammation is essential. Most current strategies for treatment of unrestrained inflammation are based on direct suppression of pro-inflammatory cytokines or cytokine activity. The identification of the cholinergic anti-inflammatory pathway now suggests several new approaches to modify cytokines and inflammatory responses to therapeutic advantage. Such potential new approaches include electrical stimulation of the vagus nerve, which may represent a novel strategy to inhibit the production of TNF and to protect against pathological inflammation. In this regard it is important to realize that permanently implanted vagus nerve stimulators are clinically approved devices for treatment of epilepsy and depression [34–37]. So far, more than 15000 patients have been implanted with a vagus nerve stimulator for these indications with only moderate side effects [38]. It is conceivable to treat patients with inflammatory diseases, severe infections and overshoot inflammatory syndromes, such as sepsis and the systemic inflammatory response syndrome (SIRS), with vagus nerve stimulation. Especially in TNF-α mediated diseases, such as Crohn's disease, rheumatoid arthritis and sepsis, vagus nerve stimulation alone or as a supplement to treatment with anti TNF-α strategies might be a valuable treatment. Since the anti-inflammatory effects of the vagus nerve are carried out through nicotinic acetylcholine receptors of the $\alpha7$ subtype, pharmacological stimulation of the $\alpha7$ subunit of the nicotinic acetylcholine receptor may be another approach to modulate inflammatory disorders. We have obtained proof of principle that compounds specifically stimulating the $\alpha7$ subunit of the nicotinic acetylcholine receptor can inhibit endotoxin-induced TNF release by macrophages *in vitro* and in mice *in vivo*. A third target might be the development of small molecules, such as CNI-1493, that stimulate proximal components of the cholinergic anti-inflammatory pathway in the CNS and induce vagal efferent firing. Of note, many anti-inflammatory drugs such as aspirin, indomethacin and ibuprofen have also been shown to increase vagus nerve activity which may indeed contribute to their mode of action [39]. Finally, it is intriguing to note that the functions of the autonomic nervous system are carried out involuntarily and often in a reflex like manner, however, due to the connections of the autonomic nervous system with the cerebral cortex a certain amount of conscious control is possible. An elegant example for this is the control certain individuals can exert over their heart rate and blood pressure in deep meditation, which exceeds the amount of maximal change observed during sleep or hypnosis. Knowledge of the link between the vagus nerve and regulation of the inflammatory response makes it conceivable that inhibition of vagal activity, which for example may be associated with chronic stress, contributes to the development of mild inflammatory syndromes. On the other hand, one might postulate that behavioral techniques that induce vagal activity could be effective as an anti-inflammatory treatment.

▌ Conclusion

The CNS and the immune system are tightly linked through humoral, endocrine and hard wired connections. The autonomic nervous system provides the CNS with real time information on the status of immunological activation in the body and the

CNS responds to this information by generating a series of generalized behavioral and endocrine (fever, anorexia, ACTH release) as well as hard wired responses. These hard wired responses include the release of epinephrine and norepinephrine through the sympathetic nervous system as well as through activating efferent activity in the vagus nerve. Both systems function to suppress inflammation in order to prevent inflammatory responses to become generalized. The vagus nerve, in particular, is an essential neural circuit for immunomodulation since its efferent activity is stimulated upon the detection of inflammation and subsequently inflammation is controlled in a reflex like manner by the anti-inflammatory effects of acetylcholine on immune cells. Knowledge of these newly discovered connections between the nervous system and the immune system, and especially of the cholinergic anti-inflammatory pathway, provides new insights in the regulation of the immune response and may pave the way for new options for the treatment of inflammatory diseases.

References

1. Janeway CA Jr, Medzhitov R (2002) Innate immune recognition. Annu Rev Immunol 20:197–216
2. van der Poll T, van Deventer SJ (1999) Cytokines and anticytokines in the pathogenesis of sepsis. Infect Dis Clin North Am 13:413–426
3. van der Poll T (2001) Immunotherapy of sepsis. Lancet Infect Dis 1:165–174
4. van Deventer SJ (1997) Tumour necrosis factor and Crohn's disease. Gut 40:443–448
5. van Dullemen HM, van Deventer SJ, Hommes DW, et al (1995) Treatment of Crohn's disease with anti-tumor necrosis factor chimeric monoclonal antibody (cA2). Gastroenterology 109:129–135
6. Steinman L (2004) Elaborate interactions between the immune and nervous systems. Nat Immunol 5:575–581
7. Roth J, Harre EM, Rummel C, Gerstberger R, Hubschle T (2004) Signaling the brain in systemic inflammation: role of sensory circumventricular organs. Front Biosci 9:290–300
8. Marvel FA, Chen CC, Badr N, Gaykema RP, Goehler LE (2004) Reversible inactivation of the dorsal vagal complex blocks lipopolysaccharide-induced social withdrawal and c-Fos expression in central autonomic nuclei. Brain Behav Immun 18:123–134
9. Berthoud HR, Neuhuber WL (2000) Functional and chemical anatomy of the afferent vagal system. Auton Neurosci 85:1–17
10. Maier SF, Goehler LE, Fleshner M, Watkins LR (1998) The role of the vagus nerve in cytokine-to-brain communication. Ann NY Acad Sci 840:289–300
11. Fleshner M, Goehler LE, Schwartz BA, et al (1998) Thermogenic and corticosterone responses to intravenous cytokines (IL-1beta and TNF-alpha) are attenuated by subdiaphragmatic vagotomy. J Neuroimmunol 86:134–141
12. Watkins LR, Goehler LE, Relton JK, et al (1995) Blockade of interleukin-1 induced hyperthermia by subdiaphragmatic vagotomy: evidence for vagal mediation of immune-brain communication. Neurosci Lett 183:27–31
13. Goehler LE, Gaykema RP, Hansen MK, Anderson K, Maier SF, Watkins LR (2000) Vagal immune-to-brain communication: a visceral chemosensory pathway. Auton Neurosci 85:49–59
14. Ishizuka Y, Ishida Y, Jin QH, et al (1998) Abdominal vagotomy attenuates interleukin-1 beta-induced nitric oxide release in the paraventricular nucleus region in conscious rats. Brain Res 789:157–161
15. Hansen MK, Daniels S, Goehler LE, Gaykema RP, Maier SF, Watkins LR (2000) Subdiaphragmatic vagotomy does not block intraperitoneal lipopolysaccharide-induced fever. Auton Neurosci 85:83–87
16. Hansen MK, Nguyen KT, Goehler LE, et al (2000) Effects of vagotomy on lipopolysaccharide-induced brain interleukin-1beta protein in rats. Auton Neurosci 85:119–126
17. Pavlov VA, Wang H, Czura CJ, Friedman SG, Tracey KJ (2003) The cholinergic anti-inflammatory pathway: a missing link in neuroimmunomodulation. Mol Med 9:125–134

18. Brattsand R, Linden M (1996) Cytokine modulation by glucocorticoids: mechanisms and actions in cellular studies. Aliment Pharmacol Ther 10 (Suppl2):81–90
19. Felten DL, Felten SY (1988) Sympathetic noradrenergic innervation of immune organs. Brain Behav Immun 2:293–300
20. Borovikova LV, Ivanova S, Zhang M, et al (2000) Vagus nerve stimulation attenuates the systemic inflammatory response to endotoxin. Nature 405:458–462
21. Wang H, Yu M, Ochani M, et al (2003) Nicotinic acetylcholine receptor alpha7 subunit is an essential regulator of inflammation. Nature 421:384–388
22. van der Poll T (2001) Effects of catecholamines on the inflammatory response. Sepsis 4: 159–167
23. Leceta J, Gomariz RP, Martinez C, Abad C, Ganea D, Delgado M (2000) Receptors and transcriptional factors involved in the anti-inflammatory activity of VIP and PACAP. Ann NY Acad Sci 921:92–102
24. Steinman L, Conlon P, Maki R, Foster A (2003) The intricate interplay among body weight, stress, and the immune response to friend or foe. J Clin Invest 111:183–185
25. Ishizuka Y, Ishida Y, Kunitake T, et al (1997) Effects of area postrema lesion and abdominal vagotomy on interleukin-1 beta-induced norepinephrine release in the hypothalamic paraventricular nucleus region in the rat. Neurosci Lett 223:57–60
26. Hasko G, Shanley TP, Egnaczyk G, et al (1998) Exogenous and endogenous catecholamines inhibit the production of macrophage inflammatory protein (MIP) 1 alpha via a beta adrenoceptor mediated mechanism. Br J Pharmacol 125:1297–1303
27. Prass K, Meisel C, Hoflich C, et al (2003) Stroke-induced immunodeficiency promotes spontaneous bacterial infections and is mediated by sympathetic activation reversal by poststroke T helper cell type 1-like immunostimulation. J Exp Med 198:725–736
28. Tracey KJ (2002) The inflammatory reflex. Nature 420:853–859
29. Benhammou K, Lee M, Strook M, et al (2000) [(3)H]Nicotine binding in peripheral blood cells of smokers is correlated with the number of cigarettes smoked per day. Neuropharmacology 39:2818–2829
30. Matsunaga K, Klein TW, Friedman H, Yamamoto Y (2001) Involvement of nicotinic acetylcholine receptors in suppression of antimicrobial activity and cytokine responses of alveolar macrophages to Legionella pneumophila infection by nicotine. J Immunol 167:6518–6524
31. Bernik TR, Friedman SG, Ochani M, et al (2002) Cholinergic antiinflammatory pathway inhibition of tumor necrosis factor during ischemia reperfusion. J Vasc Surg 36:1231–1236
32. Guarini S, Altavilla D, Cainazzo MM, et al (2003) Efferent vagal fibre stimulation blunts nuclear factor-kappaB activation and protects against hypovolemic hemorrhagic shock. Circulation 107:1189–1194
33. Borovikova LV, Ivanova S, Nardi D, et al (2000) Role of vagus nerve signaling in CNI-1493-mediated suppression of acute inflammation. Auton Neurosci 85:141–147
34. George MS, Rush AJ, Sackeim HA, Marangell LB (2003) Vagus nerve stimulation (VNS): utility in neuropsychiatric disorders. Int J Neuropsychopharmacol 6:73–83
35. George MS, Nahas Z, Bohning DE, et al (2002) Vagus nerve stimulation therapy: a research update. Neurology 59:S56–S61
36. Marangell LB, Rush AJ, George MS, et al (2002) Vagus nerve stimulation (VNS) for major depressive episodes: one year outcomes. Biol Psychiatry 51:280–287
37. Sackeim HA, Rush AJ, George MS, et al (2001) Vagus nerve stimulation (VNS) for treatment-resistant depression: efficacy, side effects, and predictors of outcome. Neuropsychopharmacology 25:713–728
38. Ben Menachem E (2002) Vagus-nerve stimulation for the treatment of epilepsy. Lancet Neurol 1:477–482
39. Arai I, Hirose H, Muramatsu M, Okuyama S, Aihara H (1985) Possible involvement of nonsteroidal anti-inflammatory drugs in vagal-mediated gastric acid secretion in rats. Jpn J Pharmacol 37:91–99

Sepsis: Clinical Aspects

Severe Sepsis in the Elderly

T.D. Girard, S.M. Opal, and E.W. Ely

▌ Introduction

Over 750 000 patients develop severe sepsis annually in the United States [1], and over 60% of these patients are 65 years of age or older [1]. With the number of octogenarians expected to double by the year 2030 [2], severe sepsis in older patients is a major public health concern. In this chapter we will review important differences between older and younger patients with severe sepsis, with special attention to treatment strategies and their application in older patients. The chapter is structured to address these important questions regarding the interaction of age and severe sepsis:

- ▌ Is severe sepsis a disease of the elderly?
- ▌ How does the immune system change with aging?
- ▌ What other factors place older patients at increased risk for sepsis?
- ▌ Is the pathophysiology of sepsis altered in older patients?
- ▌ What challenges are associated with the diagnosis of sepsis in older patients?
- ▌ What management strategies are appropriate in older patients with sepsis?
- ▌ What is the prognostic significance of increasing age in sepsis?

▌ Is Severe Sepsis a Disease of the Elderly?

Unlike many disease processes, sepsis occurs across all age groups. However, there is a clearly documented rise in its incidence with increasing age. An abrupt decline occurs after the neonatal period, after which the incidence of sepsis increases steadily throughout adulthood (Fig. 1). Angus et al. reported the annual incidence of severe sepsis across all age groups to be 3.0 cases per 1000 population [1]. The incidence rises dramatically with age such that in those over 85 years of age sepsis occurs annually at a rate of 26.2 per 1000 population. Martin et al. analyzed data from the National Hospital Discharge Survey and similarly reported the annual incidence of sepsis to be 2.4 per 1000 population [3]. Their data indicate that the average age of patients with sepsis is increasing over time. Nearly two-thirds of patients with sepsis each year are over 65 years of age [1].

While sepsis is not a disease unique to the elderly, the rising incidence of sepsis in this portion of the population and the increasing age of patients with sepsis contributes significantly to national health care costs. Greater than 52% ($ 8.7 billion) of the total national hospital cost attributable to the care of patients with sepsis in 1995 went to those patients over 65, and 30.8% ($ 5.1 billion) went to those 75 years or older [1].

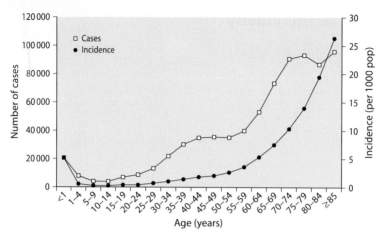

Fig. 1. National age-specific number and incidence of cases of severe sepsis. From [1] with permission. Pop: population

▮ How does the Immune System Change with Aging?

Aging of the immune system is generally referred to as immunosenescence. While some components of the inflammatory response are well-maintained, even in centenarians, other components of the immune response are markedly impaired with increased age, and alterations of inflammatory responses with aging accelerate the risk of systemic infection and severe sepsis [4]. There are numerous explanations for this increased risk, with derangements in the immune response being prominent [5].

The pathophysiologic mechanisms that underlie the aging process of the immune system are complex and multifactorial, but several common features characterize immunosenescence. The major elements of the innate immune system (neutrophils, macrophages, dendritic cells, natural killer [NK] cells, etc.) are well preserved with aging, but the adaptive immune response is significantly impaired with increased age [5]. Defects in cell-mediated immune responses are the earliest findings indicative of aging of the immune system, with CD8$^+$ cells more profoundly affected than CD4$^+$ cells [6, 7]. B cell responses and other elements of humoral immunity are also affected by age [7].

As thymus tissue is gradually replaced by fatty infiltration with aging, the rate of generation of naive T cells falls off dramatically. T cells in the elderly generate less interleukin-2 (IL-2), have limited proliferative capacity, and have impaired signal transduction after engagement with antigen presenting cells [8]. Due to reduced cell-mediated immune function, aging is associated with a markedly increased risk for infection with invasive intracellular pathogens, e.g., West Nile virus, severe acute respiratory syndrome (SARS), and *Listeria monocytogenes* [5].

The B cell population gradually shrinks with age while the plasma cell population and immunoglobulin levels increase. B cell responses show intact anamnestic responses to recall antigens, but the humoral response to neoantigens is significantly impaired in older patients [5]. The major problem with B cell function in the elderly is the relative absence of helper T cell function. The expression of three co-stimulatory molecules vital to the interaction between B cells and T cells (CD40 ligand, CD28, and OX40L) is impaired in aged T cells. This is demonstrated in the blunted antibody responses to immunizations and invasive microbial pathogens noted in older patients [9].

While cytokine and chemokine generation in older patients depends upon multiple factors, e.g., gender, nutritional status, concomitant illnesses, and exposure to various medications, elderly patients generally produce normal or elevated levels of IL-1, IL-3, IL-4, IL-6, tumor necrosis factor (TNF), interferon gamma (IFNγ), and chemokines [4]. IL-10 synthesis may be increased in elderly patients as well, indicating an exaggerated TH2-type cytokine response. This high IL-10/TNF ratio, or anti-inflammatory to pro-inflammatory ratio, has been demonstrated in older patients with severe sepsis and was associated with increased mortality [10].

What other Factors place Older Patients at Increased Risk for Sepsis?

In addition to the increased risk for infection and sepsis due to immunosenescence, other important factors place the elderly population at greater risk for sepsis. These include co-morbid illnesses, exposure to instrumentation and procedures, institutionalization, malnutrition, and poor performance status [11–14]. Significantly higher rates of co-morbidities – e.g., hypertension, myocardial infarction, cardiomyopathy, chronic obstructive pulmonary disease, malignancy, and recent surgery – were noted in those over 75 years of age compared to younger patients in a recent sepsis trial [11]. Those over age 65 in another sepsis study were twice as likely to have at least one co-morbid medical condition as younger sepsis patients [15]. Management of such conditions often necessitates instrumentation (urinary catheters, tracheotomies, and central venous catheters, etc.) that compromises the natural barriers of innate immunity and creates a portal of entry for infection. Additionally, up to one-third of patients older than 80 reside in long-term care facilities where bacterial flora demonstrate a higher level of resistance than that seen in the community [12, 16]. Institutionalization is associated with oropharyngeal colonization with Gram-negative bacilli, and this, combined with depressed cough and mucociliary transport function, leads to increased rates of nosocomial pneumonia [13]. Additionally, malnutrition is commonplace in the elderly as a result of inactivity, poor mobility, functional limitation, poor or restricted diets, chronic disease, dementia, depression, poor dentition, and polypharmacy [14].

Is the Pathophysiology of Sepsis Altered in Older Patients?

Ongoing research has revealed that sepsis is a complex interaction of both inflammatory and anti-inflammatory responses, as well as disturbed hemostasis and thrombosis; thus, a review of the pathophysiology of sepsis is warranted. Primary cellular injury may result directly from infection but more often occurs when a toxic microbial stimulus (e.g., lipopolysaccharide, peptidoglycan, and other pattern recognition molecules) launches a deleterious host response initiated by the generation of inflammatory mediators, including TNF-α, IL-1, and other cytokines and chemokines that activate leukocytes, promote leukocyte-vascular endothelium adhesion, and induce endothelial damage [17]. As a result of this endothelial damage,

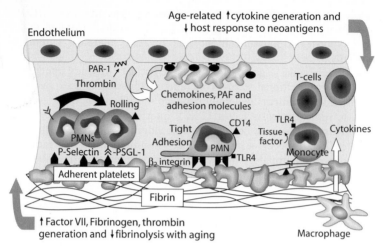

Fig. 2. Age-related increased levels of clotting factors – particularly Factor VII, Factor VIII and fibrinogen – and impaired fibrinolysis from excess plasminogen activator inhibitor-1 produce a propensity towards thrombus formation. The impaired ability to effectively clear neoantigens and the progressive, low-grade inflammation that accompanies aging leads to inefficient clearance of microbes and excess cytokine and chemokine synthesis. The bi-directional interactions between fibrin generation and inflammation adversely affect the microcirculation in older patients with sepsis. Thrombin activates leukocytes, platelets, and endothelial cells via protease activated receptor-1 (PAR-1), upregulating IL-6, IL-8, platelet activating factor (PAF), and P selectin synthesis. Neutrophils and monocytes bind to fibrin, fibrinogen, and P-selectin by P-selectin glyoprotein ligand-1 (PSGL-1). Activated myeloid cells express the pattern recognition molecules CD14 and Toll-like receptor 4 (TLR 4). The innate inflammatory reaction upregulates tissue factor expression and suppresses endogenous anticoagulant activity promoting further thrombus propagation

tissue factor is expressed, and the tissue factor-dependent clotting cascade is activated, resulting in the formation of thrombin such that microaggregates of fibrin, platelets, neutrophils, and red blood cells impair capillary blood flow, decreasing oxygen and nutrient delivery [18].

Multiple studies have noted important alterations in the pathophysiology of sepsis in older patients, as compared to that in younger patients. Levels of TNF-α were significantly higher in septic patients over 80 years of age than in younger septic patients in one study [19], and increased concentrations of soluble adhesion molecules – markers for activated or damaged endothelium – have been observed in older septic patients compared to younger septic patients [20]. Additionally, the monocytes of healthy elderly adults demonstrate increased intracellular levels of TNF-α, IL-1, and IL-6 [21], and increasing age is associated with rising circulating levels of IL-6 and D-dimer [22], activated Factor VII, and other coagulation factors [23], indicating activation of inflammatory and coagulation pathways even in the absence of acute illness (Fig. 2).

What Challenges are Associated with the Diagnosis of Sepsis in Older Patients?

Older patients with suspected infection may pose particular challenges in the diagnosis of sepsis. As such, a careful evaluation for signs of systemic inflammatory response syndrome (SIRS) [24] is essential, keeping in mind that the frequency of these signs in sepsis is altered by increased age. For example, fever may be blunted or absent in older patients with infection. In one study, fever was absent in 25 (13%) of 192 bacteremic patients 65 years of age and older compared to only 5 (4%) of 128 patients less than 65 years (p < 0.01) [25]. Another study found that half of the elderly patients evaluated had a blunted fever response to infection (< 38.3 °C), but one-quarter of these patients had a significant change in temperature above a low baseline [26]. Additionally, while the incidences of tachycardia and hypoxemia were significantly lower among septic patients over age 75 compared to younger patients in one large study, tachypnea and altered mental status were more common in the older group [27]. Confusion or altered mental status, best thought of as delirium [28] or septic encephalopathy [29], is noted to occur in the majority of septic patients [28]; therefore, clinicians must be aware of such nonspecific clinical expressions of infection in the elderly. Other common symptoms include weakness, anorexia, malaise, urinary incontinence, and falls [12].

In addition to the variation in inflammatory signs and symptoms seen in the elderly, other diagnostic difficulties may include difficulty obtaining blood, sputum, body fluids, or tissue samples in patients who are cognitively impaired, debilitated, dehydrated, or frail [12], and positioning patients for high-quality chest radiographs may be problematic, compromising the diagnostic value of these studies.

What Management Strategies are Appropriate in Older Patients with Sepsis?

Clinical practice guidelines, such as the recently published Surviving Sepsis Campaign guidelines, outline key recommendations regarding the management of patients with severe sepsis and septic shock [30]. While guidelines can serve as the foundation of management in the care of patients with sepsis, there are some differences between older and younger patients in the implementation of these strategies. However, most of the guidelines should be employed similarly regardless of age and thus serve as the basis of this section of the chapter. In fact, some therapies actually provide larger absolute risk reductions in older patients as compared to younger patients.

Initial Resuscitation and Hemodynamic Support

Although special care must be taken to avoid excess fluid accumulation in older patients, under-resuscitation is more likely in severe sepsis due to increased capacitance of the vasculature, and the initial resuscitation of any patient with severe sepsis or septic shock should begin early with a goal of maintaining adequate tissue perfusion (Grade B evidence, see Table 1), as indicated by blood pressure, central venous pressure (CVP), urine output, etc. Such early goal-directed therapy improved survival in 130 patients (with an average age of 67.1 years) randomly as-

Table 1. The 2004 Surviving Sepsis Campaign Clinical Practice Guidelines evidence-based grading system. Adapted from [30]

Recommendation grade
A. Supported by two or more large, randomized trials with unambiguous results
B. Supported by one large, randomized trial with unambiguous results
C. Supported by one or more small, randomized trials with uncertain results
D. Supported by one or more non-randomized trials with non-historical controls
E. Supported by non-randomized trials using historical controls, uncontrolled trials, case series, and/or expert opinion

signed to the intervention group in a recent study [31]. Liberal amounts of intravenous fluids (crystalloid or colloid) should be used during initial resuscitation. Vasopressor therapy with norepinephrine or dopamine may be necessary when appropriate fluid challenge fails to restore adequate tissue perfusion or during life-threatening hypotension (Grade E). Vasopressin may be added at 0.01–0.04 units/min intravenously if hypotension and/or tissue hypoperfusion persists despite these measures (Grade E).

Source Control and Antibiotics

Regardless of low strength of evidence grades due to the absence of randomized, controlled trials in this area, source control and timely antibiotic administration are two vital components of sepsis management. Diagnostic studies directed at identifying the source of infection should be performed without delay when possible (Grade E), and source control measures should be instituted early when necrotic skin, lung, or other tissues; abscesses or empyemas; infected devices; or infected catheters are identified (Grade E).

Empiric antibiotic therapy should be initiated within one hour of recognition of sepsis (Grade E) after cultures have been taken from the blood and other suspected sites of infection (Grade D). As inadequate initial antibiotic therapy is independently associated with poor outcomes across age groups [32, 33], initial empiric therapy should be broad, having activity against all probable pathogens (Grade D). This is particularly important in older patients, as co-morbid illnesses, immunocompromised states, residence in nursing homes, repeated hospitalizations, and the increased prevalence of intra-abdominal and soft tissue infections increase the likelihood of repeated antimicrobial exposure [34]. This increases the propensity of older patients to accumulate multidrug-resistant microbial flora, necessitating a broader spectrum of empiric antibiotics. As such, rapid reduction to monotherapy active against causative organisms, once identified, should be the standard approach to antibiotic therapy in older patients with sepsis [30].

The pharmacokinetics and pharmacodynamics of antimicrobial agents can be significantly altered in older patients with sepsis due to age-related decrements in renal function, reduced lean body mass, and shock-induced reduction in hepatic blood flow [35]. Therefore, these patients are at high risk of experiencing adverse effects of antibiotics [12], and clinicians must be familiar with possible side effects and monitor for them carefully. Careful therapeutic drug monitoring is recommended in the management of older patients with severe sepsis due to the rapidly changing metabolic and hemodynamic parameters notable in severe sepsis [30, 36].

Steroids

Replacement dose hydrocortisone is recommended in patients with refractory shock (Grade C). Treatment with hydrocortisone (50 mg intravenous bolus every 6 hours for 7 days) and fludrocortisone improved mortality in one important study of 300 patients with relative adrenal insufficiency and an average age of 61 years [37]. However, the use of steroids in sepsis remains a source of controversy, as steroids may result in poor glucose control, immunosuppression (at high doses), poor wound healing, and critical illness myoneuropathy. Therefore, caution and appropriate dosing are imperative, and avoidance of high-dose corticosteroid therapy is recommended (Grade A). The benefit of steroids was only seen in the subgroup of patients with relative adrenal insufficiency – defined as < 9 g/dl increase in cortisol 30 to 60 minutes post-ACTH – [37], and a subsequent study showed that total serum cortisol can be abnormally low at the same time that free cortisol is normal [38].

Drotrecogin Alfa (Activated)

Activated protein C is an endogenous protein with anti-inflammatory, antithrombotic, profibrinolytic, antiapoptotic, and endothelial regulatory effects. Recombinant human activated protein C (rhAPC, drotrecogin alfa [activated], Xigris; Eli Lilly) was evaluated in a randomized, double-blind, placebo-controlled, multicenter trial that enrolled a high percentage of older patients. Of 850 patients randomized to receive rhAPC, 48.6% were 65 years of age or older and 24.1% were 75 years of age or older. Treatment with rhAPC resulted in an absolute reduction in the risk of death of 6.1%, compared with placebo (p = 0.005) [39]. Additionally, planned subgroup analysis revealed that treatment with rhAPC in the nearly 400 patients 75 years of age or more resulted in a 15.5% reduction in the absolute risk of 28-day mortality [11]. Among older patients the incidences of serious adverse bleeding in the rhAPC and placebo groups were 3.9% and 2.2%, respectively (p = 0.34). Additionally, older and younger patients treated with rhAPC had similar rates of serious bleeding (p = 0.97) [11]. Treatment with rhAPC should be considered in patients at high risk of death from severe sepsis regardless of their age – e.g., those with septic shock requiring vasopressors despite fluid resuscitation, sepsis-induced acute respiratory distress syndrome (ARDS) requiring mechanical ventilation, or any two sepsis-induced dysfunctional organs (Grade B). The drug is contraindicated in the presence of active bleeding, with other anticoagulant drugs, platelet counts less than 30 000/μl, and in patients with other risks of uncontrollable bleeding.

Transfusion Strategies

For older patients without coronary artery disease, active hemorrhage, or ongoing tissue hypoperfusion (marked by hypotension or lactic acidosis), red blood cell (RBC) transfusion strategies should be approached conservatively, with a default hemoglobin transfusion threshold of 7 mg/dl (Grade B). A large, randomized trial demonstrated that a target hemoglobin of 7.0–9.0 g/dl resulted in no additional mortality compared to the traditional target of 10.0 g/dl [40]. Indeed, there was a trend toward improved outcomes in the conservatively transfused group. Of note, the patients who were not enrolled were statistically older than those who were enrolled (p = 0.04), possibly due to the high prevalence of coronary artery disease in older patients and a bias of physicians that such patients should not be studied. An 80 000-patient study by Wu et al. showed that older patients with myocardial infarction had higher survival rates when the hemoglobin was maintained at 10–11 g/dl [41].

Mechanical Ventilation

A significant proportion of older patients with severe sepsis require mechanical ventilation. A lung-protective strategy of ventilation – utilizing low tidal volumes (6 ml/kg predicted body weight) – resulted in a significant reduction in mortality in a randomized, controlled trial that enrolled 861 patients with acute lung injury (ALI) or ARDS (Grade B) [42]. In the 173 patients 70 years of age or older, ventilation with low tidal volumes resulted in an absolute risk reduction in 28-day mortality of 9.9% [43]. To reduce the risk of ventilator-associated pneumonia (VAP), mechanically ventilated patients should have the head of the bed raised to 45 degrees (Grade C) [44]. Additionally, a protocol-driven ventilator weaning strategy is proven to reduce the duration of mechanical ventilation. The spontaneous breathing trial is essential to such a strategy (Grade A), and has been found to result in a reduction in the duration of mechanical ventilation in randomized clinical trials [45].

Sedatives and Analgesics

Older patients are particularly at risk for anxiety, pain, and delirium, often experienced by critically ill septic patients. Protocols (Grade B) utilizing a sedation goal [46] or daily interruption of sedatives (Grade B) [47] and a standardized sedation scale [48] have been proven to reduce the duration of mechanical ventilation. The use of intermittent bolus sedation rather than continuous infusions (Grade B) [49] also results in a shorter duration of mechanical ventilation.

Miscellaneous Issues

Other important aspects of the management of sepsis are applicable in older patients and should not be overlooked, including deep vein thrombosis prophylaxis via the use of low-dose unfractionated heparin, low-molecular weight heparin, or mechanical prophylactic devices (Grade A); H2-receptor blockers or proton pump inhibitors to prevent stress ulcers (Grade A); and tight glucose control (Grade D). Hyperglycemia is common in severe sepsis patients and may impair antimicrobial defense mechanisms and worsen the pathophysiologic coagulopathy of sepsis [50]. Intensive insulin therapy with a goal of maintaining blood glucose levels between 80 and 110 mg/dL resulted in reduced mortality in a large randomized, controlled trial [51].

End-of-Life Planning

As severe sepsis results in the death of approximately one-third of older patients, practitioners must be prepared and equipped to provide quality end-of-life care. In some of these cases, it may be in the patient's best interest to withhold or withdraw support (Grade E). Although the probability of limiting life-sustaining treatment increases with advancing age [52], futility is infrequently the justification for decisions to limit support [53]. Instead, the basis for such decisions is often a complex interaction of patient- and family-centered decision making, requiring communication within the medical team and with patients and families. In difficult situations, the hospital ethics team may provide assistance in achieving resolution to controversial decisions regarding potentially unbeneficial life-sustaining treatments [54].

▌ What is the Prognostic Significance of Increasing Age in Sepsis?

Multiple retrospective and prospective studies have shown increasing age to be associated with high mortality from sepsis, independent of severity of illness and comorbid conditions. Angus et al. reported an overall mortality from sepsis of 28.6% while the rate among patients 85 and older was 38.4% (Fig. 3) [1]. Knaus et al. studied 58 737 patients and reported that increasing age was independently associated with a higher 28-day mortality, yet the association between increasing severity of illness and mortality appeared to be much stronger [55]. Gogos et al. prospectively evaluated 139 patients with severe sepsis and reported that age was an independent predictor of poor outcome [56].

However, other investigators have found that mortality rates for critically ill older and younger patients are similar after controlling for co-morbidities and severity of illness [32]. In a recent study of 406 patients with sepsis, age was a risk factor for in-hospital mortality on univariate analysis, but on multivariate analysis this association was no longer seen [33]. Multivariate analyses in studies evaluating patients with Pseudomonas bacteremia [57] and Gram-negative bacteremia [58] also failed to show that age was independently associated with mortality due to sepsis.

As health care costs continue to rise, some have suggested that rationing of limited health care resources is inevitable and that age should be used as a criteria for such rationing [59]. A proven association between increasing age and rising mortality due to sepsis may be used by some to support such health care policy. How-

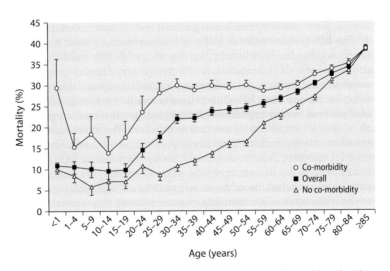

Fig. 3. National age-specific mortality rates for all cases of severe sepsis and for those with and without underlying co-morbidity. From [1] with permission

ever, if the patient, family, and health care team conclude that the patient has the right mix of baseline health, individual preference for aggressive care, and reversible acute illness, the health care team should treat the patient no differently than they do younger patients.

Data regarding post-discharge survival and quality of life after sepsis will help determine health care policy as the population ages and the incidence of sepsis increases [1]. As demonstrated in a recent sepsis trial, a high percentage of older patients who survive sepsis require nursing home care; of the 222 patients 75 years of age and older who survived to hospital discharge, 45% were transferred to a nursing home, 11% to another hospital, and only 42% were discharged home [11].

■ Conclusion

This chapter has reviewed many important differences between older and younger patients with severe sepsis. Advanced age profoundly alters the function of the immune system, accelerating the risk of infection and severe sepsis in older patients. High rates of co-morbid illness, instrumentation, institutionalization, and malnutrition further contribute to the markedly increased incidence of severe sepsis in the elderly population. Alterations in the pathophysiology of sepsis may be responsible, in part, for the increase in mortality due to severe sepsis associated with advanced age. However, despite the rising incidence and significant mortality of sepsis in older patients many elderly patients respond remarkably well to the evidence-based diagnostic and management strategies reviewed here. Ongoing research is evaluating other promising sepsis-specific treatments. Additional studies are needed to investigate important issues such as post-discharge survival and health-related quality of life in older patients after severe sepsis.

References

1. Angus DC, Linde-Zwirble WT, Clermonte G, Carcillo J, Pinsky MR (2001) Epidemiology of severe sepsis in the United States: analysis of incidence, outcome, and associated costs of care. Crit Care Med 29:1303–1310
2. Hobbs FB, Damon BL (1995) Sixty-five plus in the United States. Washington, DC, US Dept of Commerce, Economics and Statistics Administration, Bureau of the Census
3. Martin GS, Mannino DM, Eaton S, Moss M (2003) The epidemiology of sepsis in the United States from 1979 through 2000. N Engl J Med 348:1546–1554
4. Grubeck-Loebenstein B, Berger P, Saurwein-Teissl M, Zisterer K, Wick G (1998) No immunity for the elderly. Nat Med 4:870
5. Grubeck-Loebenstein B, Wick G (2002) The aging of the immune system. Adv Immunol 80:243–284
6. Fry TJ, Mackall CL (2002) Current concepts of thymic aging. Semin Immunopathol 24:7–22
7. Weksler ME, Goodhardt M, Szabo P (2002) The effect of age on B cell development and humoral immunity. Semin Immunopathol 24:35–52
8. Douek DC, Koup RA (2000) Evidence for thymic function in the elderly. Vaccine 18:1638–1641
9. Franceschi C, Bonafe M, Valensin S (2000) Human immunosenescence: the prevailing of innate immunity, the failing of clonotypic immunity, and the filling of immunological space. Vaccine 18:1717–1720
10. van Dissel JT, van Langevelde P, Westendorp RG, Kwappenberg K, Frolich M (1998) Anti-inflammatory cytokine profile and mortality in febrile patients. Lancet 351:950–953

11. Ely EW, Angus DC, Williams MD, Bates B, Qualy R, Bernard GR (2003) Drotrecogin alfa (activated) treatment of older patients with severe sepsis. Clin Infect Dis 37:187–195
12. Rajagopalan S, Yoshikawa TT (2001) Antimicrobial therapy in the elderly. Med Clin North Am 85:133–147
13. Valenti WM, Trudell RG, Bentley DW (1978) Factors predisposing to oropharyngeal colonization with gram-negative bacilli in the aged. N Engl J Med 298:1108–1111
14. Jensen GL, McGee M, Binkley J (2001) Nutrition in the elderly. Gastroenterol Clin North Am 30:313–334
15. Martin GS, Mannino DM, Moss M (2003) Effect of age on the development and outcome with sepsis. Am J Respir Crit Care Med 167:A837 (abst)
16. Nicolle LE (2000) Infection control in long-term care facilities. Clin Infect Dis 31:752–756
17. Wheeler AP, Bernard GR (1999) Treating patients with severe sepsis. N Engl J Med 340:207–214
18. Opal SM, Esmon CT (2003) Bench-to-bedside review: functional relationships between coagulation and the innate immune response and their respective roles in the pathogenesis of sepsis. Crit Care 7:23–38
19. Marik PE, Zaloga GP, NORASEPT II Study Investigators (2001) The effect of aging on circulating levels of proinflammatory cytokines during septic shock. J Am Geriatr Soc 49:5–9
20. Boldt J, Muller M, Heesen M, Papsdorf M, Hempelmann G (1997) Does age influence circulating adhesion molecules in the critically ill? Crit Care Med 25:95–100
21. O'Mahony L, Holland J, Jackson J, Feighery C, Hennessy TP, Mealy K (1998) Quantitative intracellular cytokine measurement: age-related changes in proinflammatory cytokine production. Clin Exp Immunol 113:213–219
22. Cohen HJ, Harris T, Pieper CF (2003) Coagulation and activation of inflammatory pathways in the development of functional decline and mortality in the elderly. Am J Med 114:180–187
23. Mari D, Mannucci PM, Coppola R, Bottasso B, Bauer KA, Rosenberg RD (1995) Hypercoagulability in centenarians: the paradox of successful aging. Blood 85:3144–3149
24. Bone RC, Balk RA, Cerra FB, et al (1992) Definitions for sepsis and organ failure and guidelines for the use of innovative therapies in sepsis. The ACCP/SCCM Consensus Conference Committee. American College of Chest Physicians/Society of Critical Care Medicine. Chest 101:1644–1655
25. Gleckman R, Hibert D (1982) Afebrile bacteremia. A phenomenon in geriatric patients. JAMA 248:1478–1481
26. Castle SC, Norman DC, Yeh M, Miller D, Yoshikawa TT (1991) Fever response in elderly nursing home residents: are the older truly colder? J Am Geriatr Soc 39:853–857
27. Iberti TJ, Bone RC, Balk R, Fein A, Perl TM, Wenzel RP (1993) Are the criteria used to determine sepsis applicable for patients >75 years of age? Crit Care Med 21:S130
28. Ely EW, Shintani A, Truman B, et al (2004) Delirium as a predictor of mortality in mechanically ventilated patients in the intensive care unit. JAMA 291:1753–1762
29. Eidelman LA, Putterman D, Putterman C, Sprung CL (1996) The spectrum of septic encephalopathy: definitions, etiologies, and mortalities. JAMA 275:470–473
30. Dellinger RP, Carlet JM, Masur H, et al (2004) Surviving Sepsis Campaign guidelines for management of severe sepsis and septic shock. Crit Care Med 32:858–873
31. Rivers E, Nguyen B, Havstad S, et al (2001) Early goal-directed therapy in the treatment of severe sepsis and septic shock. N Engl J Med 345:1368–1377
32. Harbarth S, Garbino J, Pugin J, Romand JA, Lew D, Pittet D (2003) Inappropriate initial antimicrobial therapy and its effect on survival in a clinical trial of immunomodulating therapy for severe sepsis. Am J Med 115:529–535
33. Garnacho-Montero J, Garcia-Garmendia JL, Barrero-Almodovar A, Jimenez-Jimenez FJ, Perez-Paredes C, Ortiz-Leyba C (2003) Impact of adequate empirical antibiotic therapy on the outcome of patients admitted to the intensive care unit with sepsis. Crit Care Med 31:2742–2751
34. El Solh AA, Pietrantoni C, Bhat A, Bhora M, Berbary E (2004) Indicators of potentially drug-resistant bacteria in severe nursing home-acquired pneumonia. Clin Infect Dis 39:474–480
35. McCue JD (1999) Antibiotic use in the elderly: issues and nonissues. Clin Infect Dis 28:750–752

36. Stalam M, Kaye D (2004) Antibiotic agents in the elderly. Infect Dis Clin North Am 18:533–549
37. Annane D, Sebille V, Charpentier C, et al (2002) Effect of treatment with low doses of hydrocortisone and fludrocortisone on mortality in patients with septic shock. JAMA 288:862–871
38. Hamrahian AJ, Oseni TS, Arafah BM (2004) Measurements of serum free cortisol in critically ill patients. N Engl J Med 350:1629–1638
39. Bernard GR, Vincent JL, Laterre PF, et al (2001) Efficacy and safety of recombinant human activated protein C for severe sepsis. N Engl J Med 344:699–709
40. Hebert PC, Wells G, Blajchman M, et al (1999) A multicenter, randomized, controlled clinical trial of transfusion requirements in critical care. N Engl J Med 340:409–417
41. Wu W, Rathore SS, Wang Y, Radford MJ, Krumholz HM (2001) Blood transfusion in elderly patients with acute myocardial infarction. N Engl J Med 345:1230–1236
42. The acute respiratory distress syndrome network (2000) Ventilation with lower tidal volumes as compared with traditional tidal volumes for acute lung injury and the acute respiratory distress syndrome. N Engl J Med 342:1301–1308
43. Ely EW, Wheeler AP, Thompson BT, Ancuklewicz M, Steinberg KP, Bernard GR (2002) Recovery rate and prognosis in older persons who develop acute lung injury and the acute respiratory distress syndrome. Ann Intern Med 136:25–36
44. Drakulovic MB, Torres A, Bauer TT, Nicolas JM, Nogue S, Ferrer M (1999) Supine body position as a risk factor for nosocomial pneumonia in mechanically ventilated patients: a randomised trial. Lancet 354:1851–1858
45. Ely EW, Baker AM, Dunagan DP, et al (1996) Effect on the duration of mechanical ventilation of identifying patients capable of breathing spontaneously. N Engl J Med 335:1864–1869
46. Brook AD, Ahrens TS, Schaiff R, et al (1999) Effect of a nursing implemented sedation protocol on the duration of mechanical ventilation. Crit Care Med 27:2609–2615
47. Kress JP, Pohlman AS, O'Connor MF, Hall JB (2000) Daily interruption of sedative infusions in critically ill patients undergoing mechanical ventilation. N Engl J Med 342:1471–1477
48. Ely EW, Gautam S, May L, et al (2001) A comparison of different sedation scales in the ICU and validation of the Richmond Agitation Sedation Scale (RASS). Am J Respir Crit Care Med 163:A954 (abst)
49. Kollef MH, Levy NT, Ahrens T, Schaiff R, Prentice D, Sherman G (1999) The use of continuous IV sedation is associated with prolongation of mechanical ventilation. Chest 114:541–548
50. Rao AK, Chouhan V, Chen X, Sun L, Boden G (2002) Activation of the tissue factor pathway of blood coagulation during prolonged hyperglycemia in young healthy men. Diabetes 48:1156–1161
51. Van Den Berghe G, Wouters P, Weekers F, et al (2001) Intensive insulin therapy in critically ill patients. N Engl J Med 345:1359–1367
52. Hamel MB, Teno JM, Goldman L, et al (1999) Patient age and decisions to withhold life-sustaining treatments from seriously ill, hospitalized adults. Ann Intern Med 130:116–125
53. Halevy A, Neal RC, Brody BA (1996) The low frequency of futility in an adult intensive care unit setting. Arch Intern Med 156:100–104
54. Schneiderman LJ, Gilmer T, Teetzel HD, et al (2003) Effect of ethics consultations on nonbeneficial life-sustaining treatments in the intensive care setting: a randomized controlled trial. JAMA 290:1166–1172
55. Knaus WA, Harrell FE, Fisher CJ Jr, et al (1993) The clinical evaluation of new drugs for sepsis. A prospective study design based on survival analysis. JAMA 270:1233–1241
56. Gogos CA, Lekkou A, Papageorgiou O, Siagris D, Skoutelis A, Bassaris HP (2003) Clinical prognostic markers in patients with severe sepsis: a prospective analysis of 139 consecutive cases. J Infect 47:300–306
57. Hilf M, Yu VL, Sharp J, Zuravleff JJ, Korvick JA, Muder RR (1989) Antibiotic therapy for Pseudomonas aeruginosa bacteremia: outcome correlations in a prospective study of 200 patients. Am J Med 87:540–546
58. Uzun O, Akalin HE, Hayran M, Unal S (1992) Factors influencing prognosis in bacteremia due to gram-negative organisms: evaluation of 448 episodes in a Turkish university hospital. Clin Infect Dis 15:866–873
59. Shaw AB (1996) Age as a basis for healthcare rationing. Support for agist policies. Drugs Aging 9:403–405

Extravascular Lung Water in Sepsis

M. Y. Kirov, V. V. Kuzkov, and L. J. Bjertnaes

▌ Introduction

Sepsis is a frequent cause of morbidity and mortality in critically ill patients [1, 2]. It is well established that during the course of sepsis, infectious agents induce a release of inflammatory mediators that may enhance pulmonary microvascular pressure and permeability. These changes promote accumulation of extravascular lung water (EVLW), formation of microthromboses, and morphological damage to the lungs [3–5]. As a result, sepsis affects the lungs in 25–42% of the cases, making it one of the most common predisposing conditions for acute lung injury (ALI) and acute respiratory distress syndrome (ARDS) [6]. Moreover, in severe sepsis complicated by septic shock, the incidence of ARDS is estimated to be 30–60% [7].

Clinically, sepsis-induced ALI is manifested by pulmonary edema, decreased lung compliance, increased venous admixture, and arterial hypoxemia, causing mortality in excess of 40% [6, 8]. Recent data show that restriction of fluid therapy, aiming to counteract pulmonary edema, positively influences the course of illness and improves outcome in patients with ALI [8]. However, a frequently occurring combination of septic shock with lung edema hampers adequate fluid resuscitation and restoration of tissue perfusion. Thus, the balance and maintenance of cardiac preload and vital organ perfusion weighed against the deleterious effect of a worsening pulmonary edema remains a challenging problem. Consequently, reliable tools for monitoring lung fluid balance are increasingly asked for in modern intensive care.

The amount of edema fluid is, however, difficult to estimate at the bedside. Clinical examination, chest radiography, and blood gases have proven to be of limited significance in quantifying pulmonary edema [6, 9, 10]. Therefore, several techniques have been developed to assess EVLW. Among the various methods, thermo-dye dilution and single transpulmonary thermodilution have been used most frequently both in experimental and clinical settings with promising results [10–13]. In addition to EVLW, these techniques simultaneously display a number of hemodynamic variables that can give valuable guidance to the treatment of diseases affecting cardiopulmonary functions, like severe sepsis. However, a debate is still ongoing regarding the role and the value of EVLW measurements for treatment of critically ill patients. Thus, the goal of this review is to discuss the application of methods for assessment of EVLW and the place for these methods in the management of patients with severe sepsis.

▮ Methods for the Determination of Extravascular Lung Water

A variety of techniques have been suggested for the early detection of EVLW accumulation, which may culminate in lung edema. These methods are listed in Table 1 accompanied by brief comments concerning their accuracy, clinical value, and comparative costs. In this chapter, we will discuss more extensively the thermo-dye dilution and the single thermodilution techniques.

The thermo-dye dilution technique is based on the simultaneous detection of two indicators with different properties: a freely diffusible indicator ('cold') and a dye (indocyanine green, ICG), which binds to plasma albumin. Both intravenously administered indicators are contained in the same solution and injected simultaneously. In contrast to the cold indicator, ICG is believed to remain in the intravascular space. It does not equilibrate with the interstitium. Thus, based on the Stewart-Hamilton principle, 'cold' and dye allow the calculation of the intrathoracic thermal volume (ITTV) and the intrathoracic blood volume (ITBV), respectively. The difference between the two distribution volumes is used to estimate the EVLW (EVLW = ITTV–ITBV) [11, 14]. The thermo-dye dilution method has been evaluated in animal models of lung edema, by comparing with postmortem gravimetry, which is supposed to be the 'gold standard' for EVLW measurement [15–17]. These studies have shown a high degree of correlation between the two methods. In addition, in humans EVLW determined with thermo-dye dilution has been validated against techniques employing isotopes [18]. In critically ill patients, fluid management guided by measurements of EVLW with thermo-dye dilution has been associated with improved clinical outcome [19]. Hence, it has been suggested that EVLW plays a role as an independent predictor of prognosis and course of illness [13, 16, 19]. However, the thermo-dye dilution technique is relatively time consuming, cumbersome and expensive. For those reasons, the method has not gained general acceptance, thus, motivating the search for a reasonable bedside alternative [11, 12, 15].

Employing a technique based on injection of a single thermo-indicator that can be detected with an indwelling arterial thermodilution catheter, was an appealing idea. In brief, the single thermodilution method is based on the calculation of ITTV according to the following formula:

$$ITTV = Cardiac\ Output(CO) \times Mean\ Transit\ time\ of\ the\ thermo\text{-}indicator\ (MTt).$$

ITTV consists of the pulmonary thermal volume (PTV) and the sum of the end-diastolic volumes of all cardiac chambers (Fig. 1). PTV can be derived from the dilution curve, based on the assumption that in a series of several mixing chambers with identical flow the largest compartment mainly determines the decay of the curve. This variable can be calculated as PTV = CO×DSt where DSt is the exponential downslope time of the thermodilution curve in the aorta. Accordingly, the global end-diastolic volume (GEDV), which is the sum of the right and left heart end-diastolic volumes, is derived as GEDV = ITTV–PTV. After the estimation of GEDV, ITBV is calculated as equal to 1.25×GEDV. The coefficient 1.25 has been derived from critically ill patients using regression analysis and assuming that in the formula ITBV = GEDV + PBV, the pulmonary blood volume (PBV) is 20% of ITBV [20]. This coefficient was determined specifically for humans and requires reconsideration when applied to experimental animals that may vary in weight and age as well

Table 1. Techniques used for measurements of extravascular lung water (EVLW): Comparative characteristics

Technique	Accuracy	Clinical value	Cost	References
Gravimetry	Postmortem gravimetry is used as the reference technique for determination of EVLW in the experimental setting.	Since gravimetry is possible only in non-survivors, the clinical value of this method is low.	Low	25, 26
Chest radiography (CR)	An approx. 35% increase in EVLW is required for the diagnosis of pulmonary edema. Absence of CR signs virtually rules out significant pulmonary edema.	As a non-quantitative method, CR has been shown to be a relatively poor indicator of pulmonary edema of various etiologies. The results depend on a variety of uncontrollable factors.	Relatively low	9
Computer tomography (CT)	CT may provide more detailed information about regional lung density changes that correlates with localized pulmonary edema.	Cannot be used at the bedside. Changes are non-specific. High radiation dose makes the CT inappropriate for frequently repeated measurements.	High	34
Magnetic resonance imaging (MRI)	MRI has significant advantages over CT and plain CR. EVLW cannot be subtracted from the intravascular volume.	Cannot be used at the bedside. No radiation but long image acquisition time and difficulties of frequently repeated measurements in ICU patients.	High	35
Positron emission tomography (PET)	EVLW can be separated from total water by ^{15}O labeled carbon monoxide.	PET requires radioactive tracers and is not intended for repeated measurements. Available in outstanding scientific centers only.	Very high	36
Bioimpedance plethysmography	The technique does not differentiate the intrathoracic fluid. Absolute values cannot be obtained.	Method has not attained wide clinical use but is a non-invasive alternative to indicator dilution techniques.	Low	37
Multiple gas technique	The method measures only EVLW that is accessible to the airways.	Method has not attained wide clinical use.	Relatively low	38
Double thermo-dye indicator dilution	Details are expounded in this review. One of the modifications uses heavy water (D_2O) as a thermo-indicator that increases the accuracy of the method.	Invasive method. Details are expounded in this review. Method is relatively cumbersome and sophisticated. Hepatic failure may affect clearance of dye-indicator (indocyanine green).	Relatively high	10, 11
Single (thermal) indicator dilution	Acceptable. Use of thermal indicator alone has been shown to have approximately the same sensitivity as double dilution.	This invasive method is intended for repeated measurements at the bedside. Details are expounded in this review.	Relatively low	20

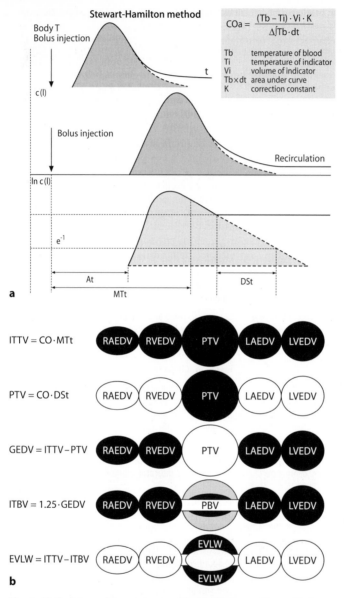

Fig. 1. Methodology of transpulmonary thermodilution. **a** Thermodilution curves and Stewart-Hamilton equation. **b** Intrathoracic volumes. T: temperature; CO: cardiac output (arterial thermodilution); MTt: mean transit time of indicator; DSt: downslope time of indicator; At: indicator appearance time; c(I): concentration of indicator; ITTV: intrathoracic thermal volume; PTV: pulmonary thermal volume; RAEDV: right atrium end-diastolic volume; RVEDV: right ventricle end-diastolic volume; LAEDV: left atrium end-diastolic volume; LVEDV: left ventricle end-diastolic volume; GEDV: global end-diastolic volume; ITBV: intrathoracic blood volume; PBV: pulmonary blood volume; EVLW: extravascular lung water

Table 2. Parameters measured by single transpulmonary thermodilution and pulse contour analysis

Parameter	Calculation	Normal range
▌ Cardiac Index (CI)	Area under transpulmonary thermodilution curve	3.0–5.0 l/min/m^2
▌ Extravascular Lung Water Index (EVLWI)	EWLVI = (ITTV–ITBV)/BW	3.0–7.0 ml/kg
▌ Intrathoracic Blood Volume Index (ITBVI)	ITBVI = 1.25 × GEDV/BW	850–1000 ml/m^2
▌ Pulmonary Vascular Permeability Index (PVPI)	PVPI = EVLW/PBV	1–3
▌ Cardiac Function Index (CFI)	CFI = CI/GEDV	4.5–6.5 min^{-1}
▌ Global Ejection Fraction (GEF)	GEF = 4 × SV/GEDV	25–35%
Transpulmonary cardiac output and pulse contour analysis derived parameters		
▌ Cardiac Index (CI)	Integral calculation of the area under curve	3.0–5.0 l/min/m^2
▌ Stroke Volume Index (SVI)	SVI = CI/HR	40–60 ml/m^2
▌ Stroke Volume Variations (SVV)	SVV = (SVmax–SVmin)/SVmean	≤10%
▌ Pulse Pressure Variations (PPV)	PPV = (PPmax–PPmin)/PPmean	≤10%
▌ Left ventricle contractility index (dPmax)	Analysis of arterial pulse contour (max. velocity of systolic part increase); dPmax = d(P)/d(t)	1200–2000 mmHg
▌ Systemic Vascular Resistance Index (SVRI)	SVRI = 80 × (MAP-CVP)/CI	1200–2000 dyne×s×cm^{-5}/m^2

ITTV: intrathoracic thermal volume; BW: body weight; GEDV: Global end diastolic volume; EVLW: extravascular lung water; PBV: pulmonary blood volume; SV: stroke volume; HR: heart rate; PP: pulse pressure; P: pressure; t: time; MAP: mean arterial pressure; CVP: central venous pressure

as between species. Thus, in our own experiments in sheep, where ITBV and PBV were measured directly using thermo-dye dilution, we found the 'ovine' coefficient to be 1.34 [21].

In analogy with the thermo-dye dilution technique, EVLW determined by single thermodilution (EVLW$_{STD}$) can be calculated as EVLW$_{STD}$ = ITTV–ITBV$_{STD}$. The combination of single thermodilution with pulse contour analysis of cardiac output offers the possibility of displaying a diversity of cardiopulmonary variables, in addition to those determined with thermo-dye dilution. After calibration, the single thermodilution technology allows cardiac index and derived parameters to be continuously recorded in a 'beat-to-beat' manner (Table 2), thus expanding the options for hemodynamic monitoring of the critically ill patient.

Recent experimental and clinical studies have shown that EVLW assessed by single thermodilution demonstrates good reproducibility and close agreement with the double indicator technique (Fig. 2) [20, 22]. Compared with both thermo-dye dilution and right heart catheterization, single thermodilution is simpler to apply, less invasive, and more cost-effective, all factors making it more suitable for use at the bedside. Recently, this new method has been validated against gravimetry in experimental models of cardiogenic and non-cardiogenic pulmonary edema [21, 23]. These studies have shown that single thermodilution correlates closely with EVLW

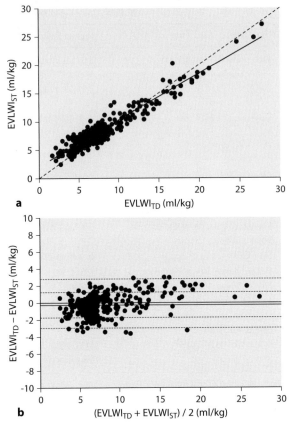

Fig. 2. Relationship between extravascular lung water index (EVLWI), measured by transpulmonary single thermodilution (ST) and thermo-dye dilution (TD) in 209 critically ill patients. **a** Linear regression analysis between $EVLWI_{TD}$ and $EVLWI_{ST}$. $EVLWI_{ST} = (0.83 \times EVLWI_{TD}) + 1.6$, $r = 0.96$, $p < 0.0001$, line of identity is dashed. **b** Agreement between $EVLWI_{TD}$ and $EVLWI_{ST}$. The bold line indicates the value for the mean difference between $EVLWI_{TD}$ and $EVLWI_{ST}$ (bias) and each dashed line indicates one standard deviation. Mean difference $EVLWI_{TD} - EVLWI_{ST} = -0.2$ ml/kg (standard deviation 1.4 ml/kg). From [20] with permission

determined with post mortem gravimetry ($EVLWI_G$). However, $EVLWI_{STD}$ overestimates $EVLWI_G$ by 3–5 ml/kg with the degree of overestimation increasing with the severity of the disease condition (Fig. 3). This difference can be explained by heat exchange of the thermal indicator with extravascular intrathoracic structures, such as the walls of the large vessels and the myocardium [16, 21].

In contrast to single thermodilution, thermo-dye dilution risks underestimating EVLW in comparison with gravimetry [11]. This underestimation increased during ALI caused by instillation of hydrochloric acid into the airways and has been explained by redistribution of pulmonary blood flow away from the edematous areas. The redistribution is thought to prevent indicator diffusion, and consequently, to obscure edema from being detected [15].

The detection of EVLW by thermodilution methods can be impaired by a number of factors such as, for instance, severe changes in cardiac output and positive

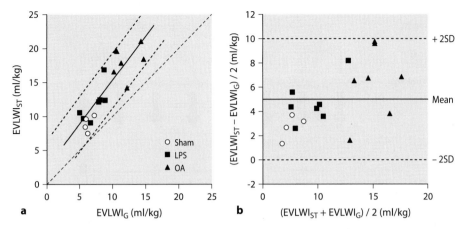

Fig. 3. Relationship between extravascular lung water index (EVLWI) measured by transpulmonary single thermodilution (ST) and postmortem gravimetry (G) in 18 sheep. Experimental groups: sham-operated (Sham), lipopolysaccharide (LPS), oleic acid (OA). **a** Linear regression analysis between $EVLWI_{ST}$ and $EVLWI_G$. $EVLWI_{ST} = (1.30 \times EVLWI_G) + 2.32$, $r = 0.85$, $p < 0.0001$. Line of identity is dashed, 95% confidence intervals are indicated by solid lines. **b** Bland-Altman plot for $EVLWI_{ST}$ and $EVLWI_G$. The x-axis shows the mean of EVLWI measurements by ST and G. The y-axis shows the difference between the methods. The bold line indicates the value for the mean difference between $EVLWI_{ST}$ and $EVLWI_G$ (bias) and each dashed line indicates two standard deviations. Mean difference $EVLWI_{ST} - EVLWI_G = 4.91$ ml/kg (standard deviation 2.54 ml/kg). From [21] with permission

end-expiratory pressure (PEEP) during mechanical ventilation [16, 24]. Thus, both thermo-dye dilution and single thermodilution require repeated measurements. In addition, the accuracy of EVLW measurements using these techniques can be influenced by inhomogeneous pulmonary edema, accumulation of chest exudates, and changes in the pulmonary blood volume [15, 16, 21].

Postmortem gravimetry used as the reference method for evaluation of pulmonary edema also has its limitations [25, 26]. The method allows only one measurement and cannot be used to follow variations over time. Consequently, gravimetrically determined EVLW is limited almost exclusively to experimental studies. Comparison of the gravimetric measurements with other techniques for determination of EVLW can be influenced by the time elapsing from euthanasia to removal of the lungs, and by pathophysiological changes in the lung circulation following cardiac arrest. Thus, the gravimetric technique can underestimate the real value of EVLWI because of partial reabsorption of edema fluid before the lungs are excised.

Summarizing the information regarding different techniques for determination of EVLW, thermo-dye dilution and single thermodilution are potentially promising methods in terms of their application at the bedside of critically ill patients.

Extravascular Lung Water Measurements in Patients with Sepsis

Several categories of ICU patients, both pediatric and adult, may benefit from monitoring of EVLW [19]. In this regard, the main pathophysiological changes prompting a need for controlling EVLW include the risk of contracting pulmonary edema,

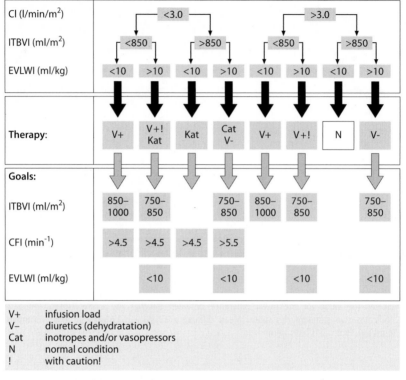

Fig. 4. Decision tree for hemodynamic monitoring. CI: cardiac index; ITBVI: intrathoracic blood volume index; EVLWI: extravascular lung water index; CFI: cardiac function index

massive fluid shifts, and severe changes in microvascular permeability. The latter changes are among the hallmarks of critical conditions like severe sepsis, burns, non-cardiogenic (ALI and ARDS) and cardiogenic lung edema, multiple trauma with severe blood loss, ischemia-reperfusion injury, etc. [10, 27]. Thus, we can consider any critical illness resulting in shock and tissue hypoperfusion that is refractory to fluid resuscitation, as a valid subject for EVLW monitoring. In addition, the method may be of value in patients undergoing major surgical procedures, particularly, cardiothoracic surgery and organ transplantation [28, 29]. In all these conditions, measurement of EVLW can support the diagnosis and may even improve the clinical outcome when used cautiously in combination with treatment protocols that are known to hasten the resolution of pulmonary edema (Fig. 4) [19, 30].

A number of studies have focused on the role of controlling hemodynamics and EVLW as a guide to the diagnosis and treatment of critically ill patients including those with sepsis [10, 13, 14, 16, 19, 30, 31]. In septic shock, invasive cardiovascular monitoring with arterial catheterization and 'beat-to-beat' analysis facilitate the administration of large quantities of fluids, vasopressor/inotrope support, and ventilatory settings. Hence, such monitoring has recently been recommended as one of the guiding parameters for hemodynamic support in sepsis [8].

During sepsis-induced pulmonary edema, accumulation of EVLW occurs before any changes in blood gases, chest radiogram and, eventually, also in pressure vari-

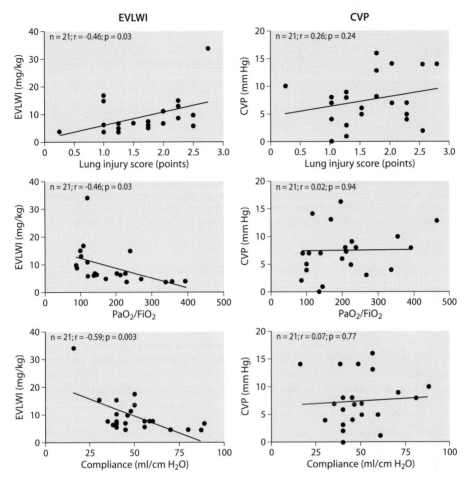

Fig. 5. Correlation of extravascular lung water index (EVLWI) and central venous pressure (CVP) with markers of lung injury in human septic shock (modified from [31] with permission)

ables. In addition, the latter variables are non-specific diagnostic tools and influenced by a variety of factors [9, 11, 12, 16]. Recently, Boussat et al. demonstrated that in sepsis-induced ALI commonly used filling pressures such as pulmonary artery occlusion pressure (PAOP) and right atrial pressure (RAP) are poor indicators of pulmonary edema. These authors rather recommend direct measurement of EVLW [10]. Consistently, we found [32] that in human septic shock, EVLW, in contrast to central venous pressure (CVP), correlates with markers of lung injury such as the oxygenation ratio, the lung compliance, and the lung injury score (Fig. 5). Interestingly, at Day 1 after the onset of severe sepsis, EVLW correlates negatively with the platelet count, thus demonstrating a role of platelet sequestration in the development of lung edema [31]. In addition, the increase in EVLW during sepsis-induced ALI is accompanied by an increment in the plasma concentration of endothelin-1, a potent mediator with vasoconstrictor properties, which also can contribute significantly to the increase in pulmonary microvascular permeability.

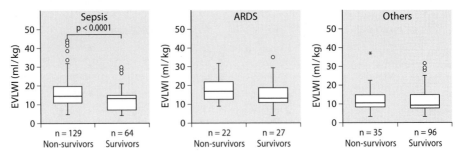

Fig. 6. Extravascular lung water and outcome. Box plot for the different subgroups of patients (i.e., sepsis, ARDS, and all others). Bold lines indicate medians, box plots indicate 25 to 75th percentiles, and bars indicate the 1.5-fold of the whole box length. Circles indicate values between 1.5-fold to threefold of the whole box length, and outliers (outside threefold of the whole box length) are indicated by asterisks. The bold asterisk indicates statistical significance (Mann-Whitney *U* test). From [13] with permission

Therefore, in sepsis, EVLW serves as a marker of ALI, provides a valid estimate of the interstitial water content in the lungs and might become an alternative to RAP in the management of fluid resuscitation.

EVLW has the most significant prognostic value in septicemic patients compared with other subpopulations of critically ill patients (Fig. 6). Thus, in subjects in whom EVLW was >15 ml/kg, the mortality rate was 65% [13]. Being an independent predictor of survival, EVLW can represent a landmark in fluid and hemodynamic management with the aim of preventing the development of pulmonary edema. When evaluated in combination with other cardiopulmonary parameters, EVLW might provide useful guidance in the process of weaning the patient off the respirator, thereby reducing the duration of mechanical ventilation, and shortening ICU and hospital stays [19, 30, 33]. Moreover, some authors have demonstrated that monitoring of EVLW can reduce mortality in critically ill patients [30]. Thus, bedside monitoring of EVLW appears to be an appropriate way of managing pulmonary edema. However, to fully evaluate EVLW$_{STD}$, further clinical trials are warranted that involve comparison with thermo-dye dilution in different categories of patients including those with sepsis.

▌ Conclusion

In sepsis, the inflammatory process in the lungs may increase the microvascular pressure and permeability, causing accumulation of EVLW and development of ALI and pulmonary edema. Among the various methods for measurement of EVLW at the bedside, both thermo-dye dilution and single transpulmonary thermodilution may be useful. In the experimental setting, these techniques correlate closely with gravimetric measurements over a wide range of changes. However, compared with postmortem gravimetry, single transpulmonary thermodilution overestimates the absolute values of EVLW. This necessitates correction of the therapeutic algorithm. Nevertheless, the dynamic changes in EVLW are of obvious clinical value allowing close monitoring of pulmonary edema at the bedside. Recent clinical studies have shown that in sepsis EVLW correlates with the severity of lung injury and appears to have a prognostic value. Thus, monitoring EVLW can be a useful additional tool in the goal-oriented therapy of severe sepsis and sepsis-induced ALI.

References

1. Hotchkiss RS, Karl IE (2003) The pathophysiology and treatment of sepsis. N Engl J Med 348:138–150
2. Bone RC (1991) The pathogenesis of sepsis. Ann Intern Med 115:457–469
3. Noda H, Noshima S, Nakazawa H, et al (1994) Left ventricular dysfunction and acute lung injury induced by continuous administration of endotoxin in sheep. Shock 1:291–298
4. Perkowski SZ, Sloane PJ, Spath JA Jr, et al (1996) TNF-alpha and the pathophysiology of endotoxin-induced acute respiratory failure in sheep. J Appl Physiol 80:564–573
5. Pittet JF, Mackersie RC, Martin TR, Matthay MA (1997) Biological markers of acute lung injury: prognostic and pathogenetic significance. Am J Respir Crit Care Med 155:1187–1205
6. Martin GS, Bernard GR (2001) Airway and lung in sepsis. Intensive Care Med 27:S63–S79
7. Hollenberg SM, Ahrens TS, Annane D, et al (2004) Practice parameters for hemodynamic support of sepsis in adult patients: 2004 update. Crit Care Med 32:1928–1948
8. Ware LB, Matthay MA (2000) The acute respiratory distress syndrome. N Engl J Med 342:1334–1349
9. Halperin BD, Feeley TW, Mihm FG, Chiles C, Guthaner DF, Blank NE (1985) Evaluation of the portable chest roentgenogram for quantitating extravascular lung water in critically ill adults. Chest 88:649–652
10. Boussat S, Jacques T, Levy B, et al (2002) Intravascular volume monitoring and extravascular lung water in septic patients with pulmonary edema. Intensive Care Med 28:712–718
11. Pfeiffer UJ, Backus G, Blumel G, et al (1990) A fiberoptic-based system for integrated monitoring of cardiac output, intrathoracic blood volume, extravascular lung water, O_2 saturation, and a-v differences. In: Lewis FR, Pfeiffer UJ (eds) Practical Applications of Fiberoptics in Critical Care Monitoring. Springer, Berlin, pp 114–125
12. Boldt J (2002) Clinical review: hemodynamic monitoring in the intensive care unit. Crit Care 6:52–59
13. Sakka SG, Klein M, Reinhart K, et al (2002) Prognostic value of extravascular lung water in critically ill patients. Chest 122:2080–2086
14. Sakka SG, Meier-Hellmann A (2000) Estimation of cardiac output and cardiac preload. In: Vincent JL (ed) Yearbook of Intensive Care and Emergency Medicine. Springer, Heidelberg, pp 671–679
15. Roch A, Michelet P, Lambert D, et al (2004) Accuracy of the double indicator method for measurement of extravascular lung water depends on the type of acute lung injury. Crit Care Med 32:811–817
16. Bock J, Lewis FR (1990) Clinical relevance of lung water measurement with the thermal-dye dilution technique. In: Lewis FR, Pfeiffer UJ (eds) Practical Applications of Fiberoptics in Critical Care Monitoring. Springer, Berlin, pp 129–139
17. Kirov MY, Evgenov OV, Kuklin VN, Bjertnaes LJ (2003) Extravascular lung water assessed by thermal-dye dilution correlates with gravimetric technique. Intensive Care Med 29:S167 (abst)
18. Sturm JA (1984) Entwicklung und Bedeutung der Lungenwassermessung in Klinik und Experiment. In: Bergmann H, Gilly H, Steinbereithner K, et al (eds) Beiträge zur Anästhesiologie und Intensivmedizin. Verlag Wilhelm Maudrich, Vienna, pp 15–39
19. Mitchell JP, Schuller D, Calandrino FS, Schuster DP (1992) Improved outcome based on fluid management in critically ill patients requiring pulmonary artery catheterization. Am Rev Respir Dis 145:990–998
20. Sakka SG, Ruhl CC, Pfeiffer UJ, et al (2000) Assessment of cardiac preload and extravascular lung water by single transpulmonary thermodilution. Intensive Care Med 26:180–187
21. Kirov MY, Kuzkov VV, Kuklin VN, Waerhaug K, Bjertnaes LJ (2004) Extravascular lung water assessed by transpulmonary single thermodilution and postmortem gravimetry in sheep. Crit Care 8:R451–R458
22. Neumann P (1999) Extravascular lung water and intrathoracic blood volume: double versus single indicator dilution technique. Intensive Care Med 25:216–219

23. Katzenelson R, Perel A, Berkenstadt, et al (2004) Accuracy of transpulmonary thermodilution versus gravimetric measurement of extravascular lung water. Crit Care Med 32:1550–1554
24. Groeneveld ABJ, Verheij J (2004) Is pulmonary edema associated with a high extravascular thermal volume? Crit Care Med 32:899–901
25. Pearce ML, Yamashita J, Beazell J (1965) Measurement of pulmonary edema. Circ Res 16: 482–488
26. Fernandez-Mondejar E, Castano-Perez J, Rivera-Fernandez R, et al (2003) Quantification of lung water by transpulmonary thermodilution in normal and edematous lung. J Crit Care 18:253–258
27. Kuntscher MV, Czermak C, Blome-Eberwein S, Dacho A, Germann G (2003) Transcardiopulmonary thermal dye versus single thermodilution methods for assessment of intrathoracic blood volume and extravascular lung water in major burn resuscitation. J Burn Care Rehabil 24:142–147
28. Hachenberg T, Tenling A, Rothen HU, Nystrom SO, Tyden H, Hedenstierna G (1993) Thoracic intravascular and extravascular fluid volumes in cardiac surgical patients. Anesthesiology 79:976–984
29. Krenn CG, Plochl W, Nikolic A, et al (2000) Intrathoracic fluid volumes and pulmonary function during orthotopic liver transplantation. Transplantation 69:2394–2400
30. Eisenberg PR, Hansbrough JR, Anderson D, Schuster DP (1987) A prospective study of lung water measurements during patient management in an intensive care unit. Am Rev Respir Dis 136:662–668
31. Kirov MY, Kuzkov VV, Bjertnaes LJ, Nedashkovsky EV (2003) Monitoring of extravascular lung water in patients with severe sepsis. Anesteziol Reanimatol 4:41–45
32. Kirov MY, Kuzkov VV, Waerhaug K, Kuklin VN, Bjertnaes LJ (2003) Extravascular lung water correlates with acute lung injury and outcome in human septic shock. Acta Anaesth Scand 47 (Suppl):31 (abst)
33. Zeravik J, Borg U, Pfeiffer UJ (1990) Efficacy of pressure support ventilation dependent on extravascular lung water. Chest 97:1412–1419
34. Forster BB, Muller NL, Mayo JR, Okazawa M, Wiggs BJ, Pare PD (1992) High-resolution computed tomography of experimental hydrostatic pulmonary edema. Chest 101:1434–1437
35. Hayes CE, Case TA, Ailion DC, et al (1982) Lung water quantitation by nuclear magnetic resonance imaging. Science 216:1313–1315
36. Wollmer P, Rhodes CG (1988) Positron emission tomography in pulmonary edema. J Thorac Imaging 3:44–50
37. Nierman DM, Eisen DI, Fein ED, Hannon E, Mechanick JI, Benjamin EJ (1996) Transthoracic bioimpedance can measure extravascular lung water in acute lung injury. Surg Res 65:101–108
38. Friedman M, Wilkins SA Jr, Rothfeld AF, Bromberg PA (1984) Effect of ventilation and perfusion imbalance on inert gas rebreathing variables. J Appl Physiol 56:364–369

Procalcitonin on the Dusty Way to the Holy Grail: A Progress Report

M. Christ-Crain and B. Müller

▌ What is Procalcitonin?

Procalcitonin (PCT) is a precursor peptide from the hormone calcitonin [1] (Fig. 1). After translation from calcitonin messenger RNA (mRNA), PCT is cleaved enzymatically into smaller peptides, finally to yield the thirty-two amino acid mature calcitonin [2]. All these calcitonin precursor peptides, including PCT, are found in the serum of normal persons.

Mature calcitonin, named after its hypocalcemic effect, was originally thought to be a hormone exclusively of thyroidal C-cell origin and to play an important role in skeletal homeostasis [3, 4]. However, provided that thyroid hormone is replaced, thyroidectomy in humans has no important pathologic consequences: calcium homeostasis remains intact and bone density is not decreased [5, 6]. Calcitonin possibly once had an important evolutionary role in the context of establishing and

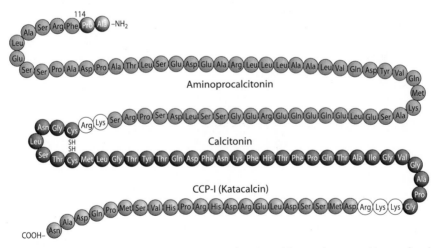

Fig. 1. Schematic illustration of human procalcitonin. Procalcitonin and its constituent peptides, are found in the free form in normal human serum. Initially, procalcitonin, consisting of 116 aminoacids, is secreted. Due to rapid cleavage by dipeptidases, 114 aminoacid long procalcitonin is found in the circulation. Additional cleaving leads to circulating aminoprocalcitonin, immature calcitonin and calcitonin carboxypeptide-I (CCP-I), previously known as katacalcin. In sepsis, these peptides are variably increased, often to huge levels due to ubiquitous expression and secretion. However, in this condition, serum levels of mature calcitonin, which is only produced by thyroidal C-cells, remain normal or are only slightly increased

protecting the skeleton under conditions of calcium stress. Thereafter, changes in amino acid sequence during evolution were responsible for a loss of activity, as fish calcitonin is about 40 times as potent as human calcitonin. Thus, mature calcitonin may have been useful to survival in seawater fish, but the presence of the parathyroid gland and other evolutionary changes occurring in tetrapods suggest that the function of the mature calcitonin hormone in humans is no longer essential [7].

Conversely, in microbial infections and in various forms of severe systemic inflammation, circulating levels of *several* calcitonin precursors, including PCT but not mature calcitonin, increase up to several-thousand-fold, and this increase, and especially the course, correlates with the severity of the condition and with mortality [8–11]. Critical analyses of the world literature have confirmed a superior diagnostic utility of serum levels of PCT in sepsis and their greater reliability in following the course of illness, as compared to other markers [1, 11–13].

▌ How to Measure PCT Levels

For the diagnosis of infections, the diagnostic accuracy of PCT and its optimum cut-offs are completely dependent on use of a sensitive assay in an appropriate clinical setting (Fig. 2). Ideally, an ultra-sensitive PCT assay should reliably measure circulating concentrations of this molecule in all healthy individuals. A rapid assay assures that results can be timely incorporated into clinical decision making. Importantly, as is the case for all diagnostic tests, a serum PCT concentration must always be interpreted with proper respect to the clinical context. In bacterial infections, the extent to which any specific calcitonin precursor peptide is increased relative to the others varies; indeed, the levels of procalcitonin NH2-terminal cleavage peptide (N-PCT) and calcitonin:calcitonin carboxyterminal peptide-I (CCP-I) may be even higher than the PCT values [14].

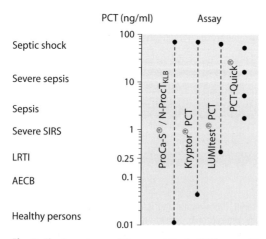

Fig. 2. The importance of the procalcitonin (PCT) assay. The diagnostic accuracy of PCT and its optimum cut-offs are dependent on the assay used in an appropriate clinical setting. Details of the different tests are described in the text. AECB: acute exacerbations of chronic bronchitis; LRTI: lower respiratory tract infections; SIRS: systemic inflammatory response syndrome

For example, an ultra-sensitive N-PCT assay (Becker K. L., et al., Washington D.C., USA), with a functional assay sensitivity of below 0.02 ng/ml and, thus, capable of measuring calcitonin precursor peptides in normal persons, utilizes an antibody to N-PCT, as the free peptide and within the PCT molecule [9, 15]. Using this assay, healthy blood donors have PCT levels of 0.03 ± 0.02 ng/ml (mean ± SD). This assay is available for research purposes.

Another ultra-sensitive assay, ProCa-S® (BRAHMS, Hennigsdorf, Germany) is available for research use. However, for the time being, this assay is manual and, therefore, not suitable for the routine day and night setting in an emergency or intensive care unit (ICU).

We recently evaluated a newly developed PCT assay to guide antimicrobial therapy in lower respiratory tract infections (LRTI) [16, 17]. This commercially available assay takes advantage of a time-resolved amplified cryptate emission (TRACE) technology (Kryptor® PCT). It is based on a sheep polyclonal anti-calcitonin antibody and a monoclonal anti-katacalcin antibody, which bind to the calcitonin and katacalcin sequence of calcitonin precursor molecules. The assay has a functional assay sensitivity of 0.06 ng/ml, i.e., 3 to 5-fold above normal mean values [18]. Assay time is 19 minutes and in clinical routine results can be obtained within one hour using 20 to 50 μl of plasma or serum [19].

Another commercially available two-site assay (LUMItest® PCT, BRAHMS, Hennigsdorf, Germany), measures both PCT and the conjoined calcitonin:CCP I by means of a luminometer. This assay is useful to detect markedly elevated calcitonin precursor levels in severe, systemic bacterial infections, i.e., in sepsis. However, this manual assay has the disadvantage of a relative insensitivity, with an accurate detection limit of ~0.3 to 0.5 ng/ml [9, 14]. Thus; the LUMItest® assay is not sensitive enough to detect mildly or moderately elevated PCT levels, which limits its diagnostic use in conditions other than overt sepsis.

A colorimetric bedside test (PCT®-Q, BRAHMS, Hennigsdorf, Germany) has the advantage of rapid determination of circulating calcitonin precursor levels in 30 minutes. Unfortunately, the assay is only semi-quantitative and is not sensitive enough to detect mildly or moderately elevated calcitonin precursor levels [20].

▌ Respiratory Tract Infections and Sepsis: Vicious Cycle of Antibiotic Overuse and Emerging Multi-resistance

LRTI, e.g., acute bronchitis, acute exacerbations of chronic obstructive pulmonary disease (COPD) or asthma, and pneumonia, account for almost 10% of the worldwide burden of morbidity and mortality [21]. As much as 75% of all antibiotic doses are prescribed for acute LRTIs, in spite of their predominantly viral etiology [21]. Due to the diagnostic uncertainty, there are large differences in the prescription pattern of antibiotics, overall and for LRTI, between countries and between different healthcare providers in the same country [22, 23]. Countries like France and especially the US have a high antibiotic resistance rate, consistent with a relatively high overall antibiotic use [17, 24]. This excessive use of antibiotics is believed to be the main cause of the spread of antibiotic-resistant bacteria [25, 26]. Thus, decreasing the excess use of antibiotics is essential to combat the increase of antibiotic-resistant microorganisms [27, 28]. A reduction in antibiotic use results in fewer side effects, lower costs, and, in the long-term, leads to decreasing drug resistance [29].

To limit antibiotic use, a rapid and accurate differentiation of clinically relevant bacterial LRTI from other, mostly viral, causes is pivotal. After obtaining the medical history, physical examination, laboratory results, and chest x-ray, the clinician is often left with diagnostic uncertainty, because signs and symptoms of bacterial and viral infections widely overlap [30, 31]. For example, bacteria can be isolated from sputum in up to 50% of patients with acute exacerbations COPD, but whether this finding represents colonization or infection is controversial [32, 33]. The lack of specific markers or a gold standard of clinically relevant bacterial infections contributes to the overuse of antibiotics in LRTI, especially in elderly patients with comorbidities or critically ill patients.

Most sepsis is caused by pulmonary infections. Independent of an infection, critically ill patients often manifest a systemic inflammatory response syndrome (SIRS) characterized by a white blood count > 12,000 or < 4,000 cells/μl; a heart rate > 90 beats/min; a respiratory rate > 20 breaths/min, and a body temperature > 38 or < 36 °C. When SIRS is present, and infection is proven or suspected, the term sepsis is used. Again, traditional clinical signs of infection and the routine laboratory tests in sepsis (e.g., C-reactive protein [CRP] or white blood cell count) are not specific and sometimes misleading. In severe infection, most classical pro-inflammatory cytokines (e.g., tumor necrosis factor [TNF]-α, interleukin [IL]-1β or IL-6) are increased only briefly or intermittently, if at all. Most sepsis is caused by pulmonary infections [34]. In this context, bacterial respiratory tract infections can be viewed as sepsis precursors. Despite the use of new treatment modalities [35], the mortality of sepsis remains high, often due to delayed diagnosis and treatment. Therefore, antimicrobial therapy in pneumonia must be promptly initiated, because a delay of > 4 to 8 h in treatment is associated with increased mortality due to progression to severe sepsis and shock [36]. In view of this diagnostic and therapeutic dilemma, an unequivocal test for the differential diagnosis of infection and sepsis and to guide antibiotic treatment would be very useful.

❚ PCT as a Tool to Guide Antimicrobial Therapy in Lower Respiratory Tract Infections

In the 'ProResp' Study we recently assessed the capability of a sensitive PCT assay (Kryptor® PCT) to identify bacterial LRTIs requiring antimicrobial treatment [16]. In a prospective, cluster-randomized, controlled, single-blinded intervention trial we compared the routine use of antimicrobial therapy versus PCT-guided antimicrobial treatment for LRTI (Fig. 3). Patients who presented with cough and/or dyspnea at the medical emergency department were assessed for eligibility. The criterion for inclusion in the study was a suspected LRTI as the main diagnosis, i.e., acute bronchitis, acute exacerbations of COPD or asthma, and pneumonia. Excluded were severely immunocompromised patients. Assessment included complete history, physical examination, measurement of body temperature, blood sampling for hematology and blood-chemistry including CRP, as well as chest x-ray. Sputum and blood collection for microbiological culture, blood gases, spirometry, and bronchoscopy with bronchoalveolar lavage (BAL), consultation of an infectious disease specialist and pulmonary care specialist were performed as needed in both groups. All

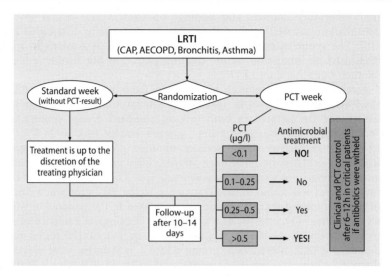

Fig. 3. 'ProResp' – Study Design [16]. Two hundred and forty-three patients admitted with suspected lower respiratory tract infections (LRTIs) were randomly assigned standard care (standard group; n=119) or procalcitonin (PCT)-guided treatment (PCT group; n = 124). On the basis of serum PCT concentrations, use of antibiotics was more or less discouraged (PCT <0.1 ug/l or <0.25 ug/l) or encouraged (≥0.5 ug/l or ≥0.25 ug/l). Reevaluation was possible after 6–24 h in both groups and mandatory in sick patients if antimicrobial therapy was withheld. CAP: community acquired pneumonia, AECOPD: acute exacerbations of chronic obstructive pulmonary disease

patients filled in a visual analog scale and a quality of life (QOL) questionnaire on admission as well as at the follow-up [37].

The diagnostic procedures, therapeutic regimen and final decision to initiate antimicrobial therapy was in all cases left to the discretion of the treating physician. In the PCT group, all physicians had to specify their intention to prescribe antibiotic therapy before they became aware of the serum PCT level, referred to as "antibiotic prescription foreseen". Thereafter, in the PCT group, the physician was advised to follow the antibiotic treatment algorithm based on the PCT value [15, 38–40]. A serum PCT level of ≤ 0.1 ng/ml was considered to indicate the absence of bacterial infection and the use of antibiotics was strongly discouraged, also in the presence of impaired pulmonary reserve in COPD [15]. A PCT value of 0.1 to 0.25 ng/ml was considered to indicate that bacterial infection was unlikely, and the use of antibiotics was discouraged. A serum PCT level between 0.25 and 0.5 ng/ml was considered to indicate a possible bacterial infection and the treating physician was advised to initiate antimicrobial therapy. A PCT value of ≥0.5 ng/ml was considered to be suggestive of the presence of bacterial infection and antibiotic treatment was strongly recommended [38]. In patients on antimicrobial therapy at the time of admission, discontinuation of antibiotics was recommended if PCT values were below 0.25 ng/ml. In both groups, a re-evaluation 6 to 24 hours after admission was possible in those patients in whom antibiotics were withheld, including clinical and laboratory work-up and re-measurement of serum PCT levels in the PCT group.

Baseline characteristics were similar in the standard group compared to the PCT group. Specifically, history, clinical signs and symptoms of respiratory tract infection, laboratory markers and findings on chest-X-ray, further investigations and consultations as well as final diagnoses were similarly distributed in both groups [16]. The group classified as "others" consisted of 24 patients in whom LRTI was diagnosed on admission by the treating physician but further evaluation revealed another diagnosis than LRTI.

Overall, bacterial cultures were grown from sputum and/or BAL in 51 cases (21.0%) and from blood in 16 cases (6.6%). A similar percentage of microorganisms could be cultured in both groups: standard group: sputum and/or BAL in 20.2%; blood in 8.4%; PCT group: sputum and/or BAL in 21.8%; blood in 4.8% (p = ns for respective comparisons of standard group versus PCT group, The most frequently isolated bacteria were *Streptococcus pneumoniae*, *Haemophilus influenzea*, enterobacteriaceae, and *Pseudomonas* spp. The highest fraction of positive sputum cultures was found in COPD patients; in the PCT group in a similar percentage of patients treated with antibiotics as compared to the patients in whom antibiotics were withheld (54.5 versus 61.1%, p = 0.73). Serological evidence of acute infection using the novel sensitive assay, was found in 141 of 175 tested patients (80.6%; Standard group: 77.3%, PCT group: 83.9%). IgM levels were elevated in 121 patients. Multiple viral infections were found in 26.3% of patients. Parainfluenza virus type 3 (n = 44), influenza B (n = 37) and adenovirus (n = 29), parainfluenza virus type 1 (n = 19) and respiratory syncytial virus (RSV) (n = 18) were the most frequent viral infections. There was serological evidence of *Mycoplasma pneumoniae* infection in three cases.

The outcome after a mean of 13.0 ± 5.4 days was similar in both groups. The four deaths in the standard group were due to sepsis (2), myocardial infarction (1), and an unknown cause after discharge (1). Both patients dying with septicemia suffered from pulmonary co-morbidities (lung cancer, lung fibrosis). None of the four deaths in the PCT group was due to delayed or withheld antimicrobial therapy, but to myocardial infarction (2) (one with advanced lung cancer and pneumonia) acute renal failure (1), and sepsis (1) (despite immediate and appropriate antimicrobial therapy based on elevated PCT levels).

Importantly, the rate of antibiotic prescriptions foreseen by the treating physician was similar in both groups. In contrast, in the PCT group the percentage of patients with LRTI who received antibiotic therapy was reduced by 46.6%, as compared to the standard group (p < 0.001). After adjusting for potential confounding factors and possible cluster-effects, the relative risk of antibiotic exposure in the PCT group was 0.49 (95% CI, 0.44–0.55, p < 0.001). Antibiotic use could be significantly reduced in all diagnostic subgroups (Fig. 4). In most patients with community-acquired pneumonia, circulating PCT levels were markedly elevated (standard group: 3.9 ± 6.2 ng/ml; PCT group: 4.6 ± 12.9 ng/ml, p = 0.29). In the PCT group, in 9% of the community-acquired pneumonia patients antibiotics were withheld based on low serum PCT levels; all had a favorable outcome with hospital stays from one to 18 days. On admission, 44.8 and 17.2% of patients with acute exacerbation of COPD had serum PCT levels of >0.1 ng/ml and >0.25 ng/ml, respectively.

In the standard group, the odds of being treated with antibiotics increased by 6.5% with each additional year of age (95% CI: 3.4% to 9.8%, p < 0.001). Conversely, in the PCT group, no such age relation was found (95% CI: –1.2 to 2.4%, p = 0.53).

Most respiratory tract infections are viral [41]. Accordingly, serological evidence of viral infection was found in almost 80% of assessed cases using a new, sensitive enzyme immunoassay (EIA) screening test. Parainfluenza, influenza, and adenovirus infections accounted for the majority of infections. Thus, the greater part of

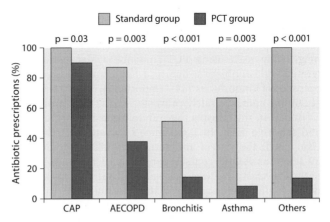

Fig. 4. Use of antibiotics in different subgroups. Antibiotic prescriptions in different subgroups of LRTI were compared between the standard group and the PCT group. CAP: community-acquired pneumonia; AECOPD: acute exacerbation of chronic obstructive pulmonary disease

patients in our study, performed during the winter, had suffered from common cold or flu preceding hospital admission. By damaging the respiratory epithelium, respiratory viruses facilitate secondary bacterial infection of the airways [42]. It is difficult to separate viral from bacterial infection based on clinical evaluation, serology and bacterial culture. Based on our data, in LRTI, low serum PCT levels of <0.1 to <0.25 ng/ml can identify patients without clinically relevant bacterial infections; in these patients antimicrobial therapy can be safely withheld.

Pneumonia is defined as inflammation of the pulmonary parenchyma, often caused by a bacterial agent, mirrored in markedly elevated PCT levels [38, 39]. Antimicrobial therapy must be promptly initiated, because a delay of >8h in treatment is associated with increased mortality [36]. Unfortunately, bacteria are usually identified in less than 50% of cases and a positive viral serology does not rule out complicating bacterial infection. In the clinical context of community-acquired pneumonia, the primary value of PCT is not the reduction of antibiotic prescription, but to facilitate the differential diagnosis of new or progressing infiltrates. Accordingly, PCT-guidance could markedly lower the number of antibiotic courses in patients with infiltrates on chest x-ray unrelated to pneumonia.

It is estimated that only 25% of patients with acute exacerbation of COPD benefit from the addition of antibiotic therapy [33]. The appearance of new strains and persistence of bacterial infection may contribute to acute exacerbations of COPD and disease progression, respectively [43]. The majority of patients with acute exacerbations of COPD in our study had positive sputum culture results. In the PCT group this rate was similar in patients in whom antibiotics were given or withheld, as was the outcome. This illustrates the limited diagnostic use of sputum cultures in acute exacerbations of COPD. Most of the patients in whom the PCT-guided treatment algorithm was overruled were in the acute exacerbation of COPD subgroup. It remains hypothetical whether these patients indeed profited from antibiotic therapy. Nevertheless, since patients with COPD have an impaired pulmonary reserve and the infection might be locally restricted, a PCT of <0.1 ng/ml as a cutoff level to withhold antibiotics is advisable in patients with severe acute exacerbations of COPD.

In acute exacerbations of asthma, there is no scientific evidence for antibiotic use and in acute bronchitis, vitamin C used as placebo, is as effective as antimicrobial therapy [37]. Accordingly, in these two subgroups of LRTI, antibiotics were only rarely used using PCT-guidance. Older patients with LRTI are more often treated with antibiotics, due to a higher morbidity and mortality especially in the presence of comorbities [44]. Importantly, this age-related overuse of antibiotic prescriptions could be safely prevented in the PCT group.

Hence, in this prospective, randomized trial including 243 patients, using a rapid and sensitive assay, PCT guidance substantially reduced antibiotic overuse in LRTI. Using PCT, the risk of antibiotic exposure was reduced by 50%, which equated to 39 fewer antibiotic courses per 100 patients with LRTI. Importantly, withholding antibiotic treatment was safe and did not compromise clinical and laboratory outcome. It must be emphasized that the diagnostic accuracy of PCT and its optimal cut-offs are completely dependent on using a sensitive assay in an appropriate clinical setting. PCT is not a substitute for a careful history and physical examination. Yet, as a surrogate marker it provides important additional information and questions the currently used 'gold standards' for the clinical diagnose of bacterial LRTI. Ideally, an ultra-sensitive PCT assay should reliably measure circulating concentrations of PCT in all healthy individuals. A rapid assay assures that results can be incorporated into the clinical decision making, which was the case in our study. However, as is the case for all diagnostic tests, a serum PCT level must always be evaluated and re-evaluated, respectively, with proper regard to the clinical context. Circulating PCT levels can be increased in non-infectious conditions, and may remain relatively low even in sepsis [15, 40].

▌ PCT – More than Just a Marker in Bacterial Infections?

Importantly, PCT, likely together with other calcitonin precursors, contributes to the deleterious effects of systemic infection. The administration of PCT to septic hamsters with peritonitis doubled their death rate, reaching levels exceeding 90%. Furthermore, treatment with PCT-reactive antiserum increased the survival of septic hamsters [45–47]. In addition, a one-hour intravenous immunoneutralization using an antiserum reacting specifically with porcine PCT, improved the physiologic and metabolic parameters of septic pigs, and greatly increased their short-term survival (from 0 to 80%) [48]. Furthermore, recent experiments have demonstrated that such immunoneutralization is effective even when administered after the animals are moribund [49].

Thus, several observations indicate that PCT is not only a necessary precursor to the biosynthesis of mature calcitonin, but also, at the high concentrations occurring in the setting of sepsis, is a potentially harmful mediator involved in the septic response. It was shown, that PCT acts as a modulator of the inflammatory/immunologic host reaction [50]. Furthermore, ionized hypocalcemia is more pronounced with increasing severity of infection, and occurs in parallel with the marked increase in calcitonin precursors [51]. In contrast, as mentioned above, serum levels of mature calcitonin are normal or only minimally elevated in sepsis [9, 10, 51].

Several characteristics of PCT favor this hormokine molecule as a therapeutic target in sepsis. In contrast to the transiently increased classical cytokines, for which immunoneutralization trials in humans have been disappointing, the massive increase of circulating calcitonin precursors persists for several days [52]. Furthermore, calcitonin precursors are very frequently increased in overt sepsis, with an early onset (within 3 hr), and the diagnostic accuracy of the measurement should greatly improve patient selection for any study of the therapeutic efficacy of PCT immunoneutralization in humans.

▮ ProCT – Where Does it come From?

Calcitonin precursors, including PCT, emanate from the calcitonin I (CALC-I) gene on chromosome 11. In the traditional endocrine view, mature calcitonin is produced mostly in the neuroendocrine C-cells of the thyroid. In the absence of infection, the extra-thyroidal transcription of the CALC-I gene is suppressed and is restricted to a selective expression in neuroendocrine cells found mainly in thyroid and lung. In these neuroendocrine cells, the mature hormone is processed and stored in secretory granules [4, 53].

Interestingly, a microbial infection induces a ubiquitous increase of CALC-I gene-expression and a constitutive release of calcitonin precursors from all parenchymal tissues and cell types throughout the body [54] (Fig. 5). Thus, under septic circumstances, the entire body could be viewed as being an endocrine gland. Indeed, the transcriptional expression of calcitonin mRNA is more uniformly up-regulated in sepsis than are the mRNAs of the classical cytokines (e.g., TNF-α and

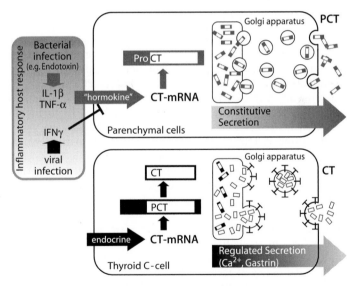

Fig. 5. Schematic diagram of CALC I expression in adipocytes and thyroidal C cells. In the classical neuroendocrine paradigm, the expression of calcitonin (CT) mRNA is restricted to neuroendocrine cells, mainly C cells of the thyroid. Initially, the 116-amino acid prohormone procalcitonin (PCT) is synthesized and subsequently processed to the considerably smaller mature CT. In sepsis and inflammation, pro-inflammatory mediators induce CT mRNA. In contrast to thyroid cells, parenchymal cells (e.g., liver, kidney, adipocytes and muscle) lack secretory granules, and hence, unprocessed PCT is released in a non-regulated, constitutive manner. INF: interferon; TNF: tumor necrosis factor; IL: interleukin

IL-6). There is a relatively low and only transient expression of calcitonin precursors in white blood cells [54–56]. No calcitonin gene expression is found if these cells are harvested from septic patients with markedly elevated serum PCT levels. In whole blood, lipopolysaccharide (LPS)-stimulation is unable to induce any detectable PCT production by leukocytes. Moreover, in septic patients, high serum PCT levels, even after near-complete eradication of the leukocyte population by chemotherapy, suggest that these cells are not a major source of PCT. Parenchymal cells (including liver, kidney, adipocytes, and muscle) provide the largest tissue mass and principal source of circulating PCT in sepsis [53]. The greater calcitonin precursor mRNA induction and calcitonin precursor peptide release from parenchymal cells in comparison to circulating cells, appears to indicate a tissue based, rather than a leukocyte based mechanism of host defense. Thus, the authors advance the hypothesis that CALC-gene products are a prototype of hormokine mediator and can follow either a classical hormonal expression or, alternatively, a cytokine-like expression pathway [54]. The production of hormokines is mediated by as yet unknown factors, and might be induced either directly via microbial toxins or indirectly via a humoral or cell-mediated host response. In sepsis, the predominance of calcitonin precursors as opposed to mature calcitonin is indicative of a constitutive pathway within cells lacking secretion granules and, hence, a bypassing of much of the enzymatic processing [53]. Consequently, as is the case for most cytokines, there is very little intracellular storage of calcitonin precursors in sepsis [54].

▌ How do Calcitonin Peptides, including PCT, Mediate their Effects?

Molecular and animal studies are only beginning to unravel the pathophysiological mechanisms of calcitonin precursor action in sepsis (Fig. 6). In this disease, several calcitonin precursors are increased, including PCT and other precursor peptides, any of which may have agonistic, antagonistic, or neutral effects [14, 47].

Furthermore, there are several members of the calcitonin gene family of peptides which comprise a functional unity [4]. The CALC-I gene, by alternative processing of the primary RNA transcript, gives rise to two different so-called mature peptides: calcitonin and calcitonin gene–related peptide I (CGRP-I). Similarly to calcitonin, CGRP-I is initially biosynthesized as a larger prohormone, which is subsequently cleaved into smaller precursors. It is of pertinence that CGRP-II, amylin, and adrenomedullin, also members of the calcitonin gene family of peptides, are encoded on the CALC-II, -IV, and -V genes, respectively. In sepsis, mRNA for CGRP-I, CGRP-II and adrenomedullin also appear to be ubiquitously expressed [57]. Based on structural homologies, different members of these calcitonin-gene family peptides have different profiles of bioactivities, which they exert by binding to the same family of receptors.

There are two subgroups of receptors for the calcitonin-gene family: calcitonin receptors (CRs) and calcitonin receptor-like receptors (CRLRs). Each member of the calcitonin-gene family of peptides binds with differing affinities to these receptors. Accessory proteins act upon these receptors, thus altering their specific responsiveness and hence the physiologic profile of action of the calcitonin-gene peptides. These accessory proteins, which are called receptor-activity-modifying proteins (RAMPs), alter the phenotype of the receptors; they act on the CRs by modifi-

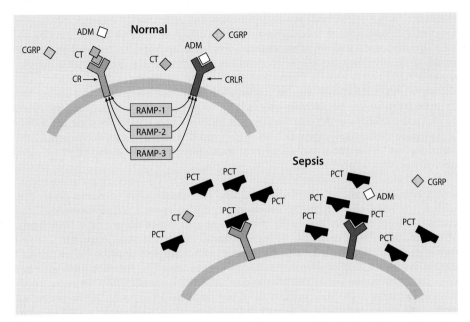

Fig. 6. Receptors for calcitonin (CT)-peptides. Based on the structural homologies, different CT-peptides have overlapping bioactivities, which they exert by binding to the same family of receptors. There are two subgroups of these G protein-coupled receptors with seven transmembrane domains: calcitonin receptors (CR) and calcitonin receptor-like receptors (CRLR). Three accessory proteins, which are called receptor-activity-modifying proteins (RAMP 1–3), act upon these receptors, thus altering their specific responsiveness and ligand affinity and hence modifying the physiologic profile of the calcitonin-peptide superfamily. Depending on which of the different RAMPs is associated with the receptor, each member of the calcitonin-gene family of peptides binds with differing affinities. In sepsis, the circulating levels of calcitonin precursors, including procalcitonin (PCT), by far exceed the levels of the other calcitonin peptides. Thus, a competitive antagonistic effect of PCT is conceivable, however, experimental data on the binding of PCT are lacking

cation of their genes, and on the CRLRs by influencing transport to the plasma membrane. The presence, concentration, and/or timing of one or more of the three RAMPs (RAMP-1, -2, and -3) determines the specific cellular phenotype of the receptor that is ultimately expressed on the cell surface [58]. The profile of RAMP expression and activity is altered by the local milieu and is subject to humoral influences. This elegant system allows for a diversification of receptor function, hence modulating the action of the calcitonin-gene products according to ambient needs. Thus, both in health and disease, a response to different peptides of the calcitonin gene family of peptides occurs in a dynamic and varying manner [4].

▊ Epilogue – How to Dance with Porcupines

As with all porcupines, careful dancing is advisable. An ideal marker for bacterial infections should allow an early diagnosis and should inform about the course and prognosis of the disease. PCT covers these features better as compared to other markers, namely CRP and pro-inflammatory cytokines [13]. Beyond doubt, the diagnosis of infections will continue to require a high level of suspicion, careful patient history, dedicated physical examination, and appropriate cultures in all patients. In this context, the use of PCT can further improve the accuracy of a diagnosis of clinical sepsis [59]. A superior diagnostic performance of PCT has also been shown in other infections, e.g., in meningitis, fulminant bacterial endocarditis [60, 61], pancreatitis [61–64], among others [65]. In pancreatitis, plasma concentrations of PCT may reflect the derangement in gut barrier function (rather than the extent of systemic inflammation) and may hence predict those patients in whom the translocation of bacteria and fungi into dead pancreas with consecutive infected necrosis is more likely [63, 66].

Nevertheless, some patients without any apparent clinical symptomatology of sepsis manifest high serum PCT levels, and conversely, some patients presenting with a syndrome that meets the commonly accepted criteria for sepsis or localized bacterial infections later eventually progressing into sepsis do not have high levels. Moreover, the clinical diagnosis of sepsis often is subjective and, hence, not uncommonly is uncertain. For example, the patient with SIRS and positive blood cultures clearly justifies a clinical diagnosis of sepsis, although a patient with SIRS who has consistently negative blood cultures and a localized bacterial infection (e.g., pneumonitis or pyelonephritis), may or may not be considered to be septic. Thus, an evaluation of the reliability of a marker for infections is contingent upon the accuracy of the clinical diagnosis. Importantly, any observational study investigating the diagnostic accuracy of a given marker is biased by the choice of the 'gold-standard'. In infections this gold-standard does not exist, and thus, all studies are prone to a potential bias. Importantly, interventional studies, in which the antimicrobial therapy is guided by the marker and in which the gold-standard is the outcome, have the potential to resolve this dilemma. For PCT, initial attempts in LRTI and meningitis have shown promising results [16, 67]. The time has arrived to conduct more interventional studies for other sites of infection (e.g., endocarditis, diverticulits, urinary tract infections, among others), using more sensitive PCT assays to tackle the vicious cycle of antibiotic overuse and emerging multi-resistance.

Furthermore, in addition to being a marker for sepsis, PCT plays a critical role as a mediator in systemic infections and contributes markedly to the deleterious effects of systemic infection. It is an extremely potent actor in the pathophysiology of sepsis. Importantly, its ease of measurement and its prolonged persistence in the serum during sepsis makes it feasible to immunoneutralize either very early or later in the course of illness. Recently, it was shown that this therapy is effective even if the septic animal is moribund [68]. Clearly, further elucidation of the biological actions of PCT in sepsis will open new therapeutic avenues.

▮ Conclusion

Serum calcitonin precursor levels, including PCT, are elevated in bacterial infections and have emerged as reliable markers and important mediators of sepsis. Most sepsis is caused by LRTIs. Conversely, LRTIs are often treated with antibiotics without evidence of clinically relevant bacterial disease. We evaluated a PCT-based therapeutic strategy to reduce antibiotic usage in LRTI, using a new rapid and sensitive assay and showed that PCT-guidance substantially and safely reduced antibiotic usage in LRTI. The optimal duration of antibiotic therapy in patients with pneumonia is being investigated. Our findings question currently used gold standards for the clinical diagnosis of bacterial LRTIs. Clearly, the further elucidation of the regulation and biological actions of PCT in infections will open new therapeutic avenues.

Acknowledgments. We thank The Brakers for providing an outstanding research environment, the staff of the emergency unit, and the department of clinical chemistry, notably Mrs. Fausta Chiaverio and Maya Kunz, for most helpful support during the study. We thank B.R.A.H.M.S. AG, Hennigsdorf, Germany and Orgenium Laboratories, Turku, Finland for providing assay material and partial support of our investigator initiated projects. Additional support for our research was granted by the Freiwillige Akademische Gesellschaft (FAG) Basel, Switzerland, and funds from the department of internal medicine, and the divisions of endocrinology and pneumology. Pharmaceutical companies selling antibiotics declined to support our research, despite the fact that antibiotic use is the most important risk factor for the emergence of antibiotic resistance.

References

1. Becker KL, Nylen ES, White JC, Muller B, Snider RH Jr (2004) Clinical review 167: Procalcitonin and the calcitonin gene family of peptides in inflammation, infection, and sepsis: a journey from calcitonin back to its precursors. J Clin Endocrinol Metab 89:1512–1525
2. Weglohner W, Struck J, Fischer-Schulz C, et al (2001) Isolation and characterization of serum procalcitonin from patients with sepsis. Peptides 22:2099–2103
3. Copp DH, Davidson AGP (1961) Evidence for a new parathyroid hormone which lowers blood calcium. Proc Soc Biol Med 107:342–344
4. Becker KL, Muller B, Nylen ES, Cohen R, Silva OL, Snider RH (2001) Calcitonin gene family of peptides. In: Becker KL (ed) Principles and Practice of Endocrinology and Metabolism. Vol. 3rd edition. J.B. Lippincott Co, Philadeplphia, pp 520–534
5. Zaidi M, Moonga BS, Abe E (2002) Calcitonin and bone formation: a knockout full of surprises. J Clin Invest 110:1769–1771
6. Hoff AO, Catala-Lehnen P, Thomas PM, et al (2002) Increased bone mass is an unexpected phenotype associated with deletion of the calcitonin gene. J Clin Invest 110:1849-1857
7. Hirsch PF, Baruch H (2003) Is calcitonin an important physiological substance? Endocrine 21:201–208
8. Nylen ES, O'Neill W, Jordan MH, et al (1992) Serum procalcitonin as an index of inhalation injury in burns. Horm Metab Res 24:439–443
9. Whang KT, Steinwald PM, White JC, et al (1998) Serum calcitonin precursors in sepsis and systemic inflammation. J Clin Endocrinol Metab 83:3296–3301
10. Assicot M, Gendrel D, Carsin H, Raymond J, Guilbaud J, Bohuon C (1993) High serum procalcitonin concentrations in patients with sepsis and infection. Lancet 341:515–518
11. Muller B, Becker KL, Schächinger H, et al (2000) Calcitonin precursors are reliable markers of sepsis in a medical intensive care unit. Crit Care Med 28:977–983
12. de Werra I, Jaccard C, Corradin SB, et al (1997) Cytokines, nitrite/nitrate, soluble tumor necrosis factor receptors, and procalcitonin concentrations: comparisons in patients with septic shock, cardiogenic shock, and bacterial pneumonia. Crit Care Med 25:607–613
13. Simon L, Gauvin F, Anre K, Saint-Louis P, Lacroix J (2004) Serum Procalcitonin and C-Reactive Protein Levels as Markers of Bacterial Infection: A Systematic Review and Meta-analysis. Clin Infect Dis 39:206–217
14. Snider RH Jr, Nylen ES, Becker KL (1997) Procalcitonin and its component peptides in systemic inflammation: immunochemical characterization. J Investig Med 45:552–560
15. Nylen ES, Muller B, Becker KL, Snyder RH (2003) The future diagnostic role of procalcitonin levels: the need for improved sensitivity. Clin Infect Dis 36:823–824

16. Christ-Crain M, Jaccard-Stolz D, Bingisser R, et al (2004) Effect of procalcitonin-guided treatment on antibiotic use and outcome in lower respiratory tract infections: cluster-randomised, single-blinded intervention trial. Lancet 363:600–607

17. Albrich W, Monnet D, Harbarth S (2004) Antibiotic selection pressure and resistance in Streptococcus pneumoniae and Streptococcus pyogenes. Emerg Infect Dis 10:514–517

18. Snider RH Jr, Nylen ES, Becker KL (1997) Procalcitonin and its component peptides in systemic inflammation: immunochemical characterization. J Investig Med 45:552–560

19. Meisner M (2002) Pathobiochemistry and clinical use of procalcitonin. Clin Chim Acta 323:17–29

20. Meisner M, Brunkhorst FM, Reith HB, Schmidt J, Lestin HG, Reinhart K (2000) Clinical experiences with a new semi-quantitative solid phase immunoassay for rapid measurement of procalcitonin. Clin Chem Lab Med 38:989–995

21. Macfarlane JT, Colville A, Guion A, Macfarlane RM, Rose DH (1993) Prospective study of aetiology and outcome of adult lower respiratory tract infections in the community. Lancet 341:511–514

22. Ortqvist A (1995) Antibiotic treatment of community-acquired pneumonia in clinical practice: a European perspective. J Antimicrob Chemother 35:205–212

23. Halls GA (1993) The management of infections and antibiotic therapy: a European survey. J Antimicrob Chemother 31:985–1000

24. Stephenson J (1996) Icelandic researchers are showing the way to bring down rates of antibiotic-resistant bacteria. JAMA 275:175

25. Wenzel RP, Wong MT (1999) Managing antibiotic use–impact of infection control. Clin Infect Dis 28:1126–1127

26. Chen DK, McGeer A, de Azavedo JC, Low DE (1999) Decreased susceptibility of Streptococcus pneumoniae to fluoroquinolones in Canada. Canadian Bacterial Surveillance Network. N Engl J Med 341:233–239

27. Gonzales R, Steiner JF, Lum A, Barrett PH Jr (1999) Decreasing antibiotic use in ambulatory practice: impact of a multidimensional intervention on the treatment of uncomplicated acute bronchitis in adults. JAMA 281:1512–1519

28. Guillemot D, Courvalin P (2001) Better control of antibiotic resistance. Clin Infect Dis 33:542–547

29. Ball P, Baquero F, Cars O, et al (2002) Antibiotic therapy of community respiratory tract infections: strategies for optimal outcomes and minimized resistance emergence. J Antimicrob Chemother 49:31–40

30. Halm EA, Teirstein AS (2002) Clinical practice. Management of community-acquired pneumonia. N Engl J Med 347:2039–2045

31. Gonzales R, Sande MA (2000) Uncomplicated acute bronchitis. Ann Intern Med 133:981–991

32. Sethi S, Murphy TF (2001) Bacterial infection in chronic obstructive pulmonary disease in 2000: a state-of-the-art review. Clin Microbiol Rev 14:336–363

33. Anthonisen NR, Manfreda J, Warren CP, Hershfield ES, Harding GK, Nelson NA (1987) Antibiotic therapy in exacerbations of chronic obstructive pulmonary disease. Ann Intern Med 106:196–204

34. Muller B, Becker KL, Schachinger H, et al (2000) Calcitonin precursors are reliable markers of sepsis in a medical intensive care unit. Crit Care Med 28:977–983

35. Bernard GR, Vincent JL, Laterre PF, et al (2001) Efficacy and safety of recombinant human activated protein C for severe sepsis. N Engl J Med 344:699–709

36. Marik PE (2000) The clinical features of severe community-acquired pneumonia presenting as septic shock. Norasept II Study Investigators. J Crit Care 15:85–90

37. Evans AT, Husain S, Durairaj L, Sadowski LS, Charles-Damte M, Wang Y (2002) Azithromycin for acute bronchitis: a randomised, double-blind, controlled trial. Lancet 359:1648–1654

38. Muller B, Becker KL, Becker KL, et al (2000) Calcitonin precursors are reliable markers of sepsis in a medical intensive care unit. Crit Care Med 28:977–983

39. Nylen ES, Snider RH Jr, Thompson KA, Rohatgi P, Becker KL (1996) Pneumonitis-associated hyperprocalcitoninemia. Am J Med Sci 312:12–18

40. Muller B, Becker KL (2001) Procalcitonin: how a hormone became a marker and mediator of sepsis. Swiss Med Wkly 131:595–602

41. Gonzales R (2003) A 65-year-old woman with acute cough illness and an important engagement. JAMA 289:2701–2708
42. Hament JM, Kimpen JL, Fleer A, Wolfs TF (1999) Respiratory viral infection predisposing for bacterial disease: a concise review. FEMS Immunol Med Microbiol 26:189–195
43. Sethi S, Evans N, Grant BJ, Murphy TF (2002) New strains of bacteria and exacerbations of chronic obstructive pulmonary disease. N Engl J Med 347:465–471
44. Strausbaugh LJ, Sukumar SR, Joseph CL (2003) Infectious disease outbreaks in nursing homes: an unappreciated hazard for frail elderly persons. Clin Infect Dis 36:870–876
45. Steinwald PM, Whang KT, Becker KL, Snider RH, Nylen ES, White JC (1999) Elevated calcitonin precursor levels are related to mortality in an animal model of sepsis. Crit Care 3:11–16
46. Nylen ES, Whang KT, Snider RH Jr, Steinwald PM, White JC, Becker KL (1998) Mortality is increased by procalcitonin and decreased by an antiserum reactive to procalcitonin in experimental sepsis. Crit Care Med 26:1001–1006
47. Whang KT, Vath SD, Becker KL, et al (2000) Procalcitonin and proinflammatory cytokine interactions in sepsis. Shock 14:73–78
48. Wagner KE, Vath SD, Snider RH, et al (2002) Immunoneutralization of elevated calcitonin precursors markedly attenuates the adverse response to sepsis in pigs. Crit Care Med 30:2313–2321
49. Martinez JM, Becker KL, Muller B, et al (2001) Late immunoneutralization of procalcitonin arrests the progression of lethal porcine sepsis. Surgical Inf 2:193–201
50. Hoffmann G, Czechowski M, Schloesser M, Schobersberger W (2002) Procalcitonin amplifies inducible nitric oxide synthase gene expression and nitric oxide production in vascular smooth muscle cells. Crit Care Med 30:2091–2095
51. Muller B, Becker KL, Kränzlin M, et al (2000) Disordered calcium homeostasis of sepsis: associated with calcitonin precursors. Eur J Clin Invest 30:823–831
52. Preas HL, 2nd, Nylen ES, Snider RH, et al (2001) Effects of anti-inflammatory agents on serum levels of calcitonin precursors during human experimental endotoxemia. J Infect Dis 184:373–376
53. Linscheid P, Seboek D, Nylen ES, et al (2003) In vitro and in vivo calcitonin I gene expression in parenchymal cells: a novel product of human adipose tissue. Endocrinology 144:5578–5584
54. Muller B, White JC, Nylen E, Snider RH, Becker KL, Habener JF (2001) Ubiquitous expression of the calcitonin-1 gene in multiple tissues in response to sepsis. J Clin Endocrinol Metab 86:396–404
55. Monneret G, Laroche B, Bienvenu J (1999) Procalcitonin is not produced by circulating blood cells. Infection 27:34–35
56. Linscheid P, Seboek D, Schaer DJ, Zulewski H, Keller U, Muller B (2004) Expression and secretion of procalcitonin and calcitonin gene-related peptide by adherent monocytes and by macrophage-activated adipocytes. Crit Care Med 32:1715–1721
57. Suarez Domenech V, White JC, Nylen ES, et al (2001) Calcitonin gene-related peptide: messenger RNA in bacterial sepsis: Postulation of microbial infection-specific response elements (MISRE) within the Calc-I gene promoter. J Invest Med 49:514–521
58. McLatchie LM, Fraser NJ, Main MJ, et al (1998) RAMPs regulate the transport and ligand specificity of the calcitonin- receptor-like receptor. Nature 393:333–339
59. Harbarth S, Holeckova K, Froidevaux C, et al (2001) Diagnostic value of procalcitonin, interleukin-6, and interleukin-8 in critically ill patients admitted with suspected sepsis. Am J Respir Crit Care Med 164:396–402
60. Mueller C, Huber R, Laifer G, Mueller B, Buerkle G, Perruchoud AP (2004) Procalcitonin and the early diagnosis of infective endocarditis. Circulation 109:1707–1710
61. Rau B, Steinbach G, Gansauge F, Mayer JM, Grunert A, Beger HG (1997) The potential role of procalcitonin and interleukin 8 in the prediction of infected necrosis in acute pancreatitis. Gut 41:832–840
62. Kylanpaa-Back ML, Takala A, Kemppainen E, Puolakkainen P, Haapiainen R, Repo H (2001) Procalcitonin strip test in the early detection of severe acute pancreatitis. Br J Surg 88:222–227

63. Ammori BJ, Becker KL, Kite P, et al (2003) Calcitonin precursors: early markers of gut barrier dysfunction in patients with acute pancreatitis. Pancreas 27:239–243
64. Ammori BJ, Becker KL, Kite P, et al (2003) Calcitonin precursors in the prediction of severity of acute pancreatitis on the day of admission. Br J Surg 90:197–204
65. Muller B, Becker KL (2001) Procalcitonin: how a hormone became a marker and mediator of sepsis. Swiss Med Wkly 131:595–602
66. Bihari D (2004) Monitoring procalcitonin is of value in acute pancreatitis. BMJ 329:232
67. Marc E, Menager C, Moulin F, et al (2002) [Procalcitonin and viral meningitis: reduction of unnecessary antibiotics by measurement during an outbreak]. Arch Pediatr 9:358–364
68. Becker KL, Nylen ES, Snider RH, Muller B, White JC (2003) Immunoneutralization of procalcitonin as therapy of sepsis. J Endotoxin Res 9:367–374

Statins in Critical Illness

P. Kruger, K. Kostner, and B. Venkatesh

Introduction

The 3-hydroxy, 3-methylglutaryl coenzyme A (HMG-CoA) reductase inhibitor class of drugs (statins) was introduced into clinical practice in the 1980s. The most recent data (for the year 2001) indicate that in Australia statin drugs were first and second on the list of all prescription medicines for both numbers used and cost [1] and a similar trend is seen worldwide.

Patients with coronary artery disease, stroke, and even subgroups such as high risk elderly patients, patients having major surgery, and patients with normal lipid levels benefit from statin therapy [2–5]. Some beneficial effects of statins seem to be independent of their lipid lowering ability and include effects on endothelial function, apoptosis, plaque stabilization and are mainly due to anti-inflammatory, anti-oxidant and immunomodulatory roles [6, 7].

Current prescribing guidelines recommend that statin therapy be discontinued in patients with an acute illness such as severe infection, major surgery, trauma or severe electrolyte, metabolic or endocrine disorders [8]. There is a paucity of data on the pharmacology and safety of statins in critically ill patients, though rhabdomyolysis and liver dysfunction are described in high risk patients [8, 9]

At least 15% of patients requiring admission to hospital are on established statin therapy from the community (Kruger et al., unpublished data) [7, 10]. The increasing level of use, together with a rapidly expanding understanding of potential beneficial effects beyond the alterations in lipid profile, especially in patients with sepsis, indicate a need for the reappraisal of the therapeutic indications of these drugs in critically ill patients. In this chapter, we review the therapeutic role of statins in the management of cardiovascular and other systemic diseases, discuss the pharmacology of statins, and critically evaluate their role in the management of septic and inflammatory states.

Statin Use in Cardiovascular Disease

HMG-CoA reductase inhibitors (statins) are first line therapy to reduce low density lipoprotein (LDL) concentrations. There is unequivocal evidence from prospective clinical trials that HMG-CoA reductase inhibitors can effectively lower the incidence of cardiovascular events in primary and secondary prevention [2, 11, 12]. However their role in acute coronary syndromes is still debated. Published data from the MIRACL [13] and PROVEIT [14] trials support the use of statins in acute coronary syndromes. Both studies demonstrated a significant reduction in the event rates.

However, Phase Z of the A to Z trial [15], to date the largest randomized trial testing the effects of aggressive statin therapy in acute coronary syndromes did not show the same benefit with regards to the primary composite end point of cardiovascular death, myocardial infarction, readmission for acute coronary syndromes, or stroke during the first 4 months. Of concern the high-dose simvastatin regimen was associated with an unusually high rate of myopathy. It is difficult to relate the outcomes of these studies to critically ill patients as each study often excluded high risk patients such as those likely to get early operations, angiographic intervention or those at risk of rhabdomyolysis.

Even though there is no doubt that reduction in LDL is the sentinel pharmacological effect of statins, evidence is accumulating that statins may confer beneficial effects through other mechanisms. These include the improvement of endothelial function, anti-oxidative, anti-inflammatory, plaque-stabilizing, and anti-coagulant effects.

∎ The Effect of Statins in Other Diseases

Stroke

Statin therapy has been demonstrated to significantly lower the risk of stroke in several studies in patients with coronary heart disease [2, 11, 16]. Whether statins prevent strokes in patients without heart disease is currently under evaluation in several trials. Because cholesterol is often not elevated in stroke patients [17] the benefit of statins in stroke patients may be an effect independent of cholesterol lowering. This is supported by recent data from Laufs and coworkers [18] who demonstrated that atorvastatin in mice up-regulates nitric oxide synthase (NOS), decreases platelet activation, and protects from cerebral ischemia.

Transplantation

Statin use is associated with improved function and survival of lung allografts. Following lung transplantation, statin recipients had a lower incidence of acute rejection, and obliterative bronchiolitis and an improved spirometry and 6-year survival as compared to those who did not receive statins [19]. A meta-analysis of statins and survival in *de novo* cardiac transplantation has also reduced one year mortality for heart transplant recipients [20]. Although the mechanism for these benefits has not been fully elucidated, it is being attributed to an immunomodulatory effect of statins.

Inflammatory Diseases

Recent reports postulate a beneficial role for statins in other inflammatory diseases such as rheumatoid arthritis, systemic lupus erythematosus, and multiple sclerosis [21]. Simvastatin has been shown to reduce the inflammation associated with hyperimmunoglobulinemia D and periodic fever syndrome [22]. Statin therapy has also been associated with reductions in C-reactive protein (CRP) concentrations, which is a marker of inflammation. Attenuation of inflammation might be mediated through reductions in serum concentrations of adhesion molecules and interleukin (IL)-6 [23].

Oncology

A recent population based, nested case control study involving 3 129 patients matched with 16 976 controls revealed statin use was associated with a risk reduction of cancer of 20% (adjusted odds ratio 0.80; 95% CI 0.66 to 0.96) [24]. Several experimental studies have suggested antineoplastic effects through inhibition of angiogenesis [25], effects on tumor cell apoptosis [26, 27] and reduced tumor progression [28] and metastasis [29].

Miscellaneous

Statins are increasingly being realized to have effects in a wide variety of disease states including an impact on bone turnover [30], multiple sclerosis, dementia, kidney disease.

Sepsis

Our group has recently completed a study of the potential beneficial role of statins in more than 400 adult patients requiring hospital care for bacteremia (Kruger et al., unpublished data). There was a significant reduction in all cause mortality (1.8% vs. 23.1%, p=0.002) and death attributable to bacteremia (1.8 vs 18.3%, p=0.018) in patients who were receiving statins that were continued at the time of their bacteremia. This survival difference persisted after controlling for differences between the groups (odds ratio 0.08, 95% CI 0.01, 0.57, p=0.012). A previous retrospective review by Liappis et al. [31] of statin use in 388 bacteremic patients also showed a dramatic decrease in deaths from bacteremia (3 vs 20%, p=0.01) and all cause mortality (6 vs 28%, p=0.002) in patients taking statins. The reduction in mortality persisted in a multivariate analysis (OR 7.6 CI 1.01–57.5). The difference in mortality rate observed between bacteremic patients on statins and those not on statins is striking. Inherent bias or between group differences that cannot be controlled or modeled limit the interpretation of retrospective data. A prospective observational cohort study has also concluded that prior statin therapy is associated with a decreased rate of severe sepsis and may reduce intensive care unit (ICU) admissions [10]. A recent animal study has demonstrated that simvastatin pre-treatment profoundly improves survival in a murine model of sepsis [32].

The above data allow us to generate the hypothesis that statins represent a therapeutic enhancement of the treatment for sepsis or that statin use favorably modulates the inflammatory response to sepsis. This would challenge the current prescribing guidelines to withhold statins in acutely ill patients and warrants further prospective investigation.

▌ Potential Mechanisms by Which Statins may Improve Mortality in Sepsis?

In addition to their main effect on LDL-cholesterol, statins also exhibit a wide range of other biological effects. These effects are often termed pleiotropic (greek: many turnings) and include actions on cell proliferation, endothelial function, immune modulatory effects, antioxidant effects, and effects on coagulation. Since all statins lower LDL-cholesterol and LDL plays an important role in many of these pleiotropic effects, it is difficult to show that these effects are not related to LDL lowering.

Emerging research on these pleiotropic effects provides potential scientific basis for an association of an outcome benefit with statin therapy in sepsis [33, 34]. Some of the potential beneficial effects in sepsis are outlined below and summarized in Figure 1.

Increase or Alterations in High Density Lipoprotein (HDL)

Significant changes in lipid metabolism occur in sepsis. Published data and work from our group indicate that total cholesterol and HDL cholesterol are decreased in sepsis and the magnitude of changes seems to reflect the severity of inflammation [35, 36]. Both the amount and the composition of HDL change in sepsis [37] and this may have an effect on the inflammatory cascade and outcome [35]. Bacterial endotoxin (lipopolysaccharide, LPS) elicits dramatic responses in the host including elevated plasma lipid levels due to the increased synthesis and secretion of triglyceride (TG)-rich lipoproteins by the liver, and the inhibition of lipoprotein lipase. This cytokine-induced hyperlipoproteinemia, clinically termed the 'lipemia of sepsis', was customarily thought to represent the mobilization of lipid stores to fuel the host response to infection. However, since lipoproteins can also bind and neutralize LPS it is postulated that TG-rich lipoproteins (very low density lipoproteins

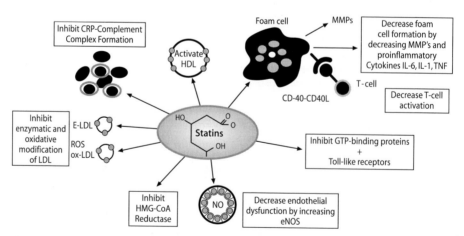

Fig. 1. A summary of the potential interactions of statins in the inflammatory cascade. LDL: low density lipoprotein, HDL: high density lipoprotein; IL: interleukin; ROS: reactive oxygen species; MonP: metalloproteinase; ox-LDL: oxidatively modified LDL; eNOS: endothelial nitric oxide synthase

[VLDL] and chylomicrons) are also components of an innate, non-adaptive host immune response to infection [40]. In general statin therapy increases HDL levels in addition to the LDL lowering effects [41, 42]. The effect of statin therapy on the lipid profile in sepsis remains poorly clarified but it may be that alterations in the lipoprotein balance have profound effects on inflammation.

Direct Antioxidant Mechanisms

Sepsis and the systemic inflammatory response syndrome (SIRS) are associated with leukocyte activation and the release of several pro-inflammatory mediators, including oxygen-free radicals. Oxygen-free radicals are involved in the pathogenesis and manifestations of sepsis as they react with various biological substrates, especially polyunsaturated fatty acids, to induce membrane dysfunction, tissue damage, and organ injury [43]. Some pleiotropic effects of statins could be attributed to their ability to suppress the synthesis of isoprenoid intermediates such as geranyl pyrophosphate or farnesyl pyrophosphate 45 and by this mechanism they may decrease oxidative stress.

Immunomodulatory Effects of Statins

It appears that statins are able to influence the inflammatory processes at several levels.
1. Pathogen-associated molecular recognition is the complex process by which phagocytosed invading pathogens are presented by a variety of immune cells to subsequently initiate and mediate components of the inflammatory response. Statins may interfere with this receptor ligand interaction, blunting the first step in the activation of the cellular cascade. Lovastatin has been shown to reduce the adhesiveness of monocytes to the vascular endothelium [45]. They have also been reported to directly inhibit the main β-integrin leukocyte function antigen (LFA)-1 [46].
2. In addition, statins deplete isoprenoids, which are important non-sterol cholesterol precursors. These precursors are essential for the farnesylation and geranylation of membranal G proteins which play a pivotal role in the signal transduction pathways that regulate cellular migration and proliferation [47].
3. Acute phase response: Several studies have shown that statin therapy either lowers circulating concentrations of CRP or reduces the risk associated with systemic inflammation, in some cases independently of the reduction in cholesterol [48].
4. Statins have been shown to inhibit elements of the inflammatory cascade induced by *Escherichia coli* endotoxin [49] and *Staphylococcus aureus* alpha toxin [50].
5. The complement system is effective in protecting the host both from autoimmunity and from invading microbes. However, the persistent activation of complement may be detrimental because it may trigger and sustain inflammation. Furthermore, enzymatic modification of LDL mediated by the complement system could be a crucial step in atherogenesis [51]. Statins have been shown to reduce complement activation *in vitro* and in animal models [52] and humans (Kostner et al. unpublished results).

Improvement in Vascular Function: the Role of Nitric Oxide

Endothelial cells play an important role in the control of vascular tone, permeability, blood flow, coagulation, thrombolysis, inflammation, tissue repair, and growth [53]. It is thought that endothelial activation, dysfunction, and apoptosis play a crucial role in the pathogenesis of sepsis and subsequent multiple organ dysfunction. Considerable research has focused on the mechanisms by which statins enhance endothelial anticoagulant and fibrinolytic properties. These studies show that statins increase expression and enhance activity of endothelial NOS [19], upregulate prostacyclin [54] and tissue-type plasminogen activator [55], and downregulate tissue factor, endothelin-1, and plasminogen activator inhibitor-1 (PAI-1) [56].

The bulk of evidence on statins points to a pro-apoptotic effect of statins. Kaneta et al. [57] suggest apoptosis is induced by hydrophobic statins (atorvastatin, lovastatin, Simvastatin, fluvastatin and cerivastatin) but the hydrophilic drug pravastatin did not induce cell apoptosis. They suggest that endothelial cell apoptosis is underlying an improvement of endothelial dysfunction. However, Almog [7] comments on the potential anti-apoptotic effects (postulated due to increased eNOS expression [18]). The pro-apoptotic effects of statins on the endothelium and vascular smooth muscle are thought to be one of the mechanisms of statin-induced protection in the stability of the atherosclerotic plaque. One important consideration is that, if a cell is committed to die, suppression of apoptosis may simply push the cell's demise in the direction of necrosis. Necrosis typically evokes an inflammatory response thus potentially exacerbating the deleterious effects of sepsis. Thus the pro-apoptotic effect of statins might induce a protective effect by suppressing inflammation. This hypothesis is also consistent with the other anti-inflammatory effects of statins described above.

▌ Prescribing Statins in the Critically Ill: Caveats

Pharmacology

Understanding how organ dysfunction can alter the pharmacology of drugs is a vital aspect of therapy and no work has been done describing the pharmacokinetics of statins in critically ill patients. It is unknown to what extent statin drugs affect the altered lipid profiles seen in sepsis and what impact this may have on the inflammatory response. When considering the pharmacodynamics of statins in patients with sepsis it is important to evaluate several possible mechanisms of action including lipid changes, alterations in inflammatory markers and changes in vascular reactivity.

When should Statins be Stopped (or Administered) in Critically Ill Patients?

There is a paucity of data on the safety of statins in the critically ill. In the general population, the statins have been proven to be a very well tolerated class of drugs [58] with reversible dose dependant rises in liver function tests in less than 1% of those treated. Cessation of treatment for adverse effects on the liver is rarely required. Myopathy is perhaps the best known and most feared complication of statin therapy [57]. Myopathy is uncommon and frank rhabdomyolysis is rare [59]. The mechanism for rhabdomyolysis has not been elucidated but may relate to depletion of secondary metabolic intermediates formed during cholesterol synthesis [60]. It is important to remember that much of the epidemiology of statin related myopathy is in a very different patient group to those discussed in this chapter. An increased incidence in at risk patients has been reported which has led to recommendations to avoid these drugs in physiologic situations that increase the risk for rhabdomyolysis, such as severe acute infection, hypotension, major surgery, trauma, severe metabolic disturbance, endocrine or electrolyte disorders, and uncontrolled seizures [8, 9].

Retrospective and observational prospective data suggest continuing statin therapy during an episode of sepsis increases any protective effect. It is unclear at present if commencing statin therapy once a patient has sepsis is safe or confers any benefit. If we are to consider continuing or commencing statin therapy in this group of critically ill patients we must completely evaluate both the efficacy and safety profile of these agents.

Interestingly, it is in some of these high-risk patient groups that possible benefits to statin therapy are emerging. An improved mortality rate and no reported adverse events appears in several of the recent publications expanding the use statin therapy [4, 10, 31]. More work is required to elucidate the impact of continued statin therapy in critically ill patients particularly with respect to possible side effects, the relative merits of each of the available statin agents, and appropriate dosing regimens.

All patients on statins should be monitored with blood tests including serum transaminases and creatinine kinase (CK). Drug administration should cease if CK levels are markedly elevated for any reason (>10 times upper limit of normal) or if serum transaminases become elevated (>3 times upper limit of normal).

HMG-CoA reductase inhibition results in inhibition of ubiquinone or coenzyme Q10. It is reported this can rarely predispose to the development of lactic acidosis due to paralysis of mitochondrial metabolism [61]. The true relevance of this interaction may become apparent as these agents are increasingly investigated in critically ill patients.

Potential Drug Interactions

Most statin drugs are metabolized by hepatic cytochromes. Lovastatin, simvastatin and atorvastatin are metabolized via P450 3A4, fluvastatin via 2C9, cerivastatin via 3A4 and 2C8. Pravastatin is metabolized via sulfation and not via the cytochrome enzymes [41]. Newer agents are metabolized to a lesser extent with only 10% of rosuvastatin metabolized (mainly via p-450 2C9 and 2C19), and only 10% of pitavastatin metabolized (mainly via 2C9 and 2C8). This has the potential benefit of limiting the impact of drug interactions altering serum levels.

Concern exists over a variety of potential drug interactions that may alter therapeutic effects of commonly used drugs. Of greater importance are the interactions that enhance toxicity. Caution needs to be exercised with a variety of drugs that may interact with hepatic cytochromes (Table 1). Changes in metabolism with a potential elevation in serum levels of statins can enhance toxicity and would dictate a reduction in dose at the very least and perhaps temporary cessation of statin therapy.

Table 1. Drugs or foods that may potentiate the toxicity of statins

Interference at the cytochrome level
▌ Cyclosporine
▌ Triazole antifungals
▌ Macrolide antibiotics – erythromycin, clarithromycin
▌ Selective serotonin reuptake inhibitors
▌ Calcium channel blockers – verapamil, diltiazem
▌ Protease inhibitors (HIV therapy)
▌ Amiodarone
▌ Cimetidine
▌ Warfarin
▌ Digoxin
▌ Grapefuit juice

Non-cytochrome mediated
▌ Fibrates – likely a pharmacodynamic effect rather than altered metabolism

Are all Statins Equivalent?

These agents contain a characteristic statin pharmacophore although other aspects of their chemical structure may differ. Varying statins have different effects on lipid profiles and possibly differing effects on inflammation or pleiotropic effects. Rosu-vastatin, simvastatin, lovastatin, and atorvastatin have the highest hepatic excretion and pravastatin the lowest. Apart from pravastatin all statins are more than 90% albumin bound. Except for pravastatin and rosuvastatin all statins are lipophilic. Whether this has any impact on differences in pleiotropic effects remains to be established.

Individual agents clearly differ in their propensity to cause rhabdomyolysis as illustrated by the withdrawal of cerivastatin from the market in 2001 due a cluster of fatal cases of rhabdomyolysis [60].

Route of Administration

Statins are given orally and the high first pass uptake in the liver serves a useful purpose as the enzymes they effect are in the liver and therefore the best place to modify cholesterol metabolism (and hopefully limit the side effects). Food intake increases the bioavailability of lovastatin but decreases the bioavailability of all other statins. It is known that time of dosing in relation to food does affect plasma levels of these drugs but has limited effect on changes in lipid profile. Oral bio-availability and the relationship of drug administration to enteral feeding have not been assessed in the critically ill patient population. The place or safety of paren-teral administration is unclear and no intravenous preparations of these agents are marketed.

What Does the Future Hold?

This is a rapidly growing field of fascinating experimental biology. Current evidence suggests a need to evaluate the safety and efficacy of statins in critically ill patients before we can update prescribing guidelines. Sepsis continues to be a major cause of morbidity and carries a 20 to 50% mortality rate [62, 63]. Besides the use of antibiotics, source control and activated protein C, no other therapy has been shown to improve outcome in sepsis. The evidence presented above would suggest that statins might have a potentially beneficial role in patients with sepsis. Statins are significantly cheaper than other therapies that have been shown to improve outcome in sepsis and the demonstration of a mortality benefit with statins would have enormous cost benefit implications for society. Further investigation of the biology of statins in inflammation and sepsis, particularly in the critically ill, is warranted.

References

1. Australian Institute of Health and Welfare (2002) Statistics on drug use in Australia 2002. Available at: *http://www.aihw.gov.au/publications/phe/sdua02/sdua02.pdf* Accessed December 2004
2. The Long-Term Intervention with Pravastatin in Ischaemic Disease (LIPID) Study Group (1998) Prevention of cardiovascular events and death with pravastatin in patients with coronary heart disease and a broad range of initial cholesterol levels. N Engl J Med 339:1349–1357
3. Ko DT, Mamdani M, Alter DA (2004) Lipid-lowering therapy with statins in high-risk elderly patients: the treatment-risk paradoxI. JAMA 291:1864–1870
4. Poldermans D, Bax JJ, Kertai MD, et al (2003) Statins are associated with a reduced incidence of perioperative mortality in patients undergoing major noncardiac vascular surgery. Circulation 107:1848–1851
5. Lindenauer PK, Pekow P, Wang K, Gutierrez B, Benjamin EM (2004) Lipid-lowering therapy and in-hospital mortality following major noncardiac surgery. JAMA 291:2092–2099
6. Kwak BR, Mach F (2001) Statins inhibit leukocyte recruitment: new evidence for their anti-inflammatory properties. Arterioscler Thromb Vasc Biol 21:1256–1258
7. Almog Y (2003) Statins, inflammation, and sepsis: hypothesis. Chest 124:740–743
8. MIMS Online Australia (2004) Prescribing information Atorvastatin, Simvastatin. At: http://www.mims.hcn.net.au. Accessed August 12th 2004
9. Adverse Drug Reactions Adivsory Committee 2004) Risk factors for myopathy and rhabdomyolysis with the statins. Australian Adverse Drug Reactions Bulletin 23:2
10. Almog Y, Shefer A, Novack V, et al (2004) Prior statin therapy is associated with a decreased rate of severe sepsis. Circulation 110:880–885
11. The Scandinavian Simvastatin Survival Study (1994) Randomised trial of cholesterol lowering in 4444 patients with coronary heart disease. Lancet 344:1383–1389
12. Sacks FM, Pfeffer MA, Moye LA, et al (1996) The effect of pravastatin on coronary events after myocardial infarction in patients with average cholesterol levels. Cholesterol and Recurrent Events Trial investigators. N Engl J Med 335:1001–1009
13. Schwartz GG, Olsson AG, Ezekowitz MD, et al (2001) Effects of atorvastatin on early recurrent ischemic events in acute coronary syndromes: the MIRACL study: a randomized controlled trial. JAMA 285:1711–1718
14. Cannon CP, Braunwald E, McCabe CM, et al (2004) Intensive versus moderate lipid lowering with statins after acute coronary syndromes. N Engl J Med 350:1495–1504
15. de Lemos JA, Blazing MA, Wiviott SD, et al (2004) Early intensive vs a delayed conservative simvastatin strategy in patients with acute coronary syndromes: phase Z of the A to Z trial. Jama 292:1307–1316

16. Hess DC, Demchuk AM, Brass LM, Yatsu FM (2000) HMG-CoA reductase inhibitors (statins): a promising approach to stroke prevention. Neurology 54:790–796
17. Prospective studies collaboration (1995) Cholesterol, diastolic blood pressure, and stroke: 13 000 strokes in 450 000 people in 45 prospective cohorts. Lancet 346:1647–1653
18. Laufs U, Gertz K, Huang P, et al (2000) Atorvastatin upregulates type III nitric oxide synthase in thrombocytes, decreases platelet activation, and protects from cerebral ischemia in normocholesterolemic mice. Stroke 31:2442–2449
19. Johnson BA, Iacono AT, Zeevi A, McCurry KR, Duncan SR (2003) Statin use is associated with improved function and survival of lung allografts. Am J Respir Crit Care Med 167: 1271–1278
20. Raval NY, Mehra MR (2004) Metaanalysis of statins and survival in de novo cardiac transplantation. Transplant Proc 36:1539–1541
21. Fischetti F, Carretta R, Borotto G, et al (2004) Fluvastatin treatment inhibits leucocyte adhesion and extravasation in models of complement-mediated acute inflammation. Clin Exp Immunol 135:186–193
22. Simon A, Drewe E, van der Meer JW, et al (2004) Simvastatin treatment for inflammatory attacks of the hyperimmunoglobulinemia D and periodic fever syndrome. Clin Pharmacol Ther 75:476–483
23. Nawawi H, Osman NS, Yusoff K, Khalid BA (2003) Reduction in serum levels of adhesion molecules, interleukin-6 and C-reactive protein following short-term low-dose atorvastatin treatment in patients with non-familial hypercholesterolemia. Horm Metab Res 35:479–485
24. Graaf MR, Beiderbeck AB, Egberts AC, Richel DJ, Guchelaar HJ (2004) The risk of cancer in users of statins. J Clin Oncol 22:2388–2394
25. Park HJ, Kong D, Iruela-Arispe L, Begley U, Tang D, Galper JB (2002) 3-hydroxy-3-methylglutaryl coenzyme A reductase inhibitors interfere with angiogenesis by inhibiting the geranylgeranylation of RhoA. Circ Res 91:143–150
26. Wong WW, Dimitroulakos J, Minden MD, Penn LZ (2002) HMG-CoA reductase inhibitors and the malignant cell: the statin family of drugs as triggers of tumor-specific apoptosis. Leukemia 16:508–519
27. Feleszko W, Mlynarczuk I, Olszewska D, et al (2002) Lovastatin potentiates antitumor activity of doxorubicin in murine melanoma via an apoptosis-dependent mechanism. Int J Cancer 100:111–118
28. Sumi S, Beauchamp RD, Townsend CM Jr, Pour PM, Ishizuka J, Thompson JC (1994) Lovastatin inhibits pancreatic cancer growth regardless of RAS mutation. Pancreas 9:657–661
29. Kusama T, Mukai M, Iwasaki T, et al (2002) 3-hydroxy-3-methylglutaryl-coenzyme a reductase inhibitors reduce human pancreatic cancer cell invasion and metastasis. Gastroenterology 122:308–317
30. Berthold HK, Unverdorben S, Zittermann A, et al (2004) Age-dependent effects of atorvastatin on biochemical bone turnover markers: a randomized controlled trial in postmenopausal women. Osteoporos Int 15:459–467
31. Liappis AP, Kan VL, Rochester CG, Simon GL (2001) The effect of statins on mortality in patients with bacteremia. Clin Infect Dis 33:1352–1357
32. Merx MW, Liehn EA, Janssens U, et al (2004) HMG-CoA reductase inhibitor simvastatin profoundly improves survival in a murine model of sepsis. Circulation 109:2560–2565
33. Blanco-Colio LM, Tunon J, Martin-Ventura JL, Egido J (2003) Anti-inflammatory and immunomodulatory effects of statins. Kidney Int 63:12–23
34. Tai SC, Robb GB, Marsden PA (2004) Endothelial nitric oxide synthase: a new paradigm for gene regulation in the injured blood vessel. Arterioscler Thromb Vasc Biol 24:405–412
35. Bonville DA, Parker TS, Levine DM, et al (2004) The relationships of hypocholesterolemia to cytokine concentrations and mortality in critically ill patients with systemic inflammatory response syndrome. Surg Infect (Larchmt) 5:39–49
36. Gui D, Spada PL, De Gaetano A, Pacelli F (1996) Hypocholesterolemia and risk of death in the critically ill surgical patient. Intensive Care Med 22:790–794
37. van Leeuwen HJ, Heezius EC, Dallinga GM, van Strijp JA, Verhoef J, van Kessel KP (2003) Lipoprotein metabolism in patients with severe sepsis. Crit Care Med 31:1359–1366
38. Gordon BR (2004) Poor outcomes associated with low lipid and lipoprotein levels. Crit Care Med 32:878–879

39. Gordon BR, Parker TS, Levine DM, et al (1996) Low lipid concentrations in critical illness: implications for preventing and treating endotoxemia. Crit Care Med 24:584–589
40. Harris HW, Gosnell JE, Kumwenda ZL (2000) The lipemia of sepsis: triglyceride-rich lipoproteins as agents of innate immunity. J Endotoxin Res 6:421–430
41. Knopp RH (1999) Drug treatment of lipid disorders. N Engl J Med 341:498–511
42. Vaughan CJ, Gotto AM Jr (2004) Update on statins: 2003. Circulation 110:886–892
43. Yu BP (1994) Cellular defenses against damage from reactive oxygen species. Physiol Rev 74:139–162
44. Goldstein JL, Brown MS (1990) Regulation of the mevalonate pathway. Nature 343:425–430
45. Weber C, Erl W, Weber KS, Weber PC (1997) HMG-CoA reductase inhibitors decrease CD11b expression and CD11b-dependent adhesion of monocytes to endothelium and reduce increased adhesiveness of monocytes isolated from patients with hypercholesterolemia. J Am Coll Cardiol 30:1212–1217
46. Weitz-Schmidt G, Welzenbach K, Brinkmann V, et al (2001) Statins selectively inhibit leukocyte function antigen-1 by binding to a novel regulatory integrin site. Nat Med 7:687–692
47. Frenette PS (2001) Locking a leukocyte integrin with statins. N Engl J Med 345:1419–1421
48. Ridker PM, Rifai N, Clearfield M, et al (2001) Measurement of C-reactive protein for the targeting of statin therapy in the primary prevention of acute coronary events. N Engl J Med 344:1959–1965
49. Rice JB, Stoll LL, Li WG, et al (2003) Low-level endotoxin induces potent inflammatory activation of human blood vessels: inhibition by statins. Arterioscler Thromb Vasc Biol 23:1576–1582
50. Pruefer D, Makowski J, Schnell M, et al (2002) Simvastatin inhibits inflammatory properties of Staphylococcus aureus alpha-toxin. Circulation 106:2104–2110
51. Kostner K (2004) Activation of the complement system: A crucial link between inflammation and atherosclerosis? Eur J Clin Invest 34:800–802
52. Mason JC, Ahmed Z, Mankoff R, et al (2002) Statin-induced expression of decay-accelerating factor protects vascular endothelium against complement-mediated injury. Circ Res 91:696–703
53. Cines DB, Pollak ES, Buck CA, et al (1998) Endothelial cells in physiology and in the pathophysiology of vascular disorders. Blood 91:3527–3561
54. Seeger H, Mueck AO, Lippert TH (2000) Fluvastatin increases prostacyclin and decreases endothelin production by human umbilical vein endothelial cells. Int J Clin Pharmacol Ther 38:270–272
55. Essig M, Nguyen G, Prie D, Escoubet B, Sraer JD, Friedlander G (1998) 3-Hydroxy-3-methylglutaryl coenzyme A reductase inhibitors increase fibrinolytic activity in rat aortic endothelial cells. Role of geranylgeranylation and Rho proteins. Circ Res 83:683–690
56. Hernandez-Perera O, Perez-Sala D, Navarro-Antolin J, et al (1998) Effects of the 3-hydroxy-3-methylglutaryl-CoA reductase inhibitors, atorvastatin and simvastatin, on the expression of endothelin-1 and endothelial nitric oxide synthase in vascular endothelial cells. J Clin Invest 101:2711–2719
57. Kaneta S, Satoh K, Kano S, Kanda M, Ichihara K (2003) All hydrophobic HMG-CoA reductase inhibitors induce apoptotic death in rat pulmonary vein endothelial cells. Atherosclerosis 170:237–243
58. Pishvaian AC, Trope BW, Lewis JH (2004) Drug-Induced liver disease in 2003. Curr Opin Gastroenterol 20:208–219
59. Thompson PD, Clarkson P, Karas RH (2003) Statin-associated myopathy. JAMA 289:1681–1690
60. Jamal SM, Eisenberg MJ, Christopoulos S (2004) Rhabdomyolysis associated with hydroxymethylglutaryl-coenzyme A reductase inhibitors. Am Heart J 147:956–965
61. Goli AK, Goli SA, Byrd RP Jr, Roy TM (2002) Simvastatin-induced lactic acidosis: a rare adverse reaction? Clin Pharmacol Ther 72:461–464
62. Angus DC, Linde-Zwirble WT, Lidicker J, Clermont G, Carcillo J, Pinsky MR (2001) Epidemiology of severe sepsis in the United States: analysis of incidence, outcome, and associated costs of care. Crit Care Med 29:1303–1310
63. Vincent JL, Abraham E, Annane D, Bernard G, Rivers E, Van den Berghe G (2002) Reducing mortality in sepsis: new directions. Crit Care 6(Suppl3):S1–18

Blood Transfusions

Anemia in Critically Ill Patients

E. Potolidis, E. Vakouti, and D. Georgopoulos

Introduction

Anemia is a common problem in critically ill patients. Indeed it has been shown that at intensive care unit (ICU) admission the mean hemoglobin concentration (Hb) of critically ill patients is ~ 11 g/dl, while in 60% and 30% of such patients, the mean Hb is less than 12 and 10 g/dl, respectively [1, 2]. It is of interest to note that in these patients the rate of hemoglobin decline is approximately 0.5 g/dl/day during the first days after ICU admission and continues to decline, particularly in patients with severe illness [1]. Thus the majority of critically ill patients exhibit anemia on ICU admission, which persists throughout the duration of their ICU stay.

Causes of Anemia in Critically Ill Patients

Several factors contribute to anemia in critically ill patients. The withdrawal of large amounts of blood for diagnostic reasons is an important but largely ignored factor for development of anemia in patients in ICUs [3]. Smoller and Kruskall showed that one half of patients who received blood transfusions had blood losses from phlebotomy that exceeded the equivalent of one unit of blood [4]. A recent European multicenter study (the ABC study) demonstrated that in critically ill patients the blood loss through blood sampling for diagnostic purposes is considerable, averaging 41 ml/day [1]. Nguyen and colleagues [5] also documented that the mean volume of blood drawn daily for laboratory studies was approximately 40 ml. Considering only septic patients this amount increased to 49 ml. In patients undergoing renal replacement therapies the blood loss due to blood sampling may be in the range of 60 ml per day [6]. Obviously this type of blood loss has an impact on blood transfusion. Indeed, Corwin et al. showed a positive relationship between the number of phlebotomies performed for diagnostic purposes and the amount of red blood cell (RBC) transfusions [7]. Furthermore, in the ABC study [1] a positive correlation was observed between organ dysfunction and the number of blood draws and total volume drawn.

We should note that in the process of blood sampling the ICU health care worker has to discard a significant blood volume in order to obtain accurate results. This volume depends on medical practice and may vary from 2 to 10 ml [5]. It is recommended that the discard volume should not be greater than twice the catheter dead-space [8, 9].

Occult bleeding is another important factor that may contribute to anemia in critically ill patients [3]. Stress gastritis (stress ulcer) is a potential source for blood loss. Surgical patients often have anemia in the postoperative period and should be monitored carefully. Blood loss into the retro-peritoneal space should be suspected and carefully investigated in patients with abdominal trauma who exhibit acute decline in hemoglobin.

An important cause of anemia in critically ill patients is functional iron deficiency [10, 11]. Typically, critically ill patients have elevated serum ferritin concentrations, low transferrin saturation, and low serum iron concentration [11, 12]. Therefore, the low serum iron levels are not able to support the heme biosynthesis and the erythropoiesis. Systemic inflammatory response syndrome (SIRS) may be the pathogenic mechanism for this pattern. Cytokines that are released during the inflammation process, like tumor necrosis factor (TNF)-α and interleukin (IL)-6, may induce the transcription and translation of ferritin and are able to down-regulate transferrin receptor messenger mRNA (iron uptake) [13]. In addition, it has been reported that nitric oxide (NO), which is increased in vasodilator shock, has the ability to reduce the ferrochelatase activity [14], thus contributing to the functional iron deficiency.

Ineffective erythropoiesis in patients with critical illness could be the result of vitamin B12 or folic acid deficiency. Data in the literature indicate that these deficiencies do not play an important role in the pathogenesis of the anemia in these patients. Indeed, a recent study showed that 2% of critically ill patients were deficient in vitamin B12 and another 2% were deficient in folic acid [15]. Nevertheless, these deficiencies are rapidly correctable causes of ineffective erythropoiesis.

It has been shown that IL-6 and TNF-α are both able to decrease the life span of RBCs [16, 17]. In addition to the reduced RBC life span due to proinflammatory cytokines, the erythrocytes of critically ill patients show decreased deformability [18]. Reactive oxygen species, increased concentrations of 2,3-DPG into the RBCs, and alterations in intracellular calcium content could be factors responsible for the decreased RBCs deformability [18]. The decrease in RBC deformability may play a role in disturbances in microcirculation, observed in critically ill patients.

Inflammatory mediators released during SIRS may also influence the differentiation of erythroid progenitor cells. It is well known that cytokines are able to inhibit the differentiation of erythroid progenitor cells [19]. In addition, interferon (IFN)-γ is able to induce apoptosis of the human erythroid colony forming cells via Fas expression and caspase activation [19]. Papadaki et al. reported that patients with rheumatoid arthritis (anemia of chronic disease which shares similar characteristics to that of critical illness) exhibit reduced apoptosis of erythroid cells in the bone marrow after treatment with anti-TNF-α antibodies [20].

Histiocytic hyperplasia with hemophagocytosis (HHH), a syndrome observed during sepsis or malignancies, may contribute to anemia in critically ill patients. The syndrome is characterized by single cytopenia (anemia, neutropenia or thrombocytopenia) or pancytopenia. Strauss et al. [21], in a postmortem clinico-pathologic study investigated 107 patients who were hospitalized and died in the ICU, showed that histiocytic hyperplasia with hemophagocytosis was present in 69 patients (64.5%). Predictors of histiocytic hyperplasia syndrome were treatment intensity and non-cardiovascular cause of death. This study demonstrated that sepsis and blood transfusion were triggering factors with a possible synergistic effect [21].

Peritubular interstitial cells in the renal cortex and parenchymal liver cells produce a glycoprotein hormone named erythropoietin (EPO). This hormone binds to the EPO receptor on erythroid progenitor cells and promotes their maturity, while on the other hand it decreases their apoptosis. Several studies have shown that EPO also has a neuroprotective effect [22, 23]. In patients with iron deficiency anemia, EPO concentration and Hb levels have a negative semilogarithmic correlation [24]. This is not the case in critically ill patients. It has been shown that in these patients for a given hematocrit (Hct) or hemoglobin, EPO plasma levels are significantly lower than those observed in patients with iron-deficiency anemia [25] (Fig. 1). von Ahsen et al. [12] calculated the erythropoietin response ($\Delta\log/\Delta Hb$) in ICU patients and noted that it was on average half of the response of patients with uncomplicated non-renal anemia. This phenomenon is referred to as blunted erythropoietic response. Studies have shown that the inappropriate low levels of erythropoietin significantly contribute to anemia in critically ill patients [26]. The blunted erythropoietic response is thought to result from decrease of erythropoietin gene expression by inflammatory mediators, such as TNF-a, IL-1 and IL-6 [3].

▌ RBC Transfusion

Anemia in critically ill patients results in significant RBCs transfusions. Approximately 40% of critically ill patients receive at least one unit of RBCs, relatively early after ICU admission [1, 2]. The mean number of RBC units transfused approaches five, while the pre-transfusion Hb is $\sim$8.5 g/dl, indicating that the large number of transfusions is not due to a very high Hb transfusion threshold [1, 2]. Corwin et al., investigated the transfusion practice of their tertiary care center and found that 85% of critically ill patients with an ICU length of stay greater than one week, received blood transfusions, with a mean of approximately 9.5 units per patient [7]. It follows that the rate of blood transfusions in these patients is very high [7, 25].

The amount of oxygen delivered to the whole blood (DO$_2$) is given by the following equation:

$$DO_2 = CO \times CaO_2$$

where CO is cardiac output (CO=SV×HR, SV is stroke volume and HR is heart rate) and CaO$_2$ is the oxygen concentration of arterial blood (CaO$_2$=1.36 Hb×SaO$_2$+0.003×PaO$_2$). It is apparent that Hb reduction decreases the amount of oxygen delivered to tissues and under certain circumstances may result in tissue hypoxia. It follows that the main goal of RBC transfusion in anemic patients is to prevent or reverse tissue hypoxia by increasing the oxygen-carrying capacity of the blood. We should note however, that in critically ill patients regional blood flow is an important determinant of oxygen supply to cells; severe tissue hypoxia may ensue despite a normal value of Hb and global DO$_2$ [28, 29].

RBC transfusion is associated with numerous adverse events (Table 1), including infection transmission [30], transfusion associated immunosuppression [27, 31–33], transfusion related acute lung injury (TRALI) [34], disturbances in microcirculation due to blood storage [35, 36], and allergic reactions [33].

The first reported cases of transfusion-associated human immunodeficiency virus (HIV) transmission occurred in 1982. Since then cases of HIV transmission have decreased due to development of antibody detection and p24 antigen detection [27, 37]. Hepatitis B virus (HBV) infection due to transfusion decreased after the introduction of screening tests for HbsAg in 1975 and the risk of transfusion trans-

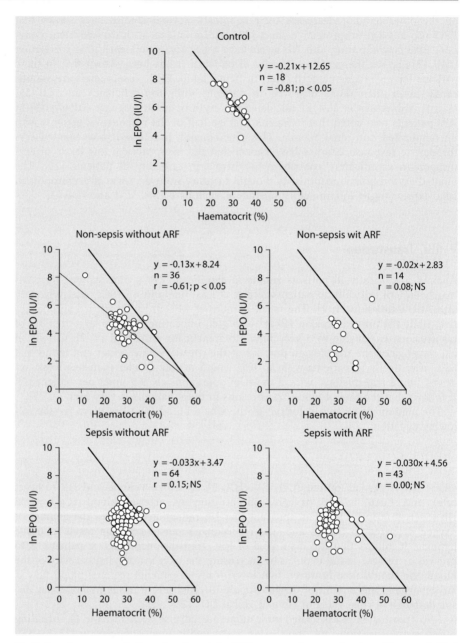

Fig. 1. Log plasma concentration of erythropoietin (EPO) concentration as a function of hematocrit (Hct) in patients with uncomplicated iron deficiency anemia (control) and in various groups of critically ill patients. Observe that the in patients with critical illness the relationship has been shifted to the left of that in control group (solid line). This phenomenon is referred to as a blunted erythropoietic response. (From [25] with permission)

Table 1. Potential hazards of red blood cell transfusion

▌ Infection transmission
▌ Transfusion-associated immunosuppression
▌ Transfusion related acute lung injury (TRALI)
▌ Disturbances in microcirculation
▌ Allergic reactions

mitted hepatitis C virus (HCV) is currently 1 in 103000 transfusions [38]. Transmission of B19 parvovirus can occur, but is not significant except in patients with hemolytic diseases, immunosuppression, and in pregnancy. Human T-cell lymphotropic virus types I and II (HTLV-I, II) have been associated with myelopathy and adult T cell leukemia. Infection will occur in 20 to 60% of recipients of blood infected with HTLV-I, II [39].

Bacterial contamination of the RBCs is another transfusion-associated risk. *Yersinia enterocolitica* is often implicated, but other Gram-negative organisms have been reported also [40]. Theakston et al. reported that the rate of contamination by *Yersinia enterocolitica* was 1 per 65000 red cell units transfused [41]. Transfusion mediated transmission of *Trypanosoma cruzi* is possible in Central and South America where this type of infection is endemic [42]. Potential infectious threats are also malaria and babesiosis [42]. The latter may occur particularly in immunocompromised and asplenic individuals. West Nile virus, a flavirus which cause encephalitis and meningitis, could be transmissed by RBCs transfusions. This virus was first recognized in 1999, in an outbreak of encephalitis in New York [43]. Mosquito bites permit the transmission from birds to humans.

Hemolytic reactions to RBC transfusion are often due to ABO incompability. Delayed reaction to transfusion may also occur, and its incidence is estimated to be 1 for 1000 patients [44].

TRALI is a noncardiogenic pulmonary edema with a significant morbidity and mortality. The frequency of this adverse event has been estimated to be 1 in 5000 transfusions [34, 45]. However, the actual incidence of this syndrome may be higher since the association of acute lung injury (ALI) and RBC transfusion may not always be recognized. The syndrome may occur within a few hours after transfusion. The pathogenesis of TRALI may be explained by a 'two-hit' hypothesis, with the first 'hit' being a predisposing inflammatory condition commonly present in the operating room or ICU [34]. The second hit may involve the passive transfer of neutrophil or HLA antibodies from the donor or the transfusion of biologically active lipids from older, cellular blood products. Treatment is supportive, with a prognosis substantially better than most causes of ALI. However, TRALI remains the third most common cause of transfusion-associated death [34].

In recent years, accumulating evidence has indicated that RBC transfusion alters the immune system of the host (transfusion related immunomodulation, TRIM) [32, 46]. Although the exact pathogenetic mechanism underlying this immunomodulation is not known, recent evidence suggests that transfusion of white blood cells may be responsible. It has been reported that white blood cells from the donor may persist in the recipient blood for up to 18 months [47, 48]. It is suggested that TRIM is able to cause cancer recurrences, although this issue is currently highly controversial [47]. More importantly, it is thought that TRIM may increase the risk

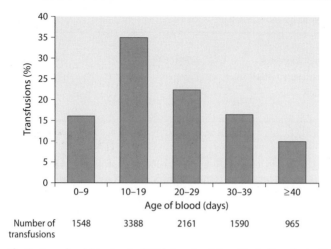

Fig. 2. Age of red blood cells (RBCs) transfused in critically ill patients. Notice that in the majority of transfusions the transfused blood is older than 10 days. (From [35] with permission)

of nosocomial infections [47]. Taylor et al. investigated whether critically ill patients who received RBC transfusion were at increased risk of acquiring infections and showed that the transfusion group was six times more likely to develop nosocomial infections compared to the non-transfusion group [49]. They further demonstrated that for each unit of RBCs transfused, the odds of developing nosocomial infection were increased by a factor of 1.5 [49]. Shorr et al. in a multicenter, prospective observational study showed that RBC transfusion was independently associated with an increase risk for ventilator associated pneumonia (VAP) [50].

Finally, it should be kept in mind that stored blood is often 'old' blood. Indeed, it has been shown that in the majority of transfusions, the age of blood is > 10 days (Fig. 2). This may have an adverse effect on the microcirculation. Marik and Sibbald showed that critically ill patients receiving old transfused RBCs (> 10 days) developed evidence of tissue hypoxia, as indicated by a significant decrease in gastric intramucosal pH (pHi) [35] (Fig. 3).

It follows that RBC transfusion is not without risk and may considerably increase morbidity and mortality. This is particularly true for critically ill patients. Large observational studies in these patients have shown that RBC transfusion is an independent risk factor for increased mortality [1, 2] (Fig. 4). Vincent et al. [1] demonstrated that receipt of a blood transfusion increased the risk of dying by a factor of 1.4 (all other variables being equal). Although the mechanism through which RBC transfusion may increase mortality is currently unknown, it is believed that the likely factors contributing to mortality are related to immunosuppression and disturbances in microcirculation as opposed to allergic reaction or infectious transmission [35, 49–50].

For several years a Hb concentration of 10 g/dl and Hct of 30% were the transfusion thresholds. Considering the risks associated with RBC transfusion it would be appropriate to explore whether lower transfusion triggers may be used in critically ill patients. In a multicenter, randomized controlled clinical trial involving 838 critically ill patients, Hebert et al. [51] showed that a restrictive transfusion strategy was at least as effective and possibly superior to the strategy of liberal transfu-

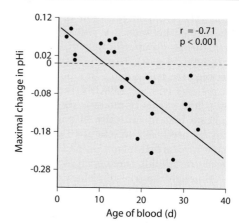

Fig. 3. Relationship between the age of transfused RBCs and the change in gastric intramucosal pH. (From [35] with permission)

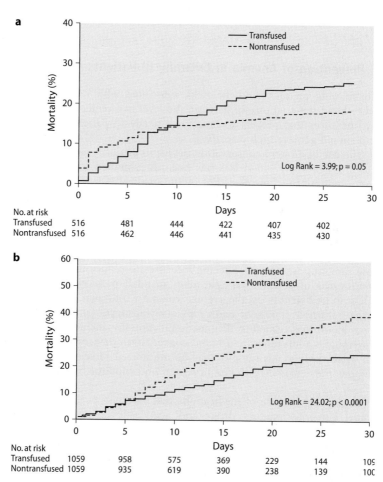

Fig. 4. Survival analysis by transfusion status among propensity-matched critically ill patients. **a** Data from [1] with permission. **b** Data from [2] with permission

sion. The Hb concentration of patients assigned to the restrictive strategy was maintained between 7–9 g/dl (transfusion threshold 7 g/dl), whereas in the liberal transfusion group Hb was maintained in the range of 10–12 g/dl (transfusion threshold 10 g/dl). This study showed that 30-day all-cause mortality did not differ between the two groups. In a post-hoc analysis, the investigators demonstrated that in patients with an APACHE II score less than 20 and in patients younger than 55 years, the mortality rate was significantly lower in restrictive group. These findings indicate that in critically ill patients a transfusion triggering threshold of 7 g/dl may be preferable to one of 10 g/dl. This, however, may not apply in patients with acute myocardial infarction and unstable angina, in whom higher transfusion triggering thresholds may be appropriate.

Although the trial of Hebert et al. [51] defined an appropriate transfusion practice for critically ill patients, physicians dealing with these patients are reluctant to follow these rules. Indeed, a recent large observational study [1] found that mean pretransfusion Hb levels remain substantially higher (8.4 g/dL for all patients transfused, and 8.5 g/dL for those without active bleeding) than the threshold suggested by the findings of the study of Hebert et al.

▌ Prevention of Anemia in Critically Ill Patients

Considering on one hand the risks associated with RBC transfusion and on the other hand the relationship between the level of anemia and morbidity and mortality, measures that prevent anemia in critically ill patients are of great importance and should achieve high priority.

The use of a blood conservation device in critically ill patients to minimize diagnostic phlebotomy blood loss has been documented to be efficacious. A prospective, randomized, controlled trial in 100 medical ICU patients confirmed that there was significant blood conservation with a device incorporated into the arterial pressure monitoring system [52]. In a recent postal survey of arterial blood sampling practices in 280 ICUs of England and Wales it was found that few measures were taken to minimize blood losses from arterial sampling in adult intensive care patients [53]. The average volume of blood withdrawn to clear the arterial line before sampling was 3.2 ml. Specific measures to reduce the blood sample size by the routine use of pediatric sample tubes in adult patients occurred in only 9.3% of ICUs. In pediatric ICUs, the average volume withdrawn was 1.9 ml, which was routinely returned in 67% of units. Obviously strategies should be implemented to reduce blood loss related to diagnostic phlebotomy, including use of pediatric tubes, low-volume adult tubes, and blood conservation devices [54]. In addition, the need for arterial blood gas samples may be minimized in selected patients by using continuous pulse oximetry to monitor SaO_2 and capnometry to monitor end-tidal CO_2 [55–57].

Decreasing the use of medications that result in perioperative bleeding (nonsteroidal anti-inflammatory drugs and acetylsalicylic acid) might also be helpful. Stress ulcer prophylaxis may be warranted in patients at high risk, such as those receiving mechanical ventilation [58]. Nevertheless, the use of stress ulcer prophylaxis in all critically ill patients should be avoided since it may increase the risk of nosocomial pneumonia [59]. Iron therapy can help to optimize EPO treatment (see below) since iron deficiency may be a contributing factor to the resistance to EPO treatment in critically ill patients [60, 61]. Moreover, adjuvant therapy, such as ascorbic acid, to increase oral iron absorption and physiologic utilization, has been widely used and should be studied in critically ill patients [62]. The use of antifibrinolytics has been found to reduce perioperative RBC transfusions and the need for re-operation because of bleeding [63]. Clotting factors such as activated factor VII are under investigation.

Selective use of salvage and autotransfusion in critically ill patients with very large postoperative recoverable blood loss may be effective at limiting the acute development of anemia and transfusion requirements [64, 65]. Acute normovolemic hemodilution describes the removal of whole blood from a patient immediately before surgery and concurrent replacement of that volume with crystalloids or colloids [27]. The blood is later re-transfused. It is not known if this may be applicable in critically ill patients.

Exogenous administration of recombinant human erythropoietin (rHuEPO) in patients with critical illness is a preventive strategy that has attracted much attention in recent years. The rational for rHuEPO therapy in critically ill patients is that increased erythropoiesis will result in higher Hb levels and subsequently will reduce the need for RBC transfusion. It is considered that critically ill patients have a limited ability to compensate for the fall in Hb concentration [66, 67]. Indeed in these patients, anemia is associated with increased morbidity and mortality, particularly in patients with pre-existing cardiac disease [66, 67]. Preventing anemia by administration of rHuEPO on one hand minimizes the risks of anemia without on the other hand, exposing the critically ill to the deleterious effects of RBC transfusion.

Van Iperen et al. [68] in a randomized open trial studied three groups of critically ill patients. One group received intravenous folic acid daily from days 1 to 14 (control group), a second group received i.v. folic acid and iron (iron group), and a third group received folic acid, iron and rHuEPO, administered subcutaneously on study days 1, 3, 5, 7 and 9 in a dose of 300 IU/Kgr. The study clearly showed that rHuEPO increased the concentration of reticulocytes and serum transferrin receptors (Fig. 5). Similarly Gabriel et al. [69] showed in patients with multiple organ failure, that rHuEPO therapy (600 units/kg) stimulated erythropoiesis. These findings indicate that the bone marrow of critically ill patients is able to respond to exogenous EPO and this therapy might be useful in increasing Hb level and reducing the need for RBC transfusion. Two randomized, double blind, placebo controlled studies have documented that this is the case. Corwin et al. [70] randomized 160 critically ill patients to receive either rHuEPO (300 units/kg of rHuEPO for 5 consecutive days and then every other day to achieve a hematocrit concentration >38%) or placebo. This study showed that rHuEPO therapy resulted in an almost 50% reduction in RBC transfusions as compared with placebo. It is of interest to note that despite receiving fewer RBC transfusions, patients in the rHuEPO group had a significantly greater increase in hematocrit. The same group of investigators, in a second larger study [71], randomized 1302 patients to receive either rHuEPO or placebo. rHuEPO was given weekly at a fixed dose of 40000 units. All patients received three weekly doses, and patients who remained in the ICU on study day 21 received a fourth dose. Treatment with rHuEPO resulted in a 10% reduction in the number of patients receiving any RBC transfusion (60.4% with placebo versus 50.5% with rHuEPO) and a 20% reduction in the total number of RBC units transfused (1963 units with placebo versus 1590 units with rHuEPO) (Fig. 6).

The optimal dose of rHuEPO therapy is not known. In a just completed randomized multicenter trial in critically ill patients, we found that the transfusion require-

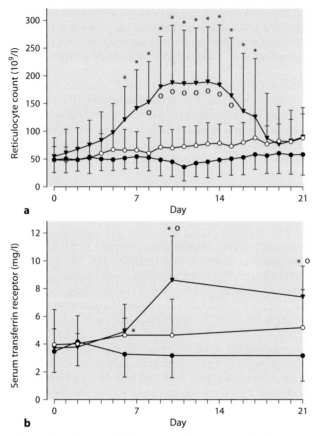

a

b

Fig. 5. a Reticulocytes and **b** serum transferrin receptors in three groups of critically ill patients receiving folic acid (control group, closed circles), folic acid and iron (iron group, open circles) and folic acid, iron and recombinant human erythropoietin (rHuEPO group, closed triangles). (From [68] with permission)

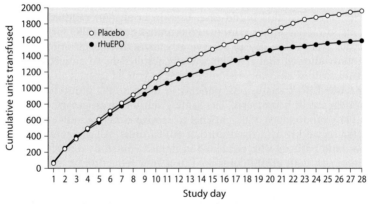

Fig. 6. Cumulative units of red blood cells transfused in patients randomized to receive recombinant human erythropoietin (rHuEPO) or placebo. The difference between the two groups was significant. (From [71] with permission)

ments were not influenced by two dosing regimes of rHuEPO (40 000 units once or three times per week), whereas there was a clear dose response of Hb and Hct to rHuEPO (unpublished data). These results indicate that dose of rHuEPO in critically ill patients should be titrated depending on the desired goal (decrease transfusion requirements or increase in Hb).

Although rHuEPO therapy considerably decreases the exposure of critically ill patients to allogenic RBCs, it seems that the outcome of critically ill patients is not influenced by this therapy. In the large study of Corwin et al. [72] neither morbidity nor mortality differed significantly between groups. The interpretation of these results is however complicated by the fact that the majority of patients receiving rHuEPO were anemic by the end of the study and the Hb level differed slightly between groups (approximately 0.3 g/dl). Considering the relationship between the level of anemia and morbidity and mortality [66, 67] the inability of this rHuEPO regimen to increase Hb to normal levels may have an impact on morbidity and mortality data. Further studies are needed to resolve this issue.

▌ Conclusion

The majority of critically ill patients exhibit anemia at some time during the course of their illness, resulting in multiple RBC transfusions. The pathogenesis of anemia in these patients is multifactorial, with blood loss and blunted erythropoietic response being the most important contributors. Although RBC transfusion remains a common practice in critically ill patients, it is associated with significant risks, such as disturbances in microcirculation and immunosuppresion. Because of these risks, transfusion practice is currently under systematic scrutiny and transfusion benefits are being critically re-evaluated. Measures to prevent rather than to treat anemia in critically ill patients should achieve high priority. Strategies to decrease blood loss, such as the development of simple techniques to decrease the blood volume withdrawn for diagnostic purposes, should be implemented in every ICU. Administration of rHuEPO in selected ICU patients may significantly decrease RBC transfusion requirements, although the impact of this therapy on patient outcome needs further study.

References

1. Vincent JL, Baron JF, Reinhart K, et al (2002) Anemia and blood transfusion in critically ill patients. JAMA 288:1499–1507
2. Corwin HL, Gettinger A, Pearl RG, et al (2004) The CRIT Study: Anemia and blood transfusion in the critically ill–current clinical practice in the United States. Crit Care Med 32:39–52
3. Vincent JL, Sakr Y, Creteur J (2003) Anemia in the intensive care unit. Can J Anaesth 50:S53–59
4. Smoller BR, Kruskall MS (1986) Phlebotomy for diagnostic laboration tests in adults: pattern of use and effect on transfusion requirements. N Engl J Med 314:1233–1236
5. Nguyen BV, Bota DP, Melot C, Vincent JL (2003) Time course of hemoglobin concentration in nonbleeding intensive care unit patients. Crit Care Med 31:406–410
6. Andrews T, Waterman H, Hillier V (1999) Blood gas analysis: a study of blood loss in intensive care. J Adv Nursing 30:851–857
7. Corwin HC, Parsonnet KC, Gettinger A (1995) RBC transfusion in the ICU: Is there a reason? Chest 108:767–771

8. Richard CM, Couchman BA, Schmidt SJ, Dank A, Purdie DM (2003) A discard volume of twice the vascular line deadspace ensures clinically accurate arterial blood gases and electrolytes and prevents unnecessary blood loss. Crit Care Med 31:1654–1658

9. Fowler RA, Berenson M (2003) Blood conservation in the intensive care unit. Crit Care Med 31:715–720

10. Scharte M, Fink MP (2003) Red blood cell physiology in critical illness. Crit Care Med 31:651–657

11. Weiss G (2002) Pathogenesis and treatment of anemia of chronic disease. Blood Rev 16:87–96

12. von Ahsen N, Muller C, Serke S, Frei U, Eckardt KU (1999) Important role of nondiagnostic blood loss and blunted erythropoietic response in the anemia of medical intensive care patients. Crit Care Med 27:2630–2639

13. Rogers JT (1996) Ferritin translation of IL-1 and IL-6: The role of sequences upstream of the start codons of the heavy and light subunit genes. Blood 87:2525–2537

14. Furukawa T, Kohuo H, Tokunaga R, Takenani S (1995) NO-mediated inactivation of mammalian ferrochelatase in vivo and in vitro:possible involvement of the iron sulphur cluster of the enzyme. Biochem J 310:533–538

15. Rondriguez RM, Corwin HL, Gettinger A, Corwin MJ, Gubler D, Pearl RG (2001) Nutritional deficiencies and blunted erythropoietin response as causes of the anemia of critical illness. J Crit Care 16:36–41

16. Salvarani C, Casali B, Salvo D, et al (1991) The role of IL-1, erythropoietin and red blood cell bound immunoglobulins in the anemia of rheumatoid arthritis. Clin Exp Rheumatol 9:241–246

17. Moldawer LL, Marano MA, Wei H, et al (1989) Cachektin/TNF-a alters the red blood cell kinetics and induces anemia in vivo. FASEB J 3:1637–1643

18. Baskurt OK, Gelmont D, Meiselman HJ (1998) Red blood cell deformability in sepsis. Am J Respir Crit Care Med 157:421–427

19. Dai CH, Krantz SB, Kollar K, Price JO (1995) Stem cell factor can overcome inhibition of highly purified human burst forming units erythroid by INF-γ. J Cell Physiol 165:323–332

20. Papadaki HA, Kritikos HD, Valatas V, Boumpas DT, Eliopoulos GD (2002) Anemia of chronic disease in rheumatoid arthritis is associated with increased apoptosis of bone marrow erythroid cells improvement following anti TNF-a antibody therapy. Blood 100:474–482

21. Strauss R, Neureiter D, Westenburger B, Wahler M, Kirchner T, Hahn EG (2004) Multifactorial risk analysis of bone marrow histiocytic hyperplasia with hemophagocytosis in critically ill medical patients-A postmortem clinicopathologic analysis. Crit Care Med 32:1316–1321

22. Digicaylioglu M, Lipton SA (2001) Erythropoietin mediated neuroprotection involves cross talk between Jak-2 and NF-kB signalling cascades. Nature 412:641–647

23. Lipton SA (2004) Erythropoietin for neurologic protection and diabetic neuropathy. N Engl J Med 350:2516–2517

24. Erlev AJ, Wilson J, Caro J (1987) Erythropoietin titers in anemic, nonuremic patients. J Lab Clin Med 109:429–433

25. Rogiers P, Zhang H, Leeman M, et al (1997) Erythropoietin response is blunted in critically ill patients. Intensive Care Med 23:159–162

26. Krafte-Jacobs B (1997) Anemia of critical illness and erythropoietin deficiency. Intensive Care Med 23:137–138

27. Goodnough LT, Brecher ME, Kanter MH, AuBuchon JP (1999) Transfusion medicine. First of two parts–blood transfusion. N Engl J Med 340:438–447

28. Rangel-Frausto MS, Pittet D, Costigan M, Hwang T, Davis CS, Wenzel RP (1995) The natural history of the systemic inflammatory response syndrome (SIRS): a prospective study. JAMA 273:117–123

29. Hinds C, Watson D (1995) Manipulating hemodynamics and oxygen transport in critically ill patients. N Engl J Med 333:1074–1075

30. Stevens CE, Aach RD, Hollinger FB, et al (1984) Hepatitis B virus antibody in blood donors and the occurrence of non-A, non-B hepatitis in transfusion recipients. An analysis of the Transfusion-Transmitted Viruses Study. Ann Intern Med 101:733–738

31. Spence RK, Cernaianu AC, Carson J, DelRossi AJ (1993) Transfusion and surgery. Curr Probl Surg 30:1101–1180
32. Blumberg N, Heal JM (1994) Effects of transfusion on immune function. Cancer recurrence and infection. Arch Pathol Lab Med 118:371–379
33. Brunson ME, Alexander JW (1990) Mechanisms of transfusion-induced immunosuppression. Transfusion 30:651–658
34. Looney MR, Gropper MA, Matthay MA (2004) Transfusion-related acute lung injury: a review. Chest 126:249–258
35. Marik PE, Sibbald WJ (1993) Effect of stored-blood transfusion on oxygen delivery in patients with sepsis. JAMA 269:3024–3029
36. Fitzgerald RD, Martin CM, Dietz GE, Doig GS, Potter RF, Sibbald WJ (1997) Transfusing red blood cells stored in citrate phosphate dextrose adenine-1 for 28 days fails to improve tissue oxygenation in rats. Crit Care Med 25:726–732
37. Goodnough LT (2003) Risks of blood transfusion. Crit Care Med 31:S678–685
38. Schreiber GB, Busch MP, Kleinman SH, Korelitz JJ (1996) The risk of transfusion transmitted viral infections. N Engl J Med 334:1685–1690
39. Centers of Disease control and prevention, U. S. P. H. S. working group (1993) Guidelines for counselling persons infected with HTLV-I and HTLV-II. Ann Intern Med 118:448–454
40. National Report (1997) Red blood cells transfusion contaminated with Yersinia enterocolitica United States 1991–1996, and initiation of a national study to detect bacteria associated transfusion reactions. MMWR Morb Mortal Wkly Rep 46:553–555
41. Theakston EP, Morris AJ, Streat SJ, Baker BW, Woodfield DG (1997) Transfusion transmitted Yersinia enterocolitica infection in New Zealand Aust N Z J Med 27:62–67
42. Dellinger EP, Anaya DA (2004) Infectious and immunologic consequences of blood transfusion. Crit Care 8 (suppl 2):S18–S23
43. Sampathkumar P (2003) West Nile virus: Epidemiology, clinical presentation, diagnosis and prevention. Mayo Clin Proc 78:1137–1143
44. Ness PM, Shirley RS, Thoman SK, Buck SA (1990) The differentiation of delayed serologic and delayed hemolytic transfusion reactions:incidence, long-term serologic findings, and clinical significance. Transfusion 30:688–693
45. Popovsky MA, Moore SB (1985) Diagnostic and pathogenetic considerations in transfusion-related acute lung injury. Transfusion 25:573–574
46. Blajchman MA, Dzik S, Vamvakas EC, Sweeney J, Snyder EL (2001) Clinical and molecular basis of transfusion-induced immunomodulation: summary of the proceedings of a state-of-the-art conference. Transfus Med Rev 15:108–135
47. Vamvakas EC, Blajchman MA (2001) Deleterious clinical effects of transfusion- associated immunomodulation: fact or fiction? Blood 97:1180–1195
48. Lee TH, Stromberg RR, Heitman J, Tran K, Busch MP (1994) Quantitation of residual white cells in filtered blood components by polymerase chain reaction amplification of HLA DQ-A DNA. Transfusion 34:986–994
49. Taylor RW, Manganaro L, O'Brien J, Trottier SJ, Parkar N, Veremakis C (2002) Impact of allogenic packed red blood cell transfusion on nosocomial infection rates in the critically ill patient. Crit Care Med 30:2249–2254
50. Shorr AF, Duh MS, Kelly KM, Kollef MH, CRIT Study Group (2004) Red blood cell transfusion and ventilator-associated pneumonia: A potential link? Crit Care Med 32:666–674
51. Hebert PC, Wells G, Blajchman MA, et al (1999) A multicenter, randomized, controlled clinical trial of transfusion requirements in critical care. N Engl J Med 340:409–417
52. Peruzzi WT, Parker MA, Lichtenthal PR, Cochran-Zull C, Toth B, Blake M (1993) A clinical evaluation of a blood conservation device in medical intensive care unit patients. Crit Care Med 21:501–506
53. O'Hare D, Chilvers RJ (2001) Arterial blood sampling practices in intensive care units in England and Wales. Anaesthesia 56:568–571
54. Barie PS (2004) Phlebotomy in the intensive care unit: strategies for blood conservation. Crit Care 8 (Suppl 2):S34–S36
55. Merlani P, Garnerin P, Diby M, Ferrin M, Ricou B (2001) Quality improvement report: Linking guideline to regular feedback to increase appropriate requests for clinical tests: blood gas analysis in intensive care. BMJ 323:620–624

56. Schmitz BD, Shapiro BA (1995) Capnography. Respir Care Clin N Am 1:107–117
57. Jubran A, Tobin MJ (1996) Monitoring during mechanical ventilation. Clin Chest Med 17: 453–473
58. Spirt MJ (2004) Stress-related mucosal disease: risk factors and prophylactic therapy. Clin Ther 26:197–213
59. Torres A, El-Ebiary M, Soler N, Monton C, Fabregas N, Hernandez C (1996) Stomach as a source of colonization of the respiratory tract during mechanical ventilation: association with ventilator-associated pneumonia. Eur Respir J 9:1729–1735
60. Lapointe M (2004) Iron supplementation in the intensive care unit: when, how much, and by what route? Crit Care 8 (Suppl 2):S37–S41
61. Horl WH (2002) Non-erythropoietin-based anaemia management in chronic kidney disease. Nephrol Dial Transplant Suppl 11:35–38
62. Tarng DC, Wei YH, Huang TP, Kuo BI, Yang WC (1999) Intravenous ascorbic acid as an adjuvant therapy for recombinant erythropoietin in hemodialysis patients with hyperferritinemia. Kidney Int 55:2477–2486
63. Henry DA, Moxey AJ, Carless PA, et al (2001): Anti-fibrinolytic use for minimizing perioperative allogeneic blood transfusion. Cochrane Database Syst Rev CD001886
64. Schaff HV, Hauer JM, Bell WR, et al (1978) Autotransfusion of shed mediastinal blood after cardiac surgery: a prospective study. J Thorac Cardiovasc Surg 75:632–641
65. Eng J, Kay PH, Murday AJ, et al (1990) Postoperative autologous transfusion in cardiac surgery: A prospective, randomised study. Eur J Cardiothorac Surg 4:595–600
66. Hebert PC, Wells G, Tweeddale M, et al (1997) Does transfusion practice affect mortality in critically ill patients? Am J Respir Crit Care Med 155:1618–1623
67. Nelson AH, Fleisher LA, Rosenbaum SH (1993) Relationship between postoperative anemia and cardiac morbidity in high-risk vascular patients in the intensive care unit. Crit Care Med 21:860–866
68. van Iperen CE, Gaillard CA, Kraaijenhagen RJ, Braam BG, Marx JJ, Van de Weil A (2000) Response of erythropoiesis and iron metabolism to recombinant human erythropoietin in intensive care unit patients. Crit Care Med 28:2773–2778
69. Gabriel A, Kozek S, Chiari A, et al (1998) High-dose recombinant human erythropoietin stimulates reticulocyte production in patients with multiple organ dysfunction syndrome. J Trauma 44:361–367
70. Corwin HL, Gettinger A, Rodriguez RM, et al (1999) Efficacy of recombinant human erythropoietin in the critically ill patient: a randomized, double blind, placebo-controlled trial. Crit Care Med 27:2346–2350
71. Corwin HL, Gettinger A, Pearl RG, et al (2002) Efficacy of recombinant human erythropoietin in critically ill patients: a randomized controlled trial. JAMA 288:2827–2835
72. Corwin HL (2004) Anemia and blood transfusion in the critically ill patient: role of erythropoietin. Crit Care 8 (Suppl 2):S42–44

Physiology, Benefits and Risks of Red Blood Cell Transfusion

C. Marcucci, C. Madjdpour, and D. R. Spahn

▌ Introduction

Since Adams and Lundy recommended the "10/30 rule" as a guide for transfusion of red blood cells (RBC) in 1942 [1], understanding of the pathophysiology of anemia and insights into the risks of transfusion have, or should have, considerably changed transfusion policy. In addition, large trials have failed to show any benefit of transfusion with hemoglobin levels as low as 7 g/l for most patients, and for selected patient groups, transfusion might even worsen outcome. The pivotal study published by Hebert and his coworkers in 1999 is a landmark on the path to new standards of patient care [2]. Increasing costs and decreasing RBC availability will augment the pressure on physicians to follow more restrictive transfusion guidelines. This chapter gives an overview of the different elements which should result in a rational and balanced transfusion strategy.

▌ Physiology of Oxygen Transport and Pathophysiology of Anemia

Oxygen Transport

Oxygen supply must match tissue oxygen needs to ensure aerobic cell respiration. Whole body oxygen delivery (DO_2) is the product of blood flow or cardiac output and arterial oxygen content (CaO_2):

$$DO_2 = \text{cardiac output} \times CaO_2$$

Where DO_2 is expressed in ml/min, cardiac output in l/min and CaO_2 in ml/l. CaO_2 is the sum of hemoglobin-bound and dissolved oxygen:

$$CaO_2 = (SaO_2 \times k_1 \times [Hb]) + (k_2 \times PaO_2)$$

where SaO_2 (%) is the arterial oxygen saturation, k_1 represents the oxygen-carrying capacity of hemoglobin which is 1.34 ml/g, [Hb] is the hemoglobin concentration (g/l), k_2 reflects the plasma oxygen dissolution coefficient at body temperature (0.23 ml/l/kPa) and PaO_2 equals the partial pressure of oxygen of arterial blood (kPa). The complete formula describing DO_2 thus reads as follows:

$$DO_2 = CO \times ((SaO_2 \times k_1 \times [Hb]) + (k_2 \times PaO_2))$$

Under physiologic conditions, DO_2 (800 to 1200 ml/min) exceeds oxygen consumption (VO_2) up to 4 times, resulting in an oxygen extraction ratio ($O_2ER = VO_2/DO_2$) of 20 to 30%. Consequently, even a marked isolated decrease in hemoglobin concentration will still result in a sufficient DO_2 to meet tissue oxygen requirements. However, below a critical hemoglobin concentration there will not only be a decrease in DO_2 but also in VO_2. This relationship of VO_2 and DO_2 is referred to as the concept of critical DO_2 (DO_2crit): above DO_2crit, tissue oxygenation is sufficient as represented by a constant VO_2 which is thus 'DO_2-independent'. In contrast, below DO_2crit body oxygen demands are no longer met resulting in a decrease of VO_2. This state is characterized by a 'VO_2/DO_2-dependency' and the development of tissue hypoxia [3].

Physiologic Adaptation to Normovolemic Anemia

In normovolemic anemia, several physiological mechanisms compensate for the decrease in hemoglobin concentration, in order to maintain DO_2 above DO_2crit. The key adaptation mechanisms to anemia are:
▌ an increase in cardiac output,
▌ redistribution of blood flow between organs, and
▌ an increase in O_2ER [4].

Cardiac output increases mainly through two mechanisms: reduced blood viscosity and increased sympathetic stimulation of the heart. The decrease in blood viscosity due to the lower hematocrit leads to an increased venous return and thus to an increased preload. Another consequence of the lower blood viscosity is a decrease in systemic vascular resistance (SVR) and afterload [5]. Increased sympathetic activity leads to an increase in myocardial contractility that contributes significantly to increased cardiac output [6]. An increase in the heart rate in response to increased sympathetic activity is only relevant in unmedicated humans [3, 7]. In contrast, in anesthetized humans, heart rate does not seem to respond to anemia [3, 7, 8]. The increase in cardiac output as a response to normovolemic anemia in anesthetized patients is therefore primarily due to an augmented stroke volume, and an increase in heart rate should be considered as a sign of hypovolemia.

Blood redistribution from non-vital to vital organs such as the heart and brain is mediated by the adrenergic system. This is especially important for the myocardium that has a high basal O_2ER with a relatively small oxygen extraction reserve. In contrast to the brain, which is able to significantly increase O_2ER, DO_2 to the heart is primarily increased by augmenting coronary blood flow. In addition, in response to the elevated blood flow to the microcirculation, the homogeneity of the capillary bed is augmented. This happens both with respect to changes over time (temporal heterogeneity) and to differences between vessels (spatial heterogeneity) as only about one third of capillaries is perfused under normal conditions. The resulting homogeneity leads to an increased O_2ER [4]. Finally, due to increased synthesis of 2,3-diphosphogylcerate (2,3-DPG) in red cells, the oxyhemoglobin dissociation curve shifts to the right thus allowing more hemoglobin-bound oxygen to be released at a given partial pressure of oxygen [5].

Tolerance to Anemia: How Low can You go?

In experimental settings, healthy volunteers have been shown to tolerate hemoglobin levels of 5 g/l under normovolemic conditions [9]. In a case report of an 84-year-old Jehovah's Witness patient, the hemoglobin concentration at which DO_2crit was reached (Hbcrit), was about 4 g/l. A review of the literature on Jehovah's Witness patients identified 134 medical and surgical patients with a hemoglobin concentration ≤8 g/l or a hematocrit ≤24% [10]. Among these 134 patients, 50 deaths were reported of which 23 were attributed exclusively or primarily to anemia. All these patients – with the exception of three patients with cardiac disease who died after cardiac surgery and two patients with missing laboratory data – died with a hemoglobin concentration ≤5 g/l or an equivalent hematocrit. Notably, this value was also found in 27 of the survivors. The effect of progressive anemia on morbidity and mortality in a surgical population has been described in a retrospective cohort study of 300 patients who refused blood transfusions for religious reasons, with a postoperative hemoglobin level of 8 g/l or less [11]. The odds ratio (OR), for mortality and morbidity, was 2.2 for each gram decrement in hemoglobin, but all patients in the group with a postoperative hemoglobin level of 7.1 to 8.0 g/l group survived. In the 6.1 to 7.0 g/l group 8.9% of patients died. Mortality increased steadily, reaching 100% in patients with 1.1 to 2.0 g/l of hemoglobin.

These findings further support the most recent recommendations that define a hemoglobin concentration ≤6 g/l as a transfusion trigger, which is quite close to the Hbcrit that can be presumed from the available literature [12]. Furthermore, in the range of 6 to 10 g/l, individual assessment of each patient's risk for complications of inadequate oxygenation is warranted. A number of clinical risk factors that may decrease a patient's tolerance to anemia and thus increase Hbcrit have been identified [13]. Patients with coronary artery disease may be particularly at risk as an adequate increase of the coronary blood flow in response to a decrease in hemoglobin concentration is not possible and myocardial ischemia may develop. In addition, impaired myocardial contractility may limit the compensatory increase in cardiac output. A retrospective cohort study in 1958 patients who declined blood transfusions due to religious reasons corroborated this hypothesis [14]. It was found that below a preoperative hemoglobin concentration of about 10 to 11 g/l the mortality increased in patients with and without cardiovascular disease, but more in those with cardiovascular disease. Conversely, the analysis of a subgroup of patients with cardiovascular disease in the TRICC trial (Transfusion Requirements in Critical Care) conducted by Hebert, showed no differences in mortality rate between a restrictive and a liberal transfusion strategy in patients with cardiovascular disease [15]. Although the authors were aware of the possible limitations of this subgroup analysis, they suggested a transfusion trigger of 7 g/l to be safe in critically ill patients with cardiovascular disease [15]. Possible exceptions were patients with acute myocardial infarction and unstable angina. Recent reviews on this topic have concluded that transfusion triggers for patients with cardiovascular disease should not differ substantially from patients without cardiovascular disease but may be mildly elevated [16, 17]. Nevertheless, in healthy patients, as in patients with concomitant diseases, RBC transfusion should be guided by clinical signs of inadequate oxygenation [12, 16]. In the case of patients with cardiovascular disease, new ST-segment depression >0.1 mV, new ST-segment elevations >0.2 mV, or new wall motion abnormalities in transesophageal echocardiography (TEE) may represent signs of inadequate oxygenation of the myocardium [16].

▌ Rationale and Efficacy of RBC Transfusions: Why Transfuse?

Rationale of RBC Transfusion

The goal of RBC transfusion should be the increase in VO_2, thereby restoring adequate tissue oxygenation, or to alleviate signs of inadequate tissue oxygenation [18]. Increasing DO_2 without a concomitant increase in VO_2 would indicate the absence of VO_2/DO_2-dependency and thus any increase in DO_2 would be of questionable relevance [18]. Out of eighteen studies examining the effect of RBC transfusions on oxygenation parameters, 14 showed an increase in DO_2 associated with transfusion but in only 5 of them was this coupled to a parallel increase in VO_2 [19]. This lack of increase in VO_2 after RBC transfusion could be explained by the absence of an oxygen debt prior to infusion. Alternatively, dysfunction of stored RBC could be a reason for the lack of increase in VO_2 after RBC transfusion [18]. During storage, RBCs undergo different changes which are summarized under the term 'storage lesions' [20]. These include a decrease in 2,3-DPG, ATP depletion, and the release of pro-inflammatory substances. This results in a left shift of the oxyhemoglobin dissociation curve (i.e., increased oxygen affinity), impaired RBC deformability and inflammatory reactions in the transfusion recipient [20, 21]. The decrease in 2,3-DPG levels and RBC deformability, in particular, would imply decreased efficacy of 'old' RBC and thus no increase in VO_2 after transfusion. In addition, changes in nitric oxide (NO) biology cause a gradual depletion of NO in stored RBCs. NO is essential for oxygen exchange and the transfused RBCs may act as "NO-sinks" provoking vasoconstriction, platelet aggregation, and ineffective DO_2 [22].

How can we identify the patients who will increase VO_2 after RBC transfusion? Casutt and co-workers examined 67 cardiovascular surgery patients who were transfused with a total of 170 RBC transfusions [23]. Hemodynamic and oxygen consumption parameters were measured approximately 5 hours before and after transfusion. Pretransfusion hemoglobin, preoperative ejection fraction and age were found to be unrelated to individual responses in cardiac index (CI), DO_2 and VO_2 after RBC transfusion. In contrast, DO_2 and VO_2-related variables correlated well with and allowed better prediction of individual responses to RBC transfusions. In particular, a low VO_2 index correlated very well to an increase in VO_2 after transfusion. Similarly, a study evaluating whole-body O_2ER as a parameter for guiding transfusions [24] included 70 patients undergoing coronary artery bypass graft (CABG) surgery with a postoperative hematocrit $\leq 25\%$. O_2ER was monitored without influencing transfusion decisions. A retrospective analysis showed that if an $O_2ER \geq 45\%$ had been used as a transfusion trigger, it would have influenced transfusion therapy. Only 7 out of 41 transfused patients reached this transfusion trigger, as did 3 out of 35 patients who were not transfused. Thus, it was concluded that whole-body O_2ER may be a helpful parameter in a transfusion algorithm [24].

Efficacy of RBC Transfusion

It seems very hard to prove whether transfusion of RBC in patients with hemoglobin values above the critical level has any benefit at all. Moreover, more and more studies suggest that blood transfusion might do more harm than good in selected patient groups with hemoglobin values of more than 7 g/dl. The information emerging from these data is often hard to interpret because of methodological differences and biases. For example, in a retrospective analysis of 1222 consecutive patients undergoing hepatectomy, perioperative blood transfusion was an independent risk factor for hospital morbidity and mortality in a multivariate risk analysis [25]. But, the advances in surgical technique, leading to an important reduction in blood loss and hence transfusion requirements, are likely to be the underlying cause for both the improved survival and the reduction in RBC transfusion. Various large observational studies have examined the effect of RBC transfusion on mortality and morbidity in intensive care settings with often contradictory results. The CRIT study (Anemia and blood transfusion in the critically ill – Current clinical practice in the United States) enrolled 4892 patients from August 2000 to April 2001 [26]; 44.1% of the patients were transfused with one or more RBC unit. The mean pre-transfusion hemoglobin was 8.6 ± 1.7 g/dl. The number of RBC units transfused was an independent risk factor for mortality and hospital length of stay (LOS). In addition, patients who were transfused experienced more complications. The ABC study (Anemia and blood transfusion in the critically ill), was performed in European intensive care units (ICUs) [27]. Similar to the CRIT study, 37.0% of the 3534 patients included (enrolment from November 15 to November 29, 1999) were transfused with mean pre-transfusion hemoglobin of 8.4 ± 1.7 g/dl. Mortality was higher for transfused patients compared to non-transfused patients with similar organ dysfunction as assessed by the Sequential Organ Failure Assessment (SOFA) score. After matching patients by propensity scores (i.e. probability) for being transfused (and thus controlling amongst other variables for SOFA and APACHE II score), 28-day mortality was significantly higher in patients with transfusions (22.7% vs. 17.1%, p = 0.02). The most recently conducted study, the SOAP study, enrolled 3147 patients between May 1 and May 15, 2002 [28]; 33% received RBC transfusion. Patients receiving transfusions were older and generally sicker, and higher transfusion rates were associated with higher mortality. However, after propensity-matching mortality rates were the same in transfused and non-transfused patients with a tendency towards better survival in transfused patients.

To date, only one randomized controlled trial has sufficient power to evaluate the effect of transfusions on mortality and morbidity in the ICU. From 1994 to 1997, Hébert et al. enrolled 838 patients who were admitted to the ICU with an initial hemoglobin concentration of ≤9 g/dl [2]. The patients were randomized to either a restrictive transfusion strategy with a transfusion trigger of 7 g/dl (target hemoglobin 7 to 9 g/dl) or a liberal transfusion strategy with a transfusion trigger of 10 g/dl (target hemoglobin 10 to 12 g/dl). Thirty-day mortality was slightly lower in the restrictive transfusion group (18.7 vs. 23.3%), although statistical significance was not reached (p = 0.11). Even for patients with cardiovascular disease there seemed to be no benefit of transfusion if hemoglobin levels were 7 g/dl or more. However, subgroup analyses of patients less than 55 years of age or patients who where less acutely ill, as defined by an APACHE II score, showed significantly lower 30-day mortality in the restrictive transfusion group. As mentioned before, the authors state that patients with active coronary syndromes might be an exception, and that higher hemoglobin based transfusion triggers might be justified in this subgroup.

Initially, this view seemed to be confirmed by a report by Wu et al. [29] of a retrospective study on 78974 patients of more than 65 years with acute coronary infarction. They categorized the patients according to hematocrit on admission and determined whether there was an association between the transfusion of RBCs and

30-day mortality. They found a beneficial effect of allogeneic blood transfusion if the hematocrit on admission was lower than 30%. On the contrary, if initial hematocrit was higher than 36%, transfusion was associated with increased mortality. This study, however, has an important bias in that patient characteristics and treatment varied significantly between patients with a low and patients with a high admission hematocrit [16]. A very recent report on the relationship of blood transfusion and outcome in patients with acute coronary syndromes (ACS), however, reaches the opposite conclusion. Rao and co-workers pooled the study populations of three large international trials (GUSTO IIb, PURSUIT, and PARAGON b) on patients presenting with ACS and assessed the association of RBC transfusion and outcome [22]. The data of 24 112 patients were examined on the propensity to bleed or receive transfusion and on the association between transfusion and 30-day death. After adjustment for baseline characteristics, blood transfusion was associated with a hazard ratio for death of 3.54 and after adjustment for baseline characteristics, bleeding, transfusion propensity, and nadir hematocrit blood transfusion was still independently associated with a hazard ratio for death of 3.94. There was no significant association between transfusion and 30-day mortality in patients with a nadir hematocrit of 25% or less, but at a nadir hematocrit above 25% RBC transfusion was linked to a higher 30-day mortality. Compared to the trial conducted by Wu, who used the hematocrit value on admission only, Rao's team based their comparison on the nadir hematocrits measured during hospitalization. Further, patients under 65 years of age and patients undergoing heart surgery were excluded in the study by Wu [29], whereas all patients regardless of age, bleeding events, or procedures were included by Rao et al. They concluded that, in the setting of ACS, blood transfusion was associated with an increased risk of 30-day mortality for patients with a hematocrit above 25%, even after adjustment for patient characteristics, baseline and nadir hematocrit, bleeding, and in-hospital procedures.

How should we interpret the results of these randomized controlled and observational trials? The validity of the observational studies is not clear because sicker patients are more likely to be transfused [30]. Although retrospective propensity analysis tries to control for potentially confounding factors, this adjustment can only be done for factors recorded. It is thus possible that unmeasured confounders bias the results. Consequently, we can only draw conclusions about statistical associations between factors and not about causality.

But what explains the overtly contradicting results between some of these trials? The GUSTO IIb, PURSUIT, and PARAGON b trials were all conducted between July 1994 and January 1996. And it was not until 1998 that the Blood Product Advising Committee of the US Food and Drug Administration voted for universal leukoreduction [31]. At the time of inclusion of the patients for the ABC study, universal leukoreduction had not been implemented in Germany, Holland, Norway, or Finland, accounting for about one third of the 3534 patients, while other participating countries were just completing it [32]. By the time the SOAP-study ran, leukoreduction was much more common. Universal leukoreduction is the subject of substantial debate. One unit of blood (approximately 500 ml) contains about 2 billion white blood cells (WBC). After processing, 90% of these are found in the RBC aliquot, primarily as granulocytes [31]. Leukoreduction aims to reduce this amount of WBC by 99.995%, leaving 5000 residual leukocytes. Leukocytes present in RBCs are held responsible for transfusion-associated immunomodulation (TRIM), febrile transfusion reactions, and transmission of intracellular pathogens such as cytomegalovirus (CMV), human T-cell lymphotropic virus (HTLV)-I and HTLV-II, Epstein-Barr virus (EBV), Herpes viruses, parasites, and prions [31]. A before-and-after cohort study in Canada found a reduction in mortality, post-transfusion fevers and antibiotic use after implementation of a universal leukoreduction program [33]. A recent prospective cohort-controlled study observed a decrease in hospital LOS in open-heart surgery with leukoreduced blood transfusions [34]. In contrast, a before-and-after study in the UK observed no impact on hospital LOS and post-operative infection in orthopedic and cardiac surgery [35].

Finally, the age of RBC units may be another important factor influencing the efficacy of RBC transfusion as outlined above. Although highly controversial, this parameter might explain some of the observed differences between the trials [20].

▌ Transfusion-related risks. Why not Transfuse?

Transfusion-related risks can be divided into transfusion-transmissible infections, immunologic risks, and mistransfusion.

Infectious Risks

RBC transfusions in Western countries have probably never been safer than today with respect to transfusion-transmissible viruses such as human immunodeficiency virus (HIV), hepatitis B virus (HBV) and hepatitis C virus (HCV) [36]. The estimated risks of infection have dramatically decreased over recent years because increased test sensitivity has reduced infectious window periods [37]. Estimates of current risk are shown in Table 1.

In contrast to Western countries, viral and parasitic transfusion-transmissible infections are a major problem in countries with a low human development index (HDI, an index based on life expectancy, literacy, enrolment into scholarly education, and per capita income) (Table 1). A high seroprevalence of these diseases in the general population of these countries, poorly organized blood donation systems, and poor sensitivity of pathogen testing are important factors [36]. The future transfusion practice in low HDI countries will strongly depend on international investment to guarantee an appropriate transfusion safety [38].

Compared to viral transfusion-transmissible infections, there is currently much more concern about transfusion-transmitted bacterial infections and post-transfusion sepsis [39] in high HDI (Western) countries. Because of the high platelet storage temperature of 20–24°C, which favors bacterial growth, contamination of platelets is more common than contamination of RBC units. Best risk estimates of transfusion-transmitted bacterial infections from a Canadian study gave values in the range of about 1:2000 to 1:8000 (13 to 44 per 100000) for platelet pools and 1:28000 to 1:143000 (0.7 to 3.6 per 100000) for transfused RBC units [40]. Notably, when comparing the incidence of transfusion-transmitted bacterial infections from different studies, the different diagnostic criteria of transfusion-transmitted bacterial infections should be considered [40].

Recently, the first possible cases of transfusion-transmitted variant Creutzfeld-Jakob disease (vCJD) have been reported [41, 42]. The probability that the first case of vCJD was not due to transfusion-transmitted vCJD ranged between 1:15000 to 1:30000. The hypothesized incubation period of transfusion-transmitted vCJD was

Table 1. Transfusion-associated risks (modified from [35])

Type of Risk Infections	Estimate of current risk (infection rate per unit)	
	High HDI countries	Low HDI countries
INFECTION		
Viruses		
▌Human immunodeficiency virus (HIV)	1:1468000–1:4700000	1:50–1:2578
▌Hepatitis B virus (HBV)	1:31000–1:205000	1:74–1:1000
▌Hepatitis C virus (HCV)	1:1935000–1:3100000	1:2578
Bacteria (contamination)	1:2000–1:8000 (platelet pools)/ 1:28000–1:143000 (red cells)	?
Parasites		
▌Malaria	1:4000000	up to 1:3
Prions		
▌Variant Creutzfeld-Jacob disease	first two possible transmissions described	?
IMMUNOLOGIC REACTIONS		
Hemolytic Transfusion Reactions		
▌Acute Hemolytic	1:13000	?
▌Delayed Hemolytic	1:9000	?
▌Alloimmunization	1:1600	?
▌Autoimmunization	? (recently identified as risk)	?
▌Immunosuppression	1:1	?
▌Transfusion-related acute lung injury	1:70000	?
▌Mistransfusion	1:14000–1:18000	?

6.5 years [41]. Britain's second transfusion-transmitted case of vCJD may have been caused by a blood transfusion dating back to 1999 [42]. This patient died of causes unrelated to vCJD. Identical to the first case, this patient was the recipient of non-leukodepleted RBCs from a donor who developed symptoms of vCJD after donation. A post-mortem examination revealed the presence of prion proteins in the patient's spleen and cervical lymph node, but not in gut-associated lymphoid tissue and tonsils which suggests an intravenous rather than an oral route of transmission [42]. An incubation period of 6.5 years in asymptomatic vCJD patients could represent a significant source of iatrogenic infection by blood donation or by contamination of surgical instruments [42]. This led the UK government to take precautionary measures, deferring blood from an important part of the donor pool (see further). Interestingly, it has been shown that leukoreduction is efficacious in reducing but fails to eliminate white-cell-associated transmission of spongiform encephalopathies [43]. In addition, some infectivity of transmissible spongiform encephalopathies is assumed to be plasma-associated [43]. Therefore, the policy of leukoreduction aimed at reducing transmissible spongiform encephalopathy infectivity may require re-evaluation.

Immunologic Risks

In contrast to low HDI countries that are very concerned with transfusion-transmissible infections, immunologic transfusion reactions are generally more frequently encountered in high HDI countries [36] (Table 1).

As mentioned, RBC transfusions seem to have an immunomodulatory effect, the causes of which remain unclear. Although several studies have suggested that WBCs cause immunomodulation, the blood components that may mediate this effect are still not defined. It goes beyond the scope of this review to discuss all other immunological risks in detail, the reader is therefore referred to a very comprehensive review on risks associated with RBC transfusions in Canada [40]. However, transfusion related acute lung injury (TRALI) is a controversial issue that should be mentioned. Estimates of the incidence vary from 0.2 per 100 000 [44] to 1 per 5 000 RBC units transfused [45]. These discrepancies are thought to be caused by underreporting [40, 46] due to a lack of awareness or misdiagnosis. The symptoms and signs of TRALI do resemble other conditions associated with transfusion and volume overload such as adult respiratory distress syndrome (ARDS) or congestive heart failure (CHF). Therefore, standardized criteria for the definition and diagnosis of TRALI are needed to calculate the incidence and allow for comparison between hospitals and transfusion policies [46].

Mistransfusion

Mistransfusion is associated with significant morbidity and mortality [47] and is unfortunately estimated to occur in one of 14 000–18 000 transfusions. It represents the transfusion hazard with the highest incidence in high HDI countries [37, 40, 47].

■ Societal Cost and Donor Selection

The societal cost for one unit of allogeneic RBCs transfused to in-patients cared for in emergency departments, ICUs, general medicine wards, and operating rooms in Canada was calculated to be US\$ 264.81 [48]. The calculation comprised the costs for collection of blood (including the donor's cost of time) production, distribution, delivery, and administration of blood products, and the costs for transfusion reaction management. Compared to 1995, when the cost of a unit of RBC was US\$ 157.17, this is a nearly two-fold increase. A large proportion of this increase is due to the implementation of nucleic acid testing (NAT) for HCV and HIV I/II, universal leukoreduction, other quality-assurance programs, and associated labor- and non-labor related costs. A cost simulation exercise showed that the cost might increase to US\$ 317.77 assuming that the cost of hemovigilance, new quality tests, etc. would increase the mean cost by 20%. New tests for vCJD, West Nile Virus, microbial infections, and inactivation of pathogens will further increase production related costs.

Finally, these newly discovered transfusion transmissible pathogens are not only responsible for a probable increase in cost, but have already led to a dramatic decrease in the number of potential donors. In 1997, the concern about potential transmission of vCJD led to three blood withdrawals of products linked to vCJD donors. In 1998, the UK decided to import all their plasma requirements and leukoreduce their blood, since the prion seemed to be primarily located in WBCs. Soon after, Canada and the US decided to defer all blood products from individuals who had lived in the UK for 6 months between 1980 and 1996. France introduced a deferral policy for all donors who had lived in the UK for one year and implemented universal leukoreduction. In April 2004, the UK decided to defer all donations from individuals who have been transfused since 1980 [49]. The ban on these blood products reduced the number of donors in the UK by 3.3% [50]. And finally, when confirming the second case of transfusion transmission of vCJD in July 2004, the UK Committee on the Microbiological Safety of Blood and Tissue advised to extend the ban to donors who are unsure whether they have had a blood transfusion and to apheresis donors who have previously had a blood transfusion. The impact of the extended ban, which will become effective from April 2005, remains to be seen.

∎ Conclusion

The transfusion of RBCs has been used for decades to improve the oxygen transport capacity and oxygen consumption related parameters of anemic patients. New insights into the pathophysiology of allogeneic blood transfusions question the capacity of stored RBC to improve these factors in most patients. Although class A evidence is lacking, most survey's have found no benefit whatsoever of RBC transfusions in patients with hemoglobin levels above 7 g/dl and, for selected patient groups, it could even compromise outcome. It seems that the WBCs present in units of packed RBCs are, at least partially, responsible for some of the complications associated with transfusion. Generalized application of leukoreduction might shift the balance in favor of transfusion, but it is too early to draw any definitive conclusions on this subject. Future trials will provide some of the answers and doubtless raise new questions. Meanwhile, increasing costs and shrinking pools of donors are a supplemental driving force to rationalize transfusion practice.

References

1. Adams RC, Lundy JS (1942) Anesthesia in cases of poor surgical risk. Some suggestions for decreasing the risk. Surg Gyn Obst 74:1011–1019
2. Hebert PC, Wells G, Blajchman MA, et al (1999) A multicenter, randomized, controlled clinical trial of transfusion requirements in critical care. N Engl J Med 340:409–417
3. Jamnicki M, Kocian R, van der Linden P, Zaugg M, Spahn DR (2003) Acute normovolemic hemodilution: physiology, limitations, and clinical use. J Cardiothorac Vasc Anesth 17:747–754
4. Morisaki H, Sibbald WJ (2004) Tissue oxygen delivery and the microcirculation. Crit Care Clin 20:213–223
5. Hebert PC, van der Linden P, Biro G, Hu LQ (2004) Physiologic aspects of anemia. Crit Care Clin 20:187–212
6. Habler O, Kleen M, Podtschaske A, et al (1996) The effect of acute normovolemic hemodilution (ANH) on myocardial contractility in anesthetized dogs. Anesth Analg 83:451–458
7. Weiskopf RB, Feiner J, Hopf H, et al (2003) Heart rate increases linearly in response to acute isovolemic anemia. Transfusion 43:235–240
8. Spahn DR, Leone BJ, Reves JG, Pasch T (1994) Cardiovascular and coronary physiology of acute isovolemic hemodilution: a review of nonoxygen-carrying and oxygen-carrying solutions. Anesth Analg 78:1000–1021
9. Weiskopf RB, Viele MK, Feiner J, et al (1998) Human cardiovascular and metabolic response to acute, severe isovolemic anemia. JAMA 279:217–221

10. Viele MK, Weiskopf RB (1994) What can we learn about the need for transfusion from patients who refuse blood? The experience with Jehovah's Witnesses. Transfusion 34:396–401
11. Carson JL, Noveck H, Berlin JA, Gould SA (2002) Mortality and morbidity in patients with very low postoperative hemoglobin levels who decline blood transfusion. Transfusion 42:812–818
12. American Society of Anesthesiologists Task Force on Blood Component Therapy (1996) Practice Guidelines for blood component therapy. Anesthesiology 84:732–747
13. McLellan SA, McClelland DB, Walsh TS (2003) Anaemia and red blood cell transfusion in the critically ill patient. Blood Rev 17:195–208
14. Carson JL, Duff A, Poses RM, et al (1996) Effect of anaemia and cardiovascular disease on surgical mortality and morbidity. Lancet 348:1055–1060
15. Hebert PC, Yetisir E, Martin C, et al (2001) Is a low transfusion threshold safe in critically ill patients with cardiovascular diseases? Crit Care Med 29:227–234
16. Spahn DR, Dettori N, Kocian R, Chassot PG (2004) Transfusion in the cardiac patient. Crit Care Clin 20:269–279
17. Fakhry SM, Fata P (2004) How low is too low? Cardiac risks with anemia. Crit Care 8 (Suppl 2): S11–14
18. Spahn DR (1999) Benefits of red blood cell transfusion: Where is the evidence? TATM 1:6–10
19. Hebert PC, McDonald BJ, Tinmouth A (2004) Clinical consequences of anemia and red cell transfusion in the critically ill. Crit Care Clin 20:225–235
20. Offner PJ (2004) Age of blood: does it make a difference? Crit Care 8 (Suppl 2):S24–26
21. Napolitano LM, Corwin HL (2004) Efficacy of red blood cell transfusion in the critically ill. Crit Care Clin 20:255–268
22. Rao SV, Jollis JG, Harrington RA, et al (2004) Relationship of blood transfusion and clinical outcomes in patients with acute coronary syndromes. JAMA 292:1555–1162
23. Casutt M, Seifert B, Pasch T, Schmid ER, Turina MI, Spahn DR (1999) Factors influencing the individual effects of blood transfusion on oxygen delivery and oxygen consumption. Crit Care Med 27:2194–2200
24. Sehgal LR, Zebala LP, Takagi I, Curran RD, Votapka TV, Caprini JA (2001) Evaluation of oxygen extraction ratio as a physiologic transfusion trigger in coronary artery bypass graft surgery patients. Transfusion 41:591–595
25. Poon RT, Fan ST, Lo CM, et al (2004) Improving perioperative outcome expands the role of hepatectomy in management of benign and malignant hepatobiliary diseases. Ann Surg 240:698–710
26. Corwin HL, Gettinger A, Pearl RG, et al (2004) The CRIT Study: Anemia and blood transfusion in the critically ill-Current clinical practice in the United States. Crit Care Med 32:39–52
27. Vincent JL, Baron JF, Reinhart K, et al (2002) Anemia and blood transfusion in critically ill patients. JAMA 288:1499–1507
28. Vincent J-L, Sakr Y, Le Gall J-R, et al (2003) Is red blood cell transfusion associated with worse outcome? Results of the SOAP Study. Chest 124:125S (abst)
29. Wu WC, Rathore SS, Wang Y, Radford MJ, Krumholz HM (2001) Blood transfusion in elderly patients with acute myocardial infarction. N Engl J Med 345:1230–1236
30. Spahn DR, Marcucci C (2004) Blood management in intensive care medicine: CRIT and ABC – what can we learn? Crit Care 8:89–90
31. Shapiro MJ (2004) To filter blood or universal leukoreduction: what is the answer? Crit Care 8 (Suppl 2):S27–30
32. Wortham ST, Ortolano GA, Wenz B (2003) A brief history of blood filtration: clot screens, microaggregate removal, and leukocyte reduction. Transfus Med Rev 17:216–222
33. Hebert PC, Fergusson D, Blajchman MA, et al (2003) Clinical outcomes following institution of the Canadian universal leukoreduction program for red blood cell transfusions. JAMA 289:1941–1949
34. Fung MK, Rao N, Rice J, Ridenour M, Mook W, Triulzi DJ (2004) Leukoreduction in the setting of open heart surgery: a prospective cohort-controlled study. Transfusion 44:30–35
35. Llewelyn CA, Taylor RS, Todd AA, Stevens W, Murphy MF, Williamson LM (2004) The effect of universal leukoreduction on postoperative infections and length of hospital stay in elective orthopedic and cardiac surgery. Transfusion 44:489–500

36. Marcucci C, Madjdpour C, Spahn DR (2004) Allogeneic blood transfusions: benefit, risks and clinical indications in countries with a low or high human development index. Br Med Bull 70:15–28
37. Goodnough LT (2003) Risks of blood transfusion. Crit Care Med 31:S678–686
38. Allain JP, Owusu-Ofori S, Bates I (2004) Blood transfusion in sub-saharan Africa. TATM 6:16–23
39. Wagner SJ (2004) Transfusion-transmitted bacterial infection: risks, sources and interventions. Vox Sang 86:157–163
40. Kleinman S, Chan P, Robillard P (2003) Risks associated with transfusion of cellular blood components in Canada. Transfus Med Rev 17:120–162
41. Llewelyn CA, Hewitt PE, Knight RS, et al (2004) Possible transmission of variant Creutzfeldt-Jakob disease by blood transfusion. Lancet 363:417–421
42. Peden AH, Head MW, Ritchie DL, Bell JE, Ironside JW (2004) Preclinical vCJD after blood transfusion in a PRNP codon 129 heterozygous patient. Lancet 364:527–529
43. Gregori L, McCombie N, Palmer D, et al (2004) Effectiveness of leukoreduction for removal of infectivity of transmissible spongiform encephalopathies from blood. Lancet 364:529–531
44. Serious Hazards of Transfusion Annual Report 2003. The Serious Hazards of Transfusion Steering Group, available at http://www.shotuk.org/SHOT%20Report%202003.pdf
45. Goodnough LT, Brecher ME, Kanter MH, AuBuchon JP (1999) Transfusion medicine. First of two parts–blood transfusion. N Engl J Med 340:438–447
46. Webert KE, Blajchman MA (2003) Transfusion-related acute lung injury. Transfus Med Rev 17:252–262
47. Williamson LM, Lowe S, Love EM, et al (1999) Serious hazards of transfusion (SHOT) initiative: analysis of the first two annual reports. BMJ 319:16–19
48. Amin M, Fergusson D, Wilson K, et al (2004) The societal unit cost of allogeneic red blood cells and red blood cell transfusion in Canada. Transfusion 44:1479–1486
49. Wilson K, Ricketts MN (2004) The succes of precaution? Managing the risk of transfusion transmission or variant Creutzfeld-Jacob disease. Transfusion 44:1475–1478
50. Annual report of the Chief Medical Officer 2003, available at http://www.publications.doh.gov.uk/cmo/annualreport2003/index.htm

The Microvasculature

The Microcirculation during Wound Healing after Oral and Maxillofacial Surgical Procedures

J. A. H. Lindeboom, K. R. Mathura, and C. Ince

▌ Introduction

Good wound healing following surgery and prevention of pressure sores form important clinical targets in intensive care medicine. A functioning microcirculation providing adequate tissue oxygenation is an essential pre-requisite for such wound healing [1]. Monitoring the progress of wound healing and assessing its response to therapy however remains a challenge today mainly due to the unavailability of suitably sensitive techniques to observe and monitor the cellular and microcirculatory determinants of wound healing.

Recently a new *in vivo* microscopic technique, called orthogonal polarization spectral (OPS) imaging, has been introduced to the clinical observation of the microcirculation of internal organs and has allowed first time observations of a large number of microcirculatory properties in human health and disease [2]. It has had a special impact in critical medicine whereby oral microcirculation, mainly sublingual, has provided sensitive information about the severity of sepsis, response to therapy and recently also about outcome [3–5]. Besides OPS imaging, sublingual [6] and more recently buccal tonometry have been used in critical care medicine to provide sensitive information about the (dys-)function of the microcirculation.

Oral and maxillofacial wounds provide a unique environment for the study of human internal wounds because they are an easily accessible compartment allowing the progress of natural wound healing to be monitored in a sterile and natural environment. Such wounds form a good example of internal surgical wounds being distinguished from surface wounds where dermis formation dominates. Thus study of such predominantly epithelial wounds allows identification of the determinants of internal wound healing and their response to therapy. In this chapter, we review the properties and determinants of wound healing in oral and maxillofacial wounds and introduce the use of OPS imaging to the study of the microcirculation of such wounds.

▌ Methods for Assessment of Oral and Maxillofacial Wound Microcirculation

The microcirculation in oral and maxillofacial surgery has always been the essential factor in wound healing after surgical procedures. The abundance of microcirculation in the oral mucosa has made it possible to challenge the boundaries of vascular regeneration potential, although non-healing wounds and flap necrosis can easily occur in the vascularly compromised surgical patients. In addition, conditions diminishing this regeneration potential, such as radiotherapy, may have detrimental effects on wound healing and thereby on surgical outcome. Infections form a further important factor in poor surgical wound healing [1].

Healthy gingiva is characterized by a subepithelial vascular plexus consisting of a capillary network with loops arching toward the epithelium. As gingival surgery compromises vascular integrity, adequate revascularization is essential for wound healing. A variety of methods have been used in the past for measuring gingival and oral mucosal blood flow, but most are invasive, indirect or are not applicable for use in humans. Perfusion of carbon black (Pelican ink), for example, has been used in several experimental animal studies as a method to identify small vessels. Kon et al. [7] observed the wound healing process and behavior of the blood vessels after periodontal curettage and injected carbon black into the carotid arteries of young adult mongrel dogs, after which the perfusion technique was carried out at different time intervals shortly before the animals were sacrificed. Of course such a technique gives excellent images of the microcirculation, but for obvious reasons is not applicable in human subjects. A popular technique to assess oral blood flow has been laser Doppler flowmetry as it evaluates changes in blood flow through non-invasive measurement methods [8]. Doppler sonography is widely used to assess blood flow in most large arteries and several of the smaller arteries in the body. It provides a non-invasive way to assess blood flow in an artery in real time. The presence or absence of flow can be fairly easily confirmed with a Doppler flow meter, and this technique has been extensively used in microvascular research for the past decade. Its non-invasiveness and ease of handling makes it a favorable method for assessment of tissue perfusion on a routine clinical basis. Recordings of flux from adjacent measuring positions, however, often show considerable variations, even with minimal alterations in probe position [8]. This influences reproducibility making single measurements not acceptable and requiring mean values for a set of data in individuals or populations. Under such conditions, reproducible measurements can be made, provided that a sufficient number of repeated measurements are carried out [9]. Many studies have used few or inhomogeneous numbers of replicated measurements in the samples presented, which may have affected the validity of the results. Flow data acquired with laser Doppler cannot be attributed to specific microvessels and provides no information on microvascular morphology. Furthermore functional capillary density in terms of density of perfused microvessels cannot be obtained by laser Doppler measurements.

Information concerning the human microcirculation can also be obtained by use of intravital microscopy for the diagnosis and treatment of peripheral vascular disease, diabetes, hypertension, and other vascular diseases. Capillary microscopy (capillaroscopy) has been the only technique available for study of the human circulation at the microscopic level in vivo. The capillary microscopy setup consists of an intravital microscope, which restricts its use in humans to the skin and other easy accessible sites like the lip and the bulbar conjunctiva [10]. For oral applications, intravital microscopy has not been very practical due to the thick gingival keratinized tissue and problems of accessibility especially in the posterior parts of the oral cavity [11]. Also, the need for invasive procedures to provide for transillumination has limited its practical use in vivo.

OPS imaging, originally described by Slaaf et al. [12], and applied in a hand type of microscope [13] has allowed microcirculatory abnormalities to be observed in a large number of clinical disorders in a simple and non-invasive way. Measurements made using OPS imaging provide information on the kinetics and architecture of the microcirculation. OPS imaging uses green (550 nm) polarized light which is guided through a set of lenses. The light is absorbed by the hemoglobin in the erythrocytes, which appear as dark moving structures in the image. The light reflected from the surface of the tissue retains its polarization and is filtered by an orthogonally placed polarizer in front of the video camera. The light that has scattered inside the tissue has lost its polarization and passes the orthogonal polarizer thus allowing observation of the flowing red blood cells (RBCs) of the underlying microcirculation by placement of a video camera in the light pathway. The image quality is remarkably clear and the microcirculation can be observed in great detail. The objective of the device is covered by a sterile cap allowing observations under various clinical settings and on internal organ surfaces not accessible to intravital microscopy settings. To validate the OPS technique for clinical studies, a study was performed comparing OPS imaging with conventional capillary microscopy [10]. OPS provided similar values for RBC velocity and capillary diameter as the images obtained with capillaroscopy. However, with OPS imaging, better image quality was obtained. We then introduced OPS imaging to neurosurgery and observed abnormal brain morphology in brain tumors [14] and abnormal kinetics in brain cortex microcirculation during subarachnoid hemorrhage [15]. Sublingual use of OPS imaging has been used in the identification of microcirculatory abnormalities in sepsis [3] and microcirculatory recruitment maneuvers during the treatment of sepsis [16]. Here we discuss the application of OPS to the study of the microcirculation during oral and maxillofacial procedures.

▌ Normal Gingival and Oral Mucosal Microcirculation

The blood supply of the gingiva is derived chiefly from branches of arteries that run along the outer surface of the alveolar bone. These vessels anastomose with branches of arteries from the periodontal ligament as well as arteries that emerge from the crest of the alveolar bone [18]. Capillary loops in the gingiva consist of an ascending arterial limb and a descending venular limb. In the oral mucosa, larger vessels in the submucosa divide into smaller branches that enter the lamina propia. These branches form one or more layers of vessels at the base of the lamina propia forming the submucosal vascular plexus. The vascular network consists primarily of capillary loops whose characteristic shape resembles a hairpin or horseshoe [18].

Using OPS imaging we were able to visualize the gingival, buccal/oral mucosa and sublingual microcirculation. Figure 1 shows a characteristic image of the capillary loops seen in the gingiva, as well as the characteristic image of the sublingual microcirculation. Blocking nerve conduction is the basic object of all local anesthetics, and the principle of action is the same for all types of anesthetic solutions. Local anesthetic solutions prevent the normal passage of ions through the nerve membrane, without which there can be no conduction of impulses. Infiltration anesthesia in the buccal fold involves injection into a high vascular region, which causes rapid transport of the injected solution away from the site of deposition. Conditions are different in regional block anesthesia (e.g., mandibular anesthesia). Owing to the large diameter of the nerve, an effective concentration takes more time to build up here. The region where the solution is deposited in a mandibular

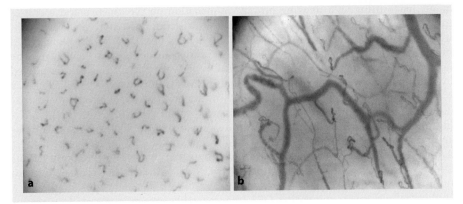

Fig. 1. An OPS image of the **a** gingival and **b** sublingual microcirculation

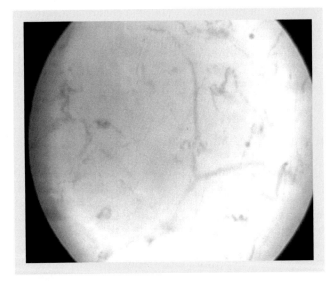

Fig. 2. The gingival microcirculation after injection of local anesthesia

block injection is less vascular than the buccal fold, although there are several large vessels passing through that area. To achieve anesthesia and hemostasis routinely, a local anesthetic with a vasoconstrictor is administered before an oral and maxillo-facial surgical procedure. Injection of an epinephrine containing local anesthetic results in a marked and significant drop I, gingival capillary density and capillary flux as is shown in the OPS image (Fig. 2). This underscores the effects of vasoconstrictor agents on the microcirculation.

▌ The Microcirculation in Oral and Maxillofacial Surgical Flaps

Adequate microvascular regeneration is fundamental for adequate wound healing, remodeling of bone, microvascular ingrowth in grafts and tissue injury repair. Several types of wounds in oral surgical procedures can be distinguished ranging from mucosal defects healing by secondary intention to several vascularized based flaps. In oral and maxillofacial procedures surgical access is mainly obtained by raising a full or partial thickness mucosal flap. This destroys a large number of vessels but the flap remains viable as a result of the microcirculation at the base of the flap. In implant dentistry, a buccal full thickness flap is frequently used for osseous access. By elevating the flap, the mucosa is cut from the periosteal and palatal or lingual microcirculation, leaving the flap to rely on the buccal mucosal capillary perfusion. Due to atraumatic surgical handling of the flap in the majority of cases the abundance of microcirculation leads to uneventful mucosal healing. However, prior surgical procedures, excessive scarring as in the patient with cleft lip and palate, and radiotherapy can jeopardize the viability of the flap leading to compromised wound healing. Soft tissue handling has become a keyword in osseointegrated implant rehabilitation and different soft tissue management techniques are used to increase esthetic outcome of implant surgery. However, there is a scarcity of information on the vascular dynamics of gingival circulation in health and disease. As soft-tissue healing has become a key issue in functionally and esthetically oriented implant dentistry, proper peri-implant tissue management must be determined, to maintain and improve gingival microvascular architecture.

Since subperiosteal soft tissue flap elevation leads to impairment of alveolar blood supply, survival of a soft tissue flap and (neo)vascularization of the underlying bone or graft depend on the integrity and adequacy of blood supply. Monitoring of the microvascular development therefore could form an important tool in assessing this process. To this end we applied the OPS technique to evaluate healing in patients undergoing reconstructive implant reconstruction in healthy human subjects. The changes in microvascularization were visualized using OPS imaging before surgery and at different time-frames after surgery until complete healing [19]. The changes in microvascular architecture and capillary flux could be clearly observed using OPS imaging and consisted of a decrease in capillary density and increase in capillary diameter immediately after surgery to an almost complete normalization of the microcirculation to preoperative levels within 3 weeks as seen in Figure 3. OPS provided images of sufficient quality to monitor describe and assess the microvascular changes in gingival flaps before, during, and after surgery.

Distraction osteogenesis is an accepted treatment for the correction of bone deficiencies. Basic principles of distraction osteogenesis include a low power osteotomy, maximum preservation of blood supply, an adequate duration of the latency period to allow optimum development of the fracture callus, a precise rate and rhythm of distraction, and a consolidation period for calcification of the newly regenerated bone before unrestrained functional loading. The key to ossification is the vascular change into the callus because osteogenesis follows after angiogenesis. We observed this process using the OPS imaging. At day 1 postoperatively until the end of consolidation, microvascular regeneration was assessed by monitoring changes in capillary density and RBC flux. We observed an increase in vascular response mainly in the early stages of active distraction [20].

Success rates of free tissue transfer in head and neck reconstruction have improved dramatically and most centers report flap survival rates between 90–95%.

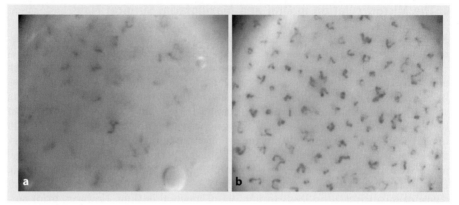

Fig. 3. Change of microcirculation in wound healing of gingival flap on **a** day 3 and **b** 3 weeks after surgery

Partial necrosis of pedicled flaps, however, remains a significant problem in reconstructive surgery. Flap failure is the result of deleterious effects of prolonged ischemia and inadequate blood perfusion, which leads to detrimental changes in vascularization and subsequent flap necrosis. Interoperative and postoperative evaluation of flap viability has primarily been dependent on clinical judgment. Of the available instrumental techniques, laser Doppler flowmetry is the most commonly used; however, clinical acceptance is moderate. This is mainly due to calibration difficulties and problems associated with movement artifacts as mentioned above.

Intravital fluorescence microscopy provides direct assess to the microvessels allowing quantitative analysis of the microcirculation, but the necessity for fluorescent dyes and the possible phototoxic reactions make this method clinically unusable. In an experimental study by Olivier et al. [21] three types of skin flaps were evaluated in a rat model using clinical examination and OPS imaging. Areas of the flap determined to be non-viable were measured and marked. As expected, clinical assessment underestimated the actual amount of flap necrosis, while OPS assessment of microcirculatory stasis correlated well with the subsequent development of necrosis. The authors concluded that OPS imaging was an excellent predictor of eventual flap necrosis and much more accurate than clinical examination ($p > 0.001$). Langer et al. [22] confirmed these findings in a mouse model, and concluded that OPS monitoring of free transferred flaps could be successfully used in humans. We applied OPS in the assessment of flaps in patients and found the technique useful in intra-operative and postoperative assessment of the viability of the flap.

∎ The Microcirculation in Pre-malignant and Malignant Oral Lesions

The diagnosis of a dysplastic premalignant lesion of the oral cavity cannot be made solely on the basis of clinical findings. Histological evaluation of a representative biopsy is needed to support the clinical suspicion. As there is no reliable method applicable to replace a biopsy for a more definitive diagnosis of oral cancer, alternative methods may be used to select the most appropriate area for biopsy. Gynther et al. [23] using direct oral microscopy studied vascular changes in mucosal lesions to select the most appropriate biopsy site. They used criteria for vascular changes as described in colposcopic literature to select biopsy sites. Criteria included vascular pattern, intercapillary distance, surface pattern, color tone, and opacity, as well as the clarity of demarcation of the mucosal lesion. In their study, 40% of the biopsy specimens selected with direct microscopy appeared to be more representative of the histological finding than those selected with routine clinical examination (p=0.01). With OPS imaging the selection of a biopsy site based on a suspected vascular pattern may be achieved more readily. Problems with fine focusing as encountered during direct oral microscopy are not present in the OPS technique since focusing is more easily applied with the hand held device. Furthermore, using direct oral microscopy microscopic examination of posterior intra-oral areas can be difficult to perform. With OPS imaging, all the oral sites can be reached with ease. OPS imaging, therefore, might be used to determine biopsy sited in premalignant mucosal lesions and to follow mucosal lesions and detect progression by evaluating vascular changes.

There is evidence from *in vivo* and *in vitro* studies that tumor growth is dependent upon neovascularization [24]. This applies to both benign and malignant tumors and becomes critical after the tumor has increased beyond approximately 2 mm. In tumors the pathological structure of the vascular network facilitates abnormal circulatory conditions and likely perpetuates hypoxia driven angiogenesis that could also mediate the dominance of positive regulators over negative ones. The pathophysiological conditions of the tumor are based on an abnormal vascular network that is derived from pathological mechanisms of vessel formation and growth [24]. The latter could likely be the consequence of tumor cell invasion of blood vessel walls and the subsequent replacement of endothelial cells by peri-endothelial tumor cells. Folkman's [24, 25] pioneering work showed a strong correlation between tumor growth and microvessel density, and they found a statistically significant relationship between tumor angiogenesis and recurrence in breast cancer. Studies of head and neck cancer at varying sites and stages demonstrated a correlation between increased microvessel density and tumor metastasis. However,

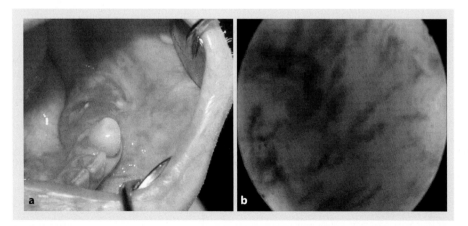

Fig. 4. Clinical picture (**a**) and an OPS image of the microcirculation (**b**) of oral squamous cell carcinoma

studies in the oral cavity have yielded conflicting data. Gleich et al. [26] examined microvessel density in T1 oral tumors and found high vascularity but no correlation with tumor behavior. In a later study, Gleich et al. [27] used Factor VIII antigen and CD-31 staining to determine microvessel density in oral T2–T3 squamous cell carcinoma but failed to demonstrate a significant correlation between tumor angiogenesis and either tumor metastasis or patient survival. A reproducible model for assessment of angiogenesis would therefore be of value in a variety of clinical situations, such as testing the efficacy of a proangiogenic therapy for improving repair in chronic or acute wounds or an antiangiogenic therapy in cancer patients.

Using OPS imaging in selected patients with T1–T2 tongue and buccal squamous cell tumors we made an assessment of the microcirculatory changes in oral tumors [28]. In all patients studied, abnormal microvascular architecture and capillary density could be observed using OPS imaging. These changes consisted of an increase in capillary density and a total disorientation of microcirculatory architecture with several fields of bleeding inside the tumor (Fig. 4).

∎ Conclusion

In this chapter, we introduce the potential use of OPS imaging in the assessment of oral capillary density, microvasculature architecture, and blood flow following surgery. The technique is straightforward and can be easily used in clinical practice to assess oral wound healing processes. In addition, measurements of the other side of the mouth can be used to identify differences between the operated and the control side. Moreover, assessment of soft tissue transferred flaps by OPS imaging may provide a more accurate method of predicting flap survival and influence clinical decisions. The oral cavity is easily accessible and repeated measurements are possible without disturbing patient comfort. As a model for wound healing or for disease processes based on disturbances in the microcirculation, the oral cavity provides an extremely useful compartment for understanding similar physiologic and patho-physiologic processes in the human body as well as providing an important clinical site for monitoring the functional state of the microcirculation in patients.

References

1. Gottrup F (2004) Oxygen in wound healing and infection. World J Surg 28:312–315
2. Mathura KR, Alic L, Ince C (2001) Initial clinical experience with OPS imaging. In: Vincent JL (ed) Yearbook of Intensive Care and Emergency Medicine. Springer, Heidelberg, pp 233–244
3. De Backer D, Creteur J, Preiser JC, et al (2002) Microvascular blood flow is altered in patients with sepsis. Am J Respir Crit Care Med 166:98–104
4. Spronk PE, Ince C, Gardien MJ, et al (2002) Nitroglycerin in septic shock after intravascular volume resuscitation. Lancet 360:1395–1396
5. Sakr Y, Dubois MJ, De Backer D, Creteur J, Vincent JL (2004) Persistent microcirculatory alterations are associated with organ failure and death in patients with septic shock. Crit Care Med 32:1825–1831
6. Weil MH, Nakagawa Y, Tang W, et al (1999) Sublingual capnometry: a new noninvasive measurement for diagnosis and quantitation of severity of circulatory shock. Crit Care Med 27:1225–1229
7. Kon S, Noveas AB, Ruben MP, Goldman HM (1969) Visualization of microvascularization of the healing periodontal wound. II. Curettage. J Periodontol 40:96–105

8. Salerud EG, Nilsson GE (1986) An integrating probe for tissue laser Doppler flowmetry. Med Biol Eng Comput 24:415–19
9. Line PD, Mowinckel P, Lien B, Kvernebo K (1992) Repeated measurements variation and precision of laser Doppler flowmetry measurements. Microvasc Res 43:285–293
10. Mathura KR, Vollebregt KC, Boer K, de Graaf JC, Ubbink DT, Ince C (2001) Comparison of OPS imaging and conventional capillaroscopy to study human microcirculation. J Appl Physiol 91:74–78
11. Miller FN, Collins JG, Feldhoff PA (1989) Non-invasive intravital fluorescent microscopy of the hamster gingiva. J Periodont Res 24:261–266
12. Slaaf DW, Tangelder GJ, Reneman RS, Jager K, Bollinger A (1987) A versatile incident illuminator for intravital microscopy. Int J Microcirc Clin Exp 6:391–397
13. Groner W, Winkelman JW, Harris AG, et al (1999) Orthogonal polarization spectral imaging: a new method for study of the microcirculation. Nat Med 5:1209–1212
14. Mathura KR, Bouma GJ, Ince C (2001) Abnormal microcirculation in brain tumors during surgery. Lancet 17:1698–1699
15. Pennings FA, Bouma GJ, Ince C (2004) Direct observation of the human cerebral microcirculation during aneurysm surgery reveals increased arteriolar contractility. Stroke 35:1284–1288
16. De Backer D (2003) OPS techniques. Minerva Anestesiol 69:388–391
17. Spronk PE, Ince C, Gardien MJ, et al (2002) Nitroglycerin in septic shock after intravascular volume resuscitation. Lancet 360:1395–1396
18. Kishi Y, Takahashi K, Trowbridge H (1990) Vascular network in papillae of dog oral mucosa using corrosive resin cast with scanning electron microscopy. Anat Rec 226:447–459
19. Lindeboom JA, Mathura KR, Ince C (2004) OPS imaging: a new in vivo technique to assess changes in microvascularization in gingival flaps. AO 16:15a (abst)
20. Lindeboom JA, Mathura KR (2001) Microvascular changes in alveolar distraction osteogenesis. Clin Oral Impl Res 12:407 (abst)
21. Olivier WA, Hazen A, Levine JP, Soltanian H, Chung S, Gurtner GC (2003) Reliable assessment of skin flap viability using orthogonal polarization imaging. Plast Reconstr Surg 112:547–555
22. Langer S, Biberthaler P, Harris AG, Steinau HU, Messmer K (2001) In vivo monitoring of microvessels in skin flaps: Introduction of a novel technique. Microsurgery 21:317–324
23. Gynther GW, Rozell B, Heimdahl A (2000) Direct oral microscopy and its value in diagnosing mucosal lesions. A pilot study. Oral Surg Oral Med Oral Pathol Oral Radiol Endod 90:164–170
24. Folkman J (1994) Angiogenesis and breast cancer. J Clin Oncol 12:441–443
25. Folkman J (1995) The influence of angiogenesis research on management of patients with breast cancer. Breast Cancer Res Treat 36:109–118
26. Gleich LL, Biddinger PW, Pavelic ZP, Gluckman JL (1996) Tumor angiogenesis in T1 oral cavity squamous cell carcinoma: role in predicting tumor aggressiveness. Head Neck 18:343–346
27. Gleich LL, Biddinger PW, Duperier FD, Gluckman JL (1997) Tumor angiogenesis as a prognostic indicator in T2–T4 oral cavity squamous cell carcinoma: a clinico-pathologic correlation. Head Neck 19:276–280
28. Lindeboom JAH, Mathura KR, Ince C (2002) Orthogonal spectral polarization imaging in oral squamous cell carcinomas. AAOM 56:3a (abst)

Modulation of Microcirculatory Disorders by Coagulatory Inhibitors

J. N. Hoffmann, J. M. Fertmann, and M. D. Menger

▌ Introduction

Activation of the coagulation system is frequently observed in patients with sepsis and severe sepsis [1]. In these patients a mismatch between pro-coagulatory and anti-coagulatory substances leads to coagulation disorders that can sometimes be clinically recognized as thromboses or bleeding disorders, and may become clinically evident as disseminated intravascular coagulation (DIC). After intravenous injection of microorganisms or bacterial wall products (e.g., endotoxin), systemic activation of coagulation can be observed within minutes [2]. In addition, systemically released inflammatory cytokines can increase coagulatory activation [3]. Tumor necrosis factor (TNF)-α, interleukin (IL)-1, IL-6, and IL-8 can stimulate tissue factor expression, and inhibit the synthesis of thrombomodulin that limits thrombin activity. In addition TNF *per se* activates synthesis of plasminogen activator inhibitor (PAI)-1 which is known to be a highly effective fibrinolysis inhibitor [4]. Besides, procoagulatory processes can directly augment inflammation without involving other cell types [5]. Increased coagulatory activation combined with a downregulation in the fibrinolytic system results in an overall pro-coagulant state leading to the formation of microthrombi and intravascular thrombosis [1, 6]. Thus, thrombin generation is highly injurious and promotes multiple humoral and cellular pro-inflammatory processes [7–10].

Excessive released intravascular thrombin has pro-inflammatory actions at the microcirculatory level by interacting with protease activated receptors (PARs). PARs may be an important link between tissue injury and endothelial cell activation. Thus, PAR-1 induces leukocyte adhesion to the endothelium via nuclear factor kappa B (NF-κB) activation and endothelial intracellular adhesion molecule 1 (ICAM-1) expression. Interestingly, PAR deficiency protected against leukocyte infiltration and renal damage in a mouse model of antibody-mediated glomerulonephritis [11]. Leukocytic responses (e.g., leukocyte rolling) were significantly delayed in the cremaster muscle preparation from PAR-deficient mice.

▌ Reversal of Microcirculatory Disorders by Endogenous Coagulatory Inhibitors

Septic multiple organ dysfunction syndrome represents the main cause of death in patients treated in postoperative intensive care units (ICUs) [12]. The interaction of leukocytes with the endothelium comprises the central step of the inflammatory reaction and can lead to decreased microvascular perfusion [13, 14]. Leukocyte adhesion to the endothelium is mediated by a complex system of adhesion molecules, the leukocyte adhesion cascade. Transmigration and immigration of leukocytes in the inflamed tissue is a central part of the generalised inflammatory reaction. Activated leukocytes do not only mediate septic multiple organ failure, but also represent key players of post-ischemic reperfusion injury and transplant organ rejection [14, 15]. This chapter will focus on the microcirculatory actions of antithrombin and activated protein C (APC), since these inhibitors are well characterized, and can be clinically used in the treatment of sepsis and during transplantation (antithrombin).

∎ Antithrombin's Microcirculatory Effects

During Ischemia-reperfusion Injury

Ischemia-reperfusion injury is clinically important in the view of organ transplantation, but also during clamping of organs for resection (e.g., extended liver resections) [16]. Post-ischemic interaction of neutrophils with the endothelium decreases capillary perfusion and, thereby, aggravates organ dysfunction [17]. Antithrombin improved hepatic blood flow and decreased liberation of liver enzymes in a clinically relevant rat model of hepatic ischemia-reperfusion injury. Myeloperoxidase measurements clearly indicated decreased leukocyte infiltration in the liver [18, 19]. Simultaneously, intrahepatic prostacyclin concentrations in liver tissue were increased. Antithrombin-induced prostacyclin release from vascular endothelial cells is likely to represent one important mechanism of action [20]. Prostacyclin not only modulates leukocyte adhesion and platelet aggregation, but is also known to be a strong vasodilator [21]. Oezden and co-workers showed that prophylactic antithrombin administration, when given before occlusion of the mesentery artery, reduced lipid peroxidation (malondialdehyde concentrations) via a prostacyclin-dependent mechanism [22]. Also myeloperoxidase activity, a marker of leukocyte infiltration was significantly reduced by antithrombin. In addition, antithrombin reduced post-ischemic tissue injury (histology findings). The first group who investigated the effects of antithrombin on post-ischemic reperfusion injury by intravital microscopy reported a highly significant reduction in post-ischemic leukocyte adherence to the endothelium with antithrombin administration [23]. The downregulation of leukocyte adherence corresponded to decreased venular leakage in this cat model of mesenteric microcirculation. In addition, antithrombin also reduced thrombin-induced rolling in flow chamber experiments. Whereas histamine-induced rolling was not influenced by antithrombin, thrombin-mediated rolling was clearly inhibited [23]. A very recent study showed an antithrombin-related inhibition of local and systemic derangement of coagulation and inflammation following intestinal ischemia-reperfusion injury that was comparable to the effects of APC [24].

In addition, antithrombin has also been used in models of acute transplant rejection [25]. In a rat xenotransplantion model, xenograft survival was significantly prolonged by a combination therapy with soluble complement receptor type I and antithrombin [26]. Moreover, antithrombin induced indefinite survival in a fully allogenic rat model of heart transplantation [27]. First results of antithrombin application during human allogenic kidney transplantation indicate a clear reduction of post-transplant ischemic injury [28]. During human simultaneous pancreas-kidney transplantation, antithrombin reduced postoperative lipase release indicating a reduction in reperfusion pancreatitis. In addition, there was a clear reduction in the incidence of pancreas graft thrombosis, which is mainly due to post-ischemic injury producing stasis of blood and microthrombosis [Hoffmann JN et al., unpublished results].

During Endotoxemia

By using intravital microscopy, our group could, for the first time, show a highly significant reduction in endotoxin-induced leukocyte adherence in postcapillary venules by prophylactic intravenous antithrombin administration [29]. Antithrombin led to a highly effective reduction in leukocyte adhesion. Interestingly, antithrombin administration did not reduce the amount of rolling leukocytes when compared to a control group. Therefore, some speculations about the mechanism of antithrombin action are possible: The microcirculatory effects of antithrombin seem not to be mediated by an inhibition of adhesion molecules from the selectin family. On the contrary, antithrombin downregulates endothelial adhesion molecules of the IgG super family (ICAM-1, VCAM-1) and leukocytic β integrins (CD11/CD18). It is highly important to point out that antithrombin action is critically dependent on an intact antithrombin-endothelial cell interaction [30]. In analogy to Harada's finding during hepatic ischemia-reperfusion injury, tryptophan 49-blocked antithrombin did not reduce leukocyte adherence and could not prevent capillary perfusion failure despite its conserved anticoagulatory activity. Also isolated thrombin inhibition by recombinant hirudin did not induce protection from endotoxin-induced microcirculatory disorders [31]. Since thrombin inhibition did not produce comparable effects, it is highly unlikely that antithrombin's microcirculatory potential is mainly mediated by thrombin inhibition [32].

After the first description of antithrombin's anti-adhesive actions during endotoxemia by our group, other authors also reproduced these findings. Thus, intravital microscopy studies in a rat mesentery model with systemic endotoxin application showed a highly significant reduction in leukocyte adhesion by application of recombinant antithrombin. Simultaneously, endotoxin-mediated leakage was significantly reduced by recombinant antithrombin [33]. Leithäuser and co-workers confirmed reduction of mesenteric leukocyte recruitment in endotoxemia that was related to less venular leakage [34]. In an elegant model of endotoxin-induced uveitis in rats, the inhibitory effects of antithrombin against leukocyte rolling and leukocyte infiltration became obvious [35].

During November 2000, the data from an intravital microscopic study in the mesentery were published by Woodman and co-workers [10]. These data seemed to be in contradiction to our results. When endotoxin was superfused over a cat mesentery preparation, antithrombin administration did not produce anti-adhesive effects. When carefully analyzing the methods section in the publication of this study, a highly probable reason for the missing antithrombin effect in this experimental model was detected, which provides additional highly important information about antithrombin action: Before the preparation of the mesentery, unfractionated heparin in a very high concentration had been given intravenously. It has been speculated that this high-dose heparin administration could have prevented antithrombin-endothelial cell interaction and subsequent antithrombin actions. In-

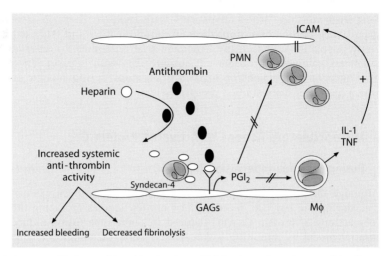

Fig. 1. Heparin is known to bind to antithrombin, thereby multiplying its anticoagulatory activity. Heparin-bound antithrombin, however, cannot interact with the vascular endothelium, and may be responsible for an increase in bleeding events and less fibrinolysis. Heparin also directly binds to glycosaminoglycans (GAGs) on endothelial cells, and to the antithrombin receptor on polymorphonuclear cells (syndecan 4), thereby preventing antithrombin–endothelial cell interaction, and subsequent anti-inflammatory antithrombin activities. In addition, systemic administration of very low amounts of heparin interferes with antithrombin-endothelial cell binding. PMN: polymorphonuclear neutrophil; ICAM: intercellular adhesion molecule; IL-1: interleukin-1; TNF: tumor necrosis factor; PGI2: prostacyclin; Mφ: macrophage

deed, in an important cell culture study, antithrombin-induced prostacyclin release was inhibited by heparin application [36].

This heparin-antithrombin antagonism at the endothelial cell level could be characterized in more detail also concerning microhemodynamic and cellular effects [37]. Heparin massively increases thrombin-antithrombin binding and the production of thrombin-antithrombin complexes (Fig. 1). Moreover, heparin binding to glycosaminoglycans (GAGs) on the endothelial cell surface prevents antithrombin-GAG binding. Direct anti-inflammatory effects of antithrombin on leukocytes are highly likely to be at least in part be mediated by syndecan 4. It has been elegantly demonstrated that antithrombin-syndecan 4 interaction is also inhibited by heparin [32, 38]. This heparin and low-molecular weight heparin adverse effect on microcirculatory antithrombin actions indicates that heparin should be avoided if antithrombin is used to modulate the inflammatory response.

The heparin-related downregulation of positive microcirculatory antithrombin effects corresponds with the results from early clinical studies, where concomitant heparin administration during antithrombin therapy induced significantly more bleeding, and did not improve survival [39]. In a recent placebo controlled multi-center trial (KyberSept trial) that tested the influence of high-dosed antithrombin therapy in more than 2300 patients with severe sepsis, this negative heparin effect obviously occurred again: antithrombin only reduced 90-day mortality in the subgroup of patients who did not concomitantly receive heparin during the 4-day treatment period [40]. Thus, exogenously applied heparin significantly interferes with antithrombin by different mechanisms of action. It is not astonishing that antithrombin administration during severe sepsis did not result in a reduction of long-term mortality when all patients were analyzed (heparin is widely used for deep venous thrombosis prophylaxis in European ICUs and was used in 60% of the study population). In fact, the KyberSept trial represents a non-randomized analysis of a combination treatment of antithrombin with heparin. These observations also question the benefit of heparin application during human sepsis and DIC, which has never been studied prospectively.

▌ Microcirculatory Actions of Activated Protein C

During Ischemia-reperfusion Injury

Although the anticoagulatory effects of protein C have been extensively characterized during the last two decades, there are few studies analyzing the microcirculatory actions of protein C. APC reduced ischemia-reperfusion-induced renal injury in a rat model by inhibiting leukocyte activation. Histological changes observed in control animals after non-crushing microvascular clamping for 60 minutes were nearly completely omitted after APC administration. Simultaneously, APC significantly inhibited the ischemia-reperfusion-induced decrease in renal tissue blood flow and the increase in the vascular permeability [41]. Since only APC significantly inhibited these post-ischemic changes, but not a specific factor Xa inhibitor or heparin, Mizutani et al. suggested that APC protects against ischemia-reperfusion renal injury not by inhibiting coagulation abnormalities, but by directly inhibiting activation of leukocytes. Other groups described a combination of anti-inflammatory and anticoagulatory actions, that provided protection [24]. Since leukopenia also reduced ischemia-reperfusion induced renal injury in their model, the authors hypothesized that APC inhibited neutrophil adhesion, and, thereby, reduced neutrophil elastase and free oxygen radical release, both increasing vascular permeability. In another experimental study the role of APC was investigated in a model of ischemia-reperfusion injury in rat livers [42]. Before inducing liver ischemia by occlusion of the portal ring with a microvascular clip for 30 minutes, APC was applied. The serum concentrations of cytokine-induced neutrophil chemoattractants (CINC) were significantly reduced by APC application. Simultaneously, lower myeloperoxidase activities in hepatic tissue during APC application indicated less neutrophil accumulation into the liver. Interestingly, an inactive derivative of factor Xa (a selective inhibitor of thrombin generation), was also effective in decreasing CINC concentrations and could prevent leukocyte accumulation, indicating that in this case hepatic microcirculatory disturbances were induced by microthrombotic occlusion in a thrombin-dependent mechanism.

During Endotoxemia

In a rabbit model of meningococcal endotoxin-induced shock, a prospective, blinded, placebo-controlled animal trial was performed. In these animals, APC was administered as a continuous infusion [43]. Interestingly, APC administration could not prevent the endotoxin-mediated decrease in mean arterial pressure (MAP) and the increase in heart rate. However, despite lacking effects on macrohemodynamics, survival was significantly improved from 45 to 75%. The authors concluded that microcirculatory APC effects were highly probable. In a model of endotoxin-induced acute respiratory distress syndrome (ARDS), APC attenuated endotoxin-induced pulmonary vascular injury by inhibiting pulmonary leukocyte infiltration [44]. Therefore, a direct effect of APC on the microcirculation also during endotoxemia was highly likely. Our group recently published findings with APC in a sepsis model that allows observation of the microcirculation under non-invasive and normotensive conditions [45]. Macrohemodynamic disturbances could be excluded by careful analysis of macrohemodynamic and microhemodynamic parameters in this model [46]. We found, that APC significantly reduced endotoxin-induced leukocyte rolling in arterioles and venules. Also, the next step in the leukocyte endothelial cell interaction, namely leukocyte adherence, was significantly inhibited in arterioles and venules [47]. Moreover, endotoxin-mediated deterioration of microvascular perfusion was effectively counteracted by intravenous APC administration. Because leukocyte rolling is predominantly mediated by adhesion molecules of the selectin family, the reduction of leukocyte rolling by APC may indicate a modulation of selectin expression. This finding corresponds to in vitro data obtained by vascular endothelial cell culturing, where human plasma-derived and human cell-produced protein C blocked E-selectin-mediated cell adhesion [48]. From our study it is highly likely that a specific anti-inflammatory interaction of APC with the endothelium is responsible for microcirculatory protection. Since thrombin inhibition alone obviously did not reduce leukocyte rolling and adhesion [31], anticoagulatory APC activities – namely inhibition of factor Va and VIIIa that would result in less thrombin formation – are most unlikely to be responsible for the protective effects of APC on the microcirculation during endotoxemia.

▌ Conclusion

The protein C and antithrombin anticoagulant pathways represent major mechanisms in controlling microvascular dysfunction during ischemia/reperfusion injury and sepsis. Local and systemic antithrombin and protein C deficiencies augment the pro-inflammatory response and, thereby, contribute to increased endothelial cell activation and subsequent endothelial dysfunction. The obvious reduction in the endogenous inhibitor potential represents the rationale to exogenously supplement both inhibitors in specific clinical situations. Many experimental trials provide evidence for high efficacy of both substances in terms of sepsis therapy. A recent phase III trial using APC in patients with severe sepsis found a significant reduction in 28-day mortality when compared to placebo [49]. Antithrombin administration reduced mortality from severe sepsis in a prospectively defined subgroup of patients not receiving concomitant heparin. When considering antithrombin anti-inflammatory activity, a substantial antithrombin-heparin interaction at the cellular level has to be taken in account. and low-dose heparin has to be omitted in these scenarios to allow antithrombin to become effective. Further experimental studies should also investigate the potential for APC and antithrombin to prevent patients from developing venous thrombosis.

References

1. Levi M, ten Cate H, van der Poll T, van Deventer SJ (1993) Pathogenesis of disseminated intravascular coagulation in sepsis. JAMA 270:975–979
2. Tanaka T, Tsujinaka T, Kambayashi J, Higashiyama M, Sakon M, Mori T (1989) Sepsis model with reproducible manifestations of multiple organ failure (MOF) and disseminated intravascular coagulation (DIC). Thromb Res 54:53–61

3. Lorente JA, Garcia Frade LJ, Landin L, et al (1993) Time course of hemostatic abnormalities in sepsis and its relation to outcome. Chest 103:1536–1542

4. Opal SM (2000) Phylogenetic and functional relationship between coagulation and the innate immune response. Crit Care Med 28:S77–S80

5. Johnson K, Aarden L, Choi Y, De Groot E, Creasey AA (1996) The proinflammatory cytokine response to coagulation and endotoxin in whole blood. Blood 87:5051–5060

6. Levi M, de Jonge E, van der Poll T, ten Cate H (2000) Novel approaches to the management of disseminated intravascular coagulation. Crit Care Med 28:S20–S24

7. Glusa E (1992) Vascular effects of thrombin. Semin Thromb Hemost 18:296–304

8. Lo SK, Lai L, Cooper JA, Malik AB (1988) Thrombin-induced generation of neutrophil activating factors in blood. Am J Pathol 130:22–32

9. Takahashi H, Tatewaki W, Wada K, Hanano M, Shibata A (1990) Thrombin vs plasmin generation in disseminated intravascular coagulation associated with various underlying disorders. Am J Hematol 33:90–95

10. Woodman R, Teoh D, Payne D, Kubes P (2000) Thrombin and leukocyte recruitment in endotoxemia. Am J Physiol 279:H1338–H1345

11. Cunningham MA, Rondeau E, Chen X (2000) Protease-activated receptor 1 mediates thrombin-dependen, cell-mediated renal inflammation in crescentic glomerulonephritis. J Exp Med 191:455–462

12. Guidici D, Baudo F, Palareti G, Ravizza A, Ridolfi L, D'Angelo A (1999) Antithrombin replacement in patients with sepsis and septic shock. Haematologica 84:452–460

13. Granger DN, Kubes P (1994) The microcirculation and inflammation: modulation of leukocyte-endothelial cell interaction. J Leukoc Biol 55:662–675

14. Harris NR, Russell JM, Granger DN (1994) Mediators of endotoxin-induced leukocyte adhesion in mesenteric postcapillary venules. Circ Shock 43:155–160

15. Grisham MB, Everse J, Janssen HF (1988) Endotoxemia and neutrophil infiltration in vivo. Am J Physiol 254:H1017–H1022

16. Land W, Messmer K (1996) The impact of ischemia/reperfusion injury on specific and non-specific, early and late chronic events after organ transplantation. Transplant Rev 10:236–253

17. Nolte D, Dehning B, Flemisch S, Muller WA, Galanos C, Messmer K (1997) Blockade of platelet-endothelial cell adhesion molecule 1 (PECAM-1, CD 31) reduces endotoxin induced microvascular leak syndrome in striated skin muscle of the BALB/c mouse. Langenbecks Arch Chir 639–641

18. Harada N, Okajima K, Kushimoto S, Isobe H, Tanaka K (1999) Antithrombin reduces ischemia/reperfusion injury of rat liver by increasing the hepatic level of prostacyclin. Blood 93:157–164

19. Mizutani A, Okajima K, Uchiba M, et al (2003) Antithrombin reduces ischemia/reperfusion-induced renal injury in rats by inhibiting leukocyte activation through promotion of prostacyclin production. Blood 101:3029–3036

20. Maria Riva C, Morganroth ML, Ljungman AG, et al (1990) Iloprost inhibits neutrophil-induced lung injury and neutrophil adherence to endothelial monolayers. Am J Respir Cell Mol Biol 3:301–309

21. Armstrong JM, Chapple D, Dusting GJ, Highes R, Moncada S, Vane JR (1977) Cardiovascular actions of prostacyclin in chloralose anesthetized dogs. Br J Pharmacol 61:136

22. Ozden A, Tetik C, Bilgihan A, et al (1999) Antithrombin III prevents 60 min warm intestinal ischemia reperfusion injury in rats. Res Exp Med 198:237–246

23. Ostrovsky L, Woodman R, Payne D, Teoh D, Kubes P (1997) Antithrombin III prevents and rapidly reverses leukocyte recruitment in ischemia/reperfusion. Circulation 96:2302–2310

24. Schoots IG, Levi M, van Vliet AK, Maas AM, Rossink EH, van Gulik TM (2004) Inhibition of coagulation and inflammation by activated protein C or antithrombin reduces intestinal ischemia/reperfusion injury in rats. Crit Care Med 32:1375–1383

25. Takeshita K, Arakawa K, Okamoto M (1996) The anticoagulant effect of antithrombin III on hyperacute xenograft rejection. Transplant Proc 28:631–632

26. Fujiwara I, Nakajima H, Arakawa K, Akioka K, Takeshita K, Oka T (1996) Prolongation of xenograft survival by soluble complement receptor type 1 and antithrombin III combination therapy. Transplant Proc 28:685–686

27. Arakami O, Takayama T, Yokoyama T, et al (2003) High dose of AT induces indefinite survival of fully allogenic cardiac grafts and generates regulatory cells. Transplantation 75:217–220

28. Hoffmann JN, Arbogast HP, Fertmann J, et al (2002) High dose antithrombin therapy reduces ischemia/reperfusion injury during human allogenic kidney transplantation: first results of a randomized controlled clinical trial. Transplantation 74:394–395 (abst)

29. Hoffmann JN, Vollmar B, Inthorn D, Schildberg FW, Menger MD (2000) Antithrombin reduces leukocyte adhesion during chronic endotoxemia by modulation of the cyclooxygenase pathway. Am J Physiol 279:C98–C107

30. Hoffmann JN, Vollmar B, Roemisch J, Inthorn D, Schildberg FW, Menger MD (2002) Antithrombin effects on endotoxin-induced microcirculatory disorders are mainly mediated by its interaction with microvascular endothelium. Crit Care Med 30:218–225

31. Hoffmann JN, Vollmar B, Inthorn D, Schildberg FW, Menger MD (2000) The thrombin antagonist hirudin fails to inhibit endotoxin-induced leukocyte/endothelial cell interaction and microvascular perfusion failure. Shock 14:528–534

32. Roemisch J, Gray E, Hoffmann JN, Wiedermann CJ (2002) Antithrombin: A new look at the actions of a serine protease inhibitor. Blood Coagul Fibrinolysis 13:1–14

33. Neviere R, Tournoys A, Mordon S, et al (2001) Antithrombin reduces mesenteric venular leukocyte interactions and small intestine injury in endotoxemic rats. Shock 15:220–225

34. Leithäuser B, Lendemans S, Schumacher J, Tillmanns H, Matthias FR (2000) Antithrombin (AT) improves inflammation induced microcirculatory disturbances in rat mesentery. Crit Care 4:S15 (abst)

35. Yamashiro K, Kiryu J, Tsujikawa A, et al (2001) Inhibitory effects of antithrombin III against leukocyte rolling and infiltration during endotoxin-induced uveitis in rats. Invest Ophtalmol Vis Sci 42:1553–1560

36. Horie S, Ishii H, Kazama M (1990) Heparin-like glycosaminoglycan is a receptor for antithrombin III-dependent but not for thrombin-dependent prostacyclin production in human endothelial cells. Thromb Res 59:895–904

37. Hoffmann JN, Vollmar B, Laschke M, et al (2002) Adverse effect of heparin on antithrombin action during endotoxemia: microhemodynamic and cellular mechanisms. Thromb Haemost 88:242–252

38. Dunzendoerfer S, Kaneider N, Rabensteiner A, et al (2001) Cell-surface heparan sulfate proteoglycan-mediated regulation of human neutrophil migration by the serpin antithrombin III. Blood 97:1079–1085

39. Blauhut B, Kramar H, Vinazzer H, Bergmann H (1985) Substitution of antithrombin III in shock and DIC: a randomized study. Thromb Res 39:81–89

40. Warren BL, Eid A, Singer P, et al (2001) High-dose antithrombin III in severe sepsis a randomized controlled trial. JAMA 286:1869–1878

41. Mizutani A, Okajima K, Uchiba M, Noguchi T (2000) Activated protein C reduces ischemia/reperfusion-induced renal injury in rats by inhibiting leukocyte activation. Blood 95:3781–3787

42. Yamaguchi Y, Hisama N, Okajima K, et al (1997) Pretreatment with activated protein C or active human urinary thrombomodulin attenuates the production of cytokine-induced neutrophil chemoattractant following ischemia reperfusion. Hepatology 25:1136–1140

43. Roback MG, Stack AM, Thompson C, Brugnara C, Schwarz HP, Saladino RA (1998) Activated protein C concentrate for the treatment of meningococcal endotoxin shock in rabbits. Shock 9:138–142

44. Murakami K, Okajima K, Uchiba M (1996) Activated protein C attenuates endotoxin-induced pulmonary vascular injury by inhibiting activated leukocytes in rats. Blood 87:642–647

45. Hoffmann JN, Vollmar B, Inthorn D, Schildberg FW, Menger MD (1999) A chronic model for intravital microscopic study of microcirculatory disorders and leukocyte / endothelial cell interaction during normotensive endotoxinemia. Shock 12:355–364

46. Hoffmann JN, Vollmar B, Laschke M, Inthorn D, Schildberg FW, Menger MD (2002) Hydroxyethyl starch (130 kD) but not crystalloid volume support improves microcirculation during normotensive endotoxemia. Anesthesiology 97:460–470

47. Hoffmann JN, Vollmar B, Laschke M, et al (2004) Microhemodynamic and cellular mechanisms of activated protein C action during endotoxemia. Crit.Care Med 32:1011–1017
48. Grinnell BW, Herman RB, Yan SB (1994) Human protein C inhibits selectin-mediated cell adhesion: role of unique fucosylated oligosaccharid. Glycobiology 4:221–224
49. Bernard GR, Vincent J-L, Laterre P-F, et al (2001) Efficacy and safety of recombinant human activated protein C for severe sepsis. N Engl J Med 344:699–709

Sublingual Capnometry in Pedatric Patients

N. M. Mehta and J. H. Arnold

▌ Introduction

Bedside, real time hemodynamic monitoring of critically ill patients provides early prediction of outcome and may be used to guide therapy by incorporation of these monitoring variables into decision-making algorithms. Clinicians have long relied on a combination of invasive and non-invasive monitoring tools as surrogates for tissue perfusion. Most of these variables reflect global tissue oxygenation. Recent interest in the microcirculation in regional tissue beds, combined with significant technological advances, has led to the development of regional hemodynamic monitoring tools such as gastric tonometry, transcranial Doppler monitoring, and near infra red spectroscopy (NIRS). Sublingual capnometry, developed as an extension of the gastric tonometry principles applied to the most accessible part of the gastrointestinal system, is thought to be an early indicator of splanchnic low flow state and perhaps an indicator of impending global hypoperfusion. It has been validated clinically and is now available for application in various clinical areas. The promise for this new device is to be able to provide clinicians with a reliable and sensitive marker of tissue hypoperfusion and an end-point for resuscitation in hemodynamically unstable critically ill patients. The following review will trace some of the important events in the development of this novel technology. We will discuss the device in its current form, highlight the published sublingual capnometry studies and discuss its application in children.

▌ Goal-directed Therapy in Critical Care

Early recognition and reversal of organ hypoperfusion remains the cornerstone of the management of shock. Low flow states and tissue dysoxia are major factors in the development of multiple organ failure (MOF) and current treatment strategies for shock are aimed at re-establishing adequate tissue oxygen delivery (DO_2). The concept of oxygen debt and the strategy of attaining supranormal oxygen transport variables as a means to repay this debt have come under scrutiny in recent years. In their meta-analysis of seven relevant studies, which enrolled a total of 1106 patients, Heyland et al. concluded that interventions to attain such supraphysiologic goals did not significantly improve outcomes [1]. Gattinoni et al. made similar observations in a controlled clinical trial that involved a screened population of 10726 patients in 56 intensive care units (ICUs). In this study, 762 patients were randomized to: a) increasing cardiac index to supranormal values, b) normalizing mixed venous oximetry, or c) control group. There were no significant differences in morbidity or mortality between these groups [2]. True supply dependency in critically ill adults was demonstrated by Yu et al. using indirect calorimetry to estimate oxygen consumption (VO_2), in an attempt to eliminate the concept of mathematical coupling seen when VO_2 was calculated in earlier studies [3]. However, this supply dependency was convincingly demonstrated in only a subset of critically ill patients. The use of supranormal levels of cardiac index, DO_2 index and VO_2 index, as endpoints in the resuscitation of trauma victims or critically ill patients, can no longer be generally recommended in any group of critically ill patients.

The timing of intervention remains critical to resuscitation from shock. Early goal directed therapy was shown to improve outcomes in adults with sepsis and septic shock by Rivers et al. [4]. Normalization of central venous oxygen saturation ($ScvO_2$), hematocrit, and mean arterial pressures (MAP) was achieved by using crystalloid and/or blood transfusion in the early goal directed arm of this study, within 6 h of admission to a specialized unit in an adult emergency department. In-hospital mortality rates, 28-day and 60-day mortality rates were significantly lower in the early-treatment group of this study. Kern and Shoemaker reviewed 21 randomized controlled trials to evaluate various goal-directed treatment strategies aimed at achieving supranormal tissue oxygenation variables that may contribute to outcome [5]. The studies, which included patients undergoing high-risk elective surgery or managed during an episode of trauma or sepsis, were divided into two groups based on the timing of the implementation of goals: a) Early goal directed studies (8–12 hrs post-op or before organ failure was expected) and b) studies with late implementation of therapies (after onset of organ failure). The meta-analysis showed that studies where supranormal goals were achieved early and aggressively had a reduced mortality and reduced incidence of organ failure. Goal-directed therapy to achieve optimal goals is thought to be ineffective in the late stages after onset of organ failure, and may even be harmful. Oxygen debt may be irreversible at this stage and attempts at increasing oxygen transport are futile. Early goal-directed therapy has been shown to be least effective in patients with lower predicted mortality and in patients with chronic illness [5]. The quality and the timing of resuscitation appear to be important variables when comparing outcomes in interventional studies in shock. One of the rate limiting steps in instituting early goal-directed therapies is the availability of robust, reliable and sensitive diagnostic or monitoring tools at the bedside. Current markers of tissue perfusion such as central venous pressure, urinary output, vital signs, arterial lactate, blood gases and mixed venous saturation are non-specific, global variables that are not organ specific. The tremendous heterogeneity of microcirculatory dynamics occurring at the organ and cellular level has been elegantly shown in shock states. Early detection of changes due to low flow states in specific tissue beds may provide clinicians with an opportunity to restore regional perfusion and avoid organ damage due to cell death. For many years, organ or tissue-specific monitoring has been largely unavailable and/or difficult to use. Gastric tonometry was one of the earliest tissue specific tools shown to be a sensitive and reliable indicator of poor perfusion and hence an effective surrogate for dysoxia in the splanchnic tissue bed [6, 7]. The emergence of newer imaging techniques has highlighted the striking microcirculatory derangements in the entire gastrointestinal tract, including the sublingual region [8].

▌ Gastric Tonometry

The splanchnic circulation is thought to be highly sensitive to hemodynamic altera-tions and the gastrointestinal tract has been called the 'canary' of the human body [9]. Gastrointestinal mucosal perfusion reflects the splanchnic circulation and is susceptible to diminished tissue perfusion and oxygenation. Higher critical DO_2 re-quirements in comparison to other organs and the mucosal counter-current micro-circulation renders the villi particularly vulnerable to ischemia, which may occur early in the course of shock. Chiara et al. [10] demonstrated reduced superior mes-enteric artery blood flow, relative to renal blood flow in a porcine model of acute hemorrhagic shock. The early disruption of the intestinal mucosal barrier function following ischemia is postulated to allow transluminal bacterial translocation into the blood stream [11]. This might trigger the inflammatory cascade responsible for MOF. Multiple investigators have studied splanchnic regional flow dynamics using direct imaging or indirect (tonometry and capnometry) techniques.

In 1964, Begrofsky demonstrated an *in vivo* system of measuring gas tensions (O_2 and CO_2) in tissues such as urinary bladder and gall bladder [12]. He sampled liquids instilled into hollow viscera after they were allowed to reach gaseous equi-librium with the surrounding tissue. This concept of 'tonometry' was utilized by Fiddian-Green et al. [6] who developed a clinically relevant model of tonometry to estimate the gastrointestinal intramucosal pH (pHi). The partial pressure of carbon dioxide (PCO_2) in the gastric mucosa is allowed to equilibrate across a gas-perme-able silicone balloon filled with saline, until it reaches a steady state in 30–90 min. The PCO_2 in the balloon now reflects gastric mucosal PCO_2. pHi is then calculated using the Henderson-Hasselbalch equation. Subsequent studies showed the correla-tion between pHi and mesenteric blood flow and in 1991, Doglio et al. validated the use of gastric tonometry as a marker of severity of shock and adequacy of re-suscitation [7]. In their cohort of 80 consecutive patients admitted to two adult ICUs, pHi was lower than 7.35 in 32.5% of cases on admission. Mortality was sig-nificantly higher in the low pHi group (65.4 vs. 43.6%, $p < 0.4$) and in those with persistently low pHi 12 h after admission (86.7 vs. 26.8%, $p < 0.001$). These impor-tant clinical findings established pHi derived from gastric tonometry as a useful, relatively non-invasive monitoring tool in the adult ICU.

The calculation of pHi using the Henderson-Hasselbalch equation assumes that PCO_2 in the saline-filled balloon accurately reflects the gastric intramucosal PCO_2 and the measured arterial bicarbonate accurately reflects the intramucosal bi-carbonate level. Using acid-suppressing drugs (antacids) may avoid extraneous CO_2 entering the saline filled balloon by back-diffusion. Intramucosal bicarbonate levels may not be accurately reflected by arterial bicarbonate, especially in experimental settings of low flow [13]. These assumptions seriously compromise the reliability of gastric tonometry. Furthermore, gastric mucosal CO_2 is influenced by changes in arterial CO_2 induced by ventilation. The gap between $PgCO_2$ and arterial PCO_2 may, in fact, be a more sensitive sign of gastric/splanchnic hypoperfusion.

Gastric Tonometry Studies in Pediatrics

In 1995, Krafte-Jacobs et al. examined the efficacy of gastric tonometry as a marker of outcome in pediatric septic shock [14]. The tonometrically obtained pHi value was a poor indicator of global perfusion in this study and did not help predict con-current or subsequent adverse events. In a subsequent study, Ivatury et al. examined the role of gastric tonometry as an organ-specific marker of splanchnic circulation in 57 patients with trauma [15]. Low pHi was associated with increased incidence of MOF and was correlated with mortality. Persistently low pHi was associated with an increased incidence of systemic or intra-abdominal complications and discriminated between survivors and non-survivors. The tissue – arterial PCO_2 gradient (delta CO_2 or DCO_2) was significantly elevated in non-survivors in a cohort of pediatric ICU patients requiring extracorporeal life support for cardiac or respiratory failure [16]. However, in a group of children with sepsis and septic shock, Duke et al. showed no added benefit from DCO_2 values obtained by tonometry, in predicting clinical outcome. Similar observations were made by Wippermann et al., in a group of five infants where tonometrically obtained pHi was measured after cardiac surgery. Intraoperative gastric tonometry using an automated gas analysis was found to be sensitive in monitoring children undergoing cardiac surgery in a study by Bichel et al. [17]. Retrospective analysis showed a lower pHi that persisted after separation from cardiopulmonary bypass in patients who developed early life-threatening complications. However, the variable was not found to be helpful for the management of these patients in the post-operative period [18]. Values for pHi did not correlate with PRISM scores, hemodynamic complications or mortality in another cohort of thirty critically ill children [19]. Thorburn et al. have demonstrated the effect of gastric feeding on gastric intramucosal CO_2 (P_iCO_2), DCO_2 and pHi measured using recirculating gas tonometry. $PiCO_2$ and DCO_2 were decreased and pHi increased in comparison to these values in the fasting state [20].

The above studies show equivocal benefit of gastric tonometry in pediatric critical care as well as significant practical shortcomings (Table 1). Despite its popularity in the adult ICU, gastric tonometry has met with considerable skepticism in the pediatric care setting. The change in the ethos of pediatric critical care towards early initiation and maintenance of enteral feeds conflicts with the use of this technique. The placement of a nasogastric tube and its radiological confirmation with interruption of enteral feeds and the need to start antacid medications, are all viewed as relatively invasive procedures in critically ill children. The unpopularity of the technique in pediatric critical care and the observations of tissue hypercarbia, as a universal indicator of low flow state in a variety of tissue beds, provided the impetus to search for less invasive and easily accessible areas for regional tissue monitoring devices. Esophageal capnometry and then sublingual capnometry were evaluated in an attempt to identify more accessible areas of the gastrointestinal tract for perfusion monitoring.

Table 1. Problems with gastric tonometry in pediatric patients

▌ Fasting/interruption of enteral feeds
▌ Invasive technique
▌ Radiographic confirmation of the gastric tube required
▌ Interruption of gastric decompression
▌ H_2 blocker drugs required (gastric pH > 4.0)
▌ Equilibration time of 30–90 min
▌ Splanchnic microcirculatory heterogeneity seen in pediatric septic shock may affect interpretation of regional pHi

Microcirculation – From Global to Regional Tissue Perfusion

The integrity of the microcirculation is essential for efficient DO_2 at the cellular level. The microcirculation may be the first to manifest derangements during sepsis and may herald the onset of MOF [21]. The capillary leak syndrome is a well-known manifestation of the endothelial dysfunction induced by the inflammatory cascade in sepsis. Other manifestations of the vascular dysregulation include coagulopathy, leukocyte activation, altered rheology [22], opening of arteriovenous shunts, intravascular pooling, and altered viscosity [21]. Altered vascular autoregulatory mechanisms and rheological changes may be responsible for the heterogeneous blood flow distribution seen in sepsis [23]. Hypoxic and inflammatory changes in sepsis also affect the subcellular structures such as membranes and mitochondria resulting in cytopathic hypoxia [24]. These changes may proceed eventually to cell death and organ dysfunction.

The microcirculation and its function may be an important endpoint for resuscitation from septic shock. Recent technologic advances have allowed visualization of the dynamic and heterogeneous nature of the microcirculation. Green polarized light was first used by Slaaf et al. to visualize the microcirculation *in vivo* [25]. The technology was subsequently incorporated into a practical, bedside hand-held microscope (orthogonal polarization spectral [OPS] imaging) by Groner et al. [26]. The device has allowed real-time imaging of the dynamic changes in the microcirculation at tissue beds such as sublingual, cerebral and gastrointestinal mucosa, in various models of shock [27–29].

Sublingual Microcirculation

De Backer and colleagues studied in great detail the dynamic changes in the sublingual microcirculation during sepsis [28]. Their study demonstrated microcirculatory hypoperfusion despite normal systemic hemodynamic parameters. Decreased vascular density (more severe in smaller vessels), increased number of hypoperfused and nonperfused small vessels and marked heterogeneity was noted in the microcirculation. The severity of these alterations was directly correlated to outcome. In a subsequent clinical study, these investigators described the evolution of sublingual microcirculatory alterations over a period of time during treatment of septic shock [29]. In this cohort of 46 patients in septic shock, microcirculatory alterations were similar on Day 1 of septic shock, but persistence of these changes (i.e., the failure of the small vessel perfusion to improve after 24 h of treatment) was associated with the development of multiple organ system dysfunction and higher mortality. Global hemodynamic parameters and oxygen variables did not discriminate between survivors and non-survivors. These studies further emphasized the importance of the microcirculation as a potential endpoint for resuscitation during septic shock and the sublingual space as a potential area for early detection of these changes.

If the sublingual space is indeed reflective of the microcirculatory changes in other important tissue beds, it has the potential for providing easy access to studying the microcirculatory hemodynamics. The development of sublingual capnometry as a surrogate for tissue perfusion may provide clinicians with an objective endpoint for resuscitation at the regional level.

■ Sublingual Capnometry

In the 1980s, a series of important observations by Weil et al., during resuscitation of patients in circulatory failure, showed the association between tissue hypercarbia and low flow states. Disproportionately high PCO_2 levels were seen in cardiac vein, liver parenchyma, kidney, and cerebral cortex of patients with low-flow states during cardiopulmonary resuscitation [30–33]. Elevated tissue PCO_2 levels were also seen in the gastric mucosa during hemorrhagic, anaphylactic, and septic shock [34–36]. Meanwhile, Gutierrez et al. had shown that gastric mucosal pHi, using gastric tonometry, was a sensitive index of tissue perfusion and oxygenation [37, 38].

Based on their observations and studies, Weil and colleagues argued that high PCO_2 was a universal indicator of critical tissue hypoperfusion. Noc et al. showed that gastric luminal PCO_2 (from saline filled balloon allowed to equilibrate with the surrounding tissue) reflected gastric wall PCO_2 during hemorrhagic shock [34]. Subsequent studies showed that esophageal tonometry and capnometry were equally sensitive as monitoring tools during hemorrhagic shock [39]. This led to the hypothesis that the sublingual space, the most proximal and easily accessible part of the gastrointestinal tract, may be a feasible area for capnometry.

Impaired DO_2 induces anaerobic metabolism, which results in decreased tissue pH due to the accumulation of intracellular H^+ ions. These H^+ ions are buffered by the HCO_3^- ions in the tissue to generate CO_2 [40]. This increase in tissue PCO_2 generation and possibly decreased washout during low-flow states produces tissue hypercarbia, which is thought to be a good indicator of tissue hypoxia. Following their initial study in an animal model, [41] Weil et al. measured the sublingual mucosal carbon dioxide tension ($P_{SL}CO_2$), using a microelectrode CO_2 sensor in 5 healthy volunteers and 46 patients with life-threatening injuries or illness [42]. $P_{SL}CO_2$ was shown to be a more sensitive marker of shock and correlated better with outcome, when compared with MAP and arterial blood lactate. In serial measurements on patients with hemorrhagic and septic shock, $P_{SL}CO_2$ was as sensitive as blood lactate to decreased perfusion and also responded dramatically to improving perfusion after treatment. In this first study on human subjects, the microelectrode was shown to be feasible for use in adults able to tolerate the response time, which ranged from 2–8 min.

In a swine model of hemorrhagic shock, Povoas et al. showed a strong correlation between the time-coincident values of $P_{SL}CO_2$ and gastric CO_2 measured by gastric tonometry ($r=0.91$; $p<0.0001$) [43]. The study also showed the delay in normalization of lactate during the reinfusion of blood when MAP, mixed venous arterial CO_2 gradient and the $P_{SL}CO_2$ returned to initial ranges (Figs. 1 and 2).

Marik [44] compared $P_{SL}CO_2$ measurements with gastric-tonometrically obtained intramucosal CO_2 (P_iCO2) and with other hemodynamic and oxygenation parameters, as markers of tissue oxygenation, in ICU patients with hemodynamic instability. In this prospective, clinical validation study, $P_{SL}CO_2$ was shown to correlate with P_iCO_2 ($r=0.78$; $p<0.001$) and the limits of agreement between the methods were 16.1 to –11.9 mmHg. The relative ease of the sublingual measurement, rapid result, and the non-interference with enteral feeding were perceived as major advantages over gastric tonometry. The study did not aim to examine the prognostic value of $P_{SL}CO_2$. The initial $P_{SL}CO_2$–$PaCO_2$ gap was higher in non-survivors and correlated with the initial mixed venous-arterial CO_2 gradient. Initial values of lactate, $P_{SL}CO_2$, and systemic DO_2 were poor discriminators of mortality. These data support the value of sublingual capnometry as a surrogate for tissue dysoxia at the bedside.

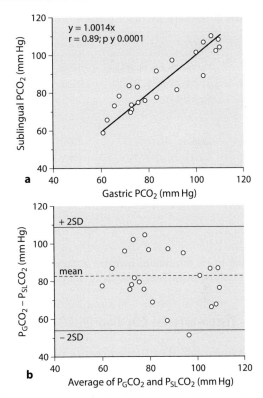

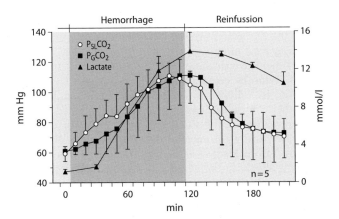

Fig. 1. a The relationship between simultaneous P_GCO_2 and $P_{SL}CO_2$ measurements. **b** Bland-Altman analysis demonstrating differences between the first sublingual measurement and the first gastric tonometric measurement ($P_{SL}CO_2$–P_GCO_2). From [43] with permission

Fig. 2. Comparisons among $P_{SL}CO_2$, P_GCO_2 and$_{lactate}$ levels before, during and after reversal of hemorrhagic shock (reinfusion). From [43] with permission

Table 2. Pre-clinical and clinical studies of sublingual capnometry

	Study	Year	Subjects	Model
1	Nakagawa Y et al. [41]	1998	10 rats	Hemorrhagic shock
2	Povoas HP et al. [43]	2000	5 domestic pigs	Hemorrhagic shock
3	Weil MH et al. [42]	1999	46 patients, 5 healthy volunteers, ER and MSICU	Shock n = 26
4	Marik PE [44]	2001	22 patients, 76 datasets	PAC placement
5	Rackow EC et al. [52]	2001	50 patients M/S/ Cardiac ICU	Circ shock n = 25, cardiac failure, n = 6, septic shock n = 19
6	Marik PE and Bankov [53]	2003	54 patients in a MSICU	PAC placement Septic shock (39%)

Due to its minimally invasive nature and rapid measurement, the device has been examined in various models of shock and in multiple clinical settings (Table 2).

▌ Tissue-arterial CO_2 Gap $(P_{SL}CO_2-PaCO_2)$

Having established tissue hypercarbia as a sensitive marker of severity of low flow states, investigators noted that hypocarbia due to hyperventilation and hypercarbia due to hypoventilation were likely to influence the magnitude of the tissue CO_2 change. Pernat et al. extended these observations in an animal model of hemorrhagic shock where they showed directional and quantitatively comparable changes in tissue CO_2 when acute changes in $PaCO_2$ were induced by hyperventilation and hypoventilation [45]. In the clinical setting, the decreased $PaCO_2$ seen due to the concomitant hyperventilation that might accompany shock could dilute the magnitude of the tissue CO_2 increase due to hypoperfusion in shock state.

In an attempt to account for the influence of total arterial CO_2, the difference between the tissue and arterial CO_2 (the $P_{SL}CO_2-PaCO_2$ gap) has been examined and shown to be a more sensitive parameter for detecting the severity of the low flow state [16]. The calculation of the $P_{SL}CO_2-PaCO_2$ gap numerically magnifies the $P_{SL}CO_2$ value by compensating for the acute CO_2 changes induced by ventilation. However, its validity in patients with chronic and compensated respiratory failure and other clinical settings remains to be examined.

The validity of the PCO_2 gap as a predictor of severity of tissue dysoxia (or more specifically gut mucosal dysoxia) has been challenged by several recent observations. Van der Meer et al. demonstrated ileal mucosal acidosis, in a porcine model of septic shock, in the absence of hypoxia and ischemia [46]. They postulated that a variety of cellular derangements (such as uncoupling of oxidative-phosphorylation, mitochondrial cytopathy and decreased oxidative substrates) and possibly decreased CO_2 clearance in the setting of endotoxemia-related shock with increased cellular metabolism were factors responsible for mucosal acidosis. This finding in Gram-negative septicemia potentially limits the applicability of gastric mucosal pH and hypercarbia as markers of tissue hypoxia and endpoints of resuscitation during septic shock. Animal studies have shown the differential effects of hypoxic hypoxia (with flow maintained) and ischemic hypoxia (due to low flow) on the PCO_2 gap [47, 48]. In the absence of decreases in tissue perfusion, PCO_2 gap may underestimate the severity of tissue dysoxia. It is likely that changes in tissue and venous CO_2 concentrations during dysoxia reflect primarily alterations in vascular perfusion and not scarcity in cellular energy supply. Furthermore, heterogeneous flow in the intestinal microvilli has been demonstrated in the ileal mucosa, with the help of intravital video imaging using OPS imaging [49]. In this porcine model of septic shock, Tugtekin et al. showed impaired and heterogeneous perfusion of the microvilli with a concomitant increase in PCO_2 gap. Therefore, sampling of the intramucosal PCO_2 and pH from one site could be misleading in the presence of such heterogeneity.

∎ Capnoprobe Sublingual System – Nellcor

The most recent sublingual capnometry device is the Nellcor(R) CapnoProbe$^{(TM)}$ N-80 Sublingual (SL) System (Nellcor Tyco Healthcare, Pleasanton, CA). The system consists of a disposable sublingual sensor equipped with a semipermeable membrane located at its tip (Fig. 3). Mucosal CO_2 diffuses across this membrane into a pH sensitive fluorescent dye solution in the sensor. Carbonic acid is produced as CO_2 enters the dye, which emits light proportional to the amount of pH change or the amount of CO_2 present (Fig. 4). This light is radiometrically quantified using fiberoptic technology by the handheld N80 device.

The device displays $P_{SL}CO_2$ in the range of 30–150 mmHg (4–20 kPa) with a resolution of 1 mmHg or 0.1 kPa. The accuracy of the CapnoProbe is within 10% for

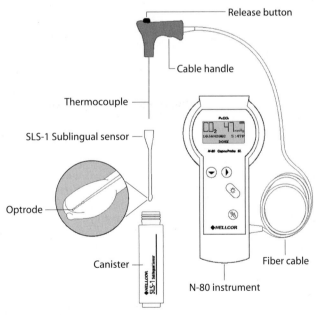

Fig. 3. The CapnoProbe^{TM} SL system consists of 2 components: The SLS1 sublingual sensor and the N80 CapnoProbe^{TM} SL monitoring device

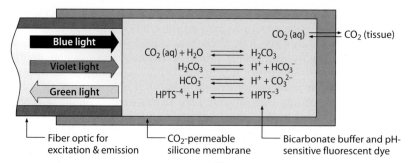

Fig. 4. Fiberoptic technology in the CapnoProbe™ sublingual sensor tip. Fluorescent intensity of the dye in the solution is directly proportional to the pH, which is lowered by the tissue CO_2 entering the solution through the semipermeable membrane

$P_{SL}CO_2$ values above 50 mmHg. The device performs optimally within a temperature range of 28 to 42 °C.

Encouraged by its application in the adult critical care population, investigators have examined the role of sublingual capnometry using the CapnoProbe device in children. Kapklein et al. presented their findings after a clinical evaluation of $P_{SL}CO_2$ and $P_{SL}CO_2$–$PaCO_2$ gap in 18 critically ill children [50]. A $P_{SL}CO_2$–$PaCO_2$ gap higher than 15 mmHg reliably detected children in shock (sensitivity of 69% and specificity of 100%). Sublingual capnometry correlated well with other indicators of shock in this study and was simple to perform. Wohrley applied sublingual capnometry in a group of 15 children undergoing cardiopulmonary bypass during repair of congenital heart disease [51]. Cardiogenic shock was determined in a subset of patients based on clinical exam and inotropic requirement. Mean $P_{SL}CO_2$ and $P_{SL}CO_2$–$PaCO_2$ gap were significantly higher in children in cardiogenic shock. These initial reports on the use of sublingual capnometry in children have been reassuring and the current generation of the sublingual capnometry device is being further evaluated by our group and others.

■ Limitations of Sublingual Capnometry: Directions for the Future

Sublingual PCO_2 measurement holds the promise of yet another monitoring tool for tissue hypoperfusion during shock. It provides a number of advantages over gastric mucosal pH measurement and has been applied in hemorrhagic, cardiogenic, and post-operative low flow states as a reliable and sensitive marker of tissue hypoperfusion. The reliability of the technique in other shock states (septic shock) and in the pediatric population is currently under investigation. If tissue hypercarbia is indeed more sensitive to ischemic than non-ischemic hypoxia, more studies will need to examine its role in endotoxin-mediated shock. The heterogeneity of the gastrointestinal microcirculation during sepsis/septic shock and its alteration by therapeutic interventions (such as catecholamines) may compromise the ultimate impact of this technology in this subgroup of patients. Sublingual capnometry is at best a surrogate for the mucosal blood flow and oxygen delivery to the gastrointestinal circulation. This tissue bed may be an important and early marker of global tissue dysoxia during shock states. The ultimate challenge for sublingual capnometry will be to demonstrate improvements in clinical outcomes following its incorporation into goal directed, decision-making algorithms.

In its current form, certain technological constraints may limit its applicability to pediatric patients, especially young infants. Technological alterations in the next generation of this device will enhance its application in this age group. The probe size and shape may need to be altered in an attempt to tailor it to the wide range of sizes of the sublingual space in pediatric practice. The area of contact of the probe and the sublingual surface remains a critical determinant of the repeatability and the accuracy of measurements. This makes the measurement user-dependent and this variable may be a problem when using the current (one-size-fits-all probe) in young infants. The sensor placement is expected to remain unchanged during the calibration time required for obtaining the final reading. This period may vary from 60–90 s and requires patient co-operation. The current probe has been extensively tested in adults and has been well tolerated. The measurement is comparable to placement of an oral temperature probe, although placement of the probe in the sublingual space to maintain contact with the mucosa requires some dexterity and practice and may be challenging in children who are awake. We have not seen any physiological adverse events during sublingual capnometry in children who are mechanically ventilated and sedated on the ICU. In this subgroup of patients, sensor contact and repeatability of measurement were optimal in our experience.

The ability of future generations of the device to measure $P_{SL}CO_2$ continually at the bedside is desirable. The current probe will need some modifications in its design to allow placement in the sublingual space for extended periods of time. Research into other areas of probe placement and tissue PCO_2 sampling may be relevant for allowing continuous measurement of this parameter. Other desirable modifications to the current probe include decreased calibration and measurement times to enhance patient cooperation, an objective indicator of optimal tissue contact with sensor and increased device memory for storage of multiple readings. Furthermore, the ability of future generations of this device to interface with continuous or contemporaneous arterial CO_2 values may allow real time display of the $P_{SL}CO_2$–$PaCO_2$ gap at the bedside. The technological sophistication required of these upgrades will have to be evaluated for its utility at the bedside and cost-effectiveness.

▌ Final Thoughts … Conclusion

In critically ill children with hemodynamic alterations, a surrogate for tissue hypoperfusion that is sensitive, non-invasive, and technically simple would be desirable. Early goal-directed therapy, guided by a reliable measure of tissue dysoxia at the regional microcirculatory level, may prevent cellular injury and multi-organ dysfunction. The sublingual tissue bed has been shown to be altered in models of shock and microcirculatory changes in this region may reflect impending changes in other important organs. This would make it an ideal non-invasive monitoring tool and sublingual capnometry may be a useful end-point for resuscitation in critically ill children with hemodynamic alterations.

Further studies are required to examine the effect of the microcirculatory heterogeneity, acid-base states, vasoactive medications and dysoxia with normal flow, on the reliability of sublingual capnometry. Pediatric data are currently being collected and will clarify the potential of this device in monitoring in the pediatric ICU. The accuracy of the sublingual capnometry device needs to be shown in neonates and infants. Technological modifications of the current generation of device may enhance its applicability to children.

References

1. Heyland DK, Cook DJ, King D, Kernerman P, Brun-Buisson C (1996) Maximizing oxygen delivery in critically ill patients: a methodologic appraisal of the evidence. Crit Care Med 24:517–524
2. Gattinoni L, Brazzi L, Pelosi P, et al (1995) A trial of goal-oriented hemodynamic therapy in critically ill patients. SvO_2 Collaborative Group. N Engl J Med 333:1025–1032
3. Yu M, Burchell S, Takiguchi SA, McNamara JJ (1996) The relationship of oxygen consumption measured by indirect calorimetry to oxygen delivery in critically ill patients. J Trauma 41:41–48
4. Rivers E, Nguyen B, Havstad S, et al (2001) Early goal-directed therapy in the treatment of severe sepsis and septic shock. N Engl J Med 345:1368–1377
5. Kern JW, Shoemaker WC (2002) Meta-analysis of hemodynamic optimization in high-risk patients. Crit Care Med 30:1686–1692
6. Fiddian-Green RG, Pittenger G, Whitehouse WM Jr (1982) Back-diffusion of CO_2 and its influence on the intramural pH in gastric mucosa. J Surg Res 33:39–48
7. Doglio GR, Pusajo JF, Egurrola MA, et al (1991) Gastric mucosal pH as a prognostic index of mortality in critically ill patients. Crit Care Med 19:1037–1040
8. De Backer D, Dubois MJ (2001) Assessment of the microcirculatory flow in patients in the intensive care unit. Curr Opin Crit Care 7:200–203
9. Dantzker DR (1993) The gastrointestinal tract. The canary of the body? Jama 270:1247–1248
10. Chiara O, Pelosi P, Segala M, et al (2001) Mesenteric and renal oxygen transport during hemorrhage and reperfusion: evaluation of optimal goals for resuscitation. J Trauma 51:356–362
11. Deitch EA, Bridges W, Berg R, Specian RD, Granger DN (1990) Hemorrhagic shock-induced bacterial translocation: the role of neutrophils and hydroxyl radicals. J Trauma 30:942–951
12. Bergofsky EH (1964) Determination of tissue O_2 tensions by hollow visceral tonometers: effect of breathing enriched O_2 mixtures. J Clin Invest 43:193–200
13. Antonsson JB, Boyle CC, 3rd, Kruithoff KL, et al (1990) Validation of tonometric measurement of gut intramural pH during endotoxemia and mesenteric occlusion in pigs. Am J Physiol 259:G519–G523
14. Krafte-Jacobs B, Carver J, Wilkinson JD (1995) Comparison of gastric intramucosal pH and standard perfusional measurements in pediatric septic shock. Chest 108:220–225
15. Ivatury RR, Simon RJ, Islam S, Fueg A, Rohman M, Stahl WM (1996) A prospective randomized study of end points of resuscitation after major trauma: global oxygen transport indices versus organ-specific gastric mucosal pH. J Am Coll Surg 183:145–154
16. Duke T, Butt W, South M, Shann F (1997) The DCO_2 measured by gastric tonometry predicts survival in children receiving extracorporeal life support. Comparison with other hemodynamic and biochemical information. Royal Children's Hospital ECMO Nursing Team. Chest 111:174–179
17. Bichel T, Kalangos A, Rouge JC (1999) Can gastric intramucosal pH (phi) predict outcome of paediatric cardiac surgery? Paediatr Anaesth 9:129–134
18. Perez A, Schnitzler EJ, Minces PG (2000) The value of gastric intramucosal pH in the postoperative period of cardiac surgery in pediatric patients. Crit Care Med 28:1585–1589
19. Calvo C, Ruza F, Lopez-Herce J, Dorao P, Arribas N, Alvarado F (1997) Usefulness of gastric intramucosal pH for monitoring hemodynamic complications in critically ill children. Intensive Care Med 23:1268–1274
20. Thorburn K, Durward A, Tibby SM, Murdoch IA (2004) Effects of feeding on gastric tonometric measurements in critically ill children. Crit Care Med 32:246–249
21. Hinshaw LB (1996) Sepsis/septic shock: participation of the microcirculation: an abbreviated review. Crit Care Med 24:1072–1078

22. Piagnerelli M, Boudjeltia KZ, Vanhaeverbeek M, Vincent JL (2003) Red blood cell rheology in sepsis. Intensive Care Med 29:1052–1061
23. Groeneveld AB, van Lambalgen AA, van den Bos GC, Bronsveld W, Nauta JJ, Thijs LG (1991) Maldistribution of heterogeneous coronary blood flow during canine endotoxin shock. Cardiovasc Res 25:80–88
24. Fink MP (2002) Bench-to-bedside review: Cytopathic hypoxia. Crit Care 6:491–499
25. Slaaf DW, Reneman RS, Wiederhielm CA (1987) Cessation and onset of muscle capillary flow at simultaneously reduced perfusion and transmural pressure. Int J Microcirc Clin Exp 6:215–224
26. Groner W, Winkelman JW, Harris AG, et al (1999) Orthogonal polarization spectral imaging: a new method for study of the microcirculation. Nat Med 5:1209–1212
27. Mathura KR, Bouma GJ, Ince C (2001) Abnormal microcirculation in brain tumours during surgery. Lancet 358:1698–1699
28. De Backer D, Creteur J, Preiser JC, Dubois MJ, Vincent JL (2002) Microvascular blood flow is altered in patients with sepsis. Am J Respir Crit Care Med 166:98–104
29. Sakr Y, Dubois MJ, De Backer D, Creteur J, Vincent JL (2004) Persistent microcirculatory alterations are associated with organ failure and death in patients with septic shock. Crit Care Med 32:1825–1831
30. Grundler W, Weil MH, Rackow EC (1986) Arteriovenous carbon dioxide and pH gradients during cardiac arrest. Circulation 74:1071–1074
31. Gudipati CV, Weil MH, Gazmuri RJ, Deshmukh HG, Bisera J, Rackow EC (1990) Increases in coronary vein CO_2 during cardiac resuscitation. J Appl Physiol 68:1405–1408
32. Weil MH, Rackow EC, Trevino R, Grundler W, Falk JL, Griffel MI (1986) Difference in acid-base state between venous and arterial blood during cardiopulmonary resuscitation. N Engl J Med 315:153–156
33. Desai VS, Weil MH, Tang W, Yang G, Bisera J (1993) Gastric intramural PCO_2 during peritonitis and shock. Chest 104:1254–1258
34. Noc M, Weil MH, Sun S, Gazmuri RJ, Tang W, Pakula JL (1993) Comparison of gastric luminal and gastric wall PCO_2 during hemorrhagic shock. Circ Shock 40:194–199
35. Tang W, Weil MH, Sun S, Noc M, Gazmuri RJ, Bisera J (1994) Gastric intramural PCO_2 as monitor of perfusion failure during hemorrhagic and anaphylactic shock. J Appl Physiol 76:572–577
36. Desai VS, Weil MH, Tang W, Gazmuri R, Bisera J (1995) Hepatic, renal, and cerebral tissue hypercarbia during sepsis and shock in rats. J Lab Clin Med 125:456–461
37. Gutierrez G, Bismar H, Dantzker DR, Silva N (1992) Comparison of gastric intramucosal pH with measures of oxygen transport and consumption in critically ill patients. Crit Care Med 20:451–457
38. Gutierrez G, Palizas F, Doglio G, et al. (1992) Gastric intramucosal pH as a therapeutic index of tissue oxygenation in critically ill patients. Lancet 339:195–199
39. Sato Y, Weil MH, Tang W, et al (1997) Esophageal PCO_2 as a monitor of perfusion failure during hemorrhagic shock. J Appl Physiol 82:558–562
40. Johnson BA, Weil MH, Tang W, Noc M, McKee D, McCandless D (1995) Mechanisms of myocardial hypercarbic acidosis during cardiac arrest. J Appl Physiol 78:1579–1584
41. Nakagawa Y, Weil MH, Tang W, et al (1998) Sublingual capnometry for diagnosis and quantitation of circulatory shock. Am J Respir Crit Care Med 157:1838–1843
42. Weil MH, Nakagawa Y, Tang W, et al (1999) Sublingual capnometry: a new noninvasive measurement for diagnosis and quantitation of severity of circulatory shock. Crit Care Med 27:1225–1229
43. Povoas HP, Weil MH, Tang W, Moran B, Kamohara T, Bisera J (2000) Comparisons between sublingual and gastric tonometry during hemorrhagic shock. Chest 118:1127–1132
44. Marik PE (2001) Sublingual capnography: a clinical validation study. Chest 120:923–927
45. Pernat A, Weil MH, Tang W, et al (1999) Effects of hyper- and hypoventilation on gastric and sublingual PCO(2). J Appl Physiol 87:933–937
46. VanderMeer TJ, Wang H, Fink MP (1995) Endotoxemia causes ileal mucosal acidosis in the absence of mucosal hypoxia in a normodynamic porcine model of septic shock. Crit Care Med 23:1217–1226

47. Dubin A, Murias G, Estenssoro E, et al (2002) Intramucosal-arterial PCO_2 gap fails to reflect intestinal dysoxia in hypoxic hypoxia. Crit Care 6:514–520

48. Vallet B, Teboul JL, Cain S, Curtis S (2000) Venoarterial CO(2) difference during regional ischemic or hypoxic hypoxia. J Appl Physiol 89:1317–1321

49. Tugtekin IF, Radermacher P, Theisen M, et al (2001) Increased ileal-mucosal-arterial PCO_2 gap is associated with impaired villus microcirculation in endotoxic pigs. Intensive Care Med 27:757–766

50. Kapklein MJ (2002) Abstract #75273616. Oral capnometry for quantification of shock in children. APS/SPR Conference, May 4–7. Baltimore, MD

51. Worhley JD (2004) Abstract #216. Sublingual capnometry in pediatric cardiovascular surgery patients. SCCM – 3rd Critical Care Congress, Feb 20–25. Orlando, FL

52. Rackow EC, O'Neil P, Astiz ME, Carpati CM (2001) Sublingual capnometry and indexes of tissue perfusion in patients with circulatory failure. Chest 120:1633–1638

53. Marik PE, Bankov A (2003) Sublingual capnometry versus traditional markers of tissue oxygenation in critically ill patients. Crit Care Med 31:818–822

Cardiorespiratory Monitoring

New Echocardiographic Parameters of Fluid Responsiveness in Ventilated Patients

A. Vieillard-Baron and F. Jardin

▌ Introduction

It is now well known that intravascular pressures reflecting ventricular preload, i.e., central venous pressure (CVP) and pulmonary artery occlusion pressure (PAOP), are inaccurate in predicting fluid responsiveness and in diagnosing adequate or inadequate volume status in ventilated patients. This has been demonstrated in severe sepsis by Michard et al. [1], and has since been re-emphasized in several studies [2, 3]. One of the reasons concerns an inability to know in which part of the Frank-Starling curve the pressure is [4]. This depends on the preload level but also on cardiac systolic function. A high incidence of right (RV) and left ventricular (LV) systolic dysfunction has been reported in severe sepsis [5], rendering hazardous the use of intravascular pressures for monitoring fluid requirement.

Since the publication of several studies, some reporting the uselessness of right heart catheterization in improving the prognosis [6, 7], and others demonstrating the ability of echocardiography to non-invasively assess cardiac function in intensive care patients [8, 9], echocardiography could appear as a perfect tool in the intensive care unit (ICU). However, until now, its main limitation was probably the absence of reliable and simple parameters of hypovolemia and of fluid responsiveness. Indeed, LV end-diastolic dimensions were not reported as reliable enough [2]. Furthermore, non-invasive assessment of PAOP by using Doppler at the mitral annulus or at the pulmonary vein may lead to the same misinterpretations as invasive measurement.

Echocardiography is also able to visualize the vena cavae either by a subcostal route for the inferior vena cava (IVC) [10] or by a transesophageal route for the superior vena cava (SVC) [11]. Cardiologists and some intensivist have long used IVC and SVC diameters, unfortunately only to evaluate CVP [12, 13]. Recently, three studies, done in part by our team, took an interest in vena cava size variations related to tidal volume in predicting requirement for blood volume expansion [14–16]. These studies examined the predictive value of the collapsibility index of the SVC and of the distensibility index of the IVC. Providing that the patient is mechanically ventilated without any spontaneous breathing effort, these new echocardiographic indices of fluid responsiveness seem to be accurate [14–16].

▌ The SVC during Mechanical Ventilation

By systematically performing transesophageal echocardiography (TEE) in patients with hypotension, we previously observed significant variations in SVC diameter during mechanical ventilation [11]. A maximal diameter is always observed during

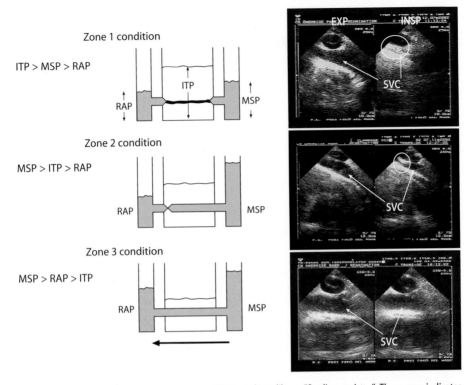

Zone 1 condition

ITP > MSP > RAP

Zone 2 condition

MSP > ITP > RAP

Zone 3 condition

MSP > RAP > ITP

Fig. 1. Illustration of the superior vena cava (SVC) working like a "Starling resistor". The arrow indicates the direction of the blood towards the right atrium. Schematic left panels represent different working conditions of a "Starling resistor". The opposite right panels demonstrate SVC diameter at expiration (EXP) and at inflation (INSP). On the lower panels, during inflation, mean systemic pressure (MSP) is higher than right atrial pressure (RAP), which is higher than intra-thoracic pressure (ITP); no variation in SVC diameter is visualized; this is a zone 3 condition. In the middle panel, MSP is still higher than RAP during inflation but ITP becomes higher than RAP; a localized collapse of SVC at the entry in the right atrium is observed (*circle*); this is a zone 2 condition. This setting is illustrated in a patient after clamping the inferior vena cava, a procedure which suddenly decreases RAP, but does not change MSP. Finally, on the top panels, ITP is higher than MSP and than RAP; a complete collapse all along the vessel is observed (*circle*); this is a zone 3 condition. This setting is illustrated in a hypovolemic patient, exhibiting a low MSP

expiration, and a minimal diameter during inflation. Tidal ventilation increases pleural pressure, which is the surrounding pressure of SVC, thus leading to a decrease in the distending pressure of SVC, i.e., the intravascular pressure minus pleural pressure, and so in its diameter. To be open, SVC, like all the venous vessels, requires a distending pressure above its closing pressure [17]. In certain conditions like hypovolemia, increase in pleural pressure is enough to lower the SVC distending pressure to below its closing pressure, thus inducing a partial or complete collapse of the vessel. In this way, the SVC could probably be compared to a "Starling resistor", as illustrated in Figure 1.

Complete or partial collapse of the SVC during inflation has several hemodynamic consequences. First, we reported a close correlation between decrease in SVC diameter and drop in RV stroke index (RVSI) related to tidal volume [11]. The

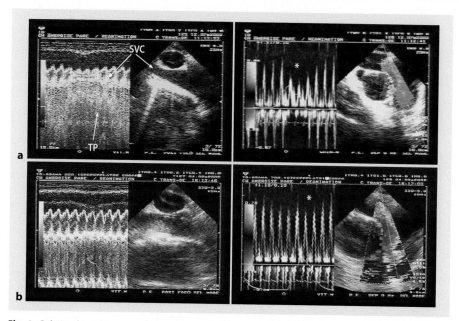

Fig. 2. Relationship between variations in superior vena cava (SVC) diameter during tidal ventilation (*left panel*) and right ventricular (RV) ejection measured using pulsed Doppler in the pulmonary artery (PA, *right panel*). In patient **a**, a complete collapse of SVC during inflation induced a marked fall in RV ejection (*asterisk*). In patient **b**, no significant changes in SVC size were observed, leading to a less marked drop in RV ejection (*asterisk*). TP: tracheal pressure

more marked the SVC diameter variations, the greater the decrease in RV ejection (Fig. 2) [11]. This has been previously suggested in animals by Fessler et al. who demonstrated that decrease in systemic venous return observed during tidal ventilation was probably induced by increase in venous resistance and not by decrease in the pressure gradient of the venous return, i.e., the mean systemic pressure minus atrial pressure [18]. Indeed, when pleural pressure is transmitted to atrial pressure, it is also transmitted to the same extent to the mean systemic pressure [18]. Second, we also demonstrated that the greater the SVC diameter variations related to tidal volume, the more significant the 'ΔDown' [19]. The ΔDown has been described as the expiratory decrease in systolic arterial pressure [20], reflecting in part the decrease in LV ejection during expiration [21]. It was proposed as a parameter of central blood volume insufficiency [22]. By inducing significant decrease in SVC diameter, tidal ventilation is responsible for a drop in RV ejection, and thus for a decrease in blood volume in the pulmonary capillaries, i.e., the preload reserve of the left ventricle [23], and finally for a drop in LV ejection at expiration, regarding the time of transit of blood throughout the lung.

Recently, we reported, in sixty-six mechanically ventilated patients in septic shock, the value of the SVC collapsibility index in predicting fluid responsiveness [14]. The SVC collapsibility index was calculated before blood volume expansion as the maximal diameter at expiration minus the minimal diameter at inspiration/maximal diameter (Fig. 3). It is very important for such a measurement to obtain a long-axis view of the SVC and to couple the time-motion study to the two-dimen-

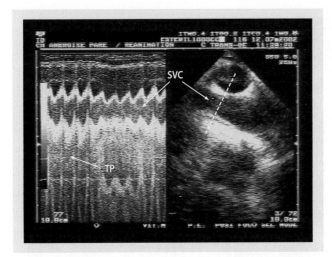

Fig. 3. Example of measurement of superior vena cava (SVC) collapsibility index in a mechanically venti-lated patient. The two-dimensional mode is coupled with the time-motion study. SVC is visualized in a long-axis view. Arrows indicate the maximal and minimal diameters of the vessel. TP: tracheal pressure

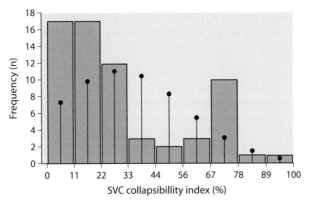

Fig. 4. Bimodal distribution of superior vena cava (SVC) collapsibility index in 66 septic patients. Most pa-tients exhibited an index below 33% or above 56%. Bars indicate the normal distribution

sional mode (Fig. 3) [24]. At baseline, the distribution of the SVC collapsibility in-dex was not normal, but demonstrated a bimodal distribution with two particular ranges of values, below 33% (46 patients) and above 56% (15 patients) (Fig. 4) [14], suggesting that SVC obeys in part the all or nothing law. This is in accordance with our hypothesis comparing SVC to a "Starling resistor". We also demonstrated that a collapsibility index above 36% could predict significant increase in cardiac output after blood volume expansion with a sensitivity of 90% and a specificity of 100% [14]. An example is given in Figure 5.

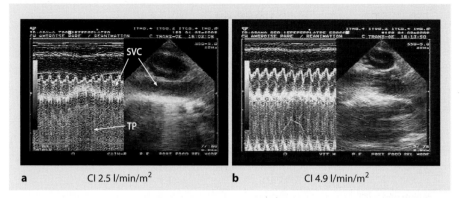

Fig. 5. Variations of superior vena cava (SVC) diameter in a septic patient exhibiting shock. At baseline **a**, TEE demonstrated a complete collapse of SVC at each inflation. After blood volume expansion **b**, the collapse disappeared and the cardiac index significantly increased. CI: cardiac index; TP: tracheal pressure

▌ The IVC during Mechanical Ventilation

Because TEE cannot be performed in certain conditions, and so SVC diameter cannot be obtained, we also studied the variations of IVC size in ventilated septic patients in prediction of fluid responsiveness. IVC may be visualized using transthoracic echocardiography (TTE) by a subcostal approach. The IVC is not submitted to intra-thoracic pressure like the SVC, but to intraabdominal pressure (IAP). IVC diameter depends in part on the relation between its surrounding pressure, i.e., the IAP, and its backward pressure, i.e., the right atrial pressure [25]. This was previously demonstrated during acute asthma in spontaneously breathing patients, where the IVC collapsed at each inspiration because of a marked fall in the atrial pressure induced by a marked decrease in intra-thoracic pressure [26]. In mechanically ventilated patients, during inflation, increase in intra-thoracic pressure is transmitted to the right atrium, thus increasing the IVC backward pressure. At the same time, the rise in IAP is less, since only about 20% of the intra-thoracic pressure is transmitted to the abdominal cavity [27]. This leads to an increase in transmural pressure of the IVC, i.e., right atrial pressure minus IAP, and thus in its diameter if the compliance of the vessel allows it.

Our hypothesis was that variations in IVC diameter related to tidal ventilation should be able to predict fluid responsiveness. The more compliant the vessel, as probably observed in hypovolemia, the more it should be distended [28]. This is illustrated in Figure 6, using the relationship at expiration between CVP and IVC diameter in 108 mechanically ventilated patients in our ICU. From a certain intravascular pressure, IVC appears unable to distend any more because of a fall in its compliance.

Finally, we recently reported in 23 mechanically ventilated septic patients without spontaneous breathing effort, the value of the IVC distensibility index in predicting fluid responsiveness [15]. The IVC distensibility index was calculated as maximal diameter at inflation minus minimal diameter at expiration/minimal diameter (Fig. 7). For this, the IVC was visualized on a long-axis view and diameters were measured just upstream of the origin of the supra-hepatic vein. We

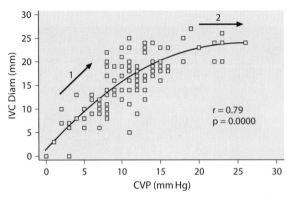

Fig. 6. Correlation between central venous pressure (CVP) and inferior vena cava diameter (IVC Diam) at expiration in 108 patients. The curve has two portions, the first (1) with a steep slope, reflecting a compliant vessel, and the second (2) with a flat slope, reflecting a non-compliant vessel unable to distend anymore. From [24] with permission

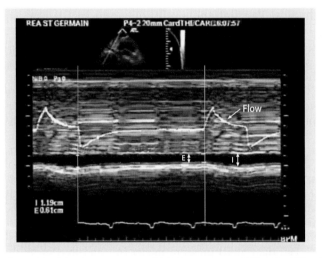

Fig. 7. Example of measurement of inferior vena cava (IVC) collapsibility index in a mechanically ventilated patient. The two-dimensional mode is coupled with the time-motion study. IVC is visualized in a long axis view. Arrows indicate the maximal and minimal diameters of the vessel. E: expiration; I: inflation

demonstrated that a distensibility index above 18% could predict significant increase in cardiac output after blood volume expansion with a sensitivity of 90% and a specificity of 90% [15]. Similar results were published by Feissel and co-workers [16]. However, we re-emphasize the importance of IAP in the variations of IVC size. Our study was performed in medical patients with only a slight increase in IAP [15], and the value of IVC diameter variations remains to be validated in conditions where IAP is elevated. This is a potential limitation in current use of IVC studies.

▌ Conclusion

Studying vena cavae in mechanically ventilated patients is probably of great interest in assessing fluid responsiveness and volemic status. Moreover, SVC and IVC studies appear to be complementary. Whereas the first needs TEE to be visualized, the second only requires TTE and so may be used when an esophageal probe is unavailable or when TEE is contraindicated. Finally, intensivists must remember that, to be correctly interpreted, variations in vena cava size related to tidal volume must be measured in patients without spontaneous breathing effort.

References

1. Michard F, Boussat S, Chemla D, et al (2000) Relation between respiratory changes in arterial pulse pressure and fluid responsiveness in septic patients with acute circulatory failure. Am J Respir Crit Care Med 162:134–138
2. Tavernier B, Makhotine O, Lebuffe G, Dupont J, Scherpereel P (1998) Systolic pressure variation as a guide to fluid therapy in patients with sepsis-induced hypotension. Anesthesiology 89:13–21
3. Michard F, Teboul JL (2002) Predicting fluid responsiveness in ICU patients: a critical analysis of the evidence. Chest 121:2000–2008
4. Braunwald E, Sonnenblick EH, Ross J (1988) Mechanisms of cardiac contraction and relaxation. In: Braunwald E (ed) Heart Disease. WB Saunders company, Philadelphia, pp 389–425
5. Vieillard-Baron A, Schmitt JM, Beauchet A, et al (2001) Early preload adaptation in septic shock? A transesophageal echocardiographic study. Anesthesiology 94:400–406
6. Richard C, Warszawski J, Anguel N, et al (2003) Early use of the pulmonary artery catheter and outcomes in patients with shock and acute respiratory distress syndrome: a randomized controlled trials. JAMA 290:2713–2720
7. Sandham J, Hull R, Brant R, et al (2003) A randomized, controlled trial of the use of pulmonary-artery catheters in high-risk surgical patients. N Engl J Med 384:5–14
8. Vieillard-Baron A, Prin S, Chergui K, Dubourg O, Jardin F (2002) Echo-Doppler demonstration of acute cor pulmonale at the bedside in the medical intensive care unit. Am J Respir Crit Care Med 166:1310–1319
9. Vieillard-Baron A, Prin S, Chergui K, Dubourg O, Jardin F (2003) Hemodynamic instability in sepsis. Bedside assessment by Doppler echocardiography. Am J Respir Crit Care Med 168:1270–1276
10. Mintz GS, Kotler MN, Parry WR, Iskandrian AS, Kane SA (1981) Real-time inferior vena cava ultrasonography: normal and abnormal findings in its use in assessing right-heart function. Circulation 64:1018–1025
11. Vieillard-Baron A, Augarde R, Prin S, Page B, Beauchet A, Jardin F (2001) Influence of superior vena caval zone condition on cyclic changes in right ventricular outflow during respiratory support. Anesthesiology 95:1083–1088
12. Lichtenstein D, Jardin F (1994) Appréciation non invasive de la pression veineuse centrale par la mesure échographique du calibre de la veine cave inférieure en réanimation. Réan Urg 3:79–82
13. Chergui K, Peyrouset O, Prin S, Rabiller A, Jardin F, Vieillard-Baron A (2003) Ability of superior and inferior vena cava diameter to predict central venous pressure. Intensive Care Med 29 (Suppl 1):S129 (abst)
14. Vieillard-Baron A, Chergui K, Rabiller A, et al (2004) Superior vena caval collapsibility as a gauge of volume status in ventilated septic patients. Intensive Care Med 30:1734–1739
15. Barbier C, Loubières Y, Schmit C, et al (2004) Respiratory changes in inferior vena cava diameter are helpful in predicting fluid responsiveness in ventilated septic patients. Intensive Care Med 30:1740–1746
16. Feissel M, Michard F, Faller JP, Teboul JL (2004) The respiratory variation in inferior vena cava diameter as a guide to fluid therapy. Intensive Care Med 30:1834–1837

17. Permutt S, Riley RL (1963) Hemodynamics of collapsible vessels with tone: the vascular waterfall. J Appl Physiol 18:924–932
18. Fessler II, Brower R, Wise R, Permutt S (1991) Effects of positive end-expiratory pressure on the gradient for venous return. Am Rev Respir Dis 145:19–24
19. Vieillard-Baron A, Chergui K, Augarde R, et al (2003) Cyclic changes in arterial pulse during respiratory support revisited by Doppler echocardiography. Am J Respir Crit Care Med 168:671–676
20. Coyle JP, Teplick RS, Long MC, Davison JK (1983) Respiratory variations in systemic arterial pressure as an indicator of volume status. Anesthesiology 59:A53 (abst)
21. Jardin F, Farcot JC, Gueret P, Prost JF, Ozier Y, Bourdarias JP (1983) Cyclic changes in arterial pulse during respiratory support. Circulation 68:266–274
22. Perel A, Pizov R, Cotev S (1987) Systolic blood pressure variation is a sensitive indicator of hypovolemia in ventilated dogs subjected to graded hemorrhage. Anesthesiology 67:498–502
23. Versprille A (1990) The pulmonary circulation during mechanical ventilation. Acta Anaesthesiol Scand 34:51–62
24. Vieillard-Baron A, Jardin F (2005) Authors' reply to Dr Miranda. Intensive Care Med (in press)
25. Takata M, Wise RA, Robotham JL (1990) Effect of abdominal pressure on venous return: abdominal vascular zone conditions. J Appl Physiol 69:1961–1972
26. Jardin F, Dubourg O, Margairaz A, Bourdarias JP (1987) Inspiratory impairment in right ventricular performance during acute asthma. Chest 92:789–795
27. Van Den Berg PC, Jansen JRC, Pinsky MR (2002) Effect of positive pressure on venous return in volume-loaded surgical patients. J Appl Physiol 92:1223–1231
28. Comolet R (1984) Biomécanique Circulatoire. Abrégé Masson, Paris, pp 36–53

Echo and PiCCO: Friends or Foe?

F. Michard

▌ Pulmonary Artery Catheter: The Swan's Song

The past few years have been marked by controversy regarding the benefit/risk ratio of pulmonary artery catheterization. After the study by Connors et al. [1] we have been recently reassured by two randomized controlled trials [2, 3]: the pulmonary artery catheter (PAC) does not increase mortality! However, its use is time-consuming [4], may increase morbity (thrombotic, infectious, and rhythmic complications) [2, 3, 5], and certainly does increase the cost of ICU care. The above mentioned studies [2, 3], which failed to demonstrate any beneficial effect in using the PAC, could be interpreted as a plea for giving up any form of hemodynamic monitoring.

However, in critically ill patients with hemodynamic instability, physical signs like hypotension, tachycardia, mottling, and low urine output, are unfortunately not specific of any pathophysiological disorder (e.g., hypovolemia, vasoplegia, or heart failure) [6–8]. In other words, in this particular context, relying only on clinical experience to determine therapy (e.g., volume loading, norepinephrine, or dobutamine) may too often consist of "making the same mistakes with increasing confidence over an impressive number of years"[1] . This is the reason why, even if hemodynamic monitoring has not been shown to be life-saving by a randomized controlled trial [9], most physicians still believe that information regarding cardiac preload, contractility, and output are of great value for the management of patients with shock. Therefore, they have turned their eyes towards two main alternative hemodynamic technologies: echocardiography-Doppler and transpulmonary thermodilution.

At first sight, these two techniques are quite different: echocardiography is non-invasive (transthoracic) or poorly-invasive (transesophageal) whereas transpulmonary thermodilution requires a central venous access and the cannulation of a big artery, usually femoral. Echo is particularly convenient for a snapshot of the hemodynamic situation at a given time but not appropriate for repetitive evaluations, i.e. for monitoring, while transpulmonary thermodilution measurements can be repeated as often as is necessary. Echo requires the experience of a skilled physician or technician (in the US) while transpulmonary thermodilution is definitely accessible to all caregivers (shooting a cold saline bolus through a central venous line does not require any specific training).

---

[1] The definition of clinical experience by O'Donnel M, in «A sceptic's medical dictionary», BMJ Publishing group, London, 1997, pp 27

Table 1. Comparison of echo with PiCCO

	ECHO	PiCCO
1. Invasiveness	–	± (depends on the context)
2. Reproducibility of measurements	–/+/++ (operator-dependent)	+++
3. Measurement of cardiac output	+++	+++
4. Volumetric assessment of cardiac preload	+++ (LVEDA)	++ (GEDV)
5. Prediction of fluid responsiveness	+++ (ΔVpeak, ΔD_{IVC})	+++ (PPV, SVV)
6. Cardiac function/contractility	++ (LVEF)	++ (GEF)
7. Detection of intracardiac shunts	+++ (contrast echo, color Doppler)	+++ (shape of the dilution curve)

LVEDA: left ventricular end-diastolic area; GEDV: global end-diastolic volume; ΔVpeak; respiratory changes in aortic peak velocity; ΔD_{IVC}: respiratory changes in inferior vena cava diameter; PPV: arterial pulse pressure variation; SVV: pulse contour stroke volume variation; LVEF: left ventricular ejection fraction; GEF: global ejection fraction

In fact, both technologies allow the assessment of cardiac output, the volumetric assessment of cardiac preload (a major step forward as compared to cardiac filling pressures), an accurate prediction of fluid responsiveness during mechanical ventilation, an estimation of cardiac function/contractility and the detection of intracardiac shunts (Table 1, Fig. 1).

The differences and similarities between echocardiography-Doppler and transpulmonary thermodilution are discussed in the present chapter before proposing an integrated use of both techniques.

▌ Invasive *versus* Non-invasive Technologies: The Wrong Debate?

Any hemodynamic monitoring technology requiring the use of either a central venous or an arterial access is considered as invasive, i.e., dangerous because it brings a risk of hemorrhagic, thrombotic and infectious complications, sometimes life-threatening. Transthoracic echocardiography is the perfect example of non-invasive technology since its use does not require the cannulation of any vessel. However, we must consider that most hemodynamically unstable patients are instrumented with a central venous line (e.g., for vasoactive agent administration) and with an arterial line for blood pressure monitoring and multiple blood samples, even if their hemodynamic evaluation is done by transthoracic echocardiography! Therefore, in this context, using transpulmonary thermodilution instead of echo does not bring any additional invasiveness. The only possible additional risks brought by the use of transpulmonary thermodilution could be the necessity to canulate a big artery and the extra-manipulations of the central venous line for cold bolus injections [10]. In fact, in contrast to venous access, there is no evidence that

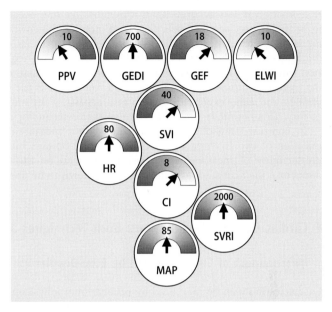

Fig. 1. Hemodynamic parameters provided by transpulmonary thermodilution. Arrows indicate normal values (white zone). PPV: pulse pressure variation (%); GEDI; global end-diastolic volume index (%); GEF: global ejection fraction (%); ELWI: extravascular lung water index (ml/kg); SVI: stroke volume index (ml/m^2); HR: heart rate (b/min); CI: cardiac index (l/min/m^2); SVRI: systemic vascular resistance index (dyne/cm^5/m^2); MAP: mean arterial pressure (mmHg). Preload (GEDI) and ejection fraction (GEF) determine stroke volume; stroke volume and heart rate determine cardiac output; cardiac output and vascular tone (SVRI) determine mean arterial pressure

femoral arterial access is associated with more frequent complications than other sites (radial, axillary) [11, 12]. The use of closed systems for cold saline injections (already currently used with PACs) should settle the potential risk of increasing infectious complications by manipulating the central venous line.

Feasibility and Reproducibility of Measurements: A Big Issue

Everybody recognizes the invaluable information and loves the direct and crystal clear (with transesophageal images) visualization of the heart provided by echocardiography-Doppler. However, an echo apparatus is not available in all intensive care units (ICUs). This seems to be particularly true in the US, where, for obvious billing reasons, many ICUs are not allowed to perform echo themselves and have to call the echo department. Moreover, everybody is not able to record echo parameters with a good reproducibility. Indeed, the use of this technology requires a specific and long training. Finally, it is now clearly recognized that even skilled operators cannot simply 'guesstimate' e.g., left ventricular ejection fraction (LVEF) [13]. Indeed, it has been shown that the 'eyeball' method for ejection fraction estimation carries normal subjects into the abnormal range, abnormal into the normal, and severely depressed into the moderate [13]! It is not surprising that a qualitative ejection fraction is less accurate than a quantitative one because echo has been found to be highly precise when specific two-dimensional algorithms are used [14]. Qualitative methods are further disadvantaged by the practice of enlarging and shrinking images to fit the screen that prevents readers from acquiring a sense of proportion from which to even roughly estimate left ventricular size [13]. In other words, the main limitations for using echo on a routine basis are the availability of the apparatus and echo experts, and the time necessary for an echo evaluation of good quality. This definitely precludes the use of this technology as a monitoring device.

In contrast, transpulmonary thermodilution measurements simply require the injection of two to three 10–20 ml cold saline boluses into a central vein. The reproducibility of measurements does not depend on the operator (who can be a nurse or a medical student), and has been shown to be about 4–5% [15, 16].

▌ Cardiac Output Measurement: Both Techniques are Accurate

Measurement of Cardiac Output by Echo-Doppler

Cardiac output can be measured by echocardiography-Doppler in a number of ways that can be divided into volumetric and Doppler-based methods [17]. Using measurements of left ventricular volume made at end systole and end diastole, the stroke volume (end-diastolic minus end-systolic volume) and hence the cardiac output can be estimated. The two main limitations of the volumetric method are resolution and geometry. The resolution of two-dimensional echocardiography is about 1 mm [17]. In a comparison of echocardiography-derived stroke volume with thermodilution, a 10% change in stroke volume corresponded to only a 0.7 mm change in ventricular radius [18]. Geometric assumptions rely on smooth circular or elliptical shapes. The ventricle is assumed to contract uniformly, which may not occur, even without regional wall motion abnormalities. Extrapolation from areas to volumes adds further errors. These are probably the reasons why volumetric-based methods showed only a poor agreement with Doppler methods [19]. Several studies have investigated the value of Doppler methods for measurement of cardiac output at the level of each of the valves. All of these techniques require measurement of the diameter at a particular cardiac level and Doppler measurements to obtain the time-velocity integrals. Cardiac output measurements at the level of the left ventricular outflow tract have generally been easier to obtain and are accurate [20–22]. Measurements are obtained by placing the sample volume in the middle of the outflow tract immediately proximal to the leaflets of the aortic valve. The diameter (D) of the left ventricular outflow tract is also measured and the cross-sectional area calculated as $\pi \times (D/2)^2$. By integrating blood velocity over time (time-velocity integral) and multiplying this parameter by the cross-sectional area, one obtains stroke volume. The product of stroke volume by heart rate gives cardiac output. In patients whose lungs are mechanically ventilated, significant (>20%) beat-by-beat variations in aortic blood flow can be observed during the respiratory cycle. In this context, the mean cardiac output will be more accurately estimated if all time-velocity integrals are considered over a single respiratory cycle. Indeed, taking into account the highest time-velocity integral (as frequently done) would result in a significant overestimation of cardiac output. Alternative methods have been proposed to measure cardiac output at the level of the mitral or pulmonary valves. Doppler determination of cardiac output with the use of mitral velocity recordings assumes a circular shape of the mitral orifice and constant area during diastole; both of these assumptions may cause considerable inaccuracy [23]. The lack of clear visual definition of the pulmonic valve hampers accurate measurement of its diameter and limits its utility in the determination of cardiac output; moreover, the considerable change in pulmonary valve cross-sectional area seen during systole partly accounts for the inaccuracy of cardiac output measurements at the level of this valve [24].

Measurement of Cardiac Output by Transpulmonary Thermodilution

After injection of a cold saline bolus central venously, a thermistor in the tip of the arterial catheter (usually femoral) is used to measure the downstream temperature changes. The cardiac output is then calculated by the analysis of the thermodilution curve using a modified Stewart-Hamilton algorithm. The measurement of cardiac output by transpulmonary thermodilution has been validated by many clinical studies as compared to pulmonary artery thermodilution and the Fick method both in children and adult patients [25–31].

Compared to echocardiography, thermodilution has frequently been criticized because of the possible influence of tricuspid regurgitation on the accuracy of measurements [32]. However, most validation studies [20–22] of cardiac output measurements by echo-Doppler have been performed against the pulmonary thermodilution technique and showed excellent agreement between the two techniques! Moreover, a recent *in vivo* study clearly showed that neither the accuracy nor the precision of thermal dilution cardiac output measurements is altered by acute tricuspid regurgitation [33]. Similar findings are therefore expected regarding cardiac output measurements by transpulmonary thermodilution in case of valvular insufficiency.

▌ Cardiac Preload: Both Techniques Provide Volumetric Parameters

Because the so-called cardiac filling pressures (central venous pressure [CVP], right atrial pressure, pulmonary artery occlusion pressure [PAOP]) are influenced by external positive end-expiratory pressure (PEEP), intrinsic PEEP, abdominal pressure, and myocardial compliance, they cannot be used to accurately assess cardiac preload, i.e., the volume of blood contained by both ventricles at end-diastole. Echocardiography provides information regarding left ventricular preload while transpulmonary thermodilution provides information regarding the filling of the whole heart.

Assessment of Cardiac Preload using Echo

The left ventricular end-diastolic area (LVEDA) is the most common parameter used to assess left ventricular preload at the bedside [34, 35]. The normal values range between 5 and 15 cm^2/m^2. Clements et al. [36] have reported a good relationship (r = 0.86) between LVEDA and left ventricular end-diastolic volume (LVEDV) assessed by radionuclide angiography while in contrast, Urbanowicz et al. [37] concluded that LVEDA does not provide a reasonable estimate of LVEDV. Conflicting results have also been published regarding the accuracy of LVEDA changes to track effective changes in preload. In patients undergoing cardiac surgery, Cheung et al. [38] showed that LVEDA is a parameter very sensitive to acute graded hemorrhage in patients undergoing surgery, whereas Axler et al. [39] failed to detect any significant change in LVEDA in response to typical rapid volume infusions in critically ill patients.

Assessment of Cardiac Preload using Transpulmonary Thermodilution

It has been known for a long time that when an indicator is injected into a system composed of several mixing chambers, the mathematical analysis of a dilution curve recorded at the system's exit allows the calculation of the total and the largest volumes of distribution of the indicator [40, 41]. Indeed, the product of the mean transit time of the indicator by the flow crossing the system gives the total volume of the system; the product of the exponential downslope time by the flow gives the volume of the largest mixing chamber [40, 41]. Applying these mathematical concepts to human physiology allows the estimation of a fraction of the intrathoracic blood volume, called the global end-diastolic volume (GEDV). Details regarding the calculation of this volume have been described elsewhere [16, 42]. The normal values for the GEDV index range between 600 and 800 ml/m^2. Importantly, the GEDV has been shown to behave as a true indicator of cardiac preload: it increases with fluid loading but not with dobutamine, and its increase following fluid loading is correlated with the increase in stroke volume (consistent with the physiological relationship between preload and stroke volume) [16, 43, 44]. Because the GEDV depends not only on ventricular blood volumes, but also on atrial and aortic blood volumes, supranormal values are observed in patients with left atrial dilation or aortic aneurysm [45].

▌ Prediction of Fluid Responsiveness: Both Techniques Provide Dynamic Parameters

Volumetric indicators of cardiac preload (LVEDA and GEDV) are useful to assess the effects of therapeutic interventions (e.g., fluid loading) on preload [46] but not to predict the effects of a preload change on stroke volume and cardiac output [47]. In contrast, dynamic parameters, e.g., the respiratory variation in arterial pulse pressure induced by mechanical ventilation, have been shown to be very helpful in identifying patients who may benefit from volume expansion [48–50] or may experience the deleterious hemodynamic effects of PEEP [51].

Prediction of Fluid Responsiveness using the PiCCO

The arterial pulse pressure variation (PPV) over a short period of a few seconds, a parameter very close to the respiratory changes in arterial pulse pressure, is automatically calculated and displayed by the PiCCO monitor. In addition, the PiCCO monitor directly measures the left ventricular stroke volume by pulse contour analysis [52]. The algorithm used analyses the shape and the area under each stroke and uses mean stroke volume derived from transpulmonary thermodilution cardiac output (the so-called calibration) to calculate the actual patient specific arterial compliance and impedance. Then compliance, impedance and the incremental changes of arterial pressure waveform yield beat-by-beat pulse contour stroke volume and continuous cardiac output. Thus, the PiCCO monitor is able to provide the continuous calculation of the stroke volume variation (SVV), which is defined as the percentage change in stroke volume over a floating period of 7.5 seconds. The pulse contour SVV has been shown to be related to the hemodynamic effects of volume expansion (the higher the SVV, the greater the increase in cardiac output) in patients undergoing brain surgery [53], in the post-operative period of cardiac surgery [54–56] and in patients with septic shock [57]. Which parameter (PPV or SVV) should be used preferentially to predict fluid responsivenss remains to be determined: from a physiological point of view SVV should be better than a surrogate like PPV, but until now better results have been reported using PPV [58].

Prediction of Fluid Responsiveness using Echo-Doppler

The respiratory variation in peak velocity of aortic blood flow (ΔVpeak) can be quantified at the level of the aortic annulus using transesophageal echocardiography (TEE) [59]. This dynamic parameter has been shown to be very useful in discriminating between responder (in whom ΔVpeak is usually greater than 12%) and non-responder (in whom ΔVpeak is usually lower than 12%) patients to a volume load [59]. During TEE, the respiratory variation in superior vena cava diameter can be quantified and is also a good predictor of fluid responsiveness [50]. A much more simple method consists of assessing the respiratory variation in inferior vena cava diameter (ΔD_{IVC}) using transparietal time-motion echocardiography [60]. In mechanically ventilated patients with septic shock, we recently demonstrated that

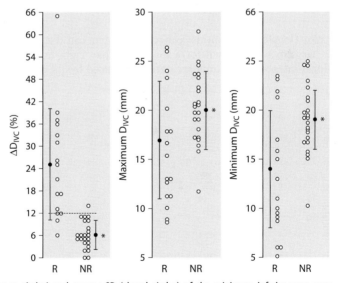

Fig. 2. Individual values (open circles) and mean$\pm$SD (closed circles) of the minimum inferior vena cava diameter (D_{IVC}), maximum D_{IVC} and respiratory variation in D_{IVC} (ΔD_{IVC}) before volume loading in responder (R) and non-responder (NR) patients. ΔD_{IVC} differentiated responders and non-responders while maximum and minimum D_{IVC} did not. * $p < 0.05$ R vs NR. From [60] with permission

when the ΔD_{IVC} is greater than 12%, a positive response to volume expansion is very likely. Conversely, when ΔD_{IVC} is lower than 12%, a positive response is very unlikely (Fig. 2) [60].

∎ Estimation of Cardiac Function/contractility

Accurate bedside assessment of cardiac contractility has recently been compared to the Graal quest since all hemodynamic parameters are more or less dependent on afterload and preload conditions [61]. Nevertheless, the ventricular ejection fraction, which is the ratio of stroke volume to ventricular end-diastolic volume, is commonly used to assess ventricular function [62]. Using echocardiography, the LVEF can be measured by estimating the end-diastolic (LVEDV) and end-systolic (LVESV) volumes as LVEF = (LVEDV–LVESV)/LVEDV. Because ventricular volumes are frequently extrapolated from area, the fractional area of change (FAC), calculated as (LVEDA–LVESA)/LVEDA is also widely used to assess left ventricular function at the bedside. Transpulmonary thermodilution allows the simultaneous measurement of stroke volume and GEDV. The ratio of stroke volume to a quarter of the GEDV (since the GEDV is the volume of blood virtually contained in four heart chambers) has been called global ejection fraction (GEF) of the heart. This parameter, automaticaly calculated and displayed by the PiCCO monitor, may be used to identify patients with right or/and left ventricular dysfunction. A recent study by Combes et al. [63] showed, in patients free of right ventricular dysfunction, that the GEF is closely correlated with the left ventricular FAC. In this study, a GEF greater than 18% was useful to identify patients with a FAC greater than 40% with a sensitivity of 88% and a specificity of 79% (Fig. 3).

∎ Detection of Intracardiac or Vascular Shunts

Color Doppler and contrast echocardiography can diagnose intracardiac shunt [64]. It has also been known for a long time than right-to-left, left-to-right, or bidirectional intracardiac shunts are easily evidenced by the visual inspection of transpul-

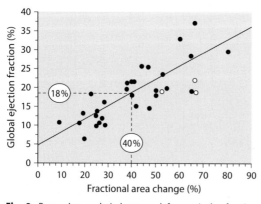

Fig. 3. Regression analysis between left ventricular fractional area change assessed by echocardiography (x axis) and the global ejection fraction assessed by transpulmonary thermodilution. Most patients with left ventricular dysfunction (FAC < 40%) have a GEF lower than 18%. From [63] with permission

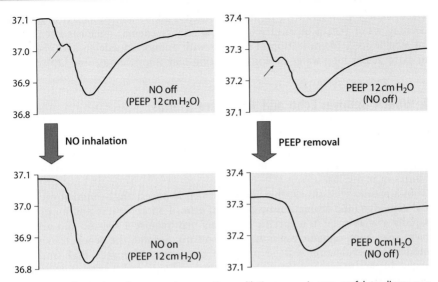

Fig. 4. The mere observation of a transpulmonary thermodilution curve is very useful to diagnose a right-to-left intracardiac shunt (small black arrow, premature hump indicating a right-to-left intracardiac shunt) and to monitor the effects of nitric oxide (NO) inhalation and positive end-expiratory pressure (PEEP) removal on this phenomenon. From [67] with permission

monary indicator dilution curves: most congenital heart diseases have been described using the dilution of indocyanine green [65]! In case of right-to-left intracardiac shunting (usually due to the opening of a patent foramen ovale), one part of the indicator passes through the atrial septum and rapidly reaches the femoral arterial thermistor. As a result, the transpulmonary dilution curve appears prematurely and becomes biphasic (Fig. 4). A left-to-right intracardiac shunt is responsible for early recirculation of the indicator, and a bidirectional shunt induces both early appearance and early recirculation of the indicator (premature and triphasic curve) [66]. Early recognition of a right-to-left shunt may have therapeutic implications such as nitric oxide (NO) inhalation or PEEP decrease/removal [67]. The efficacy of these maneuvers can be immediately assessed using a single cold saline bolus (Fig. 4) [67]. Formulas have been proposed to quantify right-to-left intracardiac shunt from the mathematical analysis of transpulmonary dilution curves [66] and hopefully will be implemented on the PiCCO monitor in the near future.

Extra-features

This chapter has deliberately focused on 7 major features of echo and PiCCO technologies (Table 1) [68]. However, other valuable parameters and information are provided by both technologies. I will simply mention the fact that echo provides invaluable anatomical and functional information regarding pericardial and valvular diseases, thrombo-embolic processes, and left ventricular wall motion abnormalities. In some instances, this information can lead to specific and urgent treatments (e.g., thrombolysis for acute massive pulmonary embolism, surgery for endocarditis). Regarding transpulmonary thermodilution, I will mention the fact that the mathematical analysis of the dilution curve also allows an estimation of extravascular lung water (i.e., a quantification of pulmonary edema), that has been shown to be reliable [69]. Identification of patients with pulmonary edema and manipulation of extravscular lung water in this population may improve outcome [70].

■ What I Believe: Echo and PiCCO are friends

A decision tree for the hemodynamic evaluation of critically ill patients using echo and PiCCO is proposed in Figure 5. This strategy takes into account not only the respective advantages of both technologies but also the logistic and realistic possibilities of many ICUs.

In a patient with shock, the cause of which is uncertain, I would suggest starting the hemodynamic evaluation by doing an echo if an apparatus and an operator are rapidly available. First, a specific diagnosis may require a specific and urgent treatment (e.g., tamponnade, pulmonary embolism). Second, the echocardiographic hemodynamic evaluation will be useful to discriminate between high and low flow states; in case of low flow state, between hypovolemia and heart failure; and in case of heart failure between right and left ventricular dysfunction. If monitoring is required after this first evaluation, PiCCO technology will be very useful to assess cardiac output, cardiac preload, fluid responsiveness and GEF (that will be interpretated in the light of echo findings) as often as is necessary.

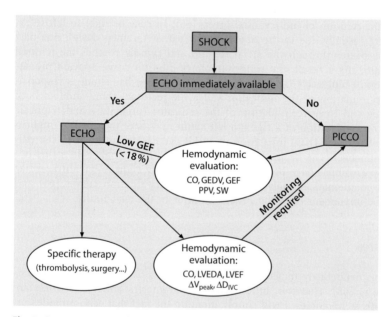

Fig. 5. Proposal of decision tree for the hemodynamic evaluation and monitoring of patients with shock (which cause is uncertain) using Echo and transpulmonary thermodilution (PiCCO). PPV: pulse pressure variation; GEDV: global end-diastolic volume; GEF: global ejection fraction; SVV: stroke volume variation; CO: cardiac output; SVRI: systemic vascular resistance index (dyne/cm^5/m^2); MAP: mean arterial pressure (mmHg)

If an echo is not rapidly available, PiCCO technology will be useful to identify patients who may benefit from a agonists (high cardiac output = vasoplegic states), volume loading (low GEDV ± high PPV), and β agonists (low GEF). Even if β agonists may be useful both in right and left ventricular failure, if the GEF is low, an echo can be useful to identify the cause of ventricular dysfunction and improve the therapeutic strategy (e.g., pulmonary vasodilators or/and less aggressive mechanical ventilation in case of right ventricular failure, systemic vasodilators or/and coronary reperfusion in case of left ventricular failure). After the identification of heart failure mechanism, GEF trends will be useful to monitor the effectiveness of the selected therapy.

In other words, echo appears to be the best diagnostic tool while PiCCO is the best monitoring tool: echo and PiCCO are friends and can/should be used in combination.

References

1. Connors AF Jr, Speroff T, Dawson NV, et al (1996) The effectiveness of right heart catheterization in the initial care of critically ill patients. SUPPORT Investigators. JAMA 276:889–897
2. Sandham JD, Hull RD, Brant RF, et al (2003) A randomized, controlled trial of the use of pulmonary artery catheters in high-risk surgical patients. N Engl J Med 348:5–14
3. Richard C, Warszawski J, Anguel N, et al (2003) Early use of the pulmonary artery catheter and outcomes in patients with shock and acute respiratory distress syndrome. JAMA 290:2713–2720
4. Lefrant JY, Muller L, Bruelle P, et al (2000) Insertion time of the pulmonary artery catheter in critically ill patients. Crit Care Med 28:355–359
5. Polanczyk CA, Rohde LE, Goldman L, et al (2001) Right heart catheterization and cardiac complications in patient undergoing noncardiac surgery: an observational study. JAMA 286:309–314
6. Shippy CR, Appel PL, Shoemaker WC (1984) Reliability of clinical monitoring to assess blood volume in critically ill patients. Crit Care Med 12:107–112
7. Wo CC, Shoemaker WC, Appel PL, Bishop MH, Kram HB, Hardin E (1993) Unreliability of blood pressure and heart rate to evaluate cardiac output in emergency resuscitation and critical illness. Crit Care Med 21:218–223
8. Michard F, Ruscio L, Teboul JL (2001) Clinical prediction of fluid responsiveness in acute circulatory failure related to sepsis. Intensive Care Med 27:1238
9. Smith GCS, Pell JP (2003) Parachute use to prevent death and major trauma related to gravitational challenge: systematic review of randomized controlled trials. BMJ 327:1459–1461
10. Polderman KH, Girbes AR (2002) Central venous catheter use. Part 2: infectious complications. Intensive Care Med 28:18–28
11. Gurman GM, Kriemerman S (1985) Cannulation of big arteries in critically ill patients. Crit Care Med 13:217–220
12. Scheer BV, Perel A, Pfeiffer UJ (2002) Clinical review: complications and risk factors of peripheral arterial catheters used for haemodynamic monitoring in anaesthesia and intensive care medicine. Crit Care 6:199–204
13. Schiller NB (2003) Ejection fraction by echocardiography: the full monty or just a peep show? Am Heart J 146:380–382
14. Weiss JL, Eaton LW, Kallman CH, Maughan WL (1983) Accuracy of volume determination by two-dimensional echocardiography: defining requirements under controlled conditions in the ejection canine left ventricle. Circulation 67:889–895
15. Godje O, Peyerl M, Seebauer T, Dewald O, Reichart B (1998) Reproducibility of double indicator dilution measurements of intrathoracic blood volume compartments, extravascular lung water, and liver function. Chest 113:1070–1077
16. Michard F, Alaya S, Zarka V, Bahloul M, Richard C, Teboul JL (2003) Global end-diastolic volume as an indicator of cardiac preload in patients with septic shock. Chest 124:1900–1908

17. Brown JM (2002) Use of echocardiography for hemodynamic monitoring. Crit Care Med 30:1361–1364

18. Axler O, Tousignant C, Thompson CR, et al (1996) Comparison of transesophageal echocardiographic, fick, and thermodilution cardiac output in critically ill patients. J Crit Care 11:109–116

19. Axler O, Megarbane B, Lentschener C, et al (2003) Comparison of cardiac output measured with echocardiographic volumes and aortic Doppler methods during mechanical ventilation. Intensive Care Med 29:208–217

20. Stoddard MF, Prince CR, Ammash N, et al (1993) Pulsed Doppler transesophageal echocardiographic determination of cardiac output in human beings: comparison with thermodilution technique. Am Heart J 126:956–962

21. Feinberg MS, Hopkins WE, Davila-Roman VG, Barzilai B (1995) Multiplane transesophageal echocardiographic Doppler imaging accurately determines cardiac output measurements in critically ill patients. Chest 107:769–773

22. Descorps-Declere A, Smail N, Vigue B, et al (1996) Transgastric, pulsed Doppler echocardiographic determination of cardiac output. Intensive Care Med 22:34–38

23. Ormiston JA, Shah PM, Tei C, et al (1981) Size and motion of the mitral valve annulus in man. I. A two-dimensional echocardiographic method and findings in normal subjects. Circulation 64:113–120

24. Stewart WJ, Jiang L, Mich R, Pandian N, Guerrero JL, Weyman AE (1985) Variable effects of changes in flow rate through the aortic, pulmonary and mitral valves on valve area and flow velocity: impact on quantitative Doppler flow calculations. J Am Coll Cardiol 6:653–662

25. Sakka SG, Reinhart K, Meier-Hellmann A (1999) Comparison of pulmonary artery and arterial thermodilution cardiac output in critically ill patients. Intensive Care Med 25:843–846

26. Goedje O, Hoeke K, Lichtwarck-Aschoff M, et al (1999) Continuous cardiac output by femoral arterial thermodilution calibrated pulse contour analysis: comparison with pulmonary arterial thermodilution. Crit Care Med 27:2407–2412

27. Goedje O, Seebauer T, Peyerl M, Pfeiffer UJ, Reichart B (2000) Hemodynamic monitoring by double-indicator dilution technique in patients after orthotopic heart transplantation. Chest 118:775–781

28. McLuckie A, Marsh M, Murdoch I, et al (1996) A comparison of pulmonary and femoral artery thermodilution cardiac indices in paediatric intensive care patients. Acta Paediatr 85:336–338

29. Tibby SM, Hatherill M, Marsh MJ, et al (1997) Clinical validation of cardiac output measurements using femoral artery thermodilution with direct Fick in ventilated children and infants. Intensive Care Med 23:987–991

30. Sakka SG, Reinhart K, Wegscheider K, et al (2000) Is the placement of a pulmonary artery catheter still justified solely for the measurement of cardiac output. J Cardiothorac Vasc Anesth 14:119–124

31. Pauli C, Fakler U, Genz T, et al (2002) Cardiac output determination in children: equivalence of the transpulmonary thermodilution method to the direct Fick principle. Intensive Care Med 28:947–952

32. Jardin F (1997) PEEP, tricuspid regurgitation, and cardiac output. Intensive Care Med 23:806–807

33. Buffington CW, Nystrom EUM (2004) Neither the accuracy nor the precision of thermal dilution cardiac output measurements is altered by acute tricuspid regurgitation in pigs. Anesth Analg 98:884–890

34. Thys DM, Hillel Z, Goldman ME, Mindich BP, Kaplan JA (1987) A comparison of hemodynamic indices derived by invasive monitoring and two-dimensional echocardiography. Anesthesiology 67:630–634

35. Tousignant CP, Walsh F, Mazer CD (2000) The use of transesophageal echocardiography for preload assessment in critically ill patients. Anesth Analg 90:351–355

36. Clements FM, Harpole DH, Quill T, Jones RH, McCann RL (1990) Estimation of left ventricular volume and ejection fraction by two-dimensional transoesophageal echocardiography: comparison of short axis imaging and simultaneous radionuclide angiography. Br J Anaesth 64:331–336

37. Urbanowicz JH, Shaaban MJ, Cohen NH, et al (1990) Comparison of transesophageal echo-cardiographic and scintigraphic estimates of left ventricular end-diastolic volume index and ejection fraction in patients following coronary artery bypass grafting. Anesthesiology 72:607–612

38. Cheung AT, Savino JS, Weiss SJ, et al (1994) Echocardiographic and hemodynamic indexes of left ventricular preload in patients with normal and abnormal ventricular function. Anesthesiology 81:376–387

39. Axler O, Tousignant C, Thompson CR, et al (1997) Small hemodynamic effect of typical rapid volume infusions in critically ill patients. Crit Care Med 25:965–970

40. Meier P, Zierler KL (1954) On the theory of indicator-dilution method for measurement of blood flow and volume. J Appl Physiol 6:731–744

41. Newman EV, Merrel M, Genecin A, et al (1951) The dye dilution method for describing the central circulation. An analysis of factors shaping the time-concentration curves. Circulation 4:735–746

42. Sakka SG, Rühl CC, Pfeiffer UJ, et al (2000) Assessment of cardiac preload and extravascular lung water by single transpulmonary thermodilution. Intensive Care Med 26:180–187

43. Wiesenack C, Prasser C, Keyl C, et al (2001) Assessment of intrathoracic blood volume as an indicator of cardiac preload: single transpulmonary thermodilution technique versus assessment of pressure preload parameters derived from a pulmonary artery catheter. J Cardiothorac Vasc Anesth 15:584–588

44. Reuter DA, Felbinger TW, Moerstedt K, et al (2002) Intrathoracic blood volume index measured by thermodilution for preload monitoring after cardiac surgery. J Cardiothorac Vasc Anesth 16:191–195

45. Sakka SG, Meier-Hellmann A (2001) Extremely high values of intrathoracic blood volume in critically ill patients. Intensive Care Med 27:1677–1678

46. Michard F (2004) Do we need to know cardiac preload? In: Vincent JL (ed) Yearbook of Intensive Care and Emergency Medicine. Springer, Heidelberg, pp 694–701

47. Michard F, Teboul JL (2002) Predicting fluid responsiveness in ICU patients. A critical analysis of the evidence. Chest 121:2000–2008

48. Michard F, Boussat S, Chemla D, et al (2000) Relation between respiratory changes in arterial pulse pressure and fluid responsiveness in septic patients with acute circulatory failure. Am J Respir Crit Care Med 162:134–138

49. Bendjelid K, Suter PM, Romand JA (2004) The respiratory change in preejection period: a new method to predict fluid responsiveness. J Appl Physiol 96:337–342

50. Vieillard-Baron A, Chergui K, Rabiller A, et al (2004) Superior vena caval collapsibility as a gauge of volume status in ventilated septic patients. Intensive Care Med 30:1734–1739

51. Michard F, Chemla D, Richard C, et al (1999) Clinical use of respiratory changes in arterial pulse pressure to monitor the hemodynamic effects of PEEP. Am J Respir Crit Care Med 159:935–939

52. Goedje O, Hoeke K, Goetz AE, et al (2002) Reliability of a new algorithm for continuous cardiac output determination by pulse-contour analysis during hemodynamic instability. Crit Care Med 30:52–58

53. Berkenstadt H, Margalit N, Hadani M, et al (2001) Stroke volume variation as a predictor of fluid responsiveness in patients undergoing brain surgery. Anesth Analg 92:984–989

54. Reuter DA, Kirchner A, Felbinger TW, Schmidt C, Lamm P, Goetz AE (2002) Optimising fluid therapy in mechanically ventilated patients after cardiac surgery by on-line monitoring of left ventricular stroke volume variations: a comparison to aortic systolic pressure variations. Br J Anesth 88:124–126

55. Reuter DA, Felbinger TW, Schmidt C, et al (2002) Stroke volume variations for assessment of cardiac responsiveness to volume loading in mechanically ventilated patients after cardiac surgery. Intensive Care Med 28:392–398

56. Reuter DA, Kirchner A, Felbinger TW, et al (2003) Usefulness of left ventricular stroke volume variation to assess fluid responsiveness in patients with reduced cardiac function. Crit Care Med 31:1399–1404

57. Marx G, Cope T, McCrossan L, et al (2004) Assessing fluid responsiveness by stroke volume variation in mechanically ventilated patients with severe sepsis. Eur J Anaesth 21:132–138

58. Michard F, Schmidt U (2004) Prediction of fluid responsiveness: searching for the Holy Grail. J Appl Physiol 97:790–791
59. Feissel M, Michard F, Mangin I, et al (2001) Respiratory changes in aortic blood velocity as an indicator of fluid responsiveness in ventilated patients with septic shock. Chest 119:867–873
60. Feissel M, Michard F, Faller JP, et al (2004) The respiratory variation in inferior vena cava diameter as a guide to fluid therapy. Intensive Care Med 30:1834–1837
61. Nitenberg A (2004) Evaluation of left ventricular performance: an insolvable problem in human beings? The Graal quest. Intensive Care Med 30:1258–1260
62. Robotham JL, Takata M, Berman M, et al (1991) Ejection fraction revisited. Anesthesiology 74:172–183
63. Combes A, Berneau JB, Luyt CE, et al (2004) Estimation of left ventricular systolic function by single transpulmonary thermodilution. Intensive Care Med 30:1377–1383
64. Konstadt SN, Louie EK, Black S, et al (1991) Intraoperative detection of patent foramen ovale by transesophageal echocardiography. Anesthesiology 74:212–216
65. Swan HJC, Zapata-Diaz J, Wood EH (1953) Dye dilution curves in cyanotic congenital heart disease. Circulation 8:70–81
66. Krovetz LJ (1974) Detection and quantification of intracardiac and great vessel shunts. In: Bloomfield DA (ed) Dye Curves: The Theory and Practice of Indicator Dilution. University Park Press, Baltimore, pp 119–143
67. Michard F, Alaya S, Medkour F (2004) Monitoring right-to-left intracardiac shunt in acute respiratory distress syndrome. Crit Care Med 32:308–309
68. Miller G (1956) The magical number seven, plus or minus two: some limits on our capacity for processing information. Psychol Rev 63:81–97
69. Katzenelson R, Perel A, Berkenstadt H, et al (2004) Accuracy of transpulmonary thermo-dilution versus gravimetric measurement of extravascular lung water. Crit Care Med 32:1550–1554
70. Mitchell JP, Schuller D, Calandrino FS, et al (1992) Improved outcome based on fluid management in critically ill patients requiring pulmonary artery catheterization. Am Rev Respir Dis 145:990–998

Lithium Dilution Cardiac Output and Arterial Pulse Power Analysis

J. Maynar, M. Jonas, and F. Labaien

▌ Introduction

Clinicians frequently have to deal with the hemodynamics of unstable patients and commonly rely on the measurement of blood pressure to give an index of cardiac output and perfusion. The fact that blood pressure is used as a surrogate for flow, despite the absence of a correlation between observed changes in blood pressure and changes in cardiac output, is a testament to the ease of measuring blood pressure and the technical difficulty of estimating cardiac output. These difficulties create the common problem of delivering a treatment on the basis of a guess of the actual blood flow. Arterial pressure measurements, in combination with clinical and laboratory assessment are frequently employed as surrogates for cardiac output measurement in sick patients. The effects of using this hemodynamic strategy with respect to clinical outcome are now becoming clearer in the critically ill and underline the clinician's problem: Does the patient require filling or inotropic drugs, vasodilators or vasoconstrictors?

This inability to guess the global cardiac output accurately without actually measuring it has lead to research and the development of less complicated methods to measure cardiac output. The critical issue for any cardiac output measurement device is the additional risk to the patient to obtaining a flow measurement. This is the major factor generating concern over pulmonary artery catheterization [1, 2] and also the motivation behind the development of alternative, less invasive techniques. This chapter will describe the pulse power analysis method of cardiac output estimation which relies on lithium dilution to calibrate the arterial waveform analysis algorithm.

In the late 19th century, Adolph Fick described how the changes in the concentration of a substance dissolved in blood could be used as an indicator for determining the blood flow. The concept of determining blood flow over time (cardiac output) by measuring the dilution of a known substance in the blood has become known as the Fick principle. Historically, indocyanine green (ICG) was the dye that was used, but this technique for many reasons was never adopted into clinical practice. In the early 1970s, Bradley developed the concept of pulmonary artery thermodilution which was subsequently commercialized by Swann and Ganz [3, 4]. Pulmonary artery catheterization and cardiac output measurement using the thermodilution technique remains the most common approach in use today. This is largely due to its longevity in the critical care arena and it is because of this familiarity that the pulmonary artery catheter (PAC) is considered to be the 'gold standard' against which newer devices are assessed. It is a technique not without risk and the measurements have poor repeatability [5]. Numerous complications of

Table 1. Properties of the ideal monitor

▌ Minimally invasive and therefore widely applicable
▌ Accurate
▌ Real time: beat-to-beat cardiac output
▌ Real time: preload + afterload
▌ Real time: oxygen delivery
▌ Nurse driven
▌ Clear data display and interpretation
▌ Bedside information management
▌ Neonates to adults

PACs have been described and include arterial puncture, pneumothorax, dysrhythmias, perforation of chamber of the heart, tamponade, valve damage, pulmonary artery rupture, and catheter knotting [6, 7]. Randomized controlled clinical trials relating to the usage of PACs have been equivocal and suspicions remain that these catheters may be related to an increase in mortality [3]. It is difficult to formally assess whether some reports of excess mortality are due to the catheters themselves or as a result of the treatment based on the measurements obtained, although evidence is accumulating that the catheter is probably not the cause, but the way the data is interpreted. In a recent study investigating the use of diuretics in the ICU population, the PAC was identified as a possible independent variable that may improve the prognosis of critically ill patients with acute renal failure [8].

The importance of early and close monitoring of the critically ill, and the outcome benefits of early goal-directed resuscitation [9], supports the clinical consensus for the need to develop new cardiac output technology which is safe, reliable, reproducible, and simple to use. Such a device would have significant advantages over the use of PACs and provides the concept of the ideal monitor (Table 1).

Currently no monitor fulfils all these criteria but novel technologies have been developed which are less invasive and utilize existing vascular access and biodynamic data. The LiDCO™*plus* system (LiDCO Ltd, Cambridge, UK) is such a device. The arterial line waveform is analyzed using a proprietary algorithm, which is calibrated using a novel indicator dilution technique.

▌ Scientific Basis

LiDCO™*plus* is a minimally invasive continuous cardiac output monitor, which uses an indicator (Lithium Dilution Cardiac Output) dilution technique to calibrate an arterial waveform analysis algorithm. The technique is quick and simple, requiring only an arterial line and central, or peripheral, venous access. These lines would probably already have been inserted in critical care patients.

A small dose of lithium chloride is injected as an intravenous bolus and cardiac output is derived from the dilution curve generated by a lithium-sensitive electrode attached to the arterial line. Studies in humans and animals have shown good agreement compared to results obtained by other techniques and its efficacy in pediatrics has also been proven. Compared with thermodilution, lithium dilution showed closer agreement in clinical studies with electromagnetic flow measurement. The lithium dilution technique is then used to calibrate an algorithm, which provides beat-to-beat cardiac output from analysis of the arterial waveform. This algorithm is not morphology dependent but rather calculates nominal stroke volume from a pressure-volume transform of the entire waveform. The nominal stroke volume is converted to actual stroke volume by calibration of the algorithm with LiDCO.

▌ Lithium Indicator Dilution Cardiac Output

The use of lithium as the indicator for the dilution technique for the measurement of cardiac output was first described in 1993 [10] and has now been extensively validated [11]. Isotonic lithium chloride (150 mM) is injected as a bolus (0.002–0.004 mmol/kg) via the central, or peripheral venous route and a concentration-time curve generated by an arterial ion selective electrode attached to the arterial line manometer system. The cardiac output is calculated from the lithium dose and the area under the concentration time curve prior to recirculation [12] using equation 1.

$$\text{Cardiac output} = \text{lithium dose} \times 60/\text{Area} \times (1 - \text{PCV})\ \text{l/min} \tag{1}$$

where lithium dose is in mmol, the area is the integral of the primary curve, and PCV is the packed cell volume which can be calculated as hemoglobin concentration (g/dl)/34 (this correction is needed because lithium is distributed in the plasma).

Lithium is safe, non-toxic in small doses, and easy to measure using an ion selective electrode. The operating characteristics of ion-sensitive electrodes enables the use of an extremely small dose of lithium, since the voltage response is to percentage change of ion concentration and lithium is not normally present in the plasma. Lithium chloride also satisfies a critical boundary condition for indicator dilution theory as there is no significant first pass loss from the circulation and it is rapidly redistributed. A study in patients comparing measurements of LiDCO using right or left atrial injection of lithium showed that there was no significant loss of lithium during its passage through the pulmonary circulation. [13]. The pharmacokinetics of intravenous lithium chloride have been closely investigated. [13]. The bolus dose of lithium for cardiac output determination (0.15–0.3 mmol in adults) is too small to have a pharmacological effect and the manufacturer's maximum recommended total dose (3 mmol) would have to be exceeded many times before toxic levels are achieved.

The basic component of the lithium indicator dilution system is the sensor (Fig. 1), which comprises a lithium sensitive electrode situated in a flow-through cell. This electrode is disposable and sterilized by gamma irradiation. It is attached to the arterial manometer line via a three way tap (Fig. 2) which when open allows blood to flow through the sensor assembly at 4 ml/min. This is rate limited by a peristaltic, battery-powered pump. The flow-through cell is made of polycarbonate and designed with an eccentric inlet so that blood swirls past the tip of the electrode. The electrode contains a membrane, which is selectively permeable to lithium. The voltage across the membrane is related by the Nernst equation to the plasma lithium concentration. A correction is applied for plasma sodium concentration because in the absence of lithium the baseline voltage is determined by the

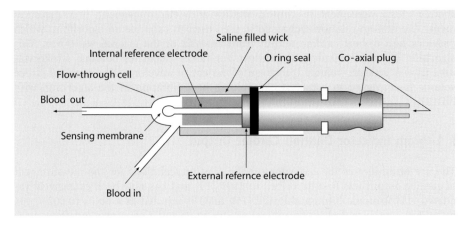

Fig. 1. The lithium selective electrode in the flow-through cell

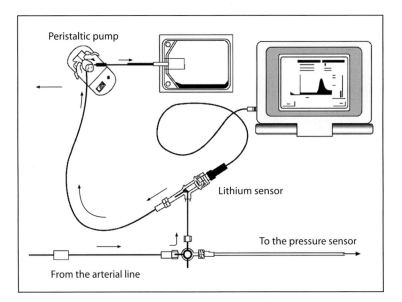

Fig. 2. Extracorporeal layout necessary for calibration

sodium concentration. The electrode is made of polyurethane with a central lumen. A wick, which is soaked in heparinized saline when the cell is first primed, makes the electrical connection between the blood at the tip of the electrode and the remote reference. The voltage is measured using an isolated amplifier, digitalized, and analyzed on-line.

▌ Assessment of Lithium Indicator Dilution

Insertion of an arterial catheter is widely used in critical care to facilitate obtaining frequent blood samples and the pulse pressure waveform for measuring blood pressure. The arterial pulse pressure waveform can also be used for measuring beat-to-beat cardiac output by using computers and mathematical algorithms. The LiDCO plus machine uses a three-step transformation of the arterial pressure waveform.

▌ **Step 1** – Arterial Pressure Transformation into a Volume-time Waveform
A non-linear look-up table is used as the basis for calculating the arterial volume changes with respect to blood pressure. This table was devised using physiological data derived from human aortic tissue.

▌ **Step 2** – Deriving Nominal Stroke Volume and the Heartbeat Duration
In order to obtain cardiac output as volume per unit time, the algorithm needs to calculate the duration of the cardiac cycle and the stroke volume, or a value proportional to it (the nominal stroke volume). The mathematical technique of autocorrelation is used to calculate a value proportional to the nominal stroke volume and the duration of the cardiac cycle. Autocorrelation can then be used to derive the root mean squared values of the blood pressure waveform, i.e., a power function that is linearly related to the stroke volume. Hence this technique of arterial waveform derivation of cardiac output is referred to as pulse power analysis as distinct from pulse contour analysis (see below)

▌ **Step 3** – Calibration of the Nominal Stroke Volume
The algorithm derived stroke volume and therefore cardiac output are initially uncalibrated. They are converted to actual values by multiplying the nominal stroke volume by a calibration factor. This is a patient-specific correction factor generated by the algorithm when the nominal data are corrected to actual data by a LiDCO calibration.

Several studies have evaluated the lithium dilution technique of cardiac output measurement, most frequently in comparison with thermodilution using the PAC. Several peer-reviewed studies have been published both in cardiac patients [14, 15] as well as in critically ill pediatric patients [16] and the accumulated evidence in animal and human studies suggest a good correlation with thermodilution using the PAC. However, whether thermodilution can be regarded as a 'gold standard' of cardiac output measurement is dubious. It is estimated that a 22% change in cardiac output is necessary before any difference is detected by this technique [12]. There is a large body of evidence supporting the accuracy of the lithium dilution technique in a variety of clinical circumstances including further validation in critically ill adults. Our findings supported these studies. We compared the LiDCO system with thermodilution data in critically ill, mainly septic, patients admitted to our general ICU. We found that over the first 12 hours the linear correlation analysis was good with a highly significant agreement ($R^2 = 0.844$, $p < 0.001$); similarly the coefficient of determination was still highly significant over the subsequent 12 hours ($R^2 = 0.839$; $p < 0.001$).

Because the concentration change of lithium is used to calculate the cardiac output, this technique cannot be used in patients receiving lithium therapy for hypomania, since the increased background lithium concentration causes an overestimation of cardiac output. The electrode may also drift in the presence of certain muscle relaxant infusions and so cause inaccurate measurements. Therefore, calibrations have to be avoided during these treatments. Also bolus techniques of administration can be used.

As with all indicator dilution techniques, intra-cardiac shunts will cause errors in the determination of cardiac output by distortion of the dilution curve. A right-left shunt will cause distortion of the initial part of the dilution curve and a left-right shunt will result in the right ventricular output being higher than the flow into the aorta.

▮ Preload Evaluation and Prediction of Fluid Responsiveness

In mechanically ventilated patients, blood pressure can develop changes from interactions between the heart and lungs during positive pressure ventilation. This is the rationale behind pulse contour analysis monitors: a continuous minimally invasive method of measuring cardiac output and preload.

The arterial pressure waveform is translated in a beat-to-beat value for stroke volume. Changes in arterial pressure during the respiratory cycle can match different fluid status predictors: systolic pressure variation (SPV) (Fig. 3), pulse pressure variation (PPV) (Fig. 4), and stroke volume variation (SVV) (Fig. 5).

Systolic pressure variation (SPV)

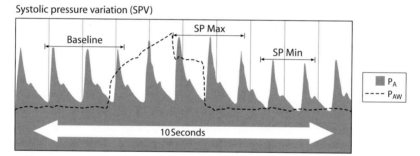

Fig. 3. Systolic pressure (SP) variation. A 10-second graph is used to reliably capture the maximum and minimum systolic values in at least one respiratory cycle

Pulse pressure variation (PPV)

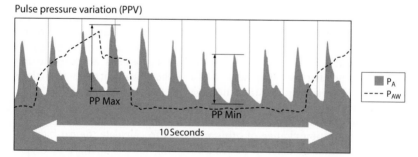

Fig. 4. Pulse pressure variation. A 10-second window is used to reliably capture the maximum and minimum values in at least one respiratory cycle. The maximal value is during inspiration (PPmax) and minimal value is in early expiration (PPmin)

Stroke volume variation (SVV)

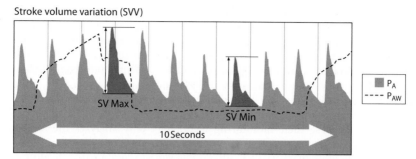

Fig. 5. Stroke volume variation. SVmax is the maximum stroke volume; SVmin is the minimum stroke volume

Physicians can now evaluate the intravascular blood volume from the heart lung interactions and these parameters may be more accurate than pressure based measures [17–24]. Information from SPV, PPV, and SVV may give also an indication of volume administration responsiveness. The heart lung interaction based parameters have mathematical expressions that are explained in the next equations and figures.

SPV (Fig. 3) is the difference between the maximum and minimal systolic blood pressure (SBP) following a positive pressure breath.

- SPV = ΔUp + ΔDown (normal value < 10 mmHg)
  ΔUp increase is related to left ventricular afterload.
- ΔUp = SBP max – apneic baseline (Normal value < 5 mmHg)
  ΔDown reflects right ventricular preload and volume responsiveness in a patient.
- ΔDown = apneic baseline – SBP min (normal value < 5 mmHg)

PPV (Fig. 4) is the maximum pulse pressure less the minimum pulse pressure divided by the average of these two pressures.

- PPV = PPmax–PPmin/(PPmax + PPmin/2) (normal value < 13%)

SVV (Fig. 5) is the difference between the maximum and minimal stroke volume (SV) following a positive pressure breath.

- SVV = SVmax–SVmin/(SVmax + SVmin/2)

A value under 10% implies that probably the patient does not need volume administration and a value over 15% implies that the patient probably needs volume expansion.

The published data suggest that these parameters can be used to predict the volemic status of high risk and critically ill patients. Studies indicate that SPV and ΔDown identify hypovolemia more closely than central venous pressure (CVP) in humans with hemorrhage [18]. Furthermore, in critically ill patients with sepsis and hypotension, SPV predicts response to volume better than echocardiography [19]. ΔDown appears closely related to pulmonary arterial occlusion pressure (PAOP) [20] and is considered a better predictor of left ventricular preload than PAOP [21]. For the PPV, a value of 13% or more enabled discrimination between patients likely to respond to volume and non-responding patients [22]. Michard again confirmed that PPV accurately predicts the hemodynamic effects of volume expansion (with the same value of 13% to discriminate volume responders to non-responders). He concluded that changes in PPV could be used to assess the hemodynamic effects of volume expansion [23]. SVV can also be used as a predictor of volume responsiveness; it was more sensitive than either CVP or systolic blood pressure as an indicator of hemodynamic changes to 100 ml colloid boluses in a study undertaken in neurosurgical patients [22]. This study identified a threshold of 9.5% for SVV with a sensitivity of 79% and a specificity of 93%. Other authors disagree with these results, finding a lack of correlation between ΔSVV at baseline and SVI after volume administration [24]. Wiesenack and co-workers [24] explain their data because their monitoring technology only analyzes the systolic portion of the arterial pressure wave.

These dynamic markers of fluid responsiveness, combined with more traditional parameters, may permit more appropriate fluid management in the ventilated patient. However, variations in stroke volume or pulse pressure may not be as readily attributed to hypovolemia in the spontaneously breathing patient or in the presence of an irregular cardiac rhythm. As a result, these parameters may not be reliable in a large proportion of critical care patients.

▌ Conclusion

The LiDCO™plus system is a safe and reliable minimally invasive device for hemodynamic monitoring. The technique obviates the need for pulmonary artery catheterization with its attendant risks and complications. The LiDCO™plus system derives beat-to-beat information about cardiac performance and its determinants, i.e., vascular resistance and preload. The absolute cardiac output used to calibrate the system is derived by lithium dilution, an extensively validated and accurate indicator dilution method [11]. The preload status is based on ventilator provoked heart-lung interactions characterized by SPV, PPV, and SVV. These parameters appear able to predict volume responsiveness better than traditional pressure measurements (e.g., CVP, PAOP) in mechanically ventilated patients [25]. The use of these variables however requires more research as the clinical consensus is not universal and there is some controversy over the interpretation of the arterial pressure variation analysis [26].

The LiDCOplus monitor provides a continuous record of hemodynamic changes and can be used to detect early and subtle changes in the cardiovascular state of the critically ill patient. Clinical use in our institutions is now directed at answering the clinician's problem: Does the patient require fluid filling or inotropic drugs, vasodilators, or vasoconstrictors? Future studies should then perhaps concentrate on the impact of using these monitored variables on the length of ICU patient stay, reduction in complications, and finally survival benefits.

References

1. Connors AF Jr, Speroff T, Dawson NV, et al (1996) The effectiveness of right heart catheterisation in the initial care of critically ill patients. JAMA 276:889–897
2. Boyd KD, Thomas SJ, Gold J, et al (1983) A prospective study of complications of pulmonary artery catheterisations in 500 consecutive patients. Chest 84:245–249
3. Branthwaite MA, Bradley RD (1968) Measurement of cardiac output by thermal dilution in man. J Appl Physiol Mar 24:434–438
4. Stetz CW, Miller RG, Kelly GE, Raffin TA (1982) Reliability of the thermodilution method in the determination of cardiac output in clinical practice. Am Rev Respir Dis 126:1001–1004

5. Boyd KD, Thomas SJ, Gold J, Boyd AD (1983) A prospective study of complications of pulmonary artery catheterizations in 500 consecutive patients. Chest 84:245–249
6. Horst HM, Obeid FN, Vij D, Bivins BA (1984) The risks of pulmonary artery catheterization. Surg Gynecol Obstet 159:229–232
7. Sandham JD, Hull RD, Brant RF, et al (2003) A randomized, controlled trial of the use of pulmonary-artery catheters in high-risk surgical patients. N Engl J Med 348:5–14
8. Shigehiko U, Gordon S, Bellomo R, et al (2004) Diuretics and mortality in acute renal failure. Crit Care Med 32:1669–1677
9. Rivers E, Nguyen B, Havstad S, et al (2001) Early goal-directed therapy in the treatment of severe sepsis and septic shock. N Engl J Med 345:1368–1377
10. Linton R, Band D, Haire K (1993) A new method of measuring cardiac output in man using lithium dilution. Br J Anaesth 71:262–266
11. Linton RAF, Band DM, O'Brien T, et al (1998) Lithium dilution cardiac output measurement – a brief review. In: Ikeda K, Doi M, Kazama T (eds) State-of-the-Art Technology in Anaesthesia and Intensive Care. Elsevier Science, Amsterdam, pp 61–66
12. Band DM, Linton RA, Jonas MM, et al (1997) The shape of indicator dilution curves used for cardiac output measurement in man. J Physiol 498:225–229
13. Jonas MM, Linton RA, O'Brien TK, et al (2001) The pharmacokinetics of intravenous lithium chloride in patients and normal volunteers. Journal of Trace Elements and Microprobe Techniques 19:313–320
14. Linton RAF, Band DM, O'Brien T, Jonas MM (1997) Lithium dilution cardiac output measurement: A comparison with thermodilution. Crit Care Med 25:1796–1800
15. Kurita T, Morita K, Kato S, Kikura M, Horie M, Ikeda K (1997) Comparison of the accuracy of the lithium dilution technique with the thermodilution technique for measurement of cardiac output. Br J Anaesth 79:770–775
16. Linton RA, Jonas MM, Tibby SM, et al (2000) Cardiac output measured by lithium dilution and transpulmonary ther-modilution in a paediatric intensive care unit. Intensive Care Med 26:1507–1511
17. Della Rocca D, Pompei L, Costa MG, et al (2001) Stroke volume variation during anaesthesia. ASA Annual Meeting Abstracts A243 (abst)
18. Rooke GA, Schwid HA, Shapira Y (1995) The effect of graded hemorrhage and intravascular volume replacement on systolic pressure variation in humans during mechanical and spontaneous ventilation. Anesth Analg 80:925–932
19. Tavernier B, Makhotine O, Lebuffe G, Dupont J, Scherpereel P (1998) Systolic pressure variation as a guide to fluid therapy in patients with sepsis-induced hypotension. Anesthesiology 89:1313–1321
20. Marik PE (1993) The systolic blood pressure variation as an indicator of pulmonary capillary wedge pressure in ventilated patients. Anaesth Intensive Care 21:405–408
21. Coriat P, Vrillon M, Perel A, et al (1994) A comparison of systolic blood pressure variations and echocardiographic estimates of end-diastolic left ventricular size in patients after aortic surgery. Anesth Analg 78:46–53
22. Berkenstadt H, Margalit N, Hadani M, et al (2001) Stroke volume variation as a predictor of fluid responsiveness in patients undergoing brain surgery. Anesth Analg 92:984–989
23. Michard F (2000) Relationship between respiratory changes in arterial pressure and fluid responsiveness in septic patients with acute circulatory failure Am J Respir Crit Care Med 162:134–138
24. Wiesenack C, Prasser C, Rödig G, Keyl C (2003) Stroke volume variation as an indicator of fluid responsiveness using pulse contour analysis in mechanically ventilated patients. Anesth Analg 96:1254–1257
25. Michard F, Teboul JL (2002) Predicting fluid responsiveness in ICU patients: a critical analysis of the evidence. Chest 121:2000–2008
26. Pinsky MR (2003) Probing the limits of arterial pulse contour analysis to predict preload responsiveness Anesth Analg 96:1245–1247

Venous Ultrasonography in Medical Intensive Care

S. Samy Modeliar, M. A. Sevestre-Pietri, and M. Slama

▌ Introduction

Medical intensive care is a young and rapidly growing specialty, supported by increasingly sophisticated technology. However, intensive care patients are often difficult to transport and may not be able to access all of these technologies (magnetic resonance imaging [MRI], positron emission tomography [PET] scan, etc.).

Over recent years, compact, portable, easy-to-use ultrasound machines have been released onto the market. The use of such machines can facilitate the management of intensive care patients. Leaving to one side the controversy concerning systematic ultrasound-guided central venous catheter placement, portable ultrasound machines can also have other applications (search for thromboses, clinicopathological studies, etc.).

In this chapter, we summarize the studies performed with this type of apparatus, as well as studies evaluating its contribution to central venous catheter placement.

▌ Ultrasound and Deep Vein Thrombosis (DVT)

Medical intensive care patients often present several concomitant diseases carrying a high risk of thromboembolism [1]. The various risk factors (immobilization, clotting disorders, dehydration, endothelial lesions, etc.) are cumulative [2, 3]. The diagnosis of DVT is difficult in the intensive care setting: patients often present several risk factors and are often unable to report suggestive symptoms. Clinical examination also has poor sensitivity and specificity (non-occlusive DVT are clinically silent) [2, 4, 5]. Meyer et al. [6], in 1995, in a retrospective study conducted in 183 multiple trauma patients, emphasized the limited clinical signs of DVT in traumatological intensive care. He reported an ultrasound DVT rate in the lower limbs of 16%, despite a thromboembolic prophylaxis rate of 100%. Durbec et al. [7], in 1997, performed venography in 80 intensive care patients after removal of a femoral central venous catheter (CVC). He detected DVT in 8.5% of patients, all of whom were asymptomatic.

Venous ultrasonography is the first-line examination in the case of suspected DVT. The only essential criterion is incompressibility of the vein studied. The addition of a flow criterion or Doppler signal does not increase the diagnostic yield of this examination compared to the incompressibility criterion alone [8].

In 2001, we performed a prospective study in our medical intensive care unit (ICU) in order to determine the frequency of DVT, as the incidence of DVT is well

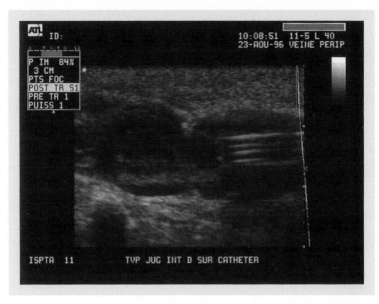

Fig. 1. Longitudinal view of internal right jugular vein in a patient with venous thrombus attached to central venous catheter

documented in surgical intensive care, but has been less extensively evaluated in medical intensive care. Thirty consecutive patients over the age of 18 years and admitted to the ICU for more than 48 hours were included. A single operator performed internal jugular and femoral vein ultrasonography in each patient, on admission and then weekly and at the time of discharge. A 7.5 MHz transducer was used. Positive ultrasound criteria for the presence of thrombosis were the presence of spontaneous intraluminal echogenic material and vessel incompressibility. Seventeen percent of patients developed a DVT during their stay in the ICU. Risk factors for DVT were the presence of a central venous catheter, duration of immobilization (15.2 days versus 4.5) and mechanical ventilation, absence of drug prophylaxis, duration of central venous catheterization, and administration of parenteral nutrition via this catheter. All these DVT were asymptomatic and situated in the internal jugular vein. A review of the literature revealed an incidence of 30% of DVT in intensive care patients in the absence of prophylaxis and an incidence of 10 to 34% in the presence of prophylaxis (depending on the study) [9–14]. This study confirmed the frequency of clinically silent DVT, already emphasized by previous studies. It also confirmed the value of systematic venous ultrasonography looking for DVT in high-risk patients.

In a second study performed in 2004, we prospectively studied the incidence of internal jugular and femoral DVT in 60 consecutive patients over the age of 18 years admitted to the ICU, during the 48 hours following their admission. A single operator performed ultrasonography of the internal jugular and femoral veins (Sonosite 180 plus apparatus, 7 MHz transducer) in each patient. The criterion defining DVT was the absence of complete compressibility of the vein. Internal jugular and femoral DVT, not suspected clinically, were revealed in 8% of patients.

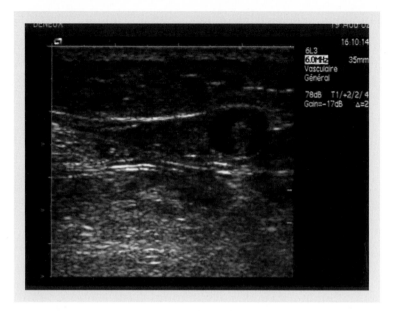

Fig. 2. Short axis of internal jugular vein with occlusive thrombus

All these studies demonstrate the considerable rate of clinically silent femoral or internal jugular DVT, supporting the use of venous ultrasonography before central venous catheter placement to avoid catheterization of a partially or completely thrombosed vessel [6, 7, 15] (Figs. 1, 2).

The presence of a central venous catheter also predisposes to the formation of DVT in 2 to 26% of patients [9, 15–17]. The incidence of DVT varies as a function of the site of central venous catheter placement (subclavian central venous catheters appear to be associated with a lower DVT rate), and the emboligenic potential of these DVT is unknown [18–20]. Systematic venous ultrasonography of catheterized vessels would allow early detection of these central venous catheter-related DVT and would allow appropriate treatment (removal of the catheter).

▍ Ultrasound, Vascular Anatomy, and Dynamic Procedures

Internal jugular and femoral veins present marked anatomical variations [21]. In many cases, the real site of the vessel does not correspond to external anatomical landmarks. This phenomenon is partly responsible for the difficulties encountered during central venous catheter placement, which can be accentuated when the catheter is inserted into a small vessel. Slama et al. [22], in 1997, in a series of 79 patients, demonstrated that vessels with a diameter less than 5 mm are particularly difficult to catheterize and that the successful catheterization rate was very significantly increased for vessels larger than 10 mm in diameter. According to Gordon et al. [23], the success of the first catheterization attempt is correlated with the diameter of the internal jugular vein in adults.

In this context, we studied the size and depth of internal jugular and femoral veins in medical intensive care patients and the effect of postural maneuvers on the diameter of small vessels (diameter less than 5 mm). Sixty consecutive patients over the age of 18 years admitted to the ICU for more than 48 hours were prospectively included. A single operator performed ultrasonography of internal jugular and femoral veins in a strict supine position, and then in a Trendelenburg position (–20°), and then in the reverse Trendelenburg position (+20°) for each patient. The transducer was positioned over the usual sites of catheterization of these vessels (Boullenger's anterior approach for internal jugular veins, and subfemoral for femoral veins), perpendicular to the skin and exerting minimal pressure to avoid deforming the vein.

The depth of the vessels, defined as the distance between the skin and the most superficial wall of the vein, was correlated with the body mass index (BMI) in the internal jugular and femoral veins. The angle of catheterization increases with the depth of the vessel, making catheterization of these vessels more and more difficult, justifying the use of ultrasound-guided catheter placement in obese patients.

Two-thirds of patients included had asymmetric internal jugular veins (predominant right internal jugular vein), which confirms the results of previous studies performed in healthy subjects [24], and which can probably be explained by a more direct course to the heart on the right side (embryological origin). Previous studies have reported a higher success rate and a lower complication rate for central venous catheter placement in the right internal jugular vein compared to the left internal jugular vein [24, 25]. This result, attributed to the fact that operators are predominantly right-handed, can also be explained by the asymmetry of internal jugular veins. The inconstant predominance of the right internal jugular vein constitutes an additional argument in favor of venous ultrasonography before central venous catheter placement in order to catheterize the predominant vessel.

Postural maneuvers induce a significant variation of the cross-sectional area of the internal jugular veins and femoral veins. In the Trendelenburg position, the cross-sectional area of the internal jugular veins increases and that of the femoral veins decreases. In contrast, in the reverse Trendelenburg position, the cross-sectional area of the internal jugular veins decreases and that of the femoral vein increases. These postural variations of the size of the vessels corroborate the results of previous studies conducted in healthy subjects [26, 27] or in anesthetized subjects [28]. In view of the diameter of the needles used (1 to 2 mm) to catheterize these vessels, changes in the size of veins, even as little as one millimeter, can be important.

No femoral veins were smaller than 5 mm in diameter, but 16% of internal jugular veins had a diameter less than 5 mm. Overall, the diameter of all of these vessels increases when the patient is placed in the Trendelenburg position. Twenty one percent of these veins even have a diameter greater than 10 mm. The Trendelenburg maneuver is therefore particularly useful for small internal jugular veins. However, it cannot be applied to all patients. It must be limited in coronary patients in whom it increases myocardial oxygen consumption, in patients with a low pulmonary reserve, in patients with intracranial hypertension, etc. The optimal slope inducing maximal increase of internal jugular veins diameter has yet to be determined and no consensus has been reached concerning postural maneuvers facilitating catheterization of internal jugular and femoral veins.

Variations in the depth of internal jugular and femoral veins and internal jugular vein asymmetry argue in favor of ultrasound-guided central venous catheter placement. This technique also allows detection of small internal jugular veins, in which the Trendelenburg position could facilitate catheterization.

▌ Ultrasound-guided Central Venous Catheter Placement

A number of studies support systematic ultrasound guidance for central venous catheter placement. In 1993, Denys et al. [29] prospectively compared internal jugular central venous catheter placement using external anatomical landmarks versus ultrasound-guided placement with 302 patients for each technique and concluded that the ultrasound-guided procedure was superior in terms of catheterization success rate, procedure time, and complication rate.

The meta-analysis by Randolph et al. [30] was designed to evaluate ultrasound-guided central venous catheter placement compared to the conventional method based on external anatomical landmarks. Eight published, randomized and controlled studies were selected from the database. Two studies concerned internal jugular veins, one concerned subclavian veins and two others concerned internal jugular and subclavian veins. Data concerning the population, interventions, outcome, and methodological quality were extracted by two investigators (discordant results were resolved by consensus). Data synthesis demonstrated the superiority of ultrasound-guided placement compared to the conventional method in terms of complication rate during catheter placement, catheter placement failure rate and number of catheter placement attempts. No time gain was demonstrated for ultrasound-guided placement (variable results according to the studies). However, certain reservations can be expressed in relation to this study. In particular, the definition of placement failure varied from one study to another.

The meta-analysis by Hind et al. [31] analyzed 18 studies (1646 patients) to evaluate ultrasound-guided central venous catheter placement. Eleven of these studies compared central venous catheter placement using two-dimensional ultrasound guidance, six used Doppler ultrasound guidance, and one used a combination of two-dimensional and Doppler ultrasound guidance, compared to anatomical landmark-guided placement. In adults, two-dimensional ultrasound decreased the relative risk of catheter placement failure by 86% in the internal jugular and subclavian veins and by 71% in the femoral vein (compared to the landmark method). It also decreased the relative risk of complications by 57% and the risk of failure of the first attempt at placement by 47%. Identical results were observed in children. In adults, Doppler ultrasound guidance increases the probability of cannulation of the vein by the first attempt (compared to the landmark method). However, the Doppler ultrasound results for cannulation of the subclavian vein were in favor of the landmark method. No studies in children with sufficient statistical power are available to conclude on the value of Doppler ultrasound guidance for central venous catheter placement.

In the absence of studies comparing Doppler ultrasound and two-dimensional ultrasonography, the authors compared the relative risks of the two techniques. The relative risk for failed catheter placement was 0.36 in favor of two-dimensional ultrasonography for internal jugular vein procedures and 0.09 for subclavian vein procedures.

Overall, ultrasound-guided internal jugular vein catheter placement decreases the number of placement attempts, the procedure time, the failure rate, and the complication rate, but the superiority of this technique in the femoral vein has not been demonstrated.

Subsequent studies have refined and extended these results. In particular, Gann and Sardi [32] reported the success of ultrasound-guided Port-a-Cath placement and the impact on patient management of performing venous ultrasonography before catheterization (change of therapeutic approach for 14% of patients investigated by venous ultrasonography).

A number of studies have expressed several reservations concerning the systematic use of ultrasound guidance for central venous catheter placement. A study by Martin et al. [33] tried to determine whether the availability of an ultrasound machine in the department had an impact on the number and the type of complications observed during internal jugular central venous access placement. This study reported the same complication rate before and after the availability of venous ultrasonography. The number and type of complications were the same with ultrasound-guided and landmark-guided central venous catheter placement. All central venous catheters were inserted by residents, who received a one-hour training in the ultrasound technique. The authors concluded that availability of ultrasonography did not improve internal jugular vein central venous catheter placement and that the good results observed in previous studies could be due to the fact that the procedure was performed by operators experienced in ultrasound. These results are therefore no longer relevant if they cannot be extrapolated to everyday medical practice.

No cost analysis of ultrasound-guided central venous catheter placement has been published. However, the apparatus itself is expensive (the Site Ride apparatus costs about 9500 euros) to which must be added the cost of sterile transducer sheaths (23 euros per kit) and the technique learning time [34]. There are also no published studies concerning the long-term outcome of patients catheterized by this technique.

As serious complications during central venous catheter placement are rare, no study has sufficient statistical power to confirm that ultrasound-guided central venous catheter placement decreases the incidence of serious complications. For example, the incidence of catheter-related infections following this technique is unknown. Another limitation to the use of ultrasound guidance is the small size of the screen, which does not allow fine analysis of anatomical variants. Systematic use of the ultrasound guidance technique could also decrease the operator's ability to insert central venous catheter by using the anatomical landmark method, as this technology is not always continuously available and the landmark technique would remain essential in certain emergency situations.

▌ Conclusion

Venous ultrasonography, when available, is a valuable technique in medical intensive care. It is an aid to the diagnosis of DVT, frequently observed in intensive care patients and often clinically silent. It provides considerable assistance for central venous catheter placement, as it is able to detect small vessels, anatomical variants and precisely locate the vein to be cannulated. On the basis of the two published meta-analyses, ultrasound-guided central venous catheter placement appears to be useful in the internal jugular and subclavian veins, but less so in the femoral vein.

The ultrasound technique is particularly useful in subjects who are difficult to catheterize, although further studies are required to resolve a number of questions (cost of the technique, impact on infections, etc.). Ultrasound-guided central venous catheter placement requires adequate training, but this investment appears to be justified. However, all operators must be trained in the conventional landmark technique for those emergency situations in which ultrasonography is not available. For all of these reasons, systematic use of the ultrasound-guided technique still raises a number of problems.

In the absence of systematic ultrasound-guidance, a simple ultrasound examination prior to catheter placement can provide a wealth of information (detection of asymmetric vessels, DVT, etc.), improving the management of those patients needing a central venous catheter.

Ultrasonography prior to central venous catheter placement is now possible with the arrival of good quality and easy to use portable ultrasound machines on the market. In units in which this type of machine can be purchased or easily shared, the investment is cost-effective, hence the importance of training young physicians in venous ultrasonography techniques, possibly with a senior specialist opinion, whenever necessary.

References

1. Samama CM, Orliaguet G, Sztark F, Perrotin D (2001) Prévention de la maladie thromboembolique en réanimation: méthodes mécaniques et moyens médicamenteux; indications et contre-indications. Réanimation 10:436–472
2. Hoyt DB, Swegle JR (1991) Deep venous thrombosis in the surgical intensive care unit. Surg Clin North Am 71:811–830
3. Emmerich J (1996) Mécanismes et facteurs de risque de la maladie veineuse thromboembolique. Rev Prat 46:1203–1210
4. Hirsh J (1990) Diagnosis of venous thrombosis and pulmonary embolism. Am J Cardiol 65:45C–49C
5. Becker F (1996) Thromboses veineuses superficielles des membres inférieurs. Rev Prat 46:1225–1228
6. Meyer CS, Blebea J, Davis K Jr, Fowl RJ, Kempczinski RF (1995) Surveillance venous scans for deep venous thrombosis in multiple trauma patients. Ann Vasc Surg 9:109–114
7. Durbec O, Viviand X, Potie F, Vialet R, Albanese J, Martin C (1997) A prospective evaluation of the use of femoral venous catheters in critically ill adults. Crit Care Med 25:1986–1989
8. Kearon C, Ginsberg JS, Hirsh J (1998) The role of venous ultrasonography in the diagnosis of suspected deep venous thrombosis and pulmonary embolism. Ann Intern Med 129:1044–1049
9. Hirsch DR, Ingenito EP, Goldhaber SZ (1995) Prevalence of deep venous thrombosis among patients in medical intensive care. JAMA 274:335–337
10. Cade JF (1982) High risk of the critically ill for venous thromboembolism. Crit Care Med 10:448–450
11. Marik PE, Andrews L, Maini B (1997) The incidence of deep venous thrombosis in ICU patients. Chest 111:661–664
12. Shorr AF, Trotta RF, Alkins SA, Hanzel GS, Diehl LF (1999) D-dimer assay predicts mortality in critically ill patients without disseminated intravascular coagulation or venous thromboembolic disease. Intensive Care Med 25:207–210
13. Kollef MH, Zahid M, Eisenberg PR (2000) Predictive value of a rapid semiquantitative D-dimer assay in critically ill patients with suspected venous thromboembolic disease. Crit Care Med 28:414–420
14. Fraisse F, Holzapfel L, Couland JM, et al (2000) Nadroparin in the prevention of deep vein thrombosis in acute decompensated COPD. Am J Respir Crit Care Med 161:1109–1114

15. Trottier SJ, Veremakis C, O'Brien J, Auer AI (1995) Femoral deep vein thrombosis associated with central venous catheterization: results from a prospective, randomized trial. Crit Care Med 23:52–59

16. Moser KM, Fedullo PF, LitteJohn JK, Crawford R (1994) Frequent asymptomatic pulmonary embolism in patients with deep venous thrombosis. JAMA 271:223–225

17. Huisman MV, Buller HR, ten Cate JW, et al (1989) Unexpected high prevalence of silent pulmonary embolism in patients with deep venous thrombosis. Chest 95:498–502

18. Harris LM, Curl GR, Booth FV, Hassett JM Jr, Leney G, Ricotta JJ (1997) Screening for asymptomatic deep vein thrombosis in surgical intensive care patients. J Vasc Surg 26:764–769

19. Di Costanzo J, Sastre B, Choux R, Kasparian M (1988) Mechanism of thrombogenesis during total parenteral nutrition: role of catheter composition. JPEN J Parenter Enteral Nutr 12:190–194

20. Efsing HO, Lindblad B, Mark J, Wolff T (1983) Thromboembolic complications from central venous catheters: a comparison of three catheter materials. World J Surg 7:419–423

21. Kahle W, Leonhardt H, Platzer W (1993) Anatomie, Volume 2 – Viscères. Flammarion-Médecine-Sciences, Paris

22. Slama M, Novara A, Safavian A, Ossart M, Safar M, Fagon JY (1997) Improvement of internal jugular vein cannulation using an ultrasound-guided technique. Intensive Care Med 23:916–919

23. Gordon AC, Saliken JC, Johns D, Owen R, Gray RR (1998) US-guided puncture of the internal jugular vein: complications and anatomic considerations. J Vasc Interv Radiol 9:333–338

24. Lobato EB, Sulek CA, Moody RL, Morey TE (1999) Cross-sectional area of the right and left internal jugular veins. J Cardiothorac Vasc Anesth 13:136–138

25. Verghese ST, Nath A, Zenger D, Patel RI, Kaplan RF, Patel (2002) The effects of the simulated Valsalva maneuver, liver compression, and/or Trendelenburg position on the cross-sectional area of the internal jugular vein in infants and young children. Anesth Analg 94:250–254

26. Armstrong PJ, Sutherland R, Scott DH (1994) The effect of position and different manoeuvres on internal jugular vein diameter size. Acta Anaesthesiol Scand 38:229–231

27. Cirovic S, Walsh C, Fraser WD, Gulino A (2003) The effect of posture and positive pressure breathing on the hemodynamics of the internal jugular vein. Aviat Space Environ Med 74:125–131

28. Hayashi H, Ootaki C, Tsuzuku M, Amano M (2000) Respiratory jugular venodilation: its anatomic rationale as a landmark for right internal jugular vein puncture as determined by ultrasonography. J Cardiothorac Vasc Anesth 14:425–427

29. Denys BG, Uretsky BF, Reddy PS (1993) Ultrasound-assisted cannulation of the internal jugular vein. A prospective comparison to the external landmark-guided technique. Circulation 87:1557–1562

30. Randolph AG, Cook DJ, Gonzales CA, Pribble CG (1996) Ultrasound guidance for placement of central venous catheters: a meta-analysis of the literature. Crit Care Med 1996 24:2053–2058

31. Hind D, Calvert N, Mcwilliams R, et al (2003) Ultrasonic locating devices for central venous cannulation: meta-analysis. BMJ 327:361

32. Gann M, Sardi A (2003) Improved results using ultrasound guidance for central venous access. Am Surg 69:1104–1107

33. Martin MJ, Husain, Piesman M, et al (2004) Is routine ultrasound guidance for central line placement beneficial? A prospective analysis. Curr Surg 61:71–74

34. Sessler CN (2004) Preventing mechanical and infectious complications of central venous catheterization. In: Vincent JL (ed) Yearbook of Intensive Care and Emergency Medicine. Springer, Heidelberg, pp 544–557

Mixed and Central Venous Oxygen Saturation

R.M. Pearse and A. Rhodes

▌ Introduction

Central venous oxygen saturation ($ScvO_2$) and mixed venous oxygen saturation (SvO_2) have been used in the assessment and management of the critically ill for many years. $ScvO_2$ refers to hemoglobin saturation of blood in the superior vena cava and SvO_2 refers to the same measurement in blood from the proximal pulmonary artery. The earliest clinical reports of the use of such data were of $ScvO_2$ in the coronary care unit [1]. Following the introduction of the pulmonary artery catheter (PAC) in 1970 [2], the routine clinical use of both $ScvO_2$ and SvO_2 became possible.

Since that time various authors have utilized SvO_2 and $ScvO_2$ as therapeutic goals in clinical trials, initially without success [3]. However, as our understanding of the clinical relevance of $ScvO_2$ and SvO_2 has improved, use of these parameters has been associated with marked improvements in outcome [4]. As a result, there is renewed interest in the use of venous saturation, in particular as a hemodynamic goal in the use of goal-directed therapy. The aim of this chapter is to give an account of the physiology of SvO_2 and $ScvO_2$ in health and disease, describe the relationship between the two and explore the use of these parameters in interventional trials.

▌ Techniques of Measurement of SvO_2 and $ScvO_2$

Venous saturation of blood can be measured in one of two ways. Either a sample of blood from the correct anatomical position can be taken and the venous saturation then measured (intermittent) or a continuous invasive catheter is used that measures the saturation of blood *in vivo*.

Intermittent Blood Sampling

The saturation of hemoglobin with oxygen is measured by spectrophotometry. The pattern of light absorption differs for oxygenated and de-oxygenated hemoglobin. The relative concentrations of each form may be calculated from absorption of light comprising two or more discrete wavelengths and a measurement of hematocrit. This technique, known as a co-oximetry, is employed in modern blood gas analyzers and allows the presence of methemoglobin and carboxyhemoglobin to be quantified as well.

Co-oximetry is a reliable technique, the main sources of error being the use of a diluted or unhomogenized blood sample. Blood sampling from the distal port of a 'wedged' PAC may provide a sample of pulmonary capillary rather than mixed venous blood [5]. Prior to the introduction of spectrophotometry, PvO_2 and $PcvO_2$ were measured and SvO_2 and $ScvO_2$ then calculated with the use of a nomogram [6]. This technique does not take account of changes either in hemoglobin affinity for oxygen or the presence of carboxyhemoglobin and methemoglobin, which may be clinically significant in the critically ill. Some older studies describing $ScvO_2$ and SvO_2 are therefore subject to a greater margin of error than subsequent research which utilized spectrophotometric techniques.

Indwelling Fiberoptic Catheter

By incorporating optical fibers into pulmonary artery and central venous catheters, the oxygen saturation of venous blood may be measured continuously without the need for intermittent blood sampling. The use of light of three wavelengths appears to be more reliable [7]. The main sources of error with this approach are malposition of the catheter and the catheter tip abutting a vessel wall. The latter is indicated by a signal on the display provided by some continuous spectrophotometry systems.

▌ Physiology of SvO_2 and $ScvO_2$

Basic Determinants of SvO_2 and $ScvO_2$

The main determinants of the oxygen content of venous blood are the delivery of oxygen to the tissues (DO_2) and its consumption by the tissues (VO_2). DO_2 is determined by the oxygen content in arterial blood and cardiac output, whilst VO_2 is affected by a range of factors which relate to tissue respiration. This relationship may be expressed by re-arranging the Fick equation:

$$CvO_2 = CaO_2 - \frac{VO_2}{CO}$$

Where CvO_2 and CaO_2 are the oxygen contents in venous and arterial blood; these are determined by the concentration of oxgenated hemoglobin and the dissolved

Table 1. Factors influencing mixed and central venous oxygen saturation

Factors affecting oxygen delivery	Factors affecting oxygen consumption
Cardiac output	**Cytopathic hypoxia**
▌ Cardiogenic shock	▌ Sepsis
▌ Reduced circulating blood volume	▌ Cyanide poisoning
▌ Exercise	
	Increased consumption
Oxygen content	▌ Pyrexia
▌ Hypoxia/O_2 therapy	▌ Exercise
▌ Hyperbaric O_2 exposure	▌ Shivering
▌ Anemia/hemorrhage	
▌ Carbon monoxide poisoning	**Reduced consumption**
	▌ Sedation/anesthesia

oxygen content. Because at standard atmospheric pressure, the quantity of dissolved oxygen is very small it is acceptable and more convenient simply to measure hemoglobin saturation. SvO_2 and $ScvO_2$ reflect the physiology of the entire body and are global indicators of tissue oxygenation and function. It is important therefore to realize that regional changes in venous saturation may occur without an overall change in SvO_2.

A diverse range of factors may affect SvO_2 (Table 1) and it is important to emphasize the need to assess the cause of any derangement before initiating treatment based on an abnormal value. The presence of intra-cardiac shunt will greatly limit the significance of changes in either SvO_2 or $ScvO_2$.

What are the Normal Values of SvO₂ and ScvO₂?

The normal value of SvO_2 has been quoted as 70% [8], however the measurement of SvO_2 and $ScvO_2$ is invasive in nature and few data exist to describe normal values. Only two studies, of which we are aware, document values for these parameters in young healthy individuals. The first is one of the earliest studies of venous saturation and provides a detailed description of hemoglobin saturation in the superior and inferior vena cavae, right atria, right ventricles and pulmonary arteries of 26 healthy subjects breathing air. The mean values were 76.8% (SD±5.2%) in the superior vena cava and 78.4% (SD±2.6%) in the pulmonary artery [9]. The second assessed trends in $ScvO_2$ in response to orthosatatic hypotension and described a median baseline $ScvO_2$ of 75% (range 69–78%) in nine subjects [10].

The most useful indicator of normal values of venous saturation in clinical practice involved the measurement of $ScvO_2$ prior to induction of anesthesia in 23 patients scheduled for major abdominal surgery. This study suggests a median value of 69% (Range 53%–83%) rising to 72% (range 66%–83%) after fluid administration [11]. These recordings were taken breathing room air but one hour after oral diazepam given as premedication for anesthesia.

All other available data describe SvO_2 and $ScvO_2$ values during major surgery or intensive care unit (ICU) admission, frequently providing little or no data regarding FiO_2, depth of anesthesia or sedation. It is more logical therefore, to assume a normal range for these parameters rather than one discrete value. Taking into account the above data and the normal value for PvO_2 which is quoted as 5 kPa [6], SvO_2 and $ScvO_2$ would be expected to vary between 70% and 80% in healthy subjects. However, values may be as low as 65% in hospital in-patients who are not critically ill.

▌ Relationship between SvO₂ and ScvO₂

The relationship between these two parameters is complex. The differences in VO_2 and DO_2 between the upper and lower regions of the body vary in health and disease. Drainage of coronary venous blood directly into the cardiac chambers via the coronary sinus and Thebesian veins also changes with myocardial work. Complete mixing of venous blood is not thought to occur until it reaches the right ventricle and, as a result, it is generally accepted that for reliable measurement of SvO_2, blood must be sampled from the pulmonary artery.

In healthy individuals, $ScvO_2$ is slightly lower than SvO_2 (76.8% vs 78.4%) [9], but this relationship changes in periods of cardiovascular instability. Scheinman and co-workers performed the earliest comparison of $ScvO_2$ and SvO_2 in both hemodynamically stable and shocked patients [12]. In stable critically ill patients, $ScvO_2$ was similar to SvO_2 ($ScvO_2$ 54.7% SD$\pm$19.92% vs SvO_2 56.9% SD$\pm$21.16%, p>0.1). In patients with heart failure, $ScvO_2$ was slightly higher than SvO_2 ($ScvO_2$ 61.8% SD$\pm$8.76% vs SvO_2 58.2% SD$\pm$8.74%, p<0.1), whilst in shock patients the pattern was even more pronounced ($ScvO_2$ 58.0% SD$\pm$13.05% vs SvO_2 47.5% SD$\pm$15.11%, p<0.001). The only other study to compare hemodynamically stable patients to those with shock describes similar findings [13]. In a more detailed study of a carefully defined group of patients with circulatory shock, mean $ScvO_2$ was again greater than SvO_2 although the range of values was large ($ScvO_2$ 74.2% SD$\pm$12.5% vs SvO_2 71.3% SD$\pm$12.7%) [14]. The largest series reported so far was a retrospective analysis of 3296 patients undergoing cardiac catheterization. Data were analyzed to identify the frequency of patients in whom $ScvO_2$ was more than 5% greater than SvO_2. This 'step-down' was identified in only 177 patients (5.4%). Whilst cardiac output was similar between the two groups, pulmonary artery pressure, pulmonary artery occlusion pressure (PAOP) and serum creatinine were all significantly greater in the step-down group. The authors concluded that poor left ventricular performance and renal dysfunction might explain these findings [15].

Most authors attribute this pattern to changes in the distribution of cardiac output that occur in periods of hemodynamic instability. In health, blood in the inferior vena cava has a high oxygen content because the kidneys do not utilize much oxygen but receive a high proportion of cardiac output [16]. As a result, inferior vena caval blood has a higher oxygen content than blood from the upper body and SvO_2 is greater than $ScvO_2$ [9, 12, 13]. In shock states, blood flow to the splanchnic and renal circulations falls, whilst flow to the heart and brain is maintained [17]. This results in a fall in the oxygen content of blood in the inferior vena cava. As a consequence in shock states the normal relationship is reversed and $ScvO_2$ is greater than SvO_2 [12-14]. In two studies in hemodynamically stable patients, $ScvO_2$ was slightly greater than SvO_2 but the differences were small [18, 19].

Some studies have aimed simply to describe the degree of correlation between $ScvO_2$ and SvO_2 but do not stratify patients according to hemodynamic status. Because of the influence of changes in the distribution of cardiac output in critical illness these trials simply report a poor correlation and are difficult to interpret [20-22]. Experimental studies indicate a good association between these parameters, although absolute values differ [23, 24]. Two studies have utilized spectrophotometry techniques to simultaneously monitor $ScvO_2$ and SvO_2 in critically ill patients. Whilst both describe discrepancies between the two parameters, one reports useful similarity in trend between the two whilst the other suggests $ScvO_2$ to be an unreliable indicator of SvO_2 [25, 26].

The relationship between $ScvO_2$ and SvO_2 is not straightforward. In health, the two values are often similar in magnitude but this is not always the case during periods of critical illness. Many previous studies of the link between these two parameters aimed to provide a more easily obtained surrogate for SvO_2 to allow calculation of intra-pulmonary shunt (Qs/Qt) or VO_2. The relationship between $ScvO_2$ and SvO_2 is too inconsistent for this purpose. Contemporary practice involves the use of these variables not to quantify VO_2 but as therapeutic end-points in their own right. In the presence of abnormalities, absolute values for either $ScvO_2$ or SvO_2 may not be as important as trend in response to treatment. The use of $ScvO_2$ in particular, has developed renewed interest as it avoids the requirement for pulmonary artery catheterization, a technique which has been criticized in the past [27].

Right Atrial Oxygen Saturation

Where reported, the saturation of blood in the right atrium is very similar to that of the pulmonary artery [9, 12–14, 28]. As might be anticipated, there was a very poor association in children immediately following surgery for major atrial or ventricular septal defects [29]. Choice of optimal position for the tip of the central venous catheter is not straightforward. Placement of the catheter tip in the right atrium may be associated with perforation of cardiac chambers whilst not advancing the catheter far enough may be associated with a higher incidence of venous thrombo-embolism [30]. For $ScvO_2$ measurement the catheter tip should probably be situated in the superior vena cava just above the entrance to the right atrium.

▌ Venous Oxygen Saturation in Pathological States

Patterns of SvO_2 and $ScvO_2$ derangement have been described in various pathological conditions. The causes of any abnormalities and the appropriate therapies required to correct them may differ widely. It is therefore important to consider each etiological group separately. The randomized trials that have utilized these parameters as hemodynamic goals are discussed separately.

Hypovolemia

The effects of circulatory disturbance due to hypovolemia have been described in both animals and humans. Reinhart et al. demonstrated fluctuations in SvO_2 and $ScvO_2$, which closely mirrored periods of hypoxia, hyperoxia, hemorrhage and subsequent resuscitation in anesthetized dogs. Values varied between 60% at baseline to 35% during periods of hypovolemia [24]. In another experimental study, a number of cardiovascular parameters were correlated with the extent of hemorrhage in dogs [31]. Central venous pressure (CVP), PAOP, arterial pressure and heart rate proved unreliable indicators but cardiac index, SvO_2 and $ScvO_2$ correlated well with the extent of blood loss. Whilst the values of SvO_2 and $ScvO_2$ were not identical, the trends were very similar throughout periods of hemodynamic change. In other experimental studies, oxygen saturations of blood from the jugular vein of rats and the right atria of rabbits have also correlated well with hemorrhage [32, 33]. Work in humans used orthostatic hypotension as a model of the cardiovascular disturbances associated with hypovolemia [10]. Median $ScvO_2$ fell from 75% at baseline to 60% at the onset of pre-syncopal symptoms. Over the same period, cardiac output fell from 4.3 to 2.7 l/min.

Clinical studies also suggest a role for the use of SvO_2 and $ScvO_2$ in the evaluation of traumatic shock. A small clinical series described derangements of SvO_2 in victims mainly of penetrating trauma [34]. Profound reductions, frequently below 30%, are described. SvO_2 rose above 60% in all four survivors but failed to do so in five of the six non-survivors. In a series of 26 major trauma victims, a value of $ScvO_2$ below 65% was not only a useful indicator of severity of blood loss but proved more reliable than conventional observations (heart rate, blood pressure, CVP) [35]. However, correlation with the extent of blood loss was not as strong as that found in experimental studies by the same author [31].

Both SvO_2 and $ScvO_2$ were lower in patients suffering in circulatory shock of various causes than a similar group of more stable patients. The data suggest that other causes of hypovolemia also result in profound reductions in venous oxygen saturation [13]. Reductions in $ScvO_2$ to below 65% were frequent in a group of patients mainly suffering from septic shock [36]. The same author went on to show that, following initial resuscitation, a value of $ScvO_2$ below 65% combined with serum lactate greater than 2 mmol/l indicated the need for additional resuscitation [37]. In early severe sepsis, mean $ScvO_2$ at baseline was 49.2% (SD±13.3%) in the control group and 48.6% (SD±11.2%) in the intervention group of a randomized trial [4]. There is also some evidence to suggest reductions in $ScvO_2$ to below 65% are associated with a poor outcome following high-risk surgery [38].

Cardiac Failure and Myocardial Infarction

Patterns of SvO_2 and $ScvO_2$ derangement in cardiac failure and following myocardial infarction have been described extensively. The earliest clinical work on $ScvO_2$ was performed by Goldman, who correlated derangements of this parameter with severity of myocardial dysfunction and subsequent response to treatment. A 60% threshold was suggested as holding particular importance and indicated a number of patients suffering from occult heart failure. Reductions in $ScvO_2$ to below 45% were generally associated with cardiogenic shock [1, 39]. Subsequent studies have also described derangements in both $ScvO_2$ and SvO_2 in cardiac failure, cardiogenic shock and following myocardial infarction. Reductions indicate the severity of disease [12, 40], whilst trends provide an indication of cardiac output and reflect response to treatment [41–44]. One study showed reductions in PvO_2 to reflect hyperlactemia and poor outcome in severe cardiac and respiratory disease [45]. Two studies demonstrated the occurrence of abnormalities of SvO_2 in chronic heart failure and acute myocardial infarction but did not recommend the use of this parameter to guide therapy [46, 47].

Cardiopulmonary Arrest

A number of studies have employed $ScvO_2$ in the management of cardiac arrest [48–51]. Although animal studies of the relationship between $ScvO_2$ and SvO_2 during cardiopulmonary arrest are contradictory, $ScvO_2$ measurement still appears to be of value [52, 53]. In a series of 43 patients with cardiopulmonary arrest, at ten minutes after the loss of spontaneous circulation, PvO_2 was greater than 4.9 kPa in 12 out of 14 survivors, whilst all 29 non-survivors had a PvO_2 below 4.1 kPa [50]. In a series of 100 cases, $ScvO_2$ above 72% was found to be a reliable indicator of return of spontaneous circulation [51]. This is particularly helpful because clinical methods of detecting return of spontaneous circulation are known to be unreliable.

Cardiothoracic and Aortic Surgery

In cardiac surgery, studies which concentrate on SvO_2 values during surgery suggest changes occur before those of blood pressure or heart rate [54] and correlate well with changes in cardiac index (CI) [54, 55]. In a study of 19 patients undergoing cardiac or lung surgery, sustained falls in SvO_2 to below 65% were associated with a higher incidence of complications especially arrhythmias [56]. Other data suggest changes in SvO_2 during and after cardiac surgery provide a more reliable indication of VO_2 than of cardiac output [57]. This may reflect a higher variability in VO_2 in the patients studied resulting from changes in anesthesia, sedation and invasive ventilation during the post-operative period. Changes in SvO_2 reflected specific events during lung transplantation, although the series was too small to draw any conclusions regarding the value of SvO_2 monitoring in this group [58].

SvO_2 monitoring during aortic surgery has also been described [59, 60]. The pattern of SvO_2 changes during the application and removal of aortic and femoral clamps appears complex. Reperfusion of the lower body following a variable period of ischemia results in large falls in SvO_2 which do not necessarily reflect a need for a change in cardiovascular management. There are few or no data regarding the monitoring of $ScvO_2$ during either cardiac or aortic surgery.

SvO_2 in Established Critical Illness

In respiratory failure, SvO_2 provided a useful indication of unsuspected problems with respiratory function resulting from sub-optimal patient position or coughing as well as guiding the choice of positive end-expiratory pressure (PEEP) and other respiratory management [61–64]. Some studies have concluded that SvO_2 monitoring provides no clear benefit in the management of mixed groups of critically ill patients [65, 66].

■ Interventional Trials Utilizing SvO_2 and $ScvO_2$ as Hemodynamic Goals

In common with other hemodynamic goals, interventional studies utilizing SvO_2 have shown conflicting results. The largest of these was a multicenter trial in a mixed group of critically ill patients [3]. Patients were randomized 48 hours after ICU admission to receive therapy targeted at maintaining $SvO_2 \geq 70\%$, $CI \geq 4.5$ l/min/m^2 or to the control group in whom a goal of 2.5–3.5 l/min/m was set for CI. These goals were then maintained for a five-day period.

At enrolment SvO_2, CI, DO_2, mean arterial pressure (MAP), and CVP were all similar between the groups. This remained the case at the end of the study period, with the exception of CI and DO_2, which were higher in the high CI group. Mean SvO_2 was between 67.3% and 69.7% in the three groups at enrolment and between 70.7% and 72.1% at the end of the study period. Similarly, the CI in the three groups was reasonable at enrolment (3.7–3.8 l/min/m) and normal or high at the end of the study period (control group 3.9 l/min/m, CI group 4.4 l/min/m, SvO_2 group 4.1 l/min/m). These figures suggest that flow related parameters were not so sufficiently deranged that further increases would alter outcome.

In peripheral vascular surgery, pre and post-operative goal directed hemodynamic therapy to achieve an SvO_2 of 65% did not alter outcome [67]. In this study, initial values for SvO_2 were low at enrolment and responded significantly in the intervention group (initial SvO_2 59.1%, final SvO_2 68.8%), but remained similar in the control group (initial SvO_2 59.1%, final SvO_2 63.8%). The outcome in this trial cannot therefore be attributed to the adequacy of therapy.

SvO_2 has been used successfully as a hemodynamic goal in cardiac surgical patients [68]. For the first eight hours after surgery, patients received either standard care or therapy to achieve a target for SvO_2 of 70% combined with a goal for serum lactate of below 2 mmol/l. Median hospital stay was shorter in the intervention group (6 vs 7 days, p < 0.05). Morbidity was also reduced in the intervention group (1.1% vs 6.1%, p < 0.01). Mean SvO_2 was 67% in both groups on arrival in the ICU but made significantly greater improvement in the intervention group (intervention group 71%±4% vs control group 69%±5, p < 0.001).

Rivers and colleagues utilized $ScvO_2$ to guide cardiovascular management in early severe sepsis and septic shock [4]. Two hundred and sixty-three patients were randomized to receive either six hours of standard care or fluid and inotropic support to achieve a target for $ScvO_2$ of 70% prior to ICU admission. In-hospital mortality was 30.5% in the intervention group and 46.5% in the control group (p = 0.009). The authors attribute this outcome improvement to a substantial reduction in episodes of 'sudden cardiovascular collapse'. Immediately following the trial period, patients receiving goal-directed therapy had higher mean $ScvO_2$ (goal-directed therapy group 70.4% SD±10.7% vs. Control group 65.3% SD±11.4%), lower serum lactate and lower mean APACHE II scores indicating less severe organ dysfunction.

Regardless of the hemodynamic goal chosen, goal-directed therapy is generally successful when employed in the resuscitation of patients at high risk of hypovolemia. Optimal benefit seems to result from short periods of goal-directed therapy applied at an early stage in the evolution of circulatory shock. Outcome from interventional trials utilizing SvO_2 and $ScvO_2$ as hemodynamic goals are also consistent with this concept. When appropriately applied, measurement of either $ScvO_2$ or SvO_2 may provide a valuable guide to circulatory management. $ScvO_2$ monitoring is particularly convenient as it allows the use of goal-directed therapy without recourse to the PAC or other forms of cardiac output measurement.

▌ Conclusion

SvO_2 and $ScvO_2$ appear to be useful indicators of disease severity and response to treatment in cardiovascular disturbances of various causes, although the utility of venous saturation in the calculation of VO_2 and Qs/Qt has been discounted. The relationship between the two parameters is complex and varies in health and disease. However, this does not appear to prevent the use of either in the assessment and management of the critically ill. Whilst cardiac output appears to be the single most important determinant of SvO_2 and $ScvO_2$, other factors must also be taken into account. Factors which influence VO_2 are of particular relevance as considerable changes in invasive ventilation, anesthesia and sedation may be made during a period of critical illness.

A primary aim of management of the critically ill is the maintenance of adequate tissue perfusion. Because of the challenges of measuring tissue function, we employ surrogate markers of tissue perfusion and function e.g., blood pressure, cardiac output, and serum lactate, each of which has limitations. The evidence regarding the use SvO_2 and $ScvO_2$ suggests that, in carefully chosen situations, they are also effective tools in the assessment and management of tissue perfusion in the critically ill.

References

1. Goldman RH, Braniff B, Harrison DC, Spivack AP (1968) The use of central venous oxygen sturation measurements in a coronary care unit. Ann Intern Med 68:1280–1287
2. Swan HJ, Ganz W, Forrester J, Marcus H, Diamond G, Chonette D (1970) Catheterization of the heart in man with use of a flow-directed balloon-tipped catheter. N Engl J Med 283:447–451

3. Gattinoni L, Brazzi L, Pelosi P, et al (1995) A trial of goal-oriented hemodynamic therapy in critically ill patients. SvO$_2$ Collaborative Group. N Engl J Med 333:1025–1032
4. Rivers E, Nguyen B, Havstad S, et al (2001) Early goal-directed therapy in the treatment of severe sepsis and septic shock. N Engl J Med 345:1368–1377
5. Suter PM, Lindauer JM, Fairley HB, Schlobohm RM (1975) Errors in data derived from pulmonary artery blood gas values. Crit Care Med 3:175–181
6. Siggaard-Andersen O, Fogh-Andersen N, Gothgen IH, Larsen VH (1995) Oxygen status of arterial and mixed venous blood. Crit Care Med 23:1284–1293
7. Rouby JJ, Poete P, Bodin L, Bourgeois JL, Arthaud M, Viars P (1990) Three mixed venous saturation catheters in patients with circulatory shock and respiratory failure. Chest 98: 954–958
8. Morgan T, Venkatesh B (2003) Monitoring oxygenation. In: Bersten A, Soni N, Oh T (eds) Oh's Intensive Care Manual. Butterworth-Heinemann, Burlington, pp 95–106
9. Barratt-Boyes BG, Wood EH (1957) The oxygen saturation of blood in the venae cavae, right-heart chambers, and pulmonary vessels of healthy subjects. J Lab Clin Med 50:93–106
10. Madsen P, Iversen H, Secher NH (1993) Central venous oxygen saturation during hypovolaemic shock in humans. Scand J Clin Lab Invest 53:67–72
11. Jenstrup M, Ejlersen E, Mogensen T, Secher NH (1995) A maximal central venous oxygen saturation (SvO$_2$max) for the surgical patient. Acta Anaesthesiol Scand Suppl 107:29–32
12. Scheinman MM, Brown MA, Rapaport E (1969) Critical assessment of use of central venous oxygen saturation as a mirror of mixed venous oxygen in severely ill cardiac patients. Circulation 40:165–172
13. Lee J, Wright F, Barber R, Stanley L (1972) Central venous oxygen saturation in shock: a study in man. Anesthesiology 36: 472–478
14. Edwards JD, Mayall RM (1998) Importance of the sampling site for measurement of mixed venous oxygen saturation in shock. Crit Care Med 26:1356–1360
15. Glamann DB, Lange RA, Hillis LD (1991) Incidence and significance of a "step-down" in oxygen saturation from superior vena cava to pulmonary artery. Am J Cardiol 68:695–697
16. Cargill W, Hickam J (1949) The oxygen consumption of the normal and diseased human kidney. J Clin Invest 28:526
17. Forsyth R, Hoffbrand B, Melmon K (1970) Re-distribution of cardiac output durin g hemorrhage in the unanesthetized monkey. Circ Res 27:311–320
18. Ladakis C, Myrianthefs P, Karabinis A, et al (2001) Central venous and mixed venous oxygen saturation in critically ill patients. Respiration 68:279–285
19. Berridge JC (1992) Influence of cardiac output on the correlation between mixed venous and central venous oxygen saturation. Br J Anaesth 69:409–410
20. Faber T (1995) Central venous versus mixed venous oxygen content. Acta Anaesthesiol Scand Suppl 107:33–36
21. Tahvanainen J, Meretoja O, Nikki P (1982) Can central venous blood replace mixed venous blood samples? Crit Care Med 10:758–761
22. Dongre SS, McAslan TC, Shin B (1977) Selection of the source of mixed venous blood samples in severely traumatized patients. Anesth Analg 56: 527–532
23. Schou H, Perez de Sa V, Larsson A (1998) Central and mixed venous blood oxygen correlate well during acute normovolemic hemodilution in anesthetized pigs. Acta Anaesthesiol Scand 42:172–177
24. Reinhart K, Rudolph T, Bredle DL, Hannemann L, Cain SM (1989) Comparison of central-venous to mixed-venous oxygen saturation during changes in oxygen supply/demand. Chest 95:1216–1221
25. Martin C, Auffray JP, Badetti C, Perrin G, Papazian L, Gouin F (1992) Monitoring of central venous oxygen saturation versus mixed venous oxygen saturation in critically ill patients. Intensive Care Med 18:101–104
26. Reinhart K, Kuhn HJ, Hartog C, Bredle DL (2004) Continuous central venous and pulmonary artery oxygen saturation monitoring in the critically ill. Intensive Care Med 30:1572–1578
27. Soni N (1996) Swan song for the Swan-Ganz catheter? BMJ 313:763–764
28. Davies GG, Mendenhall J, Symreng T (1988) Measurement of right atrial oxygen saturation by fiberoptic oximetry accurately reflects mixed venous oxygen saturation in swine. J Clin Monit 4:99–102

29. Rasanen J, Peltola K, Leijala M (1992) Superior vena caval and mixed venous oxyhemoglobin saturations in children recovering from open heart surgery. J Clin Monit 8:44–49
30. Fletcher S, Bodenham A (2000) Editorial II: Safe placement of central venous catheters: where should the tip of the catheter lie? Br J Anaesth 85:188–191
31. Scalea TM, Holman M, Fuortes M, Baron BJ, Phillips TF, Goldstein AS, Sclafani SJ, Shaftan GW (1988) Central venous blood oxygen saturation: an early, accurate measurement of volume during hemorrhage. J Trauma 28:725–732
32. Hirschl RB, Palmer P, Heiss KF, Hultquist K, Fazzalari F, Bartlett RH (1993) Evaluation of the right atrial venous oxygen saturation as a physiologic monitor in a neonatal model. J Pediatr Surg 28:901–905
33. Shah NS, Kelly E, Billiar TR, et al (1998) Utility of clinical parameters of tissue oxygenation in a quantitative model of irreversible hemorrhagic shock. Shock 10:343–346
34. Kazarian KK, Del Guercio LR (1980) The use of mixed venous blood gas determinations in traumatic shock. Ann Emerg Med 9:179–182
35. Scalea TM, Hartnett R, Duncan A, et al (1990) Central venous oxygen saturation: a useful clinical tool in trauma patients. J Trauma 30:1539–1543
36. Rady MY, Rivers EP, Martin GB, Smithline H, Appelton T, Nowak RM (1992) Continuous central venous oximetry and shock index in the emergency department: use in the evaluation of clinical shock. Am J Emerg Med 10:538–541
37. Rady MY, Rivers EP, Nowak RM (1996) Resuscitation of the critically ill in the ED: responses of blood pressure, heart rate, shock index, central venous oxygen saturation, and lactate. Am J Emerg Med 14:218–225
38. Pearse RM, Dawson D, Rhodes A, Grounds RM, Bennett ED (2003) Low central venous saturation predicts post-operative mortality. Intensive Care Med 29:S15 (abst)
39. Goldman RH, Klughaupt M, Metcalf T, Spivack AP, Harrison DC (1968) Measurement of central venous oxygen saturation in patients with myocardial infarction. Circulation 38:941–946
40. Hutter AM, Jr., Moss AJ (1970) Central venous oxygen saturations. Value of serial determinations in patients with acute myocardial infarction. JAMA 212:299–303
41. Muir AL, Kirby BJ, King AJ, Miller HC (1970) Mixed venous oxygen saturation in relation to cardiac output in myocardial infarction. BMJ 4:276–278
42. Birman H, Haq A, Hew E, Aberman A (1984) Continuous monitoring of mixed venous oxygen saturation in hemodynamically unstable patients. Chest 86:753–756
43. Ander DS, Jaggi M, Rivers E, et al (1998) Undetected cardiogenic shock in patients with congestive heart failure presenting to the emergency department. Am J Cardiol 82:888–891
44. Creamer JE, Edwards JD, Nightingale P (1990) Hemodynamic and oxygen transport variables in cardiogenic shock secondary to acute myocardial infarction, and response to treatment. Am J Cardiol 65:1297–1300
45. Kasnitz P, Druger GL, Yorra F, Simmons DH (1976) Mixed venous oxygen tension and hyperlactatemia. Survival in severe cardiopulmonary disease. JAMA 236:570–574
46. Kyff JV, Vaughn S, Yang SC, Raheja R, Puri VK (1989) Continuous monitoring of mixed venous oxygen saturation in patients with acute myocardial infarction. Chest 95:607–611
47. Richard C, Thuillez C, Pezzano M, Bottineau G, Giudicelli JF, Auzepy P (1989) Relationship between mixed venous oxygen saturation and cardiac index in patients with chronic congestive heart failure. Chest 95:1289–1294
48. Nakazawa K, Hikawa Y, Saitoh Y, Tanaka N, Yasuda K, Amaha K (1994) Usefulness of central venous oxygen saturation monitoring during cardiopulmonary resuscitation. A comparative case study with end-tidal carbon dioxide monitoring. Intensive Care Med 20:450–451
49. Rivers EP, Rady MY, Martin GB, et al (1992) Venous hyperoxia after cardiac arrest. Characterization of a defect in systemic oxygen utilization. Chest 102:1787–1793
50. Snyder AB, Salloum LJ, Barone JE, Conley M, Todd M, DiGiacomo JC (1991) Predicting short-term outcome of cardiopulmonary resuscitation using central venous oxygen tension measurements. Crit Care Med 19:111–113
51. Rivers EP, Martin GB, Smithline H, et al (1992) The clinical implications of continuous central venous oxygen saturation during human CPR. Ann Emerg Med 21:1094–1101

52. Martin GB, Carden DL, Nowak RM, Tomlanovich MC (1985) Central venous and mixed venous oxygen saturation: comparison during canine open-chest cardiopulmonary resuscitation. Am J Emerg Med 3:495–497
53. Emerman CL, Pinchak AC, Hagen JF, Hancock D (1988) A comparison of venous blood gases during cardiac arrest. Am J Emerg Med 6:580–583
54. Jamieson WR, Turnbull KW, Larrieu AJ, Dodds WA, Allison JC, Tyers GF (1982) Continuous monitoring of mixed venous oxygen saturation in cardiac surgery. Can J Surg 25:538–543
55. Waller JL, Kaplan JA, Bauman DI, Craver JM (1982) Clinical evaluation of a new fiberoptic catheter oximeter during cardiac surgery. Anesth Analg 61:676–679
56. Krauss XH, Verdouw PD, Hughenholtz PG, Nauta J (1975) On-line monitoring of mixed venous oxygen saturation after cardiothoracic surgery. Thorax 30:636–643
57. Schmidt CR, Frank LP, Forsythe SB, Estafanous FG (1984) Continuous SvO_2 measurement and oxygen transport patterns in cardiac surgery patients. Crit Care Med 12:523–527
58. Conacher ID, Paes ML (1994) Mixed venous oxygen saturation during lung transplantation. J Cardiothorac Vasc Anesth 8:671–674
59. Powelson JA, Maini BS, Bishop RL, Sottile FD (1992) Continuous monitoring of mixed venous oxygen saturation during aortic operations. Crit Care Med 20:332–336
60. Norwood SH, Nelson LD (1986) Continuous monitoring of mixed venous oxygen saturation during aortofemoral bypass grafting. Am Surg 52:114–115
61. Heiselman D, Jones J, Cannon L (1986) Continuous monitoring of mixed venous oxygen saturation in septic shock. J Clin Monit 2:237–245
62. Baele PL, McMichan JC, Marsh HM, Sill JC, Southorn PA (1982) Continuous monitoring of mixed venous oxygen saturation in critically ill patients. Anesth Analg 61:513–517
63. Divertie MB, McMichan JC (1984) Continuous monitoring of mixed venous oxygen saturation. Chest 85:423–428
64. Fahey PJ, Harris K, Vanderwarf C (1984) Clinical experience with continuous monitoring of mixed venous oxygen saturation in respiratory failure. Chest 86:748–752
65. Jastremski MS, Chelluri L, Beney KM, Bailly RT (1989) Analysis of the effects of continuous on-line monitoring of mixed venous oxygen saturation on patient outcome and cost-effectiveness. Crit Care Med 17:148–153
66. Boutros AR, Lee C (1986) Value of continuous monitoring of mixed venous blood oxygen saturation in the management of critically ill patients. Crit Care Med 14:132–134
67. Ziegler DW, Wright JG, Choban PS, Flancbaum L (1997) A prospective randomized trial of preoperative "optimization" of cardiac function in patients undergoing elective peripheral vascular surgery. Surgery 122:584–592
68. Polonen P, Ruokonen E, Hippelainen M, Poyhonen M, Takala J (2000) A prospective, randomized study of goal-oriented hemodynamic therapy in cardiac surgical patients. Anesth Analg 90:1052–1059

Cost-effectiveness of Minimally Invasive Hemodynamic Monitoring

M. L. N. G. Malbrain, T. J. R. De Potter, and D. Deeren

▌ Introduction: Why use Less-invasive Monitoring?

Non-invasive monitoring appears at first glance to be much safer than invasive hemodynamic monitoring with a pulmonary artery catheter (PAC). However, first, are less invasive techniques with the use of central venous lines and arterial lines, transesophageal Doppler monitoring, pulse contour analysis with transpulmonary thermo- or dye-dilution as adequate or better than a careful clinical evaluation, and safer than the gold standard PAC? Second, do we need these alternatives at all? These points were nicely addressed in a recent review by Bellomo and Uchino stating that "although we do not have direct evidence of any clinical benefits from invasive hemodynamic monitoring we believe that more intensive monitoring (invasive and noninvasive) is needed to ensure the safety of acutely ill patients, otherwise we would not have [intensive care units] ICUs" [1].

A recent survey in ICUs in the United Kingdom showed that PACs are still widely used (about 50%), followed by Doppler (45%), pulse contour (35%), and other (3%) techniques. An ideal continuous cardiac output (CCO) monitoring device should be safe, reliable, accurate, and reproducible. It should provide real-time, beat-to-beat cardiac output, preload, and afterload. The new technology should be minimally, if at all, invasive and widely applicable (from neonates to adults); simple to understand and to use; showing direct measured variables instead of calculated ones on a clear data display allowing for easy interpretation and application at the bedside [2].

When it comes to evidence based medicine (EBM) four major questions (Q) need to answered [3]. First (EBM Q1), does my new monitoring device work as well as the gold standard (PAC-derived)? Second (EBM Q2), does my new monitoring device provide me with new or additional information? Third (EBM Q3), does the interpretation of new data change my decision-making and treatment and finally (EBM Q4), do the new-variable driven diagnostic and therapeutic interventions eventually affect patient outcome?

However, we all know that parachutes are widely used to prevent gravitational damage and we also know that parachute use is associated with adverse events due to failure of the equipment as well as the fact that studies of free fall do not show 100% mortality [3]. So far, no randomized controlled clinical trials on parachute use have been undertaken and the basis for their use is purely observational. Therefore, the conclusion could be that those who adhere to EBM and those who insist that all interventions need to be validated by a randomized controlled trial need to come down to earth with a bump [3]. It will probably not end up this way at the bedside and the use of any of the less invasive hemodynamic monitoring devices will probably be driven by personal and subjective motives. The purpose of this chapter is to give a brief explanation on the technique for every new device followed by an attempt to answer the four EBM questions cited above based on the available literature. For each technique, a brief summary of the major advantages and disadvantages will also be given. The last part of this chapter will be dedicated to the results of a cost-effectiveness analysis comparing the different techniques based on some suggestions from a recent workshop [4].

▌ Gold Standard: the Fick Principle

Described by Adolf Fick in 1870, the Fick principle is the oldest known method of measuring cardiac output. It is based on a special case of mass balance, basically stating that in a given compartment (the heart), what goes out (arterial rate of indicator) equals what went in (venous rate of indicator) plus the rate of indicator added. This can be represented by

$$\text{Flow} \times \text{conc[art]} = \text{Flow} \times \text{conc[ven]} + \text{conc[add]}$$

Or, after rearrangement, and using oxygen extraction as indicator removed (negatively added)

$$\text{Flow(CO)} = \frac{VO_2}{CaO_2 - CvO_2}$$

where CO is cardiac output, VO_2 is oxygen consumption rate and CaO_2 and CvO_2 represent arterial and mixed venous oxygen content, respectively. In its original form, the equation is described as the amount of oxygen picked up by the blood as it passes-through the lungs, which is equal to the amount of oxygen taken up by the patient's lungs during breathing. The amount of oxygen uptake can be measured non-invasively at the mouth, and blood oxygen concentrations are measured from mixed venous and peripheral arterial blood samples. While never actually measured by Adolf Fick himself, this constitutes the direct Fick method and is considered the gold standard for cardiac output measurements. The major disadvantages are that it is very invasive and expensive in terms of equipment and staff. It requires a cardiac catheter, central venous and arterial lines, and stable metabolic conditions.

▌ Surrogate Gold Standard: Pulmonary Artery Catheter Monitoring

Description

Flow-directed PACs were first introduced in the 1970s by Swan, Ganz, Forrester et al. [5]. Their use has revolutionized intensive care medicine and, over 30 years later, they remain the undisputed gold standard in the clinical setting. While there is ongoing debate about the risk/benefit ratio of the procedure, it remains one of the most commonly used procedures performed in the critically ill worldwide [6–8]. However, the clinician using the technique is faced with multiple pitfalls that can be related to the inherent pressure–preload relation, to technical artifacts and to special disease states such as shunts and valvulopathy that invalidate the obtained readings [9–11]. The complexity of possible variations in obtained pressure tracings has led to a large interobserver variability, together with reports of very common misinterpretation of tracings even by experienced clinicians [12–14].

The technique works by injecting a bolus of indicator (usually iced fluid) into the right atrium. The resulting indicator dilution curve is recorded by a probe (a thermistor) in the pulmonary artery. The integral of the dilution curve over time is inversely proportional to cardiac output, as described by the Stewart-Hamilton equation. Over the last decade, catheters were introduced with the ability to measure cardiac output continuously and to measure right ventricular ejection fraction (RVEF). The catheter used for our cost-effective analysis was the recently introduced CCO that also provides continuous right ventricular (RV) end-diastolic volumes (RVEDV) since we felt that it would be unfair to compare the newer minimally invasive techniques with the standard PAC.

EBM Q1: Does the New Device Work as Well as the Gold Standard?

In the clinical setting, there is no other real gold standard. The thermodilution cardiac output method has been extensively compared with the Fick method as well as with dye-dilution methods [15, 16]. All three methods can be considered as equal reference methods according to a meta-analysis [17].

EBM Q2: Does the New Device Provide Me With New or Additional Information?

The PAC in itself provides – apart from calculated variables such as systemic and pulmonary vascular resistance, left and right ventricular stroke work, and oxygen extraction ratio – a measurement of cardiac output, central venous pressure (CVP), pulmonary artery pressure (PAP), and pulmonary artery occlusion pressure (PAOP). As stated before, more recent catheters are also able to measure RVEF and to calculate RVEDV continuously in sinus rhythm conditions using:

$$SV = \frac{CO}{HR} \quad \text{and} \quad RVEDV = \frac{SV}{RVEF}$$

where SV is stroke volume and HR is heart rate.

Additionally, PACs can be used to obtain blood samples from the distal port (in the pulmonary artery position), which allow the measurement of mixed venous oxygen saturation (SvO_2). To automate this process, PACs have been introduced that monitor SvO_2 continuously using fiberoptic reflectometry calibrated *in vitro* or *in vivo*. Continuous SvO_2 monitoring allows for an insight into trends in the oxygen supply/demand ratio [18].

EBM Q3: Does the Interpretation of the New Variables Change My Decision-making and Treatment?

The need to obtain insight into the cause of organ hypoperfusion and causes of systemic shock states are the basis for hemodynamic monitoring. As stated by Karl Ludwig over 100 years ago "The fundamental problems in the circulation derive from the fact that the supply of adequate amounts of blood to the organs of the body is the main purpose of the circulation while the pressures that are necessary to achieve it are of secondary importance; but the measurement of flow is difficult while that of pressure is easy so that our knowledge of flow is usually derivatory" [19].

The hemodynamic variables obtained by PAC monitoring allow the physician to get an idea of PAOP and cardiac output which cannot be obtained clinically [11, 20]. Based on different strategies, optionally combining SvO_2 and RVEDV/RVEF data, measures can be taken to optimize cardiac output using fluid expansion or vasopressor/inotrope administration.

EBM Q4: Will My New Variable-driven Diagnostic and Therapeutic Intervention Change Patient Outcome?

No study has definitively demonstrated improved outcome in critically ill patients managed using PACs. Most classic surgical studies have been invalidated by recent prospective trials [7]. Thus, the accepted indications for pulmonary artery catheterization have been generated largely on the basis of expert opinion [21]. In particular the use of PACs has been questioned since the 1996 study by Connors et al. that showed a 39% increase in mortality in patients receiving a PAC on day 1 of admission versus matched controls [10]. Although heavily criticized, the study remained unrefuted until a recent study by Richard et al., which showed no increased mortality from PAC use; however, without showing a survival benefit either [22]. Several studies have shown a reduction in morbidity using a PAC-guided strategy [6]. In large, multicenter, prospective trials a benefit of routine PAC use in high-risk surgical patients or in shock and/or acute respiratory distress syndrome (ARDS) settings has not been shown [7, 22]. This effect might be explained by the routine use of other estimates of cardiac function and preload such as echocardiographic assessment in both groups, and the inclusion of patients in whom PACs would not be considered routinely by most physicians. Nevertheless, a clear survival benefit resulting from the use of PACs remains unproven despite the placement of over 2 million devices worldwide since its introduction. However, it has to be stated that there is no cause and effect relation between the lack of studies on outcome and the wide use of the PAC; conversely it is not because a technique is widely used that the evidence is greater (remember that there is no evidence that pulse oximetry improves outcome).

Advantages

It is the most widely available catheter. There is no added fluid and no need for calibration. The values are operator independent and continuous measurements of SvO_2 and RVEDV are available.

Disadvantages

Despite the fact that it is the most widely used tool to obtain CCO it is not a 'simple' catheter that everyone can use. It is the most invasive and a very expensive option for CCO, and it is not truly continuous since an average cardiac output is provided over 5 to 10 minute periods. It has a slow response time to changes in preload or afterload, and has a poor signal to noise ratio. Since it is often used as the gold or reference standard, the data it provides are not verifiable. In other words, we may be validating the new minimally invasive techniques with the wrong standard. In fact, studies comparing the PAC with the real gold standard Fick principle have also shown some bias between both techniques.

The PiCCO system

Description

The cardiac output is measured using a transpulmonary thermodilution technique based on the Stewart Hamilton equation. By using an algorithm based on the analysis of the arterial pulse contour it is possible to continuously monitor cardiac output since the contour of the arterial pressure curve is proportional to the stroke volume [23]. This technique allows beat-to-beat variations of stroke volume and thus cardiac output in response to changing preload conditions. Currently there is one commercially available device (PiCCO, Pulsion Medical Systems, Munich, Germany).

EBM Q1: Does the New Device Work as Well as the Gold Standard?

Many studies performed in animals and different patient groups following cardiac surgery, heart or liver transplantation, septic or hypovolemic shock and burn patients found a good correlation between cardiac output obtained with the PiCCO by transpulmonary thermodilution and the gold standard thermodilution cardiac output with the PAC. Table 1 lists some of the recent validation studies [23–36]. The mean number of study subjects was 27.9 ± 15, the mean correlation coefficient r was 0.95 ± 0.02, the cardiac output was 5.7 ± 1.9 l/min (with a reasonable range), the bias was 0.2 ± 0.3 l/min and the precision was 1 ± 0.5 l/min or the limits of agreement defined as 2 standard deviations according to the Bland and Altman analysis. The standard errors were also within an acceptable range from 15 to 23% with one outlayer of 35% [31].

There are also many studies comparing the CCO obtained with the PiCCO via pulse contour analysis and the thermodilution cardiac output or the CCO obtained with a PAC (Vigilance system) [23, 25, 37]. In these studies, the correlation coefficients r ranged from 0.88 to 0.94, the cardiac output was 5.7 ± 1.9 l/min (with a reasonable range), the bias from –0.1 to 0.3 l/min, and the precision from 0.8 to 2.5 l/min.

EBM Q2: Does the New Device Provide Me with New or Additional Information?

The PiCCO device also allows the measurement of global end-diastolic volume (GEDV) and intrathoracic blood volume (ITBV) as surrogate preload markers together with extravascular lung water (EVLW) and pulmonary vascular permeability index (PVPI) [23, 24, 38]. Determination of EVLW by single transpulmonary thermodilution depends on measurement of the intrathoracic thermal volume (ITTV), and the pulmonary thermal volume (PTV), which is the largest accessible volume

Table 1. PiCCO cardiac output vs reference gold standard (PAC)

Author	Year	N	Patients	r	Bias (L/min)	Precision (L/min)	Mean CO (L/min)
Friedman [31]	2002	17	Hypovolemic shock in pigs	0.95	0	0.8	2.3
Mc Luckie [33]	1996	9	Pediatric ICU		0.19	0.42	
Goedje [32]	1998	30	Cardiac surgery	0.96	0.16	0.62	7
Goedje [26]	1998	30	Cardiac surgery	0.96	0.26	1.4	
Zöllner [34]	1998	18	ARDS (retrospective)	0.91	0.03	2.08	
Goedje [23]	1999	36	Cardiac surgery	0.93	−0.3	1.3	7
Buhre [25]	1999	12	Cardiac surgery	0.94	−0.1	0.9	5.4
Sakka [29]	1999	37	Septic shock	0.97	0.7	1.2	7
Goedje [24]	2000	40	OHT	0.98	0.35	0.4	7
Bindels [27]	2000	45	MICU	0.95	0.5	0.9	4
Sakka [35]	2000	12	Sepsis	0.98	0.73	0.78	
Zollner [36]	2000	19	CABG	0.96	0.21	1.46	
Holm [28]	2001	23	Burn	0.97	0.3	0.6	3.9
Della Rocca [30]	2002	62	OLT	0.93	0.2	1.7	7.7
Mean		27.86		0.95	0.23	1.04	5.70
Standard deviation		15.04		0.02	0.28	0.50	1.89

PAC: pulmonary artery catheter; N: number of patients; r: correlation coefficient (all correlations were done with PAC thermodilution); CO: cardiac output; ICU: intensive care unit; ARDS: acute respiratory distress syndrome; OHT: orthotopic heart transplant; MICU: medical ICU; CABG: coronary artery bypass graft; OLT: orthotopic liver transplant

transversed by the thermal indicator ("cold"). Traditionally these volumes were obtained using a double dye indicator technique (thermal combined with indocyanine green [ICG] dilution). The ITBV is then calculated as the product of cardiac output and the mean transit time (MTT) of ICG: ITBV = cardiac output x MTT_{ICG}.

With the less invasive PiCCO system, the ITTV and PTV are calculated from the MTT and the exponential downslope time (DST) of the thermodilution curve of the cold injectate: ITTV = cardiac output×MTT and PTV = cardiac output×DST. The ITTV consists of the PTV and the sum of the end-diastolic volumes of all cardiac chambers. Accordingly, the GEDV is calculated as: GEDV = ITTV – PTV. Based on a linear relation between GEDV and ITBV, ITBV = 1.25×GEDV. Since EVLW is the difference between ITTV and ITBV, EVLWI = ITTV – ITBV. Pulmonary blood volume (PBV), PVPI, stroke volume, global ejection fraction (GEF), cardiac function index (CFI) and systemic vascular resistance (SVR) were derived from these values: PBV = ITBV – GEDV; PVPI = EVLWI/PBV; stroke volume = cardiac output/heart rate; GEF = (4×SV)/GEDV; CFI = CO/GEDV and SVR = 80× (mean arterial pressure [MAP] – CVP)/cardiac output. Absolute values for cardiac output, GEDV, ITBV, stroke volume and SVR are normalized as indexed by body surface area ([cardiac index], GEDVI, ITBVI, [stroke volume index] and SVRI) and for EVLW by body weight (EVLWI). It has to be noted that in these equations GEDV is correctly measured whereas ITBV is estimated based on the correlation obtained between the single transpulmonary and the double indicator technique. Studies performing single and double dye dilution techniques confirmed the validity of the ITBV and EVLW values obtained with the PiCCO [24, 27].

Recent studies have suggested that ITBV or GEDV are better indicators of cardiac preload than the parameters obtained with a PAC especially in case of intraabdominal hypertension (IAH) and mechanically ventilated patients [38–41]. In most cases the change in CVP or PAOP is not correlated with the change in CI whereas the change in ITBVI is well correlated [24, 42]. Before adopting these parameters in clinical practice the clinician also needs to understand possible confounding factors that might influence the measured volumes, such as mitral valve regurgitation or aortic stenosis [38].

The PiCCO system also has the possibility for functional hemodynamic monitoring. Mechanical insufflation may increase pleural pressure hence increasing left ventricular (LV) preload and decreasing LV afterload causing an increase in arterial pulse pressure (PP) during inspiration [38, 41, 43, 44]. Likewise it decreases RV venous return. Therefore RV stroke volume may decrease during inspiration leading to a LV preload reduction causing a decrease in arterial pulse pressure during expiration. These respiratory changes in LV preload induce concomitant changes in LV stroke volume.

The stroke volume variation (SVV), which is the percentage change between maximal and minimal stroke volumes divided by the average of the minimum and maximum over a floating period of 30 seconds, is continuously displayed by the PiCCO monitor. The pulse pressure variation (PPV) is calculated as the difference in maximal and minimal PP divided by the mean of the two values expressed as a percentage.

EBM Q3: Does the Interpretation of the New Variables Change My Decision Making and Treatment?

As described above, the SVV and PPV have been proposed as parameters to guide fluid loading in critical care settings [43]. Their use however is limited to completely sedated patients under controlled mechanical ventilation who are in sinus rhythm. Some years ago a study (performed with the COLD system, the predecessor of the PiCCO) nicely showed that an EVLW-guided fluid restriction regimen in patients with pulmonary edema was beneficial regarding duration of mechanical ventilation and ICU stay [45]. Since the EVLW values in the study by Mitchell et al. were obtained with the double dye-indicator technique (COLD) these landmark observations needs to be validated in a randomized controlled clinical trial with the PiCCO system (using a single thermal bolus technique to determine EVLW).

A recent study by Michard and colleagues showed that in contrast to the classic intracardiac filling pressures, a static GEDV below 600 ml/m2 was capable of correctly predicting fluid responsiveness in about 75% of patients with septic shock [39]. Baseline GEDVI values were also significantly lower in responders.

Obtaining an idea of the EVLWI together with the PVPI will help in classifying patients with or without ARDS or acute lung injury (ALI) and differentiating them from acute lung edema, atelectasis, pleural effusions, etc...

EBM Q4: Will My New Variable-driven Diagnostic and Therapeutic Intervention Change Patient Outcome?

In the above mentioned study, an EVLW-guided fluid restriction regimen in patients with pulmonary edema reduced not only duration of mechanical ventilation and ICU stay but also mortality [45]. Recent studies showed that massive fluid resuscitation and the presence of a positive fluid balance, especially in the context of capillary leak, may be detrimental [46, 47]. Therefore, a holistic approach with PiCCO guided 'volumetric' therapy avoiding unnecessary over resuscitation, may prove beneficial in the future.

In a recent study in ARDS, patients with a greater reduction in EVLWI were more likely to be alive at the end of the study [48]. In a recent paper by Sakka et al., high EVLWI was associated with higher mortality in different patient groups (sepsis, ARDS) and non-survivors had overall statistically significant higher EVLWI levels [49].

Advantages

PiCCO monitoring has several advantages over the classic PAC. First it is less invasive, second it provides a cardiac output that it is less dependent on respiratory variations [38]. It provides rapidly available parameters, that are directly clinically applicable. It is reproducible for the less experienced user, simple to operate and understand. It provides volume quantification (that is positive end-expiratory pressure [PEEP] or intraabdominal pressure [IAP] independent) and can be used in a large range of patients (from small children to adults). There is no additional chest X-ray needed. There is no loss of indicator in case of right-left shunt (as with ARDS, pulmonary hypertension). It gives real-time, beat-to-beat cardiac output and real-time, beat-to-beat fluid responsiveness and afterload. It provides additional information (volumes) and functional hemodynamics (PPV, SVV). Most of the variables are measured and not estimated. It has a short response time and can be nurse driven at the bedside. It is supported by recent literature data in humans (validation, clinical use,...) that show good correlation of intermittent and continuous transpulmonary cardiac output with gold standard. EVLWI seems to be superior to chest X-ray and is validated against dye dilution and gravimetrics. ITBVI and GEDVI have been validated against double (thermodye) indicator techniques. It can alter treatment: EVLWI directed protocols reduce length of stay and duration of mechanical ventilation [50], and it can affect outcome since an EVLWI-directed protocol reduces ICU mortality in ARDS [45]. SVV and PPV are superior to other parameters in predicting fluid responsiveness [41].

Disadvantages

Possible drawbacks of transpulmonary thermodilution are: the need for a specialized arterial catheter, (iced) solution with extra fluid, the relation between PAC thermodilution cardiac ouput and transpulmonary thermodilution cardiac output seems clinically acceptable but a good correlation coefficient is not enough and should be completed with a Bland and Altman analysis to test for a systematic bias and agreement between the two methods by plotting the difference (or bias) against the mean of the two measurements. The fact that central circulation and proximal arterial catheterization are necessary is of limited relevance since most sick ICU patients require or already have these vascular accesses.

There has also been some criticism on the volume quantification: The volumetric parameters derived from the thermodilution curve are based on the assumption that the largest mixing chamber is the pulmonary thermal volume. GEDVI is correctly measured based on this assumption whereas ITBVI is estimated by extrapolation from the double indicator technique. There are concerns with regard to the possibility of mathematical coupling (the interdependence of two variables) although Buhre et al. [51] demonstrated that cardiac output could be decreased with beta-blockers without a concomitant decrease in ITBVI and Michard et al. [39] demonstrated that dobutamine increased cardiac output while GEDVI remained unchanged, suggesting the absence of such coupling. Mathematical coupling does not negate the validity of GEDVI as a predictor of intravascular volume status. The technique is not useful in valvulopathies (mitral insufficiency or aortic stenosis), abdominal aortic aneurysm or large atria. No normal values are available (for adults or children). Volumes are underestimated in morbid obesity. The volume measurement is not automated, and not continuous. No right/left quantification (for this purpose the combination with a VoLEF catheter might give some answers).

Finally, the pulse contour calibration is performed at a given time point with a given aortic impedance at that time. The accuracy of pulse contour analysis is influenced by the location of the arterial line (being less accurate the more distal the arterial catheter). In a number of conditions, vasomotor tone changes and so will resistance. Therefore, there is a need for recalibration in patients on high doses of vasopressors since these can distort the arterial waveform [38]. In general these problems can be prevented if the device is calibrated 3 to 4 times a day [38]. The current pulse contour algorithm is also not applicable in arrhythmias or during intra-aortic balloon counterpulsation.

▌ Transpulmonary Lithium Dilution (LiDCO)

Description

Using the Stewart-Hamilton equation, cardiac output can be calculated by the use of an intravascular indicator (lithium) which is injected into a central or peripheral vein and measured in a peripheral artery using a specialized sensor probe attached to the pressure line [52]. Correct application of this equation requires three conditions to be present: a constant blood flow, a homogenous mixing of blood and indicator, and absence of loss of indicator between injection and detection. Cardiac output is calculated according to

$$CO = \frac{LiCl \times 60}{Area \times (1 - PCV)}$$

where LiCl is the dose of lithium chloride in mmol, area the area under the dilution curve, and PCV the packed cell volume (derived from hemoglobin concentration). Currently, only one commercially available lithium dilution system exists (LiDCO; LiDCO Ltd, London, UK). The cardiac output obtained with lithium dilu-

Table 2. Lithium dilution cardiac output vs reference gold standard

Author	n	Patients or subjects	Reference	r^2	Bias (L/min)	Precision (L/min)	CO range (L/min)
Kurita [78]	10	Pigs	EMF	0.9	0.11	0.36	0.3–2.7
Mason [79]	10	Dogs	TD	0.98	0.1	0.9	1.1–12.8
Gunkel [80]	6	Dogs	NiCO	0.88	0.22	1.68	
Linton [81]	48	Age 5d–9yrs	TPTD	0.96	−0.1	0.3	0.4–6
Linton [82]	200	Mixed Cardiac surgery, medical intensive care	PATD	0.94	−0.25	0.46	
Young [83]	69	Cardiac surgery	PATD		−0.53	1.28	

N: number of measurements; r^2: coefficient of determination; CO: cardiac output; EMF: electromagnetic flowmetry; TD: thermodilution; NiCO: partial rebreathing cardiac output (indirect Fick); TPTD: transpulmonary thermodilution; PATD: pulmonary artery catheter thermodilution

tion can be used for calibration of a pulse contour analysis system, commercially available as an add-on for the LiDCO system (PulseCO).

EBM Q1: Does the New Device work as well as the Gold Standard?

Multiple studies have shown good to excellent correlation of the lithium dilution technique with pulmonary or transpulmonary thermodilution, especially in surgical and pediatric settings. However, the company manufacturing the LiDCO systems lists body weight below 40 kgs as a contraindication to using the system (as well as treatment with lithium salts and during the first trimester of pregnancy). Table 2 lists some recent trials comparing the lithium dilution technique to various gold standards in humans.

EBM Q2: Does The New Device Provide Me With New or Additional Information?

While the lithium dilution method provides an indicator dilution curve similar to the thermal transpulmonary dilution, and could be used in analogy with the PiCCO system to calculate volumes of mixing chambers, no such algorithms currently exist. On their website, the LiDCO company states that such algorithms are in active development. The only additional measured parameter compared to PAC monitoring is the variation of pulse pressure and stroke volume (PPV, SVV).

EBM Q3: Does the Interpretation of the New Variables Change My Decision Making and Treatment?

As described above, the SVV and PPV have been proposed as parameters to guide fluid loading in critical care settings [43, 53]. Their use, however, is limited to completely sedated patients under controlled mechanical ventilation who are in sinus rhythm. See also under PiCCO.

EBM Q4: Will My New Variable-driven Diagnostic and Therapeutic Intervention Change Patient Outcome?

At this moment, no studies that show a difference in outcome with LiDCO technology are available.

Advantages

The technique seems less invasive and the data are rapidly available. It uses existing access, does not require central circulation catheterization, and provides real time beat-to-beat variations in cardiac output together with functional hemodynamic parameters (PPV, SVV). Data interpretation is automated and presented via a colorful nurse-friendly user interface. The algorithm for analyzing the arterial waveform is different from that of the PiCCO and site unspecific and morphology independent. There is no need for an additional chest X-ray.

Disadvantages

With lithium dilution, in contrast to the PiCCO, volume quantification is not provided and the technique cannot be used in small children or patients receiving muscle relaxants. Little is known about possible toxic effects or accumulation with long-term use of lithium especially in ICU patients with organ failure. Validation has been mainly performed in animals and human data are scarce. The ion selective electrode is delicate, expensive and needs to be replaced every three days (according to the CE mark). The disposables and the lithium needed for cardiac output calibration are also expensive. Finally it provides little or no additional information to the PAC; basically it offers the clinician no direct idea of preload and it is more expensive. Also, the 3 ml blood draw required for each calibration may contribute to anemia and increased transfusion rates.

Regarding the pulse contour analysis, the same remarks apply as for the PiCCO system.

▌ Indirect Fick (Partial CO_2 Rebreathing – NICO)

Description

The Fick principle as described above can be used with a multitude of indicators that can be added or removed from the flow that is being studied. Thus, another suitable indicator is CO_2, which is produced in the body and extracted from the bloodstream in the lungs. When using CO_2 as an indicator in the Fick formula, rearrangement yields

$$CO = \frac{VCO_2}{CvCO_2 - CaCO_2}$$

VCO_2 represents the CO_2 clearance in the lungs and is easily measured by comparing inhaled and exhaled CO_2 content. $CaCO_2$ can be estimated from end-tidal CO_2 after calibration with arterial blood gas measurement in healthy subjects. $CvCO_2$, however, is difficult to measure non-invasively. To eliminate this problem, a mathematical manipulation eliminates the need for $CvCO_2$ measurement by introducing a CO_2 rebreathing period during which elimination is inhibited. While the total CO_2 rebreathing technique, popular among exercise physiologists, is difficult to reproduce in critical care settings because of poor cooperation, a modification using partial CO_2 rebreathing has been described that is also able to calculate cardiac output from VCO_2 and end-tidal CO_2 alone [54]. Starting from the previous formula, assuming cardiac output is equal in normal and partial rebreathing conditions, we get

$$CO = \frac{VCO_{2N}}{CvCO_{2N} - CaCO_{2N}} = \frac{VCO_{2R}}{CvCO_{2R} - CaCO_{2R}}$$

combined to form the differential Fick equation (based on the law of ratios, assuming $CvCO_2$ is also equal in both conditions due to rapid diffusion):

$$CO = \frac{VCO_{2N} - VCO_{2R}}{(CvCO_{2N} - CaCO_{2N}) - (CvCO_{2R} - CaCO_{2R})}$$

$$= \frac{\Delta VCO_2}{\Delta CaCO_2} = \frac{\Delta VCO_2}{S\Delta ETCO_2}$$

where R is partial rebreathing, N is normal breathing, S is slope of CO_2 dissociation curve.

Currently, the only commercial system available is the NICO® system (NICO sensor, Novametrix medical systems, Wallingford, CT).

EBM Q1: Does the New Device Work as Well as the Gold Standard?

Few published data exist that validate the indirect Fick technique and most of the data were only published in abstract form. From a theoretical point of view, reservations can be made concerning

▌ the small difference between $PvCO_2$ and $PaCO_2$ (usually only about 6 mmHg), leading to large differences in calculated cardiac output resulting from small measurement errors

▌ the assumptions of a linear CO_2-hemoglobin dissociation curve and reliable measurement of shunt fraction with Nunn's iso-shunt tables [55].

▌ Changes in ventilation (spontaneous or controlled) and hemodynamics altering the measured values of $ETCO_2$.

▌ Changes in alveolar gas exchange influencing the measurements as shown in a sheep ARDS model [56, 57].

Table 3 lists various studies that have compared partial rebreathing to bolus thermodilution, most of which have not been published as a full paper in a peer reviewed journal. While most studies report a rather large bias and precision range, this does not *a priori* negate the usefulness of the device if the above limitations are kept in mind, considering that narrow limits of agreement are impossible to obtain if the reference method itself has a wide precision range. The mean number of study subjects was 30.4, the mean correlation coefficient r was 0.82, the bias was

Table 3. Partial rebreathing cardiac output vs reference gold standard

Author	n	Patients	Reference	r^2	Bias (L/min)	Precision (L/min)
Gunkel [80]	6	Dogs	LIDCO	0.88	0.22	1.68
de Abreu [57]	20	ARDS sheep	PATD	0.54	−1.69	1.9
Odensted [84]	15	surgery	PATD	0.96	0.04	1.72
Kotake [85]	28	Aortic surgery	PATD		−0.58	0.9
Kuck [86]	36	Cardiac surgery	PATD	0.92		
Guzzi [87]	27	CABG	PATD	0.85	−0.01	0.62
Jopling [88]	48	Unknown	PATD		−1.75	2.28
Loeb [89]	12	Cardiac surgery	PATD		−0.19	1.16
Watt [90]	5	Cardiac surgery	PATD		0.20	0.70
Kuck [91]	134	CABG	PATD	0.78	0.69	0.94
Rocco [92]	12	MV patients	PATD	0.79	−1.2	3
	6	High shunt	PATD	0.62	−2.3	2.4
	6	Low shunt	PATD	0.95	0.01	0.8
Murias [93]	22	MV patients	PATD	0.84	−0.18	2.78
Mean	30.4			0.82	−0.40	1.61
SD	34.9			0.13	0.81	0.83

N: number of patients/animals; r: correlation coefficient; ARDS: acute respiratory distress syndrome; PATD: pulmonary artery catheter thermodilution; CABG: coronary artery bypass graft; MV: mechanically ventilated

−0.4 l/min and the precision was 1.61 l/min (or the limits of agreement defined as 2 standard deviations according to the Bland and Altman analysis).

EBM Q2: Does the New Device Provide Me With New or Additional Information?

Apart from ventilator-associated data (such as full respiratory mechanics with dynamic compliance and resistance, dead space tidal volume, alveolar minute volume, endtidal CO_2,...), the NICO system provides the clinician with the CO_2 elimination rate and the pulmonary capillary blood flow (PCBF), defined as the portion of the cardiac output that is effective in gas exchange.

EBM Q3: Does The Interpretation of the New Variables Change My Decision Making and Treatment?

In a prospective clinical trial, PCBF was validated against invasive measurement (cardiac output minus venous admixture flow) [56]. PCBF values were reported to be useful in titrating PEEP aimed at improving PCBF in an ALI setting. Another study showed that the use of the NICO as a metabolic monitor helped in optimizing nutritional status in mechanically ventilated ICU patients.

EBM Q4: Will My New Variable-Driven Diagnostic and Therapeutic Intervention Change Patient Outcome?

To the knowledge of the authors, no outcome data have been published on the use of PCBF in any clinical setting.

Advantages

It is less invasive than the other techniques and is based on the gold standard Fick principle. It is rapidly available (within 3 minutes) and allows automated data interpretation of measured and calculated variables. It comes with a user-friendly interface and provides many additional parameters. There is no need for a control chest X-ray after placement and it may be cost-effective (see further).

Disadvantages

Endotracheal intubation is necessary and the technique is not well validated in different ICU patient groups. The patients need to be fully sedated and in volume controlled mode since the interpretation is unreliable in assisted ventilation (weaning phase), during hyperventilation (since $PaCO_2$ must be above 30 mmHg) and during diaphragm manipulation, so its accuracy is limited by cardiopulmonary disease. Changes in ventilator settings that alter dead space or ventilation/perfusion ratio will have an effect on the calculated variables and will hence compromise the interpretation of the absolute values. The theoretical principle is quite complex, based on a lot of assumptions and hence prone to errors. The shunt calculation may be inexact since shunted blood is not measured.

▌ Esophageal Doppler

Description

One of the most promising techniques for non-invasive assessment of cardiac output is esophageal Doppler monitoring. First described in 1971, and later refined by Singer in 1989, the basis of the technique is that flow in a cylinder can be calculated from flow velocity and cross-sectional area of the cylinder [58, 59]. With a continuous or pulsed-wave Doppler beam, blood flow velocity can be calculated from the frequency shift of the reflected ultrasound waves using the Doppler principle. By using the pulsatile nature of aortic flow, a velocity-time integral (VTI) can be constructed that is defined as the area under the flow curve from onset (t1) to end (t2) of flow. This represents the stroke distance, or the distance traveled by the red blood cells down the aorta during the stroke cycle. Stroke volume determination then comes down to volume calculation of a cylinder (the aorta), with a base defined as the cross-sectional area where flow was measured and the height the stroke distance or VTI. Cardiac output can easily be calculated from stroke volume as shown above.

$$Area = \pi r^2$$

$$Stroke\ distance = \int_{t_1}^{t_2} \frac{dV}{dT}$$

In contrast to the PAC, the esophageal Doppler probe can be inserted within minutes and after only very limited training. It has been reportedly left *in situ* for over 2 weeks without complications [60].

EBM Q1: Does The New Device Work as Well as the Gold Standard?

From the above description, it is clear that a few prerequisite assumptions are required to be true for esophageal Doppler to give an accurate estimate of cardiac output

▌ The descending aorta is assumed to be cylindrical, while in reality its shape can change depending on pulse pressure and aortic compliance.

▌ In some devices, aortic diameter is derived from a normogram based on age and body weight.

▌ The flow in the aorta is assumed to be laminar, while tachycardia, anemia and aortic valve disease can cause turbulent flow [2].

▌ Narrow alignment of the Doppler beam with the direction of aortic flow is required for accurate measurement, as is apparent from the Doppler equation [61]. Generally, an angle of less than 20° is recommended.

▌ For derivation of cardiac output from aortic flow, the fraction of blood going to the brachiocephalic and coronary arteries (30%) is assumed to be constant. However, this is variable among patients and disease states [62].

▌ Diastolic flow in the descending aorta is assumed to be negligible.

As a result, studies comparing esophageal Doppler to some reference technique have reported a wide range in reliability. Table 4 lists various studies comparing the technique *in vivo*.

EBM Q2: Does the New Device Provide Me With New or Additional Information?

Although cardiac output is probably the most valuable parameter obtained by esophageal Doppler, assessment of LV contractility and preload with esophageal Doppler have been reported using flow waveform analysis [63]. Parameters of interest

Table 4. Esophageal Doppler cardiac output vs reference gold standard

Author	n	Patients	Reference	r^2	Bias (L/min)	Precision (L/min)	CO range (L/min)
Valtier B [94]	136	ICU	PATD	0.95	0.24	1.75	1.7–14.8
Bernardin [95]	22	ICU (hypovolemic)	PATD	0.92			3.5–12.5
Baillard [96]	14	ICU	PATD	0.95	–0.1	1	2.4–13
Singer [59]	238	ICU	PATD		0.6%	14.1%	
Leather [97]	14	Surgery (prostatectomy)	PATD		0.89	1.8	3.4–7.3
Hullet [98]	20	CABG	PATD	0.62	–0.56	1.3	2.1–10.2
Dark [99]	2400	Meta-analysis	PATD		0.19		

N: number of measurements; r: correlation coefficient; CO: cardiac output; ICU: intensive care unit; PATD: pulmonary artery catheter thermodilution; CABG: coronary artery bypass graft

are the flow time, index of preload, defined as the time required from start of waveform upstroke to return to baseline, and peak flow velocity, index of contractility [59, 64]. Since flow time is heart rate dependent it is usually corrected by dividing flow time by the square root of the cycle length (FTc). Obviously, in the hands of a trained operator, complete transesophageal echocardiography provides abundant additional information, of which the discussion is outside the scope of this text.

EBM Q3: Does the Interpretation of the New Variables Change My Decision Making and Treatment?

Using FTc, Singer et al. manipulated ventricular filling in ICU patients by i.v. loading or i.v. nitrates and observed a relation between PAOP, cardiac output and FTc that seemed to indicate a use for FTc as optimal filling marker [65]. Madan and colleagues observed a better correlation between FTc and cardiac output (r = 0.52) than with PAOP and cardiac output (r = 0.2) [66]. Dobutamine and esmolol have been shown to increase and decrease the peak flow velocity respectively [65]. Both parameters could be used to optimize fluid loading and inotrope use from a theoretical point of view.

EBM Q4: Will My New-variable Driven Diagnostic and Therapeutic Intervention Change Patient Outcome?

In a prospective, randomized controlled trial, Sinclair et al. demonstrated a significantly shorter hospital stay for patients whose volume status during proximal femur fracture repair had been optimized using esophageal Doppler (goal FTc > 350 msec and optimized stroke volume vs usual care) [67]. Mythen and Webb showed a decrease in major complications, a lower incidence of gut hypoperfusion (measured by intramucosal gastric pH) and shorter length of hospital stay in an unblinded cardiac surgery trial where stroke volume was optimized perioperatively [68]. Finally Muchada showed, in a retrospective study of 110 sedated adult general surgery patients, that the use of esophageal Doppler (Hemosonic) enabled the physician to optimize therapeutic and or fluid management improving patient outcome and reducing procedure-related morbidity (Muchada et al. unpublished data).

Advantages

It provides real-time and very quick cardiac output as well as afterload data interpretation. It is less invasive than, for example, the PiCCO or LiDCO. The data interpretation is fully automated and presented via a user-friendly interface. It provides many additional parameters as well as an estimate for preload via the corrected flow time.

Disadvantages

As with any technique there is a steep learning curve. It is not a really CCO device since it is dependent on patient movement (the probe tends to move in the esophagus) and requires specialized training. The measurement is approximate (especially if there is no M-mode available to correctly measure aortic diameter) and does not measure total cardiac output but only descending aortic blood flow. Since it is operator dependent, it cannot be nurse driven at the bedside.

▌ Thoracic Electrical Bioimpedance (TEB)

Description

The technique of TEB monitoring (or impedance cardiography) applies the assumption that the thorax is a non-homogeneous conductor of injected electrical current [69]. Thoracic muscle, lung, fat, skin, bone, air and blood are conductors with different resistances. Electrical current takes the path of least resistance, the blood (130 Ω cm). Total TEB, 'Z', depends on three components: (a) baseline impedance (Z_0), indirectly proportional to thoracic fluid content (average normal value 25 Ω); (b) tidal changes in ITBV caused by respiration (changes of about 1 Ω); and (c) changes in thoracic blood volume caused by the cardiac cycle (changes of 0.1 to 0.2 Ω) [69]. The latter impedance changes are primarily due to changes in aortic volume [70].

One set of body surface electrodes (placed on upper neck and upper abdomen) is the source and sink of a constant high-frequency, low-magnitude current, creating a voltage difference that is sensed by another set of body surface electrodes (placed on lower neck and at the level of the diaphragm) that also detect electrical signals from the heart [69]. Impedance cardiography provides us with a continuous, non-invasive estimate of stroke volume (and hence cardiac output) through measurement of impedance changes over time (dZ/dt), and with the ventricular ejection time. Difficulties arise when the electrocardiogram (EKG) does not allow accurate determination of the beginning of the QRS complex; with movement artifacts; without good electrode-to-skin contact; with low Z_0 or dZ/dt; substantial thoracic fluid overload (low signal-to-noise ratio, bypassing of the aortic electrical current); tachydysrhythmias; severely abnormal thoracic anatomy [69]; cardiac valve disease, aortic dilatation and intracardiac shunts [70]. It may remain reliable for detecting trends of changes in the circulation with time [71].

There are many commercially available devices for TEB use in the ICU such as the IQ System (Renaissance Technologies, Newton, PA, USA) or the BioZ (Cardiodynamics, San Diego, CA, USA).

EBM Q1: Does the New Device Work as Well as the Gold Standard?

A recent meta-analysis (372 articles) found an overall correlation coefficient r of 0.82 between cardiac output measurements using impedance cardiography and several other 'reference' methods [72]. When the studies with repeated measurements in the same subjects (possibly creating a bias) were excluded, the correlation decreased to 0.73. The performance of impedance cardiography was similar in various groups of patients, with the exception of 'cardiac patients', in whom the correlation coefficient was 0.77 (overall) and 0.66 in studies with only one measurement per subject. Another meta-analysis (201 articles) found a correlation with other methods ranging from 0.82 to 0.93 [69]. The correlation with thermodilution was 0.81 (16 803 measurements) and with direct Fick 0.79 (587 measurements). Interestingly, the average correlation was only 0.56 (range 0.36–0.75) in patients with sepsis. In patients with a chest tube, the correlation was no more than 0.35. The considerable variations in correlation coefficients between studies can be explained by the different methods and calculations used in impedance cardiography.

EBM Q2: Does the New Device Provide Me With New or Additional Information?

Compared with the PAC, bioimpedance may allow monitoring of some extra parameters. First, it provides us with an estimation of the thoracic fluid content, which is indirectly proportional to Z_0 [2, 69]. However, we were not able to find any studies comparing this parameter with thoracic intravascular volume measurements obtained with another method. As far as EVLW is concerned, Z_0 was demonstrated to be decreased in a group of 131 patients with suspected heart failure and chest X-ray signs of cardiomegaly or pulmonary edema [73]. Z_0 also differed significantly in 26 patients in the emergency department, divided after clinical and radiographic evaluation in three groups: decreased, normal or increased thoracic fluid, corresponding to Z_0 values of 37.4 Ω, 26.5 Ω and 21.8 Ω, respectively (p < 0.02) [74]. On the other hand, there was no correlation between Z_0 and EVLW measured by double indicator dilution in 13 patients with noncardiogenic pulmonary edema (r = –0.24, p = 0.56) [74].

Second, the isovolumetric relaxation time is a measure of active ventricular relaxation and therefore of diastolic function [69]. The maximum of the second derivative of impedance $(d^2Z/dt^2)_{max}$ is a reflection of the maximum acceleration of aortic blood flow, and therefore a measure of cardiac contractility [69]. The combination of both parameters was shown to be useful for differentiating systolic and diastolic heart failure [75].

EBM Q3: Does the Interpretation of the New Variables Change My Decision Making and Treatment?

In a prospective, blinded study of 55 patients older than 65 years, presenting to the emergency department with dyspnea, unblinding of the results of the impedance cardiography resulted in a change of diagnosis in 5.3% of patients and a change of treatment in 23.6% of patients [76].

EBM Q4: Will My New Variable-driven Diagnostic and Therapeutic Intervention Change Patient Outcome?

At this time, no studies that show a difference in outcome with impedance cardiography are available.

Advantages

Together with the partial CO_2 rebreathing technique, it is the least invasive method. It has been on the market for a long period of time and a substantial number of validation studies have been performed.

Disadvantages

The estimate of cardiac output is less accurate in patients with significant fluid overload, pulmonary edema, pleural effusions, or even massive peripheral edema. The technique is very sensitive to any alteration in position or contact of the electrodes; and the technique is inaccurate in patients with atrial fibrillation/flutter or other arrhythmias with an irregular R-R interval. So, when used in the ICU, TEB may not be as accurate as the other techniques; therefore TEB was not included in the cost and effectiveness analysis.

Cost and Effectiveness

Costs

A cost estimation (in Euros) was performed for the different less or non-invasive (continuous) cardiac output measurement techniques, based on cost of the devices, chest X-ray, sterile draping, disposables, and physician and nursing time. Costs were scored based on the initial set-up, the first measurement and the evolution over time in a hypothetical situation where cardiac output measurements (or calibrations) were performed four times a day for 5 up to 15 days. It was also assumed that every patient needed an arterial and a central venous line. Costs were compared based on costs of the initial set-up and the costs of the first and next measurements as well as the costs based on the number of cardiac output calibrations per day and the duration of measurement period.

The cost evaluation was based on the following estimates and official price offers received from the different companies that produce the devices. It does not take into account special offers like free devices with the use of a specific number of disposables over a specific period of time since most of the companies have similar offers. In order to be concise and objective it is only based on official listed prices for the Belgian market: Devices: Pulsion PiCCO device: 16000.– €; LiDCO device: 17000.– €; Novametrics NICO device: 15600.– €; Edwards Vigilance monitor: 15200.– €; and the Abbott Hemosonic device: 23000.– €.

Catheters and disposables: CVC catheter 24.75 €; arterial line (seldinger technique): 20.– €; pressure transducer: 24.75 €; PiCCO catheter: 214.1 €; LiDCO initial setup (lithium sensor and connections): 125.5 €; NICO rebreathing loop: 78.– €; Hemosonic disposable: 50.– €; swan-ganz sheath: 24.85 €; CEDV Swan-Ganz catheter (=PAC with CCO and continuous right ventricular end diastolic volume measurement): 250.– €; 50ml of saline: 0.36 €; syringe: 0.36 €; needle: 0.023 €; stopcock: 0.31 €; sterile drapings: 10.– €; local anesthetic: 1.– €; chest X-ray: 21.– €; nursing costs: 25.– € per hour; and doctor costs: 100.– € per hour. Table 5 shows the initial set-up cost for the different devices while Table 6 shows the cost for the first measurement.

The cost for the initial setup was the highest for the PAC, followed by the PiCCO and LiDCO and the lowest for the Hemosonic (Table 5). Figure 1 shows bar graphs of the different cost issues for the different devices. The cost for the first measurement was the highest for the LiDCO at 6.2 €. For the other techniques the cost per measurement varied between 0.8 and 3.8 € (Table 6).

Figure 2 shows the evolution of total costs per day over time: these were between 192 to 483.– € for the first day and dropped to 17.5 to 93.4 € per day after 15 days. Figure 3 plots the evolution of the cumulative costs (in €) over time for the different devices.

The total cost score (Fig. 4) was calculated as a percentage based on the rank order for the different cost comparisons (setup, first measurement, further monitoring). The NICO and Hemosonic devices were least expensive followed by the PAC.

Table 5. Cost comparison (in €) for the initial setup for the different devices

Device	Cost of Device	Transducer (Unit price)	Transducer (n)	Transducer (Total price)	X-ray	Sheath	Disposables	CVC	Arterial line	NaCl	Sterile drapings	Local anes	Dr time	Dr cost/ hr	Dr Total cost	Total Setup Cost
PiCCO	16000	24.75	1	24.75	0	0	214.1	24.75	0	0.36	10	1	20	100	33.33	308.3
LiDCO	17000	24.75	2	49.5	0	54.7	70.8	24.75	20	0.36	10	1	20	100	33.33	291.2
NICO	15600	24.75	2	49.5	0	0	78	24.75	20	0	0	0	10	100	16.67	215.7
Hemosonic	23000	24.75	2	49.5	0	0	50	24.75	20	0	0	0	10	100	16.67	187.7
PAC	15200	24.75	3	74.25	21	24.85	250	0	20	1.17	10	1	30	100	50	480

N: number; CVC: central venous catheter; Dr: doctor; PAC: pulmonary artery catheter

Table 6. Cost comparison (in €) for the first measurement and cost per day

	Syringe	Lithium	NaCl	Nursing time	Nurse cost/hr	Nurse Total Cost	Total Cost First measurement	Total Cost Per day
▌PiCCO	0.36	0	0.29	7.5	25	3.13	3.775	15.1
▌LiDCO	0.36	3.44	0.29	5	25	2.08	6.173	24.69
▌NiCO	0	0	0	3	25	1.25	1.25	5
▌Hemosonic	0	0	0	3	25	1.25	1.25	5
▌PAC	0	0	0	2	25	0.83	0.83	3.33

The total cost per day was based on the assumption that one calibration (either with physiologic saline or lithium) was performed every 6 hours

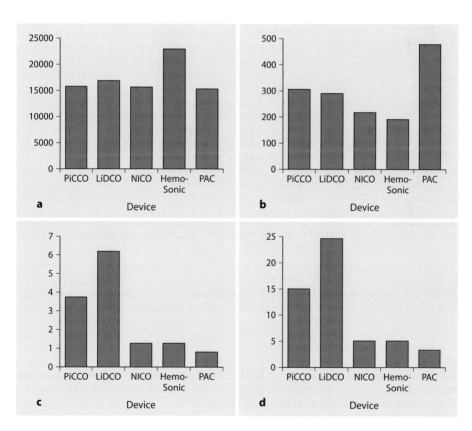

Fig. 1. Cost comparison (in €) of the different less or non-invasive hemodynamic monitoring devices. See text for explanation. **a** Comparison of the cost of the device itself; **b** Comparison of the cost for the initial set-up; **c** Comparison of the cost per measurement; **d** Comparison of the cost per day (based on the assumption that one calibration was performed every 6 hours)

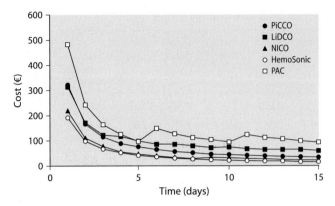

Fig. 2. Evolution of the total cost (in €) per day over time for the different devices in the hypothetical situation were hemodynamic monitoring was used for 5 up to 15 days. See text for explanation

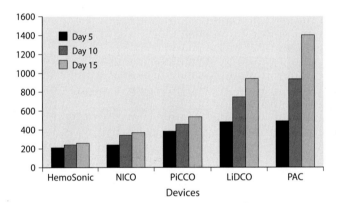

Fig. 3. Evolution of the cumulative costs (in €) over time for the different devices. Bar graph showing cost snapshots on day 5, 10 and 15, assuming that 4 calibrations per day were performed for up to 15 days and taking into account the initial setup costs

Finally the more time consuming PiCCO and LiDCO techniques were most expensive mainly due to the cost of nursing time and the lithium.

Effectiveness

Effectiveness analysis was based on the level of invasiveness, the advantages versus the disadvantages and the available literature information to answer the four evidence based medicine questions as cited above.

The total effectiveness score (Fig. 4) was calculated as a percentage based on the rank order for the different effectiveness comparisons. The PiCCO device was the most effective followed by the Hemosonic and the gold standard. Finally the NICO and LiDCO techniques were least effective mainly due to the lack of validation in clinical ICU patient populations and the fact that they do not provide the physician

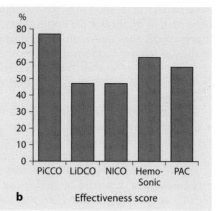

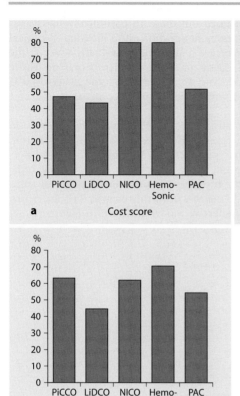

Fig. 4. Bar graphs showing the final scores (in %) for the different non-invasive hemodynamic monitoring devices. **a** Total cost score (%); **b** Total effectiveness score (%); **c** Combined cost and effectiveness score (%)

with a real preload estimate or in case of the LiDCO does not give additional information compared to the PAC.

Combined Cost and Effectiveness

The combined cost and effectiveness score was calculated as a percentage obtained by adding the cost to the effectiveness score and dividing this number by two (Fig. 4).

Cost-effectiveness is only one aspect of a possible economic analysis to compare different technologies, the others being cost minimization, cost benefit, and cost utility. And although economic evaluations are increasingly common in the critical care literature, reported approaches to their conduct are not standardized [4]. Bringing cost-effectiveness analysis from the literature to the bedside raises some major concerns. First, evidence for the effectiveness of critical care interventions is often lacking. Second, the care we provide in the ICU is often supportive rather than curative (as is the case when using less or non-invasive hemodynamic technologies). Third, critical illness is a complex process that can occur in varied, heterogeneous patient populations. Fourth, the ICU resuscitation endpoints we use (e.g., cardiac output, ejection fraction, oxygenation,...) are not suitable for a cost-effectiveness analysis. Fifth, the recommended outcomes in cost-effectiveness analyses such as quality of life and utility assessment are difficult to measure in critical illness. Sixth, the importance of end-of-life care is difficult to evaluate. Seventh, the burden of intensive care monitoring and treatment on family members is not easily captured in a cost effectiveness analysis. And finally, data on the costs of ICU therapies are often derived from sources with different practice patterns and cost structures.

Without having the ambition to be totally correct and complete we opted to do a cost effectiveness analysis for the non-invasive hemodynamic technologies from the physician's and hospital administrator's perspectives. Although the societal perspective, which represents the public interest, is the best way to look at a new technology or medication, since it provides the broadest perspective and the most comprehensive data, it would be to difficult to cover within this chapter [4]. An example of a sensitivity analysis from the cost-effective model is shown in Figure 5.

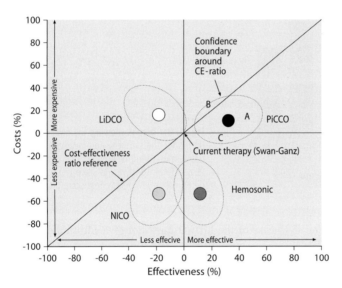

Fig. 5. Example of a sensitivity analysis from the cost-effective model. A standard cost-effectiveness ratio reference is drawn. Area A represents the likelihood that the cost-effectiveness ratio of the use of the PiCCO is more effective than the PAC reference standard. Area B represents the likelihood that the cost-effectiveness ratio of the use of the PiCCO lies above the standard threshold meaning that although it is more effective it is too expensive to justify its use and area C represents the likelihood that the use of the PiCCO is both cheaper and better than the current gold standard (PAC). Only devices which have confidence boundaries lying within the lower right quadrant and the lower triangle of the upper right quadrant are cost-effective (PiCCO and Hemosonic); the use of devices within the lower triangle of the left lower quadrant are acceptable taking into account that they may be less effective (NICO); the use of devices above the diagonal line is questionable, they could be used as an alternative provided their costs are reduced (LiDCO)

▌ Conclusion

After the scientific earthquake caused by the paper by Connors et al. [10], critical care physicians have started to use fewer PACs in their ICUs, especially in Europe [8, 10, 77]. However, not using any form of invasive monitoring may lead to a literal and figural dead-end [1]. We conclude from our cost and effectiveness analysis that less or non-invasive hemodynamic monitoring technologies are not so bad and they can be as accurate as the PAC. They can offer useful additional and new information that can help or alter our decision-making and treatment strategies. However, each technology is different, needs to be assessed on its own merits and has a steep learning curve. We also believe that costs and effectiveness will play a major role in the future, therefore we hope that this chapter will provide some answers to future users.

Volumetric estimates of preload status such as GEDVI and ITBVI are of significant value in the assessment of traumatically injured patients. This volumetric assessment is especially useful in patients with increased IAP or patients with changing ventricular compliance and elevated intrathoracic pressure in whom traditional intracardiac filling pressure measurements such as PAOP and CVP may be erroneously elevated and difficult to interpret since they are zero-referenced against atmospheric and not intrathoracic pressure [38]. Reliance on such pressures to guide resuscitation can lead to inappropriate therapeutic decisions, under- or overresuscitation, and organ failure. Pulse contour technology (LiDCO and PiCCO) has the potential to significantly improve the speed and accuracy of patient resuscitation following surgery or traumatic injury. The functional hemodynamic variables PPV and SVV may even prove to be superior if the patient is in regular sinus rhythm and fully sedated under controlled mechanical ventilation.

References

1. Bellomo R, Uchino S (2003) Cardiovascular monitoring tools: use and misuse. Curr Opin Crit Care 9:225–229
2. Chaney JC, Derdak S (2002) Minimally invasive hemodynamic monitoring for the intensivist: current and emerging technology. Crit Care Med 30:2338–2345
3. Smith GC, Pell JP (2003) Parachute use to prevent death and major trauma related to gravitational challenge: systematic review of randomised controlled trials. BMJ 327:1459–1461
4. American Thoracic Society workshop on outcomes research (2002) Understanding costs and cost-effectiveness in critical care. Am J Respir Crit Care Med 165:540–550
5. Swan HJ, Ganz W, Forrester J, Marcus H, Diamond G, Chonette D (1970) Catheterization of the heart in man with use of a flow-directed balloon-tipped catheter. N Engl J Med 283:447–451
6. Ivanov R, Allen J, Calvin JE (2000) The incidence of major morbidity in critically ill patients managed with pulmonary artery catheters: a meta-analysis. Crit Care Med 28:615–619
7. Sandham JD, Hull RD, Brant RF, et al (2003) A randomized, controlled trial of the use of pulmonary-artery catheters in high-risk surgical patients. N Engl J Med 348:5–14
8. Robin ED (1987) Death by pulmonary artery flow-directed catheter. Time for a moratorium? Chest 92:727–731
9. Kumar A, Anel R, Bunnell E, et al (2004) Pulmonary artery occlusion pressure and central venous pressure fail to predict ventricular filling volume, cardiac performance, or the response to volume infusion in normal subjects. Crit Care Med 32:691–699
10. Connors AF Jr, Speroff T, Dawson NV, et al (1996) The effectiveness of right heart catheterization in the initial care of critically ill patients. SUPPORT Investigators. JAMA 276:889–897

11. Matthay MA, Chatterjee K (1988) Bedside catheterization of the pulmonary artery: risks compared with benefits. Ann Intern Med 109:826–834
12. Jacka MJ, Cohen MM, To T, Devitt JH, Byrick R (2002) Pulmonary artery occlusion pressure estimation: how confident are anesthesiologists? Crit Care Med 30:1197–1203
13. Squara P, Bennett D, Perret C (2002) Pulmonary artery catheter: does the problem lie in the users? Chest 121:2009–2015
14. Gnaegi A, Feihl F, Perret C (1997) Intensive care physicians' insufficient knowledge of right-heart catheterization at the bedside: time to act? Crit Care Med 25:213–220
15. Branthwaite MA, Bradley RD (1968) Measurement of cardiac output by thermal dilution in man. J Appl Physiol 24:434–438
16. Olsson B, Pool J, Vandermoten P, Varnauskas E, Wassen R (1970) Validity and reproducibility of determination of cardiac output by thermodilution in man. Cardiology 55:136–148
17. Stetz CW, Miller RG, Kelly GE, Raffin TA (1982) Reliability of the thermodilution method in the determination of cardiac output in clinical practice. Am Rev Respir Dis 126:1001–1004
18. Keech J, Reed RL 2nd (2003) Reliability of mixed venous oxygen saturation as an indicator of the oxygen extraction ratio demonstrated by a large patient data set. J Trauma 54:236–241
19. Singer M (1998) Cardiac output in 1998. Heart 79:425–428
20. Eisenberg PR, Jaffe AS, Schuster DP (1984) Clinical evaluation compared to pulmonary artery catheterization in the hemodynamic assessment of critically ill patients. Crit Care Med 12:549–553
21. Mueller HS, Chatterjee K, Davis KB, et al (1998) ACC expert consensus document. Present use of bedside right heart catheterization in patients with cardiac disease. American College of Cardiology. J Am Coll Cardiol 32:840–864
22. Richard C, Warszawski J, Anguel N, et al (2003) Early use of the pulmonary artery catheter and outcomes in patients with shock and acute respiratory distress syndrome: a randomized controlled trial. JAMA 290:2713–2720
23. Goedje O, Hoeke K, Lichtwarck-Aschoff M, Faltchauser A, Lamm P, Reichart B (1999) Continuous cardiac output by femoral arterial thermodilution calibrated pulse contour analysis: comparison with pulmonary arterial thermodilution. Crit Care Med 27:2407–2412
24. Goedje O, Seebauer T, Peyerl M, Pfeiffer UJ, Reichart B (2000) Hemodynamic monitoring by double-indicator dilution technique in patients after orthotopic heart transplantation. Chest 118:775–781
25. Buhre W, Weyland A, Kazmaier S, et al (1999) Comparison of cardiac output assessed by pulse-contour analysis and thermodilution in patients undergoing minimally invasive direct coronary artery bypass grafting. J Cardiothorac Vasc Anesth 13:437–440
26. Godje O, Hoke K, Lamm P, et al (1998) Continuous, less invasive, hemodynamic monitoring in intensive care after cardiac surgery. Thorac Cardiovasc Surg 46:242–249
27. Bindels AJ, van der Hoeven JG, Meinders AE (2000) Extravascular lung water in patients with septic shock during a fluid regimen guided by cardiac index. Neth J Med 57:82–93
28. Holm C, Melcer B, Horbrand F, Henckel von Donnersmarck G, Muhlbauer W (2001) Arterial thermodilution: an alternative to pulmonary artery catheter for cardiac output assessment in burn patients. Burns 27:161–166
29. Sakka SG, Reinhart K, Meier-Hellmann A (1999) Comparison of pulmonary artery and arterial thermodilution cardiac output in critically ill patients. Intensive Care Med 25:843–846
30. Della Rocca G, Costa MG, Pompei L, Coccia C, Pietropaoli P (2002) Continuous and intermittent cardiac output measurement: pulmonary artery catheter versus aortic transpulmonary technique. Br J Anaesth 88:350–356
31. Friedman Z, Berkenstadt H, Margalit N, Sega E, Perel A (2002) Cardiac output assessed by arterial thermodilution during exsanguination and fluid resuscitation: experimental validation against a reference technique. Eur J Anaesthesiol 19:337–340
32. Godje O, Peyerl M, Seebauer T, Dewald O, Reichart B (1998) Reproducibility of double indicator dilution measurements of intrathoracic blood volume compartments, extravascular lung water, and liver function. Chest 113:1070–1077
33. McLuckie A, Murdoch IA, Marsh MJ, Anderson D (1996) A comparison of pulmonary and femoral artery thermodilution cardiac indices in paediatric intensive care patients. Acta Paediatr 85:336–338

34. Zollner C, Briegel J, Kilger E, Haller M (1998) [Retrospective analysis of transpulmonary and pulmonary arterial measurement of cardiac output in ARDS patients]. Anaesthesist 47:912–917

35. Sakka SG, Ruhl CC, Pfeiffer UJ, et al (2000) Assessment of cardiac preload and extravascular lung water by single transpulmonary thermodilution. Intensive Care Med 26:180–187

36. Zollner C, Haller M, Weis M, et al (2000) Beat-to-beat measurement of cardiac output by intravascular pulse contour analysis: a prospective criterion standard study in patients after cardiac surgery. J Cardiothorac Vasc Anesth 14:125–129

37. Haller M, Zollner C, Briegel J, Forst H (1995) Evaluation of a new continuous thermodilution cardiac output monitor in critically ill patients: a prospective criterion standard study. Crit Care Med 23:860–866

38. Malbrain ML, Cheatham ML (2004) Cardiovascular effects and optimal preload markers in intraabdominal hypertension. In: Vincent JL (ed) Yearbook of Intensive Care and Emergency Medicine. Springer, Berlin, pp 519–543

39. Michard F, Alaya S, Zarka V, Bahloul M, Richard C, Teboul JL (2003) Global end-diastolic volume as an indicator of cardiac preload in patients with septic shock. Chest 124:1900–1908

40. Malbrain ML (2004) Is it wise not to think about intraabdominal hypertension in the ICU? Curr Opin Crit Care 10:132–145

41. Michard F, Teboul JL (2002) Predicting fluid responsiveness in ICU patients: a critical analysis of the evidence. Chest 121:2000–2008

42. Reuter DA, Felbinger TW, Moerstedt K, et al (2002) Intrathoracic blood volume index measured by thermodilution for preload monitoring after cardiac surgery. J Cardiothorac Vasc Anesth 16:191–195

43. Michard F, Boussat S, Chemla D, et al (2000) Relation between respiratory changes in arterial pulse pressure and fluid responsiveness in septic patients with acute circulatory failure. Am J Respir Crit Care Med 162:134–138

44. Michard F, Chemla D, Richard C, et al (1999) Clinical use of respiratory changes in arterial pulse pressure to monitor the hemodynamic effects of PEEP. Am J Respir Crit Care Med 159:935–939

45. Mitchell JP, Schuller D, Calandrino FS, Schuster DP (1992) Improved outcome based on fluid management in critically ill patients requiring pulmonary artery catheterization. Am Rev Respir Dis 145:990–998

46. Alsous F, Khamiees M, DeGirolamo A, Amoateng-Adjepong Y, Manthous CA (2000) Negative fluid balance predicts survival in patients with septic shock: a retrospective pilot study. Chest 117:1749–1754

47. Balogh Z, McKinley BA, Cocanour CS, et al (2003) Supranormal trauma resuscitation causes more cases of abdominal compartment syndrome. Arch Surg 138:637–642

48. Davey-Quinn A, Gedney JA, Whiteley SM, Bellamy MC (1999) Extravascular lung water and acute respiratory distress syndrome–oxygenation and outcome. Anaesth Intensive Care 27:357–362

49. Sakka SG, Klein M, Reinhart K, Meier-Hellmann A (2002) Prognostic value of extravascular lung water in critically ill patients. Chest 122:2080–2086

50. Eisenberg PR, Hansbrough JR, Anderson D, Schuster DP (1987) A prospective study of lung water measurements during patient management in an intensive care unit. Am Rev Respir Dis 136:662–668

51. Buhre W, Kazmaier S, Sonntag H, Weyland A (2001) Changes in cardiac output and intrathoracic blood volume: a mathematical coupling of data? Acta Anaesthesiol Scand 45:863–867

52. Jonas MM, Tanser SJ (2002) Lithium dilution measurement of cardiac output and arterial pulse waveform analysis: an indicator dilution calibrated beat-by-beat system for continuous estimation of cardiac output. Curr Opin Crit Care 8:257–261

53. Reuter DA, Felbinger TW, Schmidt C, et al (2002) Stroke volume variations for assessment of cardiac responsiveness to volume loading in mechanically ventilated patients after cardiac surgery. Intensive Care Med 28:392–398

54. Capek JM, Roy RJ (1988) Noninvasive measurement of cardiac output using partial CO_2 rebreathing. IEEE Trans Biomed Eng 35:653–661

55. Benatar SR, Hewlett AM, Nunn JF (1973) The use of iso-shunt lines for control of oxygen therapy. Br J Anaesth 45:711–718
56. de Abreu MG, Geiger S, Winkler T, et al (2002) Evaluation of a new device for noninvasive measurement of nonshunted pulmonary capillary blood flow in patients with acute lung injury. Intensive Care Med 28:318–323
57. de Abreu MG, Quintel M, Ragaller M, Albrecht DM (1997) Partial carbon dioxide rebreathing: a reliable technique for noninvasive measurement of nonshunted pulmonary capillary blood flow. Crit Care Med 25:675–683
58. Side CD, Gosling RG (1971) Non-surgical assessment of cardiac function. Nature 232:335–336
59. Singer M, Clarke J, Bennett ED (1989) Continuous hemodynamic monitoring by esophageal Doppler. Crit Care Med 17:447–452
60. Gan TJ, Arrowsmith JE (1997) The oesophageal Doppler monitor. BMJ 315:893–894
61. Oh JK, Seward JB, Tajik JA (1999) The Echo Manual, Second Edition, Lippincott, Williams and Wilkins, pp 16–19
62. Boulnois JL, Pechoux T (2000) Non-invasive cardiac output monitoring by aortic blood flow measurement with the Dynemo 3000. J Clin Monit Comput 16:127–140
63. Singer M (1993) Esophageal Doppler monitoring of aortic blood flow: beat-by-beat cardiac output monitoring. Int Anesthesiol Clin 31:99–125
64. Wallmeyer K, Wann LS, Sagar KB, Kalbfleisch J, Klopfenstein HS (1986) The influence of preload and heart rate on Doppler echocardiographic indexes of left ventricular performance: comparison with invasive indexes in an experimental preparation. Circulation 74:181–186
65. Singer M, Allen MJ, Webb AR, Bennett ED (1991) Effects of alterations in left ventricular filling, contractility, and systemic vascular resistance on the ascending aortic blood velocity waveform of normal subjects. Crit Care Med 19:1138–1145
66. Madan AK, UyBarreta VV, Aliabadi-Wahle S, et al (1999) Esophageal Doppler ultrasound monitor versus pulmonary artery catheter in the hemodynamic management of critically ill surgical patients. J Trauma 46:607–611
67. Sinclair S, James S, Singer M (1997) Intraoperative intravascular volume optimisation and length of hospital stay after repair of proximal femoral fracture: randomised controlled trial. BMJ 315:909–912
68. Mythen MG, Webb AR (1995) Perioperative plasma volume expansion reduces the incidence of gut mucosal hypoperfusion during cardiac surgery. Arch Surg 130:423–429
69. Summers RL, Shoemaker WC, Peacock WF, Ander DS, Coleman TG (2003) Bench to bedside: electrophysiologic and clinical principles of noninvasive hemodynamic monitoring using impedance cardiography. Acad Emerg Med 10:669–680
70. Moshkovitz Y, Kaluski E, Milo O, Vered Z, Cotter G (2004) Recent developments in cardiac output determination by bioimpedance: comparison with invasive cardiac output and potential cardiovascular applications. Curr Opin Cardiol 19:229–237
71. Summers RL, Peacock WF (2004) Clinical assessment of hemodynamics using impedance cardiography. In: Vincent JL (ed) Yearbook of Intensive Care and Emergency Medicine. Springer, Heidelberg, pp 565–575
72. Raaijmakers E, Faes TJ, Scholten RJ, Goovaerts HG, Heethaar RM (1999) A meta-analysis of published studies concerning the validity of thoracic impedance cardiography. Ann NY Acad Sci 873:121–127
73. Peacock WI, Albert NM, Kies P, White RD, Emerman CL (2000) Bioimpedance monitoring: better than chest x-ray for predicting abnormal pulmonary fluid? Congest Heart Fail 6:86–89
74. Raaijmakers E, Faes TJ, Meijer JM, et al (1998) Estimation of non-cardiogenic pulmonary oedema using dual-frequency electrical impedance. Med Biol Eng Comput 36:461–466
75. Summers RL, Kolb JC, Woodward LH, Galli RL (1999) Differentiating systolic from diastolic heart failure using impedance cardiography. Acad Emerg Med 6:693–698
76. Peacock W, Summers R, Emerman C (2003) Emergent dyspnea impedance cardiography-aided assessment changes therapy: the ED-IMPACT Trial. Ann Emerg Med 42:S82
77. Trottier SJ, Taylor RW (1997) Physicians' attitudes toward and knowledge of the pulmonary artery catheter: Society of Critical Care Medicine membership survey. New Horiz 5:201–206
78. Kurita T, Morita K, Kato S, Kikura M, Horie M, Ikeda K (1997) Comparison of the accuracy of the lithium dilution technique with the thermodilution technique for measurement of cardiac output. Br J Anaesth 79:770–775

79. Mason DJ, O'Grady M, Woods JP, McDonell W (2001) Assessment of lithium dilution cardiac output as a technique for measurement of cardiac output in dogs. Am J Vet Res 62:1255–1261

80. Gunkel CI, Valverde A, Morey TE, Hernandez J, Robertson SA (2004) Comparison of noninvasive cardiac output measurement by partial carbon dioxide rebreathing with the lithium dilution method in anesthetized dogs. J Vet Emerg Crit Care 14:187–195

81. Linton RA, Jonas MM, Tibby SM, et al (2000) Cardiac output measured by lithium dilution and transpulmonary thermodilution in patients in a paediatric intensive care unit. Intensive Care Med 26:1507–1511

82. Linton R, Band D, O'Brien T, Jonas M, Leach R (1997) Lithium dilution cardiac output measurement: a comparison with thermodilution. Crit Care Med 25:1796–1800

83. Young CC, Garica-Rodrigues CR, Cassell C, et al (2000) Lithium dilution versus thermodilution cardiac output measurement in cardiac surgery patients. ASA Meeting Abstract A586. Available at: http://www.asaabstracts.com

84. Odenstedt H, Stenqvist O, Lundin S (2002) Clinical evaluation of a partial CO_2 rebreathing technique for cardiac output monitoring in critically ill patients. Acta Anaesthesiol Scand 46:152–159

85. Kotake Y, Moriyama K, Innami Y, et al (2003) Performance of noninvasive partial CO_2 rebreathing cardiac output and continuous thermodilution cardiac output in patients undergoing aortic reconstruction surgery. Anesthesiology 99:283–288

86. Kuck K, Ing D, Haryadi DG, et al (1998) Evaluation of partial re-breathing cardiac output measurement during surgery. Anesthesiology 89:A542 (abst)

87. Guzzi L, Jaffe MB, Orr JA (1998) Clinical evaluation of a new non-invasive method of cardiac output measurement: preliminary results in CABG patients. Anesthesiology 89:A543 (abst)

88. Jopling MW (1998) Noninvasive cardiac output determination utilizing the method of partial CO_2 rebreathing. A comparison with continuous and bolus thermodilution cardiac output. Anesthesiology 89:A544 (abst)

89. Loeb RG, Brown EA, DiNardo JA, et al (1999) Clinical accuracy of a new non-invasive cardiac output monitor. Anesthesiology 91:A474 (abst)

90. Watt RC, Loeb RG, Orr JA (1998) Comparison of a new non-invasive cardiac output technique with invasive bolus and continuous thermodilution. Anesthesiology 89:A536 (abst)

91. Kuck K, Orr JA, Haryadi DG, et al (1999) Evaluation of the NICO partial rebreathing cardiac output monitor. Anesthesiology 91:A560 (abst)

92. Rocco M, Spadetta G, Morelli A, et al (2004) A comparative evaluation of thermodilution and partial CO_2 rebreathing techniques for cardiac output assessment in critically ill patients during assisted ventilation. Intensive Care Med 30:82–87

93. Murias GE, Villagra A, Vatua S, et al (2002) Evaluation of a noninvasive method for cardiac output measurement in critical care patients. Intensive Care Med 28:1470–1474

94. Valtier B, Cholley BP, Belot JP, de la Coussaye JE, Mateo J, Payen DM (1998) Noninvasive monitoring of cardiac output in critically ill patients using transesophageal Doppler. Am J Respir Crit Care Med 158:77–83

95. Bernardin G, Tiger F, Fouche R, Mattei M (1998) Continuous noninvasive measurement of aortic blood flow in critically ill patients with a new esophageal echo-Doppler system. J Crit Care 13:177–183

96. Baillard C, Cohen Y, Fosse JP, Karoubi P, Hoang P, Cupa M (1999) Haemodynamic measurements (continuous cardiac output and systemic vascular resistance) in critically ill patients: transoesophageal Doppler versus continuous thermodilution. Anaesth Intensive Care 27:33–37

97. Leather HA, Wouters PF (2001) Oesophageal Doppler monitoring overestimates cardiac output during lumbar epidural anaesthesia. Br J Anaesth 86:794–797

98. Hullett B, Gibbs N, Weightman W, Thackray M, Newman M (2003) A comparison of CardioQ and thermodilution cardiac output during off-pump coronary artery surgery. J Cardiothorac Vasc Anesth 17:728–732

99. Dark PM, Singer M (2004) The validity of trans-esophageal Doppler ultrasonography as a measure of cardiac output in critically ill adults. Intensive Care Med 30:2060–2066

Gas Exchange Measurement in the ICU

T. S. Walsh and F. Monaco

▌ Introduction

Metabolic gas exchange measurements are challenging in the intensive care patient. During the 1970s to 1990s there was considerable interest in determining oxygen consumption (VO_2) in critically ill patients [1]. This interest arose from observations that lower VO_2 was associated with higher mortality, and led to the hypothesis that interventions to increase oxygen delivery (DO_2) and VO_2 might improve patient outcomes. Recent meta-analyses of these trials have suggested that interventions occurring after ICU admission, and particularly after the onset of organ failures, are not effective for most critically ill patients with regard to improving outcomes [2]. There is evidence that early interventions can have clinically and statistically significant effects on patient survival [3].

Until recently, measuring VO_2 required a pulmonary artery catheter (PAC), measurement of cardiac output and the arterial and mixed venous blood oxygen content. The reverse Fick method was used to calculate VO_2. Decreased use of the PAC, together with the results of meta-analyses suggesting lack of effectiveness of VO_2 and DO_2 targeted therapy, have decreased interest in routine determination of VO_2. The methodological issues associated with relating DO_2 and VO_2 using the PAC also contributed to the decline in interest in VO_2 determination [4].

In recent years, new technology has offered the ability to measure VO_2 and VCO_2 in mechanically ventilated critically ill patients. This chapter describes the current state of the art for metabolic monitoring and discusses potential applications that could improve the management of patients.

▌ Gas Analysis Measurement Techniques

The gas analysis techniques used in commercially available devices can broadly be classified as closed or open.

Closed Circuit Techniques

These can be considered as modifications of closed water-sealed spirometry systems, which many consider the experimental gold standard for VO_2 determination. CO_2 and water vapor are removed from recirculating gas within a closed circuit. Oxygen is added to the system in order to maintain a constant content. The oxygen added corresponds to VO_2. For VCO_2 measurement, CO_2 concentration in the expired gas and an estimate of gas flow are used. Closed system methods have rarely been used for ventilated patients because of methodological limitations. In particular, it is difficult to use these devices with modern intensive care ventilators, which are based on open circuits. Any leaks in the system, changes in resistance and gas compression, and changes in end expiratory lung volume have the potential to introduce large measurement errors. These factors, together with the necessity for frequent changes in ventilator settings in the critically ill, make closed system techniques impractical in the clinical setting.

Open Circuit Techniques

Most widely used and validated devices for use in mechanically ventilated patients are based on open circuits. This method requires the accurate measurement of inspiratory and expiratory concentrations of oxygen and carbon dioxide.

There are two possible methods of deriving VO_2 and VCO_2. If inspiratory volume (V_I) and expiratory volume (V_E) are measured, gas exchange can be calculated from the simple equations:

$$VO_2 = [FiO_2 \times V_I] - [FeO_2 \times V_E]$$

$$VCO_2 = [FiCO_2 \times V_I] - [FeCO_2 \times V_E]$$

This approach is subject to large measurement error, because the accurate measurement of flow and gas volumes are difficult in ventilated patients (see below). Most modern devices have derived ways of measuring VO_2 and VCO_2 from only one ventilatory volume (inspiratory or expiratory). Some of the most accurate devices have used dilution methods to remove the need to measure tidal or minute volume altogether. All methods that do not directly measure inspiratory and expiratory volume are based on the Haldane transformation. This uses the fact that if no other gases are present other than O_2, CO_2, and nitrogen (N_2) (assuming the 'inert gases' have insignificant and constant concentration), various substitutions into physiological equations can be carried out that remove the need to measure either inspiratory or expiratory volumes. The need to measure both inspiratory and expiratory volumes is transformed into the need to only measure one volume accurately. The important assumption with this approach is that N_2 exchange is not occurring into or from the body. Exchange of any other gases, such as nitrous oxide, also invalidate this approach. The presence of a 'steady state' is a prerequisite for metabolic gas exchange measurements with modern devices.

Methodological Issues for Gas Exchange Methods in Mechanically Ventilated Patients

Oxygen and Carbon Dioxide Measurement: The paramagnetic oxygen sensor is the standard means of measuring oxygen concentrations in modern devices; analyzers based on infrared absorption are used for CO_2 measurement. Gases are generally sampled at fixed flow rates from the ventilator circuit and drawn into the device. Accurate gas exchange measurements require two features that have largely been solved with modern devices:

▌ Rapid-response time: this is needed for breath-by-breath analysis and to detect changes in gas concentration when breathing patterns are irregular. The response time requirement depends on the respiratory rate. A simple guide relating the maximum respiratory rate for which the analyzer is accurate to the 10% to 90% response time (t_{10-90}) is:

$$RR_{max}(breaths/min) = 10/t_{10-90}(sec)$$

Most modern devices have a response time of about 0.15–0.2 seconds and are therefore accurate up to respiratory rates of 40–50 breaths/minute. This is an important consideration in tachypneic patients, for example during weaning. The validity of measurements decreases at high respiratory rates, particularly for devices that rely on breath-by-breath analysis (e.g., M-COVX^{TM}, Datex-Ohmeda, Helsinki) rather than mixing chambers (e.g., Deltatrac^{TM}, Datex-Ohmeda, Helsinki).

▌ Accuracy and linearization of measurements: Infrared CO_2 absorption measurements are non-linearly related to concentration so that corrections must be made to linearize the relationship. This must be done with high precision for gas exchange measurement; the systems used are therefore more complex than in simple capnometry. In addition, the systems rely on accurate and regular calibration. Failure to calibrate carefully in accordance with individual manufacturers guidelines can result in significant inaccuracy.

High Gas Pressures: A characteristic of mechanical ventilation is that pressure in the inspiratory limb of the breathing circuit fluctuates during the respiratory cycle. With modern ventilation techniques, positive end-expiratory pressure (PEEP) is applied to most patients in the intensive care unit (ICU). Levels of PEEP of 5–15 cmH_2O may be applied even in the absence of severe lung injury. It is therefore necessary for gas concentration measurements in the inspiratory and expiratory limbs to be made by the same analyzer under different pressure conditions. This is particularly problematic because high pressure can alter gas partial pressures. Modern devices compensate for these pressure fluctuations by measuring pressure in the sampling tubing and applying pre-determined compensation coefficients. Inaccurate pressure compensation can cause large measurement errors, particularly at high FiO_2, because the absolute error becomes large compared to the FiO_2–FeO_2 difference.

System Leaks: Most open system devices rely on collection of expired gas volume. Leaks from the patient-ventilator circuit are therefore potential sources of error. The exact nature of the systematic error introduced by a leak depends on the site at which it occurs and the device design. Common sources of leaks are around endotracheal tubes, humidifiers, and from chest drains. These may be exacerbated by the use of high inspiratory pressures or PEEP. Any suction applied to the system simulates leak and invalidates measurements. Leaks make gas exchange measurement in children with uncuffed endotracheal tubes extremely problematic, although some investigators have attempted this [5]. A leak occurring from the mixing chamber of a Deltatrac^{TM} has been described as a source of systematic error [6]. This emphasizes the need for regular calibration and servicing of devices to detect and correct machine error.

High Inspired Oxygen Concentration: Gas exchange measurements rely on the accurate measurement of gas concentrations to detect small differences between inspired and expired values. This is particularly true when the Haldane transformation is used because even small errors are magnified by the equation. This is analogous to the problem of error magnification with the inverse Fick method described above. For most mechanically ventilated patients, FiO_2–FeO_2 difference decreases as FiO_2 is increased to treat hypoxemia [7]. Gas exchange measurement error increases disproportionately above an FiO_2 of 0.6 and there are no automated devices that are reliable at $FiO_2 > 0.8$. Most commercially available devices recognize this and include rejection algorithms for conditions where the FiO_2–FeO_2 difference is too small for analysis. This is the major limitation of gas exchange measurements in the ICU, but it is worth noting that VCO_2 measurement usually remains valid.

Unstable Inspired Oxygen Concentration: Fluctuation in FiO_2 during the inspiratory cycle is a common feature of modern ventilators because of the design of oxygen blenders and the absence of a mixing chamber in most modern machines. It is most likely during spontaneous breathing modes because of breath-by-breath variation in gas delivery. This can result in unstable FiO_2–FeO_2 difference and unstable VO_2 measurements [8]. These problems are exacerbated by high inspiratory pressures and at high FiO_2 for the reasons discussed above. This problem can be difficult to solve in practice. It should be suspected if large minute-by-minute fluctuations in VO_2 are observed in apparently stable patients. Individual ventilator manuals may include information concerning FiO_2 stability. Newer systems that use breath-by-breath analysis (e.g., COV-X^{TM}) may be less subject to these inaccuracies. Various complex solutions have been suggested such as the addition of a mixing chamber or the use of additional pressure regulators [9]. Most clinicians are unlikely to consider ventilator modifications justified to increase VO_2 measurement accuracy. A simple measure that decreases fluctuation is to include an active humidifier chamber in the inspiratory limb, which improves gas mixing. Placing the monitor gas sampling line close to the patient also allows maximum mixing of inspiratory gas.

Ambient temperature, pressure and humidity: Gas volumes correlate with temperature and ambient pressure. In addition, respiratory gases contain water vapor, which contributes a partial pressure. These factors must be accounted for in accurate gas exchange measurements. Adjusting gas volumes for temperature and ambient pressure is straightforward using the gas laws. Most modern devices adjust for temperature and ambient pressure, but regular calibration of ambient pressure may be required (e.g,. Deltatrac^{TM}). Data are usually presented as standard or ambient temperature and pressure, dry gas (STPD and ATPD respectively) or at body temperature (37 °C) and pressure, gas saturated with water vapor (6.26 kPa) (BTPS). It is important to note the conditions expressed by monitors.

Most gas analyzers measure partial pressure, which means the effect of water vapor can be important [10]. This was a source of error in early devices, but is corrected for in modern automated systems. Two approaches have been used: first, sampled gas is dried prior to measurement, or second, humidities of all gases measured are equalized with ambient air humidity using special tubing material, which is selectively permeable for water vapor (e.g., Nafion^{TM}, PermaPure Inc., N.J., USA). For these reasons it is important to use the correct sampling tubing during measurement.

Flow Measurements: Devices that measure flow usually derive VO_2 and VCO_2 using the Haldane transformation from either inspiratory or expiratory volume. Highly accurate flow sensors are available that perform well under ideal conditions, namely static flow of clean dry gas. Pneumotachographs are most commonly used for this purpose. Problems arise when human respiratory flow is measured under clinical conditions. In the ICU, excessive secretions, humidity, and variable flow patterns are common in the ventilator circuit. Any interruption to flow can alter the characteristics of the flow meter, resulting in systematic errors in gas exchange measurements [11]. Filters and heat and moisture exchangers placed at an appropriate position in the inspiratory circuit can decrease the chance of this error, but it is important to check that the characteristics of the sensor are not altered. Regular checks for moisture and secretions are necessary, particularly during prolonged measurement.

Ventilators that use continuous flow pneumatic techniques can make gas exchange measurements impractical. High flow rates in the circuit dilute gas concentrations to very low levels, which result in unacceptable measurement error. Systems in which continuous flow cannot be turned off may make metabolic measurements using gas exchange devices impossible.

Lack of Steady State: For accurate VO_2 and energy expenditure determination the patient must be in a steady state for inert gases, most importantly nitrogen. The presence of small concentrations of non-inert gases, such as volatile anesthetics and nitric oxide (NO), will reduce the accuracy of measurements. At therapeutic gas concentrations the inaccuracy is small and in most cases is not clinically significant. Devices that compensate for volatile anesthetic use, which are intended for use during anesthesia, are now available. In addition, sudden changes in CO_2 steady state decrease the validity of VO_2 and energy expenditure determination until steady state is fully re-established. After changes in ventilation, complete steady state is not fully re-established for 30–60 minutes, but as the majority of change occurs in the initial minutes, clinically important inaccuracy usually only lasts for 5–10 minutes. Continuous gas exchange monitoring allows tracking of changes and visual confirmation of new steady state. Even after complex physiological disruptions, such as after liver reperfusion during transplantation, steady state is usually visually re-established within 10 minutes [12].

▌ Deltatrac™: the Current Gold Standard

Many systems for measurement of gas exchange in mechanically ventilated patients have been used in the ICU. The most widely validated system is Deltatrac™. This has undergone a number of independent laboratory and clinical validations and evaluations and is usually considered the gold standard for gas exchange measurement in the critically ill.

Mode of Action

During mechanical ventilation, inspired gas is sampled from the inspiratory circuit and all expired gas is collected via tubing from the common gas outlet of the ventilator from which it passes into a mixing chamber. The respiratory quotient (RQ) is calculated from inspiratory and expiratory gas fractions alone, using a formula derived using the Haldane transformation, from measurements made from the inspiratory limb of the circuit and from the mixing chamber:

$$RQ = \frac{1 - FiO_2}{\dfrac{FiO_2 - FeO_2}{FeCo_2} - FiO_2}$$

Gas from the mixing chamber is drawn through a highly accurate fixed flow generator. VCO_2 is calculated as the product of the constant flow and the concentration of CO_2 downstream from the mixing chamber. The VO_2 is subsequently calculated from RQ and VCO_2 using the equation:

$$VO_2 = VCO_2/RQ$$

The system therefore removes the need to measure accurate gas volumes completely, but relies on the accuracy of the gas fraction measurements and the flow generator. Water vapor in respiratory gases or dry calibration gases is balanced with ambient air using a water trap and Nafion tubing (see above). With this system the humidity of analyzed gases is equalized with ambient air prior to measurements. Thereafter, gas fractions are expressed at standard temperature and pressure.

Regular and careful calibration is required. During use, the machine performs baseline checks for CO_2 and O_2 every 10 minutes. Correction for inspired CO_2 fraction is made by assuming that the CO_2 fraction of the oxygen/air mixture decreases linearly from 0.04 to 0% as FiO_2 changes from 21 to 100%. Prior to each use the machine is calibrated against a standard gas mixture and ambient barometric pressure. Modern versions (Deltatrac II^{TM}) perform these automatically. Approximately every 3–6 months the accuracy of the flow generator should be checked using an alcohol burn. A *qualitative* alcohol burn checks the overall accuracy of the machine and is quick and simple; the RQ measured by the machine should be 0.67. A *quantitative* burn of an accurately measured volume of pure alcohol, which will produce a predictable volume of CO_2, can be used to make fine adjustment to the flow generator. The drift in flow generator calibration has been shown to be negligible over 3 months. Gas injection techniques using CO_2 and/or N_2 can also be used to simulate VCO_2 and VO_2 in order to calibrate the flow generator.

Accuracy

A number of studies have assessed the accuracy of the machine in laboratory studies and under clinical conditions. Most of these authors found negligible inaccuracy in association with increasing levels of PEEP up to about 20 cmH$_2$O. The effect of increasing FiO_2 was also small and relative errors of <5% occurred even at FiO_2 of 0.8 [13]. Using lung model simulations of increases in oxygen consumption, Ronco and Phang found the Deltatrac^{TM} could detect changes with an error of less than 1% [13]. The most detailed clinical validation in ventilated patients was carried out by Tissot and colleagues [9]. They compared VO_2 and VCO_2 by the Deltatrac^{TM} with measurements made using a mass spectrometer and with the Douglas bag method in ventilated critically ill patients. The Deltatrac^{TM} gave values that agreed closely with measurements with both methods and any disparity was clinically insignificant [9].

Deltatrac^{TM} solves many of the problems associated with gas exchange measurements in the ICU. Disadvantages are a high cost, large size, and the need for rigorous calibration procedures. Recent developments represent a trade-off between miniaturization and integration of measurement devices with routine monitoring systems, and loss of precision in comparison with Deltatrac^{TM}.

▌ New Devices

The most recently marketed device, the M-COVX^{TM} (Datex-Ohmeda, Helsinki, Finland), is a bedside module that integrates with ICU monitoring systems. The main advantages over Deltatrac^{TM} are compact size, system integration, and lower cost. The principle of measurement is different: a flow sensor located at the patient airway measures tidal volume based on the pressure drop across a turbulent flow restrictor [14], and gas fractions are determined by a standard side stream analyzer. The technical advance in the system is integrating the flow signal, which is instantaneous, with the gas fraction measurement, which has a 1–2 second delay. Complex software reconstructs the two signals and integrates them using the Haldane transformation. The system has a quoted accuracy of ± 10% up to an FiO$_2$ of about 0.7 and a respiratory rate of < 35/minute. Comparison with Deltatrac^{TM} suggests that acceptable agreement occurs, particularly at FiO$_2$ values < 0.5 [15]. The response time for detecting changes in metabolic gas exchange may be shorter with this system because it calculates breath-by-breath values rather than relying on changes in a mixing chamber. For clinical measurements in ICU patients the major source of error appears to be tidal volume inaccuracy from water condensation in the flow sensor [11].

▌ Potential Application of Gas Exchange Measurement in the Intensive Care Unit

Nutritional Assessment

Energy expenditure measurements can be used to guide the dose of either enteral or parenteral nutrition. It is uncertain what level of under- or over-nutrition in relation to measured energy expenditure has clinically important adverse effects during critical illness. It is established that over nutrition can cause hyperglycemia, which may have adverse effects during critical illness and also that excessive lipogenesis can be associated with liver injury. Several studies have clearly shown that predictive equations for energy requirements have poor agreement with measured values made using metabolic monitors in the ICU [16]. Feeding can also increase VCO$_2$ either because of high carbohydrate intake (RQ = 1) or excessive calorie intake [17]. Gas exchange measurements may be useful in the 'difficult to wean' patient in order to optimize nutrition when ventilatory failure is the principle clinical problem. New compact systems for measuring energy expenditure in the ICU make this a feasible routine monitor, but more work is needed to establish whether these measurements translate into clinical benefit.

Measuring Metabolic Stress

Inflammation is associated with increased VO$_2$ and energy expenditure. For example, patients with sepsis syndrome tend to have higher energy expenditure than patients with systemic inflammatory response syndrome (SIRS) alone or those without SIRS

[18]. Energy expenditure measurements may be particularly useful in managing conditions associated with large increases in energy expenditure, such as major burns. Higher VO_2 has also been positively correlated with higher circulating concentrations of pro-inflammatory cytokines after cardiopulmonary bypass [19]. Energy expenditure measurements are also useful in complex metabolic disorders such as fulminant hepatic failure in which metabolic rate is clinically difficult to assess [20].

Measuring VO_2 in ICU patients may contribute to clinical management by providing an indirect measure of metabolic stress. Changes in VO_2 in response to interventions such as cooling or anti-inflammatory agents may be a useful measure of efficacy [21, 22]. Conversely, routine monitoring can detect acute increases in metabolic demand that could cause patient distress or myocardial ischemia.

Oxygen Kinetics

A low VO_2 is associated with adverse outcome in many forms of critical illness, especially associated with sepsis. In addition, the inability to increase VO_2 in response to fluids and inotropic agents that increase DO_2 is a strong predictor of high mortality [23–25]. These studies used inverse Fick calculations, which are now performed infrequently in many ICUs because of concerns about the utility of PACs, adverse effects associated with their use, and the validity of VO_2 calculations [2, 26]. Non-invasive gas exchange measurement is a potential goal of resuscitation in ventilated patients, but has not been assessed in clinical trials.

Assessment of Pulmonary Physiology

The accurate measurement of CO_2 concentration, VCO_2, minute volume and $PaCO_2$ make an accurate assessment of alveolar ventilation and respiratory deadspace feasible in mechanically ventilated ICU patients. These parameters have not been integrated into commercially available systems, but are potential future applications of the technology. Changes after ventilator adjustments may be useful in the management of acute lung injury (ALI) or during difficult weaning.

Weaning from Mechanical Ventilation

Current evidence suggests that weaning outcomes can be improved through a number of strategies. The first is to have clear protocols or systems to recognize when patients are ready to start the process of weaning. Second is the process of graded reduction in mechanical support by the ventilator, and identifying patients who are capable of breathing unaided. This process is usually approached either by progressive reductions in inspiratory pressure support or regular spontaneous breathing trials, or a combination of these approaches. Third, the patient should be disconnected from the ventilator and extubated. The process of reduction of support may be amenable to weaning protocols, but for many difficult to wean patients, individual assessment of gas exchange could be helpful for assessing the reasons for weaning failure. Specifically, weaning failure is likely to be associated with increasing VO_2 due to higher respiratory muscle work, cardiac work, and the effect of anxiety and stress on metabolic rate. Conversely, dynamic assessment of VCO_2 can indicate whether the achieved alveolar ventilation is adequate to maintain normocapnia. In patients with increasing VO_2, VCO_2 would be expected to increase if respiratory acidosis is not evolving.

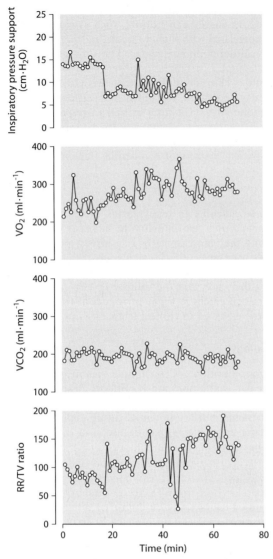

Fig. 1. Changes in metabolic gas exchange, measured with the M-COVX™ device, in a patient undergoing graded reduction in pressure support ventilation during a weaning trial (*top panel*). The patient demonstrated a significant increase in oxygen consumption (VO₂), but did not increase the carbon dioxide elimination (VCO₂). As a result there was a progressive decrease in the respiratory exchange ratio during the trial. Changes in the respiratory rate/tidal volume ratio (RR/TV) are shown for comparison (*bottom panel*). This patient suffered very prolonged weaning

Several studies have assessed the utility of VO₂ measurements during weaning trials. These studies mostly used small numbers of patients and were not carried out using recently suggesting recommendations for assessing weaning 'tests'. A common approach was to use the difference between volume controlled ventilation

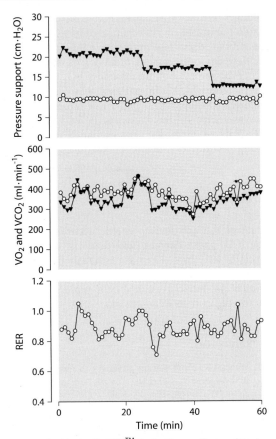

Fig. 2. Changes in metabolic gas exchange, measured with the M-COVX™ device, in a patient undergoing graded reduction in pressure support ventilation during a weaning trial (*top panel*). This patient had a high but stable VO_2 and VCO_2 during the trial and was extubated successfully later the same day. The stability in the VO_2 and VCO_2 is reflected in a stable respiratory exchange ratio (RER)

and spontaneous breathing as an index of the 'oxygen cost of breathing'. McDonald and colleagues found a correlation between higher oxygen cost of breathing and duration of weaning in 30 ventilated patients [27]. A series of studies by Shikora and colleagues also suggested that the oxygen cost of breathing predicted ventilation outcomes in patients with delayed weaning [28–30]. This finding was not reproduced in a small series of 8 patients with chronic obstructive pulmonary disease (COPD) [31] or in a series of 10 patients with a mixture of underlying diagnoses [32].

In a study of 20 short-term ventilated patients, Oh and colleagues measured the difference in VO_2 and VCO_2 between synchronized intermittent mandatory ventilation (SIMV) and continuous positive airway pressure (CPAP) ventilation [33]. These authors found a percent change in VO_2 ranging from 5% to 42% and similar wide-ranging changes in VCO_2. The authors also noted increases in plasma catecholamines, which correlated with weaning failure. These findings were thought to illustrate how metabolic stress, in addition to the oxygen cost of breathing, is a contributor to changes in metabolic gas exchange during weaning trials. Two recent trials that evaluated the utility of VO_2 changes during multiple weaning trials in ICU patients suggested that these had predictive value for successful outcomes [34, 35].

New devices, such as M-COVX^{TM}, can be used during weaning trials. We have observed significant increases in VO_2 during weaning trials, together with failure to increase VCO_2, in patients who suffer prolonged or failed weaning (Fig. 1), whereas most patients who wean rapidly exhibit either small changes in metabolic gas exchange or the increases in VO_2 are matched by increases in VCO_2 (Fig. 2). The role of metabolic gas exchange measurement for monitoring weaning trials using new devices merits further investigation.

▌ Conclusion

State of the art devices enable accurate assessment of metabolic gas exchange in the ICU. These devices have potential utility as monitoring devices for various aspects of ICU care. They are established as the best method for assessing metabolic rate and for measuring VO_2 either at steady state or during cardiorespiratory manipulation. Further work should explore the utility of these devices in settings such as the difficult to wean patient.

References

1. Walsh TS (2003) Recent advances in gas exchange measurement in intensive care patients. Br J Anaesth 91:120–131
2. Kern JW, Shoemaker WC (2002) Meta-analysis of hemodynamic optimization in high-risk patients. Crit Care Med 30:1686–1692
3. Rivers E, Nguyen B, Havstad S, et al (2001) Early goal-directed therapy in the treatment of severe sepsis and septic shock. N Engl J Med 345:1368–1377
4. Walsh TS, Lee A (1998) Mathematical coupling in medical research: lessons from studies of oxygen kinetics. Br J Anaesth 81:118–120
5. Selby AM, McCauley JC, Schell DN, O'Connell A, Gillis J, Gaskin KJ (1995) Indirect calorimetry in mechanically ventilated children: a new technique that overcomes the problem of endotracheal tube leak. Crit Care Med 23:365–370
6. Bracco D, Chiolero R, Pasche O, Revelly JP (1995) Failure in measuring gas exchange in the ICU. Chest 107:1406–1410
7. Ultman JS, Bursztein S (1981) Analysis of error in the determination of respiratory gas exchange at varying FIO2. J Appl Physiol 50:210–216
8. Browning JA, Linberg SE, Turney SZ, Chodoff P (1982) The effects of a fluctuating Fio2 on metabolic measurements in mechanically ventilated patients. Crit Care Med 10:82–85
9. Tissot S, Delafosse B, Bertrand O, Bouffard Y, Viale JP, Annat G (1995) Clinical validation of the Deltatrac monitoring system in mechanically ventilated patients. Intensive Care Med 21:149–153
10. Severinghaus JW (1989) Water vapor calibration errors in some capnometers: respiratory conventions misunderstood by manufacturers? Anesthesiology 70:996–998
11. Donaldson L, Dodds S, Walsh TS (2003) Clinical evaluation of a continuous oxygen consumption monitor in mechanically ventilated patients. Anaesthesia 58:455–460
12. Walsh TS, Hopton P, Garden OJ, Lee A (1998) Effect of graft reperfusion on haemodynamics and gas exchange during liver transplantation. Br J Anaesth 81:311–316
13. Ronco JJ, Phang PT (1991) Validation of an indirect calorimeter to measure oxygen consumption in the ranges seen in critically ill patients. J Crit Care 6:36–41
14. Merilainen P, Hanninen H, Tuomaala L (1993) A novel sensor for routine continuous spirometry of intubated patients. J Clin Monit 9:374–380

15. McLellan S, Walsh T, Burdess A, Lee A (2002) Comparison between the Datex-Ohmeda M-COVX metabolic monitor and the Deltatrac II in mechanically ventilated patients. Intensive Care Med 28:870–876
16. Chiolero R, Revelly JP, Tappy L (1997) Energy metabolism in sepsis and injury. Nutrition 13:45S–51S
17. al Saady NM, Blackmore CM, Bennett ED (1989) High fat, low carbohydrate, enteral feeding lowers PaCO2 and reduces the period of ventilation in artificially ventilated patients. Intensive Care Med 15:290–295
18. Moriyama S, Okamoto K, Tabira Y, et al (1999) Evaluation of oxygen consumption and resting energy expenditure in critically ill patients with systemic inflammatory response syndrome. Crit Care Med 27:2133–2136
19. Oudemans-van Straaten HM, Jansen PG, te Velthuis H, et al (1996) Increased oxygen consumption after cardiac surgery is associated with the inflammatory response to endotoxemia. Intensive Care Med 22:294–300
20. Walsh TS, Wigmore SJ, Hopton P, Richardson R, Lee A (2000) Energy expenditure in acetaminophen-induced fulminant hepatic failure. Crit Care Med 28:649–654
21. Manthous CA, Hall JB, Olson D, et al (1995) Effect of cooling on oxygen consumption in febrile critically ill patients. Am J Respir Crit Care Med 151:10–14
22. Oudemans-van Straaten HM, Jansen PG, Velthuis H, et al (1996) Endotoxaemia and postoperative hypermetabolism in coronary artery bypass surgery: the role of ketanserin. Br J Anaesth 77:473–479
23. Vallet B, Chopin C, Curtis SE, et al (1993) Prognostic value of the dobutamine test in patients with sepsis syndrome and normal lactate values: a prospective, multicenter study. Crit Care Med 21:1868–1875
24. Hayes MA, Timmins AC, Yau EH, Palazzo M, Watson D, Hinds CJ (1997) Oxygen transport patterns in patients with sepsis syndrome or septic shock: influence of treatment and relationship to outcome. Crit Care Med 25:926–936
25. Rhodes A, Lamb FJ, Malagon I, Newman PJ, Grounds RM, Bennett ED (1999) A prospective study of the use of a dobutamine stress test to identify outcome in patients with sepsis, severe sepsis, or septic shock. Crit Care Med 27:2361–2366
26. Heyland DK, Cook DJ, King D, Kernerman P, Brun-Buisson C (1996) Maximizing oxygen delivery in critically ill patients: a methodologic appraisal of the evidence. Crit Care Med 24:517–524
27. McDonald NJ, Lavelle P, Gallacher WN, Harpin RP (1988) Use of the oxygen cost of breathing as an index of weaning ability from mechanical ventilation. Intensive Care Med 14:50–54
28. Shikora SA, Benotti PN, Johannigman JA (1994) The oxygen cost of breathing may predict weaning from mechanical ventilation better than the respiratory rate to tidal volume ratio. Arch Surg 129:269–274
29. Shikora SA, Bistrian BR, Borlase BC, Blackburn GL, Stone MD, Benotti PN (1990) Work of breathing: reliable predictor of weaning and extubation. Crit Care Med 18:157–162
30. Shikora SA, MacDonald GF, Bistrian BR, Kenney PR, Benotti PN (1992) Could the oxygen cost of breathing be used to optimize the application of pressure support ventilation? J Trauma 33:521–526
31. Annat GJ, Viale JP, Dereymez CP, Bouffard YM, Delafosse BX, Motin JP (1990) Oxygen cost of breathing and diaphragmatic pressure-time index. Measurement in patients with COPD during weaning with pressure support ventilation. Chest 98:411–414
32. Hubmayr RD, Loosbrock LM, Gillespie DJ, Rodarte JR (1988) Oxygen uptake during weaning from mechanical ventilation. Chest 94:1148–1155
33. Oh TE, Bhatt S, Lin ES, Hutchinson RC, Low JM (1991) Plasma catecholamines and oxygen consumption during weaning from mechanical ventilation. Intensive Care Med 17:199–203
34. Miwa K, Mitsuoka M, Takamori S, Hayashi A, Shirouzu K (2003) Continuous monitoring of oxygen consumption in patients undergoing weaning from mechanical ventilation. Respiration 70:623–630
35. Mitsuoka M, Kinninger KH, Johnson FW, Burns DM (2001) Utility of measurements of oxygen cost of breathing in predicting success or failure in trials of reduced mechanical ventilatory support. Respir Care 46:902–910

Neurologic Crises

Management of Large Hemispheric Infarction

K. E. Wartenberg and S. A. Mayer

▌ Introduction: Natural History of Large Hemispheric Infarction

Large hemispheric infarctions due to middle cerebral artery (MCA) or internal carotid artery (ICA) occlusion are an important cause of morbidity and mortality in the neurological intensive care unit (ICU). Neurological deterioration occurs as a consequence of malignant cerebral edema in approximately 5–10% of hemispheric ischemic strokes [1–3], but in over two-thirds of patients when the complete MCA territory is infarcted [1, 3]. The reported mortality of these 'malignant' hemispheric infarctions varies between 42 and 80% [1–5].

Patients with complete MCA infarction are generally 10 years younger (mean age 56 years) than the average stroke patient [1]. The initial presentation usually includes contralateral conjugate gaze paresis, hemineglect, and reduced level of consciousness in addition to the expected sensorimotor and language deficits [1, 6, 7].

Most patients experience neurological decline within 48 hours [1, 3]. Of those who deteriorate, worsening occurs within 24 hours in 36% and within 48 hours in 68% [3]. The first sign of transtentorial herniation is usually drowsiness, followed by pupillary asymmetry, hyperventilation, and contralateral motor posturing [8, 9]. Autonomic abnormalities may include hyper- or hypoventilation, bradycardia, and sustained hypertension or blood pressure lability [1, 3, 5, 7]. Bilateral motor posturing and lower extremity rigidity then follows as the midbrain and diencephalon are subjected to physical distortion and compression [8]. Without life support, death typically occurs within five days [1, 3, 5] as a result of brain death, respiratory failure, cardiac arrhythmia, or pneumonia [1–3].

Infarction of the brain parenchyma and the vasculature results in a delayed break down of the blood brain barrier with extravasation of serum proteases and worsening of brain edema 24 to 72 hours after the initial infarct signs [9]. Hemispheric brain swelling leads to brain tissue shifting with subsequent brain stem distortion, bihemispheric dysfunction through mechanical displacement, vascular compression, uncal and transtentorial herniation (Fig. 1). Intracranial pressure (ICP) is usually not elevated early in the process of transtentorial herniation from large hemispheric infarction, but increases later as severe cytotoxic edema ensues. Ongoing ischemia is usually not the cause of neurological deterioration beyond 24 hours of onset, but this can result from vascular compression of the anterior and posterior cerebral arteries against the falx or tentorium, and is a universal finding in patients who become brain dead [4].

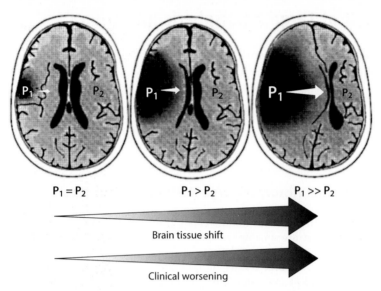

Fig. 1. Schematic diagram of the importance of tissue shifts and hypothetical significance of pressure differentials in clinical worsening from large hemispheric infarction with edema. P_1 represents the pressure in the injured hemisphere and P_2 the pressure in the uninjured hemisphere. As edema ensues, pressure differentials occur and accentuate, leading to tissue shifts and clinical worsening. From [4] with permission

▮ Etiology of Large Hemispheric Infarctions

Large hemispheric infarctions occur as the consequence of an occlusion of the distal ICA or proximal MCA trunk without sufficient collateral flow (Figs. 2 and 3). Total ICA occlusions lead to infarction of the anterior cerebral artery (ACA) and MCA territories [7].

Most patients have risk factors for vascular disease such as hypertension, diabetes, hypercholesteremia, tobacco abuse, history of transient ischemic attacks or ischemic strokes, congestive heart failure (CHF), and coronary artery disease. Atrial fibrillation is more frequent in patients with MCA and ICA territory strokes compared to the remaining stroke population [1–3, 6]. ICA dissection is a significant cause of large territory infarctions in younger patients (12%) [6]. In one series of 610 patients with large hemispheric strokes 42% were attributed to focal or general atherosclerosis and 33% to a cardioembolic source [6].

▮ Diagnosis of Early MCA Infarction

Computed tomography (CT) of the brain obtained within 6 hours of symptom onset has a sensitivity of 82% for ischemic hemispheric infarctions [10]. Early infarct signs on CT include:

▮ Hyperdense MCA sign (high contrast in the MCA that is brighter than the adjacent brain tissue and other intracranial arteries in the absence of calcification) (Fig. 4)

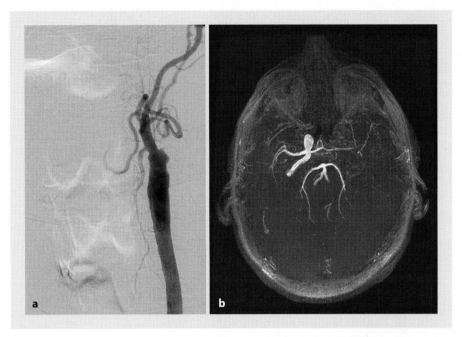

Fig. 2. a ICA occlusion after the bifurcation demonstrated by cerebral angiography with a common carotid artery injection. **b** MR Angiogram of the Circle of Willis shows no flow signal in the left ICA and crossfilling of the left MCA via the anterior communicating artery

▌ Hyperdense ICA sign distinguishable from the opposite ICA and the surrounding bone
▌ Obscuration of the lentiform nucleus defined by decreased density compared to the contralateral nucleus
▌ Effacement of the sylvian fissure with loss of grey-white matter distinction compared to the contralateral side
▌ Involvement of other vascular territories seen as hypodensity in the ACA, anterior choroidal and posterior cerebral arteries (PCA)
▌ Complete sylvian fissure obscuration and extensive effacement of the hemisphere as well as compression of the lateral ventricle demonstrating mass effect
▌ Midline shift at the level of the pineal gland and the septum pellucidum (anteroseptal shift) [2, 10]

▌ Predictors of Fatal Deterioration

Several studies have identified risk factors for secondary fatal neurological deterioration after MCA infarction. A multivariate analysis of 201 patients with large hemispheric strokes [2] identified the following predictors of fatal brain swelling:
▌ History of hypertension
▌ History of CHF
▌ An elevated white blood count (WBC)

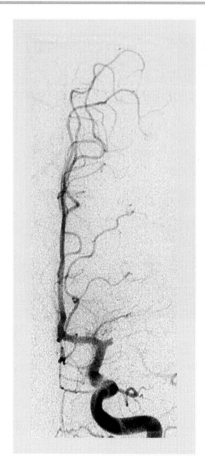

Fig. 3. MCA main stem occlusion by cerebral angiogram with left common carotid injection

▌ CT involvement of > 50% of MCA territory (Fig. 5), and
▌ CT involvement of additional territories [1, 2, 10, 11].

In a series of 37 patients with MCA stroke and proximal vessel occlusion a National Institute of Health Stroke Scale (NIHSS) on admission of 19 or greater was found to be highly predictive of severe neurological deterioration (sensitivity 96%, specificity 72%) [12].

Several studies have found that radiographic evidence of a large initial infarction volume can reliably identify those at greatest risk for neurological deterioration. In a case control study of 31 patients studied with contrast CT, attenuated corticomedullary contrast enhancement involving the entire MCA territory within 18 hours of onset was found to be the most reliable neuroradiological predictor of neurological deterioration, with a sensitivity of 87% and specificity of 97% [13]. In another study horizontal pineal displacement greater than 4 mm on CT performed within 48 hours of stroke onset was highly predictive of mortality with a specificity of 89% and a sensitivity of 46% in 127 patients [14]. In an analysis of magnetic resonance imaging (MRI) predictors, a reduction in the apparent diffusion coefficient (ADC) of greater than 82 ml was the most accurate predictor of deterioration, with

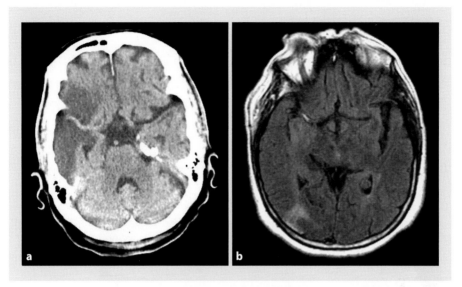

Fig. 4. a Hyperdense MCA sign (right) on CT surrounded by hypoattenuation in the right frontal and temporal regions with loss of sulci and grey-white matter differention. **b** The Fluid Attenuated Inversion Recovery (FLAIR) sequence reveals high signal in the right MCA consistent with a thrombus

a sensitivity of 87% and specificity of 91% [12]. This finding is supported by a retrospective analysis that identified a diffusion weighted imaging (DWI) lesion volume exceeding 145 ml within 14 hours of symptom onset as the best predictor of a malignant clinical course, with a sensitivity and specificity of 100% in a multivariate model [15].

Krieger et al. identified nausea and vomiting within 24 hours of stroke onset, systolic blood pressure (SBP) >180 mmHg after 12 hours, and involvement of >50% of the MCA territory on CT as independent predictors of fatal brain swelling in a multivariate analysis of 135 patients [16]. Carotid "T" occlusion was significantly associated with a fatal outcome in 74 MCA infarction patients with acute carotid artery distribution stroke [17]. Severe cerebral blood flow (CBF) reductions in the MCA territory, detected by Xenon-CT (mean CBF 8.6 ml/100 gm/minute) [18] or single photon emission CT (SPECT) [19] can also identify patients at risk for fatal brain edema.

Neurochemical monitoring with cerebral microdialysis is another interesting tool to monitor the course of MCA infarction. An increase in extracellular glutamate, glycerin and lactate concentration and an augmentation of the lactate/pyruvate ratio in peri-infarct areas was thought to reflect developing brain edema with subsequent secondary neuronal ischemia as those changes of neurochemicals preceded an increase in ICP [20–22]. Bosche et al. found significantly lower non-transmitter amino acid concentrations in the areas adjacent to the infarct in patients who developed malignant brain edema [23].

In summary, the CT criteria involvement of >50% of the MCA territory and other vascular territories, and the presence of a midline shift at the level of the pineal gland of septum pellucidum represent the most reliable predictors of fatal neurological deterioration.

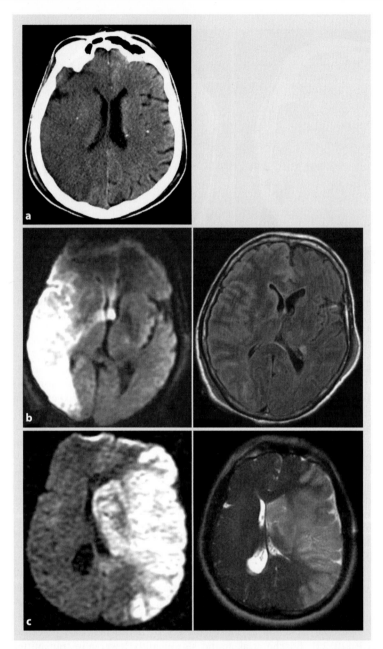

Fig. 5. a CT showing hypoattenuation in the total right MCA and ACA territory with effacement of the adjacent sulci and loss of the grey-white matter distinction. **b** Left: Diffusion-weighted MRI sequence (DWI) demonstrating restricted diffusion in the right MCA territory compatible with early acute ischemia. Right: Effacement of the sulci, loss of grey-white matter differentiation and local mass effect on the right lateral ventricle on the FLAIR sequence corresponding to panel on the left. **c** DWI (left) and T2-weighted (right) MRI sequence revealing significant cerebral edema from a left MCA territory infarction seen as hyperintense signal with effacement of the lateral ventricle and >2 cm midline shift at the level of the septum pellucidum

Acute Management

The mainstay of supportive care for large hemispheric infarction is endotracheal intubation and mechanical ventilation for airway protection and depressed level of consciousness. The costs of critical care management of stroke patients treated with mechanical ventilation has been calculated to be (1996 USD) $ 89 400 for every patient discharged alive, and $ 174 200 for each quality-adjusted life year saved. The functional status of most survivors is poor, with over 50% left severely disabled and completely dependent [24]. For this reason, aggressive efforts to attain reperfusion within an early time window or to minimize brain injury are justified. Intravenous recombinant tissue plasminogen activator (rt-PA) administered within 3 hours of onset of the first stroke symptom is the only FDA approved acute stroke treatment [25]. The PROACT trials demonstrated safety and efficacy of intra-arterially administered recombinant pro-urokinase within 6 hours of stroke onset. The recanalization rate was 66% with a 10% risk of intracerebral hemorrhage, and the likelihood of survival with a good outcome was significantly increased [26, 27]. Several other methods to potentially salvage hypoperfused but not yet infarcted brain tissue are currently under investigation, such as bridging of intravenous and intra-arterial t-PA, mechanical thrombus removal, intra-arterial abciximab, stenting, and angioplasty. Induced hypertension with norepinephrine or phenylephrine augments cerebral perfusion pressure (CPP) and mean flow velocity and may improve perfusion in areas at risk for further infarction (e.g. the ischemic penumbra) [28]. One preliminary prospective clinical report indicates that a trial of induced hypertension can result in clinical improvement of neurological signs in 54% of patients, usually within 20 minutes [29].

Intensive Care Management

Patients with large hemispheric strokes are best managed in an ICU. The mainstays of treatment for massive cerebal edema include osmotherapy and hyperventilation [7, 30]. The goal of osmotherapy is to reduce brain volume by creating an osmotic gradient between the intracellular and extracellular compartment [7].

Mannitol infusion leads to a reduction in brain water content first by creating an osmotic gradient between the interstitial and intracellular compartments and the intravascular space across the semipermeable blood brain barrier. Mannitol also reduces blood viscosity and improves microvascular CBF, which may result in reflex vasoconstriction and reduced cerebral blood volume, and has free radical scavenger properties. It has a fast onset of action, which is helpful in cases of impending transtentorial herniation. The recommended dose is 0.5–1.5 g/kg i.v. every 1 to 6 hours. Complications may include transient intravascular fluid overload, secondary volume contraction or hypokalemia resulting from the diuretic effect of repeated doses over longer intervals [7, 30]. In a series of seven patients with large hemispheric infarction the administration of a bolus of 1.5 g/kg mannitol did not have any effect on midline shift measured by MRI or neurological status [31]. It has also been suggested that mannitol might have a greater effect on normal rather than infarcted tissue due to a disruption of the blood brain barrier [4]. At least theoretically, this might result in worsening of midline shift as mannitol extravasates in the infarcted tissue and dehydrates the normal contralateral hemisphere. In clinical practice, however, this does not occur, and there are animal studies demonstrating that mannitol dehydrates infarcted tissue at least as effectively as normal brain tissue [32].

Hypertonic saline solutions improve microvascular perfusion and CPP by causing volume expansion, increases in cardiac output and systemic blood pressure, and decreased production of cerebrospinal fluid (CSF). Hypertonic saline also can modify inflammatory responses, interact with the neuroendocrine system and expand intracranial elastance. We use continuous infusion of 3% saline solution or 23.4% saline boluses for ICP control in our neurocritical ICU. There are only a few prospective clinical trials that have investigated the effect of hypertonic saline in fatal large hemispheric infarctions with conflicting results, and none of these studies have evaluated functional outcome [30]. In one study, hypertonic saline hydroxyethyl starch solution successfully decreased elevated ICP by 34% within 15 minutes in patients with space-occupying infarctions [33]. In general, the administration of hypertonic saline over a longer period seems to be safe in the absence of renal failure and CHF, though careful monitoring of central venous pressure (CVP) and fluid balance is prudent.

There is no evidence supporting the use of glucocorticoids for the treatment of brain edema from acute stroke [30]. Barbiturates decrease the cerebral metabolic rate, resulting in diminished CBF and blood volume with reduction of cerebral edema formation. The neuroprotective properties (free radical scavenging) of barbiturates make them attractive for the treatment of brain swelling related to ischemia on a theoretical basis [30], but practical experience suggests that barbiturates may in fact be harmful when used to control ICP in patients with MCA infarction. Of 60 patients with large hemispheric infarctions who were subjected to barbiturate coma with thiopental (3–5 mg/kg bolus followed by continuous infusion) to achieve burst suppression pattern on a continuous electroencephalogram (EEG) for 48 hours, only 5 patients (8%) survived. Thiopental infusion resulted in a decrease of ICP, which was not sustained and was complicated by arterial hypotension requiring vasopressors, pneumonia, sepsis and hepatic dysfunction [34]. Hypotension in this setting may have been provoked by previous dehydration from osmotherapy [7].

Hyperventilation has long been considered a mainstay of management for increased ICP and cerebral edema. Decreased PCO_2 (30–35 mmHg) is achieved by increasing the ventilation rate, leading to vasoconstriction, diminished cerebral blood volume, and lower ICP. This effect is rapid – a reduction in ICP usually occurs within 30 minutes – but may be limited by excessive vasoconstriction resulting in further cerebral ischemia if the patient is excessively hyperventilated. Normocapnia should be reinstituted slowly because of a possible rebound effect [7, 30]. Hyperventilation is a useful tool for the acute stabilization of impending herniation, but is often not effective over longer periods of time.

▋ Decompressive Surgery

Hemicraniectomy for large hemispheric infarction was first reported in 1935. Horizontal and vertical tissue shifts, and ventricular and vascular compression by massive brain edema are relieved by removal of the bone flap over the frontal, temporal and parietal lobe at the infarct site. This allows the edematous brain to expand extracranially, improves CPP and retrograde flow in the MCA, preserves CBF, and may prevent further ongoing ischemia. The diameter of the craniectomy should be at least 12 cm (14 to 15 cm anterior-posterior, and 10 to 12 cm from the temporal base to the vertex is recommended) [7]. A small diameter hemicraniectomy can result in compression and kinking of bridging veins, or mushroom-like herniation of the brain with shearing distortion and additional ischemic lesions (Fig. 6) [35].

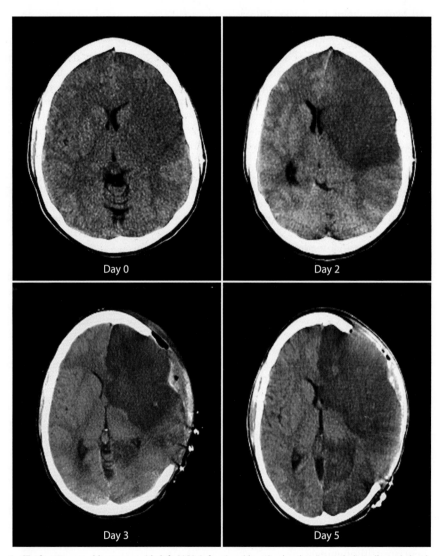

Fig. 6. CT of a 35 year old woman with left MCA infarction (day 0) who deteriorated clinically and developed additional left ACA territory infarction and significant midline shift to the right on day 2. After decompressive hemicraniectomy the CT showed slight improvement of the midline shift on day 3. On day 5 she proceeded to infarct the left PCA territory because the diameter of the hemicraniectomy was too small

After resection of the temporal bone to the skull base the dura is opened, adjusted, and a biconvex dural patch is placed into the incision (duroplasty). Resection of the infarction is not advisable as the margins between infarct and penumbra are poorly defined. The bone flap can be conserved in the abdominal subcutaneous tissue or in a cooled sterile isotonic solution. Reimplantation of the bone flap is possible 6 to 12 weeks after removal, once the swelling has resolved. Potential complications include intracranial, wound and bone flap infection, subdural and epidural hematoma, subdural CSF hygroma, paradoxical herniation after the swelling period and hydrocephalus [7, 30, 35, 36].

The first prospective but uncontrolled clinical trial of hemicraniectomy included 32 patients with a midline shift of more than 10 mm at the septum pellucidum level. Most of the patients who underwent decompressive surgery at a mean time of 39 hours after stroke onset suffered a non-dominant MCA territory infarction and did not have any medical complications. The mortality rate in the surgical group was 34%. The control group encompassed patients with more severe medical co-morbidities and inability to consent and had a mortality rate of 76% [36]. The next prospective, uncontrolled trial included 31 patients undergoing hemicraniectomy considerably earlier in the course (within the first 24 hours of symptom onset), with a mortality rate of 16% [37]. In another prospective, non-randomized series of 34 patients, mortality at 3 months was 67% in the conservatively managed group and 16% in the group receiving surgery immediately after the onset of neurological deterioration [38]. Ultra-early hemicraniectomy performed within 6 hours of stroke onset in 12 patients resulted in a mortality of 8% compared to 36% in 30 patients undergoing surgery after 6 hours of symptom onset and 80% in 10 patients managed with maximal medical therapy [39].

Hemicraniectomy is clearly a life-saving procedure. However, analysis of functional outcome of patients after hemicraniectomy has revealed conflicting results. Multiple case series, clinical trials and a metaanalysis suggest that timing of hemicraniectomy and age of the patients are crucial factors in determining outcome: Early surgery has a greater impact on reduction of mortality, and young patients (<50 years) tend to have a better outcome [37–41]. Although many clinicians are reluctant to offer hemicraniectomy to patients with dominant hemisphere infarcts, a meta-analysis found no difference in functional outcome comparing left versus right-sided [40]. A retrospective analysis of 188 patients identified age 50 years and involvement of more than one vascular territory as predictors of death among patients undergoing hemicraniectomy [42]. In another analysis of long-term outcomes, none of 36 patients who had a hemicraniectomy attained an independent outcome at a 6-month follow-up [43].

The HeaDDFIRST (Hemicraniectomy and Durotomy for Deterioration From Infarction Related Swelling Trial) was the first multicenter, prospective, randomized trial that investigated mortality and functional outcome in patients undergoing hemicraniectomy versus comprehensive standardized medical therapy. Enrollment in this study was limited to 26 randomized patients. Mortality was reduced from 46 to 27%, but this reduction was not statistically significant [44]. Two multicenter, prospective randomized trials comparing hemicraniectomy and medical management are still ongoing:

▮ DESTINY (Decompressive Surgery for the Treatment of Malignant Infarction of the Middle Cerebral Artery) and
▮ HAMLET (Hemicraniectomy After MCA infarction with Life-threatening Edema Trial).

▌ Hypothermia

Mild systemic hypothermia (33–36 °C) can be achieved with surface and intravascular cooling devices. Cooling decreases cerebral metabolism, preserves the blood brain barrier, and reduces inflammatory responses as well as excitotoxic neurotransmitter release [7, 30]. In 25 patients with large MCA territory infarcts hypothermia (33 °C) was started after an interval of 14 hours after stroke onset and maintained for 48–72 hours, which significantly reduced the ICP. The patients were subjected to passive rewarming (17 to 24 hours) which resulted in a continuous rise in ICP with subsequent herniation and death in 9 patients thought to be attributable to a hypermetabolic response (44% mortality). Complications of hypothermia included shivering, sepsis, pneumonia, thrombocytopenia, coagulopathy, and elevation of serum amylase and lipase levels. Cardiac arrhythmias, including prolongation of the PR and QT interval, ventricular ectopy and fibrillation, are adverse effects that limit cooling to levels below 32 °C [7, 45].

More gradual controlled rewarming appears to be safer than passive or active rewarming. In one series of MCA infarction patients treated with hypothermia, a mean temperature increase of 0.1 to 0.2 °C over 2 to 4 hours correlated with a more gradual increase in ICP and improved cerebral cellular and metabolic compensation mechanisms [46]. In a large prospective uncontrolled trial of 50 patients undergoing mild-to-moderate hypothermia (32–33 °C) for 72 hours after large hemispheric infarction ICP was significantly reduced [47]. In this study, passive rewarming within 16 hours was associated with a pronounced rise in ICP compared to controlled rewarming over a longer period of time (>16 hours) (Fig. 7).

The most common side effects of hypothermia in this study were arrhythmia (sinus bradycardia, prolonged PR and QT intervals), arterial hypotension, pneumonia, decreased serum potassium, decreased platelet count, and coagulopathy. Mortality was 38% overall. All patients received midazolam and propofol for sedation, morphine and fentanyl for analgesia, and neuromuscular blockade with vecuronium and atracurium during hypothermia and rewarming [47].

In summary, the use of hypothermia for control of cerebral edema in large hemispheric infarction is feasible, but the risks are prominent. It seems most likely that cooling shows greater promise as an acute intervention designed to reduce infarct volume, than a primary form of treatment for malignant brain edema.

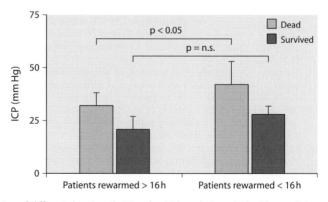

Fig. 7. ICP levels after rewarming of different durations (>16 and <16 hours). From [47] with permission

∎ Conclusion

Space-occupying edema after large hemispheric infarctions is difficult to control with conservative intensive medical management including osmotherapy, hyperventilation and barbiturate coma. It is of major importance to predict which patients may experience severe neurological deterioration from tissue shifts and edema expansion.

Decompressive surgery is extremely effective in decreasing mortality, especially when performed early in the course, but the quality of life of those who survive may be poor, particularly if the patient is older than 50 years. Hypothermia is a promising additional tool for short-term ICP control but our experience suggests that it is not as robust as hemicraniectomy as a life-saving procedure for patients with malignant edema.

Additional research is needed to develop ICU treatment strategies that minimize brain edema and the need for hemicraniectomy among victims of large hemispheric infarction.

References

1. Hacke W, Schwab S, Horn M, Spranger M, De Georgia M, von Kummer R (1996) 'Malignant' middle cerebral artery territory infarction: Clinical course and prognostic signs. Arch Neurol 53:309–315
2. Kasner SE, Demchuk AM, Berrouschot J, et al (2001) Predictors of fatal brain edema in massive hemispheric ischemic stroke. Stroke 32:2117–2123
3. Qureshi AI, Suarez JI, Abutaher MY, et al (2003) Timing of neurologic deterioration in massive middle cerebral artery infarction: A multicenter review. Crit Care Med 31:272–277
4. Frank JI (1995) Large hemispheric infarction, deterioration, and intracranial pressure. Neurology 45:1286–1290
5. Berrouschot J, Sterker M, Bettin S, Köster J, Schneider D (1998) Mortality of space-occupying ('malignant') middle cerebral artery infarction under conservative intensive care. Intensive Care Med 24:620–623
6. Heinsius T, Bogousslavsky J, Van Melle G (1998) Large infarcts in the middle cerebral artery territory: Etiology and outcome patterns. Neurology 50:341–350
7. Steiner T, Ringleb P, Hacke W (2001) Treatment options for large hemispheric stroke. Neurology 57 (Suppl 2):S61–S68
8. Ropper AH, Shafran B (1984) Brain edema after stroke. Clinical outcome and intracranial pressure. Arch Neurol 41:26–29
9. Ayata C, Ropper AH (2002) Ischaemic brain oedema. J Clin Neurosci 9:113–124
10. Von Kummer R, Nolte PN, Schnittger H, Thron A, Ringelstein EB (1996) Detectability of cerebral hemisphere ischaemic infarcts by CT within 6 h of stroke. Neuroradiology 38:31–33
11. Moulin T, Cattin F, Crepin-Leblond T, et al (1996) Early CT signs in acute middle cerebral artery infarction: Predictive value for subsequent infarct locations and outcome. Neurology 47:366–375
12. Thomalla GT, Kucinski T, Schoder V, et al (2003) Prediction of malignant middle cerebral artery infarction by early perfusion- and diffusion-weighted magnetic resonance imaging. Stroke 34:1892–1900
13. Haring HP, Dilitz E, Pallua A, et al (1999) Attenuated corticomedullary contrast: An early cerebral computed tomography sign indicating malignant middle cerebral artery infarction. A case control study. Stroke 30:1076–1082
14. Pullicino PA, Alexandrov AV, Shelton JA, Alexandrova NA, Smurawska LT, Norris JW (1997) Mass effect and death from severe acute stroke. Neurology 49:1090–1095
15. Oppenheim C, Samson Y, Mana R (2000) Prediction of malignant middle cerebral artery infarction by diffusion-weighted imaging. Stroke 31:2175–2181

16. Krieger DW, Demchuk AM, Kasner SE, Jauss M, Hantson L (1999) Early clinical and radiological predictors of fatal brain swelling in ischemic stroke. Stroke 30:287–292
17. Kucinski T, Koch C, Gryzska U, Freitag HJ, Krömer H, Zeumer H (1998) The predictive value of early CT and angiography for fatal hemispheric swelling in acute stroke. Am J Neuroradiol 19:839–846
18. Firlik AD, Yonas H, Kaufmann AM, et al (1998) Relationship between cerebral blood flow and the development of swelling and life-threatening herniation in acute stroke. J Neurosurg 89:243–249
19. Berrouschot J, Barthel H, von Kummer R, Knapp WH, Hesse S, Schneider D (1998) 99m technetium-ethyl-cysteinate-dimer single-photon emission CT can predict fatal ischemic brain edema. Stroke 29:2556–2562
20. Schneweis S, Grond M, Staub F, et al (2001) Predictive value of neurochemical monitoring in large middle cerebral artery infarction. Stroke 32:1863–1867
21. Berger C, Annecke A, Aschoff A, Spranger M, Schwab S (1999) Neurochemical monitoring of fatal middle cerebral artery infarction. Stroke 30:460–463
22. Heiss WD, Dohmen C, Sobesky J, et al (2003) Identification of malignant brain edema after hemispheric stroke by PET-imaging and microdialysis. Acta Neurochir 86:237–240
23. Bosche B, Dohmen C, Graf R, et al (2003) Extracellular concentrations of non-transmitter amino acids in peri-infarct tissue of patients predict malignant middle cerebral artery infarction. Stroke 34:2908–2915
24. Mayer SA, Copeland D, Bernardini GL, et al (2000) Cost and outcome of mechanical ventilation for life-threatening stroke. Stroke 31:2346–2353
25. The National Institute of Neurological Disorders, and Stroke rt-PA Study Group (1995) Tissue plasminogen activator for acute ischemic stroke. N Engl J Med 333:1581–1587
26. Del Zoppo GJ, Higashida RT, Furlan AJ, et al (1998) PROACT: A phase II randomized trial of recombinant pro-urokinase by direct arterial delivery in acute middle cerebral artery stroke. Stroke 29:4–11
27. Furlan AJ, Higashida RT, Wechsler LR (1999) Intra-arterial prourokinase for acute ischemic stroke: The PROACT study: A randomized controlled trial. JAMA 282: 2003–2011
28. Schwarz S, Georgiadis D, Aschoff A, Schwab S (2002) Effects of induced hypertension on intracranial pressure and flow velocities of the middle cerebral arteries in patients with large hemispheric stroke. Stroke 33:998–1004
29. Rordorf G, Koroshetz WJ, Ezzeddine MA, Segal AZ, Buonnanno FS (2001) A pilot study of drug-induced hypertension for treatment of acute stroke. Neurology 56:1210–1213
30. Hofmeijer J, van der Worp B, Kappelle J (2003) Treatment of space-occupying cerebral infarction. Crit Care Med 31:617–625
31. Manno EM, Adams RE, Derdeyn CP, Powers WJ, Diringer MN (1999) The effects of mannitol on cerebral edema after large hemispheric cerebral infarct. Neurology 52: 583–587
32. Paczynski RP, He YY, Diringer MN, Hsu CY (1997) Mulitple-dose mannitol reduces brain water content in a rat model of cortical infarction. Stroke 28:1437–1443
33. Schwarz S, Schwab S, Bertram M, Aschoff A, Hacke W (1998) Effects of hypertonic saline hydroxyethyl starch solution and mannitol in patients with increased intracranial pressure after stroke. Stroke 29:1550–1555
34. Schwab S, Spranger M, Schwarz S, Hacke W (1997) Barbiturate coma in severe hemispheric stroke: useful or obsolete? Neurology 48:1608–1613
35. Wagner S, Schnippering H, Aschoff A, Koziol JA, Schwab S, Steiner T (2001) Suboptimum hemicraniectomy as a cause of additional cerebral lesions in patients with malignant infarction of the middle cerebral artery. J Neurosurg 94:693–696
36. Rieke K, Schwab S, Krieger D, et al (1995) Decompressive surgery in space-occupying hemispheric infarction: Results of a open, prospective trial. Crit Care Med 23:1576–1587
37. Schwab S, Steiner T, Aschoff A, et al (1998) Early hemicraniectomy in patients with complete middle cerebral artery infarction. Stroke 29:1888–1893
38. Mori K, Aoki A, Yamamoto N, Horinaka N, Maeda M (2001) Aggressive decompressive surgery in patients with massive hemispheric embolic cerebral infarction associated with severe brain swelling. Acta Neurochir (Wien) 143:483–492
39. Cho DY, Chen TC, Lee HC (2003) Ultra-early decompressive craniectomy for malignant middle cerebral artery infarction. Surg Neurol 60:227–233

40. Gupta R, Connolly ES, Mayer SA, Elkind MSV (2004) Hemicraniectomy for massive middle cerebral artery territory infarction: A systematic review. Stroke 35:539–543

41. Walz B, Zimmermann C, Böttger S, Haberl RL (2002) Prognosis of patients after hemicraniectomy in malignant middle cerebral artery infarction. J Neurol 249:1183–1190

42. Uhl E, Kreth FW, Elias B, et al (2004) Outcome and prognostic factors of hemicraniectomy for space occupying cerebral infarction. J Neurol Neurosurg Psychiatry 75:270–274

43. Foerch C, Lang JM, Krause J, et al (2004) Functional impairment, disability, and quality of life outcome after decompressive hemicraniectomy in malignant middle cerebral artery infarction. J Neurosurg 101:248–254

44. Frank JI, Chyatte D, Thisted R, et al (2003) Hemicraniectomy and durotomy upon deterioration from infarction related swelling trial (HeADDFIRST): First public presentation of the primary study findings. Neurology 60 (Suppl 1):S52.004

45. Schwab S, Schwarz S, Spranger M, Keller E, Bertram M, Hacke W (1998) Moderate hypothermia in the treatment of patients with severe middle cerebral artery infarction. Stroke 29:2461–2466

46. Steiner T, Friede T, Aschoff A, Schellinger PD, Schwab S, Hacke W (2001) Effect and feasibility of controlled rewarming after moderate hypothermia in stroke patients with malignant infarction of the middle cerebral artery. Stroke 32: 2833–2835

47. Schwab S, Georgiadis D, Berrouschot J, Schellinger PD, Graffagnino C, Mayer SA (2001) Feasibility and safety of moderate hypothermia after massive hemispheric infarction. Stroke 32:2033–2035

Inducing Hypothermia in the ICU:
Practical Aspects and Cooling Methods

K. H. Polderman

▌ Introduction

Therapeutic hypothermia, the intentional lowering of a patient's body temperature with the aim of achieving neuroprotection or cardioprotection, is being used with increasing frequency in intensive care units (ICUs) worldwide. Hypothermia can be used to mitigate post-anoxic injury following cardiac arrest, to lower intracranial pressure (ICP) and prevent secondary injury in patients with severe traumatic brain injury (TBI), and to improve outcome in patients with severe stroke [1, 2]. Other potential indications include mitigation of cardiac reperfusion injury following myocardial infarction and restoration of coronary flow, perinatal asphyxia, decreasing ICP in patients with subarachnoid hemorrhage (SAH) or hepatic encepalopathy, prevention of fever in patients with neurological injury, and many others [1–4]. Levels of evidence supporting the use of hypothermia in these situations range from level I (for the cooling of selected patients with postanoxic coma following cardiac arrest) to level IV, where only animal studies and case reports are available. These issues were reviewed recently [2]. This chapter will focus on the practical aspects of inducing hypothermia, reviewing the various methods that are available with their associated advantages and drawbacks, as well as technical problems that may be encountered and methods to overcome such difficulties.

It is presumed that quick induction of hypothermia is important to achieve optimum effects, though benefits can still be realized after time periods of up to 8 hours and perhaps longer [1]. Therefore, methods for rapid induction of hypothermia, and ways to reliably maintain temperatures within relatively narrow ranges are needed to successfully apply induced hypothermia. Hypothermia is likely to be used mainly in the intensive care setting, but ideally should be initiated in the emergency room and/or in the ambulance while the patient is en route to the hospital. This means that the ideal method should not only enable quick and reliable induction of hypothermia, but preferably should be usable in all of the abovementioned settings. None of the currently available methods meets all of these specifications. One solution might be to combine different cooling methods; this is discussed further below.

▌ Mechanisms of Neurological Injury and Protective Effects of Hypothermia

In the past it was generally assumed that the protective effects of hypothermia were exclusively or mainly due to slowing of cerebral metabolism, leading to a decrease in consumption of oxygen and glucose. It has now become clear that the effect on metabolism is just one of many underlying mechanisms, and probably not the primary one. This explains why induction of mild, rather than moderate-to-deep, hypothermia can nevertheless exert protective effects, and why hypothermia can be effective even if initiated several hours after injury [1]. These mechanisms are extensively discussed elsewhere [1–3] and will be discussed only very briefly here.

An important concept in understanding the protective effects of hypothermia is that neurological injury should be viewed as a continuous and relatively protracted process, rather than as an immediate event occurring at just one specific moment (i.e., the moment of direct injury). This applies to both ischemic and traumatic brain injury; the destructive processes set in motion by (traumatic or ischemic) injury can begin immediately, in the minutes following injury, but can also begin many hours later. These processes can then continue for many hours and even days after the initial injury [1]. One of these processes, apoptosis, may be ongoing for weeks following the initial insult. These destructive sequences may be re-initiated by new events occurring at later stages, such as a rise in ICP leading to a new episode of ischemia. This can re-trigger some or all of the cascade of injurious processes listed in Table 1, leading to a vicious cycle of ever-increasing injury.

For TBI, this chain of events has come to be known as secondary injury, as opposed to the primary injury occurring directly at the moment of trauma. Primary injury is present from the moment of trauma and cannot be influenced by medical interventions; in contrast, secondary injury can (at lest in theory) be prevented or mitigated. It is well recognized that final outcome is in large part determined by secondary injury, and its prevention is thus the key goals of therapy. Although these issues have been mostly studied in the context of TBI, similar mechanisms may play out in other types of neurological injury, including global ischemia following cardiac arrest.

▌ Physiology of Temperature Regulation and Metabolic Changes during Hypothermia

The human body is usually viewed as being divided into two 'compartments': the core and the peripheral compartment. Core temperature is strictly regulated around a 'set-point' of $36.6\pm0.4\,°C$, with slight variations occurring in the course of each day. Peripheral temperature is controlled far less strictly, and may be several degrees lower than core temperature. The set-point for core temperature is influenced by a number of different factors and can change for prolonged periods, as can happen when a patient develops fever. Regardless of the precise set-point, perceived deviations will lead to a number of physiological adaptations aimed at restoring the temperature to the set value. One important method to control temperature is by limiting, or increasing, heat transfer to the peripheral body compartment, through vasodilation (leading to more heat loss) or vasoconstriction (leading to reduced heat loss). The heat transferred from core to periphery is passed on to the skin, at a speed also controlled through vasodilation or vasoconstriction (increased or decreased skin perfusion) and by adjustments in the production of sweat (evaporation). Heat loss subsequently occurs through evaporation, convection, conduction and radiation. The rate of heat loss is influenced by the temperature gradient (more heat loss in cold surroundings), area of exposed surface (less heat loss if the body is covered by clothes or blankets), and thermal conductivities (easier transfer of heat to water than to air). Under normal circumstances radiation accounts for 50–70% of heat loss; in sedated and supine patients convection becomes more important. Transfer of heat by conduction and convection is also influenced by the amount of subcutaneous fat, with less heat loss in obese individuals.

▌ Physiological Response to Induction of Hypothermia

When patients are actively cooled, the drop in temperature will be perceived as a disturbance in homeostasis, leading to immediate counter-responses. One of these changes is vasoconstriction in the skin, reducing the effectiveness of all surface cooling methods and complicating attempts to induce hypothermia. In awake or only mildly sedated patients shivering is likely to occur, with up to fourfold increase in heat generation and an increase in oxygen consumption of between 40 and 100% [4–6]. These mechanisms can be countered or suppressed by administration of various drugs, such as opiates and sedatives or anaesthetics. Sedation and anesthesia also increase peripheral blood flow, thereby facilitating the transfer of heat from the core to the periphery. Use of vasodilatory drugs such as nitroglycerin or ketanserin can further facilitate this process. If shivering is very difficult to suppress by opiates alone, use of brief-acting muscle paralyzing agents may be considered. In most cooled patients the use of paralyzing agents is unnecessary, certainly after the target temperature has been reached because counter-regulatory mechanisms including shivering diminish at temperatures ≤34 °C (Table 1).

Hypothermia generally leads to vasoconstriction of arteries and arterioles; however, cerebral blood flow is maintained. In healthy coronary arteries there is an increase in blood flow during mild hypothermia [4, 7, 8]; however, in diseased (severely atherosclerotic) coronary arteries the opposite effect may occur [8]. This difference is presumed to be caused by endothelial dysfunction associated with atherosclerosis [7]. In theory, there could, therefore, be a risk of myocardial injury during induction of mild hypothermia in patients with severe atherosclerosis of the coronary arteries. This is important because many of the patients treated with hypothermia are admitted for myocardial infarction. However, none of the clinical trials using hypothermia to achieve neuroprotection have reported problems related to hypothermia-induced myocardial ischemia. Indeed, hypothermia has been used to mitigate myocardial injury following myocardial infarction; although it remains to be determined whether hypothermia is effective for this purpose in the clinical setting (initial studies show apparent benefits in patients with anterior infarction provided target temperatures ≥35 °C were reached before reperfusion), this strongly suggests that hypothermia is surely not harmful in this situation. One of the reasons may be that hypothermia induces bradycardia in all patients when temperatures decrease below 35–35.5 °C, with a substantial reduction in metabolism and oxygen demand. In a sense hypothermia mimics a highly effective beta-blockade, with simultaneous decreases in metabolism and oxygen requirements.

Table 1. The most important consequences and physiologic changes associated with hypothermia in the temperature range of 32–34 °C, the most commonly used temperature range for induced therapeutic hypothermia. Risks are influenced by age, co-morbidity (especially cardiovascular disease) and the presence of metabolic or electrolyte disorders. The patient's temperature setpoint is assumed to be 37 °C

	Temperature	Potential effect & possible countermeasures
▌ **Shivering**	30–35 °C	Maximum at 35–35.5 °C. Decreases significantly when temperature drops below 33–33.5 °C, completely disappears below ±31 °C. *Potential countermeasures:* (not always required!): opiates, sedatives, paralysis; warming of face, hand and feet may reduce shivering threshold (evidence for this is conflicting); ketanserin, clonidine, neostigmine
	≤30 °C	'Hibernation': shivering ceases, marked decrease in rate of metabolism. *Potential countermeasures:* in general, avoid temperatures below 32 °C
▌ **Metabolism & endocrinology**	≤35 °C	Decrease 7–8% per °C; ↓O_2 consumption, ↓CO_2 production; ↑Glycerol, ↑free fatty acids, ↑ketonic acids, ↑lactate; mild metabolic acidosis (although intracellular pH rises slightly). ↓insulin sensitivity, ↓insulin secretion, ↑levels of epinephrine and norepinephrine; ↑levels of cortisol, risk of hyperglycemia *Potential countermeasures:* reduce feed; intensive insulin therapy as required; adjust ventilator settings
▌ **Gastro-intestinal**	≤35 °C	Impaired bowel function, subileus; mild pancreatitis (occurs very frequently; rarely clinically significant); ↑liver enzymes *Potential countermeasures:* reduce feed; monitor gastric retention, if required use duodenal probe for enteral feeding; intensive insulin therapy as required
▌ **Cardiovascular**	≤35 °C	Initial tachycardia at temp ≤36 °C; followed by bradycardia when temperature decreases below 35–35.5 °C. Slight increase in blood pressure, rise in CVP, decrease in CO (without decrease in mixed venous saturation). *Potential countermeasures:* Usually none required. If bradycardia is deemed unacceptable consider external pacing or isoprenalin. NB: atropine is ineffective for hypothermia-induced bradycardia Potential EKG changes (below 32–33 °C): ↑PR-interval, widening of QRS-complex, ↑QT interval. Severe arrhythmias are highly unlikely if temperatures remain ≥30 °C; mild arrhythmias, starting with atrial fibrillation may occur at temperatures below 32 °C in some patients. This should be viewed as a danger signal, and temperature decreased no further and preferably raised slightly. *Potential countermeasures:* careful EKG monitoring; avoidance of drugs that can increase EKG changes such as ↑QT interval. Avoid temperatures ≤30 °C ('overshoot'). Avoid/promptly treat electrolyte disorders

Table 1 (continued)

	Temperature	Potential effect & possible countermeasures
▮ **Renal**	≤35 °C	↑ Diuresis, tubular dysfunction, electrolyte loss & electrolyte disorders *Potential countermeasures:* Fluid loading (infusion of refrigerated fluids for cooling); monitor hourly diuresis, maintain positive fluid balance especially during cooling phase (while temperature is decreasing); frequent monitoring & prompt administration of electrolytes, especially magnesium
▮ **Hematological & immune suppression**	≤35 °C	↓ Platelet count, impaired platelet function, impaired coagulation cascade; impaired WBC function; ≤33 °C ↓ WBC count; ↓ pro-inflammatory cytokines, with increased risk of infections, especially pneumonia & wound infections. *Potential countermeasures:* Platelets/bleeding: usually none required. Consider platelet and/or FFP administration before surgery & invasive procedures. Immune function: monitor for infections (including daily blood cultures; extra attention for wound care & prevention of bed sores. Consider use of antibiotic prophylaxis/SDD
▮ **Neurological**	≤30–31 °C	↓ Consciousness, lethargy, coma. *Potential countermeasures:* (in ICU setting): none required. Avoid temperatures ≤30 °C because of risk of arrhythmias
▮ **Pharma-cokinetics**	≤35 °C	Altered clearance of various drugs, including muscle paralyzers, propofol, fentanyl, phenytoin, pentobarbital, verapamil, propanolol and volatile anesthetics (reduced clearance). No data available for many other drugs, consider likelihood of decreased clearance. Clearance of aminoglycosides and neostigmine may not be affected by hypothermia. *Potential countermeasures:* Reduce doses when necessary; use bolus doses of opiates to combat shivering rather than increasing the rates of continuous administration

EKG: electrocardiogram; WBC: white blood cell; FFP: fresh frozen plasma; SDD: selective digestive decontamination; CVP: central venous pressure

The effectiveness of the mechanisms controlling body temperature, and the precision of the set-point decrease with age; the vascular response is more effective, and counter-regulatory responses to hypothermia occur more quickly and effectively in younger than in older patients. In addition, the rate of metabolism and, often, body mass index decrease with age. Therefore, in general it is far more difficult to induce hypothermia in younger than in older patients, especially when surface cooling methods are used. Cooling may take more time, and higher doses of sedatives or opiates may be required to counteract counter-regulatory mechanisms such as shivering. Cooling also becomes more difficult if the patient is obese.

All these considerations may influence the choice of cooling techniques in general, as well as the appropriate method for individual patients. Before discussing the currently available cooling methods, the most important precautions and potential side effects as well as the most important potential physiological changes will be briefly discussed here. A number of side effects are listed in Table 1. The reader is referred to reference [4] for more extensive information on this subject.

▌ Metabolic Changes and Side Effects

Hypothermia induces a myriad of physiological changes throughout the body. Cooling will affect a patient's circulatory and respiratory parameters, metabolic rate (including drug metabolism), coagulation system, and various laboratory parameters [4]. Awareness of these physiological changes, targeted interventions to prevent potentially harmful effects, and close monitoring are the key to successful use of hypothermia in clinical practice. Some treatments frequently used simultaneously with cooling can significantly increase the risk for developing side effects. For example, cooling can cause fluid loss and hypovolemia (through hypothermia-induced diuresis), but this problem is much less severe in patients with post-anoxic injury following cardiac arrest than in patients with TBI who are simultaneously treated with cooling and drugs that can increase diuresis, such as mannitol and norepinephrine [9–10].

As explained above, the reduction in metabolic rate is not the most important mechanism for providing protection after ischemia or trauma. However, the effects of cooling on metabolism are significant, and important for other reasons. In sedated (non-shivering) patients, metabolism is reduced by ±7–8% for each °C reduction in body temperature; thus at core temperatures of 32 °C the metabolic rate is around 60–70% of the value at 37 °C.

The consequences of this include reductions in oxygen demand and in production of carbon dioxide. Indeed, induced hypothermia has been used to improve oxygenation in patients with sepsis and severe acute respiratory distress syndrome (ARDS) [11]. In addition, the reduced metabolic rate will lead to reduced feeding requirements, and various other changes [4]. Thus administration of feed should be reduced in patients treated with hypothermia, by around 8% per degree of temperature reduction. An additional and important consideration is that hypothermia frequently leads to a decrease in insulin secretion, as well as reduced insulin sensitivity. This means that there is a significant risk for development of hyperglycemia during cooling, which if unchecked may have significant detrimental effects on outcome. Strict control of glucose levels using intensive insulin therapy has been shown to decrease morbidity and mortality in the ICU [12–13], at least in surgical patients [12]. Thus glucose levels should be carefully monitored in all ICU patients, but particular attention should be paid to this when hypothermia is initiated.

Mild hypothermia decreases cardiac output by about 25%, and leads to an increase in vascular resistance and central venous pressure (CVP). Mixed venous saturation will remain unchanged, or rise slightly. All patients will develop bradycardia (after an initial episode of tachycardia when temperature decreases below 36 °C). Significant arrhythmias rarely develop unless temperature drops below 28–30 °C. The initial arrhythmia will be atrial fibrillation, which should be viewed as a serious danger signal. In this situation, ventricular fibrillation can sometimes be induced by mechanical stimulation; in addition the myocardium becomes less responsive or unresponsive to most of the commonly used anti-arrhythmic drugs. Therefore temperatures below 32 °C should be avoided when using therapeutic hypothermia, leaving a "margin" of 2 °C before the critical temperature of 28–30 °C is reached.

Hypothermia can induce 'cold diuresis' and electrolyte disorders [9–10, 14, 15]. This occurs mostly in the phase where body temperature is decreasing, and is more commonly observed in patients with TBI [10, 16]. Careful monitoring of fluid balance and electrolyte levels, especially magnesium [16–18], is an important requirement when using hypothermia. Although hypothermia has been linked to adverse outcome in trauma patients [19–20], on multivariate analysis this connection is far less clear [21–22], and the correlation observed in previous studies may have been to some extent confounded by the presence of shock. In studies using hypothermia in patients with severe TBI, as well as studies in patients with other injuries, no increase in the rate of bleeding complications was observed. However, hypothermia does induce a mild bleeding diathesis, with decreased platelet count and platelet function as well as impaired coagulation. Standard coagulation tests may show normal values, because they are usually performed at 37°C in the lab.

There is a clear and significant risk of infections (especially wound infections and pneumonia) during cooling, especially if cooling is continued for >24 hours. Use of antibiotic prophylaxis should be considered.

Shivering may be a problem insofar as it interferes with quick lowering of body temperature. The often feared increase in oxygen consumption is rarely a significant problem in mechanically ventilated patients. Shivering decreases significantly once temperatures decrease below 34°C. Some authors report that facial and airway heating increases the shivering threshold and facilitates cooling [23, 24]; however, the data on this are conflicting [25].

▌ Methods to Induce Hypothermia

Cooling strategies can be roughly divided into methods to cool the core, methods to cool the periphery, and various accessory measures (Table 2). Most are aimed at increasing heat loss through convection or conduction. Accessory measures include sedation and prevention of shivering, exposure of area's of the body not being actively cooled, applying moisture (water or alcohol) to these exposed areas, and use of anti-pyretic drugs. Unfortunately, anti-pyretics are relatively ineffective when the cause of fever is non-infectious [26].

The speed of cooling appears to increase the likelihood of realizing the desired protective effects; moreover, the risk of side effects is especially high in the cooling phase, i.e., the time period during which the patient's temperature is decreasing. Therefore it is important to decrease the patient's temperature as quickly as possible while avoiding 'overshoot', and thereafter maintaining temperatures at the desired level within as narrow a range as possible. Many of the large clinical studies dealing with hypothermia achieved only relatively slow rates of cooling, and some had difficulties in maintaining temperatures within the desired range. Times required to lower temperatures from 37 to 32°C have ranged from a minimum of 2½; hours (when several cooling methods were combined) to more than 8 hours [1–3]. Improvements in cooling techniques and the advent of new cooling devices, as well as the combination of different available methods (such as ice-water infusion and a mechanical cooling device) may enable us to significantly decrease these time intervals, thereby enabling us to further improve outcome [27].

As explained above, many factors will influence the ease and rate of cooling, including the patient's age, weight, and gender, the nature of the underlying disease or injuries, the area of skin that is cooled (when surface cooling is used), the surrounding (room) temperature, sedation and analgesia, other countermeasures to prevent shivering, etc. (reviewed in [4]). Drugs such as acetaminophen can be used

Table 2A. Cooling methods – surface cooling with cold fluids

a	Surface cooling using fluids
▌ Sponge baths, ice packs, water and alcohol sprays	Efficacy low to intermediate; easy to use, inexpensive, no technical devices required. Can be used in ambulance and ER. Drawbacks: relatively ineffective, especially at reliably maintaining the desired temperature; risk of skin lesions & burns especially with longer use of icepacks. Relatively labor intensive; patient may remain wet for prolonged periods of time.
▌ Immersion of patient in cold water	Highly effective and inexpensive. However, highly unpractical, labor-intensive, and poor at maintaining temperature in a narrow range; risk of overshoot. Cannot be used in ambulance
▌ Water-circulating cooling blankets (currently available: rubber/re-usable blankets,[1] non-reusable wrapping garments,[2,3] and hydrogel-coated 'sticky' pads[4]	Efficacy varies from fair to good (also depending on proper use and accessory methods). Influenced by heat transfer from core to periphery. Re-usable blankets have lower costs compared to most other devices; however, they can be labor intensive for nursing staff. Wrapping garments may be somewhat more effective due to better skin contact and cooling of greater body surface, but are more expensive (non-reusable). Hydrogel pads may be the most effective in heat transfer due to optimal (adhesive) contact with the skin; pads are also non-reusable. An advantage may be a reduction in nursing workload. The risk of (mild) skin lesions and burns may be slightly higher due to improved skin contact. Few comparative studies are available comparing these devices and other methods

[1] Blanketrol® II hyper-hypothermia, Cincinnati Sub-Zero company, Cincinnati, United States
[2] CritiCool/ThermoWrap™ system, MTRE advanced technologies Ltd, Or-Akiva, Israel
[3] Rapr-Round™ system, Gaymar Industries Inc, Orchard Park, United States
[4] Arctic Sun temperature management system™, Medivance Inc, Colorado, United States
ER: emergency room

as additional tools, but neurological fever usually responds poorly to drug treatment alone [26].

Induction of hypothermia and management of side effects can be most easily accomplished in the intensive care setting. An important question is whether hypothermia can also be used safely in awake patients. Preliminary studies using mild hypothermia induced by surface cooling have been performed in awake patients with stroke [28]. Brief (3-hour) periods of hypothermia have been used to mitigate reperfusion injury and decrease infarct size in awake patients undergoing percutaneous coronary intervention after myocardial infarction, in a small pilot study [29] and a larger, soon to be published clinical trial (the Cool MI study). Endovascular (core) cooling was used in these studies. External (cold air) cooling has also been used in awake patients with fever, to achieve normothermia [26]. In awake patients shivering can be treated with relatively small doses of opiates; of these, meperidine (pethidine®) may be slightly more effective, due to a disproportionately large reduction in the shivering threshold compared to other opiates [30], and a higher activity at the kappa receptor [31]. Alternatives to treat shivering include administration of clonidine, neostigmine and ketanserine; however, care should be taken to avoid adverse effects, such as hypothermia-induced bradycardia, which can be aggravated by use of clonidine.

Table 2 B. Cooling methods – surface cooling with cold air

b	Surface cooling using air
▮ Exposure of skin	Easily accomplished, inexpensive; however, ineffective. Efficacy can be improved by sedation/anesthesia, use of vasodilatory drugs, and applying moisture to the skin. Can be used in ambulance & ER.
▮ Fans/ventilators	Efficacy low to intermediate; low costs. However, associated with increased risks of infection.
▮ Air-circulating cooling blankets[1]	Efficacy low to intermediate. Relatively inexpensive. An advantage is that these devices are often already available due to their use in the ICU/OR to warm patients.
▮ Specially designed cooling beds[2]	Efficacy unknown (prototypes have been used in some clinical studies, but final version not yet commercially available, introduction expected early 2005). Potential advantages in prevention of bedsores

[1] Polar Air™ and Bair Hugger®, Augustine Medical Inc., Eden Prairie, United States
[2] Name not yet known, prototype called TheraCool; Kinetic Concepts Inc., San Antonio, United States
ER: emergency room; OR: operating room

Table 2 C. Cooling methods – core cooling with fluids

c	Core cooling
▮ Intravascular catheters (various types available)[1-3]	Effective and comparatively quick cooling ($\pm 2\,°C/hr$), highly effective and reliable for maintaining temperature within narrow specified ranges. Core cooling with associated advantage: not dependent on heat transfer to periphery, countermeasures such as peripheral vasoconstriction are thus circumvented. Disadvantage: requires invasive procedure, with some time loss and potential procedural risk; cannot be used in ambulance. Relatively expensive (one time use of catheters). Few safety data for longer-term use.
▮ Infusion of ice-cold (4 °C) fluids	Effective and very quick method to induce hypothermia ($2,5–3,5\,°C/hr$); can be used in combination with other methods. Can be easily used in the ambulance and ER. Main disadvantage: cannot be used to maintain temperature within narrow range; requires infusion of large volumes of fluid; risk of overshoot

[1] CoolLine™ and Coolgard®, Alsius Corporation, Irvine, United States
[2] Celcius Control™, Innercool therapies, San Diego, United States;
[3] SetPoint® and Reprieve, Radiant medical, Redwood City, United States
ER: emergency room

Table 2 D. Cooling methods – miscellaneous cooling methods

d	Miscellaneous
▮ Extracorporeal circulation	Highly effective and very quick method to manage temperature either cooling or re-warming). Cooling rate ($>4\,°C/hr$), reliable in maintaining temperature. Drawback: highly invasive, impractical in the ICU setting, requires OR team and transfer to OR, not practical for maintaining hypothermia for prolonged periods of time.
▮ Antipyretic agents	Efficacy varies, ineffective in "central" (neurological) fever. Low costs, little additional workload

OR: operating room

▌ Conclusion

There is increasing evidence that hypothermia can be used to protect injured cells from (additional) injury. Cooling has been used to provide neuroprotection following ischemic and traumatic injury, and is being studied for potential application as a cardioprotective. Successful application of hypothermia requires understanding of the physiological changes and potential side effects associated with hypothermia, and implementation of protocols to prevent or deal with these side effects. Treatment should be initiated as soon as possible following injury, although hypothermia can be successful even if initiated many hours later. Quick induction of hypothermia can be achieved by combining different cooling methods and initiating cooling as early as possible. By using the methods at our disposal, both in inducing hypothermia and by using our best supportive treatments and intensive care facilities to effectively prevent the side effects of cooling, after many failed or only partially successful attempts we may finally be in a position to realize hypothermia's therapeutic potential in various types of injury.

References

1. Polderman KH (2004) Application of therapeutic hypothermia in the ICU: opportunities and pitfalls of a promising treatment modality. Part 1: Indications and evidence. Intensive Care Med 30:556–575
2. Polderman KH (2004) Use of induced hypothermia for neuroprotection. In: Vincent JL (ed) Yearbook of Intensive Care and Emergency Medicine. Springer, Heidelberg, pp 830–843
3. Bernard SA, Buist M (2003) Induced hypothermia in critical care medicine: a review. Crit Care Med 31:2041–2051
4. Polderman KH (2004) Application of therapeutic hypothermia in the intensive care unit. Opportunities and pitfalls of a promising treatment modality. Part 2: Practical aspects and side effects. Intensive Care Med 30:757–769
5. Frank SM, Fleisher LA, Olson KF, et al (1995) Multivariate determinates of early postoperative oxygen consumption: the effects of shivering, core temperature, and gender. Anesthesiology 83:241–249
6. Horvath SM, Spurr GB, Hutt BK, Hamilton LH (1956) Metabolic cost of shivering. J Appl Physiol 8:595–602
7. Frank SM, Satitpunwaycha P, Bruce SR, Herscovitch P, Goldstein DS (2003) Increased myocardial perfusion and sympathoadrenal activation during mild core hypothermia in awake humans. Clin Sci (Lond) 104:503–508
8. Nabel EG, Ganz P, Gordon JB, Alexander RW, Selwyn AP (1988) Dilation of normal and constriction of atherosclerotic coronary arteries caused by the cold pressor test. Circulation 77:43–52
9. Polderman KH, Tjong Tjin Joe R, Peerdeman SM, Vandertop WP, Girbes ARJ (2002) Effects of artificially induced hypothermia on intracranial pressure and outcome in patients with severe traumatic head injury. Intensive Care Med 28:1563–1567
10. Polderman KH, Peerdeman SM, Girbes ARJ (2001) Hypophosphatemia and hypomagnesemia induced by cooling in patients with severe head injury. J Neurosurg 94:697–705
11. Villar J, Slutsky AS (1993) Effects of induced hypothermia in patients with septic adult respiratory distress syndrome. Resuscitation 26:183–192
12. van den Berghe G, Wouters P, Weekers F, (2001) Intensive insulin therapy in critically ill patients. New Engl J Med 345:1359–1367
13. Finney SJ, Zekveld C, Elia A, Evans TW (2003) Glucose control and mortality in critically ill patients. JAMA 290:2041–2047
14. Weinberg AD (1993) Hypothermia. Ann Emerg Med 22:370–377
15. Pozos RS, Danzl D (2001) Human physiological responses to cold stress and hypothermia. In: Pandolf KB, Burr RE (ed) Medical Aspects of Harsh Environments, Vol 1. Textbooks of

Military Medicine. Borden Institute, Office of the Surgeon General, US Army Medical Department, Washington, pp 351–382

16. Polderman KH, Bloemers F, Peerdeman SM, Girbes ARJ (2000) Hypomagnesemia and hypophosphatemia at admission in patients with severe head injury. Crit Care Med 28:2022–2025

17. Polderman KH, van Zanten ARH, Girbes ARJ (2003) The importance of magnesium in critically ill patients: a role in mitigating neurological injury and in the prevention of vasospasms. Intensive Care Med 29:1202–1203

18. Vink R, Cernak I (2000) Regulation of intracellular free magnesium in central nervous system injury. Front Bioscience 5:656–665

19. Jurkovich GJ, Greiser WB, Luterman A, Curreri PW (1987) Hypothermia in trauma victims: An ominous predictor of survival. J Trauma 27:1019–1024

20. Luna GK, Maier RV, Pavlin EG, Anardi D, Copass MK, Oreskovich MR (1987) Incidence and effect of hypothermia in seriously injured patients. J Trauma 27:1014–1018

21. Tisherman SA, Rodriguez A, Safar P (1999) Trauma care in the new Millennium. Therapeutic hypothermia in traumatology. Surg Clin North Am 79:1269–1289

22. Steinemann S, Shackford SR, Davis JW (1990) Implications of admission hypothermia in trauma patients. J Trauma 30:200–202

23. Iaizzo PA, Jeon YM, Sigg DC (1999) Facial warming increases the threshold for shivering. J Neurosurg Anesthesiol 11:231–239

24. Sweney MT, Sigg DC, Tahvildari S, Iaizzo PA (2001) Shiver suppression using focal hand warming in unanesthetized normal subjects. Anesthesiology 95:1089–1095

25. Doufas AG, Wadhwa A, Lin CM, Shah YM, Hanni K, Sessler DI (2003) Neither arm nor face warming reduces the shivering threshold in unanesthetized humans. Stroke 34:1736–1740

26. Mayer SA, Commichau C, Scarmeas N, Presciutti M, Bates J, Copeland D (2000) Clinical trial of an air-circulating cooling blanket for fever control in critically ill neurologic patients. Neurology 56:292–298

27. Rijnsburger ER, Girbes ARJ, Spijkstra JJ, Peerdeman SM, Polderman KH (2004) Induction of hypothermia using large volumes of ice-cold intravenous fluid: a feasibility study. Intensive Care Med 30 (Suppl 1):S143 (abst)

28. Kammersgaard LP, Rasmussen BH, Jørgensen HS, Reith J, Weber U, Olsen TS (2000) Feasibility and safety of inducing modest hypothermia in awake patients with acute stroke through surface cooling: a case-control study: the Copenhagen Stroke Study. Stroke 31:2251–2256

29. Dixon SR, Whitbourn RJ, Dae MW, et al (2002) Induction of mild systemic hypothermia with endovascular cooling during primary percutaneous coronary intervention for acute myocardial infarction. J Am Coll Cardiol 40:1928–1934

30. Ikeda T, Sessler DI, Tayefeh F, et al (1998) Meperidine and alfentanil do not reduce the gain or maximum intensity of shivering. Anesthesiology 88:858–865

31. Kurz M, Belani KG, Sessler DI, et al (1993) Naloxone, meperidine, and shivering. Anesthesiology 79:1193–1201

Metabolic Alterations

Making Strong Ion Difference the "Euro" for Bedside Acid-Base Analysis

J. A. Kellum

▍ Introduction

There are three widely used approaches to acid-base physiology using apparently different 'currency' for accounting changes in acid-base balance. In fact the currency can be easily exchanged but the persistence of different currencies makes the business of sorting out acid-base problems inefficient. A better approach would be to accept a common currency. Already, in terms of describing acid-base abnormalities and classifying them into various groups, the three widely accepted methods yield comparable results [1]. Importantly, each approach differs only in assessment of the metabolic component (i.e., all three treat PCO_2 as an independent variable). These three methods quantify the metabolic component either by using

- ▍ HCO_3^- (in the context of PCO_2);
- ▍ the standard base-excess (SBE); or
- ▍ the strong ion difference (SID).

All three yield virtually identical results when used to quantify the acid-base status of a given blood sample [2–5]. So why should we not accept a common currency?

More than 20 years have passed since the publication of Peter Stewart's landmark paper [6] and textbook [7] introducing his "physical chemical" approach to understanding acid-base physiology. While his views have remained somewhat controversial, two facts have emerged. First, while Stewart's terminology (e.g., strong ion difference) and his concepts of acid-base control (e.g., electrical neutrality and conservation of mass governing water dissociation) are certainly novel, measures of acid-base in the blood are not significantly different from what we have seen before. For example, Stewart's term SID refers to the absolute difference between completely (or near completely) dissociated cations and anions. According to the principle of electrical neutrality, this difference is balanced by the weak acids and CO_2 such that SID can be defined either in terms of strong ions or in terms of the weak acids and CO_2 offsetting it. Of note, the SID defined in terms of weak acids and CO_2, which has been subsequently termed the effective SID (SIDe) [8], is identical to the "buffer base" term coined by Singer and Hastings over half a century ago [9]. Thus changes in SBE also represent changes in SID [2]. Similarly, Stewart's term for total weak acid concentration (A_{TOT}) is defined as the dissociated (A^-) plus undissociated (AH) weak acid forms. The familiar anion gap, when normal, is actually 'caused by' A^- (see further discussion below). Therefore, the currency conversions between the 'traditional' approaches to acid-base balance using HCO_3^- or SBE and anion gap and the physical chemical approach using SID and strong ion gap (SIG) should be fairly straightforward; indeed, they are (Table 1).

Table 1. Currency exchange system for acid-base approaches

'Traditional' Variable	Physical Chemical Variable	Comment
pH	pH	
PCO_2	PCO_2	
HCO_3^-	Total CO_2	Total CO_2 includes dissolved CO_2, H_2CO_3 and CO_3^{2-} in addition to HCO_3^-. However for practical purposes, at physiologic pH, the two variables are very similar.
Buffer Base	SIDe	In the absence of unmeasured anions SIDe = SIDa = SID. However, since this rarely happens, SIDe = SID = SIDa − SIG (see text for discussion).
SBE	$SID_{PRESENT}$ − $SID_{EQUILIBRIUM}$	For blood plasma, SBE rather than ABE quantifies the amount of strong acid (or strong base if SBE is negative) that would be needed to return the SID to its equilibrium point (the point at which pH = 7.4 and PCO2 = 40). Note, that change in SBE can brought about by a change in A^- or SID, but SBE only quantifies the change in SID required to reach equilibrium. In the case of a change in A^-, the new equilibrium for SID will be different (see text).
Anion gap (normal)	A^-	Virtually all of A^- is composed of albumin and phosphate. A^- can be approximated by: 2(albumin in g/dl) + 0.5(phosphate in mg/dl).
Anion gap (abnormal)	$A^- + X^-$	The value of X^- is the actually the difference between all unmeasured anions minus all unmeasured cations. Since, typically, unmeasured anions > unmeasured cations, the sign of X^- is positive. If a 'cation gap' exists, the convention would be to term that a negative anion gap and X^- would carry a negative sign.
Anion gap − A^-	SIG	Given that anion gap − A^- = SIG and $A^- + X^-$ = anion gap, there is temptation to equate SIG and X^-. However, SIG will change if unmeasured weak acids (A_X^-) are present as well so actually SIG = $X^- + A_X^-$.
N/A	A_{TOT}	$A_{TOT} = A^- + AH$.

SID: strong ion difference (e = effecitve, a = apparent); SBE: standard base excess; SIG: strong ion gap

The second fact about the physical chemical approach is that it has become widely adopted by acid-base researchers. Although far from universal, this approach has been used by researchers in intensive care, anesthesiology, emergency medicine, traumatology, nephrology, and exercise physiology. A MEDLINE search on the terms "strong ion difference" and "strong ion gap" returns 500 articles since 1990. However, the terms "base excess" and "anion gap" each, alone, produce over 3000 for the same time period. Similarly, SID has not made it into the standard teaching of acid-base for medical students. Although most subspecialty texts in critical care and widely utilized educational programs for intensivists like the European Society of Intensive Care Medicine (ESICM) Patient-centred Acute Care Training (PACT) [10], cover SID along side more traditional approaches, there is still limited 'penetration' into medical education. An often-stated reason for this is that it is unclear how the physical chemical approach changes clinical practice. While acid-base researchers find the transparency of easily measured and derived independent variables appealing, clinicians argue that the computer chip in the blood gas machine calculates SBE for them. Who cares how it is derived? Furthermore, since few hospital laboratories report SID or SIG, it is actually much more work to use this approach.

Modern ICU 'STAT labs' and point-of-care technology have reinforced this opinion. If one were stranded on the proverbial desert island with only a single set of blood gases and serum electrolytes to work with, one could estimate the exact outcome of, for example, an infusion of sodium chloride solution using the change in SID [11]. This could also be done using the traditional approach as well, and if the patient on the desert island were a healthy subject, it would work quite well. Unfortunately if the patient were critically ill and a large volume of saline were needed, it would be a different story. First, the volume administered will change the 'bicarbonate space' which is estimated at 40–50% of total body water [12]. However, the volume of distribution (Vd) of bicarbonate changes with changes in plasma pH [13]. Worse still, bicarbonate Vd changes differently with respiratory vs metabolic acid-base derangements [14]. Compare all this to the simple elegance of examining not an imaginary bicarbonate space but rather a change in SID brought about by the administration of Na^+, Cl^-, and water [11]. However, few of us practice on desert islands and what is the value of 'simple elegance' in predicting the effects when we can measure serial blood gases and chemistry? Careful, attentive ICU monitoring will, no doubt, prove more accurate than our sagely SID. In this regard, is SID the Apple computer of the acid-base world; better in all measurable ways but impractical for the casual user? Of course, those of us entrusted with the care of the critically ill and injured are not 'casual users' of acid-base and a common currency for us to use would be of value.

▌ A Brief Primer on Leading Acid-Base Approaches

The Bicarbonate Approach

The basis of this approach is the Henderson-Hasselbalch equation:

$$pH = pKa + \log_{10}[HCO_3^-]/aPCO_2 \tag{1}$$

Where pKa is the dissociation constant for carbonic acid and a is the solubility coefficient for carbon dioxide in blood at 37°C.

By using the Henderson-Hasselbalch equation one can classify abnormalities in plasma pH as being associated with abnormalities in PCO_2 (termed respiratory) or HCO_3^- (termed metabolic). Too much PCO_2 is indicative of respiratory acidosis, while too little is termed respiratory alkalosis. Conversely, changes in pH that are not due to PCO_2 must result in changes in HCO_3^-. A metabolic acidosis results in a reduction in HCO_3^- while a metabolic alkalosis results in increase in HCO_3^-. Furthermore, changes in PCO_2 that occur in response to metabolic acid-base derangements and changes in HCO_3^- that occur in response to respiratory acid-base derangements, both termed compensation, can be predicted (Table 2). From these predictions, a

Table 2. Acid-base patterns observed in humans. From [1] with permission

Disorder	HCO$_3^-$ (mEq/L)	PCO$_2$ (mmHg)	SBE (mEq/L)
▌Metabolic acidosis	< 22	= (1.5 × HCO$_3^-$) + 8 = 40 + SBE	< -5
▌Metabolic alkalosis	> 26	= (0.7 × HCO$_3^-$) + 2 = 40 + (0.6 × SBE)	> +5
▌Acute respiratory acidosis	= [(PCO$_2$ - 40)/10] + 24	> 45	= 0
▌Chronic respiratory acidosis	= [(PCO$_2$ - 40)/3] + 24	> 45	= 0.4 × (PCO$_2$ - 40)
▌Acute respiratory alkalosis	= [(40 - PCO$_2$)/5] + 24	< 35	= 0
▌Chronic respiratory alkalosis	= [(40 - PCO$_2$)/2] + 24	< 35	= 0.4 × (PCO$_2$ - 40)

set of rules can be derived and from these complex, as well as simple, acid-base abnormalities can be diagnosed.

The Base Excess Approach

The two primary limitations of the bicarbonate approach are: 1) it requires six rules or equations to use, and 2) it does not quantify the magnitude of the metabolic component of an acid-base derangement. Because HCO$_3^-$ is also dependent on the PCO$_2$, mixed disorders will invalidate the HCO$_3^-$ concentration as a measure of metabolic acidosis or alkalosis. This problem first lead Singer and Hastings, in 1948, to propose the term "buffer base" to define the sum of HCO$_3^-$ plus the nonvolatile weak acid buffers (A$^-$) [9]. A change in buffer base corresponds to a change in the metabolic component. The methods for calculating the change in buffer base were later refined by investigators [15, 16] and refined further by others [17, 18] to yield the base excess methodology. Base excess is the quantity of metabolic acidosis or alkalosis defined as the amount of acid or base that must be added to a sample of whole blood *in vitro* in order to restore the pH of the sample to 7.40 while the PCO$_2$ is held at 40 mmHg [16]. While this calculation is quite accurate *in vitro*, inaccuracy exists when applied *in vivo* in that base excess changes with changes in PCO$_2$ [19, 20]. This effect is understood to be due to equilibration across the entire extracellular fluid space (whole blood plus interstitial fluid). When the base excess equation is modified to account for an 'average' content of hemoglobin across this entire space, a value of 5 g/dl is instead used and this defines the SBE. It should be pointed out that this value does not represent the true content of hemoglobin suspended in the volume of whole blood together with interstitial fluid, but rather an empiric estimate which improves the accuracy of the base excess. It can be argued that the entire extracellular fluid space is involved in acid-base balance since this fluid flows through blood vessels and lymphatics, mixing constantly [21]. Thus, the value of SBE is that it quantifies the change in metabolic acid-base status *in vivo*. It is of interest that base excess is only accurate *in vivo* when it assumes a constant hemoglobin concentration.

However, neither the base excess approach nor the bicarbonate approach will tell us about the mechanisms of metabolic acid-base balance. For example, the body does not 'regulate' the SBE. It is not a substance that can be excreted in the feces or reabsorbed from the proximal tubule. Similarly, any metabolic acid will titrate

HCO_3^- and changes in this variable tell us nothing anything about the nature of acid or base in question.

The Physical Chemical Approach

There are three mathematically independent determinants of blood pH:
- the difference between strong cations (e.g., Na^+, K^+) and strong anions (e.g., Cl^-, lactate) known as the SID;
- the total weak acid 'buffers' (A_{TOT}) which include mainly albumin and phosphate and lastly;
- PCO_2.

These three variables (SID, A_{TOT} and PCO_2) and only these three can independently affect plasma pH. H^+ and HCO_3^- are dependent variables whose concentrations in plasma are determined by SID, A_{TOT} and PCO_2. Changes in H^+ concentration in plasma occur as a result of changes in the dissociation of water and A_{TOT} brought about by the electrochemical forces produced by changes in SID, and PCO_2. The main difference between the physical chemical approach and other approaches is the emphasis on independent and dependent variables. Only changes in the independent variables (SID, A_{TOT} and PCO_2) can bring about changes in the dependent variables (H^+ and HCO_3^-). Movements of H^+ or HCO_3^- *per se* cannot affect their concentrations in plasma unless changes in SID, A_{TOT} and/or PCO_2 also occur. Several detailed reviews of this approach are available in the literature [1, 4–6, 22–24].

▋ Common Currencies for Acid-Base Analysis

Strong Ion Difference and Standard Base Excess

As discussed above, SID can be defined in terms of strong ions or buffer base. But are the two the same and what is the real SID? It is impractical if not impossible to measure all the strong ions in blood plasma. In health, well over 95% of all the strong cations in plasma are Na^+ ions. The rest, are ions of K^+, Ca^{++} and Mg^{++}. Although these last two are divalent, so they count twice, both are partially bound to albumin, thus the free (or ionized) concentrations of both are usually quite low (and it is only the ionized concentrations that contribute to the SID). On the anion side, the vast majority are Cl^- ions, with lactate contributing only a mEq or two per liter in health except during exercise. However, blood plasma may contain many other ions such as ketones, sulfate, citrate, acetate and many others. In the ICU, the concentration of each of these ions may reach a level that significantly affects the SID. Thus, if we measure all the Na^+, K^+, Ca^{++} and Mg^{++} and subtract all the Cl^- and lactate we still only have the apparent SID (SIDa) the actual SID may be quite different. By contrast the SIDe which is also known as buffer base is derived from PCO_2 and A^-. Importantly, however, while PCO_2 can be quite accurately measured in a blood sample, A^- is estimated from the albumin and phosphate concentrations. Conformational changes in albumin and unmeasured weak ions, especially proteins, may be present and as such, the SIDe may be quite different from the SID. The difference between the SIDa and the SIDe is the SIG – a 'gap' in the strong ion difference but composed itself of either strong or weak ions or both. Indeed, it would be possible for the sum of strong cations and weak anions (or vice versa) to cancel each other out leaving a SIG of zero but plenty of unmeasured ions still present. For practical purposes, however, most SIGs are positive (meaning anions > cations) and SIDa > SIDe. Since weak ions are indeed weak, and conformational changes in albumin are not thought to amount to very significant effects on A^-, it is likely that SIDe is closer to the true SID. However, it is not necessary that we know the 'true' SID only whether it is normal relative to that patient's acid-base equilibrium point. And for this we can safely use the SBE. SBE is mathematically equivalent to the change in SID required to restore pH to 7.4 given a PCO_2 of 40 mmHg and the prevailing A_{TOT}. Thus, a SBE of –10 mEq/L means that the SID is 10 mEq less than that required to achieve pH 7.4. What the SID actually is, is not particularly helpful. Thus, while SID appears to be a suitable common currency for evaluating the metabolic component of an acid-base abnormality, the way we measure its impact is the SBE.

The Anion Gap and the Strong Ion Gap

Metabolic acid-base disturbances can be brought about by changes in strong ions or weak ions. These ions can be routinely measured (e.g., Cl^-) or not (e.g., ketones). Those not routinely measured are referred to as unmeasured ions. Many years ago, it was impractical to measure certain ions such as lactate and it remains impractical to measure others such as sulfate. Thus, the literature contains a confusing array of information regarding the magnitude of unmeasured ions (usually anions) and techniques to estimate them.

Among these techniques the anion gap is without question the most durable. For more than 30 years the anion gap has been used by clinicians and it has evolved into a major tool to evaluate acid-base disorders [25]. The anion gap is calculated, or rather estimated, from the differences between the routinely measured concentrations of serum cations (Na^+ and K^+) and anions (Cl^- and HCO_3^-). Normally, this difference or 'gap' is made up of two components. The major component is A^-, i.e., the charge contributed by albumin, and to a lesser extent by phosphate. The minor component is made up by strong ions such as sulfate and lactate, whose net contribution is normally less than 2 mEq/L. However, there are also unmeasured (by the anion gap) cations such as Ca^{++}, and Mg^{++} and these tend to offset the effects of sulfate and lactate except when either is abnormally increased (Fig. 1). Plasma proteins other than albumin can be either positively or negatively charged but in the aggregate tend to be neutral [8] except in rare cases of abnormal paraproteins such as in multiple myeloma. In practice the anion gap is calculated as follows:

$$\text{Anion gap} = (Na^+ + K^+) - (Cl^- + HCO_3^-) \tag{2}$$

Because of its low and narrow extracellular concentration, K^+ is often omitted from the calculation. Respective normal values with relatively wide ranges reported by most laboratories are 12±4 (if K^+ is considered) and 8±4 mEq/l (if K^+ is not considered). The 'normal anion gap' has decreased in recent years following the introduction of more accurate methods for measuring Cl^- concentration [26, 27]. However, the various measurement techniques available mandate that each institution reports its own expected 'normal anion gap'.

Some authors have raised doubts about the diagnostic value of the anion gap in certain situations [28, 29]. Salem and Mujais [28] found routine reliance on the an-

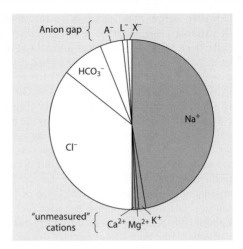

Fig. 1. Charge balance in blood plasma. Shaded area comprises cations; unshaded comprises anions. A^-, dissociated weak acid; L^-, lactate; X^-, unmeasured strong anions. The anion gap is comprised of A^-, L^- and X^-, along with any unmeasured weak acids (part of A^- but not 'seen' by the calculation) plus any variation in unmeasured cations outside their normal narrow range. By contrast strong ion gap (SIG) is comprised only of X^- plus any unmeasured part of A^-

ion gap to be "fraught with numerous pitfalls". The primary problem with the anion gap is its reliance on the use of a 'normal' range produced by albumin and to a lesser extent phosphate as discussed above. These constituents may be grossly abnormal in patients with critical illness leading to a change in the 'normal' range for these patients. Moreover, because these anions are not strong anions their charge will be altered by changes in pH. This has prompted some authors to adjust the 'normal range' for the anion gap by the patient's albumin and phosphate concentration. Each g/dl of albumin has a charge of 2.8 mEq/l at pH 7.4 (2.3 mEq/l at 7.0 and 3.0 mEq/l at 7.6) and each mg/dl of phosphate has a charge of 0.59 mEq/l at pH 7.4 (0.55 mEq/l at 7.0 and 0.61 mEq/l at 7.6). Thus a convenient way to estimate the 'normal' anion gap for a given patient is by use of the following formula [1]:

'normal' anion gap=2(albumin g/dl) + 0.5(phosphate mg/dl)   (3a)

Or for international units:

'normal' anion gap=0.2(albumin g/l) + 1.5(phosphate mmol/l)   (3b)

When this patient-specific normal range was used to examine the presence of unmeasured anions in the blood of critically ill patients, the accuracy of this method improved from 33% with the routine anion gap (normal range=12 mEq/L) to 96% [1]. This technique should only be used when the pH is less than 7.35 and even then it is only accurate within 5 mEq/l. When more accuracy is needed a slightly more complicated method of estimating A^- is required [30, 31].

Another alternative to using the traditional anion gap is to use the difference or 'gap' between the SIDa and SIDe. This is termed the strong ion gap (SIG) to distinguish it from the anion gap [30] and, unlike the anion gap, it does not change with changes in pH or albumin concentration. Because the concentration of unmeasured anions is expected to be quite low (<2 mEq/l) the SIG is expected to be quite low.

However, some investigators have found elevations in SIG, particularly in critically ill patients even when no acid-base disorder is apparent [32–35]. By contrast, results from studies in normal animals [11, 31] and from values derived from published data in exercising humans [30], put the 'normal' SIG near zero. There is even a suggestion that critically ill patients in different countries might have differences in their SIG. In the United States [33, 36], Holland [32], and Thailand [37] the SIG is about 5 mEq/l while studies from England [34] and Australia [35] report values >8 mEq/l. The difference may lie with the use of gelatins in these countries [38], which are an exogenous source of unmeasured ions [39]. In this scenario, the SIG is likely to be a mixture of endogenous and exogenous anions. Interestingly, previous studies that have failed to find a correlation between SIG and mortality were performed in countries that use gelatin based resuscitation fluids [34, 35], whereas studies of patients not receiving gelatins [33, 37] or any resuscitation at all [36] have found a positive correlation between SIG and hospital mortality. Indeed Kaplan and Kellum have recently reported that pre-resuscitation SIG predicts mortality in injured patients better than blood lactate, pH or injury severity scores [36].

Thus, the predictive value of SIG may exceed that of the anion gap but it may vary from population to population and even between institutions. As such, estimating the SIG from the anion gap, after correcting for albumin, and PO_4, and after subtracting out lactate, may be a reasonable substitute for the long hand calculation [1, 32, 38].

▌ A Common Currency Approach to the Patient with an Acid-base Abnormality

With the SBE as measure of the change in SID and the anion gap corrected for the patient's A^- in hand, one can travel though any metabolic acid-base jurisdiction. Furthermore, the approach described here will focus on the readily available clinical information and in these times of cost-containment may be more 'user friendly' than some of the more traditional approaches as well. In addition, this approach is consistent with the physicochemical principles of acid-base balance outlined above.

First, Characterize the Disorder

The first step in the approach to a patient with an acid-base imbalance is to characterize the disorder. Acid-base imbalances are usually recognized by abnormalities in the venous plasma electrolyte concentrations so it is useful to start there. Although HCO_3^- is a dependent variable, the venous HCO_3^- concentration is the easiest way to screen for acid-base disorders. However, a normal HCO_3^- concentration in no way excludes the presence of even serious acid-base derangements. Therefore, if the history and physical examination leads one to suspect a disease process that results in an acid-base imbalance, more investigation will be required. Still, the venous plasma electrolytes provide useful information. The HCO_3^- concentration is normally 22-26 mEq/l. Increases in HCO_3^- concentration occur with primary and compensatory metabolic alkaloses and decreases occur with primary or compensatory metabolic acidoses. Unfortunately, in mixed disorders, the HCO_3^- concentration may be misleading and the presence of any abnormality in HCO_3^- concentration requires further investigation. In addition to examining the HCO_3^- concentration, venous blood can be used to calculate the anion gap (equation 2) and compare it to the normal anion gap (A^-) estimated from albumin and PO_4 (equation 3a or b). If the HCO_3^- concentration is < 22 or > 26 mEq/l or the anion gap – A^- is > 2 mEq/l or if there is clinical suspicion for a mixed disorder, arterial blood should be sampled for blood gas analysis. This test will provide information on the pH, $PaCO_2$ and SBE. While simple disorders will conform to the equations presented in Table 2, 'mixed' disorders are quite common.

In patients with acidemia (arterial blood pH < 7.35), the next step is to examine the anion gap. The anion gap should also be examined when there is suspicion of an occult metabolic acidosis even in a patient with alkalemia. However, severe alkalemia will increase anion gap by 2–4 mEq/l and hence wider 'tolerance limits' should be used. Further, the presence of unexplained anions in the absence of acidosis is of uncertain clinical significance. If unmeasured anions are detected, it is a good idea to compare their amounts to the abnormality in SBE. For example, if the calculated anion gap is 5 mEq/l $>$ the estimated A^- and the SBE is –15 mEq/l, a mixed metabolic acidosis is present. The unmeasured anions (e.g., ketones) account for a SBE of –5 mEq/l while some other process is responsible for another 10 mEq/l. Such a condition could occur, for example, if very large amounts of 0.9% saline are used to treat a patient with diabetic ketoacidosis. As the ketosis resolves the acidosis persists because the SID is kept low from exogenous Cl^- administration. In any case, the SBE of –15 mEq/L means that the SID is 15 mEq less than its equilibrium point. The anion gap calculation provides information as to why. If the anion gap $= A^-$ then SIG is close to zero and the cause of the acidosis must be one (or more) of the measured ions. A quick inspection of the two most important ions (Na^+ and Cl^-) will often provide the diagnosis. However, beware of assigning too much significance to a single ion. It is the balance between strong cations and strong anions that is important. Na^+ and Cl^- make up the majority of the SID. The second pitfall is to expect a specific normal value for SID. The only normal SID is the one that occurs at the equilibrium point for that blood sample when pH is 7.40 and PCO_2 is 40 mmHg.

Second, Determine the Cause

Once the disorder has been characterized, the clinician must integrate the information obtained from the history and physical examination in order to arrive at an accurate diagnosis. However, mixed disorders continue to be problematic. Any disorder that does not fit into the classification scheme shown in Table 2 can be considered a mixed disorder. However, some mixed disorders may appear to be simple disorders when first encountered. For example, a patient with chronic respiratory acidosis and a $PaCO_2$ of 60 mmHg would be expected to have an SBE +8 mEq/l (see Table 2). If this patient develops a metabolic acidosis, the SBE will decrease and may at one point be 0 mEq/l. At this point, it may appear that the patient has a pure, acute respiratory acidosis rather that a mixed disorder. If the metabolic acidosis causes an increase in the anion gap, this may provide a clue. Another useful method is to obtain at least two blood gas analyses in order to examine for trends. However, in general, it is only by careful attention to history and physical examination that the true diagnosis can be made. In all cases using all the available information and keeping in mind the 'common currency' of SID will greatly simplify the task.

References

1. Kellum JA (2000) Determinants of blood pH in Health and Disease. Crit Care 4:6–14
2. Kellum JA, Bellomo R, Kramer DJ, Pinsky MR (1997) Splanchnic buffering of metabolic acid during early endotoxemia. J Crit Care 12:7–12
3. Schlichtig R, Grogono AW, Severinghaus JW (1998) Human PaCO2 and standard base excess compensation for acid–base imbalance. Crit Care Med 26:1173–1179
4. Corey HE (2003) Stewart and beyond: New models of acid-base balance. Kidney Int 64:777–787
5. Wooten EW (2003) Calculation of physiological acid-base parameters in multicompartment systems with application to human blood. J Appl Physiol 95:2333–2444
6. Stewart P (1983) Modern quantitative acid-base chemistry. Can J Physiol Pharmacol 61:1444–1461
7. Stewart PA (1981) How To Understand Acid-Base: A Quantitative Acid-Base Primer For Biology And Medicine, 1 edn. Elsevier, New York
8. Figge J, Mydosh T, Fencl V (1992) Serum proteins and acid-base equilibria: a follow-up. J Lab Clin Med 120:713–719
9. Singer RB, Hastings AB (1948) An improved clinical method for the estimation of disturbances of the acid-base balance of human blood. Medicine (Baltimore) 27:223–242
10. European Society of Intensive Care Medicine (ESICM) PACT (Patient-centred Acute Care Training). http://www.esicm.org/PAGE_pactprogramme
11. Kellum JA, Bellomo R, Kramer DJ, Pinsky MR (1998) Etiology of metabolic acidosis during saline resuscitation in endotoxemia. Shock 9:364–368
12. Fernandez PC, Cohen RM, Feldman GM (1989) The concept of bicarbonate distribution space: the crucial role of body buffers. Kidney Int 36:747–752
13. Garella S, Dana CL, Chazan JA (1973) Severity of metabolic acidosis as a determinant of bicarbonate requirements. N Engl J Med 289:121–126
14. Adrogue HJ, Brensilver J, Cohen JJ, Madias NE (1983) Influence of steady-state alterations in acid-base equilibrium on the fate of administered bicarbonate in the dog. J Clin Invest 71:867–883
15. Astrup P, Jorgensen K, Siggaard-Andersen O (1960) Acid-base metabolism: New approach. Lancet 1:1035–1039
16. Siggaard-Andersen O (1962) The pH-log PCO2 blood acid-base nomogram revised. Scand J Clin Lab Invest 14:598–604
17. Grogono AW, Byles PH, Hawke W (1976) An *in vivo* representation of acid-base balance. Lancet 1:499–500
18. Severinghaus JW (1976) Acid-base balance nomogram–A Boston-Copenhagen détente. Anesthesiology 45:539–541
19. Brackett NC, Cohen JJ, Schwartz WB (1965) Carbon dioxide titration curve of normal man. N Engl J Med 272:6–12
20. Prys-Roberts C, Kelman GR, Nunn JF (1966) Determinants of the in vivo carbon dioxide titration curve in anesthetized man. Br J Anaesth 38:500–550
21. Schlichtig R (1999) Acid-base balance (quantitation). In: Grenvik A, Shoemaker WC, Ayres SM, Holbrook PR (eds) Textbook of Critical Care. W.B. Saunders Co, Philadelphia, PA, pp 828–839
22. Leblanc M, Kellum JA (1998) Biochemical and biophysical principles of hydrogen ion regulation. In: Ronco C, Bellomo R (eds) Critical Care Nephrology. Kluwer Academic Publishers, Dordrecht, The Netherlands, pp 261–277
23. Jones NL (1990) A quantitative physciochemical approach to acid-base physiology. Clin Biochem 23:189–195
24. Sirker AA, Rhodes A, Grounds RM, Bennett ED (2002) Acid-base physiology: the 'traditional' and the 'modern' approaches. Anaesthesia 57:348–356
25. Narins RG, Emmett M (1980) Simple and mixed acid-base disorders: A practical approach. Medicine (Baltimore) 59:161–187
26. Sadjadi SA (1995) A new range for the anion gap. Ann Intern Med 123:807–808
27. Winter SD, Pearson R, Gabow PG, Schultz A, Lepoff RB (1990) The fall of the serum anion gap. Arch Intern Med 150:3113–3115

28. Salem MM, Mujais SK (1992) Gaps in the anion gap. Arch Intern Med 152:1625–1629
29. Gilfix BM, Bique M, Magder S (1993) A physical chemical approach to the analysis of acid-base balance in the clinical setting. J Crit Care 8:187–197
30. Kellum JA, Kramer DJ, Pinsky MR (1995) Strong ion gap: a methodology for exploring unexplained anions. J Crit Care 10:51–55
31. Kellum JA, Bellomo R, Kramer DJ, Pinsky MR (1995) Hepatic anion flux during acute endotoxemia. J Appl Physiol 78:2212–2217
32. Moviat M, van Haren F, van der Hoeven H (2003) Conventional or physicochemical approach in intensive care unit patients with metabolic acidosis. Crit Care 7:R41–R45
33. Balasubramanyan N, Havens PL, Hoffman GM (1999) Unmeasured anions identified by the Fencl-Stewart method predict mortality better than base excess, anion gap, and lactate in patients in the pediatric intensive care unit. Crit Care Med 27:1577–1581
34. Cusack RJ, Rhodes A, Lochhead P, et al (2002) The strong ion gap does not have prognostic value in critically ill patients in a mixed medical/surgical adult ICU. Intensive Care Med 28:864–869
35. Rocktaschel J, Morimatsu H, Uchino S, Bellomo R (2003) Unmeasured anions in critically ill patients: can they predict mortality? Crit Care Med 31:2131–2136
36. Kaplan L, Kellum JA (2004) Initial pH, base deficit, lactate, anion gap, strong ion difference, and strong ion gap predict outcome from major vascular injury. Crit Care Med 32:1120–1124
37. Dondorp AM, Chau TT, Phu NH, et al (2004) Unidentified acids of strong prognostic significance in severe malaria. Crit Care Med 32:1683–1688
38. Kellum JA (2003) Closing the gap on unmeasured anions. Crit Care 7:219–220
39. Hayhoe M, Bellomo R, Liu G, McNicol L, Buxton B (1999) The aetiology and pathogenesis of cardiopulmonary bypass-associated metabolic acidosis using polygeline pump prime. Intensive Care Med 25:680–685

Pulse High Volume Hemofiltration: Rationale and Early Clinical Experience

R. Ratanarat, A. Brendolan, and C. Ronco

▌ Introduction

Severe sepsis represents the leading cause of mortality and morbidity in critically ill patients world wide. Our understanding of the complex pathophysiologic alterations occuring in the sepsis syndrome is increasing, but unfortunately mortality associated with this disorder remains unacceptably high, ranging from 30–50% [1–4]. Despite these new insights, the cornerstone of therapy continues to be early recognition, prompt initiation of effective antibiotic therapy, and eliminating the source of infection. Goal-directed hemodynamic, ventilatory, and metabolic support to reach targets are also vital. To date, the adjuvant treatment of sepsis remains a major therapeutic challenge. Based on the humoral theory of sepsis, blood purification is theoretically attracting interest and would provide a broad-based restoration of humoral homeostasis thereby avoiding both excessive inflammation and counter-inflammation. High volume hemofiltration (HVHF) is an extracorporeal blood purification therapy aimed at non-selectively reducing the circulating levels and activity of both pro- and anti-inflammatory mediators involved in the sepsis syndrome and multi-organ dysfunction syndrome (MODS). Numerous *in vitro* studies have shown that hemofiltration is capable of removing nearly every known substance involved in sepsis to a certain degree, prooving its technical efficacy. Multiple animal studies have shown a beneficial effect of HVHF on survival in endotoxemic models. Recent human studies have demonstrated that HVHF improves hemodyamics with decreased vasopressor requirements and trends to improved survival of septic patients. Because of technical requirements of high blood flows, tight ultrafiltration control, and large amounts of costly sterile fluids, we proposed a "Pulse HVHF" technique which can be applied for short periods of up to 6–8 hours per day, providing intense plasma water exchange. In this chapter, we will discuss some of the basic principles and rationale of "Pulse HVHF", review animal experiments, and finally discuss the results of recent human studies and their implication.

▌ The Rationale of High Volume Hemofiltration

The sepsis syndrome is associated with an overwhelming, systemic overflow of pro- and anti-inflammatory mediators leading to generalized endothelial damage, multiple organ failure (MOF) and altered cellular immunological responsiveness. The complex inflammatory network involved is synergistic and acts like a cascade. It includes mediators with autocrine and paracrine actions as well as cellular and intracellular components. A large number of inflammatory mediators, including tumor necrosis factor alpha (TNF-α), interleukin-1 (IL-1), IL-6, platelet activating factor (PAF), and nitric oxide (NO), have a pronounced role in the cascade, but attempts to improve survival in human trials with innovative, predominantly anti-inflammatory therapeutic strategies have been extremely disappointing [5], possibly because of a discrepancy between the biological timing of the syndrome and the clinical timing of symptoms.

Nearly paralleling the surge of pro-inflammatory mediators there is a rise in anti-inflammatory substances by which a state of immunoparalysis or monocyte hyporesponsiveness can be induced [6]. Both pro- and anti-inflammatory factors become upregulated and interact with each other, leading to various rises in mediator levels that change over time. Therefore, neither single-mediator-directed nor one-time interventions seem appropriate.

Continuous renal replacement therapies (CRRT) allow extracorporeal treatment in critically ill patients with hypercatabolism and fluid overload. CRRT have commonly used three types of epurative mechanisms: convection, diffusion, and adsorption by the filtering membrane. In addition to removing excess fluid and waste products in septic patients, convective modalities have the advantage of removing higher molecular weight substances, which include many inflammatory mediators. Adsorption to the filter membrane is a saturable process wihin a timeframe of a few hours. An augmentation can be reached by increasing membrane surface area and ultrafiltration rate which probably extends the surface used for adsorption more distally into the membrane pores [7]. The removal of the broad spectrum of pathogenetic molecules identified in sepsis by convection and adsorption may be clinically beneficial, introducing the concept of blood purification [8–12].

One of the major criticisms attributed to continuous blood purification treatments in sepsis – its lack of specificity – could turn out to be a major strength. Non-specific and continuous removal of soluble mediators, be they pro- or anti-inflammatory, without completely eliminating their effect may be the most logical and adequate approach to a complex and long-running process like sepsis.

Numerous *in vitro* as well as animal and human studies have shown that synthetic filters used in continuous hemofiltration (CVVH) can extract nearly every substance involved in sepsis to a certain degree [13]. Notable examples are complement factors [14, 15], TNF-α, IL-1, IL-6 [15-17], IL-8 and PAF [18, 19]. Regarding plasma cytokine levels, their decrease appears nevertheless of minor degree. Other studies could not show any influence on cytokine plasma levels with CRRT [20–23]. On the other hand, significant clinical benefits in terms of hemodynamic improvement have been achieved even without measurable decreases in cytokine plasma levels [24]. However, when the response to sepsis is viewed in a network perspective, absolute values would be less relevant than relative ones within an array of interdependent mediators as even small decreases could induce major balance changes. This makes measurement of cytokine plasma levels debatable while more local or tissue levels should preferably be measured whenever possible. These issues are still extremely controversial. However, these data emphasize that convection and also adsorption may achieve a certain degree of 'blood purification'.

Consequently, it would be logical to try to improve the efficiency of extracorporeal treatments by increasing the amount of plasma water exchange, i.e., increasing ultrafiltration rates. This modality is so-called HVHF.

▌ HVHF: Animal Studies

Animal studies provide great support to this concept. In a landmark study, a porcine model of septic shock induced by endotoxin infusion was investigated [25]. The animals developed profound hypodynamic shock. With HVHF (at 6 l/h), right ventricular function, blood pressure and cardiac output showed a remarkable improvement compared to control and sham-filtered animals [25, 26]. The same group extended their findings in the same model by i.v. administration of ultrafiltrate from lipopolysaccharide (LPS)-infused animals into healthy animals. The animals receiving ultrafiltrate from endotoxemic animals rapidly developed hemodynamic features of septic shock while animals infused with ultrafiltrate from healthy animals showed a moderate blood pressure rise [25]. These studies established that a convection-based treatment can remove substances with hemodynamic effects resembling septic shock, when sufficiently high ultrafiltration rates are applied.

Supporting evidence is provided by recent animal studies that demonstrated significant hemodynamic benefit [27–29], improvement in immune cell hyporesponsiveness [28], and reduced mortality [28, 29] applying HVHF rates of 80–100 ml/kg/h. A study using an experimental porcine pancreatitis model compared low-volume hemofiltration and HVHF at 100 ml/kg/h of ultrafiltrate. In this study, early filter change was used to delineate the effect of cytokine removal by adsorption on the filter, and a hyperdynamic septic state was induced through an intervention that approximates the underlying conditions encountered in human sepsis. Additionally, interventions started late when the animals had already developed the clinical picture of hyperdynamic septic shock in order to simulate real clinical conditions, HVHF demonstrated survival advantages, changes in TNF-α levels as well as monocyte and polymorphonuclear neutrophil function. Of relevance, increasing ultrafiltration dose had a greater effect than frequency of filter change [29].

▌ HVHF: Human Studies

In a randomized, controlled human study in 425 critically ill patients with acute renal failure, it was shown that utrafiltration dose correlated significantly with survival [30]. With an ultrafiltration dose of 20 ml/kg/h, mortality rate was 59% compared to a mortality rate of 43% with 35 ml/kg/h and 42% with 45 ml/kg/h ultrafiltration. In septic patients (11–14% per randomization group), there was a trend of direct correlation of treatment dose with survival, even above 35 ml/kg/h in contrast to the whole group where a survival plateau was reached with that dose. This observation supports the concept of a 'septic dose' of hemofiltration contrasting to a 'renal dose' of the same treatment prescribed for acute renal failure patients without systemic inflammation.

Over the last few years, several human studies have examined the clinical effects of HVHF with ultrafiltration rates equivalent to 7–9 liters/h for a 70-kg adult. These studies demonstrated the beneficial effects on oxygenation and time to extubation in children undergoing cardiac surgery [31], improvements in hemodyamics with decreased vasopressor requirements [32–34], and trends to improved survival [34, 35]. Impressive clinical results were obtained in an evaluation of short-term HVHF in 20 patients in catecholamine-refractory septic shock [33] comprising a patient cohort with very poor expected survival. A control group was not defined. Only one four-hour session of HVHF removing 35 liters (6 l/h) of ultrafiltrate replaced by bicarbonate-containing fluid was applied as soon as mean blood pressure could not be stabilized above 70 mmHg with dopamine, norepinephrine, and epinephrine after appropriate volume resuscitation. HVHF was followed by conventional CVVH. Endpoints were increase in cardiac index, mixed venous oxygen saturation and arterial pH, and decrease in norepinephrine requirements. Eleven patients reached all predefined endpoints and showed impressively good survival (9 of 11) at 28 days. Nine patients did not reach all endpoints and had a 100% mortality rate. Apart from response to HVHF, time from ICU admission to the start of HVHF and body weight were the only factors associated with survival in the analysis. Patients with higher body weight did worse possibly because they received a smaller ultrafiltration dose per body weight as speculated by the authors. These trials still need cautious interpretation with respect to their limited design but they certainly deliver sound evidence of feasibility and efficacy to set the stage for a large-scale trial on HVHF in sepsis.

▌ "Pulse HVHF": Concept and Technique

According to previous studies, ultrafiltration rates above 50-60 ml/kg/h (60 l/day including net ultrafiltration) in continuous hemofiltration mode is considered high and can be defined as HVHF.

Technological problems and the increased costs of the therapy initially limited the clinical application of the HVHF technique, but newer CRRT machines permit a full range of treatment modes and higher pre- or post- dilution effluent flow rates, as well as being more user-friendly. These machines include some important hardware and software aspects such as high precision scales, and powerful heating systems for maintaining constant sufficiently high temperature for the high volumes of infused solution. Figure 1 shows a recently-designed CRRT machine (MultiFiltrate, Fresenius Medical Care, Bad Homburg).

In order to explore any possibility of rendering HVHF cost-benefit effective and to utilize this technique without major problems, we propose Pulse HVHF as a compromise between clinical indications and practical and technical considerations. A daily schedule of HVHF (85 ml/kg/h) for 6–8 h followed or preceded by CVVH (at 35 ml/kg/h) for the remaining time, leads to a cumulative dose of approximately 48 ml/kg/h (80 l/day in a 70 kg patient). This schedule may be changed according to the patient's hemodynamic response and needs, and to organizational needs.

To reach ultrafiltration rates of 85 ml/kg/hr, some major determinants of ultrafiltration need to be considered. High blood flow rate (as compared to conventional CRRT) requires vascular access (e.g., 14 F catheters) to attain a constant flow of at least 300 ml/min. A filtration fraction of 25% can then be set. If the catheter or cannulated vessel is too small, the resistance of the arterial lumen of the catheter creates a negative pressure before the pump, which may reach values as high as –300 mmHg, resulting in negative impact on dialyzer life. The same type of pressure may be encountered in the venous side of the circuit. The return or venous pressure may be even greater because of a hemoconcentration effect that takes place when high amounts of 'net ultrafiltration' are present. The 'net ultrafiltration' is the real amount of fluid removed from the patient after the reinfusion of the sub-

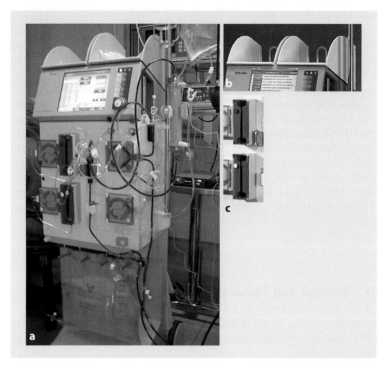

Fig. 1. a MultiFiltrate continuous renal replacement therapy (CRRT) Machine (Fresenius Medical Care, Bad Homburg); **b** replacement fluid capacity up to 24 liters hemofiltration solution; **c** two integrated heating systems (35/39 °C)

stitution fluid. Thus, despite a high exchange volume during 'pulse therapy', net ultrafiltration should be maintained as low as possible, or even at zero balance.

When high blood flows are used, anticoagulation become less critical, since the time of contact between blood and artificial surface is reduced. However, in case of high filtration fraction, blood viscosity and hematocrit may significantly increase within the filter. Adequate anticoagulation is essential to avoid clot formation and filter clotting. Pulse HVHF requires a large hemofilter with a surface area of 1.8 to 2 m^2 (in a 70 kg patient) to achieve such a high ultrafiltration rate. We recommend highly biocompatible, synthetic membranes with a permeability coefficient between 30 and 40 ml/h/mmHg. These membranes have solute sieving coefficients close to 1 for a wide spectrum of molecular weights [36]. Bicarbonate buffered hemofiltration fluid (35 mmol/l) should be administered with a combination of 33 to 50% in pre-dilution and 50 to 66% in post-dilution.

Other important aspects of general patient care with this regimen include temperature monitoring, antibiotic dose adjustments, and nutritional adjustments (derived from amino acid, phosphate, vitamin losses).

▌ "Pulse HVHF": When to Start?

At this time, evidence delineating the benefit of HVHF in patient survival is lacking. Both the 'pro' and 'con' studies lack statistical power and were performed in a restricted number of closed format ICUs. However, hemodynamic and oxygenation improvements seem to be the reasonable objectives of the adjuvant therapy of a septic/MODS patient who cannot maintain blood pressure after adequate volume resuscitation and catecholamine (dopamine, norepinephrine) administration. The initial hemodynamic improvement with HVHF seems to be maintained over 96 hours, with a significant decrease (>70%) in norepinephrine requirements [37]. One of the major questions is that of timing: when to start the treatment. Since the real benefits are still being investigated, firm criteria for initiation have not been fixed making timing of treatment more controversial. However the major indication is the presence of refractory hemodynamic instability, and thus HVHF could be indicated for the elective treatment of hemodynamically unstable patients. With recent evidence confirming the benefits of 'early goal directed therapy', we believe that HVHF treatment should be initiated as early as possible as this was clearly shown to affect survival rates [33].

▌ "Pulse HVHF": Clinical Experience

We treated 16 critically ill patients (10 male and 6 females, mean age 55.2 ± 10.2 years, mean APACHE II score 31.8) with severe sepsis using the schedule as described above. The commercial bicarbonate buffered replacement fluid was used in simultaneous pre- and post-dilution, at a different ratio on the basis of the various circuit pressures during the treatment. Our patients underwent daily pulse HVHF to evaluate its feasibility, and its effects on hemodynamics.

No treatment was prematurely discontinued because of extracorporeal circuit clotting or high pressure problems. Hemodynamic stability was improved (Table 1), allowing a decrease in vasopressor requirement (>75%) (Fig. 2). Mean daily Kt/V was 3.3. The pulse HVHF treatment was continued for 6 ± 2 days, the CVVH treatment was continued for 15 ± 4 days.

In addition, there is growing evidence for the role of apoptosis in organ injury during sepsis and inflammation in general. A recent surge of interest has been directed to apoptosis as a biological hallmark of the dysregulation of the immune system associated sepsis [38, 39]. Furthermore, activated protein C (Drotrecogin alfa [activated]), which has recently been shown to improve survival of severe sep-

Table 1. Hemodynamic changes pre and post pulse high-volume hemofiltration treatment

	Pre-treatment	Post-treatment	p-value
▌ Heart rate (bpm)	70 ± 14	80 ± 19	n.s.
▌ Mean arterial pressure (mmHg)	101 ± 28	89 ± 16	n.s.
▌ Norepinephrine dose (µg/min)	18.3 ± 11.3	5.4 ± 5.1	0.04
▌ Temperature (°C)	36.6 ± 1.4	36.5 ± 0.8	n.s.

Results shown as mean ± SD

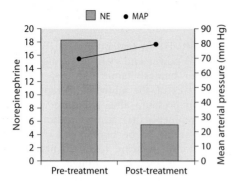

Fig. 2. Average norepinephrine (NE) doses pre and post pulse high-volume hemofiltration (HVHF) treatment. MAP: means arterial pressure

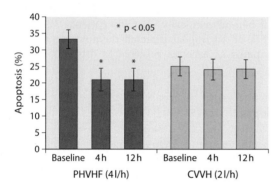

Fig. 3. Percentage of plasma pro-apoptotic activity on U937 human monocytic cells during post pulse high-volume hemofiltration (PHVHF) compared to CVVH treatment

tic patients has strong anti-apoptotic properties, in addition to its other activities [40]. In sepsis, apoptosis is accelerated in monocytes, and it might play an important role in 'monocyte hyporesponsiveness' and exposes the host to further increase in disease severity. We, therefore, also studied the effects of pulse HVHF on monocyte apoptosis. We found that septic plasma had remarkably pro-apoptotic effect on U937 human monocytic cells compared with control. Pulse HVHF but not CVVH significantly reduced the pro-apoptotic plasma activity already at 1 hr and this was maintained unvaried at 4 and 12 hr as depicted in Fig. 3. Our result demonstrates that pulse HVHF not only has hemodynamic benefits but also positive biological effects in sepsis patient.

▌ Conclusion

Sepsis is a leading cause of acute renal failure in the ICU and continues to have an alarmingly high mortality rate despite advancements in understanding the complex processes involved in the sepsis syndrome and new treatments. Selective therapeutic techniques have failed to demonstrate benefit in sepsis; thus, broader non-selective modalities may play a vital role.

Standard dose hemofiltration does not affect plasma levels of inflammatory mediators and in clinical trials failed to improve mortality. Increasing the dose has been shown to be beneficial, thus high volume hemofiltration may be a formidable option in altering the course of sepsis. The technical aspects of this modality have been demonstrated and it is safe and easy to perform with modern machines. Animal studies clearly show benefits in survival. Small uncontrolled human studies to date have been promising and we wait for the results of large properly designed clinical trials to prove its benefits.

References

1. Laupland KB, Davies HD, Church DL, et al (2004) Bloodstream infection-associated sepsis and septic shock in critically ill adults: a population-based study. Infection 32:59–64
2. Dellinger RP (2003) Cardiovascular management of septic shock. Crit Care Med 31:946–955
3. Friedman G, Silva E, Vincent JL (1998) Has the mortality of septic shock changed with time. Crit Care Med 26:2078–2086
4. Angus DC, Linde-Zwirble WT, Lidicker J, et al (2001) Epidemiology of severe sepsis in the United States: analysis of incidence, outcome, and associated costs of care. Crit Care Med 29:1303–1310
5. Wheeler AP, Bernard GR (1999) Treating patients with severe sepsis. N Engl J Med 340:207–214
6. Adib-Conquy M, Adrie C, Moine P, et al (2000) NF-kappa B expression in mononuclear cells of patients with sepsis resembles that observed in lipopolysaccharide tolerance. Am J Respir Crit Care Med 162:1877–1883
7. Langsdorf LJ, Zydney AL (1994) Effect of blood contact on the transport properties of hemodialysis membranes: a two-layer membrane model. Blood Purif 12:292-307
8. Bellomo R, Tipping P, Boyce N (1993) Continuous veno-venous hemofiltration with dialysis cytokines from the circulation of septic patients. Crit Care Med 21:522–526
9. Schetz M, Ferdinande P, Van der Berghe G, et al (1995) Removal of pro-inflammatory cytokines with renal replacement therapy: sense or nonsense? Intensive Care Med 21:169–176
10. Millar AB, Armstrong L, van der Linden J, et al (1993) Cytokine production and hemofiltration in children undergoing cardiopulmonary bypass. Ann Thorac Surg 56:1499–1502
11. Journois D, Pouard P, Greely WJ, et al (1994) Hemofiltration during cardiopulmonary bypass in pediatric cardiac surgery. Anesthesiology 81:1181–1189
12. Goldfarb S, Golper TA (1994) Proinflammatory cytokines and hemofiltration membranes. J Am Soc Nephrol 5:228–232
13. De Vriese AS, Vanholder RC, Pascual M, et al (1999) Can inflammatory cytokines be removed efficiently by continous renal replacement therapies? Intensive Care Med 25:903–910
14. Hoffmann JN, Hartl WH, Deppisch R, et al (1995) Hemofiltration in human sepsis: evidence for elimination of immunomodulatory substances. Kidney Int 48:1563–1570
15. Gasche Y, Pascual M. Suter PM, et al (1996) Complement depletion during haemofiltration with polyacrylonitrile membranes. Nephrol Dial Transplant 11:117–119
16. Kellum JA, Johnson JP, Kramer D, et al (1998) Diffusive vs. convective therapy: effects on mediators of inflammation in patients with severe systemic inflammatory response syndrome. Crit Care Med 26:1995–2000
17. Kellum JA, Bellomo R, Mehta R, Ronco C (2003) Blood purification in non-renal critical illness. Blood Purif 21:6–13
18. Ronco C, Tetta C, Lupi A, et al (1995) Removal of platelet-activating factor in experimental continuous arteriovenous hemofiltration. Crit Care Med 23:99–107
19. Mariano F, Tetta C, Guida GE, et al (2001) Hemofiltration reduces the priming activity on neutrophil chemiluminescence in septic patients. Kidney Int 60:1598–1605
20. Sander A, Armbruster W, Sander B, et al (1997) Haemofiltration increases IL-6 clearance in early systemic inflammatory response syndrome but does not alter IL-6 and TNF alpha plasma concentrations. Intensive Care Med 23:878–884
21. De Vriese AS, Colardyn FA, Philippe JJ, et al (1999) Cytokine removal during continuous hemofiltration in septic patients. J Am Soc Nephrol 10:846–853
22. Ronco C, Brendolan A, Lonnemann G, et al (2002) A pilot study on coupled plasma filtration with adsorption in septic shock. Crit Care Med 30:1250–1255

23. Cole L, Bellomo R, Hart G, et al (2002) A phase II randomized controlled trial of continuous hemofiltration in sepsis. Crit Care Med 30:100–106
24. Heering P, Morgera S, Schmitz FJ, et al (1997) Cytokine removal and cardiovascular hemodynamics in septic patients with continuous veno-venous hemofiltration. Intensive Care Med 23:288–296
25. Grootendorst AF, van Bommel EFH, van der Hoven B, et al (1992) High volume hemofiltration improves right ventricular function of endotoxin-induced shock in the pig. Intensive Care Med 18:235–240
26. Grootendorst AF, van Bommel EFH, van der Hoven B, et al (1992) High volume hemofiltration improves hemodynamics of endotoxin-induced shock in the pig. J Crit Care 7:67–75
27. Bellomo R, Kellum JA, Gandhi CR, et al (2000) The effect of intensive plasma water exchange by hemofiltration on hemodynamics and soluble mediators in canine endotoxemia. Am J Respir Crit Care Med 161:1429–1436
28. Rogiers P, Zhang H, Smail N, et al (1999) Continuous venovenous hemofiltration improves cardiac performance by mechanisms other than tumor necrosis factor-alpha attenuation during endotoxic shock. Crit Care Med 27:1848–1855
29. Yakebas EF, Eisenberger CF, Ohnesorge, et al (2001) Attenuation of sepsis-related immunoparalysis by continuous veno-venous hemofiltration in experimental porcine pancreatitis. Crit Care Med 29:1423–1430
30. Ronco C, Bellomo R, Homel P, et al (2000) Effects of different doses in continuous venovenous haemofiltration on outcomes of acute renal failure: a prospective randomised trial. Lancet 356:26–30
31. Journois D, Israel Biet D, Pouard P, et al (1996) High-volume, zero-balanced hemofiltration to reduce delayed inflammatory response to cardiopulmonary bypass in children. Anesthesiology 85:965–976
32. Cole L, Bellomo R, Journois D, et al (2001) High-volume haemofiltration in human septic shock. Intensive Care Med 27:978–986
33. Honore PM, Jamez J, Wauthier M, et al (1998) Prospective evaluation of short-term, high-volume isovolemic hemofiltration on the hemodynamic course and outcome in patients with intractable circulatory failure resulting from septic shock. Crit Care Med 28:3581–3587
34. Joannes-Boyau O, Rapaport S, Bazin R, et al (2004) Impact of high volume hemofiltration on hemodynamic disturbance and outcome during septic shock. ASAIO J 50:102–109
35. Oudemans-van Straaten HM, Bosman RJ, van der Spoe JI, et al (1999) Outcome of critically ill patients treated with intermittent high-volume haemofiltration: A prospective cohort analysis. Intensive Care Med 25:814–821
36. Uchino S, Cole L, Morimatsu H, et al (2003) Solute mass balance during isovolaemic high volume haemofiltration. Intensive Care Med 29:1541–1546
37. Honore PM, Jamez J, Wauthier M, et al (2000) Prospective evaluation of short-term, high-volume isovolemic hemofiltration on the hemodynamic course and outcome in patients with intractable circulatory failure resulting from septic shock. Crit Care Med 28:3581–3587
38. Weber SU, Schewe JC, Putensen C, et al (2004) Apoptosis as a pathomechanism in sepsis. Anaesthesist 53:59–65
39. Hotchkiss RS, Tinsley KW, Karl IE (2003) Role of apoptotic cell death in sepsis. Scand J Infect Dis 35:585–592
40. Joyce DE, Grinnell BW (2002) Recombinant human activated protein C attenuates the inflammatory response in endothelium and monocytes by modulating nuclear factor-kappa B. Crit Care Med 30 (Suppl 5):288–293

Liver Transplantation in the Management of Fulminant Hepatic Failure

M. A. Silva, E. Esmat, and D. F. Mirza

Introduction

Fulminant liver failure is characterized by a massive acute onset hepatocyte dysfunction, which leads to a cascade of events resulting in severe coagulopathy and hepatic encephalopathy that could eventually cause death. This occurs in a previously healthy individual with no known underlying liver disease [1]. The disease could evolve to a terminal stage within days or weeks and despite recent advances in intensive care and organ support techniques, mortality remains high [2]. Early deaths in fulminant liver failure are related to cerebral edema and circulatory collapse, whereas late deaths are often as a result of sepsis and multi-organ failure (MOF). The outcome of fulminant liver failure is determined by etiology, the degree of hepatic encephalopathy present on admission, and by complications. Orthotopic liver transplantation is the only treatment modality that impacts survival in fulminant liver failure with a 1-year survival of 60–90% depending on the cause of fulminant liver failure and the selection criteria applied [3–5]. Although medical management of fulminant liver failure has improved, early prediction of which patients need a liver transplant to survive is still an important task. Artificial and bioartificial support systems do not seem to increase survival in fulminant liver failure, but may act as a 'bridging mechanism' until orthotopic liver transplantation or liver regeneration can take place [6, 7]. In children, fulminant liver failure is rare, but has a mortality rate of 70% without appropriate management and/or orthotopic liver transplantation [8].

Definition of Fulminant Liver Failure

Hepatic encephalopathy is the hallmark of fulminant liver failure and clearly marks the transition from a severe condition to a deadly disease. Since the initial definition of fulminant liver failure in 1970 by Tray and Davidson [9], there have been many proposed classifications and definitions of the disease. The interval between onset of jaundice and the appearance of hepatic encephalopathy is commonly used to sub-classify acute liver failure. The classification described by O'Grady et al. in 1993 is used at our center and is widely accepted [1]. In this classification, hepatic encephalopathy between 0 to 7 days from onset of jaundice is called hyperacute liver failure. Acute liver failure refers to the onset of hepatic encephalopathy between 8 and 28 days. Hepatic encephalopathy developing between 29 and 72 days is referred to as subacute liver failure [1]. This definition, however, is not useful in pediatric fulminant liver failure since the clinical presentation may be prolonged particularly if secondary to autoimmune or metabolic liver disease [8].

▌ Etiology of Fulminant Liver Failure

There is wide geographical variation in the etiology of fulminant liver failure. In the United Kingdom the commonest cause is acetaminophen overdose (70%) followed by seronegative or non A to E hepatitis, where no identifiable cause is found. Other causes include idiosyncratic drug reactions and Wilson's disease [6, 10, 11]. In the United States, drug related hepatotoxicity accounts for more than 50% of the causes for fulminant liver failure. This includes acetaminophen toxicity (40%) and idiosyncratic drug reactions (10%) [2]. Most cases of acute viral hepatitis are caused by hepatitis A and B virus. Hepatitis B is a common cause of fulminant liver failure in the far east and hepatitis E is relevant to India [12, 13]. Hepatitis E virus can result in fulminant liver failure, especially in the third trimester of pregnancy. Current evidence indicates that hepatitis C virus infection alone does not result in fulminant liver failure commonly. There is however an increased risk for fulminant liver failure in the presence of co-infection that also involves the hepatitis C virus. In children, the etiology of fulminant liver failure varies depending on age. In neonates, inherited metabolic liver disease or infection is likely while viral hepatitis, autoimmune liver disease, or drug induced liver failure are common in older children.

▌ The Histopathology of Fulminant Liver Failure

Fulminant liver failure develops from both cytotoxic and cytopathic injury, either alone or in combination. Cytotoxic injury results from direct injury to hepatocytes by hepatotoxic viruses (hepatitis A virus), drugs or their toxic metabolites, and other toxins. Cytopathic injury is caused by an immune-mediated response to hepatocytes that express abnormal cell surface antigens, as observed in hepatitis B virus infection and idiosyncratic drug reactions. The most common histologic pattern seen in fulminant liver failure is hepatocellular necrosis with or without preservation of hepatic architecture. Lobular collapse, islands of regenerative hepatocytes, infiltration with polymorphonuclear cells, lymphocyes, plasmocytes or eosinophils with proliferation of duct like structures around portal areas could also be encountered.

▌ Clinical Presentation of Fulminant Liver Failure

Depending on the severity and etiology of the liver cell injury, the clinical presentation varies from non-specific symptoms such as nausea, vomiting and abdominal discomfort to confusion, agitation and coma. The diagnosis becomes more obvious when the results of liver biochemical tests and coagulation studies become available. Once a diagnosis is made, a formal assessment of the degree of hepatic encephalopathy is essential. This is graded from I to IV. Patients with grade I hepatic encephalopathy exhibit slow mentation with inappropriate behavior seen in grade

II, followed by permanent somnolence in III, and coma in grade IV. The overall mortalities are higher in patients who progress to grade III and IV. Cerebral edema is the primary contributory factor for such increased mortality, which is more prominent in the hyper acute and acute liver failure groups. This is probably as a result of inadequate time for the equilibration of osmotic loads associated with liver failure. Cerebral edema is estimated to occur in up to 80% of patients with fulminant liver failure [13]. In children the extent of jaundice is variable in the early stages, but all children have coagulopathy. Encephalopathy is particularly difficult to diagnose in neonates. Vomiting and poor feeding are early signs, while irritability and reversal of day/night sleep patterns indicating more established hepatic encephalopathy. In older children, hepatic encephalopathy may present with aggressive behavior or convulsions.

▌ Management of Fulminant Liver Failure

Patients with abnormal liver function tests and coagulopathy need to have their mental state under close surveillance for signs of deterioration and benefit from admission to high dependency care. Such patients with slight alteration of mental state could deteriorate rapidly and early referral to a specialist hepatobiliary unit with liver transplant facilities is essential. In these patients a multidisciplinary input from a hepatologist, liver intensivist, and a liver transplant surgeon is crucial since progression to multi-organ dysfunction could be rapid.

Special considerations:
▌ Prevention of complications such as nutritional derangement, cerebral edema, sepsis, coagulopathy, and MOF
▌ Assessment of prognosis and selection for liver transplantation
▌ Provision of hepatic support

Specific therapy for acetaminophen overdose in the form of N-acetylcysteine (NAC) is of value if given within 8–10 hours following consumption. It replenishes glutathione stores and thus prevents the development of hepatotoxicity. The effectiveness of NAC diminishes with time, but it may be of use up to 72 hours after acetaminophen ingestion.

▌ Prevention and Management of Complications

Fluid and Nutrition

Fulminant liver failure is a catabolic state, and protein calorie malnutrition develops rapidly. Enteral nutrition is preferred to parenteral nutrition. Glycemia needs strict control especially in patients with deep hepatic encephalopathy and constant infusion with 10 to 20% glucose is preferred to bolus administration to maintain glucose levels above 4 mmol/l. Fluid restriction with 75% of maintenance is optimal to prevent cerebral edema. There is a tendency to avoid excessive sodium in patients with chronic liver disease and this is translated into the care of patients with fulminant liver failure. Correction of hypomagnesemia, hypokalemia, or hypophosphatemia may also be required. H_2 receptor antagonists and proton-pump inhibitors are also used to reduce the incidence of stress ulceration of the gastrointestinal tract.

Cerebral Edema

Cerebral edema resulting in raised intracranial pressure (ICP) is associated with the risk of brain herniation and death. An arterial ammonia level higher than 200 µg/dl in patients with advanced hepatic encephalopathy has been reported as a strong indicator of imminent brain herniation [14]. Monitoring ICP has, however, not been shown to increase survival in these patients and therefore should be limited to specialized units and to patients awaiting orthotopic liver transplantation. Most centers prefer epidural to subdural or intraparenchymal transducers when monitoring ICP as a result of lower rate of complications [13]. Monitoring of jugular bulb oxygen saturation with a reversed jugular venous catheter is also used to guide interventions to reduce intracranial hypertension. Patients should be nursed at 20° head up tilt position in order to improve jugular venous outflow. If ICP remains above 25 mmHg for longer than 10 minutes indicating a sustained rise, 0.5–1 g/kg of 20% solution of mannitol is given over 20 minutes. This is repeated until plasma osmolarity reaches 310 mOsm/l. Patients with oliguria and renal failure may require hemodialysis to avoid hyperosmolarity. Hyperventilation produces cerebral vasoconstriction and reduces cerebral blood flow, but its effects are usually transient. Intravenous anesthesia with thiopentone maintaining normocapnia is reserved for patients unresponsive to osmotic agents.

Subclinical seizures and overt seizures are difficult to recognize in sedated and ventilated patients. They may, however, be suspected in patients with elevated ICP and low jugular bulb saturation, which reflects an increased oxygen consumption by the brain. Anti-convulsants used in this setting have been shown to decrease ICP and improve jugular bulb saturations [15]. There is some evidence that moderate hypothermia (32–33 °C) in humans reduces ICP and improves cerebral blood flow (CBF) [16].

Coagulation Support

Coagulation parameters are a reliable method of assessing liver function especially in patients where evaluation of mental state is not possible. Administration of fresh frozen plasma and platelets needs to be done judiciously since there is no evidence that this increases survival and fluid overload is a risk. Thus correction of coagulopathy is not indicated unless bleeding occurs or invasive procedures are planned. Recombinant activated factor VII offers advantages of shorter half-life and avoidance of fluid overload. The use of factor VIIa, however, is yet to be established and results of multicenter studies are still awaited [17].

Prevention of Sepsis

Fever and leukocytosis are absent in up to 30% of infected patients with fulminant liver failure [13]. Infection must therefore be suspected in the presence of any sudden clinical or biochemical deterioration. This is especially so in the presence of improving liver functions. There are no generally acceptable guidelines regarding the use of prophylactic antibiotics in fulminant liver failure, but the use of broad-spectrum antibiotics and antifungal agents are beneficial.

Organ Support

A hyperdynamic circulation is characteristic of fulminant liver failure, with systemic and splanchnic arterial vasodilation resulting in an increased cardiac output and decreased arterial pressure. Repositioning of volume is required to correct arterial hypotension, with normal blood pressures being achieved only rarely. This should be guided by central venous pressures which should be maintained between 8–12 mmHg. The use of a pulmonary artery catheter enables better monitoring of cardiovascular status. Blood, colloid, or albumin is preferred over crystalloids for volume expansion. Epinephrine or norepinephrine are the preferred vasopressors, but should be used with caution since they impair tissue perfusion and produce unwanted increase in CBF.

Intubation and mechanical ventilation is required in patients with agitation or deep hepatic encephalopathy, to avoid surges of ICP rise and pulmonary aspiration. If dialysis is needed, continuous hemofiltration is preferred over intermittent hemodialysis to avoid rapid fluid shifts that may aggravate cerebral edema.

▌ Prognostication and Selection of Transplantation Candidates

The only therapeutic intervention of proven benefit for patients with advanced fulminant liver failure is orthotopic liver transplantation. An accurate and early assessment of the individual patient is critical in deciding whether liver transplantation is indicated. This is a decision that often needs to be taken with limited clinical and background information, in the presence of rapid clinical deterioration, where delay could result in the patient becoming un-transplantable due to clinical contra-indications. The risks of an emergency orthotopic liver transplantation in the context of evolving or established MOF must be balanced against the possibility of survival with continued medical supportive care alone.

Survival of patients with fulminant liver failure is 40 to 80% depending on factors including etiology, patient age, severity of liver dysfunction, degree of liver necrosis, number and nature of complications, and duration of illness [18]. Patients with grade II hepatic encephalopathy have a mortality of 30%; those who progress to grade IV have a mortality rate greater than 80%. In general, survival tends to be better in cases with acute hepatitis and acetaminophen overdose (40%). In contrast, patients with fulminant liver failure caused by idiosyncratic drug reactions, toxins, hepatitis B and D virus co-infection, and idiopathic etiologies have mortality rates approaching 80 to 90% [18].

Several prognostic systems have been developed for fulminant liver failure to help determine the likelihood of spontaneous recovery and to select patients who would require emergency orthotopic liver transplantation. Like all diagnostic tests, the best evidence to support the use of a particular criteria is from the confirmation of its performance in validation studies [19]. However, selection criteria and methodology in validation studies done to date are questionable. The very nature of the condition under investigation introduces bias, which makes the design of studies difficult. The numbers of patients in such studies are relatively small, the studies usually being unblinded, and retrospective. The studies also span over decades, during which medical supportive management has changed substantially. Further bias is introduced by inclusion of transplanted patients as 'non survivors', an assumption that could be flawed. These bias' tend to overestimate the accuracy

Table 1. The King's College Criteria

Acetaminophen etiology

▌Arterial pH < 7.3 after volume resuscitation or

Concurrent findings of;

▌Grade III encephalopathy or above

▌Creatinine > 300 µmol/L

▌INR > 6.5

Non-acetaminophen etiology

▌INR > 6.7 or

Any three of;

▌Unfavorable etiology (idiosyncratic drug, seronegative)

▌Age < 10 or > 40 years

▌Acute/subacute presentation

▌Bilirubin > 300 µmol/L

▌INR > 3.5

of selection criteria under study [19]. The prognostic criteria that are used commonly in the management of patients with fulminant liver failure should be therefore applied to individual patients with these limitations in mind.

▌ The King's College Criteria

The King's College criteria (KCH) have been the most widely used worldwide and are different for acetaminophen and non-acetaminophen induced fulminant liver failure (Table 1). These criteria have been evaluated subsequently and have been found to be relatively effective in predicting death and the need for transplantation. However, failure to fulfill the KCH criteria does not predict survival [20, 21]. Also more published data exist to support the use of the acetaminophen than the non-acetaminophen criteria. The KCH criteria have a clinically acceptable specificity, and the patient who fulfills the criteria is very likely to die without transplantation. Survival with medical management alone in this group is between 10 to 15% [19]. The sensitivity of the KCH criteria is relatively limited in that a proportion of patients die without fulfilling criteria and thus without prior identification and consideration as potential orthotopic liver transplantation candidates. The clinical deterioration is so great in almost 50% of patients who fulfill the criteria, that orthotopic liver transplantation is never a realistic option either due to the presence of contra-indications to orthotopic liver transplantation at the time of fulfilling criteria or to their development while waiting for a graft.

▌ Alternative Prognostic Markers

Several other prognostic markers have been proposed in order to overcome the problems with the established criteria and to improve selection. A wide variety of blood markers have been proposed including factor V, and factor VIII/V ratio [22], serum levels of Gc protein, serial prothrombin times, and arterial ketone body ratio

[23–25]. None have, however, proved better than the KCH criteria. A liver volume of less than 1000 ml on CT scanning is associated with very poor survival [26]. Although reducing liver volume is accepted as a poor prognostic indicator in children as well [8], CT imaging of such an ill patient is not always practical. Liver biopsy may, while confirming the etiology of fulminant liver failure, help determine the degree of hepatocyte necrosis, with a biopsy showing more than 70% necrosis associated with more than a 90% mortality without orthotopic liver transplantation [27]. Even in the setting of coagulopathy, a transjugular biopsy could be of value in helping the process of prognostication and decision for early orthotopic liver transplantation [27]. The addition of serum lactate levels and phosphate levels to the KCH criteria have been shown to increase its sensitivity and reduce the time taken to arrive at a decision regarding listing a patient for orthotopic liver transplantation [28, 29]. Recent reports have, however, disputed the usefulness of serum phosphate levels in this role [30].

▌ Prognostic Factors in Children

Prognostic factors for survival with fulminant liver failure in children are not well established. In general, children with metabolic liver disease or severe coagulopathy are unlikely to recover without an orthotopic liver transplantation [31]. Children with a history of acetaminophen poisoning or hepatitis have a better outlook for spontaneous recovery [8]. In children, a poor prognosis and a need for immediate referral for orthotopic liver transplantation is usually indicated by the following factors [8]:

▌ Prothrombin time > 60 s
▌ Decreasening transaminase levels
▌ Raising bilirubin levels > 300 mmol/L
▌ Decreasing liver size
▌ Acid-base pH < 7.3
▌ Hypoglycemia with increasing dextrose requirement
▌ Hepatic coma grade II or III

The presence of irreversible multi-organ dysfunction, which includes mitochondrial disorders and erythrophagocytosis, or obvious cerebral damage on computed tomography (CT) or magnetic resonance imaging (MRI) are contraindications for orthotopic liver transplantation [8].

▌ Liver Transplantation for Fulminant Liver Failure

Liver transplantation is the only measure that can radically influence the course of fulminant liver failure. Since its introduction, results of orthotopic liver transplantation in patients with fulminant liver failure have improved significantly (Fig. 1). The outcome however still remains worse than that of those transplanted for chronic liver disease. This is primarily as a result of the high early post-operative mortality in patients transplanted for fulminant liver failure. Most deaths in this period occur as a result of sepsis and MOF [19]. Early deaths secondary to a raised ICP are less common due to improved management of cerebral edema.

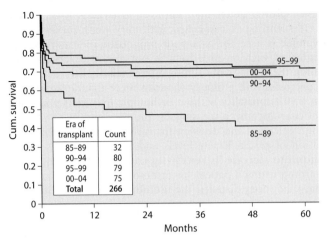

Fig. 1. Survival curves of liver transplant recipients for fulminant hepatic failure at the Liver Unit, Queen Elizabeth Hospital, Birmingham, United Kingdom, showing improvement in survival with progression of time

The severity of the pre-transplant fulminant liver failure and the nature of the graft used are inextricably linked and influence the outcome of the transplant. The critically ill recipient is particularly vulnerable and will not tolerate initial poor function of a transplanted graft. The more unwell a patient is, either in terms of fulminant liver failure or MOF, the greater the prospect of poor outcome following orthotopic liver transplantation. The severity of MOF at the time of orthotopic liver transplantation in patients with fulminant liver failure has been shown to be the single best predictor of patient survival in a study done by the King's College group [32]. In a series from KCH, 45% of patients fulfilling the KCH criteria with acetaminophen related disease had such severe MOF that listing for orthotopic liver transplantation was not an option with 90% of these patients dying [33]. A further 35% of the patients listed for transplantation did not undergo orthotopic liver transplantation with the majority of cases developing clinical contraindications while awaiting a graft [33].

A successful outcome with orthotopic liver transplantation is more likely when a sick recipient is matched to an optimal graft. The difficulty lies with striking a balance between the risk of delaying an orthotopic liver transplantation until an optimal graft is available with the likelihood of further clinical deterioration, and the early acceptance of a suboptimal graft.

Auxiliary Segmental Liver Transplantation

The liver is an organ that has the unique ability of regeneration following an acute and self-limiting injury. Due to this, auxiliary segmental liver transplantation has a theoretically attractive role in fulminant liver failure. This is by placing a partial liver graft while leaving all or part of the native liver in situ. This procedure was first done as a heterotopic graft and later as an auxiliary partial orthotopic procedure. With resolution of the insult causing the fulminant liver failure, the native liver may regenerate sufficiently to return to pre-insult functional status. This would allow withdrawal of immunosuppression, which usually results in auxiliary graft rejection and atrophy. This improves quality of life of the patient with no long-term side effects and reduced costs. Another potential advantage with auxiliary liver transplantation in fulminant liver failure is its use in the setting of live donors. Adult living related transplantation is an option given the urgency of the requirement for transplantation and the availability of organs. In order to overcome the problems of a small for size graft, right sided auxiliary partial liver transplantation in adults and left sided grafts for children have been proposed [34].

Auxiliary segmental liver transplantation is however a technically more demanding procedure which has a high rate of anastomotic complications, neurological sequelae and graft loss due to non function [35, 36]. The procedure should therefore be considered only in patients with a high chance of liver regeneration. Prediction of those patients in whom regeneration of the native liver is likely is difficult, and bears little relation to the histological extent of hepatic necrosis, the presence of fibrotic or regenerative nodules. Better results have been observed with younger patients (<40 years), with hyperacute liver failure (rather than sub acute liver failure), and in fulminant liver failure due to hepatitis A and B viral hepatitis and acetaminophen poisoning [34]. A reappraisal of the procedure in a single large center using a case controlled model recently concluded that on an intent-to treat basis, the efficacy of auxiliary partial liver transplantation is low and careful consideration is needed in the light of increased risks of technical complications and graft loss. However, when using optimal grafts, survival rates are similar to orthotopic liver transplantation if initial problems could be overcome [36]. There have also been recent reports of successful use of auxiliary liver transplantation in fulminant liver failure using grafts in the setting of non-heart beating donors [37].

▌ Living Donor Liver Transplantation for Fulminant Liver Failure

When patients with fulminant liver failure are managed in large volume liver transplant centers, the transplant rate approaches 40–70%, but the median waiting time is 5 days, once being listed as a orthotopic liver transplantation candidate [38]. While waiting for a graft, the patient may deteriorate beyond a stage where transplantation is possible. When faced with a choice of using a marginal graft, which has a poor outcome in patients with fulminant liver failure, the option of a living donor liver transplantation, with a more optimal graft which will usually have a shorter cold ischemia time, seems better. The use of grafts from living donors is established practice in the treatment of fulminant liver failure in children in the USA, most European and far eastern centers [39]. Even though a timely procedure, for fulminant liver failure in children, the outcomes with living donor liver transplantation remain inferior to cadaveric orthotopic liver transplantation [40]. Transplantation of the right lobe of the liver from living adults is also being practiced with increased frequency although the procedure remains controversial [39].

A graft to recipient weight ratio more than 0.8% is optimal under elective conditions, when calculations for adequate liver volume are made. In the setting of fulminant liver failure, a value greater than 1% is usually required. This is easily obtained with a left lateral liver segment using an adult donor in a recipient child. It is near impossible to achieve the same with a left lateral segment for an adult recipient. This could result in a small for size graft and eventual graft loss. Living donor liver transplantation was successfully extended to adults with the introduction of the right lobe graft in 1996 [41]. The potential advantage of living donor liver transplantation in adults with fulminant liver failure is in the increased speed of availability of high quality organs. The ethical considerations are, however, more complex than those with pediatric transplantation where the graft is most frequently from a parent and utilizes a left lateral segment which carries a low risk for the donor. With living donor liver transplantation in adults, utilization of the right lobe entails donation of approximately 65% of liver volume which results in a higher risk for the donor. Complications in the donor include biliary complications that require intervention in 6%, reoperation in 4.5%, and death in 0.2% [39]. These are also more frequent in centers performing fewer living donor liver transplantation. Due to this it is unclear whether this technique will find a place where rapid procurement of cadaveric grafts is already possible [19].

▋ Liver Support Systems

Orthotopic liver transplantation is the only established treatment for fulminant liver failure with allied treatment involving supportive care focusing on bridging patients until either orthotopic liver transplantation or spontaneous recovery. Liver support systems include artificial and bioartificial systems. The role of artificial liver support encompasses removal of toxins (e.g., aromatic amino acids, and ammonia), synthesis of products (e.g., coagulation factors, albumin), and reversal of the inflammatory process in the liver [7]. The early support systems used hemodialysis, hemofiltration, and hemoperfusion. These systems were strictly artificial and directed against removal of water-soluble and protein bound toxins. Hemodialysis requires a semipermeable dialysis membrane through which fluid and small solutes pass via diffusion. Hemoperfusion removes toxins and low molecular weight molecules by using different absorbents (e.g., charcoal). The more recently developed artificial systems use hemodiasorption, which combines hemodialysis with absorption using charcoal or albumin. These systems include the BioLogic-DT®, and the molecular absorbent recirculating system known as MARS.

Biological components are now also included into these support systems. These bioartificial support systems utilize living hepatocytes housed within a bioreactor through which the patient's blood or plasma is pumped in an extracorporeal circuit. The hepatocytes may be human or xenogenic. Data from randomized trials, however, do not show a significant reduction of mortality with the use of support systems compared to standard medical therapy [7]. Patients with acute on chronic liver failure may however benefit from the use of artificial support systems, with the evidence related to bioartificial support systems being less conclusive. Reviews also indicate that both artificial and bioartificial systems are associated with several serious (e.g., bleeding, systemic infection, disseminated intravascular coagulation [DIC], allergic shock), and non-serious (e.g., minor bleeding, increased ICP, hypotension and hypersensitivity) adverse effects. Currently there are no published data to support the use of either biological or non-biological systems in the treatment of fulminant liver failure outside the setting of randomized controlled trials.

The use of hepatocyte transplantation has also been proposed for a supportive role in the management of fulminant liver failure. In this technique, human hepatocytes are infused into the splenic or hepatic portal vascular beds to provide adjuvant hepatic function for the failing liver. Isolated reports have shown the practicality of the technique but the clinical benefit is yet to be established.

▌ Conclusion

Despite a multidisciplinary approach and maximal supportive intensive care treatment, mortality of fulminant liver failure ranges between 40–80%. An etiological diagnosis when made early is of benefit and the geographical area in which the patient acquired the disease is also of importance. Improved medical and intensive care management over the last decade with more therapies targeting specific complications have been developed. Early prognostication remains a vital aspect of patient care. Orthotopic liver transplantation is the only treatment modality that radically alters the course of fulminant liver failure and there are measures to reduce waiting time for a donor liver once a patient with fulminant liver failure is listed for transplantation. These are the use of living donor liver transplantation and auxiliary segmental orthotopic liver transplantation. The use of auxiliary segmental orthotopic liver transplantation needs however to be reevaluated in light of early results. Published series on this modality of transplantation are small and the emergence of controlled clinical trials in this context are unlikely. There have been promising experiences with artificial and bioartificial liver assist devices, but these are yet to show impact on survival and remain as bridging measures for those patients who will eventually require orthotopic liver transplantation.

References

1. O'Grady JG, Schlam SW, Williams R (1991) Acute liver failure: redefining the syndrome. Lancet 342:273–275
2. Lee WM (2003) Acute liver failure in the United States. Semin Liver Dis 23:217–226
3. Adam R, Cailliez V, Majno P, et al (2000) Normalised intrincic mortality risk in liver transplantation: European liver transplant registry study. Lancet 356:621–627
4. Roberts MS, Angus DC, Bryce CL, Valenta Z, Weissfeld L (2004) Survival after liver transplantation in the United States: A disease-specific analysis of the UNOS database. Liver Transpl 10:886–897
5. Mirza DF, Mohamed R, Mutimer DJ, McMaster P (1995) Timing and candidacy for transplantation in acute liver failure: the European experience. Liver Transpl Surg 1:182–186
6. Dowling DJ, Mutimer DJ (1999) Artificial liver support in acute liver failure. Eur J Gastroenterol Hepatol 11:991–996
7. Lui JP, Gluud LL, Als-Nielsen B, Gluud C (2004) Artificial and bioartificial support systems for liver failure. Cochrane Database Syst Rev 1:CD003628
8. Kelly DA (2002) Managing liver failure. Postgrad Med J 78:660–667
9. Trey C, Davidson CS (1970) The management of fulminant hepatic failure. Prog Liver Dis 3:282–298
10. Mohamed R, Hubscher SG, Mirza DF, Gunson BK, Mutimer DJ (1997) Posttransplantation chronic hepatitis in fulminant hepatic failure. Hepatology 25:1003–1007
11. Williams R (1996) Classification, etiology, and considerations of outcome in acute liver failure. Semin Liver Dis 16:343–348
12. Acharya SK, Dasarathy S, Kumer TL, et al (1996) Fulminant hepatitis in a tropical population: clinical course, cause, and early predictors of outcome. Hepatology 23:1448–1455
13. Vaquero J, Blei AT (2003) Etiology and management of fulminant hepatic failure. Curr Gastroenterol Rep 5:39–47

14. Clemmesen JO, Larsen FS, Kondrup J, Hansen BA, Ott P (1999) Cerebral herniation in patients with acute liver failure is correlated with arterial ammonia concentration. Hepatology 29:648–653
15. Ellis AJ, Wendon JA, Williams R (2000) Subclinical seizure activity and prophylactic phenytoin infusion in acute liver failure: a controlled clinical trial. Hepatology 32:536–541
16. Jalan R, Olde Damink SW, Deutz NE, et al (2003) Moderate hypothermia prevents cerebral hyperemia and increase in intracranial pressure in patients undergoing liver transplantation for acute liver failure. Transplantation 75:2034–2039
17. Silva MA, Muralidharan V, Mirza DF (2004) The management of coagulopathy and blood loss in liver surgery. Semin Hematol 41:132–139
18. Gill RQ, Sterling RK (2001) Acute liver failure. J Clin Gastroenterol 33:191–198
19. Bernal W, Wendon J (2004) Liver transplantation in adults with acute liver failure. J Hepatol 40:192–197
20. Shakil AO, Kramer D, Mazariegos GV, Fung JJ, Rakela J (2000) Acute liver failure: clinical features, outcome analysis, and applicability of prognostic criteria. Liver Transpl 6:163–169
21. Anand AC, Nightingale P, Neuberger JM (1997) Early indicators of prognosis in fulminant hepatic failure: an assessment of the King's criteria. J Hepatol 26:62–68
22. Pereira LM, Langley PG, Hayllar KM, Tredger JM, Williams R (1992) Coagulation factor V and VIII/V ratio as predictors of outcome in paracetamol induced fulminant hepatic failure: relation to other prognostic indicators. Gut 33:98–102
23. Lee WM, Galbraith RM, Watt GH, et al (1995) Predicting survival in fulminant hepatic failure using serum Gc protein concentrations. Hepatology 21:101–105
24. Harrison PM, O'Grady JG, Keays RT, Alexander GJ, Williams R (1990) Serial prothrombin time as prognostic indicator in paracetamol induced fulminant hepatic failure. BMJ 301: 964–966
25. Saibara T, Onishi S, Sone J, et al (1991) Arterial ketone body ratio as a possible indicator for liver transplantation in fulminant hepatic failure. Transplantation 51:782–786
26. Shakil AO, Jones BC, Lee RG, et al (2000) Prognostic value of abdominal CT scanning and hepatic histopathology in patients with acute liver failure. Dig Dis Sci 45:334–339
27. Donaldson BW, Gopinath R, Wanless IR, et al (1993) The role of transjugular liver biopsy in fulminant liver failure: relation to other prognostic indicators. Hepatology 18:1370–1376
28. Bernal W, Donaldson N, Wyncoll D, Wendon J (2002) Blood lactate as an early predictor of outcome in paracetamol-induced acute liver failure: a cohort study. Lancet 359:558–563
29. Schmidt LE, Dalhoff K (2002) Serum phosphate is an early predictor of outcome in severe acetaminophen-induced hepatotoxicity. Hepatology 36:659–665
30. Ng KL, Davidson JS, Bathgate AJ (2004) Serum phosphate is not a reliable early predictor of outcome in paracetamol induced hepatotoxicity. Liver Transpl 10:158–159
31. Bhaduri BR, Mieli-Vergani G (1996) Fulminant hepatic failure: pediatric factors. Semin Liver Dis 16:349–355
32. Devlin J, Wendon J, Heaton N, Tan KC, Williams R (1995) Pretransplantation clinical status and outcome of emergency transplantation for acute liver failure. Hepatology 21:1018–1024
33. Bernal W, Wendon J, Rela M, Heaton N, Williams R (1998) Use and outcome of liver transplantation in acetaminophen-induced acute liver failure. Hepatology 27:1050–1055
34. Boudjema K, Bachellier P, Wolf P, Tempe JD, Jaeck D (2002) Auxiliary liver transplantation and bioartificial bridging procedures in treatment of acute liver failure. World J Surg 26:264–274
35. van Hoek B, de Boer J, Boudjema K (1999) Auxillary versus orthotopic liver transplantation for acute liver failure. J Hepatol 30:699–705
36. Azoulay D, Samuel D, Ichai P, et al (2001) Auxiliary partial orthotopic versus standard orthotopic whole liver transplantation for acute liver failure: a reappraisal from a single center by a case-control study. Ann Surg 234:723–731
37. Muiesan P, Girlanda R, Baker A, Rela M, Heaton N (2003) Successful segmental auxiliary liver transplantation from a non-heart-beating donor: implications for split-liver transplantation. Transplantation 75:1443–1445
38. Liu CL, Fan ST, Lo CM, Yong BH, Fung AS, Wong J (2002) Right-lobe live donor liver transplantation improves survival of patients with acute liver failure. Br J Surg 89:317–322

39. Brown RS Jr, Russo MW, Lai M, et al (2003) A survey of liver transplantation from living adult donors in the United States. N Engl J Med 348:818–825
40. Liu CL, Fan ST, Lo CM, et al (2003) Live donor liver transplantation for fulminant hepatic failure in children. Liver Transpl 9:1185–1190
41. Lo CM, Fan ST, Liu CL, et al (1997) Adult-to-adult living donor liver transplantation using extended right lobe grafts. Ann Surg 226:261–269

Sedation

Sedation Strategies in the Critically Ill

S. Mehta

▌ Introduction

Patients in the intensive care unit (ICU) often require life-saving treatments such as mechanical ventilation and dialysis, and devices such as central venous catheters. To aid the healing process, facilitate use of life support technology, and relieve anxiety and pain, sedative drugs are commonly administered. Evidence is now emerging that how much sedation we give, and when and how we stop it, are very important in determining patient outcome. Two recent randomized trials have started to lay the scientific foundation for this important therapy: a trial evaluating a nurse-driven sedation protocol [1], and an article in the *New England Journal of Medicine* on daily sedation cessation [2]. The importance of this topic is further highlighted by an executive report of practice variables for intravenous sedation by a multidisciplinary task force from the Society of Critical Care Medicine (SCCM) [3]. Because of the frequent use of sedative medications, the methods of administration available to the clinician, as well as their impact on outcome, this is an important area of research in the ICU.

▌ Risks of Under- and Over-sedation (Table 1)

Both inadequate and excessive sedation may have deleterious effects on the critically ill patient. Undertreated pain results in physiologic responses (hypercoagulability, immunosuppression, persistent catabolism) that are associated with poor outcomes [4]. Pain increases sympathetic activity and catecholamine release, placing additional demands on the cardiovascular system in the critically ill. Prolonged pain can result in severe anxiety and even delirium. Anxiety or agitation associated with insufficient sedation may increase the risk of adverse events such as self-extubation, loss of venous catheters, and self-injury or injury to clinicians. Finally, inadequate sedation may leave patients with traumatic memories of the ICU.

On the other hand, excessive sedation can also lead to complications, including respiratory depression, hypotension, bradycardia, ileus, and venous thromboembolism. Excessive sedation can make evaluation of a patient's neurological status difficult, and may prevent recognition of acute neurologic events. Observational studies have identified sedation as an independent risk factor for ventilator associated pneumonia (VAP) [5]. Delayed recovery related to over-sedation may prolong the duration of mechanical ventilation, as well as ICU and hospital stay, and may increase hospital costs. Finally, over-sedation may also have long-term emotional

Table 1. The delicate balance between under-sedation and over-sedation

Potential dangers of under-sedation
▍ Agitation
▍ Sleep deprivation
▍ Myocardial ischemia
▍ Ventilator asynchrony
▍ Self-extubation
▍ Post-traumatic stress disorder

Potential dangers of over-sedation
▍ Respiratory depression, hypotension, ileus
▍ Prolonged alteration in consciousness
▍ Increased duration of mechanical ventilation
▍ Increased duration of ICU and hospital stay
▍ Increased medication costs

effects, as one study has suggested that an inability to recall experiences during a critical illness leads to psychological distress after recovery [6].

▍ Choice of Sedative and Analgesic Agents

Guidelines for intravenous (i.v.) sedation produced by a multidisciplinary task force from the SCCM have been published recently [3]. These guidelines include recommendations regarding the preferred agents for analgesia and sedation in the ICU. Benzodiazepines are the preferred agents for anxiolysis and relief of agitation, and morphine is the preferred analgesic, with fentanyl as an alternative for patients with hemodynamic instability or morphine allergy. However, these guidelines are based on contradictory results from very few randomized trials in diverse ICU populations. The paucity of data available on the choice of sedatives in the ICU was highlighted in a systematic review by Ostermann and coworkers [7], who found that only a minority of sedative agents used in the ICU have been evaluated rigorously by more than 1 or 2 randomized controlled trials, and most of these trials were not double-blinded.

The report recommends midazolam and propofol as the preferred agents for short-term sedation (< 24 h) and lorazepam for long-term sedation (> 24 hr) [3]. However, published studies are controversial, and many do not support these recommendations. McCollam and coworkers compared the safety, efficacy, and cost of infusions of lorazepam, midazolam, and propofol in critically ill patients, and found that although lorazepam was the most cost-effective, over-sedation occurred more commonly with lorazepam than with the other two agents [8]. They concluded that midazolam is the most titratable drug, avoiding both over-sedation and undersedation. Similar results were observed in a study which used sophisticated modeling techniques to compare the pharmacokinetics and pharmacodynamics of lorazepam and midazolam administered as continuous infusions [9]. These investigators found significant delays in emergence from sedation with lorazepam as compared with midazolam.

Even when guidelines based on reputable evidence are available, it is clear that wide variation in clinical practice exists [10]. Surveys of sedation and analgesic administration in North American and British ICUs reveal widely varying practice patterns with regard to type of medications, route of administration (intermittent versus continuous), and sedation monitoring [11–15].

Continuous Infusions versus Bolus Administration

Because intermittent bolus injection of sedatives results in peaks and troughs of effect, as well as potential periods of anxiety and agitation, many intensivists believe that continuous infusion of sedatives produces more predictable and reliable anxiolysis, maximizing the therapeutic benefit and minimizing side effects [16]. Conversely, time to awakening after discontinuation of sedative infusions can occasionally be delayed for greater than 24 h [16], presumably due to drug accumulation. In addition, one retrospective study found a correlation between the use of continuous sedative infusions and prolonged duration of mechanical ventilation, as well as ICU stay, even when adjusting for age and severity of illness [17]. However, given the retrospective design, it is difficult to make any conclusions regarding causality.

There are no randomized trials comparing continuous versus intermittent administration of sedatives to ICU patients. In practice, continuous infusions are very frequently used, as revealed in US [12, 14], British [18] and Danish [13] surveys, for the following reasons. First, many patients have difficulty communicating their sedative/analgesic requirements because of the presence of an endotracheal tube or an altered level of consciousness. Second, the maintenance of an adequate, continuous, opioid blood concentration improves patients' analgesia [19]. Finally, there is increasing evidence that the continuous administration of opioid decreases morbidity [20], and may decrease mortality [21], compared with intermittent administration.

Sedation Scoring Systems

There are currently no guidelines available for assessing the adequacy of analgesia or sedation [3]. Whereas there are validated methods for the subjective scoring of pain (linear or visual analog scale), a standard scoring system for sedation has been difficult to develop and implement [22]. In a study evaluating factors affecting ICU nurses' delivery of sedatives, Weinert and coworkers found that conflicts arose between physicians and nurses when explicit and shared goals of sedation were lacking [23]. One way of encouraging a more uniform approach to sedation would be to agree on a common terminology for describing patients' depth of sedation.

Assessing the degree of sedation can be difficult in mechanically ventilated patients, with whom communication is invariably limited. The use of sedation scales is the most frequently used method of quantifying the sedative effect. More than 25 sedation instruments have been described, yet none is universally accepted. A systematic review elegantly highlighted the need for more information regarding the measurement properties of sedation scales [24]. Of the published sedation scales, six developed in adult ICU patients [25–30] have been tested for reliability and validity, and only three of these have been tested for responsiveness, defined as the ability to detect change in sedation status over time [28–30]. Nevertheless, what appears to be important is not so much the precise scale used, as the routine incorporation of a measurement tool into sedation practice.

The use of sedation scales reduces the risk of over- and under-sedation. However, over-sedation is more difficult to detect. An under-sedated patient shows signs of agitation and distress, whereas an over-sedated patient may look comfortable. In addition, deeply sedated patients are less demanding in terms of physical management and emotional needs. Perhaps most disturbing is the observation in some hospitals that the intensity of sedation varies inversely with the number of nurses on a shift, suggesting that 'compliant' patients permit understaffing of ICUs [31]. Recognition of over-sedation with a sedation scale should trigger a reduction in drug dose. Indeed, Detriche et al. found that the number of patients who were excessively sedated was significantly reduced with the introduction of a simple 5-point sedation scale [32]. A Norwegian quality improvement observational study found that implementation of a locally developed sedation protocol and the Motor Activity Assessment scale [27] led to reductions in total duration of mechanical ventilation and length of stay [33].

Despite the availability of easy-to-use sedation scales, their use is not widespread. A British survey found that 67% of adult ICUs employ scoring systems [11], while a Danish survey found that only 16% of respondents use a sedation scale [13]. In a US survey, 78% of intensivists "monitor sedative use" [14], but 43% use the Glasgow coma score, which is not technically a sedation scoring system. In a recent Canadian survey [15], 49% of intensivists report using a sedation scale, and the majority employ the Ramsay scale [25].

▌ The Use of Sedation Protocols

The use of detailed protocols to manage clinical problems is becoming more common in the ICU [10]. Protocols are currently being used to manage mechanical ventilation, ventilator weaning, and antibiotic decision making. Protocols promote a multi-disciplinary approach to patient care, and enhance efficiency by making the clinical plan explicit to all care providers. Nurses, therapists and physicians thereby achieve a level of uniformity of approach and goals for the patient, reducing within-patient variability of decision-making. In addition, protocols enhance efficiency by allowing non-physician care providers to proceed with clinical decision-making without the need for continuous physician input. In this regard, protocolized weaning from mechanical ventilation directed by nurses and respiratory therapists has been shown to lead to more rapid extubation than physician-directed weaning, as well as significant cost savings [34].

Sedation protocols are algorithms by which nurses adjust sedative and analgesic doses based upon written guidelines and assessment of the patient's level of sedation. Use of sedation protocols has been shown to decrease the duration of mechanical ventilation, promote the judicious use of therapeutic agents, reduce variability in prescribing, and decrease sedative costs in critically ill patients [1, 35–38].

Brook and coworkers performed a randomized trial comparing a nursing-implemented sedation protocol with usual sedation care in 322 adults requiring mechanical ventilation [1]. Patients assigned to the intervention group were managed using a protocol in which nurses titrated the sedative/analgesic agents according to the patient's level of sedation as measured by the Ramsay scale [25]. According to the protocol the patient's sedation level was assessed every 4 h, and the infusion rate was turned down if the level was adequate, or increased if it was inadequate. In the control group all decisions regarding sedation were made by the ICU team. The primary outcome was the duration of mechanical ventilation, and secondary outcomes included ICU and hospital length of stay, and tracheostomy rate. The investigators controlled for important co-interventions with the use of a weaning protocol in all patients. They found that the use of a sedation protocol reduced the duration of ventilation by 1.5 days (p = 0.003) compared with the usual care group. They also demonstrated a reduction in ICU stay (5.7 vs 6.5 days, p = 0.013) and hospital stay (14.0 vs 19.9 days, p < 0.001), and a lower tracheostomy rate in the intervention group. This study was generally methodologically sound, but there are several limitations, which should be addressed in future studies. Recognizing that blinding is very difficult with this type of study, the lack of blinding may have resulted in bias favoring the treatment group. The performance of this study in a single center with previous experience in sedation research raises the issue of generalizability. Additionally this study enrolled only medical ICU patients, and thus the applicability of this protocol to surgical patients is unknown.

Despite compelling evidence that use of sedation protocols improves outcome and reduces costs, only a minority of ICUs have adopted their use. A multicenter survey of critical care pharmacists found that sedation, pain or paralytic protocols were used in only 26% of respondents' practices, and health professional-generated pain/sedation scores were used to assess dosing needs in only 25% of the practices [39]. In a recent survey of Canadian intensivists, 29% responded that they employ a sedation protocol [15].

In summary, guidelines that minimize unnecessary variability in practice, prevent excessive medication, and emphasize individual patient management improve the effective utilization of sedatives and analgesics. Use of standardized protocols may also increase clinician satisfaction. The potential impact of guidelines/protocol on nursing satisfaction was highlighted by a survey that we recently completed [40]. We surveyed ICU nurses at three Canadian University Hospitals regarding their satisfaction with current sedation and analgesia practice. Only 51% were satisfied with current practice, and cited physician inconsistency in choice of sedatives and dosing as the major reason for their dissatisfaction. Almost all respondents thought a nursing-directed sedation protocol combined with a sedation/agitation scoring system would be valuable to patient care (91%), by reducing inconsistency in practice, and allowing individualized dosing based on the nursing assessment. Finally, 94% of respondents reported that a protocol would enhance professional nursing practice, by providing greater autonomy, promoting consistency between nurses, and serving as a valuable communication and assessment tool.

▌ Daily Interruption of Sedative Infusions

Daily interruption of sedative infusions, allowing patients to awaken daily, has recently been shown to have notable advantages [2]. Kress et al. performed a randomized trial that enrolled 128 ventilated patients who were receiving continuous i. v. sedation. Patients randomized to the intervention group had their sedative infusion interrupted on a daily basis. During the interruption, patients were observed closely by a research nurse who contacted a study physician when the patient awakened or became agitated. The physician then decided whether or not to resume the sedative infusion, and if so, it was restarted at half the previous rate and re-titrated to achieve sedation at a Ramsay score of 3–4 [25]. The control group was managed by the ICU team in a usual care fashion. A sedation protocol was not used in either group.

With their simple intervention, the authors demonstrated a significant reduction in the duration of mechanical ventilation in the treatment group (median 4.9 vs 7.3 days, p=0.004) and an accompanying decrease in lengths of stay in ICU (6.4 vs 9.9 days, p=0.02) and in hospital (13.3 vs 16.9, p=0.19). In addition, fewer patients in the intervention group required neurological diagnostic testing to assess changes in mental status. In summary, daily interruption of sedative infusions allows more informative evaluation of a patient's neurological status, is helpful to determine whether the current targeted level of sedation is still necessary or if less sedative medication is adequate, and reduces the likelihood of over-sedation with delayed recovery.

The main concern with the internal validity of this trial relates to the undisclosed cointerventions, which have a powerful impact on outcome. For example, a standardized ventilator weaning protocol was not used (which we know can shorten the duration of ventilation), and no details regarding the methods of weaning are provided (which also influence the duration of the weaning period and the ultimate success of weaning). These factors, in addition to the lack of blinding, raise the possibility that bias may have been introduced if the intervention group was weaned from the ventilator more aggressively than the control group. Another issue weakening the inferences from this trial is generalizability, as the study enrolled only medical patients in a single ICU. The applicability of these results to surgical patients and the translation of this benefit to other ICUs is unclear. In addition, while the intervention in this trial may be technically easier to reproduce than the sedation protocol used in the Brook study [1], it is also significantly more demanding in terms of human resources. A dedicated nurse who observed the patient for signs of awakening or agitation was present whenever the infusions were stopped in the intervention group. The safety and efficacy of this protocol in the average ICU where many other demands are placed upon nurses' time are unknown.

Two subsequent publications from the same study identified other benefits of daily sedative interruption. One reported that daily sedative interruption did not result in adverse psychological outcomes, reduced symptoms of posttraumatic stress disorder, and may be associated with reduced posttraumatic stress disorder [41]. The other publication reported that daily sedative interruption was associated with reductions in the incidence of six common ICU complications: VAP, bacteremia, barotrauma, venous thromboembolic disease, cholestasis, and sinusitis [42].

▌ Delirium in ICU Patients

Delirium in the ICU is common, with an estimated incidence of 20%. Delirium in critically ill patients is of particular concern to the intensivist because of its associated morbidity [43]. In one study, delirium was associated with an increased incidence of self-extubation and removal of catheters, and opiate use was identified as a risk factor for its development [43]. Ely and coworkers found that the occurrence of delirium was an independent predictor of higher 6-month mortality and longer hospital stay, and was associated with a higher incidence of cognitive impairment at hospital discharge [44].

The SCCM guidelines recommend routine assessment for the presence of delirium in ICU patients [3]. However, in the ICU population, the frequent inability to conduct an interview makes diagnosis of delirium difficult, and until recently, there was no easily applicable assessment tool for delirium. There are now two scales designed specifically to assess delirium in the ICU population. Bergeron and colleagues developed and evaluated a screening checklist of eight items based on DSM criteria and features of delirium [45]. The sensitivity and specificity of this checklist for the diagnosis of delirium in ICU patients were 99 and 64%, respectively. The screening checklist can be applied by a clinician in under 5 minutes. The CAM-ICU is another delirium assessment tool which demonstrates excellent reliability and validity in this population [46]. It is clear that delirium can have a great impact on important patient outcomes, thus routine screening may provide valuable information. In addition, once delirium in diagnosed in the ICU, the optimal treatment, whether it be pharmacologic or non-pharmacologic, is not known.

The Impact of Sedation Strategies on Health-related Quality of Life

Whereas in the past, intensivists may have tried to achieve a deeply sedated, unresponsive state, clinician preferences are moving toward caring for sleepy patients who are easily awakened, and who are pain and anxiety-free. To add to the drawbacks of deep sedation mentioned above, one study has suggested that an inability to recall experiences during a critical illness leads to psychological distress after recovery [6]. However, the psychological ramifications of keeping patients lightly sedated are not known, and need to be determined in future studies.

Patients surviving their ICU stay often have reduced health-related quality of life and post-traumatic stress disorder (PTSD) [47], especially if acute lung injury was present [48]. However, there is very limited information available regarding the impact of sedation on health-related quality-of-life outcomes. In this regard, Nelson et al. observed a significant correlation between the number of days of sedative administration in the ICU, and both depressive symptoms and PTSD at follow-up [49]. However, because of the small sample size and retrospective design of the study, they were unable to draw any conclusions about causality.

Conclusion

It is clear that the manner in which sedatives are used in the ICU is important, in terms of meaningful clinical and cost-related outcomes such as duration of mechanical ventilation and lengths of hospital and ICU stay. The management of sedation in critically ill patients may be equally or more important than the choice of which sedative drug to use. Because there is no risk-free sedative medication, recent efforts to improve outcomes for patients in the ICU have shifted toward investigations of the manner in which sedatives are administered.

Many important questions regarding sedation in the ICU remain unanswered. It is clear that intensivists need better methods of ensuring that the lowest effective doses of the most appropriated sedative, analgesic, and tranquilizing drugs are given for the shortest time to critically ill patients receiving mechanical ventilation.

References

1. Brook AD, Ahrens TS, Schaiff R, et al (1999) Effect of a nursing-implemented sedation protocol on the duration of mechanical ventilation. Crit Care Med 27:2609–2615
2. Kress JP, Pohlman AS, O'Connor MF, et al (2000) Daily interruption of sedative infusions in critically ill patients undergoing mechanical ventilation. N Engl J Med 342:1471–1477
3. Sedation and Analgesia Task Force of the American College of Critical Care Medicine (ACCM) of the Society of Critical Care Medicine (2002) Clinical practice guidelines for the sustained use of sedatives and analgesics in the critically ill adult. Crit Care Med 30:119–141
4. Lewis K, Whipple J, Michael K, Quebbeman EJ (1994) Effect of analgesic treatment on the physiological consequences of acute pain. Am J Hosp Pharm 51:1539–1554
5. Rello J, Diaz E, Roque M, et al (1999) Risk factors for developing pneumonia within 48 h of intubation. Am J Respir Crit Care Med 159:1742–1746
6. Griffiths RD, Jones C (2001) Filling the intensive care memory gap? Intensive Care Med 27:344–346
7. Ostermann ME, Keenan SP, Seiferling RA, Sibbald WJ (2000) Sedation in the intensive care unit. A systematic review. JAMA 283:1451–1459
8. McCollam JS, O'Neil MG, Norcross D, Byrne TK, Reeves ST (1999) Continuous infusion of lorazepam, midazolam, and propofol for sedation of the critically ill surgery trauma patient: a prospective randomized comparison. Crit Care Med 27:2454–2458
9. Barr J, Zomorodi K, Bertaccini EJ, Shafer SL (2001) A double-blind, randomized comparison of IV lorazepam versus IV midazolam for sedation of ICU patients via a pharmacologic model. Anesthesiology 95:286–298
10. Morris AH (2000) Developing and implementing computerized protocols for standardization of clinical decisions. Ann Intern Med 132:373–383
11. Murdoch S, Cohen A (2000) Intensive care sedation: a review of current British practice. Intensive Care Med 26:922–928
12. Hansen-Flaschen JH, Brazinsky S, Basile C, Lanken PN (1991) Use of sedating drugs and neuromuscular blocking agents in patients requiring mechanical ventilation for respiratory failure. JAMA 266:2870–2875
13. Christensen BV, Thunedborg LP (1999) Use of sedatives, analgesics and neuromuscular blocking agents in Danish ICUs 1996/97. Intensive Care Med 25:186–191
14. Rhoney DH, Murry KR (2003) National survey of the use of sedating drugs, neuromuscular blocking agents, and reversal agents in the intensive care unit. J Intensive Care Med 18:139–145
15. Mehta S, Burry L, Martinez C, et al (2003) A comprehensive survey of Canadian physicians regarding the use of sedatives and analgesics in mechanically ventilated adults in the ICU. Am J Respir Crit Care Med 167:A909 (abst)
16. Pohlman A, Simpson K, Hall J (1994) Continuous intravenous infusions of lorazepam versus midazolam for sedation during mechanical ventilatory support: a prospective, randomized study. Crit Care Med 22:1241–1247
17. Kollef M, Levy N, Ahrens TS, Schaiff R, Prentice D, Sherman G (1998) The use of continuous IV sedation is associated with prolongation of mechanical ventilation. Chest 114:541–548
18. Bion JF, Ledingham IM (1987) Sedation in intensive care: a postal survey. Intensive Care Med 13:215–216
19. Bennett RL, Batenhorst RL, Bivins BA, et al (1982) Patient-controlled analgesia. A new concept of postoperative pain relief. Ann Surg 195:700–705
20. Mangano DT, Siliciano D, Hollenberg M, et al (1992) The Study of Perioperative Ischemia (SPI) Research Group. Postoperative myocardial ischemia. Therapeutic trials using intensive analgesia following surgery. Anesthesiology 76:342–353

21. Anand KJS, Phil D, Hickey PR (1992) Halothane-morphine compared with high-dose sufentanil for anesthesia and postoperative analgesia in neonatal cardiac surgery. N Engl J Med 326:1–9

22. Young C, Knudsen N, Hilton A, Reves JG (2000) Sedation in the intensive care unit. Crit Care Med 28:854–866

23. Weinert CR, Chlan L, Gross C (2001) Sedating critically ill patients: factors affecting nurses' delivery of sedative therapy. Am J Crit Care 10:156–165

24. De Jonghe B, Cook D, Appere-De-Vecchi C, Guyatt G, Meade M, Outin H (2000) Using and understanding sedation scoring systems. Intensive Care Med 26:275–285

25. Ramsay MA, Savege TM, Simpson BR, Goodwin R (1974) Controlled sedation with alphaxalone-alphadolone. BMJ 2:656–659

26. Riker RR, Fraser GL, Cox PM (1994) Continuous infusion of haloperidol controls agitation in critically ill patients. Crit Care Med 22:433–440

27. Devlin JW, Boleski G, Mlynarek M (1999) Motor Activity Assessment Scale: a valid and reliable sedation scale for use with mechanically ventilated patients in an adult surgical intensive care unit. Crit Care Med 27:1271–1275

28. De Lemos J, Tweeddale M, Chittock D, for the Sedation Focus Group (2000) Measuring quality of sedation in adult mechanically ventilated critically ill patients: the Vancouver Interaction and Calmness Scale. J Clin Epidemiology 53:908–919

29. Ely EW, Truman B, Shintani A, et al (2003) Monitoring sedation status over time in ICU patients. Reliability and validity of the Richmond Agitation-Sedation Scale (RASS). JAMA 289:2983–2991

30. De Jonghe B, Cook D, Griffith L (2003) Adaptation to the intensive care environment (ATICE): Development and validation of a new sedation assessment instrument. Crit Care Med 2344–2354

31. Shelly MP (1992) Intensive care sedation: progress towards decreasing mortality rate. Br J Intensive Care 4:323–332

32. Detriche O, Berre J, Massaut J, Vincent J-L (1999) The Brussels sedation scale: use of a simple clinical sedation scale can avoid excessive sedation in patients undergoing mechanical ventilation in the intensive care unit. Br J Anaesth 83:698–701

33. Brattebo G, Hofoss D, Flaatten H, Muri AK, Gjerde, Plsek PE (2002) Effect of a scoring system and protocol for sedation on the duration of patients' need for ventilator support in a surgical intensive care unit. BMJ 324:1386–1389

34. Kollef MH, Shapiro SD, Silver P, et al. (1997) A randomized, controlled trial of protocol-directed versus physician-directed weaning from mechanical ventilation. Crit Care Med 25:567–574

35. Watling SM, Johnson M, Yanos J (1996) A method to produce sedation in critically ill patients. Ann Pharmacother 30:1227–1231

36. MacLaren R, Plamondon JM, Ramsay KB, Rocker GM, Patrick WD, Hall RI (2000) A prospective evaluation of empiric versus protocol-base sedation and analgesia. Pharmacotherapy 20:662–672

37. Devlin JW, Holbrook AM, Fuller HD (1997) The effect of ICU sedation guidelines and pharmacist interventions on clinical outcomes and drug cost. Ann Pharmacother 31:689–695

38. Saich C, Manji M, Dyer I, Rosser D (1999) Effect of introducing sedation guidelines on sedative costs per bed day. Br J Anaesth 82:792–793

39. Watling SM, Dasta JF, Seidl EC (1997) Sedatives, analgesics, and paralytics in the ICU. Ann Pharmacother 31:148–153

40. Burry L, Hynes-Gay P, Cook D, Meade M, Gibson J, Mehta S (2003) A survey of ICU nurses regarding the use of sedatives and analgesics in mechanically ventilated adults. Am J Respir Crit Care Med 167:A659 (abst)

41. Kress JP, Gehlbach B, Lacy M, Pliskin N, Pahlman AS, Hall JB (2003) The long-term psychological effects of daily sedative interruption on critically ill patients. Am J Respir Crit Care Med 168:1457–1461

42. Schweickert WD, Gehlbach BK, Pohlman AS, Hall JB, Kress JP (2004) Daily interruption of sedative infusions and complications of critical illness in mechanically ventilated patients. Crit Care Med 32:1272–1276

43. Dubois M-J, Bergeron N, Dumont M, Dial S, Skrobik Y (2001) Delirium in an intensive care unit: a study of risk factors. Intensive Care Med 27:1297–1304
44. Ely EW, Shintani A, Truman B (2004) Delirium as a predictor of mortality in mechanically ventilated patients in the intensive care unit. JAMA 291:1753–1762
45. Bergeron N, Dubois M-J, Dumont M, Dial S, Skrobik Y (2001) Intensive care delirium screening checklist: evaluation of a new screening tool. Intensive Care Med 27:859–864
46. Ely EW, Inouye SK, Bernard GR, et al (2001) Delirium in mechanically ventilated patients. Validity and reliability of the confusion assessment method for the intensive care unit (CAM-ICU). JAMA 286:2703–2710
47. Davidson TA, Caldwell ES, Curtis JR, Hudson LD, Steinberg KP (1999) Reduced quality of life in survivors of acute respiratory distress syndrome compared with critically ill control patients. JAMA 281:354–360
48. Schelling G, Stoll C, Haller M, et al (1998) Health-related quality of life and posttraumatic stress disorder in survivors of the acute respiratory distress syndrome. Crit Care Med 26:651–659
49. Nelson BJ, Weinert CR, Bury CL, et al (2000) ICU drug use and subsequent quality of life in acute lung injury patients. Crit Care Med 28:3626–3630

Delirium in the Intensive Care Unit

E. W. Ely

▌ Introduction

Historically, two words were used to describe confused patients. One was the Roman word 'delirium', which referred to an agitated and confused person (think of hyperactive delirium). The other was from the Greek word 'lethargus', which was used to describe a quietly confused person (think of hypoactive delirium). Intensive care unit (ICU) patients commonly demonstrate both of these motoric subtypes as they progress through different stages of their illness and therapy. In either case, the patient's brain is not functioning normally. It therefore makes sense that the original derivation of delirium comes from the Latin word *deliria*, which literally means to 'be out of your furrow'. For greater clarity and to avoid misuse of terms such as dementia and delirium, basic definitions of some commonly referred to cognitive syndromes are shown in Table 1.

Table 1. Highlights regarding cognitive syndromes. From [66] with permission

▌ **Confusion:** A characteristic occurring in delirium resulting in an altered state of consciousness, and characterized by deficits in attention, memory, visuconstructional ability, and executive functions (also defined as reduced mental clarity, coherence, comprehension, and reasoning). *Think*: disturbed orientation with respect to person, place, and time.

▌ **Delirium:** A disturbance of consciousness characterized by an *acute* onset and fluctuating course of impaired cognitive functioning, so that a patient's ability to receive, process, store, and recall information is strikingly impaired. Delirium develops over a short period of time (hours to days), is usually reversible, and is a direct consequence of a medical condition, substance intoxication or withdrawal, use of a medication, toxin exposure, or a combination of these factors. *Think*: rapid onset, clouded consciousness (bewildered/confused), often worse at night, fluctuating.

▌ **Dementia:** Development of a state of generalized cognitive deficits in which there is a deterioration of previously acquired intellectual abilities usually developing over weeks and months. The deficits include memory impairment and at least one of the following: aphasia, apraxia, agnosia, or a disturbance in executive functioning. The cognitive deficits must be sufficiently severe to cause impairment in occupational or social functioning, and they may be progressive, static, or reversible depending on the pathology and the availability of effective treatment. *Think*: gradual onset, intelectual impairment, memory disturbance, personality/mood change, no clouding of consciousness.

▌ **Psychosis:** A major mental disorder characterized by hallucinations, delusions, or the inability to tinguish reality from fantasy, which lead to an inability to maintain interpersonal relations and t compromised daily functioning. *Think*: hallucinations/delusions, impaired reality testing, inappropr mood and impulse control, no clouding of consciousness.

In the ICU we aggressively monitor many organ systems for the development of dysfunction or failure. For example, we use pulse oximetry and blood gases to monitor for pulmonary dysfunction, blood pressure and electrocardiography to monitor for cardiac dysfunction, and urine output and serum creatinine to monitor for renal dysfunction. Health care professionals in the ICU have traditionally used inadequate monitoring devices to detect dysfunction in arguably the most important organ of all – the brain. Delirium, acute central nervous system (CNS) dysfunction resulting from any number of common insults that ICU patients experience, has largely been overlooked in critical care research until the past few years. Recent discussions of encephalopathy and organ dysfunction secondary to sepsis fail to mention delirium as one of the clinical manifestations of CNS dysfunction [1, 2].

The ICU literature often refers to delirium as 'ICU psychosis' [3, 4], which represents a potentially dangerous misnomer. The development of delirium often goes unnoticed in the ICU because we think of it as 'part of the scenery', or an expected and inconsequential outcome of mechanical ventilation and other therapies necessary to save lives in the ICU. A series of investigations has recently been conducted that provided validated means of detecting delirium by non-psychiatrists (e.g., internists, nurses, or respiratory therapists). The CNS monitoring instruments and observations from these investigations are leading to a change of culture and practice in the ICU whereby we more closely follow patients for the development of delirium and modify their care to help prevent this potentially disastrous complication. Indeed, the most recent clinical practice guidelines of the Society of Critical Care Medicine (SCCM) [5] have recommended routine (daily) monitoring of delirium in all mechanically ventilated patients, which will be discussed later in this chapter.

▌ Pathophysiology and Etiology of Delirium

Delirium is thought to be related to imbalances in the synthesis, release, and inactivation of neurotransmitters modulating the control of cognitive function, behavior, and mood [6, 7]. Three of the neurotransmitter systems involved in the pathophysiology of delirium are dopamine, gama-aminobutyric acid (GABA), and acetylcholine [8, 9]. While dopamine increases excitability of neurons, GABA and acetylcholine decrease neuronal excitability [8]. An imbalance of one or multiple of these neurotransmitters results in neuronal instability and unpredictable neurotransmission. In general, an excess of dopamine and depletion of acetylcholine are two major physiological problems felt to be central to delirium. In addition to these neurotransmitter systems, others are thought to be involved in the development of delirium such as serotonin imbalance, endorphin hyperfunction, and increased central noradrenergic activity [7, 9].

A number of causal factors lead to neurotransmitter imbalance including reduction in cerebral metabolism, primary intracranial disease, systemic diseases, secondary infection of the brain, exogenous toxic agents, withdrawal from substances of abuse such as alcohol or sedative-hypnotics agents, hypoxemia, metabolic disturbances, and the administration of psychoactive medications such as benzodiazepines and narcotics [10]. Since the cerebral concentrations of these neurotransmitters are sensitive to many organic and biochemical changes, many things can result in their imbalance [9, 10]. Cognitive neuroscience and psychopharmacology are active areas of research, which will hopefully yield advances in our understanding and treatment of delirium.

▌ 'Confusion' Regarding Delirium Terminology

There are over 25 terms in the literature used to refer to delirium such as 'subacute befuddlement' and 'toxic confusional state'. Others simply refer to delirium as confusion or neurological impairment. The neurology literature tends to use the term 'delirium' exclusively to refer to the hyperactive subtype [11], while referring to hypoactive delirium as encephalopathy. These subtypes are discussed in the next section of this chapter. As mentioned above, 'ICU psychosis' is a potentially dangerous misnomer that refers to delirious patients who are demonstrating increased psychomotor activity and hallucinations (i.e., hyperactive delirium) [12].

▌ The Occurrence of Delirium in the ICU and its Subtypes

The prevalence of delirium in ICU cohort studies has been reported as 20 [13], 70 [14], or 80% [15] depending upon the characteristics of the patient population and the instrument used. Its incidence is likely to increase in future years as older persons more frequently receive ICU care. Two major developments that are frequently linked during an older person's ICU course are the need for mechanical ventilation and the development of profound and possibly persistent cognitive impairment [16]. Almost every patient in the ICU receives either narcotics or benzodiazepines at some point during their stay, yet physicians rarely modify the quantity or dosing intervals of these drugs based on patient age. Patients on mechanical ventilation are frequently sedated to the point of stupor or coma in order to improve oxygenation, alleviate agitation, and to prevent them from removing support devices. However, age is only rarely factored into complex decisions regarding how to dose these potent medications, or when to remove sedatives and liberate patients from mechanical ventilation. The result is that it is now commonplace in the ICU to find most elderly patients receiving mechanical ventilation in a drug-induced state of 'suspended animation'.

The motoric subtypes of delirium are hypoactive, hyperactive, and mixed. Peterson et al. [17] recently reported on delirium subtypes from a cohort of 613 ventilated and non-ventilated ICU patients in whom delirium was monitored over 20,000 observations. These investigators found that among patients who developed delirium, pure hyperactive delirium was rare (<5%), while hypoactive and mixed types of delirium were the predominant subtypes (~45% each). Interestingly, the hypoactive subtype was significantly more common in older patients than in the young. The risk factors for and clinical implications of these meteoric subtypes are the subject of ongoing investigations.

The period surrounding cessation of sedation represents a typical scenario in the ICU setting in which delirium may either be easily recognized or completely missed by clinicians. Patients emerging from the effects of sedation may do so peacefully or in a combative manner. On one extreme are the 'peaceful' patients, who are often erroneously assumed to be thinking clearly. Delirium in this context is referred to as 'hypoactive delirium' and is characterized by decreased mental and physical activity and inattention [12]. Such mental status changes could lead to adverse outcomes such as reintubation, which itself has been shown to increase tenfold the risk of nosocomial pneumonia and death. In addition, hypoactive delirium is associated with aspiration, pulmonary embolism, decubitus ulcers, and other complications related to immobility.

On the other extreme are agitated or combative patients (i.e., hyperactive delirium), who are at risk not only for self-extubation and subsequent reintubation, but also pulling out central venous access and even falling out of bed. These patients are most often given higher doses of sedatives that commit them to at least another day of mechanical ventilation. This places patients at risk for being left in a cognitively impaired state and on mechanical ventilation unnecessarily [18]. Because of this difficult cycle, it is important for health care professionals to avoid overuse of psychoactive medications and to develop better methods of assessing cognitive function, especially during the transition from drug-induced or metabolic coma to wakefulness.

▮ Missing the Diagnosis of Delirium

The above-mentioned 'quiet' or hypoactive delirium is frequently overlooked by physicians and nurses. Delirium remains unrecognized by the clinician in as many as 66 to 84% of patients experiencing this complication [19, 20], and it may be attributed incorrectly to dementia, depression, or just an 'expected' occurrence in the critically ill, elderly patient [19]. Many clinicians expect delirium to present with agitation or hallucinations, features that are not required for the diagnosis. Other reasons for the lack of recognition of delirium include infrequent cognitive assessments and the fluctuating nature of delirium. It has been shown that the very development of delirium is associated with fewer interactions and less time spent by nurses and physicians in direct patient care [21, 22].

▮ Geriatric ICU Concerns and Pre-existing Cognitive Impairment

It is estimated that over the next three decades the cost of care for those over 65 will increase ten-fold [23]. These data have been used to argue for limiting ICU care provided to the elderly in order to conserve resources [24]. However, a recent report from Angus et al. documented that nearly 60% of all ICU days were incurred by patients older than 65 years [25]. In fact, adults <65 had 37 ICU days per year per 1,000 person-years vs. 240 for those over 75 years. The incidence of acute respiratory failure requiring mechanical ventilation rises 10-fold from the age of 55 to 85 [26], resulting in greater numbers of elderly patients being treated in our ICUs [27].

Because of these age-related demographics and the relationship between pre-existing cognitive impairment and development of delirium, clinicians are likely to discover an increased burden of delirium among hospitalized patients across the country. It has been shown that advanced age and cognitive decline lead to reductions in the level of interactions and potentially life-saving therapeutic interventions from clinicians and caregivers [28, 29]. Despite this, we know that more and more elderly patients are being admitted to the ICU than ever before, and certainly this will include older patients with pre-existing cognitive impairment ranging from mild to overt dementia. A cohort investigation by Pisani et al. [30] studied the impact of pre-existing cognitive impairment (mostly mild) on ICU outcomes and found that those with and without cognitive impairment had similar outcomes in terms of both ICU and hospital length of stay and mortality. However, the persistence of delirium symptoms in such patients could strongly affect discharge rates to nursing homes following hospitalization.

Prognostic Significance of Delirium

Reports indicate that CNS organ dysfunction is associated with complications of mechanical ventilation including aspiration, nosocomial pneumonia, reintubation, and self-extubation. It has also been shown in mechanically ventilated neurosurgical patients that the strongest predictor of failed extubation was an abnormal Glasgow coma score [31]. In medical ICU patients, Salam et al. [32] showed that there were important interactions between cognitive dysfunction and the likelihood of failed extubation.

In non-ICU populations, the development of delirium in the hospital is associated with an in-hospital mortality of 25 to 33%, prolonged hospital stay, and three times the likelihood of discharge to a nursing home [16, 33, 34]. In a three-site study of medical non-ICU patients, delirium was found to be an independent predictor of the combined outcome of death or nursing home placement [35]. Francis and Kapoor [36] found that two-year mortality in patients having experienced delirium was 39% vs 23% in controls, but multivariate analysis showed that this was largely explained by baseline cognitive and functional status. Perhaps the most convincing report of the independent association between delirium and mortality among *non*-ICU patients was published by McCusker and colleagues [37], showing an adjusted hazard of dying of 2.11 associated with the development of delirium. This mortality increase has now been shown independent of dementia status [38].

Among ICU patients, we now have evidence that delirium is a predictor of mortality (Fig. 1) [39]. In fact, the development of delirium is associated with a threefold increase in risk of death after controlling for pre-existing comorbidities, severity of illness, coma, and the use of sedative and analgesic medications. These data also showed that delirium is not simply a transition state from coma to normal, as delirium occurred just as often among those who never developed coma as it did among those with coma and persisted in 11% of patients at the time of hospital discharge. Furthermore, three recent prospective studies found that delirium was associated with an increased risk for dementia over 2 to 3 years [40-42]. In light of these findings, future studies should determine whether or not prevention or treatment of delirium changes clinical outcomes including mortality, length of stay, cost of care, and long-term neuropsychological outcomes among survivors of critical illness.

Costs Associated with Delirium in the ICU Patient

Delirium complicates the hospital stay of more than 2 to 3 million elderly patients per year in the USA, involving over 17.5 million in-patient days and accounting for over $ 4 billion in Medicare expenditures [43]. In the only study to date reporting

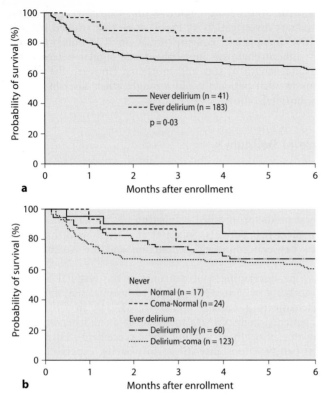

Fig. 1. Delirium versus six-month survival. These Kaplan-Meier plots show the relationship between delirium and 6-month survival. **a** Never vs. ever Delirium (according to whether or not the patient ever developed delirium in the ICU), **b** Clinical Severity (subdividing the never and ever delirium groups in order to better understand the phenomenology of delirium). The never delirium group, composed of those who were always). Normal and those who were Coma-Normal (e.g., deeply sedated and then normal when drugs stopped) had higher survival than the ever delirium group, which was composed of those with Delirium Only and Delirium-Coma. From [39] with permission

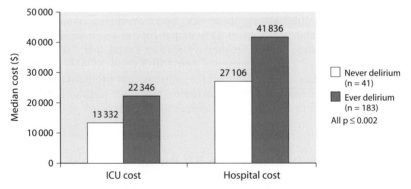

Fig. 2. Median ICU and hospital cost per patient. This histogram shows cost according to clinical categorization of 'ever delirium' vs. 'never delirium'. Delirium was significantly associated with increased ICU and hospital cost. From [44] with permission

on costs associated with delirium in the ICU, Milbrandt and colleagues [44] found that median ICU and hospital costs were significantly higher for those with at least one episode of delirium vs. those with no delirium (Fig. 2). Even after controlling for important potentially confounding variables, such as baseline comorbidities and severity of illness, delirium was associated with a 40% relative increase in ICU and total hospital costs. In addition, the data demonstrated a 'dose-response' in which cumulative delirium severity was associated with incrementally greater cost.

The associated annual cost of ICU delirium could be enormous. In the study by Milbrandt mentioned above [44], delirium occurred in 82% of mechanically patients and was associated with an incremental increase in ICU cost of over $ 9000 per patient. In the United States, there are approximately 880,000 to 2 760 000 ICU admissions annually for respiratory failure requiring mechanical ventilation. Therefore, the estimated number of cases of ICU delirium could range from 721,600 to 2 263 200 per year with an associated increase in health care costs ranging between $ 6.5 and $ 20.4 billion. If we use the incidence of delirium from a less severely ill ICU cohort in which delirium occurred in only 19% of patients [45], the estimated annual costs would still be in the range of $ 1.5 to $ 4.7 billion. Since some of the additional cost associated with delirium could be attributable to unmeasured differences between patient groups, these estimates represent the upper limit of the cost attributable to ICU delirium. However, even if only 20% of the difference in costs between patients with and without delirium were in fact due to delirium, this would still be a significant public health concern with $ 300 million to $ 4 billion in annual attributable costs.

▌ Risk Factors for Delirium

Only a few studies of ICU patients have assessed risk factors for delirium, though many investigations over the past decade, using a variety of non-ICU cohorts, have identified numerous risk factors for the development of delirium [34]. Patients who are highly vulnerable to delirium may develop the disorder following only minor physiologic stressors, whereas those with low baseline vulnerability require a more noxious insult to become delirious [46]. It is possible to stratify patients into risk groups depending on the number of risk factors present [19, 46-48]. Three or more risk factors increase the likelihood of developing delirium to around 60% or higher, and it is a rare patient in the ICU who would not be in the high-risk group. In fact, most ICU patients have over 10 risk factors for delirium [15, 49].

In practical terms, the risk factors can be divided into three categories: 1) host factors; 2) the acute illness itself; and 3) iatrogenic or environmental factors (Table 2). Issues that are ripe for study in terms of prevention or intervention have been marked with an asterisk in the table, which is obviously not meant to be exhaustive. In the only ICU cohort risk factor study published to date [45], factors related to the medical history included hypertension and smoking (raising one's awareness of the risks of relative under-perfusion of the brain or nicotine withdrawal). During the ICU stay, a dose-dependent risk was found for patients having been treated with opiates.

Psychoactive medications are the leading iatrogenic risk factors for delirium. Benzodiazepines, narcotics, and other psychoactive drugs are associated with a 3 to 11 times increased relative risk [33], and the number and rate of adding psychoac-

Table 2. Risk factors for delirium

Host Factors	Acute Illness*	Iatrogenic or Environmental
▌ Elderly	Severe sepsis*	Sedative and analgesic use*
▌ Underlying comorbidities (e.g., heart, liver, or renal failure, diabetes, hypertension)	Acute respiratory distress syndrome*	Immobilization (e.g., restraints or catheters)*
▌ Pre-existing cognitive impairment or dementia	Multiple organ dysfunction syndrome	Total parenteral nutrition*
▌ Hearing or vision impairment*	Drug overdose or illicit drugs	Sleep deprivation*
▌ Neurologic disease (stroke or seizure)	Acquisition of nosocomial infection*	Malnutrition*
▌ Alcoholism and smoking*	Metabolic disturbance*	Anemia (phlebotomy)*

*Potentially modifiable factors through specific interventions or avoidance

tive medications increase the risk of delirium by 4 to 10 times [33]. Coupling these data with knowledge regarding the extreme variability in the pharmacokinetics of sedatives and analgesics according to age, ethnicity, drug metabolizing ability and other factors, perhaps the most promising delirium interventions could be centered on delivery patterns of these medications.

▌ Combining Sedation and Delirium Assessments at the Bedside

The SCCM guidelines suggest that all critically ill patients be simultaneously monitored for level of sedation and for delirium [5]. Bedside critical care nurses and the rest of the ICU team need to utilize data obtained from well-validated, reliable, objective, yet brief assessment tools to monitor for both components of consciousness (arousal level and content of consciousness) [50]. Neurological monitoring in the ICU can be streamlined using a two-step approach to sedation and delirium.

The first step in neurologic assessment of ICU patients is to assess a patient's level of consciousness/sedation using an objective sedation assessment. The recommended standard of care is to use objective assessment scales in order to avoid over-sedation and to promote earlier liberation from mechanical ventilation. Sedation scales help provide common language for the multidisciplinary team to use when discussing goals and treatments for patients. While the Ramsay Scale [51] has been the most widely used instrument for decades in both clinical practice and the published literature [52], other recently developed instruments such as the sedation-agitation scale (SAS) [53] and Richmond agitation-sedation scale (RASS) [54, 55] have been better validated and are being widely implemented [15, 56]. It is important to emphasize again the importance of using these instruments to guide patient-targeted or goal-directed sedation. The concept of using sedation scales over time within patients was addressed in the second RASS validation study [55], in which emphasis was placed on the fact that gone should be the days of giving potent psychoactive medications without a specific agreed upon target level of effect.

The second step in assessing the brain's function in critically ill ICU patients builds on the level of arousal assessment discussed above and involves the delirium

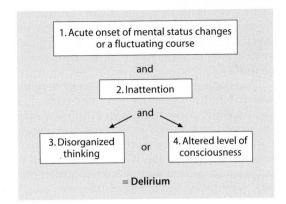

Fig. 3. Definition of delirium as per the Confusion Assessment Method for the ICU (CAM-ICU) adapted from the Diagnostic Statistical Manual IV (DSM IV) of the American Psychiatric Association

assessment. All patients who are responsive to verbal stimuli should be assessed for delirium. The first delirium assessment tools designed specifically for non-verbal, intubated ICU patients were published in 2001 [13, 15, 57]. One of these instruments is the Intensive Care Delirium Screening Checklist (ICDSC) [13], which is used as a screening instrument due to its high sensitivity (99%) yet moderate specificity (64%). The other is the Confusion Assessment Method for the ICU (CAM-ICU) [15, 57], which has a sensitivity and specificity of ~95% and very high inter-rater reliability (kappa 0.96). The CAM-ICU was designed to be a serial assessment tool for use by bedside clinicians (nurses or physicians). Thus, it is easy to use, taking only 1 minute on average to complete, and requires minimal training. Delirium assessment using the CAM-ICU incorporates 4 key features that comprise the definition of delirium as taken from the Diagnostic Statistical Manual IV of the American Psychiatric Association. The four features are as follows: Feature 1: change in mental status from baseline or fluctuating course of mental status; Feature 2: inattention; Feature 3: disorganized thinking; and Feature 4: altered level of consciousness. Delirium is present when both Features 1 and 2 and either 3 or 4 are present (Fig. 3). The CAM-ICU has been translated into numerous languages and numerous aspects of neurologic monitoring are discussed and available for download via an educational website (www.icudelirium.org).

Strategies for Optimal Management of ICU Delirium

Primary Prevention and Non-pharmacological Approaches

In a trial of 852 general medical patients over the age of 70 [58], strategies for primary prevention of delirium resulted in a 40% reduction in the odds of developing delirium (15% in controls vs. 9.9% in the intervention patients). The protocol [58] focused on optimization of risk factors via the following methods: repeated reorientation of the patient by trained volunteers and nurses, provision of cognitively stimulating activities for the patient three times per day, a non-pharmacological sleep protocol to enhance normalization of sleep/wake cycles, early mobilization activities and range of motion exercises, timely removal of catheters and physical restraints, institution of the use of eyeglasses and magnifying lenses, hearing aids and earwax disimpaction, and early correction of dehydration. Unfortunately, this intervention did not show sustained benefit when the patients were followed to 6 months [59]. Other recent studies of delirium prevention were able to reproduce success only in subgroups such as those without underlying dementia [60] or not at all [61].

However, this study of primary prevention did not focus on critically ill patients, and excluded mechanically ventilated patients. Considering that ICU studies using the CAM-ICU have documented delirium rates of 70–80%, one might view the 'room for improvement' in delirium management as far greater for critically ill ICU patients. While primary prevention of delirium is preferred, some degree of delirium is inevitable in the ICU. In these cases, the above-mentioned basic tenets of patient management such as restoring sleep/wake cycles, timely removal of catheters, early mobilization, use of scheduled pain protocol, minimization of unnecessary noise/stimuli and frequent reorientation should be applied liberally. Family involvement can be very helpful in reorienting and soothing delirious patients. It is important to teach family members of the fluctuating course of delirium as well as how they can detect delirium. Preventive and management strategies for delirium in the ICU represent an important area for future investigation.

Pharmacological Therapy

Medications should be used only after giving adequate attention to correction of modifiable contributing factors (e.g., sleep disturbance, restraints, etc) as discussed above and in Table 2. It is important to recognize that delirium could be a manifestation of an acute, life-threatening problem that requires immediate attention (such as hypoxia, hypercarbia, hypoglycemia, metabolic derangements, or shock). After addressing such concerns, delirious patients should be considered for pharmacological management. It should be recognized that while agents used to treat delirium are intended to improve cognition, they all have psychoactive effects which may further cloud the sensorium and promote a longer overall duration of cognitive impairment. Therefore, until we have outcomes data that confirm beneficial effects of treatment, these drugs should be used judiciously in the smallest possible dose and for the shortest time necessary, a practice *infrequently* adhered to in most ICUs. Indeed, some patients will prove refractory to all 'cocktail' approaches to sedation and delirium therapy, and these patients should be considered for a trial of complete cessation of all psychoactive drugs.

Benzodiazepines, which are used most commonly in the ICU for sedation, are not recommended for the management of delirium because of the likelihood of over-sedation, exacerbation of confusion, and respiratory suppression. However, they remain the drugs of choice for the treatment of delirium tremens (and other withdrawal syndromes) and seizures. The amnestic qualities of benzodiazepines make these agents especially useful when noxious or unpleasant procedures are required. It is likely, however, that residual accumulation of these drugs may lead to prolonged delirium long after the drugs have been discontinued. In certain populations, particularly elderly patients with underlying dementia, benzodiazepines may lead to increased confusion and agitation. In such cases, one may try to take advantage of the sedative effects of haloperidol in lieu of continued benzodiazepines. Preliminary results from a prospective, randomized, yet unblinded trial of sedation in post-operative cardiac surgical patients showed that those treated with dexmedetomidine as compared to propofol or midazolam were less likely to develop delirium [62]. This work must be confirmed on a larger scale with documented improved outcomes prior to modifying standard sedation practices.

There are currently no drugs with FDA-approval for the treatment of delirium. The SCCM guidelines recommend haloperidol as the drug of choice, though it is acknowledged that this is based on sparse outcomes data from non-randomized case series and anecdotal reports (i.e., level C data). Nevertheless, haloperidol is a butyrophenone 'typical' antipsychotic, which is the most widely used neuroleptic agent for delirium [63]. It does not suppress the respiratory drive and works as a dopamine receptor antagonist by blocking the D_2 receptor, which results in treatment of positive symptomatology (hallucinations, unstructured thoughts patterns, etc) and produces a variable sedative effect.

In the non-ICU setting, the recommended starting dose of haldoperidol is 0.5 to 1.0 mg orally or parenterally, with repeated doses every 20 to 30 minutes until the desired effect is achieved. In the ICU setting, a recommended starting dose would be 5 mg every 12 hours (i.v. or PO), with maximal effective doses usually in the neighborhood of 20 mg/day. This dose range will usually be adequate to achieve the 'theoretically optimal' 60% D_2 receptor blockage [64], while avoiding complete D_2 receptor saturation associated with the adverse effects cited below. Because of the urgency of the situation in many ICU patients – due to the potential for inadvertent removal of central lines, endotracheal tubes, or even aortic balloon pumps – much higher doses of haloperidol are often used. Unfortunately, there are few data in the way of formal pharmacological investigations to guide dosage recommendations in the ICU. Once calm, the patient can usually be managed with much lower maintenance doses of haloperidol.

Neither haloperidol nor similar agents (i.e., droperidol and chlorpromazine) have been extensively studied in the ICU [5]. Newer 'atypical' antipsychotic agents (e.g., risperidone, ziprasidone, quetiapine, and olanzapine) may also prove helpful for delirium [65]. The rationale behind use of the atypical antipsychotics over haloperidol (especially in hypoactive/mixed subtypes of delirium) is theoretical and centers on the fact that they affect not only dopamine, but also other potentially key neurotransmitters such as serotonin, acetylcholine, and norepinephrine. Adequately powered randomized controlled trials of these agents are not available to date.

Adverse effects of typical and atypical antipsychotics include hypotension, acute dystonias, extrapyramidal effects, laryngeal spasm, malignant hyperthermia, glucose and lipid dysregulation, and anticholinergic effects such as dry mouth, constipation, and urinary retention. Perhaps the most immediately life-threatening adverse effect of antipsychotics is torsades de pointes, and these agents should not be given to patients with prolonged QT intervals unless thought to be absolutely necessary. Patents who receive substantial quantities of typical or atypical antipsychotics or co-administered arrhythmogenic drugs should be monitored closely with electrocardiography. Having mentioned these potential difficulties, antipsychotics (most experience having been accrued with haloperidol) are usually well tolerated from both the hemodynamic and respiratory standpoint.

▌ Conclusion

Critically ill patients are at great risk for the development of delirium in the ICU. However, this form of brain dysfunction is grossly under-recognized and under-treated. Delirium is mistakenly thought to be a transient and expected outcome in the ICU, and of little consequence (i.e., part of the 'ICU psychosis'). It is now recognized that delirium is one of the most frequent complications experienced in the ICU, and even after adjusting for covariates such as age, gender, race and severity of illness, delirium is an independent risk factor for prolonged length of stay and higher 6-month mortality rates. In addition many ICU survivors demonstrate persistent cognitive deficits at follow-up testing months to years later. It is essential for health care professionals to be able to recognize delirium readily at the bedside. The CAM-ICU is a valid, reliable, quick, and easy to use serial assessment tool for monitoring delirium in both ventilated and non-ventilated ICU patients. Delirium is a multi-factorial problem for ICU patients that demands an interdisciplinary approach for assessment, management and treatment. Critical care nurses and physicians should assume a position of leadership in the ICU regarding delirium monitoring, as they are the best-suited members of the ICU team to implement successfully this essential component of patient management, which is now recommended by the SCCM clinical practice guidelines. Lastly, while ongoing trials will hopefully elucidate the optimal ways to treat delirium, standard pharmacological and non-pharmacological management strategies have been reviewed.

References

1. Papadopoulos MC, Davies DC, Moss RF, Tighe D, Bennett ED (2000) Pathophysiology of septic encephalopathy: a review. Crit Care Med 28:3019–3024
2. Russell JA, Singer J, Bernard G, et al (2000) Changing pattern of organ dysfunction in early human sepsis is related to mortality. Crit Care Med 28:3405–3411
3. Granberg A, Engberg B, Lundberg D (1996) Intensive care syndrome: a literature review. Intensive Crit Care Nurse 12:173–182
4. Wilson LM (1972) Intensive care delirium: the effect of outside deprivation in a windowless unit. Arch Intern Med 130:22–23
5. Jacobi J, Fraser GL, Coursin DB, et al (2002) Clinical practice guidelines for the sustained use of sedatives and analgesics in the critically ill adult. Crit Care Med 30:119–141
6. Justic M (2000) Does "ICU psychosis" really exist? Crit Care Nurse 20:28–37
7. Meagher DJ, Trzepacz PT (2000) Motoric subtypes of delirium. Semin Clin Neuropsychiatry 5:75–85
8. Webb JM, Carlton EF, Geeham DM (2000) Delirium in the intensive care unit: Are we helping the patient? Crit Care Nurs Q 22:47–60
9. Crippen D (2001) Treatment of agitation and its comorbidities in the intensive care unit. In: Hill NS, Levy M (ed) Ventilator Management Strategies for Critical Care. Marcel Dekker, Inc., New York, pp 243–284
10. Lipowski ZJ (1989) Delirium in the elderly patient. N Engl J Med 320:578–582
11. Wijdicks,E.F.M. (2002): Neurologic Complications of Critical Illness. Oxford University Press, New York
12. Meagher DJ, Hanlon DO, Mahony EO, Casey PR, Trzepacz PT (2000) Relationship between symptoms and motoric subtype of delirium. J Neuropsychiatry Clin Neurosci 12:51–56
13. Bergeron N, Dubois MJ, Dumont M, Dial S, Skrobik Y (2001) Intensive Care Delirium Screening Checklist: evaluation of a new screening tool. Intensive Care Med 27:859–864
14. McNicoll L, Pisani MA, Zhang Y, Ely EW, Siegel MD, Inouye SK (2003) Delirium in the intensive care unit: occurrence and clinical course in older patients. J Am Geriatr Soc 51:591–598
15. Ely EW, Inouye SK, Bernard GR, et al (2001) Delirium in mechanically ventilated patients: validity and reliability of the confusion assessment method for the intensive care unit (CAM-ICU). JAMA 286:2703–2710
16. Levkoff SE, Evans DA, Liptzin B, et al (1992) Delirium: The occurrence and persistence of symptoms among elderly hospitalized patients. Arch Intern Med 152:334–340

17. Peterson JF, Truman BL, Shintani A, Thomason JWW, Jackson JC, Ely EW (2003) The prevalence of hypoactive, hyperactive, and mixed type delirium in medical ICU patients. J Am Geriatr Soc 51:S174 (abst)

18. Kollef MH, Levy NT, Ahrens T, Schaiff R, Prentice D, Sherman G (1999) The use of continuous IV sedation is associated with prolongation of mechanical ventilation. Chest 114:541–548

19. Francis J, Martin D, Kapoor WN (1990) A prospective study of delirium in hospitalized elderly. JAMA 263:1097–1101

20. Inouye SK (1994) The dilemma of delirium: clinical and research controversies regarding diagnosis and evaluation of delirium in hospitalized elderly medical patients. Am J Med 97:278–288

21. Armstrong-Esther CA, Browne KD (1986) The influence of elderly patients' mental impairment on nurse-patient interaction. J Adv Nurs 11:379–387

22. Wray NP, Friedland JA, Ashton CM, Scheurich J, Zollo AJ (1986) Characteristics of house staff work rounds on two academic general medicine services. J Med Educ 61:893–900

23. Hobbs FB, Damon BL (1995) Sixty-five plus in the United States. U.S. Dept. of Commerce, Economics and Statistics Administration, Bureau of the Census, Washington, DC

24. Sage WM, Hurst CR, Silverman JF, Bortz WM (1987) Intensive care for the elderly: outcome of elective and nonelective admissions. J Am Geriatr Soc 35:312–318

25. Angus DC, Kelly MA, Schmitz RJ, White A, Popovich J, for the committee on manpower for pulmonary and critical care societies (COMPACCS) (2000) Current and projected workforce requirements for care of the critically ill and patients with pulmonary disease: can we meet the requirements of an aging population? JAMA 284:2762–2770

26. Behrendt CE (2000) Acute respiratory failure in the United States: incidence and 31-day survival. Chest 118:1100–1105

27. Chelluri L, Grenvik A, Silverstein M (1995) Intensive care for critically ill elderly: mortality, costs, and quality of life. Review of the literature. Arch Intern Med 155:1013–1022

28. Hamel MB, Philips RS, Teno JM, et al (1996) Seriously ill hospitalized adults: do we spend less on older patients? J Am Geriatr Soc 44:1043–1048

29. Hamel MB, Teno JM, Goldman L, et al (1999) Patient age and decisions to withhold life-sustaining treatments from seriously ill, hospitalized adults. Ann Intern Med 130:116–125

30. Pisani MA, Redlich C, Ely EW, McNicoll L, Inouye S (2003) Favorable ICU outcomes in older patients with preexisting cognitive impairment. Am J Respir Crit Care Med 167:A252 (abst)

31. Namen AM, Ely EW, Tatter S, et al (2001) Predictors of successful extubation in neurosurgical patients. Am J Respir Crit Care Med 163:658–664

32. Salam A, Tilluckdharry L, Amoateng-Adjepong Y, Manthous CA (2004) Neurologic status, cough, secretions and extubation outcomes. Intensive Care Med 30:1334–1339

33. Inouye SK, Schlesinger MJ, Lyndon TJ (1999) Delirium: a symptom of how hospital care is failing older persons and a window to improve quality of hospital care. Am J Med 106:565–573

34. American Psychiatric Assoc (1999) Practice guideline for the treatment of patients with delirium. Am J Psychiatry 156:1–20

35. Inouye SK, Rushing JT, Foreman MD, Palmer RM, Pompei P (1998) Does delirium contribute to poor hospital outcomes? a three-site epidemiologic study. J Gen Intern Med 13:234–242

36. Francis J, Kapoor WN (1992) Prognosis after hospital discharge of older medical patients with delirium. J Am Geriatr Soc 40:601–606

37. McCusker J, Cole M, Abrahamowicz M, Primeau F, Belzile E (2002) Delirium predicts 12 month mortality. Arch Intern Med 162:457–463

38. Fick DM, Agostini JV, Inouye SK (2002) Delirium superimposed on dementia: a systematic review. JAGS 50:1723–1732

39. Ely EW, Shintani A, Truman B, et al (2004) Delirium as a predictor of mortality in mechanically ventilated patients in the intensive care unit. JAMA 291:1753–1762

40. Rockwood K, Cosway S, Carver D (1999) The risk of dementia and death after delirium. Age Ageing 28:551–556

41. Rahkonen T, Luukkainen-Markkula R, Paanilla S, Sulkava R (2000) Delirium episode as a sign of undetected dementia among community dwelling subjects: a 2 year follow up study. J Neurol Neurosurg Psychiatry 69:519–521

42. McCusker J, Cole M, Dendukuri N, Belzile E, Primeau F (2001) Delirium in older medical inpatients and subsequent cognitive and functional status: a prospective study. Can Med Assoc J 165:575–583
43. U.S. Bureau of the Census (1991) Statistical Abstract of the United States. 3. US Bureau of the Census, Washington, DC
44. Milbrandt E, Deppen S, Harrison P, et al (2004) Costs associated with delirium in mechanically ventilated patients. Crit Care Med 32:955–962
45. Dubois MJ, Bergeron N, Dumont M, Dial S, Skrobik Y (2001) Delirium in an intensive care unit: a study of risk factors. Intensive Care Med 27:1297–1304
46. Inouye SK, Charpentier PA (1996) Precipitating factors for delirium in hospitalized elderly persons: predictive model and interrelationship with baseline vulnerability. JAMA 275:852–857
47. Inouye SK, Viscoli C, Horwitz RI, Hurst LD, Tinetti ME (1993) A predictive model for delirium in hospitalized elderly medical patients based on admission characteristics. Ann Intern Med 119:474–481
48. Marcantonio ER, Goldman L, Mangione CM, et al (1994) A clinical prediction rule for delirium after elective noncardiac surgery. JAMA 271:134–139
49. Ely EW, Gautam S, Margolin R, et al (2001) The impact of delirium in the intensive care unit on hospital length of stay. Intensive Care Med 27:1892–1900
50. Plum F, Posner J (1980) The Diagnosis of Stupor and Coma. F.A. Davis Co., Philadelphia
51. Ramsay M, Savege TM, Simpson ER, Goodwin R (1974) Controlled sedation with aphaxalone-alphadolone. BMJ 2:656–659
52. Ostermann ME, Keenan SP, Seiferling RA, Sibbald W (2000) Sedation in the intensive care unit. JAMA 283:1451–1459
53. Riker R, Picard JT, Fraser G (1999) Prospective evaluation of the sedation-agitation scale for adult critically ill patients. Crit Care Med 27:1325–1329
54. Sessler CN, Gosnell M, Grap MJ, et al (2002) The Richmond Agitation-Sedation Scale: validity and reliability in adult intensive care patients. Am J Respir Crit Care Med 166:1338–1344
55. Ely EW, Truman B, Shintani A, et al (2003) Monitoring sedation status over time in ICU patients: reliability and validity of the Richmond Agitation-Sedation Scale (RASS). JAMA 289:2983–2991
56. Ely EW, Gautam S, May L, et al (2001) A comparison of different sedation scales in the ICU and validation of the Richmond Agitation Sedation Scale (RASS). Am J Respir Crit Care Med 163:A954
57. Ely EW, Margolin R, Francis J, et al (2001) Evaluation of delirium in critically ill patients: validation of the confusion assessment method for the intensive care unit (CAM-ICU). Crit Care Med 29:1370–1379
58. Inouye SK, Bogardus ST, Charpentier PA, et al (1999) A multicomponent intervention to prevent delirium in hospitalized older patients. N Engl J Med 340:669–676
59. Bogardus ST, Desai MM, Williams CS, Leo-Summers L, Acampora D, Inouye SK (2003) The effects of a targeted multicomponent delirium intervention of postdischarge outcomes for hospitalized older adults. Am J Med 114:383–390
60. Marcantonio ER, Flacker JM, Wright RJ, Resnick NM (2001) Reducing delirium after hip fracture: a randomized trial. JAGS 516–522
61. Cole MG, McCusker J, Bellavance F, et al (2002) Systematic detection and multidisciplinary care of delirium in older medical inpatients: a randomized trial. CMAJ 167:753–759
62. Maldonado JR, van der Starre PJ, Wysong A (2003) Post-operative sedation and the incidence of ICU delirium in cardiac surgery patients. Anesthesiology 99:A465 (abst)
63. Ely EW, Stephens RK, Jackson JC, et al (2004) Current opinions regarding the importance, diagnosis, and management of delirium in the intensive care unit: a survey of 912 healthcare professionals. Crit Care Med 32:106–112
64. Kapur S, Remington G, Jones C, et al (1996) High levels of dopamine d2 receptor occupancy with low-dose haloperidol treatment: a pet study. Am J Psychiatry 153:948–950
65. Skrobik Y, Bergeron N, Dumont M, Gottfried SB (2004) Olanzapine vs haloperidol: treating delirium in a critical care setting. Intensive Care Med 30:444–449
66. Ely EW, Siegel MD, Inouye SK (2001) Delirium in the intensive care unit: An under-recognized syndrome of organ dysfunction. Semin Respir Crit Care Med 22:115–126

Quality Issues

The Critically Ill Obese Patient: A Management Challenge

J. Varon and P. Marik

▮ Introduction

Obesity has become the 'new epidemic' in Western countries. This is a serious disorder that results in significant impairment of health [1, 2]. Indeed, obese adults are at a higher risk of morbidity and mortality from many acute and chronic medical conditions, including hypertension, dyslipidemia, coronary heart disease, diabetes mellitus, gallbladder disease, pulmonary diseases, some types of cancer, gout and arthritis [1]. Ideal body weight standards are commonly determined by age, sex and height. The majority of individuals who weigh more than 20% over their calculated ideal body weight have excessive adipose mass [1]. One useful formula for the critical care practitioner is the body mass index (BMI), which is the ratio of weight (in kilograms) to height (in meters) squared (wt/ht^2). This is the most convenient method of quantifying the degree of obesity [3]. The National Center for Health Statistics has defined overweight as a BMI of 27.8 or more in men and 27.3 or more in women. Severely overweight is defined as a BMI of 31.1 or more in men and 32.3 or more in women [3]. The lower cut-offs correspond to approximately 20% above desirable body weight in the 1983 Metropolitan Life Insurance Company mortality tables, whereas the upper cut-offs correspond to 40% above desirable body weight [3].

From an epidemiological standpoint, the National Health and Nutrition Examination Survey (NHANES) reported an alarming increase in overweight adults in the United States from 35% in 1994 to 64.9% in the year 2000 [4]. When compared to European countries, recent data have demonstrated that the prevalence of obesity is three times higher in the US than France, and one-and-a-half times that of England [5].

As obesity is such a common condition and being an important risk factor for many diseases, it is not surprising that many obese patients are treated in the intensive care unit (ICU). The critically ill obese patient presents the critical care team with many unique problems.

▮ Critical Illness and Obesity

The risk of death from all causes increases throughout the range of moderate and severe overweight for both men and women in all age groups [6]. The graphed relationship between BMI and mortality is 'J-shaped' with increased death rates with malnutrition and with increasing BMI [7, 8]. Obesity may also increase the risk of death in acutely ill patients. Landi and coworkers analyzed the association between BMI and mortality in a cohort of over 8000 hospitalized Italian patients between 1991 and 1997, reproducing the 'J-shaped' association between BMI and mortality [9].

The impact of obesity on ICU outcome has been studied only recently. In the development of the APACHE II and III or SAPS and SAPS II prognostic indices, obesity was not included as a comorbid variable. In a retrospective cohort study, El-Sohl and co-workers compared the clinical course and outcome of 117 morbidly obese critically ill patients to a group of matched ICU patients of normal body weight [10]. These authors reported a significantly longer ICU stay and hospital mortality in the morbidly obese patients. However, other authors have suggested that obesity may be 'protective' in critical illness. Marik and coauthors, utilizing the Project IMPACT database found that 38% of patients had a normal BMI, 7.1% of the patients were underweight, and 54.1% were overweight with 5.5% being morbidly obese [11]. Hospital length of stay in these patients was significantly longer at the extremes of BMI. By multivariate analysis, the SAPS II Score, a non-medical admission, sepsis on admission, and BMI group were independent predictors of hospital mortality. The analysis of this large cohort of critically ill patients suggested that obesity could be protective in overweight and obese critically ill patients, while morbid obesity appears to have little effect on outcome. This study is contrasted by that of Smith-Choban and colleagues, who reported that morbidly obese patients have an eight-fold higher mortality following blunt trauma than non-obese patients [12]. Furthermore, other authors have shown hospitalized obese patients are at an increased risk of developing respiratory and other complications (see below) [13, 14].

■ Respiratory Effects of Obesity (Table 1)

The effects of obesity on respiratory function are complex and influenced by the degree of obesity, age, and body fat distribution (central or peripheral). The expiratory reserve volume is consistently decreased in obese patients while the forced expiratory volume in one second (FEV_1) to forced vital capacity (FVC) ratio is increased [15–17]. Interestingly, the vital capacity (VC), total lung capacity (TLC), and functional residual capacity (FRC) are generally maintained in otherwise normal individuals with mild to moderate obesity but are reduced by up to 30% in morbidly obese patients [15, 16, 18]. These latter changes occur predominantly in patients with central obesity [16, 18]. A simple mechanical effect of fat distribution on lung volumes is the most likely explanation for these findings.

Table 1. Respiratory and chest wall alterations in morbidly obese patients

■ Abnormal chest elasticity
■ Abnormal diaphragmatic position
■ Increased upper airway resistance
■ Increased chest wall resistance
■ Increased airway resistance
■ Decreased expiratory reserve volume
■ Ventilation-perfusion mismatch
■ Widened alveolar-arterial oxygen gradient

Obese patients have an increased work of breathing due to abnormal chest elasticity, increased chest wall resistance, increased airway resistance, abnormal diaphragmatic position, and upper airway resistance, as well as the need to eliminate a higher daily production of carbon dioxide [15]. Patients with morbid obesity are generally hypoxemic, with a widened alveolar-arterial oxygen gradient caused by ventilation-perfusion mismatching [15, 19]. Alveolar collapse and airway closure at the bases contribute to this phenomenon. The FRC falls when assuming a supine position, further increasing ventilation-perfusion mismatching. This may result in severe arterial hypoxemia, and sudden death [20]. Anesthesia further reduces the FRC, with the encroachment of the FRC on the closing volume.

Abnormalities in the control of ventilation are commonly seen in obese patients. Vgontzas and colleagues demonstrated significant sleep apnea in 40% of men and 3% of women with a BMI greater than 45.3 [21]. Indeed, hypoventilation plays a significant role in mortality post discharge. In one study, at 18 months following hospital discharge, mortality was 23% in the obesity-associated hypoventilation group as compared with 9% in a simple obesity group [22]. These changes in pulmonary function have important implications in the management of obese patients requiring assisted mechanical ventilation [23]. As the lung volumes may be reduced and airway resistance increased, a tidal volume calculated according to the patient's actual body weight is likely to result in high airway pressures and alveolar overdistension. The initial tidal volume should therefore be based on the ideal body weight, and then adjusted according to inflation pressures and blood gases. The use of positive end-expiratory pressure (PEEP) may prevent end-expiratory airway closure and atelectasis, particularly in dorsal pulmonary regions. Weaning the obese patient from mechanical ventilation is frequently a difficult and challenging task. Burns and colleagues have demonstrated that in obese patients the reverse Trendelenburg position at 45 degrees resulted in a larger tidal volume and lower respiratory rate than the 0, or 90 degree position, and they postulated that this position may facilitate the weaning process [24]. In our practice, this position is the preferred one for weaning.

Obese patients are at particular risk for aspiration pneumonia, especially in the postoperative period [25, 26]. This risk is increased due to several factors, including a higher volume of gastric fluid, a lower than normal pH of gastric fluid in fasting obese patients, increased intraabdominal pressure, and a higher incidence of gastroesophageal reflux [26]. This is another important reason to nurse the obese patient in the semi-upright position. As noted above, obese patients have a higher incidence of postsurgical pulmonary complications [27, 28]. These acute pulmonary events are twice as likely to occur in obese as compared to non-obese patients [13]. Obese blunt trauma victims have a particularly poor outcome frequently related to respiratory failure [12]. Postoperative respiratory failure is worsened by thoracic and upper abdominal incisions. Goldhaber and colleagues have reported that obesity is the single most important risk factor for pulmonary embolism [14]. It has been shown that obese patients have a higher incidence of postoperative thromboembolic disease [29, 30]. Decreased mobility, venous stasis and an increased thrombotic potential may account for this finding. Diminished levels of antithrombin III and circulating fibrinolytic activity have been demonstrated in obese patients [31]. The high risk of thromboembolic disease in obese ICU patients warrants an aggressive approach to deep venous thrombosis (DVT) prophylaxis. In our practice subcutaneous heparin, low-molecular weight heparin or the combination of pneumatic compression and heparin is used for these high-risk patients.

Endotracheal intubation can be a challenging experience in the morbidly obese patient. In the Australian Incident Monitoring Study, obesity with limited neck mobility and mouth opening accounted for the majority of cases of difficult intubation [32]. Physicians caring for these patients must be well versed in intubation techniques as well as the use of adjuncts for intubation.

▍ Cardiovascular Effects of Obesity

Patients with morbid obesity have an increase in total blood volume and resting cardiac output. Both increase in direct proportion to the amount the patient weighs over the ideal body weight [33–35]. The cardiac and stroke index are normal in otherwise healthy obese patients [33–35]. These patients have an increase in the mean oxygen consumption (VO_2) with a normal arterio-venous oxygen difference [33–35]. The distribution of cardiac output has been reported to be similar in obese and lean individuals. Although the resting cardiac output is increased, obese patients have been demonstrated to have impaired left ventricular contractility and a depressed ejection fraction, both at rest and after exercise [34, 36, 37].

The left ventricular filling pressure is elevated in obese patients due to the combination of increased preload and reduced ventricular distensibility [33–35]. De Divitiis and colleagues reported a mean left ventricular end-diastolic pressure (LVEDP) of 16.6 mmHg in their series of patients [33]. Consequently, fluid loading is poorly tolerated in these patients. Cuff sphygmomanometry can be inaccurate in the obese patient depending on the size of the cuff used. Therefore, continuous monitoring of systemic blood pressure with an arterial cannula may be prudent in such patients.

▍ Drug Dosing in Obese Patients

Drug distribution, metabolism, protein binding, and clearance are altered by the physiological changes associated with excessive weight [38–41]. Some of these pharmacokinetic changes may, however, negate the consequences of others and the pharmacokinetic alterations may differ in the morbidly obese compared to the mildly or moderately obese [42]. However, a number of drugs used in the ICU, most notably digoxin, aminophylline, aminoglycosides, and cyclosporin, can cause drug toxicity if obese patients are dosed based on their actual body weight.

The volume of distribution of drugs in obese patients is largely dependent on the lipophilicity of the drug [41]. The volume of distribution of drugs which are weakly lipophilic (aminoglycosides, quinolones) is moderately increased when compared to normal individuals. However, the volume of distribution is normal for some weakly lipophilic drugs (theophylline, H_2-blockers, neuromuscular blockers). The volume of distribution is increased for many, but not all lipophilic drugs. Benzodiazepines, verapamil and sufentanil, have a large volume of distribution indicating distribution into adipose tissue. However, for other lipophilic drugs the volume of distribution and volume of distribution/kg are decreased (digoxin, cyclosporin, propranolol) suggesting that factors other than lipid solubility effect tissue distribution [39].

Although histologic abnormalities are common on liver biopsy in morbidly obese patients, the clearance of most drugs that are hepatically metabolized is not reduced [43]. An exception to this rule are drugs such as methylprednisolone and popranolol in which hepatic clearance is markedly reduced [39, 44]. For drugs that are renally excreted, elimination will depend on the creatinine clearance. A higher glomerular filtration rate (GFR) has been reported in obese patients with normal renal function, and this will increase the clearance of drugs which are eliminated primarily by glomerular filtration [45]. In obese patients with renal dysfunction, the creatinine clearance, as calculated using standard formulae, correlates very poorly with the measured creatinine clearance [46]. Therefore, in the obese patient with renal dysfunction, the dosing regimen of renally excreted drugs should be based on the measured creatinine clearance [47].

▌ Nutritional Requirements

Although obese individuals have excess body fat stores and large lean body stores, they are likely to develop protein energy malnutrition in response to metabolic stress, particularly if their nutritional status was poor before injury [48, 49]. Nutrition should not be withheld from the obese patient in the mistaken belief that weight reduction is beneficial during critical illness. Indeed, malnutrition is a recognized risk that is associated with all bariatric surgery [50].

Obese patients have a higher respiratory quotient than non-obese patients presumably related to a block in both lipolysis and fat oxidation, resulting in a shift to the preferential use of carbohydrates which further accelerates body protein breakdown even further to fuel gluconeogenesis [51, 52]. It is unclear as to whether the ideal body weight or total body weight should be used in these equations. The obese patient's energy expenditure should therefore be measured by indirect calorimetry [53]. If indirect calorimetry is not available, patients should receive between 20 to 25 kcal/kg of ideal body weight/day [54]. Most of the calories should be given as carbohydrates with fats given to prevent essential fatty acid deficiency. It has been suggested that critically ill obese patients receive nutritional support with a hypocaloric high-protein formulation. It has been postulated that if adequate protein is supplied and obligatory glucose requirements are met, endogenous fat stores will be used for energy [55]. Protein requirements in the obese patient may be difficult to determine because of the increased lean body mass. Current consensus recommends a level of 1.5 to 2.0 g/kg of ideal body weight to achieve nitrogen equilibrium [54, 55].

▌ Gaining Vascular Access

One of the most challenging features of the morbidly obese patient is venous and arterial access. Poor peripheral venous sites in these patients necessitate more frequent use of central venous access. A short stubby neck, loss of physical landmarks and a greater skin-blood vessel distance make internal-jugular and subclavian vein cannulation technically difficult.

Obese patients have a higher incidence of catheter malpositions and local puncture complications, with catheter related infections and thromboses. Femoral venous access may not be possible as these patients usually have severe intertrigo. The use of Doppler ultrasound-guided techniques for obtaining central venous access in these patients is recommended [56].

Radiological Procedures

Bedside radiographs are of a very poor quality in the morbidly obese patient, limiting their diagnostic value. Abdominal and pelvic ultrasonography is limited by extensive abdominal wall and intra-abdominal fat. Percutaneous aspiration and drainage of intraperitoneal and retroperitoneal collections may be hindered by the obese body habitus. Many computed tomography tables have weight restrictions (about 350 lbs) that prohibit imaging of morbidly obese patients. In many situations, the authors have sent morbidly obese patients to the local Zoo to obtain computed tomography.

Conclusion

The management of the morbidly obese critically ill patient is a challenging and formidable task. A better understanding of the pathophysiologic changes that occur with obesity and the complications unique to this group of patients may improve their outcome.

References

1. National Institutes of Health (1985) Health implications of obesity: Consensus development conference statement. Ann Intern Med 103:147–151
2. Flegal KM, Carroll MD, Ogden CL, Johnson CL (2002) Prevalence and trends in obesity among US adults, 1999–2000. JAMA 288:1723–1727
3. Najjar MF, Rowland M (1987) Anthropometric reference data and prevalence of overweight, United States, 1976–1980. Vital and Health Statistics, Series 11, No 238. DHHS Pub. No. (PHS) 87–1688. Public Health Service. US Government Printing Office, Washington
4. Kuczmarski RJ, Flegal KM, Campbell SM, Johnson CL (1994) Increasing prevalence of overweight among US adults: The National Health and Nutrition Examination Surveys, 1960–1991. JAMA 272:205–211
5. VanItalie TB (1996) Prevalence of obesity. Endocrinol Metab Clin North Am 25:887–905
6. Fontaine KR, Redden DT, Wang C, Westfall AO, Allison DB (2003) Years of life lost due to obesity. JAMA 289:187–193
7. Calle EE, Thun MJ, Petrelli JM, Rodriguez C, Heath CW Jr (1999) Body-mass index and mortality in a prospective cohort of US adults. N Engl J Med 341:1097–1105
8. National Institutes of Health (1998) Clinical guidelines on the identification, evaluation, and treatment of overweight and obesity in adults. NIH Publication No. 98–4083. National Institutes of Health, Bethesda
9. Landi F, Onder G, Gambassi G, Pedone C, Carbonon PU, Bernaberi R (2000) Body mass index and mortality among hospitalized patients. Arch Intern Med 160:2641–2644
10. El Solh A, Sikka P, Bozkanat E, Jaafar W, Davies J (2001) Morbid obesity in the medical ICU. Chest 120:1989–1997
11. Marik P, Doyle H, Varon J (2003) Is obesity protective during critical illness? An analysis of a National ICU database. Crit Care Shock 6:156–162
12. Smith-Choban P, Weireter LJ, Maynes C (1991) Obesity and increased mortality in blunt trauma. J Trauma 31:1253–1257
13. Rose DK, Cohen MM, Wigglesworth DF, DeBoer DP (1994) Critical respiratory events in the postanesthesia care unit: patient, surgical and anesthetic factors. Anesthesiol 81:410–418
14. Goldhaber SZ, Goldstein E, Stampfer ML, Manson JE, Colditz GA, Speizer EE (1997) A prospective study of risk factors for pulmonary embolism in women. JAMA 277:642–645
15. Ray C, Sue D, Bray G, Hansen J, Wasserman K (1983) Effects of obesity on respiratory function. Am Rev Respir Dis 128:501–506

16. Lazarus R, Sparrow D, Weiss ST (1997) Effects of obesity and fat distribution on ventilatory function. The normative aging study. Chest 111:891–898
17. Douglas FG, Chong PY (1972) Influence of obesity on peripheral airway patency. J Appl Physiol 33:559–563
18. Collins LC, Hoberty PD, Walker JF, Fletcher EC, Petris AN (1995) The effect of body fat distribution on pulmonary function tests. Chest 107:1298–1302
19. Holley HS, Milic-Emili J, Becklake MR, Bates DV (1967) Regional distribution of pulmonary ventilation and perfusion in obesity. J Clin Invest 46:475–481
20. Drenick EJ, Fisler JS (1988) Sudden cardiac arrest in morbidly obese surgical patients unexplained after autopsy. Am J Surg 155:720–726
21. Vgontzas AN, Tan TL, Bixler EO, Martin LF, Shubert D, Kales A (1994) Sleep apnea and sleep disruption in obese patients. Arch Intern Med 154:1705–1711
22. Nowbar S, Burkart KM, Gonzales R, et al (2004) Obesity-associated hypoventilation in hospitalized patients: prevalence, effects, and outcome. Am J Med 116:1–7
23. Marik PE, Varon J (2001) Management of the critically ill obese patient. Crit Care Clin 17:187–200
24. Burns SM, Egloff UB, Ryan B, Carpenter R, Burns JE (1994) Effect of body position on spontaneous respiratory rate and tidal volume in patients with obesity, abdominal distension and ascites. Am J Crit Care 3:102–106
25. Vaughan RW, Conaham TJI (1980) Part I. Cardiopulmonary consequences of morbid obesity. Life Sci 26:2119–2127
26. Vaughan RW, Bauer S, Wise L (1975) Volume and pH of gastric juice in obese patients. Anesthesiol 43:686–689
27. Agarwal N, Shibutani K, San Filippo JA (1982) Hemodynamic and respiratory changes in surgery of the morbidly obese. Surgery 92:226–233
28. Pasulka PS, Bistrian BR, Benotti PN (1986) The risks of surgery in obese patients. Ann Intern Med 104:540–546
29. Clayton JK, Anderson JR, McNicol GP (1976) Preoperative prediction of postoperative deep vein thrombosis. BMJ 2:910–912
30. Kakkar VV, Howe CT, Nicolaides AN, Renney JT, Clarke M (1970) Deep vein thrombosis of the leg: is there a "high-risk" group. Am J Surg 120:527–530
31. Bern MM, Bothe AJ, Bistrian B, Batist G, Haywood H, Blackburn G (1983) Effects of low-dose warfarin on antithrombin III levels in morbidly obese patients. Surgery 94:78–83
32. Williamson JA, Webb RK, Szekely S, Gillies ER, Dreosti AV (1993) The Australian incident monitoring study. Difficult intubation: an analysis of 2000 incident reports. Anaesth Intensive Care 21:602–607
33. Backman L, Freyschuss U, Hallbert D, Melcher A (1983) Cardiovascular function in extreme obesity. Acta Med Scand 149:437–439
34. De Divitiis O, Fazio S, Peteto M, Maddalena G, Contaldo F, Mancini M (1981) Obesity and cardiac function. Circulation 64:477–480
35. Rexrode KM, Manson JE, Hennekens CH (1996) Obesity and cardiovascular disease. Curr Opin Cardiol 11:490–495
36. Nakajma T, Fujioka S, Tokunaga K, Hirobe K, Matsuzawa Y, Tarui S (1985) Noninvasive study of left ventricular performance in obese patients: influence of duration of obesity. Circulation 71:481–486
37. Alpert MA, Singh A, Terry BE, Kelly DL, Villareal D, Mukerji V (1989) Effect of exercise on left ventricular systolic function and reserve in morbid obesity. Am J Cardiol:63:1478–1482
38. Abernethy DR, Greenblatt DL (1986) Drug disposition in obese humans: An update. Clin Pharmacokinet 11:199–213
39. Cheymol G (1993) Clinical pharmacokinetics of drugs in obesity: An update. Clin Pharmacokinet 25:103–114
40. Blouin RA, Kolpek JH, Man HJ (1987) Influence of obesity on drug disposition. Clin Pharm 6:706–714
41. Abernethy DR, Greenblatt DJ (1982) Pharmacokinetics of drugs in obesity. Clin Pharmacokinet 7:108–124

42. Blouin RA, Chandler MH (1992) Special pharmacokinetic consideration in the obese. In: Evans WE, Schentag JJ, Jusko WJ (eds) Applied Pharmacokinetics: Principles of Therapeutic Drug Monitoring. 3rd ed. Lippincott, Williams and Wilkins, pp 1–20

43. Anderson T, Gluud C (1984) Liver morphology in morbid obesity: a literature study. Int J Obes 8:97–106

44. Caraco Y, Zylber-Katz E, Barry EM, Levy M (1995) Antipyrine disposition in obesity: evidence for negligible effect of obesity on hepatic oxidative metabolism. Eur J Clin Pharmacol 47:525–530

45. Blouin RA, Bauer LA, Miller DD, Record KE, Griffen WO (1982) Vancomycin pharmacokinetics in normal and morbidly obese subjects. Antimicrob Agents Chemother 21:575–580

46. Snider RD, Kruse JA, Bander JJ, Dunn GH (1995) Accuracy of estimated creatinine clearance in obese patients with stable renal function in the intensive care unit. Pharmacotherapy 15:474–453

47. Erstad BL (2004) Dosing of medications in morbidly obese patients in the intensive care unit setting. Intensive Care Med 30:18–32

48. Shikora SA, Muskat PC (1994) Protein-sparing modified-fast total parenteral nutrition formulation for a critically ill morbidly obese patient. Nutrition 10:155–158

49. Ireton-Jones CS, Francis C (1995) Obesity: Nutrition support practice and application to critical care. Nutr Clin Pract 10:144–149

50. Elliot K (2003) Nutritional considerations after bariatric surgery. Crit Care Nurs Q 26:133–138

51. Jeevanandam M, Young DH, Schiller WR (1991) Obesity and the metabolic response to severe multiple trauma in man. J Clin Invest 87:262–269

52. Jeevanandam M, Ramias L, Schiller WR (1991) Altered plasma amino acid levels in obese traumatized man. Metabolism 40:385–390

53. Makk LJK, McClave DSA, Creech PW (1990) Clinical application of the metabolic cart to the delivery of total parenteral nutrition. Crit Care Med 18:1320–1327

54. Burge JC, Goon A, Choban PS, Flancbaum L (1994) Efficacy of hypocaloric total parenteral nutrition in hospitalized obese patients: a prospective, double-blind randomized trial. JPEN J Parenter Enteral Nutr 18:203–207

55. Dickerson RN, Rosato EF, Mullen JL (1986) Net protein anabolism with hypocaloric parenteral nutrition in obese stressed patients. Am J Clin Nutr 44:747–755

56. Gratz I, Afshar M, Kidwell P, Weiman DS, Sharrif HM (1994) Doppler-guided cannulation of the internal jugular vein: a prospective randomized trial. J Clin Monit 10:185–188

Computers in the ICU: Fasten Your Seatbelts!

J. Decruyenaere and K. Colpaert

∎ Introduction

The intensive care unit (ICU) has several typical characteristics that make it favorable for computerization [1]. The first is that the ICU is an extremely data-intensive environment. The amount of data generated in the ICU can be so overwhelming that it often leads to data-overload and eventually to loss of information. Morris and Gardner [2] reported more than 236 different variable categories in a medical ICU record and concluded that this far exceeds human intellectual capability. It is estimated that humans are capable of adequately managing only 5 to 9 variables [3]. A second ICU characteristic is that the diagnostic-therapeutic cycle is very short compared to other medical disciplines. The diagnostic-therapeutic cycle is the cornerstone of medical decision-making. In every medical discipline, the physician makes a diagnosis by acquiring data and transforming this data by categorization into information (the probable diagnosis). According to this diagnosis, an appropriate therapy is chosen. The effect of this therapy on the underlying disease can only be evaluated by the acquisition and interpretation of new data. For most diseases, e.g., hypertension or cancer, this cycle takes months and even years. In contrast, in the ICU, the cycle is typically short, lasting from less than a minute to a maximum of a few weeks. It is evident that in such an environment, information technology can play a pivotal role in supporting and supervising the process of medical decision making.

A third ICU characteristic relevant to computerization is the fact that intensive care medicine is extremely expensive and consumes a very large portion of available health care resources. In the US, it is estimated that ICU medicine costs around 1% of the gross domestic product [4]. An integrated computerization of the ICU could optimize the use of resources on the management level. Even small-scale optimization, guided by an efficient information technology (IT) system, could lead to substantial cost savings.

∎ History

In 1946, the world's first all-electronic computer, ENIAC, was introduced, and although being monstrous (weighing over thirty tons) it was from this prototype that most other modern computers evolved. It already embodied almost all the components and concepts of today's high-speed, electronic digital computers. Shortly thereafter, the first commercially available computer was produced, but applications in medicine only started in the late 1950s when the National Institutes of Health (NIH) investigated the possibility of computer-based problem solving.

The first reports of the use of computers in the ICU were published by Stacy and Peters in 1965 [5], Shubin and Weil in 1966 [6], and Osborn et al. in 1968 [7]. Out of these first academic systems, commercial systems were developed. The first generation commercial systems (1972–1988) used minicomputers that were able to collect various data automatically from the bedside monitor. The second generation (1988–1994) used personal computers (PCs) and had more advanced user interface screens with graphical presentations based on the paper forms in use at the time. The third generation systems, in use since the last decade, made spectacular progress mainly related to improvements in network technologies, the use of client/server configurations with the deployment of a PC for every single bed, the introduction of relational databases, and the development of more reliable and robust connections with the different bedside devices.

▌ Current Situation

The development of an Intensive Care Information System (ICIS) is now so complex and time-consuming that on-site development is nearly impossible. The only realistic option is to buy a commercially available product which can afterwards be configured and adapted to match as far as possible the local needs of your ICU. Only a few bigger companies and maybe a dozen smaller companies currently offer dedicated software solutions for the ICU. None of the available software products are perfect and although they share many common features, they differ in smaller ways, resulting in product-specific advantages and disadvantages.

All of the software products share two main functions [1]:

▌ Recording and automatic storing of all monitoring data from the different monitoring devices surrounding the patient, of all respiratory data from the mechanical ventilator, and in some systems an automatic link to capture the infusion rate of the syringe pumps.

▌ The replacement of all handwritten forms by computerized equivalents such as the Computerized Physician Order Entry (CPOE) including the electronic prescribing of medication.

Most ICIS programs offer some basic form of workflow management and some even have basic alerting properties, but advanced computer decision support is still lacking.

▌ Key Factors for a Successful Implementation

Despite all the technological advances, successful ICIS implementation is still a challenge. In our experience, some key factors have to be realized, otherwise, the implementation of an ICIS could lead to disappointments (i.e., important time delays, additional costs, poor end-user acceptance) or even complete failure.

In our local implementation team, we identified the following important success strategies (without ranking of importance):

1) Do not rely on commercial information and demos (use them to gain a 'look and feel' of the program) but focus on frequent visits to ICUs where ICISs are already in use
2) Be sure to have upper management support (hospital management and hospital IT-Department)
3) Make a realistic financial plan with an estimation of the total cost of ICIS – ownership (cf. below)
4) Choose an IT company with a strong local presence, because extensive on-site support is essential during the whole implementation period
5) Make sure the company is financially healthy
6) Create a sense of ownership among end-users by asking for continuous input; poor end-user acceptance is still one of the major obstacles to successful implementation
7) Plan a realistic but stringent implementation time frame
8) Create a multidisciplinary local implementation team (including nurses and ICU physicians) and give them specific time facilities
9) Provide extensive training of the end-users before implementation; a special ICIS simulation environment to give the end-user education is extremely helpful
10) Provide extra nursing staff in the unit during the first weeks of the 'go-live' period
11) Install a dedicated around-the-clock ICIS help desk function during the first weeks of the 'go-live' period

▌ Cost of Ownership

The implementation of an ICIS is expensive. Typically, only the costs for hardware and software are taken into account, however, they represent only a part (typically a quarter to a third) of the 'Total Cost of Ownership'. The 'Total Cost of Ownership' can be defined as the total cost of acquiring, installing, using, maintaining, changing, upgrading and disposing of an IT-system over its predicted useful lifespan. In cost/benefit analyses, 'Total Cost of Ownership' represents the cost side.

In our ICU, we implemented an ICIS in the 22 bed surgical unit. It consists of an advanced ICIS with full connections to monitors, ventilators, and syringe pumps and is also interfaced with the Hospital Information System (HIS) for administrative data and lab results. The implementation resulted in a paperless ICU. The 'Total Cost of Ownership' of this advanced 22 bed ICIS was calculated at 1 307 166 Euro over an estimated 5-year lifespan period, which corresponds to 11 883 Euro per ICU bed per year (approximately $ 15 234 per ICU bed per year) [8]. It is clear that the initial hardware and software purchase price of around 25 000 Euro per bed was only a fraction of the 'Total Cost of Ownership'.

▌ Potential Benefits

In contrast to costs, benefits of IT-systems are much harder to measure and prove. For managers only direct financial benefits are important, however, an immediate financial return of investment is – at least now – hardly achievable. Non-financial benefits can be more important, such as improving the quality of care, decreasing the length of stay in the ICU and perhaps eventually achieving a higher survival rate. In an indirect way and seen over a longer time span, this also leads to minimizing ICU costs.

Time

As far as we know, there are no reports on time utilization of ICU physicians comparing a computerized versus a traditional paper-based unit. Several studies, however, have investigated the impact on nurse time. The older studies showed no time benefit [9–11], but a recent well-designed study showed that the introduction of an ICIS in a cardiovascular unit reduced documentation time of the nurses by 29 minutes for every 8 hour shift [12]. This time was completely re-allocated to direct patient care.

We have not performed a study in our ICU, but nurses generally experience the new system as time-neutral. However, it is important to take into consideration that the computer-based ICU file is now much more complete and accurate. Concerning the ICU physicians, the workload is considerably higher, especially for physicians in training but again, the amount and quality of the patient information is substantially more valuable.

Computerized Physician Order Entry (CPOE)

In 1999, the institute of Medicine declared in their report "To Err is Human – Building a safer Health System" that at least 44 000, and perhaps as many as 98 000, patients die in US hospitals each year as a result of medical errors, of which at least 7000 are due to medication errors alone [13]. These errors are frequently a result of problems with the paper-based medical record and order entry system. As a result of this study, the Leapfrog group was founded, which strongly recommends that hospitals and other health care entities institute CPOE [14]. Not only do adverse drug events (ADE) cause patient harm, their costs are estimated by Classen et al. [15] to be at least $ 2000 per ADE. Because of the continuously increasing number of drugs available, dosing regimen complexity, changing drug indications, numerous contraindications and adverse effects, the physician's memory is not always a reliable bridge between research advances and clinical practice. And although many physicians still deny its negative effect, long working hours and sleep deprivation also can predispose medical professionals to fatigue-induced medication errors in the ICU [16].

The power of a CPOE system lies in its ability to help physicians prescribe medications by recognizing drug allergies and drug interactions, by showing relevant laboratory results, by automatically calculating the correct drug dose, by recommending dosage adjustments in renal or hepatic failure, and by showing guidelines supported by evidence-based best practices. These features help minimize human error, improve medication management, facilitate reporting, and improve resource utilization. Even in its most basic form, a CPOE system can already tremendously reduce the number of illegible or poorly written prescriptions, which can lead to the wrong drug, wrong dose or wrong route of administration. Bates et al. [17] evaluated the impact of CPOE in general wards, and found that the number of non-intercepted serious medication errors decreased by 86% after its implementation.

In another study, the same author [18] studied the impact of a modest CPOE system (general ward and ICU) and showed that it decreased non-intercepted serious medication errors by more than 55%. A reduction of time spent handling medications (dispensing and administration) demonstrates that electronic solutions can help free up time for direct patient contact and care. Implementation of a combination of CPOE with a more sophisticated computerized decision support system for prescribing antibiotics, as shown by Evans et al. [19], was associated with a significant reduction in the cost of antibiotics, total costs, and length of hospital stay. Only a few studies have been published evaluating the impact of CPOE on medication errors in the ICU, most of them being carried out in pediatric ICUs. They all showed at least a significant decrease in medication errors, and one resulted in a significant but less substantial effect on potential adverse drug events [20]. Also, the medication turn-around time and ancillary service response time was shortened tremendously. A recent prospective study conducted in our adult surgical ICU demonstrated an impressive decrease in medication prescription errors after the implementation of an ICIS (26.5 vs. 3.6%, $p<0.001$) (Fig. 1) [21]. This was mainly due to the almost complete elimination of true prescription errors and incorrect orders, which have no real potential to cause serious harm. However, there was also a three-fold decrease in the more important non-intercepted serious medication errors (Fig. 2). In particular, dosing errors in renal failure patients were significantly reduced, due to the built-in dosing prescribing aid. Although most of these reports show a positive impact on healthcare, the generalized introduction of CPOE for medication is still hampered by technological problems (e.g., unavailability of bug-free software, interfacing with the pharmacy department) and by the associated high implementation costs. However until now, impact on mortality could not be proven, since all studies were underpowered.

Decision Support and Computerized Guidelines

A good physician has the ability to make sound clinical judgments. Traditionally, medical decision-making was considered an intuitive process, however more recently, formal methods using computer-assisted medical decision-making have been applied to medical problem-solving [22].

Computer decision support in the ICU can be used in the following areas:

- Interpretation of data – for example, interpretation of respiratory or hemodynamic parameters
- Alerts – for example, notification of a possible drug interaction at the time a new drug is ordered, or – more experimental – notification of the detection of a pattern in several variables compatible with a sepsis in an early phase
- Diagnoses – for example early detection of renal dysfunction or detection of nosocomial infections
- Treatment suggestions – for example suggestions about the most effective antibiotics to order

Some ICISs already have basic alerting possibilities but sophisticated computer-based decision support is still a sort of 'Holy Grail'. The lack of computerized decision support is not only a technological problem but is also due to a lack of well-tested, effective and universally-accepted decision support models and rules for the ICU [23].

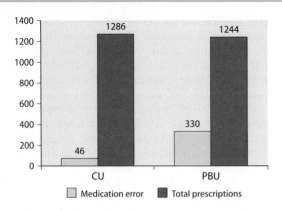

Fig. 1. Number of medication errors according to total number of prescriptions per unit. CU = Computerized Unit vs. PBU = Paper-based Unit; CU = 3.6% vs. PBU = 26.5% p < 0.001

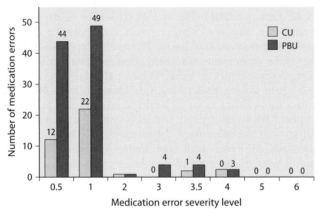

Fig. 2. Number of medication errors according to level of severity in a Computerized Unit (CU) vs. a Paper-Based Unit (PBU) excluding level 0 errors. (Level of Severity: 0 = true prescription error, incomplete order, which have limited potential to cause harm; 0.5 = potential adverse drug event, intercepted; 1 = error occurred but without harm to the patient; 2 = error which required monitoring, no harm; 3 = change in vital signs, increased need of monitoring or laboratory tests, eventually no harm; 3.5 = temporary harm, needing treatment/intervention; 4 = cf. Level 3.5, with increased length of stay; 5 = permanent harm; 6 = death)

However, Morris et al. have already developed extensive and detailed computer-based treatment guidelines. These guide the clinician by using imbedded decision rules and combining them with the actual physiological data of the patient to provide immediate bedside decision support [24, 25].

ICU Management and Research

An ICIS database is an essential tool for benchmarking, for comparing ICU performance using standardized outcomes and for controlling ICU costs [26].

An even greater potential lies in ICU research. Using large databases, which combine data from different centers, will undoubtedly lead to significant research advances and more specifically in outcome research. Problems remain in efficiently joining databases from different centers. Furthermore, there are the known problems of ensuring data quality and of querying the right data in the right way [27, 28].

▌ Future Trends

Despite all the progress and the fact that currently available ICISs have succeeded in providing a paperless ICU, many of the above mentioned benefits have yet to be realized. Many problems remain: a too rigid user-interface, the technological complexity of the systems, the poor integration of ICISs with other hospital information systems, and the high 'Total Cost of Ownership'. All these factors help to explain the fact that after decades of development, only a minority (probably less than 5%) of ICU departments currently make use of one of the available systems. Another essential factor is that current ICISs still offer no, or very limited, real-time bedside decision support.

Recently, important new insights in the design of complex and maintainable software systems such as object orientation, component-based programming, distributed systems, agent-based systems and web services have been developed. As a result, future ICISs will make use of whole collections of smaller specialized software programs, called intelligent agents [1]. By the definition of King [29], an intelligent agent is considered to be a computer surrogate for a person or a process that fulfils a stated need or activity. The surrogate entity provides decision-making capabilities that are similar to the described intentions of a human. It is important, however, to realize that software agents will provide support for physicians and will never replace them completely.

An intelligent agent has to perform a clearly defined or delimited task. In the ICU, typically tens of smaller tasks are performed simultaneously. Medications are added and changed, infusion pump rates have to be continuously adapted according to specific monitoring parameters (e.g., insulin pump according to blood glucose levels) and antibiotic therapy is guided by clinical parameters, microbiological, and radiological results. In most cases, a hierarchy of agents will be needed. In the prescription of medication, one agent can be responsible for the right dosing in renal failure, another for the right dosing in hepatic failure, another agent can check for interaction between other medications given to the patient, and a last agent can check if it is not cheaper and feasible to give the same medication by the oral or enteral routes. One of the most attractive features of an intelligent agent lies in the fact that a high level task that ICU physicians are now performing (e.g., adapting the insulin pump rate) corresponds completely with the dedicated task of the corresponding specific intelligent agent. The ICIS of the future will be far easier to understand, to maintain, and to change, when a corresponding match on a high abstract level exists between the real life task and a software component [1].

The internal implementation of the agent is encapsulated, which means that the function of the agent and the way this function is implemented is completely separated. This allows replacement of agents with newer versions performing exactly the same tasks but implemented in a completely different way (e.g., rule-based agent versus an agent working with a neuronal network algorithm). This replacement can be done without recompilation of the software application.

The best way to understand the implementation of intelligent agents (and also their variant 'web services') is to think about Lego blocks. These plastic toy bricks come in different colors, shapes, and sizes, but all Lego blocks have the same standardized studs and corresponding holes that allow them to be assembled, taken apart, and reassembled in all sorts of creative ways [30].

ICU bed decision intelligent agents can therefore be developed worldwide by several independent teams, provided agreement on a universal interface can be reached. This will accelerate considerably the development of the future ICIS and will reduce the total workload by avoiding doing the same job repeatedly in different centers.

One of the biggest hurdles for the widespread acceptance of computers in the ICU is the complexity of the technology, which demands the ICU physician to be an IT expert. This will change in the future. To quote an article in *The Economist* [30]: "Consider another complex technology like a car. Driving a car in the early 1900s required skill in lubricating various moving parts, sending oil manually to the transmission, setting the choke and knowing what to do if the car broke down, which it invariable did. People at the time hired chauffeurs, mostly because they needed to have a mechanic at hand to fix the car, just as firms today need IT staff to sort out their computers". In the next decade, complexity will of course increase, in the same way that current cars are more complex than the cars of the early 1900s, but complexity will be pushed completely to the background to make the front end for the user extremely simple.

▌ Conclusion

Computers have been used for more than thirty years in the ICU and currently available programs are now able to automatically record all monitoring data and replace all paper forms by an electronic equivalent, resulting in a paperless ICU and, already, in important quality benefits [12, 21, 31].

However, widespread implementation is still lacking due to the high implementation costs, the complexity of hardware and software configuration, interfacing problems with other hospital departments, the lack of proven benefits, the fear that computers will replace physicians in decision making, and concerns about security.

Recently, important new insights in the design of complex and maintainable software-systems such as object-orientation, component-based programming, distributed systems, agent-based systems, and web-services have been developed. This will lead to a completely new 4th generation of ICIS, which have the potential to ensure all the above mentioned benefits.

It is our conviction that within ten years, full ICU computerization including advanced real-time and bedside decision making capabilities will become essential to guarantee the highest quality of care for every patient, to optimize nurse and physician work flow, to ensure economical ICU management, and last but not least, to support advanced research by using large multicenter patient databases.

The ever-increasing complexity of the technology will become completely hidden for the end-user, as has been the case with every maturing technology. Fourth generation ICISs will be extremely user-friendly and future ICU physicians will not have to be IT-experts, but can focus completely on their core task, caring for the critically ill. Leading IT-companies worldwide have already started developing this new 4th generation of ICISs. After more than 30 years, the plane is finally taking off the runway – fasten your seatbelts!

References

1. Decruyenaere J, De Turck F, Vanhastel S, Vandermeulen F, Demeester P, De Moor G (2003) On the design of a generic and scalable multilayer software architecture for data flow management in the intensive care unit. Methods Inf Med 42:79–88
2. Morris A, Gardner R (1992) Computer applications. In: Hall J, Schmidt G, Wood L (eds) Principles of Critical Care. Mc Graw-Hill, New York, pp 500–514
3. Miller (1956) The magical number seven plus or minus two. Some limits on our capacity for processing information. Psychol Rev 63:81–97
4. Fein I (1993) The critical care unit. In search of management. Crit Care Clin 9:401–413
5. Stacy R, Peters R (1965) Computations of respiratory mechanical parameters. In: Waxman BD, Stacy R (eds) Computers in Biomedical Research. Academic Press, New York
6. Shubin H, Weil M (1966) Efficient monitoring with a digital computer of cardiovascular function in seriously ill patients. Ann Intern Med 65:453–460
7. Osborn J, Beaumont J, Raison J, et al (1968) Measurement and monitoring of acutely ill patients with digital computer. Surgery 64:1057–1070
8. Decruyenaere J, Danneels C, Verwaeren G, Myny D, Oeyen S, Colpaert K (2004) Calculation of the total cost of ownership of an intensive care information system. Crit Care Med 32 (Suppl):A116 (abst)
9. Pierpont G, Thilgen D (1995) Effect of computerized charting on nursing activity in intensive care. Crit Care Med 23:1067–1073
10. Menke J, Broner C, Campbell D, Mc Kissick M, Edwards-Beckett J (2001) Computerized clinical documentation system in the pediatric intensive care unit. BMC Med Inform Decis Mak 1:3
11. Maracovic D, Kenney C, Elliott D, Sindhusake D (1997) A comparison of nursing activities associated with manual and automated documentation in an Australian intensive care unit. Comput Nurs 15:205–211
12. Bosman R, Rood E, Oudemans-van Straaten H, Van der Spoel J, Wester J, Zandstra D (2003) Intensive care information system reduces documentation time of the nurses after cardiothoracic surgery. Intensive Care Med 29:83–90
13. Kohn L, Corrigan J, Donaldson M (1999) In: To Err is Human: Building a safer Health Care System. National Academy Press, Washington DC
14. The Leapfrog Group for Patient Safety Mission. Available at: *http://www.leapfroggroup.org*
15. Classen D, Pestotnik S, Evans R, Lloyd J, Burke J (1997) Adverse drug events in hospitalized patients: excess length of stay, extra costs, and attributable mortality. JAMA 277:301–306
16. Landrigan C, Rothschild J, Cronin J, et al (2004) Effect of reducing interns' work hours on serious medical errors in intensive care units. N Engl J Med 351:1838–1848
17. Bates D, Teich J, Lee J, Segher D (1999) The impact of computerized physician order entry on medication error prevention. J Am Med Inform Assoc 6:313–321
18. Bates D, Leape L, Cullen D, et al (1998) Effect of computerized physician order entry and a team intervention on prevention of serious medication errors. JAMA 280:1311–1316
19. Evans R, Classen D, Perstotnik S, Lundsgaarde H, Bucke J (1994) Improving empiric antibiotic selection using computer decision support. Arch Intern Med 154:878–884
20. Potts A, Barr F, Gregory D (2004) Computerized physician order entry and medication errors in a pediatric critical care unit. Pediatrics 113:59–63
21. Colpaert K, Claus B, Somers A, Vandewoude K, Oeyen S, Decruyenaere J (2004) Medication errors in the intensive care unit: comparison between computerized versus paper-based physician order entry. Crit Care Med 32 (Suppl):A351 (abst)
22. Gardner M, Shabot M (2001) Patient-monitoring systems. In: Shortliffe E, Perreault L (eds) Medical Informatics: Computer Applications in Health Care And Biomedicine. Springer, New York, pp 443–484
23. Morris A (2000) Developing and implementing computerized protocols for standardization of clinical decisions. Ann Intern Med 132:373–383
24. McKinley B, Moore F, Sailors R, et al (2001) Computerized decision support for mechanical ventilation of trauma induced ARDS: Results of a randomized clinical trial. J Trauma 50: 415–424

25. East T, Heerman L, Bradshaw R, et al (1999) Efficacy of computerized decision support for mechanical ventilation: Results of a prospective multicenter multi-center randomized trial. Proc AMIA Symp:251–255
26. Ward N, Levy M (2001) Clinical information systems in the ICU. In: Vincent JL (ed) Yearbook of Intensive Care and Emergency Medicine. Springer, Heidelberg, pp 685–694
27. Pronovost R, Angus D (1999) Using large-scale databases to measure outcomes in critical care. Crit Care Clin 15:615–631
28. Ward N (2004) Using computers for Intensive Care Unit Research. Respir Care 49:518–524
29. King J (1995) Intelligent agents: bringing good things to live. AI Expert 2:17–19
30. The Economist (2004) Make it simple: a survey of information technology. The Economist October 30th Special Issue 1–20
31. Fraenkel D, Cowie M, Daley P (2003) Quality benefits of an intensive care clinical information system. Crit Care Med 31:120–125

Reducing ICU Mortality: To what Extent?

P. H. J. van der Voort

▌ Introduction

In clinical intensive care research, mortality in the intensive care unit (ICU), or hospital mortality, including time after ICU treatment, is often used as an endpoint. Indeed, mortality is a solid endpoint and reaching this endpoint is beyond doubt. It may be seen as the best and ultimate endpoint we can have in ICU research. Around 10 to 15% of all patients admitted in Dutch ICUs will die in the ICU and another 5% after ICU discharge while still in the hospital (Fig. 1). However, the absolute mortality rate is not informative enough. For purposes of evaluation, prognostic models like APACHE, SAPS, and MPM can be used to predict in-hospital mortality. The ratio of the observed mortality to the predicted mortality creates a standardized mortality ratio (SMR). The SMR is a severity of disease adjusted mortality rate.

▌ Mortality as a Study Endpoint

The relatively high incidence of mortality in the ICU makes this endpoint valuable. Although as clinicians we try to reduce mortality, a high mortality incidence is attractive from a statistical viewpoint. For example, selective decontamination of the digestive tract (SDD) in liver transplantation does not obviously reduce mortality in single studies nor in a meta-analysis [1]. Given the in-hospital mortality rate after liver transplantation of around 10%, mortality is not a suitable endpoint for the available data in liver transplantation patients. This problem is often referred to as insufficient power. A large study population can resolve this problem but may be difficult to col-

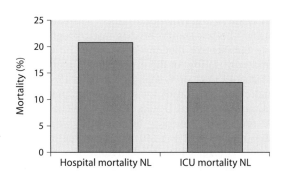

Fig. 1. Hospital and intensive care mortality in the Netherlands

Table 1. Studies on interventions shown to reduce ICU mortality

	Trial [ref.]	Patient group	Abs Mort Control group (%)	Abs Mort Treatment group (%)	Abs Mort Reduction (%)	Rel Mort Reduction (%)	OR	RR
1	SDD [2]	Mixed	31.2	24.2	7.0	22.4	0.70	0.91
2	ARDSnet [3]	Mixed	39.8	31	8.8	22	0.68	0.87
3	Intensive insulin [4]	Mixed	26.3	16.8	9.5	36.1	0.57	0.89
4	APC [5]	Severe sepsis	30.8	24.7	6.1	19.8	0.74	0.92
5	Steroids [6]	Septic shock	72	61	11	15	0.53	0.92

Abs Mort: absolute mortality; Rel Mort: relative mortality; OR: odds ratio; RR: relative risk

lect (for instance, liver transplantation patients). At present, the relatively high in-hospital mortality of 30% for septic patients or other ICU patients with multiple organ failure is attractive from an epidemiological and statistical viewpoint. An even higher mortality is reported for septic shock (Table 1). Although attractive for statisticians, clinicians would rather reduce mortality or eliminate it. Recently, several interventions have been reported that by themselves reduce mortality of ICU patients substantially. Older medications have also now been shown to reduce mortality when they are used according to new standards (steroids, insulin, SDD). In addition, a new medication is now available (activated protein C, drotrecogin alfa (activated)). An adjusted use of the mechanical ventilator can save lives compared to traditional ways of administering mechanical ventilation.

∎ Odds Ratios

The crude odds ratios and absolute (hospital) mortality reduction for these interventions from the original studies are shown in Table 1. At present, it is unknown what the effect of a combination of these interventions will be on mortality rates. It usually takes years for strategies to be implemented in daily practice. Therefore, the current incidence of mortality in a standard ICU cannot be seen as the lowest possible mortality rate. However, we can make estimations on theoretical grounds.

Principles of prognostic diagnostic tests using prior and posterior odds as well as chances and likelihood ratios can be used for other purposes as well. In that scenario, the test should be diagnostic/prognostic for death. The result of using multiple consecutive diagnostic tests can be predicted by multiplying likelihood ratios and odds ratios. In the estimation of mortality rates when applying four live saving strategies (1–4 or 1–3 plus 5 in Table 1) we should multiply odds ratios. The product of all odds ratios for severe sepsis patients is 0.20. This means that for a person admitted to the ICU with an *a priori* chance for dying of 40% it might be possible to reduce the mortality to 20% of the *a priori* mortality rate, resulting in an absolute mortality of 8% (40×0.2). For septic shock patients, the product of the odds ratios is 0.14, which might reduce mortality from 70 to 10%. It is difficult to believe that these tremendous mortality reductions can be obtained.

Odds Ratio versus Relative Risk

The answer to this doubt is that we should be aware of the fact that odds ratios overestimate the effect when a relatively high chance for the event (death) is apparent. Zhang and Yu determined the magnitude of the difference of odds ratio and relative risk in several situations [7]. Mortality rates in the treatment groups of 16 to 31% (Table 1) show that the event occurs frequently. Instead of odds ratios, a more realistic description of the effect is relative risk. In Table 1, relative risks are shown for five interventions, calculated from the original publication data. The product of four relative risks is 0.65 (1–4 or 1–3 and 5). That means that for a person entering the ICU with a chance for dying of 40% it should be possible to reduce the absolute mortality rate for severe sepsis patients to 40×0.65 = 26% and for septic shock patients (*a priori* chance for dying 72%) to 45%. In contrast, the product of odds ratios resulted in mortality rates of 8 and 10% respectively.

It is interesting to see that relative risks for all proven mortality reduction interventions are around 0.90 (while odds ratios range from 0.53 to 0.70). When the SMR is used to evaluate outcome and an SMR of 1 is basically the result of standard intensive care treatment, than it is possible to predict outcome in patients where the interventions are implemented. For instance, in an ICU where SDD and glucose regulation are implemented, roughly a SMR of 1.0×0.9×0.9 = 0.81 may be reached for the patients receiving these two interventions.

Hypothesis Testing in a Standard ICU

The hospital mortality data for the ICU in the Medical Center Leeuwarden (MCL) over time are shown in Figure 2. A gradual decrease in the SMR is shown. Over time, some of the life-saving strategies have been implemented: Steroids, SDD, low tidal volume ventilation, and intensive insulin therapy. These are all interventions that can be applied to the majority of ICU patients admitted with multiple organ

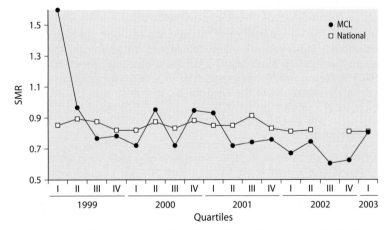

Fig. 2. Standardized mortality ratio (SMR) based on APACHE II mortality prediction for the Medical Center Leeuwarden (MCL) compared to national data over a 4-year period

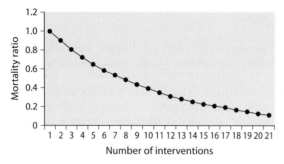

Fig. 3. The prediction of mortality ratios with an increasing number of interventions. For all interventions a relative risk of 0.9 is used for this calculation. With an increasing number of interventions the decline in mortality ratio decreases

failure. Theoretically, the SMR would be reduced to $1.0 \times 0.9 \times 0.9 \times 0.9 \times 0.9 = 0.66$. Indeed, the SMR has fallen to around 0.7. The use of activated protein C will affect severe sepsis patients but will not reduce the overall SMR substantially because the absolute number of patients being treated with activated protein C will be low.

How Far can we Reduce Mortality?

When increasingly more interventions that reduce mortality are implemented, the mortality rate will be further reduced. However, the absolute mortality rate will decrease with an increasing number of effective interventions (Fig. 3). For new trials in that situation, the *a priori* chance for dying, when mortality is the primary endpoint, is relatively low. The number of patients in new trials should be increased to show a mortality reduction leading to larger and larger trials.

Conclusion

In conclusion, all interventions recently shown to be effective have a relative risk of around 0.9. Odds ratios are not sufficient in intensive care studies with mortality is an endpoint when mortality is a common outcome. An increasing number of mortality reducing interventions will lead to a decrease in absolute mortality reduction per intervention and to the need for larger trials.

References

1. Nathens AB, Marshall JC (1999) Selective decontamination of the digestive tract in surgical patients. Arch Surg 134:170–176
2. De Jonge E, Schultz MJ, Spanjaard L, et al (2002) Effects of selective decontamination of the digestive tract on mortality and antibiotic resistance. Intensive Care Med 28 (suppl 1):S12 (Abst)
3. The Acute Respiratory Distress Syndrome Network (2000) Ventilation with lower tidal volumes as compared with traditional tidal volumes for acute lung injury and the acute respiratory distress syndrome. N Engl J Med 342:1301–1308

4. Van den Berghe G, Wouters P, Weekers F, et al (2001) Intensive insulin therapy in critically ill patients. N Engl J Med 345:1359–1367
5. Bernard GR, Vincent JL, Laterre PF, et al (2001) Efficacy and safety for recombinant human activated protein C for severe sepsis. N Engl J Med 344:699–709
6. Annane D, Sebille V, Charpentier C, et al (2002) Effect of treatment with low doses of hydrocortisone and fludrocortisone on mortality in patients with septic shock. JAMA 288:862–871
7. Zhang J, Yu KF (1998) What's the relative risk? A method of correcting the odds ratio in cohort studies of common outcomes. JAMA 280:1690–1691

Improving Palliative Care
for Patients in the Intensive Care Unit

J. R. Curtis

▮ Introduction

Because of the severity of illness, the intensive care unit (ICU) is a setting where death is common. A recent study suggests that approximately 20% of all deaths in the USA occur in the ICU which translates to approximately 540 000 Americans who die in the ICU each year [1]. This proportion varies dramatically in different parts of the world. The geographic variation in end-of-life care in the ICU reflects both cultural and religious variation in the approach of clinicians as well as variation in the availability of ICU beds [2, 3]. A recent study in Europe showed dramatic variation in the approach to end-of-life care across Europe with particular differences noted between the north and the south [2]. Undoubtedly, some component of geographic variation represents appropriate differences based on the cultural differences in different areas, while some of the variation represents an opportunity to improve the quality of care in some places.

Despite this important geographical variation, studies throughout the developed world have shown that the majority of deaths in the ICU involve withholding or withdrawing life-sustaining therapies [4–7]. Thus, the ICU represents a setting where decisions about managing the dying and death of patients are made on a frequent basis. These decisions involve a determination of the goals of care, communication among the clinicians in the ICU, and communication between clinicians and the patient and his or her family. Decision-making and communication about end-of-life care can be difficult for clinicians in many settings, but may be especially difficult in the ICU because the culture and mission of the ICU is oriented to saving lives.

Palliative care can be defined broadly as interdisciplinary care for persons with life-threatening illness or injury that addresses physical, emotional, social, and spiritual needs and seeks to improve quality of life and minimize symptoms and distress for the patient and his or her family. Using this definition, palliative care is obviously an important component of the care that we provide to all patients in all settings, including the ICU. Palliative care, more narrowly defined, is also a specialty using unique expertise and up-to-date interventions to deliver high quality care to patients with terminal or life-limiting illness or injury, especially in the setting where that illness or injury cannot be cured or reversed. There is a growing recognition that integrating palliative care into the care that we provide to all patients can enhance the experiences of care for patients and their families. In the ICU, this can and should be done in two complementary ways: training all clinicians in the skills of palliative care and using the expertise of palliative care specialists and consultants. Palliative care is much more than 'end-of-life care' or 'comfort care', although end-of-life care and comfort care are important components of palliative care. Palliative care also includes careful decision-making about the goals of care, pain and symptom management, and communication about the goals of care that should be applied to all patients with a life-threatening illness.

In the past year or two, a number of important studies have been published concerning the integration of palliative care into the ICU. This review will cover four topics important for providing high quality palliative care in the ICU setting with an emphasis on the recent advances. The topics include:

▌ decision-making about the goals of care,
▌ communication within the medical team and with patients and families
▌ symptom assessment and management, and
▌ provision of high quality care in the setting of withholding or withdrawing life-sustaining treatments.

A series of interventions in each of these four categories that can improve the quality of palliative care in the ICU are shown in Table 1.

Table 1. Interventions that can improve quality of palliative care in the ICU

Intervention	References
Decision-making about goals of care	
▌ Value end-of-life and palliative care and routinely include it on rounds and in the medical record incorporating psychological, emotional, and spiritual aspects of caring for critically ill patients	[14]
▌ Convene multi-disciplinary rounds and explicitly review the goals of care for each patient	[36]
▌ Facilitate early communication within the team and with the family to discuss goals, prognoses, and treatment options	[13, 17–19, 44]
▌ Ensure access to effective palliative or ethics consultation	[13, 17–19, 44]
Communication within the team and with the patient and family	
▌ Schedule formal family conferences with specific talking points early in ICU course	[13, 30]
▌ Educate critical care clinicians in specific aspects of communication with families including listening to family and running effective, supportive family conferences	[13, 30, 31]
▌ Liberalize family visiting hours	[51]
Pain and symptom assessment and treatment	
▌ Clearly establishing goals of care can improve symptom management in dying patients	[14]
▌ Clinicians should anticipate and treat procedure-related pain and symptoms	[37, 40]
Withholding and withdrawing life-sustaining treatments	
▌ Use protocols for withholding and withdrawing life sustaining treatments	[49]
▌ Provide nurses with documentation standards for withholding and withdrawing life sustaining treatments	[49]

▌ Decision-making about the Goals of Care

Increasingly the ICU has become the place where patients, their families, and clinicians make the difficult transition from care oriented primarily toward curing disease and prolonging life to care oriented primarily toward patient comfort and dignity. The ethical and legal principles of autonomy, beneficence, futility, surrogate decision-making, and the justification for use of medication to relieve pain even when it may unintentionally hasten death (often called the principle of "double effect") are generally well accepted in the critical care community. Despite the general agreement on these principles, there is evidence that critical care clinicians vary greatly in their approaches to decisions about the goals of care in the ICU setting. For example, using a cross-sectional survey design with a series of hypothetical scenarios, Cook and colleagues showed that critical care physicians and nurses showed tremendous variability in the goals of care they thought most appropriate for a series of different patient presentations [8]. Similarly, in a retrospective chart review, Curtis and colleagues showed dramatic geographic variation in the decisions to withhold intensive care for patients dying of human immunodeficiency virus (HIV)-related *Pneumocystis carinii* pneumonia that was not accounted for by severity of the pneumonia or the underlying HIV disease [3]. Prendergast and colleagues surveyed critical care physicians showing dramatic variation across the USA in the proportion of patients dying in an ICU who have life-sustaining treatments withheld or withdrawn [9]. Similar variability has been shown in a cross-sectional survey and a prospective observational study across Europe [2, 10].

A recent multicenter, international observational study by Cook and colleagues demonstrated that two of the most powerful predictors of the decision to withhold or withdraw life-sustaining treatments were the attending physician's prediction of the patient's probability of survival, and that physician's assessment of the patient's preferences regarding end-of-life care [11]. This study suggests that physicians bear profound responsibility to be certain that their survival predictions are sound and that their impressions of patients' preferences for end-of-life care are well founded.

One of the greatest challenges to improving palliative care in the ICU is identifying patients who should be targeted for routine 'palliative care' interventions. For example, the SUPPORT study was a randomized trial that targeted seriously ill patients with one or more of nine specific illnesses with illness-specific markers of a predicted median survival of 6–12 months [12]. A recent before-after study testing a communication intervention in the ICU focused on patients who had a predicted length of ICU stay longer than 5 days or a predicted mortality of greater than 25% as estimated by the attending physician [13]. Prognostic models, such as APACHE, could also be used to identify those patients at highest risk for death, although such models are limited in their ability to accurately predict the risk of death for an individual patient. Palliative care, using a broad definition that incorporates symptom management and communication about goals of therapy, is obviously applicable to most critically ill patients. However, identifying those patients and families who will benefit from palliative care interventions is a more challenging task and one that can be operationalized in many ways.

Decision-making in the ICU involves complex relations between physicians, nurses, and other clinical members of the critical care team, as well as interactions between these groups of clinicians and the patient and their family. Since less than 5% of ICU patients are able to communicate with clinicians at the time that these decisions are made, clinicians and/or families make most of these decisions [4].

There is tremendous geographic variation in the role of these individuals in making decisions. There are some locations where the family have no legal standing in decision-making and the goal of clinician-family communication is one of providing education and support. There are other places where clinicians ask family members to make the decisions about withdrawing life support in a way that many believe is inappropriate. There is growing consensus that some form of shared-decision-making is the most appropriate model for making decisions about withholding and withdrawing life support [14]. The degree of sharing of responsibility may vary based on cultural norms and also on patient and family preferences for role in decision-making [15]. A recent study from France showed that half the family members of critically ill patients did not want to be involved in decision-making and of those family members that did want to be involved, only a minority reported they were involved [16]. Therefore, an important role for the critical care clinician is to assess the role that family members want to play in decision-making.

There have been a number of studies during the last few years that have suggested that routine palliative care or ethics consultation for many patients in the ICU can improve the quality of care. Schneiderman and colleagues performed a randomized controlled trial of a routine ethics consultation for patients "in whom value-related treatment conflicts arose" [17]. They found that routine ethics consultation reduced the number of days that patients spent in the ICU and hospital, suggesting that these consultations reduced the prolongation of dying. In addition, families and clinicians reported a high level of satisfaction with ethics consultations, although satisfaction was not compared with the group that was randomized not to receive an ethics consultation. Similarly, in a before-after study design, Campbell and Guzman showed that routine palliative care consultation reduced the number of ICU days for patients with anoxic encephalopathy after cardiac arrest and for patients with multiple organ failure [18]. Other studies, both before-after designs and randomized trials, have also suggested the benefit of ethics or palliative care consultation in the ICU setting [19, 20]. Therefore, the weight of this recent evidence suggests that palliative care or ethics specialists may have an important role to play in the ICU setting to improve quality of care received by critically ill patients and their families. These specialists likely facilitate high quality care both by helping clarify the goals of care earlier and by helping with communication within the team and with the family.

▌ Communication with Patients and Families and within the ICU team

Several studies have shown that family members with loved ones in the ICU rate communication with the critical care clinicians as one of the most important skills for these clinicians [21]. In fact, most families of critically ill patients rate clinicians' communication skills as equally or more important than clinical skills [21]. Furthermore, observational studies suggest that ICU clinicians frequently do not meet families' needs for communication [16, 22, 23]. A study from France suggests that 50% of family members of critically ill patients have important misunderstandings of diagnosis, prognosis, or treatment after a meeting with physicians [16]. Fortunately, interventions designed in part or exclusively to improve communication within the team and with the patient and family have suggested improvement in the processes of ICU care with decreased length of stay for those patients who ultimately die [13, 17, 18].

A cross-sectional survey suggested that family members have a significant burden of symptoms of depression and anxiety [24] and a qualitative study showed that families are also working through diverse processes such as reviewing the patient's life and understanding the effect of the loss of the patient on the family relationships [25]. There are also more likely to be discordant views about appropriate treatment among ICU team members, consultants, and primary care physicians, as well as different family members. Prior research from France and the USA suggests that ICU nurses have a more critical view of the decision-making and inter-disciplinary communication around end-of-life care in the ICU than physicians [26, 27]. Because the ICU team is made up of a number of health care professionals from many disciplines, it is important that all team members directly involved in communication with patients and families be included in the process of end-of-life care in the ICU. Communication and consensus within the ICU team is a vital step in the process of making decisions about withholding or withdrawing life-sustaining therapy, as described in the prior section. It is important that all team members are informed about the medical situation and goals of therapy so that patients and families do not receive conflicting messages from different staff members [28, 29].

There has been little research on the current quality of clinician-family communication in the ICU. An observational study examined audiotapes of ICU family conferences to develop a framework for understanding the content of these discussions and the techniques used by clinicians to provide support to family members [30]. In this study, researchers found that critical care clinicians spent 70% of the time talking during family conferences and only 30% of the time listening to family members. In addition, the higher the proportion of time that clinicians spent listening, the more satisfied family members were with the family conference [31]. This study suggests that critical care clinicians may increase family satisfaction with communication about end-of-life care if they spent more time listening and less time talking.

Critical care clinicians can benefit from understanding the process of ICU family conferences and the ways these conferences can be improved. An observational qualitative study suggested that many ICU family conferences that address withholding and withdrawing life support in one area of the USA follow a similar structure [30]. It may be helpful for clinicians to review this structure and use or adapt it as appropriate. The first step of a discussion about dying and death is generally to be sure that everyone participating in the discussion has met everyone else present, since some clinicians present for the discussion may not have met all family members. It can be helpful to review the agenda for the conference with the family and ask at the beginning of the conference if there are additional agenda items that the family would like to discuss. After these opening comments and introductions there is usually a two-way information exchange during which clinicians update the family about the patient's illness and treatments and the family educate the clinicians about the patient's values and the things that are important to the patient. The conference then often turns to discussion of the future including prognosis for survival and also prognosis for quality of life if the patient does survive. This is also when the discussion of dying and what that patient's death might be like often comes up. Finally, there is often a discussion of the decisions to be made either at this conference or in the future and closing comments by the family and the clinicians.

During these discussions, it is important to discuss prognosis in an honest way that is meaningful to patients and their families. For example, median survival or percent chance of surviving the ICU may not be very meaningful to most family members. In discussing prognosis, clinicians should also be honest about the degree of uncertainty in the prognosis. Qualitative research in other settings suggests it can be very helpful to provide prognostic information in a way that makes it clear that the clinician cares for both the patient and the family and also cares about what happens to the patient [32].

Oftentimes clinicians may arrive at the decision that withdrawing life-sustaining therapy is in the patient's best interest before the family does. These situations can be a source of conflict between the ICU clinicians and the family [33]. In these situations, the family may need time to accept and understand the patient's prognosis and to come to terms with the loss of a loved one. Allowing families the time to make these adjustments can be an important use of ICU resources in some settings, while it may be a luxury that critical care clinicians can not afford when ICU beds are a scarce resource. Rushing families to make the decision to withdraw life-sustaining therapy before they are ready can set up an antagonistic relationship between clinicians and families and can erode the trust that families have in the clinicians. Once this trust is eroded, it is often difficult to regain.

ICU team members may differ in the timing with which they believe that life-sustaining therapy should be withdrawn. Oftentimes, nurses come to this decision earlier than physicians, which surveys of nurses have demonstrated can be a source of frustration for some critical care nurses [34, 35] and a source of inter-disciplinary conflict for physicians and nurses. The best way to avoid and address such conflict is to ensure that lines of communication are open between team members. A recent before-after study done in one ICU suggests that one method to improve communication within the ICU team is to have the entire team present and participating during ICU morning rounds and to explicitly review the goals of care [36]. This is a relatively simple solution that can have a profound effect on team communication, but may require reorganization of morning rounds to allow all team members to be present.

▌ Assessment and Management of Pain and other Symptoms

Evidence suggests that a patient's burden of physical and emotional suffering in the ICU during their last days is inadequately addressed. In SUPPORT, 40% of patients who died with acute respiratory failure and sepsis had severe pain and dyspnea during the last three days of life [12]. A prospective cohort study of cancer patients in the ICU showed a high burden of pain and other symptoms [37]. To provide optimal palliative care for dying patients in the ICU, it is essential for clinicians to grasp the differences in the goals of care between patients receiving comfort care and other ICU patients. Compassionate critical care requires that pain, dyspnea, nausea, and delirium be addressed in the care of all patients; however, critical care clinicians must balance the goals of comfort with other goals of intensive care. For example, weaning from mechanical ventilation, assessment of neurologic status, and hemodynamic instability sometimes prevent clinicians from providing sufficient sedation to eliminate all signs of patient discomfort. When the primary goals of care are re-oriented toward comfort, there is no need to weigh other concerns with the sole possible exception of the dying patient whose sedating medication is withheld in hopes that they will regain sufficient consciousness to interact with family members.

Current guidelines for palliative care in the ICU are built on the same medical regimens that ICU clinicians use for treating pain, agitation, and dyspnea. One common form of this regimen includes a combination of morphine or other opiate with a benzodiazepine, continually infused and titrated to the cessation of expressions of discomfort, including grimacing, agitated behavior, and autonomic hyperactivity. Some circumstances may also justify the use of barbiturates, haloperidol, or propofol [38]. Fears of "over-dosing" dying patients in the ICU should be allayed by clinician education and by documenting the specific criteria for which drugs are being used and drug doses are being increased. A recent retrospective cohort study showed that higher doses of opiate and benzodiazepines used in the setting the withdrawal of life-sustaining treatment were not associated with a decreased time from withdrawal of life support to death. On the contrary, there was a trend in the opposite direction suggesting that increased doses of benzodiazepines were associated with increased time to death [39]. This study suggests that current use of analgesics and sedatives in the ICU setting are not hastening death.

Another aspect of assessment and management of symptoms in the ICU relates to symptoms caused by medical procedures. Prospective cohort studies have shown a significant burden of symptoms associated with routine ICU procedures [37, 40]. Importantly, in addition to the procedures that most critical care clinicians would anticipate as causing symptoms, such as placement of central lines or arterial lines, other procedures associated with significant symptoms included endrotracheal suctioning and turning patients [37, 40].

Any effort to increase the use of analgesics and sedatives in the ICU must be cognizant of the recent randomized trial showing that daily interruption of analgesia and sedation by a protocol to decrease use of these medications can decrease the number of days that patients spend on mechanical ventilation and in the ICU [41]. Daily interruption of analgesics and sedatives has become a standard part of intensive care, but in the patient transitioning to comfort as the primary goal of care, such a protocol will no longer serve an important purpose and should be modified to focus on the primary goal of patient comfort.

Delirium is an important and common problem in the ICU [42] and addressing delirium is important to providing good quality palliative care. Delirium is associated with a number of adverse outcomes, including increased mortality, increased length of stay, self-extubation, and removal of catethers [42, 43]. For these reasons, it is important that all patients in the ICU be assessed for delirium on a routine basis. The Confusion Assessment Method for the ICU (CAM-ICU) is an instrument for assessing delirium in critically ill patients that has been validated recently [44], although its role in clinical practice is yet to be determined. Critically ill patients nearing the end of life have many reasons for delirium, including multisystem organ failure, sepsis, sleep deprivation, electrolyte disturbances, hepatic encephalopathy, withdrawal syndromes, and medications. In patients for whom the goals of care are to reverse the underlying critical illness, it is important to identify and treat delirium. Even in the setting of end-of-life care, if delirium is interfering with communication or causing distress, clinicians should identify treatable causes of delirium and attempt to reverse these causes.

▌ Withdrawal of Life-sustaining Treatments

Observational studies show that the vast majority of patients who die in ICUs do so after a decision to limit life sustaining-treatments [4–7]. Therefore, improving the process by which life-sustaining treatments are withdrawn is an important aspect of improving the quality of end-of-life care for patients dying in the ICU. Unfortunately, there are few data to guide clinicians in the practical aspects of withdrawing life-sustaining treatments. Practice should be guided by a thorough understanding of the goal of withdrawing life-supportive care: the goal is to remove treatments that are no longer desired or indicated and that do not provide comfort to the patient. Any treatment may be withheld or withdrawn, and most ethicists concur that there is no ethical difference between withholding or withdrawing life-supportive treatments [45].

The withdrawal of life-sustaining treatments is a clinical procedure, and as such, deserves the same preparation and expectation of quality as other procedures. Several topics should be discussed with families including explanations of how interventions will be withdrawn, how the patient's comfort will be insured, the patient's expected length of survival, and any strong family or patient preferences about other aspects of end-of-life care. Time should be spent discussing, understanding, and accommodating cultural and religious perspectives. An explicit plan for performing the procedure and handling complications should be formulated: the patient should be in the appropriate setting with irrelevant monitoring removed; the process should be carefully documented including the reasons for increasing sedation or analgesia; and outcomes should be evaluated to improve the quality of this care. There is evidence from a recent study that documentation regarding withdrawal of life support is poor [46].

Once a decision is made to withdraw life-sustaining treatments, the time-course over which a life-sustaining treatment is withdrawn should be determined by the potential for discomfort as treatment is stopped. The only rationale for tapering life-sustaining treatment in this setting is to allow time to meet the patient's needs for symptom control. There is usually no need to taper vasopressor medications, antibiotics, nutrition, or most other critical care treatments. Mechanical ventilation is one of the few life-support treatments whose abrupt termination can lead to discomfort. In a common approach of terminating mechanical ventilation, often called 'rapid terminal weaning' or 'terminal ventilator discontinuation', the inspired oxygen fraction (FiO_2) is reduced to room air and the positive end expiratory pressure (PEEP) to zero as a first step with anticipatory dosing of narcotics as needed for patient comfort. In the next step, ventilatory support is gradually reduced from baseline to zero over 5–10 minutes with dosing of narcotics or benzodiazepines as needed for manifestations of dyspnea or other symptoms. At that point the patient is placed on a T-piece with humidified air or extubated. Since the term 'weaning' suggests the goal is independent spontaneous ventilation, the phrase 'terminal ventilator discontinuation' is more appropriate. Limited data exist as to whether patients should be extubated. Small observational cohort studies have found no significant difference in patient comfort [47, 48], but these studies lack power to detect clinically important differences. Terminal ventilator discontinuation may unnecessarily prolong dying if various steps are prolonged. Typically the transition from full ventilatory support to T-piece or extubation should take less than 10–20 minutes. Families should be cautioned that death, while expected, may not be certain and that the timing can vary.

As with many aspects of critical care, a protocol for withholding life-sustaining treatments, if carefully developed and implemented, may provide an opportunity to improve the quality of care. Treece and colleagues describe the development of a "withdrawal of life support order form" for use in a critical care unit and evaluated implementation in a before-after study [49]. The order form contains four sections. The first section highlights some of the preparations prior to withdrawal of life support including discontinuing routine x-rays and laboratory tests and stopping all prior medication orders such as prophylaxis for deep venous thrombosis. The second section provides an analgesia and sedation protocol that provides for continuous infusions if medications are needed and gives nurses wide latitude for increasing the doses quickly if needed with no maximal dose. However, the order form also requires documentation of the reasons for dose escalation. The third section contains a ventilator withdrawal protocol as outlined above. The fourth section provides the principles surrounding withdrawal of life sustaining treatments. These authors showed that physicians and nurses found the order form helpful [49]. They also showed that implementation of this order form was associated with an increase in the use of benzodiazepines and opiates in the hour prior to ventilator withdrawal and the hour after ventilator withdrawal, but was not associated with any decrease in the time from ventilator withdrawal to death. These findings suggest that such an order form can result in an increase in drug use targeting patient comfort without necessarily hastening death. Institutions with considerable variability in the withdrawal of life support process or institutions where ICU nurses express frustration with this process should consider adapting and implementing such a protocol or order form.

In considering withholding and withdrawing life-sustaining treatment, it is important to incorporate culturally sensitive care by understanding that some cultures do not accept western ethical principles such as the equivalence of withholding and withdrawing life support or the definition of brain death. Therefore, it is important to anticipate these scenarios and be prepared to apply principles of culturally effective end-of-life care to these situations [50].

▌ Conclusion

Perhaps the single most important recommendation for improving palliative and end-of-life care in the ICU is for intensive care clinicians to *value* palliative and end-of-life care and make these aspects of care an important part of their rounds and documentation. Multi-disciplinary rounds that cover both the curative and palliative aspects of caring for critically ill patients should occur routinely in the ICU. It is particularly important that nurses and other ICU clinicians are part of a collaborative interdisciplinary team that takes responsibility for end-of-life decision-making and care. Every patient admitted to the ICU who has a significant risk of death or of a prolonged ICU stay should generate a meeting between the patient's family and the clinical team where the patient's condition is discussed and the patient's values about intensive care are elicited [13, 17]. Techniques to clearly and unequivocally communicate decisions about limits of life-sustaining treatment to all hospital staff should be implemented. Hospitals should try to humanize their ICUs by liberalizing visiting hours [51] and making lay or professional counselors and spiritual care providers available to families [28]. Assessment of pain and other symptoms should be a high priority for critical care clinicians. Protocols for withdrawing life sustaining treatment and forms for documenting this process should be implemented [49]. These interventions can improve the quality of palliative care provided in the ICU.

References

1. Angus DC, Barnato AE, Linde-Zwirble WT, et al (2004) Use of intensive care at the end of life in the United States: An epidemiologic study. Crit Care Med 32:638–643
2. Sprung CL, Cohen SL, Sjokvist P, et al (2003) End-of-life practices in European intensive care units: the Ethicus Study. JAMA 290:790–797
3. Curtis JR, Bennett CL, Horner RD, Rubenfeld GD, DeHovitz JA, Weinstein RA (1998) Variations in ICU utilization for patients with HIV-related Pneumocystis carinii pneumonia: Importance of hospital characteristics and geographic location. Crit Care Med 26:668–675
4. Prendergast TJ, Luce JM (1997) Increasing incidence of withholding and withdrawal of life support from the critically ill. Am J Respir Crit Care Med 155:15–20
5. Vincent JL, Parquier JN, Preiser JC, Brimioulle S, Kahn RJ (1989) Terminal events in the intensive care unit: Review of 258 fatal cases in one year. Crit Care Med 17:530–533
6. Eidelman LA, Jakobson DJ, Pizov R, Geber D, Leibovitz L, Sprung CL (1998) Foregoing life-sustaining treatment in an Israeli ICU. Intensive Care Med 24:162–166
7. Keenan SP, Busche KD, Chen LM, McCarthy L, Inman KJ, Sibbald WJ (1997) A retrospective review of a large cohort of patients undergoing the process of withholding or withdrawal of life support. Crit Care Med 22:1020–1025
8. Cook DJ, Guyatt GH, Jaeschke R, et al (1995) Determinants in Canadian health care workers of the decision to withdraw life support from the critically ill. JAMA 273:703–708
9. Prendergast TJ, Claessens MT, Luce JM (1998) A national survey of end-of-life care for critically ill patients. Am J Respir Crit Care Med 158:1163–1167
10. Vincent JL (1999) Forgoing life support in western European intensive care units: results of an ethical questionnaire. Crit Care Med 16:1626–1633
11. Cook D, Rocker G, Marshall J, et al (2003) Withdrawal of mechanical ventilation in anticipation of death in the intensive care unit. N Engl J Med 349:1123–1132
12. The SUPPORT Principal Investigators (1995) A controlled trial to improve care for seriously ill hospitalized patients: The study to understand prognoses and preferences for outcomes and risks of treatments (SUPPORT). JAMA 274:1591–1598
13. Lilly CM, De Meo DL, Sonna LA, et al (2000) An intensive communication intervention for the critically ill. Am J Med 109:469–475
14. Thompson BT, Cox PN, Antonelli M, et al (2004) Challenges in end-of-life care in the ICU: statement of the 5th International Consensus Conference in Critical Care: Brussels, Belgium, April 2003: executive summary. Crit Care Med 32:1781–1784
15. Heyland DK, Tranmer J, O'Callaghan CJ, Gafni A (2003) The seriously ill hospitalized patient: preferred role in end-of-life decision making? J Crit Care 18:3–10
16. Azoulay E, Chevret S, Leleu G, et al (2000) Half the families of intensive care unit patients experience inadequate communication with physicians. Crit Care Med 28:3044–3049
17. Schneiderman LJ, Gilmer T, Teetzel HD, et al (2003) Effect of ethics consultations on non-beneficial life-sustaining treatments in the intensive care setting: a randomized controlled trial. JAMA 290:1166–1172
18. Campbell ML, Guzman JA (2003) Impact of a proactive approach to improve end-of-life care in a medical ICU. Chest 123:266–271
19. Dowdy MD, Robertson C, Bander JA (1998) A study of proactive ethics consultation for critically and terminally ill patients with extended lengths of stay, Crit Care Med 26:252–259
20. Schneiderman LJ, Gilmer T, Teetzel HD (2000) Impact of ethics consultations in the intensive care setting: a randomized, controlled trial. Crit Care Med 28:3920–3924
21. Hickey M (1990) What are the needs of families of critically ill patients? A review of the literature since 1976. Heart Lung 19:401–415

22. Kirchhoff KT, Walker L, Hutton A, et al (2002) The vortex: families' experiences with death in the intensive care unit. Am J Crit Care 11:200–209

23. Azoulay E, Pochard F, Chevret S, et al (2001) Meeting the needs of intensive care unit patient families: a multicenter study, Am J Respir Crit Care Med 163:135–139

24. Pochard F, Azoulay E, Chevret S, et al (2001) Symptoms of anxiety and depression in family members of intensive care unit patients: Ethical hypothesis regarding decision-making capacity. Crit Care Med 29:1893–1897

25. Swigart V, Lidz C, Butterworth V, Arnold R (1996) Letting go: family willingness to forgo life support. Heart Lung 25:483–494

26. Ferrand E, Lemaire F, Regnier B, et al (2003) Discrepancies between perceptions by physicians and nursing staff of intensive care unit end-of-life decisions. Am J Respir Crit Care Med 167:1310–1315

27. Levy CR, Ely EW, Bowman C, Engelberg RA, Patrick DL, Curtis JR (2005) Quality of death in the ICU: Examining the perceptions of family and critical care clinicians, Chest (in press)

28. Abbott KH, Sago JG, Breen CM, Abernethy AP, Tulsky JA (2001) Families looking back: one year after discussion of withdrawal or withholding of life-sustaining support. Crit Care Med 29:197–201

29. Tilden VP, Tolle SW, Garland MJ, Nelson CA (1995) Decisions about life-sustaining treatment: Impact of physicians' behaviors on the family. Arch Intern Med 155:633–638

30. Curtis JR, Engelberg RA, Wenrich MD, et al (2002) Studying communication about end-of-life care during the ICU family conference: Development of a framework. J Crit Care 17:147–160

31. McDonagh JR, Elliott TB, Engelberg RA, et al (2004) Family satisfaction with family conferences about end-of-life care in the ICU: Increased proportion of family speech is associated with increased satisfaction. Crit Care Med 32:1484–1488

32. Curtis JR, Wenrich MD, Carline JD, Shannon SE, Ambrozy DM, Ramsey PG (2001) Understanding physicians' skills at providing end-of-life care: Perspectives of patients, families, and health care workers. J Gen Intern Med 16:41–49

33. Way J, Back AL, Curtis JR (2002) Withdrawing life support and resolution of conflict with families. BMJ 325:1342–1345

34. Asch DA (1996) The role of critical care nurses in euthanasia and assisted suicide. N Engl J Med 334:1374–1379

35. Meltzer LS, Huckabay LM (2004) Critical care nurses' perceptions of futile care and its effect on burnout. Am J Crit Care 13:202–208

36. Pronovost P, Berenholtz S, Dorman T, Lipsett PA, Simmonds T, Haraden C (2003) Improving communication in the ICU using daily goals. J Crit Care 18:71–75

37. Nelson JE, Meier D, Oei EJ, Nierman DM, et al (2001) Self-reported symptom experience of critically ill cancer patients receiving intensive care. Crit Care Med 29:277–282

38. Truog RD, Berde CB, Mitchell C, Grier HE (1992) Barbiturates in the care of the terminally ill. N Engl J Med 327:1678–1682

39. Chan JD, Treece PD, Engelberg RA, et al (2004) Association between narcotic and benzodiazepine use after withdrawal of life support and time to death. Chest 126:286–293

40. Puntillo KA (1990) Pain experience of intensive care unit patients. Heart Lung 19:525–533

41. Kress JP, Pohlman AS, O'Connor MF, Hall JB (2000) Daily interruption of sedative infusions in critically ill patients undergoing mechanical ventilation. N Engl J Med 342:1471–1477

42. Ely EW, Shintani A, Truman B, et al (2004) Delirium as a predictor of mortality in mechanically ventilated patients in the intensive care unit. JAMA 291:1753–1762

43. Milbrandt EB, Deppen S, Harrison PL, et al (2004) Costs associated with delirium in mechanically ventilated patients. Crit Care Med 32:955–962

44. Ely EW, Inouye SK, Bernard GR, et al (2001) Delirium in mechanically ventilated patients: validity and reliability of the confusion assessment method for the intensive care unit (CAM-ICU). JAMA 286:2703–2710

45. Council on Scientific Affairs, A. M. A. (1996) Good care of the dying patient. JAMA 275:474–478

46. Kirchhoff KT, Anumandla PR, Foth KT, Lues SN, Gilbertson-White SH (2004) Documentation on withdrawal of life support in adult patients in the intensive care unit. Am J Crit Care 13:328–334
47. Daly BJ, Thomas D, Dyer MA (1996) Procedures used in the withdrawal of mechanical ventilation. Am J Crit Care 5:331–338
48. Campbell ML, Bizek KS, Thill M (1999) Patient responses during rapid terminal weaning from mechanical ventilaion: A prospective study. Crit Care Med 27:73–77
49. Treece PD, Engelberg RA, Crowley L, et al (2004) Evaluation of a standardized order form for the withdrawal of life support in the intensive care unit. Crit Care Med 32: 1141–1148
50. Crawley LM, Marshall PA, Lo B, Koenig BA (2002) Strategies for culturally effective end-of-life care. Ann Intern Med 136:673–679
51. Berwick DM, Kotagal M (2004) Restricted visiting hours in ICUs: time to change. JAMA 292:736–737

Subject Index

Printing: Strauss GmbH, Mörlenbach
Binding: Schäffer, Grünstadt